Wrist and Elbow Arthroscopy with Selected Open Procedures

William B. Geissler

Editor

Wrist and Elbow Arthroscopy with Selected Open Procedures

A Practical Surgical Guide to Techniques

Third Edition

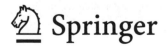 Springer

Editor
William B. Geissler
Division of Hand and Upper Extremity Surgery
Section of Arthroscopic Surgery and Sports Medicine
Department of Orthopedic Surgery and Rehabilitation
University of Mississippi Medical Center
Jackson, MS
USA

ISBN 978-3-030-78883-4   ISBN 978-3-030-78881-0   (eBook)
https://doi.org/10.1007/978-3-030-78881-0

This Springer imprint is published by the registered company Springer Nature Switzerland AG
The registered company address is: Gewerbestrasse 11, 6330 Cham, Switzerland

Preface

I cannot believe I am already writing the preface to the third edition of Springer's *Wrist and Elbow Arthroscopy with Selected Open Procedures: A Practical Surgical Guide to Techniques* so soon after the second edition. However, there have been so many new and exciting arthroscopic procedures to both the wrist and elbow that it was decided to go forward with a third edition to be able to describe all of these new, fascinating techniques. Wrist and elbow arthroscopy has continued to expand at a rapid rate, as more surgeons are exposed to this modality and then have developed their own techniques and procedures to continue to advance this field. As in the previous editions, the goal was to make this textbook as international as possible. Recognized wrist and elbow arthroscopy experts from around the world were asked to contribute to this textbook. Thought leaders from the United States, South America, Europe, and China have all contributed chapters to this third edition.

Recent advances in wrist and elbow surgery are not limited to arthroscopy. There has been a huge advancement in open surgical techniques of both the wrist and elbow. In this edition, we've added selected chapters on open techniques for wrist and elbow surgery. In these chapters, international thought experts who developed recent advances were asked to provide their input on open surgery of both the wrist and elbow. These chapters are limited in their historical content, but the main concept of their chapters was to describe exactly how they did their surgical technique, and provide tips and pearls on how to perform it. I personally believe that this is a huge contribution to the third edition as it is not limited only to arthroscopy but includes specific recent editions to open surgery of the wrist and elbow. We all know that not everything can be treated by arthroscopy alone, and it is nice to learn the tips and tricks from international experts on open techniques for specific indications of the wrist and elbow.

This current edition has more than doubled the number of chapters of the previous edition, from 34 to 76. This shows our commitment to include the most recent advancements in wrist and elbow surgery, both open and arthroscopic, in this textbook. The goals of this text were to be as international as possible and to be the most up-to-date source for both wrist and elbow surgery.

The third edition includes new and exciting advances in arthroscopic wrist techniques on arthroscopic approaches to perilunate dislocations, the evaluation and treatment of ulnar triquetrum ligament split tears, and arthroscopic repair of triangular fibrocartilage complex tears through bone tunnels. For the elbow, additional chapters have been included on arthroscopic nerve release, which is certainly a controversial topic.

For selected open techniques, multiple chapters have been included for both the wrist and elbow. New concepts in carpal instability are included, as well as multiple chapters on various techniques to address carpal instability. Further chapters have been added on the complex management of distal radius fractures, including both volar and dorsal approaches, fragment specific fixation, and management of distal radius malunions. Lastly, multiple chapters have been added regarding management of intra-articular supracondylar humerus fractures with both open reduction fixation and hemi-joint replacement. Lastly, chapters have been added on the rehabilitation of these complex hand and wrist injuries, particularly in athletes.

First, I'd like to acknowledge and thank the international group of excellent experts who have committed their expertise to author these chapters for the third edition. The tips and tricks are particularly invaluable, as they teach us how to do their procedures to help our patients in the field of wrist and elbow pathology. Doubling the number of chapters, and including open surgery, really allows this textbook to cover the field of both wrist and elbow pathology to help the surgeon treat these complex disorders. As always, I want to acknowledge my early mentors in hand surgery, including Terry Whipple, MD, who has exposed me to the techniques of wrist arthroscopy. He particularly demonstrated to me how precise and delicate arthroscopic surgery of the wrist is to be performed correctly. I need to acknowledge Alan E. Freeland, MD, who was my mentor, friend, and colleague who instructed me in hand surgery and guided my career throughout the years. He will be truly missed. I would also like to acknowledge and thank the staff of Day Surgery Center at the University of Mississippi Medical Center, including Stephanie, Lisa, Brenda, Kandi, Perry, and Mark. There are many others, but they work very long hours with very little complaining as we frequently run overtime to complete the surgeries. I need to thank my administrative team of Haylee and Trina, who work hard in the trenches to take care of our patients. I specifically need to thank Brittany, who has spent countless hours transcribing my dictations in undergoing multiple revisions for the chapters. I want to thank the nearly 30 hand and upper extremity fellows who have rotated through the years, from whom I have learned far more than I have taught.

Lastly, but certainly not least, I need to thank my family. Susan, my wife, has endured multiple hardships with my long hours and traveling to understand and promote these concepts of wrist and elbow surgery. I would like to thank my daughter, Rachel Leigh, and grandson, Jack, for showing me there is hope for the future, and for inspiring me to continue to work hard. There will be continuous evolution and change, which will lead to new and exciting procedures and, potentially, a fourth edition on wrist and elbow surgery.

Jackson, MS, USA

William B. Geissler

Contents

Contributors

Joshua M. Abzug, MD Department of Orthopaedics, University of Maryland School of Medicine, Timonium, MD, USA

Julie E. Adams, MD Department of Orthopedic Surgery, University of Tennessee College of Medicine – Chattanooga, Chattanooga, TN, USA

Laith Al-Shihabi, MD Department of Orthopaedic Surgery, Rush University Medical Center, Chicago, IL, USA

Andrea Atzei, MD Fenice HSRT Hand Surgery and Rehabilitation Team, Centro di Medicina, Treviso, Italy
Policlinico San Giorgio, Pordenone, Italy

Alejandro Badia, MD Badia Hand to Shoulder Center, OrthoNOW Orthopedic Urgent Care Centers, Doral, FL, USA

Nicole Badur, MD Hand Surgery and Surgery of Peripheral Nerves, University Hospital Bern, Bern, Switzerland

Gregory Ian Bain, MBBS, FRACS, FA (Orth) A, PhD Department of Orthopaedic Surgery, Flinders University of South Australia, Adelaide, SA, Australia

Mark E. Baratz, MD Department of Orthopedic Surgery, University of Pittsburgh Medical Center, Bethel Park, PA, USA

Jarrad A. Barber, MD Department of Orthopaedics, Harbin Clinic, Rome, GA, USA

Randy Bindra, MD, FRACS Department of Orthopaedic Surgery, Griffith University School of Medicine, Gold Coast University Hospital, Southport, QLD, Australia

Mitchell C. Birt, MD Hand and Upper Extremity Surgery, University of Kansas Medical Center, Kansas City, KS, USA

Daniel J. Brown, MBChB, MA, FRCS(Orth)(Eng) Department of Trauma and Orthopaedics, Liverpool University Hospitals NHS FT and University of Liverpool, Liverpool, UK

Michael Brown, DPT School of Health-Related Professions, Department of Physical Therapy, University of Mississippi Medical Center, Jackson, MS, USA

Jared L. Burkett, MD Alabama Orthopaedic Clinic, Mobile, AL, USA

Alvaro Motta Cardoso Jr., MD NAEON Institute, Sao Paulo, Brazil

Andrew Y. H. Chin, MBBS, FRCSEd, FAMS Singapore General Hospital, Hand and Reconstructive Microsurgery, Singapore, Singapore

Sonya M. Clark, DO Upstate Hand Center, Spartanburg, SC, USA

Tyson K. Cobb, MD Shoulder Elbow Wrist and Hand Center of Excellence, Davenport, IA, USA

Mark Steven Cohen, MD Department of Orthopaedic Surgery, Rush University Medical Center, Chicago, IL, USA

Fernando Corella, PhD Orthopedic and Trauma Department, Hospital Universitario Infanta Leonor, Madrid, Spain

Hand Surgery Unit, Hospital Universitario Quironsalud Madrid, Madrid, Spain

Gregory Couzens, MBBS, FRACS Brisbane Hand and Upper Limb Research Institute, Brisbane Private Hospital, Brisbane, QLD, Australia

Orthopaedic Department, Princess Alexandra Hospital, Woolloongabba, QLD, Australia

Institute of Health and Biomedical Innovation, Queensland University of Technology, Brisbane, QLD, Australia

Randall W. Culp, MD Department of Orthopaedic Surgery, Thomas Jefferson University Hospitals, Philadelphia Hand to Shoulder Center, King of Prussia, PA, USA

Wood W. Dale, MD Department of Orthopaedic Surgery and Rehabilitation, University of Mississippi Medical Center, Jackson, MS, USA

Pablo De Carli, MD Orthopaedic and Traumatology Department, and Hand and Upper Extremity Section, Hospital Italiano, Buenos Aires, Argentina

Associate Proffesor, Clinical Surgery, Instituto Universitario Hospital Italiano de Buenos Aires, Buenos Aires, Argentina, Buenos Aires, Argentina

Miguel Del Cerro, MD Hand Surgery Unit, Hospital Beata María Ana, Madrid, Spain

Francisco del Piñal, MD Unit of Hand-Wrist and Plastic Surgery, Private Practice and Hospital Mutua Montañesa, Santander, Spain

Mark A. Dodson, MD Department of Orthopedic Surgery and Rehabilitation, University of Mississippi Medical Center, Jackson, MS, USA

Mid State Orthopedic and Sports Medicine Center, Alexandria, LA, USA

Hand and Upper Extremity Fellow, Department of Orthopaedic Surgery and Rehabilitation, University of Mississippi Medical Center, Jackson, MS, USA

Partner, Mid State Orthopedic and Sports Medicine Center, Alexandria, LA, USA

Scott Edwards, MD Department of Orthopaedic Surgery, University of Arizona College of Medicine, Phoenix, AZ, USA

Bassem T. Elhassan, MD Department of Orthopedic Surgery, Mayo Clinic, Rochester, MN, USA

Carlos Henrique Fernandes, MD Department of Orthopedic Surgery, Universidade Federal de São Paulo, São Paulo, Brazil

John J. Fernandez, MD Midwest Orthopaedics at Rush University, Chicago, IL, USA

Larry D. Field, MD Upper Extremity, Mississippi Sports Medicine and Orthopaedic Center, Jackson, MS, USA

Alan E. Freeland, MD Department of Orthopaedic Surgery and Rehabilitation, University of Mississippi Medical Center, Brandon, MS, USA

Christina E. Freibott, MPH Department of Orthopedic Surgery, Columbia University Irving Medical Center, New York, NY, USA

Isaac D. Gammal, MD, MBA Department of Orthopedic Surgery, North Shore-LIJ Medical Center, New Hyde Park, NY, USA

Jose Carlos Garcia Jr., PhD Department of Orthopedic Surgery, NAEON Institute and Moriah Hospital, Sao Paulo, Brazil

Erich M. Gauger, MD Orthopaedic Surgery, Allina Health, Coon Rapids and St Paul, Minneapolis, MN, USA

William B. Geissler, MD Division of Hand and Upper Extremity Surgery, Section of Arthroscopic Surgery and Sports Medicine, Department of Orthopedic Surgery and Rehabilitation, University of Mississippi Medical Center, Jackson, MS, USA

Joshua A. Gillis, MD St. Joseph's Hospital, Roth McFarlane Hand and Upper Limb Centre, London, ON, Canada

Michael B. Gottschalk, MD Hand and Upper Extremity, Department of Orthopaedic Surgery, Emory University Hospital, Atlanta, GA, USA

Mathilde Gras, MD Clinique Bizet, International Wrist Center-Clinique du Poignet, Institut de la Main, Paris, France

Andrew S. Greenberg, MD Orthopaedic Associates of Manhasset, P.C., Great Neck, NY, USA

A. Jordan Grier, MD Department of Orthopaedic Surgery, Duke University Medical Center, Durham, NC, USA

Michael Hackl, MD Faculty of Medicine, University of Cologne, Cologne, Germany
University Hospital Cologne, Center of Orthopedic and Trauma Surgery, Cologne, Germany

Andreas Harbrecht, MD University of Cologne, Faculty of Medicine and University Hospital, Center for Orthopedic and Trauma Surgery, Cologne, Germany

Michael R. Hausman, MD Department of Orthopaedic Surgery, Mount Sinai Medical Center, New York, NY, USA

Rachel E. Hein, MD Division of Plastic and Reconstructive Surgery, Duke University Medical Center, Durham, NC, USA

Pak-cheong Ho, MBBS(HK), FHKCOS Department of Orthopaedics and Traumatology, Prince of Wales Hospital, Hong Kong, China

Benjamin Hope, MBBS, FRACS, FAOrthA Brisbane Hand and Upper Limb Research Institute, Brisbane, QLD, Australia
Orthopaedic Department, Princess Alexandra Hospital, Woolloongabba, QLD, Australia

Jessica M. Intravia, MD, MHA Donald and Barbara Zucker School of Medicine at Hofstra, Long Island Jewish Medical Center and North Shore University Hospital, Northwell Health Orthopaedic Institute, New Hyde Park, NY, USA

Sanjeev Kakar, MD Department of Orthopedic Surgery, Mayo Clinic, Rochester, MN, USA

Andrew Keightley, MBBS, BSc, FRCS (Tr and Orth) Royal Surrey Hospital, Department of Trauma and Orthopaedics, Guildford, Surrey, UK

Justine S. Kim, MD Department of Plastic and Reconstructive Surgery, University of Pittsburgh Medical Center, Pittsburgh, PA, USA

Steven M. Koehler, MD Department of Orthopaedic Surgery, Mount Sinai Medical Center, New York, NY, USA

Siu-cheong Jeffrey Justin Koo, MBSS(HK), FHKCOS, FHKAM Department of Orthopaedics and Traumatology, Alice Ho Miu Ling Nethersole Hospital, Hong Kong, China

Hermann Krimmer, PhD Handcenter Ravensburg, Ravensburg, Germany

Christopher G. Larsen, MD Department of Orthopaedic Surgery, Northwell Health, North Shore University Hospital/Long Island Jewish Medical Center, New Hyde Park, NY, USA

Steven J. Lee, MD Surgery of the Hand/Upper Extremity, Lenox Hill Hospital, New York, NY, USA

Nicholas Institute of Sports Medicine and Athletic Trauma, New York, NY, USA

Timothy Leschinger, MD University Hospital Cologne, Center of Orthopedic and Trauma Surgery, Cologne, Germany

Bo Liu, MD, FRCS (Orth) Department of Hand Surgery, Beijing Ji Shui Tan Hospital, The Fourth Clinical College of Peking University, Beijing, China

Jeremy Loveridge, MBBS, FRACS (Orth) Brisbane Hand and Upper Limb Research Institute, Brisbane, QLD, Australia

Riccardo Luchetti, MD Rimini Hand & Rehabilitation Center, Rimini, Italy

Timothy Luchetti, MD Department of Orthopedic Surgery, University of Pittsburgh Medical Center, Bethel Park, PA, USA

Michael L. Mangonon, DO Plancher Orthopaedics & Sports Medicine, New York, NY, USA

Noah C. Marks, MD Mississippi Sports Medicine and Orthopaedic Center, Jackson, MS, USA

Christophe Mathoulin, MD, FMH Clinique Bizet, International Wrist Center-Clinique du Poignet, Institut de la Main, Paris, France

Duncan Thomas McGuire, MBCHB, FC (Orth) (SA), MMed Department of Orthopaedic Surgery, Groote Schuur Hospital, Cape Town, South Africa

Megan Anne Meislin, MD Department of Orthopaedic Surgery, Loyola University Medical Center, Maywood, IL, USA

Lorenzo Merlini, MD Clinique Bizet, International Wrist Center-Clinique du Poignet, Institut de la Main, Paris, France

Cesar Dario Oliveira Miranda, MD Department of Hand Surgery, Hand Surgery Institute Salvador, Salvador, Bahia, Brazil

M. Christian Moody, MD Department of Orthopaedic Surgery, Division of Hand and Upper Extremity, Prisma Health System, Greenville, SC, USA

Michael J. Moskal, MD Orthopaedic Surgery Department, University of Louisville, Sellersburg, IN, USA

Lars Peter Müller, MD, PhD Faculty of Medicine, University of Cologne, Cologne, Germany University Hospital Cologne, Center of Orthopedic and Trauma Surgery, Cologne, Germany

Nicholas Munaretto, MD Department of Orthopedic Surgery, Mayo Clinic, Rochester, MN, USA

Daniel J. Nagle, MD, FAAOS, FACS Department of Orthopedics, Northwestern University Feinberg School of Medicine, Chicago, IL, USA

Michael N. Nakashian, MD Brielle Orthopaedics at Rothman Institute, Brick Township, NJ, USA

Michael J. O'Brien, MD Department of Orthopaedics, Tulane University School of Medicine, New Orleans, LA, USA

Montserrat Ocampos, MD Orthopedic and Trauma Department, Hospital Universitario Infanta Leonor, Madrid, Spain

Hand Surgery Unit, Hospital Universitario Quironsalud Madrid, Madrid, Spain

A. Lee Osterman, MD The Philadelphia Hand to Shoulder Center, P.C.,, King of Prussia, PA, USA

Meredith N. Osterman, MD Philadelphia Hand to Shoulder Center, Department of Orthopedics, Thomas Jefferson University Hospital, Philadelphia, PA, USA

Greg Packer, MBBS, FRCS(Ed), FRCS(Orth) Department of Orthopaedic Surgery, Southend University Hospital, Westcliff-on-Sea, Essex, UK

W. Cody Pannell, DPT School of Health-Related Professions, Department of Physical Therapy, University of Mississippi Medical Center, Jackson, MS, USA

Loukia K. Papatheodorou, MD, PhD Department of Orthopaedic Surgery, University of Pittsburgh School of Medicine, Pittsburgh, PA, USA

Stephanie S. Pearce, MD The Steadman Clinic and Steadman Philippon Research Institute, Vail, CO, USA

Enrique Pereira, MD Department of Hand Surgery, Penta Institute of Traumatology and Rehabilitation, Buenos Aires, Argentina

Stephanie C. Petterson, MPT, PhD Research Department, Stamford, CT, USA

Kevin D. Plancher, MD Plancher Orthopaedics & Sports Medicine, New York, NY, USA

Kevin F. Purcell, MD, MPH, MS Department of Orthopedic Surgery, University of Mississippi Medical Center, Jackson, MS, USA

Remy V. Rabinovich, MD Department of Orthopaedic Surgery, Thomas Jefferson University Hospitals, Philadelphia Hand to Shoulder Center, Philadelphia, PA, USA

Senthooran Raja, MBBS, MSc Brisbane Hand and Upper Limb Research Institute, Brisbane, QLD, Australia

Orthopaedic Department, Princess Alexandra Hospital, Woolloongabba, QLD, Australia

Valentin Rausch, MD BG University Hospital Bergmannsheil, Center for Orthopedic and Trauma Surgery, Bochum, Germany

Mark S. Rekant, MD Department of Orthopaedic Surgery, Philadelphia Hand to Shoulder Center, Thomas Jefferson University, Cherry Hill, NJ, USA

Marc J. Richard, MD Department of Orthopaedic Surgery, Duke University Medical Center, Durham, NC, USA

Matthew Richard Ricks, BSc, MBBS, MSc, MSc Wrightington Hospital, Upper Limb Unit, Wigan, Lancashire, UK

Melvin P. Rosenwasser, MD Department of Orthopedic Surgery, Columbia University Irving Medical Center, New York, NY, USA

Mark Ross, MBBS, FRACS, FAOrthA Brisbane Hand and Upper Limb Research Institute, Brisbane, QLD, Australia

Orthopaedic Department, Princess Alexandra Hospital, Woolloongabba, QLD, Australia

The University of Queensland, St. Lucia, QLD, Australia

David S. Ruch, MD Department of Orthopaedic Surgery, Duke University Medical Center, Durham, NC, USA

Felix H. Savoie III, MD Department of Orthopaedics, Tulane University School of Medicine, New Orleans, LA, USA

Steven Shin, MD, MMSc Cedars-Sinai Medical Center, Department of Orthopaedics, Cedars-Sinai Orthopaedic Center, Los Angeles, CA, USA

Department of Orthopaedics, Cedars-Sinai Orthopaedic Center, Los Angeles, CA, USA

Seth C. Shoap, BA, BS Department of Orthopedic Surgery, Columbia University Irving Medical Center, New York, NY, USA

David J. Slutsky, MD The Hand and Wrist Institute, Torrance, CA, USA

Dean G. Sotereanos, MD University of Pittsburgh Medical Center, Pittsburgh, PA, USA

Department of Orthopaedic Surgery, University of Pittsburgh School of Medicine, Pittsburgh, PA, USA

Stephanie Catherine Spence, MBChB Brisbane Hand and Upper Limb Research Institute, Brisbane, QLD, Australia

Orthopaedic Department, Princess Alexandra Hospital, Woolloongabba, QLD, Australia

Scott P. Steinmann, MD Department of Orthopedic Surgery, University of Tennessee College of Medicine – Chattanooga, Chattanooga, TN, USA

Mayo Clinic, Rochester, MN, USA

John M. Stephenson, MD Department of Orthopaedic Surgery, University of Arkansas for Medical Sciences, Little Rock, AK, USA

Aaron H. Stern, BA Weiss Orthopaedics, Sonoma, CA, USA

John R. Talley, MD Division of Plastic Surgery, Department of Surgery, Stanford University Medical Center, Palo Alto, CA, USA

Steven M. Topper, MD Colorado Hand Center, Colorado Springs, CO, USA

Leigh-Anne Tu, MD Department of Orthopedics, University of Pittsburgh Medical Center, Bethel Park, PA, USA

David V. Tuckman, MD Orthopedic Associates of Manhasset, Great Neck, NY, USA

Stephan Uschok, MD Faculty of Medicine, University of Cologne, Cologne, Germany

University Hospital Cologne, Center of Orthopedic and Trauma Surgery, Cologne, Germany

Randall W. Viola, MD Department of Hand, Wrist, Elbow, and Microvascular Surgery, The Steadman Clinic and Steadman Philippon Research Institute, Vail, CO, USA

Juntian Wang, MD Cedars-Sinai Medical Center, Department of Orthopaedics, Cedars-Sinai Orthopaedic Center, Los Angeles, CA, USA

Adam Charles Watts, MBBS, BSc, FRCS (Tr and Orth) University of Manchester, Wrightington Hospital, Upper Limb Unit, Wigan, Lancashire, UK

Kilian Wegmann, MD, PhD Faculty of Medicine, University of Cologne, Cologne, Germany

University Hospital Cologne, Center of Orthopedic and Trauma Surgery, Cologne, Germany

Noah D. Weiss, MD Weiss Orthopaedics, Sonoma, CA, USA

Daniel Williams, BSc, MBChB, FRCS Brisbane Hand and Upper Limb Research Institute, Brisbane, QLD, Australia

Orthopaedic Department, Princess Alexandra Hospital, Woolloongabba, QLD, Australia

Scott W. Wolfe, MD Hand and Upper Extremity Service, Department of Orthopedic Surgery, The Hospital for Special Surgery, New York, NY, USA

Chia H. Wu, MD, MBA Department of Orthopedic Surgery, Baylor College of Medicine, Houston, TX, USA

Feiran Wu, MA, MB, BChir Department of Orthopaedics, Queen Elizabeth Hospital, University Hospitals Birmingham, Birmingham, UK

Robert W. Wysocki, MD Department of Orthopedic Surgery, Rush University, Chicago, IL, USA

Jeffrey Yao, MD Department of Orthopaedic Surgery, Stanford University Medical Center, Redwood City, CA, USA

Robert M. Zbeda, MD Department of Orthopaedic Surgery, Lenox Hill Hospital, New York, NY, USA

Arthroscopic Wrist Anatomy and Setup

Nicole Badur, Riccardo Luchetti, and Andrea Atzei

Introduction

Arthroscopy, first described in 1918 in a cadaver knee joint and in 1962 successfully as an operative procedure [1], has equipped the orthopedic surgeon with an excellent tool to assess and treat intra-articular pathologies. After successful application on large joints, the technique has been progressively extended onto smaller sized joints as the shoulder, the hip, the ankle, the elbow, and the wrist. Wrist arthroscopy was reported first in 1979 for diagnostic purposes [2]. From the late 1980s through the 1990s, arthroscopy has become an important means in the armory of a hand surgeon and wrist arthroscopy, the so-called golden standard for diagnosing intra-articular lesions in the wrist. Since then, it has continued to evolve not only as a diagnostic but also as a therapeutic tool and indications have steadily grown. Iatrogenic complications from open wrist surgery as capsular fibrosis resulting in stiffness are reduced by arthroscopic surgery [3, 4]. Wrist arthroscopy is now an established procedure for treating many intra-articular wrist pathologies with chronic wrist pain and in acute wrist trauma [5].

The wide list of indications for wrist arthroscopy is continuously growing and includes basic treatment of soft tissue pathologies such as synovitis, ganglia, fibrosis, stiffness, management of triangular fibrocartilage complex (TFCC)

tears, scapholunate- and lunotriquetral ligament lesions, and removal of loose bodies. Osseous procedures include partial bone resections in ulnocarpal or ulnostyloid impaction syndrome and scaphotrapeziotrapezoid (STT) or triquetrohamate (TH) arthritis [6]. The method has also gained wider acceptance in more sophisticated procedures as assisting reduction of intra-articular distal radius fractures [7–13] or scaphoid fractures [14, 15] and in posttraumatic sequelae. Arthroscopically assisted osteotomy in intra-articular distal radius malunions [16, 17], treatment of scaphoid nonunions [15], and arthroscopic arthrolysis has been described [18]. Arthroscopic decompression of the lunate for Kienböck's disease [19], arthroscopic proximal row carpectomy [20], and arthroscopically assisted partial wrist fusions have been described [21].

Dedicated miniaturized instrumentation meeting the needs of a small joint, a thorough knowledge of wrist anatomy and the anatomic landmarks [22], as well as careful and skilled surgical technique are required to allow a safe and appropriate arthroscopic treatment of disorders in the wrist joint.

Setup and Equipment

Setup

Wrist arthroscopy requires standard arthroscopic equipment. An arm table, arthroscopy tower system with monitor, video recorder and printer, a scope with a camera attached, light source with fiber-optic cable, motorized shavers, radiofrequency ablators, an image intensifier, and a traction system have become the standard of care. Digital systems allow data transfer to a USB stick.

The intervention is frequently carried out under regional anesthesia (axillary block) or general anesthesia under sterile conditions in an aseptic operation theater. Although wrist arthroscopy has also been described without exsanguination

Supplementary Information The online version of this chapter (https://doi.org/10.1007/978-3-030-78881-0_1) contains supplementary material, which is available to authorized users.

N. Badur (✉)
Hand Surgery and Surgery of Peripheral Nerves, University Hospital Bern, Bern, Switzerland

R. Luchetti
Rimini Hand & Rehabilitation Center, Rimini, Italy

A. Atzei
Fenice HSRT Hand Surgery and Rehabilitation Team, Centro di Medicina, Treviso, Italy

Policlinico San Giorgio, Pordenone, Italy

W. B. Geissler (ed.), *Wrist and Elbow Arthroscopy with Selected Open Procedures*,
https://doi.org/10.1007/978-3-030-78881-0_1

[15], the use of a pneumatic tourniquet placed at the upper arm is generally recommended.

The patient is positioned supine on the operation table with the affected arm on a hand table. The arm is abducted 90° and the elbow flexed 90° allowing a vertical position of the forearm, wrist, and hand. In this position, the wrist is kept in neutral pronosupination. Horizontal wrist arthroscopy has been described [10, 23]; however, we prefer the vertical position to maintain a neutral rotation of the wrist and 360-degree access to the wrist. Traction is usually recommended to distend the wrist and improve intra-capsular vision [1]. Vertical traction across the wrist is preferably achieved using a traction tower. The arm and forearm need to be padded with towels, preventing direct skin contact with the metal of the tower, and are then stabilized to the tower. Different models of traction towers exist (Fig. 1.1).

Vertical traction is then applied by suspending the fingers with sterile finger traps and applying countertraction through a gearing mechanism at the tower that allows precise modulation. To visualize the radiocarpal joint, the finger traps are preferably placed on the index and middle finger or the index, middle, and ring finger. Other traction devises allowing traction to all fingers are also used (Fig. 1.2). The applied traction varies between 3.5 and 7 kg in patients. For visualization of the STT, joint traction can be applied by suspending only the thumb.

Advantages of traction towers such as the Whipple, Borelli, or Geissler traction tower are that they provide good stability that can be crucial for certain interventions as arthroscopic-assisted reduction of distal radius fractures. Further they can be sterilized. For some interventions, however, we need a free pronosupination as for arthroscopic sta-

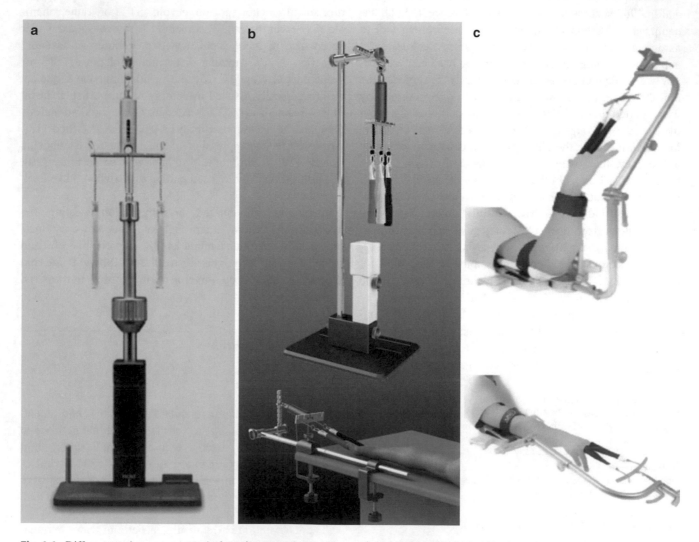

Fig. 1.1 Different traction systems. Vertical traction tower designed by Whipple (Linvatec®, Largo, FL, USA). Wrist positions can be adjusted through a ball-and-socket joint. The central rod position hinders intraoperative X-ray views (**a**). Traction tower designed by Borelli (Micai®, Genova, Italy), allowing free dorsal and volar approach to the wrist, rotation of the wrist, and easy image intensifier access with the eccentric rod position. Vertical and horizontal position of the wrist is possible (**b**). Wrist tower designed by Geissler (Acumed®, Hillsboro, Oregon, USA) that can be modified allowing different angles in wrist position and vertical or horizontal traction positioning without interference with intraoperative X-ray (**c**)

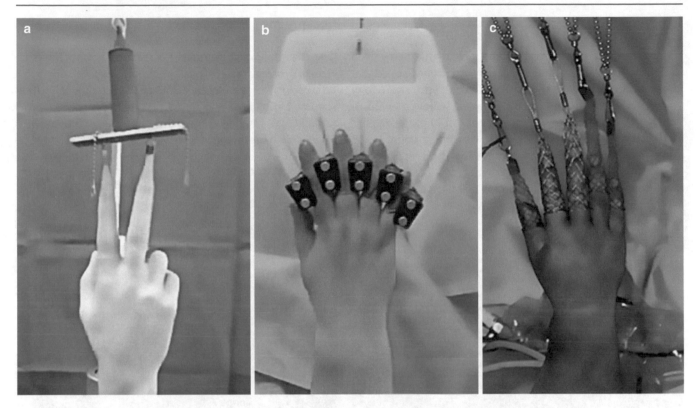

Fig. 1.2 Vertical traction is applied using Chinese finger traps at the index and middle finger (**a**). Traction on all fingers, the thumb included if needed, can be applied by special traction hands (e.g., Arthrex®, Naples, FL, USA) (**b**) and standard suspension systems (**c**). (Modified from Atzei et al. [33]. With permission from Elsevier)

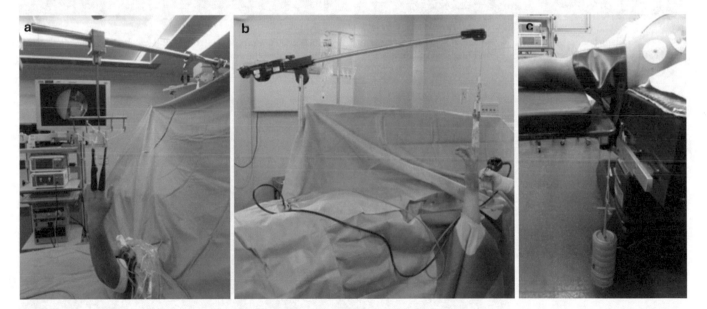

Fig. 1.3 Unconventional vertical overhead traction systems allowing rotation of the wrist and 360° access (**a** and **b**). A counter-traction band is placed around the arm proximal to the elbow. The tension can be adjusted by adding weights (**c**)

bilization of TFCC lesions, and the stability provided by the tower can hinder. Also, the central bar of some towers can interfere with the intraoperative use of an image intensifier. The fact that traction towers need to be sterilized can be a hassle if there is only one available and more wrist arthroscopies are performed within the same operating session.

If a traction tower is not available, a simple traction method can be used: a shoulder traction holder can provide overhead suspension with a countertraction band around the arm proximal to the elbow. The tension can be adjusted by adding weights (Fig. 1.3). Those systems are easy to set up and allow undisturbed intraoperative X-ray access as well as more freedom of motion than a traction tower while providing less stability (Fig. 1.4).

Anesthesia is positioned on the side of the uninvolved extremity or at the patient's head, the surgeon on the side that is awaiting surgery, at the patient's head. The arthroscopy tower and video monitor are placed at the patient's feet, usually on the opposite side of the patient. An image intensifier is positioned in the operating theater so that it is not in the way of the surgeon and rolled into the operating field as needed. The assistant and scrub nurse can position themselves depending on the intervention and the surgeon's needs which may differ in diagnostic and interventional wrist arthroscopies (Fig. 1.5).

Equipment

The most important instrument is the arthroscope (Fig. 1.6). Because of the size of the joint, arthroscopes for wrist arthroscopy are smaller in diameter than traditional arthroscopes. Different diameters of the optic are used in wrist arthroscopy, ranging from 1.9 to 2.7 mm, with either a 30-degree or less common a 70-degree viewing angle to

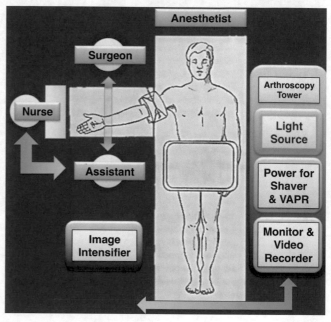

Fig. 1.4 Undisturbed intraoperative X-ray access is possible by simple overhead suspension of the wrist while providing less stability

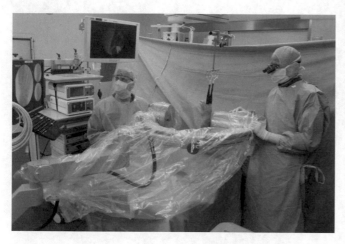

Fig. 1.5 Positioning of the patient, the surgical and anesthetic staff, and the arthroscopic equipment

Fig. 1.6 Wrist arthroscopy equipment

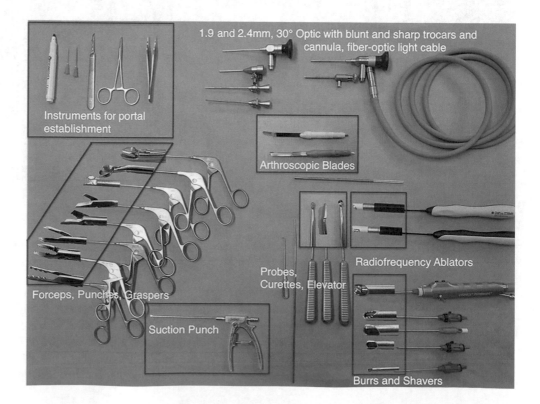

meet the needs of the different articulations in the wrist. The light source cable is also smaller in diameter. The smaller the diameter of the arthroscope, the higher is the risk of bending and damaging the fiber-optic in the cannula. Short cannulas (5–8 cm) and scopes (lever arm of 100 mm) are long enough and allow easier handling and control [24]. The 2.7 or 2.4 mm optic is ideal for the exploration of the radiocarpal and midcarpal joint as the arthroscopic vision field is bigger, but too bulky for exploration of the distal radioulnar joint (DRUJ), the scaphotrapeziotrapezoid (STT) joint, and in patients with a small wrist. In those cases, the use of an arthroscope with a diameter of 1.9 mm or smaller is more appropriate.

A blunt trocar with a trocar sleeve is important to establish the viewing and working portals of the joints to be inspected without damaging the articular cartilage.

Numerous instruments, appropriate to meet the criteria of diagnosing and treating wrist pathologies have been developed. The probe is probably the simplest but most useful diagnostic tool in wrist arthroscopy, serving as an extension of the surgeon's finger [1]. For some interventions, the use of a stronger probe as used in shoulder arthroscopy that does not bend is beneficial [16]. A variety of differently angled punches, baskets with or without the option of incorporating a suction mechanism, and grasping forceps in various sizes are useful in removing loose bodies and excising pieces of soft tissue. Small arthroscopy knives with differently shaped and retrograde blades aid in excising unstable chondral portions of the carpal bones. A freer elevator, pins, and a variety of small differently shaped osteotomes are useful tools in arthroscopically assisted correction of mal-united distal radius fractures [17].

Differently aggressive and sized motorized shavers and differently sized burrs ranging from 2.0 to 4.5 mm with integrated finger-controlled suction mechanism are powered instruments for debriding synovium or resecting bone, for example, when performing a resection of the distal pole of the scaphoid for STT arthritis or a radial styloidectomy for beginning radiocarpal arthritis as in stage 1 of scaphoid nonunion advanced collapse (SNAC I). Shavers and burrs can be operated with a foot pedal or by finger control and allow continuous or oscillating cutting.

Radiofrequency probes allow efficient soft tissue debridement and ligament or capsular shrinkage [25], but because of the risk of thermal injury, adequate fluid control must be carefully managed [26].

Traditionally, wrist arthroscopy has been carried out with constant joint irrigation for distension and improvement of intra-articular vision [27]. Lactated Ringer's solution is used for irrigation because it is rapidly reabsorbed from the soft tissues [8]. Electric fluid pumps that regulate fluid volume to avoid extravasation and decrease intraoperative bleeding may be used, but pure gravitational force is gener-

ally sufficient for the irrigation of the wrist joint. Outflow is provided via the port of the cannula with the camera or a separate needle placed into the ulnar side of the wrist or the successively established portals. While the classic (wet) wrist arthroscopy bears the disadvantage of cumbersome extra-articular water leakage into the soft tissue and the risk of serious complications as development of compartment syndrome [7, 8, 28, 29], the wrist joint can easily be inspected without the use of water, referred to as "dry arthroscopy" [30]. Synovial villi or ruptured ligament parts do not interfere with the intra-articular vision as they do not float into the field of vision and remain at their origins. In the usual joint, there is mucous fluid that does not impede vision. However, depending on the procedure to be performed, an initial washout of the joint may be useful, for example, evacuation of hematoma in acute intra-articular distal radius fractures. Debris can be cleared by injecting 10–20 ml of saline through the side valve of the scope followed by aspirating with the shaver. The wrist joint can also be dried with small neurosurgical patties inserted with a grasper. Other helpful maneuvers to keep a clear vision in dry arthroscopy are to immerse the tip of the scope into warm water to prevent condensation (fog effect) due to temperature differences outside and inside the wrist and to avoid closeness of the scope and motorized instruments, thus preventing splashing. The arthroscope can be cleaned by rubbing its tip carefully at the local soft tissue [30].

However, dry arthroscopy also has its limits. For example, when radiofrequency ablators are used, water is necessary as milieu conductor and to prevent temperature peaks and possible joint damage. Also when using a burr, the aspiration may be blocked by small cartilage and bone fragments and water facilitates the aspiration.

The equipment is completed by different utensils for specified arthroscopic procedures as ligament repair, from simple needles or longer Tuohy needles [31] to more sophisticated, commercially available ligament repair kits [32].

Surgical Technique

Certain rules need to be respected in order to obtain a good intra-articular vision and to avoid complications. It is very important that all external anatomic landmarks and portals must be marked after the traction to the wrist is applied but before starting the arthroscopic procedure so that the relationship of surface landmarks are not altered [28]. The following landmarks can be palpated if the wrist is not too swollen (Fig. 1.7):

Osseous Landmarks:
- *Dorsal*: Lister's tubercle, distal radial edge, dorsal ulnar head, index, middle, (ring), and small metacarpals

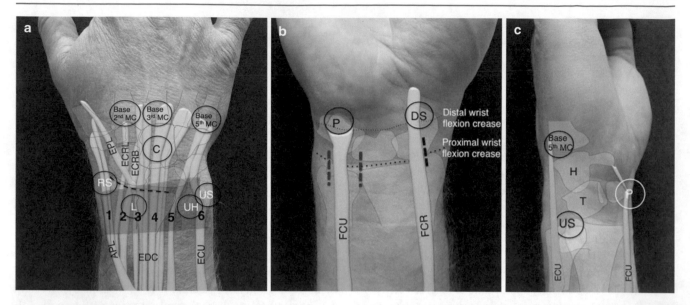

Fig. 1.7 Osseous and tendinous landmarks of the wrist from dorsal (**a**), volar (**b**), and ulnar (**c**). RS, radial styloid; L, Lister's tubercle; UH, ulnar head; US, ulnar styloid; P, pisiform; DS, distal pole of the scaphoid; APL, abductor pollicis longus; ECRL, extensor carpi radialis longus; ECRB, extensor carpi radialis brevis; EPL, extensor pollicis longus; EDC, extensor digitorum communis; ECU, extensor carpi ulnaris; FCU, flexor carpi ulnaris; FCR, flexor carpi radialis. The numbers 1–6 represent the extensor compartments. Volar incisions for the establishment of the VR and VM joint (*black line*), for the VU and V-DRUJ (*red line*), and for the 6-U and DF portal (*blue line*)

- *Radial*: Radial styloid process, trapezium, base of the first metacarpal
- *Ulnar*: Ulnar styloid, triquetrum, base of the fifth metacarpal
- *Volar*: Pisiform and distal pole of the scaphoid

Tendinous Landmarks:
- *Dorsal*: Extensor carpi radialis longus (ECRL) tendon, extensor pollicis longus (EPL) tendon, extensor digitorum communis (EDC) tendon, extensor carpi ulnaris (ECU) tendon
- *Radial*: Abductor pollicis longus (APL) tendon
- *Ulnar*: Extensor carpi ulnaris (ECU) tendon
- *Volar*: Flexor carpi radialis (FCR) tendon, flexor carpi ulnaris (FCU) tendon

Not all palpable surface landmarks need to be drawn onto the skin as orientation for establishing the portals; we mark the key structures as needed for each intervention (Fig. 1.8). Standard wrist arthroscopy includes the assessment of the radiocarpal and ulnocarpal joint, the midcarpal and STT joint, and the distal radioulnar joint (DRUJ). Numerous arthroscopic dorsal and palmar approaches have been described and are routinely used. The most commonly used dorsal radiocarpal portals are named relative to the extensor compartments between which they are located.

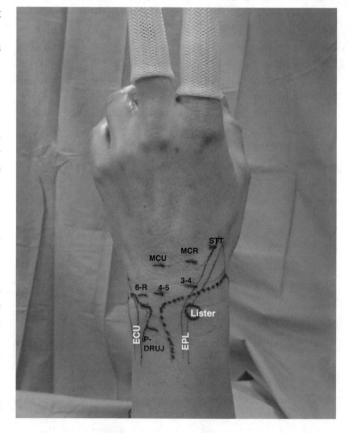

Fig. 1.8 Preoperative marking of the landmarks and dorsal portals for performing a standard wrist arthroscopy. Abbreviations are according to the previous figure

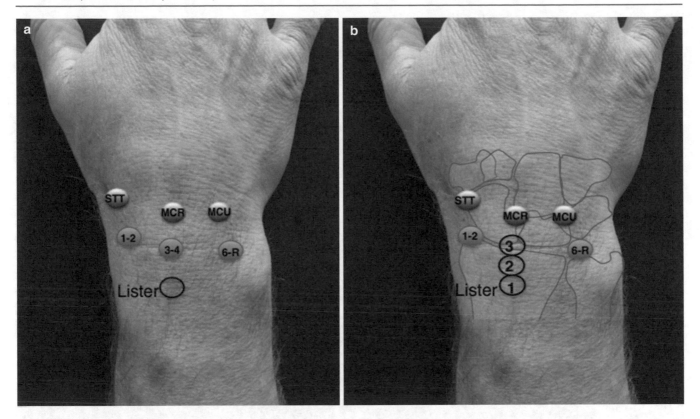

Fig. 1.9 Establishment of the 3–4 portal using the "three circles technique": a *circle* is drawn around the palpable Lister's tubercle (**a**). Two circles of the same size are then drawn distally to the first circle. The third and most distal circle lies at the level of the 3–4 portal (**b**)

The first portal to be established in almost every wrist arthroscopy is the 3–4 radiocarpal portal. It can be identified by simple palpation of the "soft spot" just distal of the dorsal rim of the radius in a vertical line with Lister's tubercle. Two methods of localizing the entry point for the 3–4 portal are used. The first method is called the "3 circle method" (Fig. 1.9). A circle is drawn around Lister's tubercle. Two other circles of the same dimension are drawn just distal to the first one in a vertical line with Lister's tubercle. The third circle is located directly over the soft spot that is the entry point of the 3–4 portal [33]. The second method is called the "rolling thumb method" (Fig. 1.10). The thumb pulp is placed on Lister's tubercle and is then rolled over the tubercle distally. The tip of the thumb is now exactly centered on the soft spot corresponding to the 3–4 portal. An 18- or 22-G needle is inserted at the soft depression into the radiocarpal joint, minding the normal inclination of the distal radius. Therefore, the needle is pointing 20–30° proximally to parallel the articular curve of the distal radius to verify correct intra-articular placement (Fig. 1.11).

Injection of a saline solution through this needle to distend the radiocarpal joint has been described. A normal uninjured wrist can contain 2–5 ml of fluid, but in the case of TFCC lesions, or lesions of the intracarpal ligaments of the proximal carpal row, up to 10–15 ml can be injected and the adjacent joints (distal radioulnar- and midcarpal joint) are

indirectly filled. As stated above, our preferred method for wrist arthroscopy is the so-called dry technique. The traction often is sufficient for obtaining a quiet good intra-articular vision. After the needle has been placed correctly, the skin is incised with a number 15 blade instead of using a number 11 blade as common for arthroscopy in other joints. Care must be taken to incise only the skin to prevent damage to superficial vessels, tendons, and cutaneous nerves. Depending on the portal to be established, the nerves can be found in very close proximity to the portals and are at risk [34–36]. Longitudinal incisions are possible and favorable if the incision needs to be enlarged in a proximal-distal direction, for example, if conversion to an open intervention needs to be performed. However, we generally prefer horizontal skin incisions on the dorsal aspect of the wrist, in line with the skin lines, thus improving the esthetic appearance of the scar. A blunt hemostat is advanced through the subcutaneous tissue by carefully spreading the branches until there is contact with the joint capsule. The capsule is then pierced with the tip of the closed hemostat (Fig. 1.12). A blunt trocar is introduced through a cannula into the joint directed volar and proximal at an approximately 30° angle, aligning the cannula with the volar inclination of the distal radius. The trocar is removed and the arthroscope is introduced through the cannula. The radial midcarpal portal can be established following the same technique, following the 10° obliquity of the

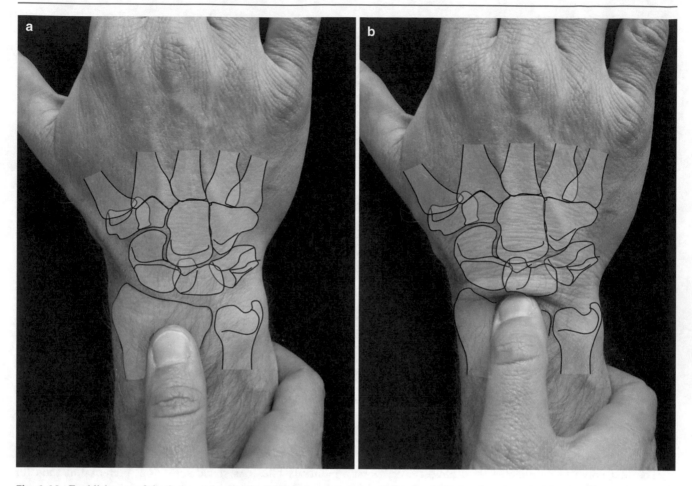

Fig. 1.10 Establishment of the 3–4 portal using the "rolling thumb technique": the thumb is placed on the palpable Lister's tubercle (**a**). The thumb is then rolled distally over the tubercle until the pulp of the surgeon's thumb feels the soft spot corresponding to the 3–4 portal (**b**)

first carpal row (see Fig. 1.11). For establishment of the other portals, we recommend to insert the needle arthroscopically controlled.

Despite the revolutionary advances in wrist arthroscopy, we have to remember that all indications to perform an arthroscopy should be based on a thorough clinical examination, aiming at detecting the origin of the intra-articular pathology and consequently avoiding inappropriate indications that would not address the true nature of the pathology [37].

The diagnostic evaluation always starts with the exploration of the radiocarpal joint, but the evaluation of the midcarpal joint should never be neglected and is considered a part of wrist arthroscopy. Arthroscopy of the DRUJ has only recently gained interest [38, 39]. It is performed in special indications and not conducted in every wrist arthroscopy.

A standardized, systematic arthroscopic examination with a routine circuit helps in visualizing all structures and not forgetting anything [4]. A few simple rules that should be followed are as follows:

- Examination of the radial side before the ulnar side
- Examination of the distal part of the articulation before the proximal part
- Examination of the volar aspect before the dorsal aspect
- Examination of the ligaments before the articular surfaces
- Simple inspection before using a probe

Rotation of the 30-degree-angle arthroscope allows the exploration of different regions of the articulation, and switching the arthroscope and the instrument within the different portals can be limited. It is crucial to stabilize the arthroscope and control the small movements of the optic within the joint in order to prevent damage to the articular cartilage. Therefore, the arthroscope should be held in a manner that allows constant contact to the skin of the wrist. The small optic is short enough to be grasped in a way that provides contact of the surgeon's index finger to the patient's wrist while larger arthroscopes need to be stabilized with the middle and ring finger (Fig. 1.13).

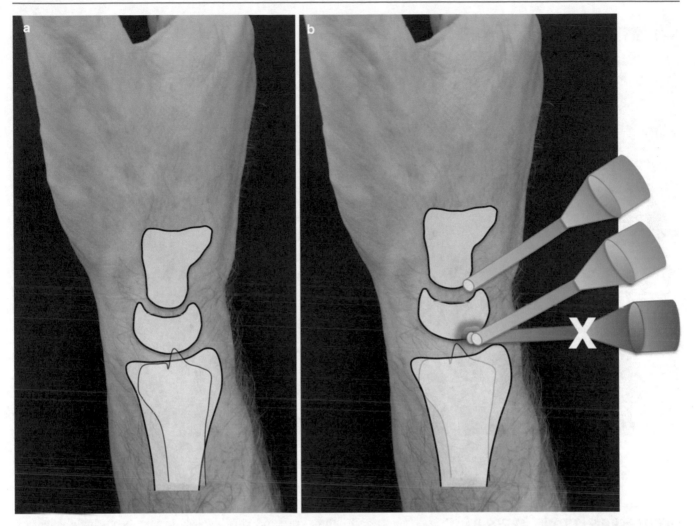

Fig. 1.11 Schematic lateral view of the wrist (**a**). External traction allows widening of the articular spaces. The arthroscope should be inserted into the radiocarpal and midcarpal joints, respectively, parallel-ing the dorsal articular slope of the joints. Horizontal introduction of the arthroscope may damage the articular cartilage of the carpal bones (**b**)

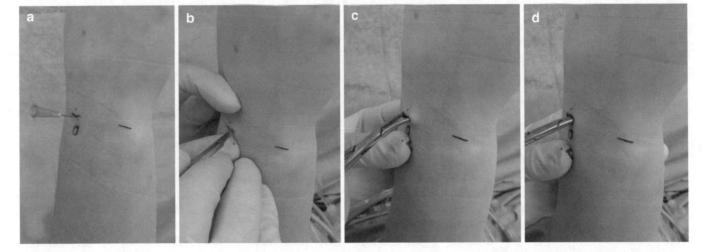

Fig. 1.12 Standard procedure for establishment of an arthroscopic wrist portal (3–4 portal), right wrist. Localization of the radiocarpal joint space with a 22-G needle (**a**). Horizontal skin incision (**b**). Spreading of the subcutaneous tissues with a blunt hemostat to the capsule (**c**). Piercing of the capsule with the closed tip of the hemostat (**d**)

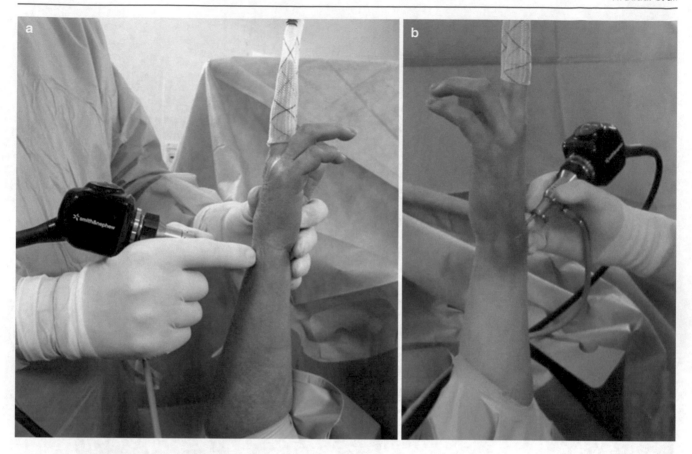

Fig. 1.13 Handling of the arthroscope. Control of minimal movements within the joint is achieved by constant finger contact to the patient's wrist with the index finger (**a**) or the middle to small finger (**b**)

Arthroscopic Portals: Approaches and Anatomy

Meticulous knowledge of the anatomy is essential for performing wrist arthroscopy (Fig. 1.14) [40]. The entry portals are numerous (Fig. 1.15) and need to be adapted to the pathology and the particular anatomy in this region [1, 28, 41]. The standard arthroscopic portals have been developed on the dorsal side of the wrist, and their localizations and names are in direct relation to the six extensor compartments. In the space between two extensor compartments, the arthroscopic portals can be established and instruments introduced without the risk of damaging the extensor tendons. On the dorsal side of the wrist, there are not many neurovascular structures that could be damaged (Fig. 1.16a–c). Volar portals have been previously reported [42, 43] but lacked popularity for a long period because they seemed to jeopardize important neurovascular structures on the volar side of the wrist (Fig. 1.16d, e). Only recently the safety of volar portals to the wrist could be shown [44–48], and it is possible to have viewing and working portals that encircle the whole wrist joint. This is called the "box concept" (Fig. 1.17) [24].

The arthroscopic exploration of the wrist is divided into three parts: proximal, volar (dorsal when using a volar portal), and distal. Then the arthroscope can be rotated to the radial and the ulnar side. We generally proceed with the arthroscopic overview from proximal to distal and from radial to ulnar (Fig. 1.18).

Dorsal Portals of the Radiocarpal Joint

Five standard dorsal portals of the radiocarpal joint are routinely used [35].

1–2 Portal
The 1–2 portal is situated between the first extensor compartment, containing the abductor pollicis longus (APL) tendon and the extensor pollicis brevis (EPB) tendon, and the second extensor compartment, containing the extensor carpi radialis longus and brevis (ECRL and ECRB) tendons. Proximally it is bordered by the distal, radial end of the radius, the radial styloid, and distally by the scaphoid. Several important structures can be found in this interval and may be endangered when establishing the 1–2 portal (Fig. 1.19). Two branches of the sensory branch of the radial

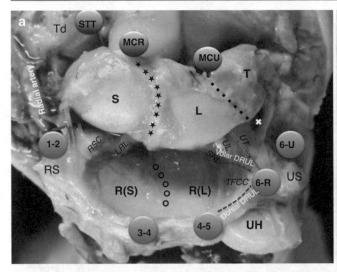
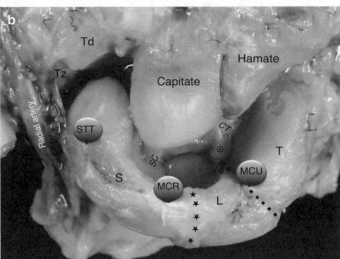

Fig. 1.14 Anatomic dissection of the radiocarpal (**a**) and midcarpal joints (**b**). The radiocarpal portals are indicated with *red circles* and the midcarpal portals with *black circles*. The proximal articular part of the radiocarpal joint is comprised by the scaphoid- and lunate fossa of the radius (R(S) and R(L)), separated by the interfosseal ridge (š) and the TFCC with its volar and dorsal distal radioulnar ligaments (DRUL). The volar radiocarpal ligaments are from radial to ulnar the radioscaphocapitate (RSC) ligament, the long radiolunate (LRL) ligament, and the short radiolunate (SRL) ligament. The volar ulnocarpal ligaments are the ulnolunate (UL) and the ulnotriquetral (UT) ligament. Ulnar and distal to the UT ligament, we find the entry to the pisotriquetral joint (°). The distal part of the radiocarpal joint is formed by the proximal articular surfaces of the scaphoid (S), the lunate (L) and the triquetrum (T). The scapholunate ligament (★) and the lunotriquetral ligament (◆)

separate the carpal bones of the first carpal row, respectively. The proximal part of the midcarpal joint is formed by the distal articular surfaces of the scaphoid, lunate, and triquetrum. The distal pole of the scaphoid and the proximal articular surfaces of the trapezium (Tz) and the trapezoid (Td) form the scaphotrapeziotrapezoid (STT) joint as a part of the midcarpal joint. The scaphoid body articulates with the capitate. The lunate, triquetrum, capitate, and hamate form the 4-bone corner. The lunate may have two distal articular facets, a major one for the capitate and a smaller one for the hamate (♯), which are separated by a longitudinal crest (❖). The volar midcarpal ligaments are radially the scaphocapitate (SC) ligament as the distal portion of the RSC ligament and ulnarly the capitotriquetral (CT) ligament, that is, usually covered by a fibroadipose structure (◉). *UH* ulnar head, *US* ulnar styloid. (Modified from Atzei et al. [33]. With permission from Elsevier)

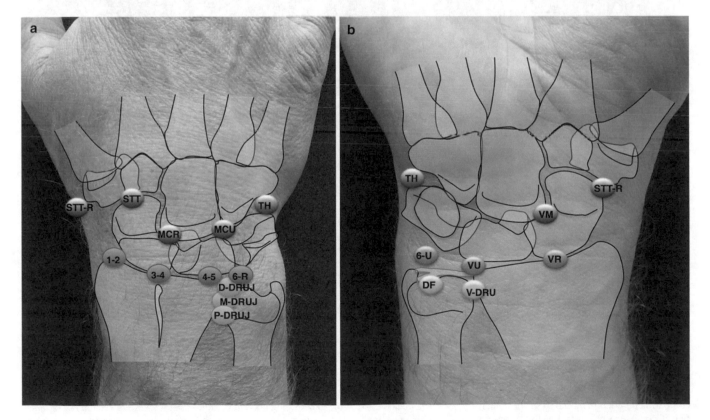

Fig. 1.15 Overview of the dorsal (**a**) and volar (**b**) portals used in wrist arthroscopy. Portals to the radiocarpal joint are marked in *red*, portals to the midcarpal joint are marked in *black*, and portals to the DRUJ are marked in *blue*

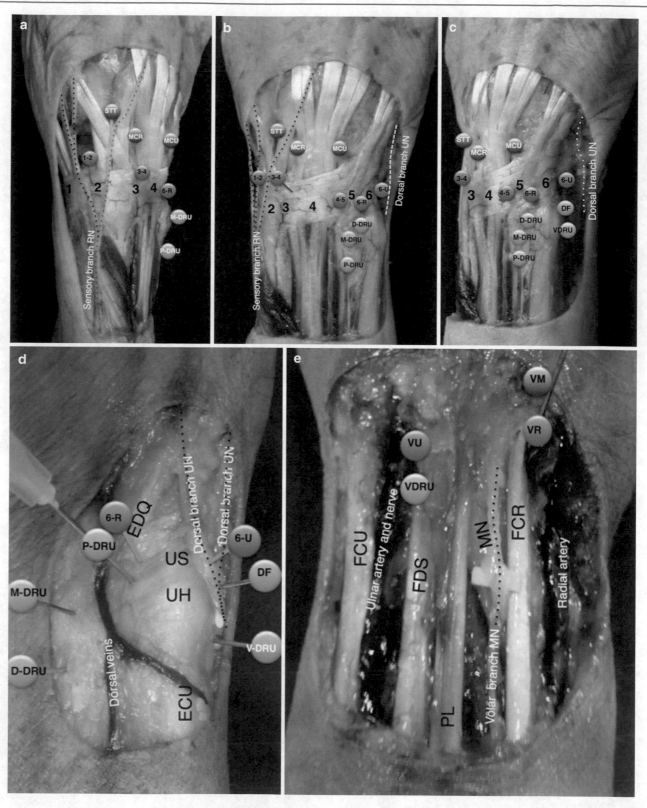

Fig. 1.16 Anatomic dissection of the wrist from dorso-radial (**a**), dorsal (**b**), dorso-ulnar (**c**), ulnar (**d**), and volar (**e**). (1) First compartment: containing the abductor pollicis longus (APL) tendon and the extensor pollicis brevis (EPB) tendon. (2) Second compartment: containing the extensor carpi radialis longus and brevis (ECRL and ECRB) tendons. (3) Third compartment: containing the extensor pollicis longus (EPL) tendon. (4) Fourth compartment: containing the extensor digitorum communis (EDC) tendons and the extensor indicis proprius (EIP) tendon. (5) Fifth extensor compartment: containing the extensor digiti quinti (EDQ) tendon. (6) Sixth extensor compartment: containing the extensor carpi ulnaris (ECU) tendon. On the radial side of the wrist, the sensitive branches of the superficial radial nerve can be visualized, and on the ulnar side, the terminal branches of the sensitive dorsal branch of the ulnar nerve. Entry portals to the radiocarpal joint and the midcarpal joint are marked in *red* or *black*, respectively. Entry portals to the DRUJ joint are marked in *blue*. ((**a–c**) Modified from Atzei et al. [33]. With permission from Elsevier)

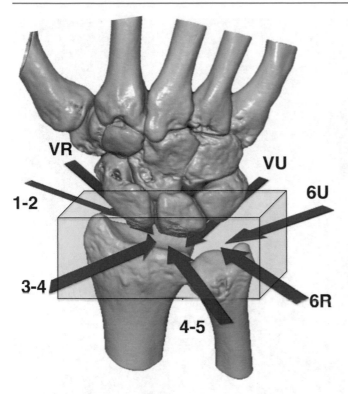

Fig. 1.17 "Box concept" of the wrist. The wrist can be thought of as a box, which can be visualized from almost every perspective. Through a combination of arthroscopic portals, it is possible to have viewing and working portals that encircle the wrist. This enables the arthroscopic surgeon to see and instrument from all directions. (Modified from Bain et al. [24]. With permission from Elsevier)

nerve (SBRN) were shown in proximity with a mean of 3 mm radial and 5 mm ulnar to the portal. The radial artery was located on average 3 mm radial to the portal [34]. In a different study, the mean distance of the SBRN was only 1.8 mm [36]. Partial or complete overlap of the lateral antebrachial cutaneous nerve (LABCN) with the SBRN is reported in up to 75% [49].

We recommend to carefully entry the joint capsule close to the tendons of the first extensor compartment and just distal to the radial styloid to avoid damage to the dorsal branch of the radial artery. Inserting the optic through this portal allows exploration of the entire dorsal capsule of the radiocarpal joint and the major part of the anterior capsule with the extrinsic ligaments. Further the proximal pole and the body of the scaphoid, the proximal pole of the lunate, the articular surface of the radius, and the dorsal rim of the radius can be visualized. This portal is mainly used as portal for instrument placement in special surgical procedures such as arthroscopic arthrolysis, resection of volar or dorsal ganglion cysts, or styloidectomy, just to mention a few.

- *Proximal*: We can observe the radial styloid and the scaphoid fossa of the radius.
- *Volar*: We identify the radioscaphocapitate (RSC) ligament and the long radiolunate (LRL) ligament that originate from the anterior margin of the radius.
- *Distal*: The most proximal 2/3 of the scaphoid and the proximal surface of the lunate can be visualized.

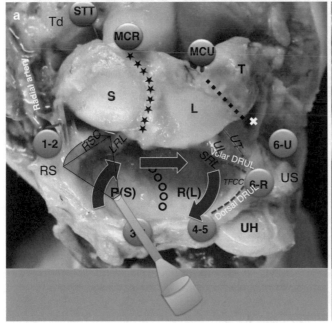

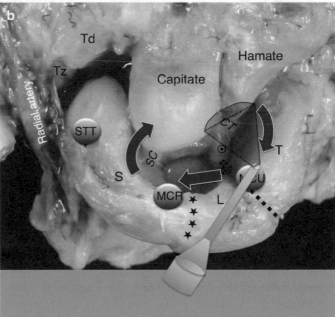

Fig. 1.18 Arthroscopic tour of the radiocarpal and midcarpal joint. For the radiocarpal joint, the primary viewing portal is the 3–4 portal, and we proceed from radial to ulnar, proximal to distal (**a**). For the midcar-pal joint, the MCU portal is the main viewing portal, and we proceed with the arthroscopic tour from ulnar to radial (**b**). Abbreviations are according to Fig. 1.14

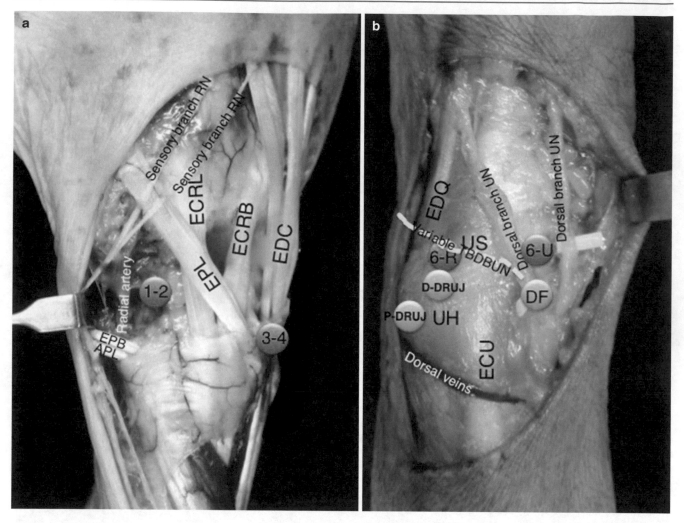

Fig. 1.19 Particular anatomy of the radial (**a**) and ulnar (**b**) aspect of the wrist. Branches of the sensitive branch of the radial nerve (SBRN) are moved radially by a retractor and the close relation of the dorsal branch of the radial artery to the 1–2 portal becomes evident. On the ulnar side, the close relation of the two dorsal branches of the ulnar nerve (UN) to the 6-U portal and the direct foveal (DF) portal is demonstrated. The terminal branching of the dorsal branch of the ulnar nerve (DBUN) is variable and a transverse branch of the DBUN (TBDBUN) can be found in some cases. ((**a**) Modified from Atzei et al. [33]. With permission from Elsevier)

- *Radial*: Rotating the arthroscope to the radial side, one is very close to the radial part of the radiolunate articulation and the vision is limited.
- *Ulnar*: Pivoting to the ulnar side, the anterior margin of the radius and the radioscapholunate (RSL) ligament (ligament of Testut) can be appreciated.
- *Dorsal*: Rotating to the dorsal side, we can see the entire dorsal part of the radiocarpal capsule with an oblique view of the dorsal radiocarpal ligament (DRCL).

3–4 Portal

The 3–4 portal is situated between the third extensor compartment, containing the extensor pollicis longus (EPL) tendon, and the fourth extensor compartment with the common finger extensor (EDC) tendons and the extensor indicis proprius (EIP) tendon (Fig. 1.20, Video 1.1). Proximally it is boarded by the distal radius and distally by the scapholunate ligament. The entry is 1 cm proximal to Lister's tubercle. The portal is considered safe with a low risk of damaging neurovascular structures. The mean distance of the SBRN is reported between 4.85 mm [36] and 16 mm radial to the portal [34]. The main risk is damaging the EPL tendon itself. We recommend to routinely establish this portal as the first portal for placement of the arthroscope. It is the main radiocarpal viewing portal as almost the complete radiocarpal articulation can be visualized through this portal:

- *Proximal*: We can observe the distal radial epiphysis with the interfosseal ridge that separates the scaphoid fossa and the lunate fossa in a sagittal direction.
- *Volar*: In the center of the field of vision, we see the RSL ligament that has the aspect of a fibro-fatty villus. It is con-

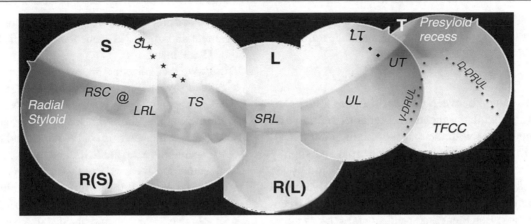

Fig. 1.20 Complete arthroscopic view of the radiocarpal joint through the 3–4 portal, from the radial styloid to the ulnar insertion of the TFCC in a right wrist. *S* scaphoid, *R(S)* scaphoid fossa of the radius, *L* lunate, *R(L)* lunate fossa of the radius, *T* triquetrum, *SL* (★-line) scapholunate ligament, *RSC* radioscaphocapitate ligament, *LRL* long radiolunate ligament, *TS* Testut (radioscapholunate) ligament, *SRL* short radiolunate ligament, *LT* (♦-line) lunotriquetral ligament, *UL* ulnolunate ligament, *UT* ulnotriquetral ligament, *V-DRUL* volar distal radioulnar ligament, *D-DRUL* dorsal distal radioulnar ligament, @ gap between RSC and LRL ligament. (Modified from Atzei et al. [33]. With permission from Elsevier)

sidered to be more of a neurovascular connective tissue than a true ligament [50]. De facto, it is the reference point for the exploration of the radiocarpal articulation. The volar radiocarpal ligaments are examined next. From radial to ulnar, we find the stout radioscaphocapitate (RSC) ligament, arising from the radial styloid, then inserting on the waist of the scaphoid and reaching the palmar part of the capitate. Ulnar to the RSC ligament, we find the long radiolunate (LRL) ligament that is wider, and its fibers are orientated more obliquely. Its insertion is mainly at the lunate while some fibers proceed to the triquetrum. The short radiolunate (SRL) ligament is the most ulnar ligament. The RSC and the LRL ligaments are separated by an interligamentous gap where volar wrist ganglions usually originate. The LRL ligament forms together with the SRL ligament, a reversed V that comprises the radioscapholunate ligament. At the apex of the V, one will find the anterior part of the scapholunate ligament.

- *Distal*: The articular surfaces of the scaphoid and the lunate and the scapholunate interosseous ligament (SLIL) between the two bones are visualized. It appears as an "indentation" and has a cartilage-like look [22]. The SLIL can be divided into a weak anterior part, a thin membranous proximal part and a strong dorsal part [51]. By slightly flexing and extending the wrist, the articular surfaces of the scaphoid and the lunate can be inspected more volarly and dorsally.
- *Radial*: Rotating the arthroscope radially, one can explore the radial compartment of the radiocarpal articulation. We can visualize the proximal pole and the body of the scaphoid, the radiocarpal ligament, the radial styloid, and the scaphoid fossa of the radius very nicely.

- *Ulnar*: Rotating the optic to the ulnar side, we can appreciate the lunate fossa of the radius and the triangular fibrocartilage complex (TFCC). Sometimes it can be difficult to see the separation between the radial margin of the TFCC and the articular surface of the lunate fossa of the radius. A probe will help in distinguishing between articular surface and TFCC. The TFCC is arranged in a three-dimensional manner into three components: the proximal triangular ligament, the distal hammock structure, and the ulnar collateral ligament (UCL) [52]. The volar and dorsal distal radioulnar ligaments (v-DRUL and d-DRUL) are thickenings of the periphery of the TFCC. They originate from the ulnar margin of the radius and insert as the proximal component of the TFCC at the ulna fovea (pc-TFCC) while the distal hammock structure and the UCL represent the distal component of the TFCC (dc-TFCC), attaching at the ulnar styloid and the ulnocarpal capsule. If the TFCC is intact, only the superficial part of the ulnar attachment of the radioulnar ligaments can be seen. In traumatic or degenerative central TFCC lesions, we can see onto the exposed ulnar head and the pc-TFCC at the fovea can be visualized. The ulnocarpal ligaments consist of the ulnolunate ligament (UL), the ulnocapitate (UC), and the ulnotriquetral ligament (UT) and originate at the anterior edge of the TFCC, the v-DRUL, and the ulnar styloid and insert on the lunate and the triquetrum, respectively. It is also possible to visualize the prestyloid recess, a synovial pouch that is located volar to the ulnar styloid. The meniscus homologue, a synovial tissue distal to the prestyloid recess that physiologically covers the tip of the ulnar styloid, can sometimes present as an indurated structure that can lead to impingement between the ulnar styloid and the triquetrum [53]. Next we analyze the complete articular surface of the lunate and the triquetrum as well as the lunotriquetral ligament.

4–5 Portal

This portal is situated between the fourth extensor compartment containing the above-mentioned tendons and the fifth extensor compartment with the extensor digiti quinti (EDQ) tendon. It is in line with the fourth metacarpal and slightly proximal to the 3–4 portal. Proximally it is bordered by the radius and distally by the lunate. Establishing the 4–5 portal does not put any particularly relevant structures at risk except from the EDC and EDQ tendons itself, dorsal sensory nerve branches are at a mean distance of 16.13 mm (range: 9.48–26.82 mm) [36]. The 4–5 portal has been the most frequently used portal for placement of the instruments; however, nowadays it is less frequently used than the 6-R portal. The 4–5 portal allows observation of the same structures as the 3–4 portal but with a more direct view onto the ulnar compartment of the wrist joint (Fig. 1.21). The possibility of exchanging the position of the arthroscope and the instruments with the 3–4 portal allows to accomplish surgical interventions in all parts of the radiocarpal articulation:

- *Proximal*: In the center of the field of vision, we see the radial insertion of the TFCC that merges with the lunate fossa on the radial side.

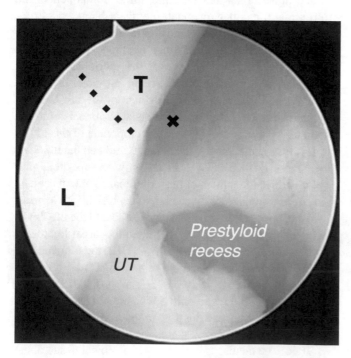

Fig. 1.21 Arthroscopic exploration of the ulnar compartment of the wrist from the 4–5 radiocarpal portal. Abbreviations and symbols are used according to the previous figure. °: entry to the pisotriquetral joint. x: entry into the pisotriquetral joint. The opening is covered by a synovial membrane (right wrist). (Modified from Atzei et al. [33]. With permission from Elsevier)

- *Volar*: Focusing on the ulnar side, we encounter the LRL ligament and the SRL ligament and the UL ligament and the UT ligament.
- *Distal*: We recognize the proximal lunate and triquetrum, separated by the lunotriquetral interosseous ligament (LTIL).
- *Radial*: Swinging the arthroscope to the radial side, we can visualize the volar rim of the radius and the ulnar part of the scaphoid fossa, the RSC, and the LRL ligaments as well as the dorsal capsule of the radiocarpal articulation. We can observe the dorsal surface of the lunate and the central, membranous part as well as the dorsal part of the scapholunate ligament and its distal attachment to the dorsal capsule.
- *Ulnar*: Rotating the arthroscope to the ulnar side, we can observe the most ulnar part of the TFCC up to the prestyloid recess and the pisotriquetral articulation. The pisotriquetral joint is part of the wrist joint. It is a diarthrosis and is enclosed in a small capsule. The pisotriquetral joint often communicates with the radiocarpal joint through a fenestration in the capsule [54].

6-R Portal

The 6-R portal is localized radial to the sixth extensor compartment that contains the extensor carpi ulnaris (ECU) tendon. Its radial border is the EDQ tendon. The portal is approximately 5 mm distal to the dorsal part of the TFCC, representing the proximal border. Distally the portal is bounded by the lunotriquetral interosseous ligament. The structure most at danger in establishing this portal is the TFCC. To avoid damage of the TFCC, this portal is established by the use of a needle under direct vision of the arthroscope (Videos 1.2 and 1.3). The structure second most at risk is the dorsal sensory branch of the ulnar nerve (DBUN) (see Fig. 1.19b). The mean distance of the DBUN to the 6-R portal has been found to be 8.2 mm [34]. A transverse branch of the DBUN (TBDBUN) has been found in 27% of dissected cadavers [55] with a very variable course. If present, it is encountered a mean of 2 mm proximal to the 6-R portal [34] (Fig. 1.22). Together with the 3–4 portal, the 6-R portal is one of the two essential portals in wrist arthroscopy as they allow to examine and access the whole radiocarpal joint. Although the 6-R portal is the main working portal, instruments and the arthroscope can easily be switched between those two portals. The 6-R portal shows the ulnocarpal compartment and is particularly useful in repairing lesions of the TFCC, the lunotriquetral ligament, or lesions of the lunate and the triquetrum (Video 1.4):

- *Proximal*: We can perfectly visualize the complete peripheral component of the TFCC up to the prestyloid recess and the opening into the pisotriquetral bursa.

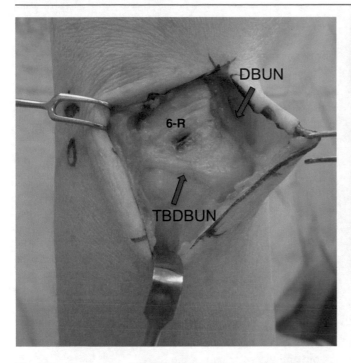

Fig. 1.22 Open approach to the DRUJ after wrist arthroscopy. Note the transverse branch of the dorsal branch of the ulnar nerve (TBDBUN) crossing 3 mm proximal to the 6-R portal

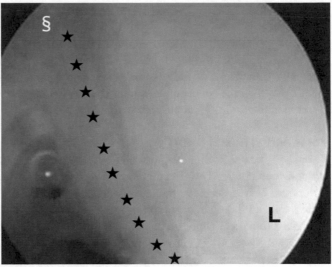

Fig. 1.23 Arthroscopic view onto the dorsal aspect of the radiocarpal joint from the 6-R portal. The dorsal, distal aspect of the lunate (L) and the scapholunate ligament (★-line) can be inspected up to the attachment of the SL ligament to the dorsal capsule (§) that separates the radiocarpal joint from the midcarpal joint (right wrist). (Modified from Atzei et al. [33]. With permission from Elsevier)

- *Volar*: The ulnolunate and ulnotriquetral ligaments (ULL and UTL), supporting the TFCC volarly, and the depression corresponding to the pisotriquetral articulation are examined.
- *Distal*: The entire articular surface of the triquetrum and the central volar part of the LTIL can be analyzed.
- *Radial*: Sweeping the arthroscope radially, we will find the TFCC, the lunate fossa of the radius, and the short radiolunate ligament. We also can explore parts of the dorsal aspect of the radiocarpal articulation (Fig. 1.23, Video 1.5).
- *Ulnar*: Rotating the arthroscope to the ulnar side, it is possible to glide into the prestyloid recess and the pisotriquetral space if the opening is not covered by a thick synovial membrane as reported in 27% [54].

6-U Portal

The 6-U portal is situated ulnar to the ECU tendon. Ulnarly it is bounded by the DBUN, proximally by the TFCC, and distally by the triquetrum. Damaging the terminal branches of the DBUN that divides itself inconsistently about 1.5 cm distal to this portal is the highest risk when establishing the 6-U portal. The frequent anatomical variations of the terminal branching of the DBUN are an additional risk. The mean distance of the DBUN from the 6-U portal is 8.3 mm if there is only one terminal branch and 1.9 mm if two terminal

branches are present. In cases where a TBDBUN is found, the mean distance is 2.5 mm proximal to the portal. In some cases, the branch is crossing directly over the portal [36]. Therefore the 6-U portal has been used for a long time predominantly as an outflow portal. Some authors, however, have shown that respecting certain rules, and keeping the possible anatomic variations of the dorsal branch of the ulnar nerve in mind, the 6-U portal can be used advantageously in diagnostic wrist arthroscopy and in treating certain pathologies [56], especially those around the ulnocarpal complex as the visualization of the ulnocarpal compartment is excellent.

- *Proximal*: We can see the ulnar and dorsal border of the TFCC and the prestyloid recess.
- *Volar*: The ULL and the UTL can be inspected.
- *Dorsal*: The dorsal ulnotriquetral ligament on the dorsal aspect of the TCFF may be visualized if not covered with synovial tissue. The ECU subsheath is a further stabilizer on the dorsal aspect of the TFCC but not visible with an intact capsule.
- *Distal*: The triquetrum can be perfectly displayed, most notably the ulnar part as well as the depression between the triquetrum and the lunate corresponding to the lunotriquetral ligament. The lunotriquetral ligament is more difficult to detect than the scapholunate interosseous ligament, and probing the ligament is the best way to localize it [57].

Volar Portals of the Radiocarpal Joint

Two volar portals to the radiocarpal joint are used. Especially the dorsal capsular structures, dorsal radiocarpal ligaments, and volar subregions of the scapholunate interosseous ligament as well as the lunotriquetral interosseous ligament are better visualized from a volar perspective [44, 45].

Volar Radial Portal (VR)

Two ways of establishing this portal have been described and are considered safe. The first method is the so-called in-out technique, first described in cadavers (Fig. 1.24) [43]: the optic is placed in an ulnar portal (4–5 or 6-R), a blunt trocar is inserted into the 3–4 portal, and pushed toward the anterior radiocarpal joint capsule. It is then pushed through the capsule between the RSC and LRL ligaments, exiting next to the flexor carpi radialis tendon where a small skin incision is made. A cannula can then be placed safely over the trocar and the arthroscope inserted from the volar side into the radiocarpal joint. The second method of establishing the volar radial portal has also been shown to be safe [44, 45]: a 1–2 cm longitudinal skin incision is made at the proximal wrist crease over the flexor carpi radialis (FCR) tendon, the tendon sheath is divided and the tendon retracted ulnarly. After identification of the radiocarpal joint space with an 18-G needle, the volar capsule is penetrated with the tip of a blunt artery forceps between the RSC ligament and the LRL ligament. A blunt trocar is inserted with a cannula, the trocar removed, and the arthroscope is introduced over the cannula. Structures at risk are the radial artery on the radial side and the volar cutaneous branch of the median nerve (VBMN) ulnarly (see Fig. 1.16d). There is a safe zone of 3 mm in all directions with respect to the mentioned structures [47].

This portal allows visualization of the complete radiocarpal articulation, particularly the dorsal capsule, the dorsal radiocarpal ligament (DRCL), the volar aspect of the bones of the first carpal row, and the volar subregions of the intercarpal ligaments. The TFCC can also be visualized (Fig. 1.25). A good surgical indication where the volar radial portal is beneficial is arthroscopic arthrolysis in cases in which complete dorsal capsulotomy for the treatment of flexion stiffness is needed:

- *Proximal*: The scaphoid and lunate fossae of the distal radius as well as the dorsal rim of the radius can be visualized.
- *Dorsal*: The dorsal capsule is inspected, the established dorsal 3–4 portal can be localized, and the radiolunotriquetral ligament is seen.
- *Distal*: We can visualize the proximal pole of the scaphoid and the volar part of the SLIL.
- *Radial*: Rotating the optic to the radial side, it is possible to visualize the radial styloid and the external part of the articular capsule.
- *Ulnar*: Swinging the optic to the ulnar side, one can visualize the entire surface of the distal radius up to the TFCC and the prestyloid recess. It is also possible to visualize the anterior part of the lunate, but the vision may be limited in cases where the radioscapholunate ligament is very voluminous.

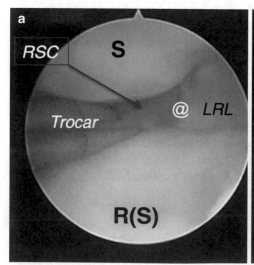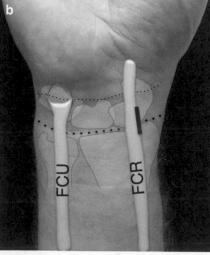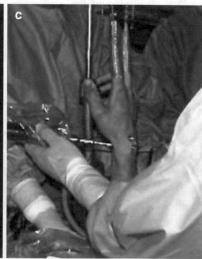

Fig. 1.24 Establishment of the volar radial radiocarpal portal with the "in-out" technique (right wrist). The optic is introduced via a dorsal ulnar portal (4–5 or 6-R): the proximal pole of the scaphoid (S) is visualized above, and we see the scaphoid fossa of the radius (R(S)) below; the trocar is introduced via the 3–4 portal and advanced through the gap (@) between the radioscaphocapitate (RSC) and the long radiolunate (LRL) ligaments and advanced volarly (**a**). On the volar radial side of the wrist, the skin incision is made at the level of the proximal wrist crease (*blue line*), radial to the flexor carpi radialis (FCR) tendon, close to the radial artery (**b**). After the blunt tip of the trocar has been advanced volarly through the joint capsule, a trocar sleeve can be placed over the trocar from the volar side, the trocar removed from the dorsal side, and the arthroscope is place into the trocar sleeve from volar (**c**). (Modified from Atzei et al. [33]. With permission from Elsevier)

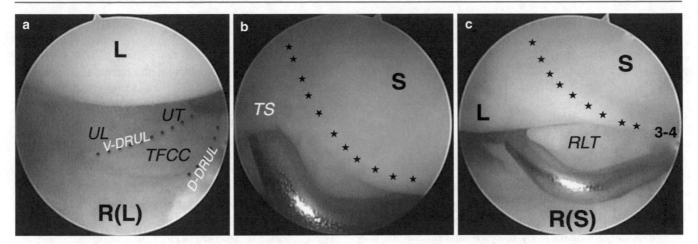

Fig. 1.25 Arthroscopic exploration of the radiocarpal joint from the volar radial portal (right wrist). Abbreviations and symbols are used according to the previous figures. Exploration of the ulnar part of the radiocarpal joint and the ulnocarpal joint: the articular surface of the lunate fossa of the radius can be examined and the corresponding proximal and volar aspect of the lunate. Further the radial insertion of the TFCC, the TFCC and the volar and especially the dorsal distal radioulnar ligaments are visualized. On the volar aspect, the UL and UT liga- ments can also be seen (**a**). With the probe in the 3–4 portal, the Testut ligament can be palpated. Especially the volar aspect of the scaphoid and the scapholunate ligament is visualized (**b**). The dorsal extrinsic radiolunotriquetral (RLT) ligament can be tested with a probe. The proximal aspect of the scaphoid, lunate, and the scapholunate ligament are inspected (**c**). (Modified from Atzei et al. [33]. With permission from Elsevier)

Volar Ulnar Portal (VU)

The volar ulnar portal of the radiocarpal joint has been described by Slutsky [46]. Like the volar radial portal, its clinical experience is still limited. The VU portal is bounded proximally by the ulnar styloid, distally by the triquetrum, ulnarly by the FCU tendon, and radially by the finger flexor tendons. A 2 cm longitudinal skin incision is centered over the proximal wrist crease along the ulnar edge of the common finger flexor tendons (see Fig. 1.7b). The tendons are retracted radially and the volar radiocarpal joint capsule is pierced with an 18-G needle. The capsule is then pierced with the tip of a blunt hemostat, followed by the insertion of a cannula and a blunt trocar. The trocar is removed and the arthroscope is inserted. The portal penetrates the ulnolunate ligament adjacent to the radial insertion of the TFCC. As for the establishment of the volar radial portal, the volar ulnar portal can also be created with the "in-out" technique with the arthroscope in the 3–4 portal. A blunt trocar is inserted into the 6-U portal and pushed toward the anterior ulnocarpal joint capsule. It is then pushed through the capsule between the UL and UT ligaments, exiting ulnar to the flexor tendons where a small skin incision is made.

Structures at risk are the flexor tendons, the ulnar artery, and ulnar nerve; however, they have been generally found more than 5 mm ulnar to the trocar (see Fig. 1.16d). The median nerve is protected by the flexor tendons. The volar cutaneous branch of the ulnar nerve is highly variable and its distal branch is at risk with a volar ulnar approach if present.

Like the VR portal, the VU portal provides a view of the dorsal articular surface of the radius and the dorsal extrinsic ligaments. Ulnar-sided structures that are more easily seen from the ulnar volar side of the wrist include the volar subre- gion of the LTIL, the dorsal distal radioulnar ligament, and the dorsal ulnar wrist capsule, containing the ECU subsheath (ECUS) [46]. Like the scapholunate interosseous ligament (SLIL), the LTIL can be divided into three parts: the volar part, the central part, and the dorsal part [58]. While the cen- tral part has more the structure of a thin membrane, the dor- sal part of the SLIL and the volar part of the LTIL are the most important subregions contributing to stability. The VU portal is especially useful for the viewing and debridement of palmar tears of the lunotriquetral ligament [46] and in assisting in reduction of distal radius fractures [24].

Arthroscopy of the Midcarpal Joint

The midcarpal joint contributes together with the radiocarpal joint to flexion-extension and radio-ulnar deviation of the wrist (see Fig. 1.14), and arthroscopy of the midcarpal joint should be routinely performed in every wrist arthroscopy.

Six portals to the midcarpal joint are used in wrist arthros- copy (see Figs. 1.15 and 1.16). Next to the two standard dor- sal midcarpal portals, one volar midcarpal portal [47], the standard ulnar STT portal, the radial STT portal [59], and the accessory triquetro-hamate (TH) portal [60] have been described. The midcarpal joint is comprised of three proxi- mal bones: the scaphoid, lunate, and triquetrum, and four distal bones: the trapezium, trapezoid, capitate, and hamate. The depth of the midcarpal joint is less than half of that of the radiocarpal joint, and the joint is tighter than the radiocarpal joint. The joint space of the scapholunate and lunotriquetral articulation can be inspected directly as there are no interosseous ligaments distally. The portal most commonly used in midcarpal arthroscopy is the ulnar midcarpal (MCU) portal.

Radial Midcarpal (MCR) Portal

The MCR portal is situated 1 cm distal to the 3–4 portal and in line with the radial margin of the third metacarpal. It is bounded radially by the ECRB tendon, ulnarly by the fourth extensor compartment, proximally by the concave surface of the scaphoid, and distally by the proximal pole of the capitate. The radial midcarpal portal is the principle midcarpal portal as it allows visualization of the complete midcarpal joint including the STT joint. Structures at risk while establishing this portal are the extensor tendons (see Fig. 1.16a–c). The SBRN is found at a mean distance of 6.65 mm [36] to 15.8 mm radial to the portal and was found in one occasion 2 mm ulnar to the portal [34]. A small transverse skin incision is made over the palpable soft spot 1 cm distal to the 3–4 portal after the entry to the joint has been triangulated with an 18-G needle. The joint capsule is pierced with a blunt hemostat, then a trocar sleeve with a blunt trocar is inserted, orientated approximately 10° proximally to parallel the dorsal midcarpal joint axis, followed by a 1.9 mm 30-degree-angle arthroscope.

The complete midcarpal articulation can be visualized (Video 1.6), the distal surface of the lunate, the triquetrum and the scaphoid (Fig. 1.26a), and the proximal surface of the hamate and the capitate. Sweeping the arthroscope over the distal pole of the scaphoid, even the proximal surface of the trapezium and trapezoid can be evaluated (Fig. 1.26b) and resection of the distal pole of the scaphoid in STT arthritis is possible. As the joint is usually tight, it is however not always possible to advance the arthroscope sufficiently volar to see the volar capsule and midcarpal ligaments [60]:

- *Proximal*: We see the concave surface of the lunate and the scaphoid, separated by a physiologic cleft corresponding to the scapholunate articulation. A fibrocartilaginous meniscus can be present in the joint, mainly at the volar aspect.
- *Volar*: When the joint is lax, we can pass the arthroscope volarly enough to visualize the distal part of the RSC ligament that forms the radial limb of the arcuate ligament anterior to the capitate.
- *Distal*: The field of vision is completely filled by the convex head of the capitate.
- *Radial*: Sweeping the arthroscope radially along the scaphoid, we can follow the complete scaphocapitate

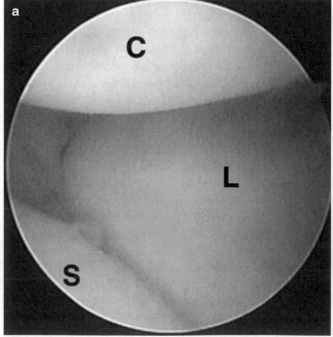 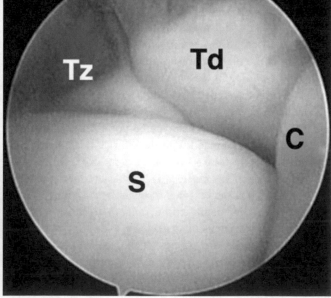

Fig. 1.26 Arthroscopic exploration of the midcarpal joint through the MCR portal (right wrist): we see the concave surface of the scaphoid (S) and the lunate (L) below, separated by a narrow gap corresponding to the scapholunate articulation. The articular surface of the round head of the capitate (C) can be inspected above (**a**). Exploration of the STT joint from the MCR portal (right wrist): the distal pole of the scaphoid (S), articulating with the trapezium (Tz) and the trapezoid (Td), can be assessed. Note that the trapezoid is encountered more dorsally than the trapezium and only the dorsal aspect of the trapezium can be visualized through this portal (**b**). (Modified from Atzei et al. [33]. With permission from Elsevier)

articulation area up to the STT joint distally. The trapezoid is found more dorsally than the trapezium, the two carpal bones are separated by a narrow groove corresponding to the trapeziotrapezoidal articulation. Sometimes the volar radial scaphotrapezial ligament can be seen, a strong structure that is reinforced by the FCR tendon sheath [60, 61].

- *Ulnar*: Rotating the scope to the ulnar side, we find the articulating corner of four carpal bones, forming a cross by the hamate, capitate, lunate, and triquetrum. We inspect carefully the lunotriquetral joint, and we can assess the distal alignment of the articulating surfaces of the two bones. A fibrocartilaginous meniscus can be present in the joint. The lunate can present with one concave, articulating only with the capitate, or two concave facets for a common articulation with the capitate and hamate. In this case, we find a longitudinal ridge at the lunate, separating the two articulation fossae to the hamate and the capitate, respectively. Viegas has classified the different types of the lunate into type I, if articulating only with the capitate, and type II, if an additional facet for the hamate is present [62] (Fig. 1.27).

Ulnar Midcarpal (MCU) Portal

The MCU portal is situated symmetrically to the above-mentioned portal in the soft depression of the four-corner intersection of the hamate, capitate, lunate, and triquetrum, on the midaxial line of the fourth metacarpal where the soft sport is easily palpable making it to the preferred portal to be established first for arthroscopy of the midcarpal joint (see Fig. 1.18b). The portal is situated approximately 1–1.5 cm distal to the 4–5 portal. It is bounded radially by the EDC tendons and ulnarly by the EDQ tendon. In type I lunates, the proximal border is the lunotriquetral joint and the distal border is the capitohamate articulation. In type II lunates, the proximal border remains the same but the distal border is the proximal pole of the hamate. The structure most at risk is the EDQ tendon. The SBRN is remote to this portal, and the branches of the DBUN are found a mean of 15.1 mm ulnar to this portal (see Fig. 1.16a–c). However, aberrant branches can run closer or directly over the portal [34]. In type II lunates, the exploration of the ulnar component of the midcarpal joint is easier via the MCU portal (Fig. 1.28); however, the visualization of the radial aspect of the midcarpal

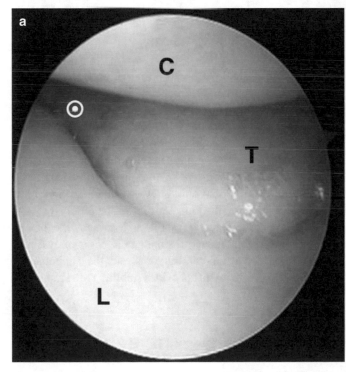
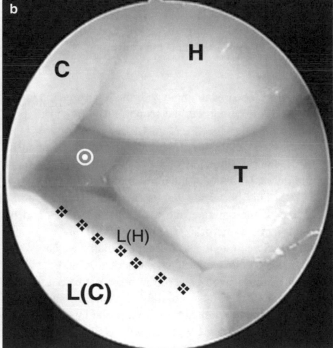

Fig. 1.27 Exploration of the corner of the four midcarpal bones (lunate, triquetrum, capitate, and hamate) via the MCR portal. Lunate type I according to Viegas with one distal articular facet, articulating with the capitate. Note the step of the triquetrum to the lunate that is a physiological finding and not a sign for lunotriquetral instability. (◉) Fibroadipose tissue, covering the capitatotriquetral ligament (**a**). Lunate type II according to Viegas with a separate distal articular facet (L(H)), articulating with the hamate (H). The facet articulating with the capitate (L(C)) is bigger. The two facets of the lunate are separated by a longitudinal crest (❖) (**b**). (Modified from Atzei et al. [33]. With permission from Elsevier)

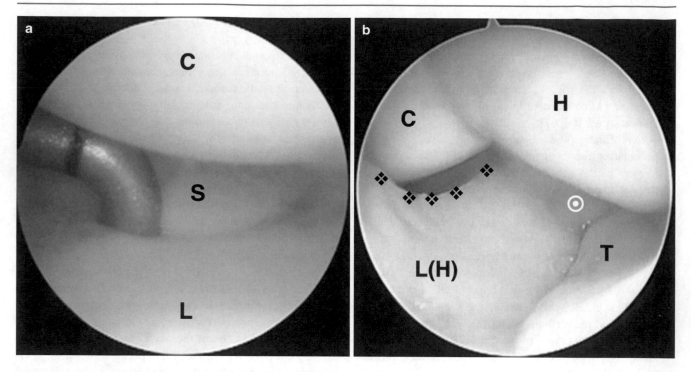

Fig. 1.28 Arthroscopic view of the midcarpal joint through the MCU portal. The scapholunate articulation is tested with a probe (**a**) and is intact as the probe cannot be protruded into the articulation. The articulation of the lunate, triquetrum, capitate, and hamate is inspected, showing a lunate type Viegas II (**b**). (Modified from Atzei et al. [33]. With permission from Elsevier)

joint is not as good as through the MCR portal, especially the exploration of the STT joint is not convenient from the MCU portal.

- *Proximal*: The distal lunate with the lunotriquetral articulation in the center and the scapholunate articulation can be visualized (Videos 1.7 and 1.8).
- *Volar*: One can identify the ulnar limb of the arcuate ligament, the continuation of the capitotriquetral ligament, and the distal fibers of the ulnocapitate ligament.
- *Distal*: This portal allows visualization of the proximal aspect of the capitate, the apex of the hamate, and the capitohamate interosseous ligament (CHIL).
- *Radial*: Sweeping the arthroscope radially, we have a better view of the scapholunate articulation and the alignment of those two bones of the proximal carpal row can be assessed. It is also possible to visualize and test the scaphocapitate articulation with a probe inserted into the MCR portal (Video 1.9), but not the STT joint.
- *Ulnar*: Looking ulnarly, we see the distal surface of the triquetrum, and it is possible to analyze the articulation between the hook-shaped tip of the hamate and the triquetrum. The saddle-shaped triquetrohamate (TH) joint is held tightly by the volar triquetrohamate and triquetrocapitate ligaments [60], and it is difficult to enter the TH articulation directly except in the setting of midcarpal instability.

Volar Midcarpal (VM) Portal

The volar midcarpal portal has been mentioned as an accessory midcarpal portal [47]; however, it lacks widespread use and we do not have any clinical experience with this portal. The topographic landmarks and skin incision are the same as for the VR portal (see Figs. 1.15b and 1.16d). The volar aspect of the midcarpal joint is identified with a 22-G needle on average 11 mm (range 7–12 mm) distal to the entry to the VR portal, and the joint entered with a cannula and a blunt trocar after piercing the joint capsule with a blunt artery forceps. The portal may be useful in assessing the palmar aspects of the capitate and the hamate in cases of avascular necrosis or osteochondral fractures and the capitohamate interosseous ligament that provides stability to the transverse carpal arch [63].

Scaphotrapeziotrapezoid (STT) Portal

The STT portal is found at the level of the STT joint in line with the radial margin of the index metacarpal just ulnar to the EPL tendon. The portal is bordered ulnarly by the ECRL tendon, proximally by the distal pole of the scaphoid, and distally by the trapezium, and the trapezoid and is localized approximately 1 cm distally to the 1–2 portal. Structures that can be jeopardized are the radial artery, the EPL tendon, and small terminal branches of the SBRN (see Figs. 1.16a, b and 1.19a). Establishing the portal on the ulnar side of the EPL tendon usually keeps the radial artery safe.

The joint is triangulated with an 18-G needle, and confirming correct placement of the needle in the STT joint under fluoroscopy can be convenient. Then a skin incision is made and the joint capsule pierced with a blunt artery forceps. A 1.9-mm 30-degree-angled arthroscope is inserted over a trocar sleeve after a blunt trocar has been introduced to the joint.

The STT joint can be inspected; however, the concavity of the distal pole of the scaphoid makes it difficult to explore the anterior part of this articulation. The portal is primarily utilized for instrumentation, particularly for arthroscopic resection of the distal pole of the scaphoid in STT arthritis.

Radial STT (STT-R) Portal

The radial STT portal is situated at the same level of the STT joint as the standard STT portal but radial to the APL tendon [59]. The radial artery is found at a mean distance of 8.8 mm radial to the portal. The terminal branches of the SBRN with individual arborization are in close vicinity of the portal and care must be taken when establishing the portal. The portal is created as described for the standard STT portal above. Together the two portals for the STT joint allow a working angle of 130°, and the radial STT portal (sometimes also called volar STT portal) serves as a better working portal for removal of the distal pole of the scaphoid in STT arthritis.

Triquetrohamate Portal (TH)

For completeness, we mention the TH portal, which is an accessory portal on the ulnar aspect of the midcarpal joint. It is located between the ECU and FCU tendon and is bordered proximally by the triquetrum and distally by the base of the fifth metacarpal and the hamate. The portal has been described for an inflow or outflow cannula and can be used as an instrument portal in assessing the triquetrohamate joint and the proximal pole of the hamate [60]. However, we do not have any experience with this portal.

Arthroscopy of the DRUJ

The DRUJ is the main articulation of the wrist allowing pronosupination. Arthroscopy of the DRUJ is the most recently introduced part in wrist arthroscopy and preserved for special indications. The anatomy of the DRUJ is complex. It is mostly described as a diarthrodial trochoid articulation com-

posed of the medial articular facet of the distal radius, the radial notch, and the distal end of the ulna. As the distal ulna not only articulates with the distal radius but also with the carpus by the ulnocarpal joint, arthroscopy of the DRUJ addresses the evaluation of pathologies of the DRUJ and the ulnocarpal articulation. In a normal wrist joint, the TFCC with its volar and dorsal distal radioulnar ligaments, merging at the insertion at the fovea, supports the DRUJ. The volar branch of the DRUL merges also with the ulnocarpal (UC) ligaments, which also contribute stability to the ulnar side of the carpus (Fig. 1.29).

In a normal wrist, the DRUJ is very narrow and hard to enter and explore; therefore, the 1.9-mm arthroscope should be used. Traction should be reduced to 3–5 kg for DRUJ arthroscopy [5] to reduce the tension. As for the radiocarpal joint arthroscopy, fluid distension is generally not necessary for DRUJ arthroscopy. If needed, we use saline to flush out the synovial liquid in intense DRUJ synovitis, then the joint is dried with suction. DRUJ arthroscopy is useful in the assessment of soft tissue disorders and the articular cartilage of the sigmoid notch or ulnar head [64].

Four portals for the DRUJ have been described: two dorsal portals [65], one volar portal (V-DRUJ) [39], and the direct foveal portal (DF) [66] (see Figs. 1.15 and 1.16).

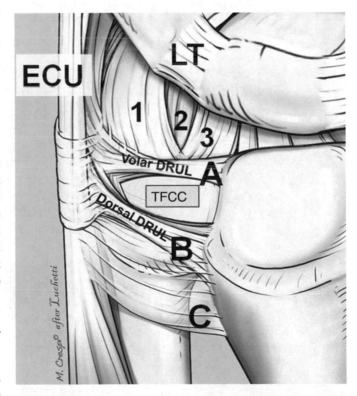

Fig. 1.29 Drawing of the DRUJ. *LT*, lunotriquetral ligament; *ECU*, extensor carpi ulnaris; 1, 2, 3, volar ulnocarpal ligaments (1: ulnotriquetral, 2: ulnocapitate, 3: ulnolunate); A, volar distal radioulnar ligament; B, dorsal distal radioulnar ligament; C, dorsal articular capsule

The two dorsal portals, the proximal DRUJ portal (P-DRUJ) and the distal DRUJ portal (D-DRUJ), are the standard portals for exploration of the DRUJ and normally utilized for the assessment of the foveal insertion of the deep component of the distal RUL as the main stabilizer of the DRUJ or for arthrolysis of the DRUJ. However, we prefer to start the DRUJ exploration through a dorsal portal located at a midpoint between the traditional P-DRUJ and D-DRUJ portals, below the radial insertion of the TFCC, at the point

where the distal profile of the ulnar head curves to parallel the sigmoid notch (Figs. 1.30 and 1.31). Through this portal, we assess the surface of the ulnar head, the TFCC with its volar and dorsal distal RUL and its foveal insertion, and the sigmoid notch. As in the radiocarpal joint, the dorsal and volar portals allow an omnidirectional evaluation of the DRUJ (Fig. 1.32).

Distal DRUJ Portal (D-DRUJ)

This portal is located in line with and about 5–8 mm proximal to the 6-R portal just under TFCC (see Fig. 1.16). With the forearm in neutral rotation, the TFCC has the least tension; however, because of the shape of the ulnar head, wrist supination facilitates the establishment of the dorsal DRUJ portals (Fig. 1.33). The DRUJ is bordered radially by the EDQ and EDC tendons and ulnarly by the ECU tendon. Proximally it is bounded by the ulnar head and distally by the TFCC (see Fig. 1.16e). The structure that can be jeopardized is the TFCC, while the only sensory nerve in proximity to the portal is the TBDBUN that has been found at a mean distance of 17.5 mm distally to the portal (Figs. 1.18b and 1.22) [34]. In the presence of a positive ulnar variance, this portal should not be used [64]. After localizing the portal with a 22-G needle, a small longitudinal skin incision is made and the dorsal capsule is pierced with a blunt artery forceps. Then a cannula with trocar is inserted, followed by a 1.9-mm

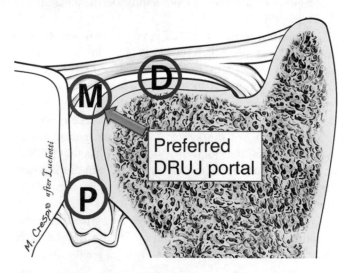

Fig. 1.30 Dorsal DRUJ portals: drawing of the dorsal portals. D, distal DRUJ portal; P, proximal DRUJ portal; M, mid–DRUJ portal (preferred dorsal portal)

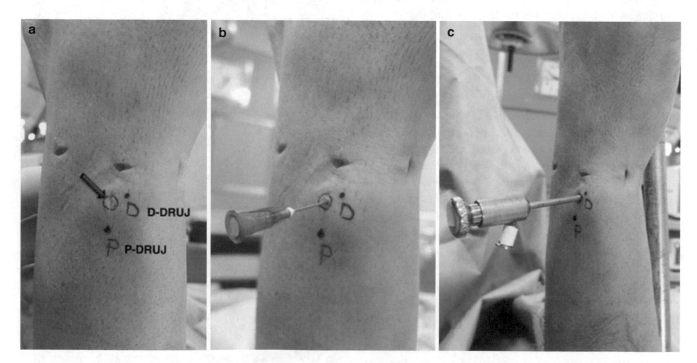

Fig. 1.31 Establishment of our preferred dorsal DRUJ portal. The *red arrow* is pointing at the entry portal and its relation to the classic proximal DRUJ portal (P-DRUJ) and distal DRUJ portal (D-DRUJ) (**a**). Verification of the correct entry point with introduction of a needle (**b**) and introduction of a blunt trocar over a trocar sleeve (**c**)

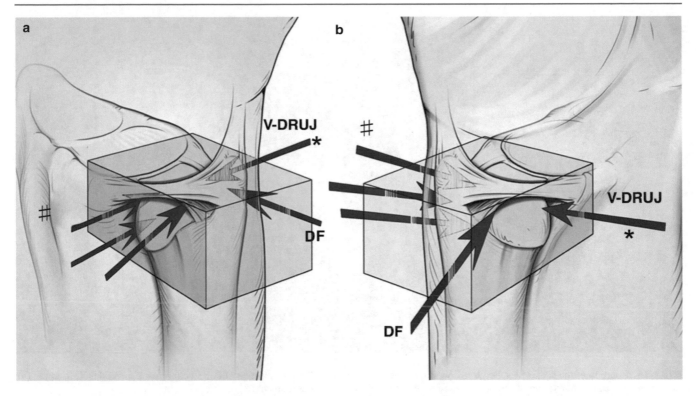

Fig. 1.32 Drawing of the "box concept" of the arthroscopic portals to the DRUJ: dorsal view (**a**) and volar view (**b**). There are three dorsal and two volar portals: ♯, preferred dorsal portal; *, preferred volar portal

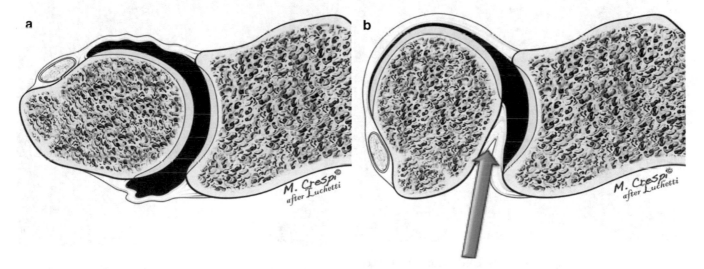

Fig. 1.33 Transverse drawing of the DRUJ in neutral rotation (**a**) and supination (**b**). Due to the osseous morphology of the ulnar head, it becomes evident that introduction of the scope through a dorsal portal into the DRUJ (*red arrow*) is easier when the wrist is fully supinated (**b**)

30-degree-angle arthroscope. We recommend starting the joint exploration by rotating the scope (Fig. 1.34), rather than moving its tip inside the joint.

- *Proximal*: The whole surface of the ulnar head can be visualized.
- *Distal*: The undersurface of the TFCC is visible.

- *Radial*: Rotating the scope radialwards, the TFCC is visualized and its radial insertion at the sigmoid notch of the radius is shown (Fig. 1.35). The DRUJ capsule attaches to the volar and dorsal distal radioulnar ligaments, and the volar capsule of the DRUJ can be seen obliquely.
- *Ulnar*: Turning the arthroscope to the ulnar side, the proximal insertion of the deep component of the distal radio-

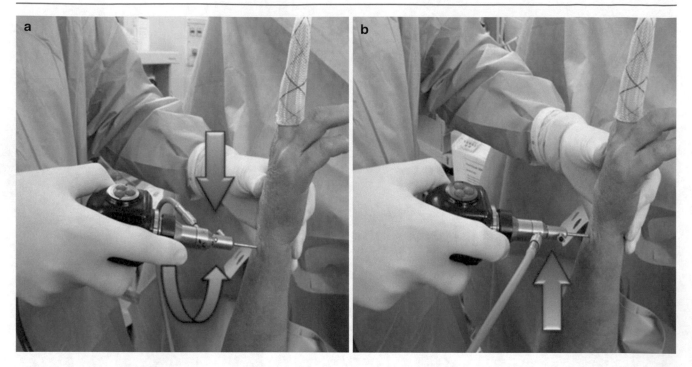

Fig. 1.34 Rotation of the scope for a better vision of the DRUJ (*red arrows*). The first position allows a better vision of the TFCC insertion (**a**); the second allows a better vision of the radial insertion of the TFCC and the sigmoid notch (**b**)

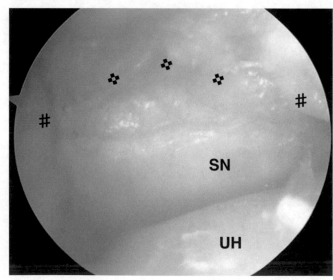

Fig. 1.35 Arthroscopic exploration of the DRUJ through the D-DRUJ portal. SN, sigmoid notch; UH, ulnar head; ❖, central insertion of the TFCC; ♯, radial insertion of the volar and dorsal branches of the TFCC

Fig. 1.36 Arthroscopic view of the undersurface of the TFCC with its volar and dorsal DRUL, merging at the insertion at the fovea (*blue arrows*)

ulnar ligaments, merging at the ulnar fovea, can be seen. A 22-G needle, introduced from the area of the DF portal, may elevate the ligament to obtain a better vision of the ulnar part of the TFCC, inserting at the fovea (Fig. 1.36).

Proximal DRUJ Portal (P-DRUJ)

The P-DRUJ portal is situated 1 cm proximal to the distal DRUJ portal. It is located at the level of the proximal soft spot

of the DRUJ, corresponding to the axilla of the joint, just proximal to the sigmoid notch of the radius and the flare of the ulnar metaphysis [64]. The portal is bordered radially by the EDQ tendon and the radial sigmoid notch, ulnarly by the ECU tendon and the neck of the ulna, and distally by the TFCC. The structure most at risk is the EDQ tendon. The P-DRUJ portal is a very narrow portal. If preferred, the joint can then be filled with saline, but the capacity of distension of this articulation is limited. A small skin incision is made, and

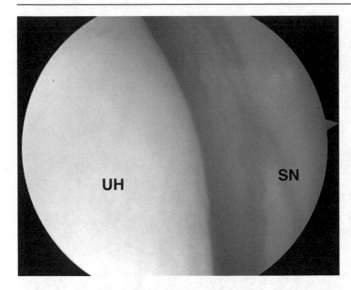

Fig. 1.37 Arthroscopic exploration of the DRUJ from the P-DRUJ portal. UH, ulna head; SN, sigmoid notch

the dorsal joint capsule is pierced with a blunt hemostat. A cannula with a blunt trocar is inserted, aiming slightly distally, then a 1.9-mm 30-degree wide-angle scope. On entry into the P-DRUJ, we can first see the sigmoid notch of the radius and the articular surface of the neck of the ulna (Fig. 1.37). Systematically, the following structures are inspected:

- *Proximal*: The palmar aspect of the capsule of the DRUJ can be visualized.
- *Distal*: The articular surface of the ulnar head can be seen on the ulnar side, and the junction of the TFCC to the sigmoid notch of the radius is visible.
- *Volar*: The volar capsule of the DRUJ can be seen and the course of the volar radioulnar ligament. The origin of the volar ulnocarpal ligaments more distally is difficult to see.
- *Radial*: The sigmoid notch of the radius can be inspected by rotating the arthroscope radially.
- *Ulnar*: The articular surface of the neck of the ulna can be visualized by turning the scope to the ulnar side.

Volar Distal Radioulnar Portal (V-DRUJ)

Two ways of establishing the V-DRUJ exist. The initial description of establishing the V-DRUJ portal uses the same landmarks as those of the VU portal (see Figs. 1.7b and 1.15b, e) [39]. After the skin incision is made, the common flexor tendons retracted radially and the FCU tendon with

the ulnar neurovascular bundle retracted ulnarly, the joint capsule is entered approximately 5–10 mm proximal to the entry to the VU radiocarpal portal. The DRUJ joint is located with a 22-G needle and the joint capsule pierced with a blunt artery forceps followed by insertion of a cannula and a blunt trocar, then the arthroscope. Our preferred method for creating the V-DRUJ portal uses a similar technique as described above for the establishment of the volar radial radiocarpal joint (Fig. 1.38). In our experience, the ulnar neurovascular bundle has never been damaged performing this technique. For the introduction of the arthroscope through the V-DRUJ portal, a switching rod can be used.

From a volar approach, the course of the dorsal radioulnar ligament can be followed, which is not possible from the dorsal DRUJ portals, until it merges with the volar radioulnar ligament and inserts at the fovea. With the instruments placed through one of the dorsal DRUJ portals, arthroscopic procedures such as the wafer partial ulnar head resection can be performed directly under the TFCC instead of through its lesion from above.

Direct Foveal Portal (DF)

The direct foveal (DF) portal as described by Atzei et al. [66] is located approximately 1 cm proximal to the 6-U portal (see Figs. 1.15b, 1.16e, 1.39). For establishment of the DF portal, the forearm is held in full supination. That way, the portal is bounded by the ulnar styloid and the ECU tendon dorsally, the flexor carpi ulnaris (FCU) tendon volarly, the ulnar head proximally, and the TFCC distally. The DBUN is at risk and is usually displaced dorsally to the portal if the forearm is held in supination (see Fig. 1.16e). A 22-G needle is inserted percutaneously just underneath the TFCC to verify the correct position. Then a small longitudinal skin incision is made between the ECU and FCU tendon. Next the extensor retinaculum is exposed and split along its fibers. The DRUJ capsule is incised longitudinally to reach the distal articular surface of the ulnar head under the TFCC.

When the surgeon is more experienced with establishing this portal and familiar with the anatomy, the DF portal can be created using the standard portal establishing technique without any clinically relevant disturbance to the DBUN.

The DF portal is used as a dedicated working portal for fixation of the TFCC to the ulnar fovea in proximal TFCC lesions. Small shavers or curettes are used to debride the torn or avulsed ligament back to healthy tissue, debride the fovea, and prepare it for suture screw or anchor insertion while the arthroscope is in the distal DRUJ portal.

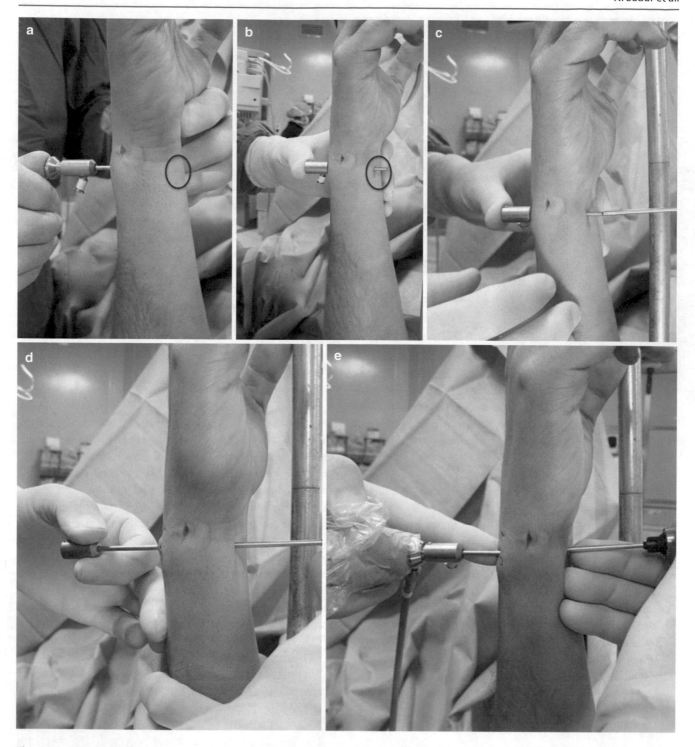

Fig. 1.38 Technical procedure to establish the volar DRUJ portal: A blunt trocar perforates the volar capsule and is pushed through the volar skin after a small skin incision is made (*red circle*) (**a** and **b**). The trocar is then used as a guide for the introduction of the shaver into the DRUJ, the trocar is pulled backwards, and the shaver advanced into the DRUJ through the volar DRUJ portal (**c** and **d**). Handling of the arthroscope and shaver. The surgeon should stay at the ulnar side of the wrist (**e**)

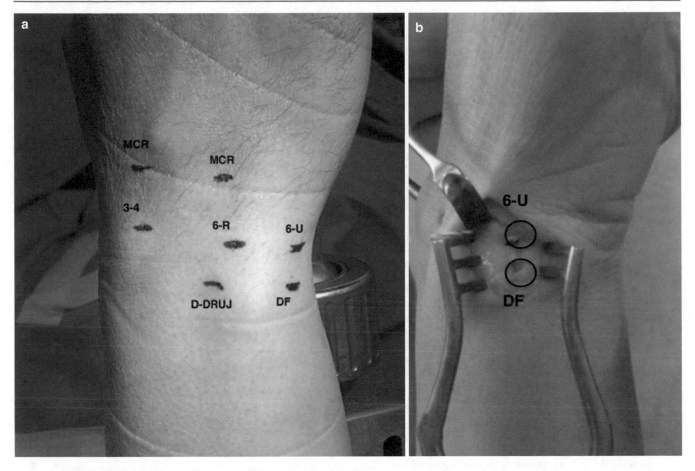

Fig. 1.39 Anatomic location of the DF portal (**a**). The DF portal is located 1 cm proximal to the 6-U portal and a skin incision can connect those two portals while leaving the retinaculum and capsule intact (**b**)

Conclusion

Wrist arthroscopy is a reasonable recently introduced technique but has continued to evolve rapidly. In its beginning, wrist arthroscopy was primarily used for diagnostic purposes. The introduction of smaller optics and miniaturized instruments however has allowed the development of more arthroscopically sophisticated surgical interventions. Nowadays, it is impossible to ignore the impact of therapeutic wrist arthroscopy that limits the iatrogenic effect of open wrist procedures, for example, as creating intra-articular fibrosis. It has been proved more reliable in assessing many wrist pathologies than even sophisticated MRI images. Step by step and adapting to the surgical needs, the portals for wrist arthroscopy have been developed. Starting with the four classic standard portals (3–4 radiocarpal, 4–5 radiocarpal, radial midcarpal, and ulnar midcarpal), an increasingly number of new portals as well as volar portals have been established and proved to be safe. However, the learning curve takes its time

and precise knowledge of the anatomy, and the pathologies of the wrist are crucial in order to limit the risk of complications or true diagnostic or therapeutic failures. Earlier teaching of wrist arthroscopy has been performed under simple observing conditions. Nowadays, the teaching is much more structured and numerous instructional courses are offered, allowing to study wrist arthroscopy and the handling of the arthroscope and instruments in cadavers. The European Wrist Arthroscopy Society (EWAS, www.wristarthroscopy.eu) has developed specific courses on fresh cadavers for a couple of years. Practicing on cadavers and examining the wrist joint from different portals and viewing angles help in understanding the three-dimensional anatomy of the wrist. Once normal arthroscopic wrist anatomy is clear, pathologic problems can be more readily identified and treated. It is without doubt that the creativity of the surgeon and the introduction of adapted miniaturized instruments will allow for realization of precise performance and continuous development of more and more sophisticated arthroscopic techniques.

References

1. Ekman EF, Poehling GG. Principles of arthroscopy and wrist arthroscopic equipment. Hand Clin. 1994;10:557–66.
2. Chen YC. Arthroscopy of the wrist and finger joints. Orthop Clin North Am. 1979;10:723–33.
3. Fontès D. Wrist arthroscopy. Current indications and results. Chir Main. 2004;23:270–83. French.
4. Mathoulin C, Levadoux M, Martinache X. Intérêt thérapeutique de l'arthroscopie du poignet: à propos de 1000 cas. E-Mémoires de l'Académie Nationale de Chirurgie. 2005;4:42–57. French.
5. Wolf JM, Dukas A, Pensak M. Advances in wrist arthroscopy. J Am Acad Orthop Surg. 2012;20:725–34.
6. Harley BJ, Werner FW, Boles SD, Palmer AK. Arthroscopic resection of arthrosis of the proximal hamate: a clinical and biomechanical study. J Hand Surg Am. 2004;29:661–7.
7. Doi K, Hattori Y, Otsuka K, Abe Y, Yamamoto H. Intra-articular fractures of the distal aspect of the radius: arthroscopically assisted reduction compared with open reduction and internal fixation. J Bone Joint Surg Am. 1999;81:1093–110.
8. Geissler WB. Arthroscopically assisted reduction of intra-articular fractures of the distal radius. Hand Clin. 1995;11:19–29.
9. Geissler WB, Freeland AE. Arthroscopically assisted reduction of intraarticular distal radial fractures. Clin Orthop Relat Res. 1996;327:125–34.
10. Lindau T. Wrist arthroscopy in distal radial fractures using a modified horizontal technique. Arthroscopy. 2001;17:E5.
11. Shih JT, Lee HM, Hou YT, Tan CM. Arthroscopically-assisted reduction of intra-articular fractures and soft tissue management of distal radius. Hand Surg. 2001;6:127–35.
12. Trumble TE, Culp RW, Hanel DP, Geissler WB, Berger RA. Intra-articular fractures of the distal aspect of the radius. Instr Course Lect. 1999;48:465–80.
13. Whipple TL. The role of arthroscopy in the treatment of intra-articular wrist fractures. Hand Clin. 1995;11:13–8.
14. Shih JT, Lee HM, Hou YT, Tan CM. Results of arthroscopic reduction and percutaneous fixation for acute displaced scaphoid fractures. Arthroscopy. 2005;21:620–6.
15. Wong WY, Ho PC. Minimal invasive management of scaphoid fractures: from fresh to nonunion. Hand Clin. 2011;27:291–307.
16. del Piñal F, García-Bernal FJ, Delgado J, Sanmartín M, Regalado J, Cerezal L. Correction of malunited intra-articular distal radius fractures with an inside-out osteotomy technique. J Hand Surg Am. 2006;31:1029–34.
17. del Piñal F, Cagigal L, García-Bernal FJ, Studer A, Regalado J, Thams C. Arthroscopically guided osteotomy for management of intra-articular distal radius malunions. J Hand Surg Am. 2010;35:392–7.
18. Luchetti R, Atzei A, Fairplay T. Arthroscopic wrist arthrolysis after wrist fracture. Arthroscopy. 2007;23:255–60.
19. Bain GI, Smith ML, Watts AC. Arthroscopic core decompression of the lunate in early stage Kienbock disease of the lunate. Tech Hand Up Extrem Surg. 2011;15:66–9.
20. Weiss ND, Molina RA, Gwin S. Arthroscopic proximal row carpectomy. J Hand Surg Am. 2011;36:577–82.
21. Ho PC. Arthroscopic partial wrist fusion. Tech Hand Up Extrem Surg. 2008;12:242–65.
22. Buterbaugh GA. Radiocarpal arthroscopy portals and normal anatomy. Hand Clin. 1994;10:567–76.
23. Huracek J, Troeger H. Wrist arthroscopy without distraction. A technique to visualise instability of the wrist after a ligamentous tear. J Bone Joint Surg Br. 2000;82:1011–2.
24. Bain GI, Munt J, Turner PC. New advances in wrist arthroscopy. Arthroscopy. 2008;24:355–67.
25. Lee JI, Nha KW, Lee GY, Kim BH, Kim JW, Park JW. Long-term outcomes of arthroscopic debridement and thermal shrinkage for isolated partial intercarpal ligament tears. Orthopedics. 2012;35:e1204–9.
26. Sotereanos DG, Darlis NA, Kokkalis ZT, Zanaros G, Altman GT, Miller MC. Effects of radiofrequency probe application on irrigation fluid temperature in the wrist joint. J Hand Surg Am. 2009;34:1832–7.
27. Botte MJ, Cooney WP, Linscheid RL. Arthroscopy of the wrist: anatomy and technique. J Hand Surg Am. 1989;14:313–6.
28. Geissler WB, Freeland AE, Weiss APC, Chow JC. Techniques of wrist arthroscopy. J Bone Joint Surg Am. 1999;81:1184–97.
29. Geissler WB. Intra-articular distal radius fractures: the role of arthroscopy? Hand Clin. 2005;21:407–16.
30. del Piñal F, García-Bernal FJ, Pisani D, Regalado J, Ayala H, Studer A. Dry arthroscopy of the wrist: surgical technique. J Hand Surg Am. 2007;32:119–23.
31. DeAraujo W, Poehling GG, Kuzma GR. New Tuohy needle technique for triangular fibrocartilage complex repair: preliminary studies. Arthroscopy. 1996;12:699–703.
32. Geissler WB. Arthroscopic knotless peripheral ulnar-sided TFCC repair. Hand Clin. 2011;27:273–9.
33. Atzei A, Luchetti R, Sgarbossa A, Carità E, Llusà M. Set-up, portals and normal exploration in wrist arthroscopy. Chir Main. 2006;25(Suppl 1):S131–44. French.
34. Abrams RA, Petersen M, Botte MJ. Arthroscopic portals of the wrist: an anatomic study. J Hand Surg Am. 1994;19:940–4.
35. Grechening W, Peicha G, Fellinger M, Seibert FJ, Weiglein AH. Anatomical and safety considerations in establishing portals used for wrist arthroscopy. Clin Anat. 1999;12:179–85.
36. Tryfonidis M, Charalambous CP, Jass GK, Jacob S, Hayton MJ, Stanley JK. Anatomic relation of dorsal wrist arthroscopy portals and superficial nerves: a cadaveric study. Arthroscopy. 2009;25:1387–90.
37. Atzei A, Luchetti R. Clinical approach to the painful wrist. In: Geissler WB, editor. Wrist arthroscopy. New York: Springer; 2005. p. 185–95.
38. Lawler EA, Adams BD. Arthroscopy of the distal radioulnar joint. In: Slutsky D, Nagle D, editors. Techniques in wrist and hand arthroscopy. Philadelphia: Churchill Livingstone Elsevier; 2007. p. 54–7.
39. Slutsky DJ. Distal radioulnar joint arthroscopy and the volar ulnar portal. Tech Hand Up Extrem Surg. 2007;11:38–44.
40. Berger RA. Arthroscopic anatomy of the wrist and distal radioulnar joint. Hand Clin. 1999;15:393–413.
41. Whipple TL, Marotta JJ, Powell JH 3rd. Techniques of wrist arthroscopy. Arthroscopy. 1986;2:244–52.
42. Levy HJ, Glickel SZ. Arthroscopic assisted internal fixation of volar intraarticular wrist fractures. Arthroscopy. 1993;9:122–4.
43. Tham S, Coleman S, Gilpin D. An anterior portal for wrist arthroscopy. Anatomical study and case reports. J Hand Surg Br. 1999;24:445–7.
44. Abe Y, Doi K, Hattori Y, Ikeda K, Dhawan V. A benefit of the volar approach for wrist arthroscopy. Arthroscopy. 2003;19:440–5.
45. Slutsky DJ. Wrist arthroscopy through a volar radial portal. Arthroscopy. 2002;18:624–30.
46. Slutsky DJ. The use of a volar ulnar portal in wrist arthroscopy. Arthroscopy. 2004;20:158–63.
47. Slutsky DJ. Clinical applications of volar portals in wrist arthroscopy. Tech Hand Up Extrem Surg. 2004;8:229–38.
48. Van Meir N, Degreef I, De Smet L. The volar portal in wrist arthroscopy. Acta Orthop Belg. 2011;77:290–3.
49. Mackinnon SE, Dellon AL. The overlap pattern of the lateral antebrachial cutaneous nerve and the superficial branch of the radial nerve. J Hand Surg Am. 1985;10:522–6.

50. Berger RA, Kauer JM, Landsmeer JM. Radioscapholunate ligament: a gross anatomic and histologic study of fetal and adult wrists. J Hand Surg Am. 1991;16:350–5.

51. Berger RA. The gross and histologic anatomy of the scapholunate interosseous ligament. J Hand Surg Am. 1996;21(2):170–8.

52. Nakamura T, Makita A. The proximal ligamentous component of the triangular fibrocartilage complex. J Hand Surg Br. 2000;25:479–86.

53. Zahiri H, Zahiri CA, Ravari FK. Ulnar styloid impingement syndrome. Int Orthop. 2010;34:1233–7.

54. Arya AP, Kulshreshtha R, Kakarala GK, Singh R, Compson JP. Visualisation of the pisotriquetral joint through standard portals for arthroscopy of the wrist: a clinical and anatomical study. J Bone Joint Surg Br. 2007;89:202–5.

55. Ehlinger M, Rapp E, Cognet JM, Clavert P, Bonnomet F, Kahn JL, Kempf JF. Transverse radioulnar branch of the dorsal ulnar nerve: anatomic description and arthroscopic implications from 45 cadaveric dissections. Rev Chir Orthop Reparatrice Appar Mot. 2005;91:208–14.

56. Luchetti R, Atzei A, Rocchi L. Incidence and causes of failures in wrist arthroscopic techniques. Chir Main. 2006;25:48–53. French.

57. Lee JH, Taylor NL, Deckman RA, Rosenwasser MP. Arthroscopic wrist anatomy. In: Geissler WB, editor. Wrist arthroscopy. New York: Springer; 2005. p. 7–14.

58. Ritt MJ, Bishop AT, Berger RA, Linscheid RL, Berglund LJ, An KN. Lunotriquetral ligament properties: a comparison of three anatomic subregions. J Hand Surg Am. 1998;23:425–31.

59. Carro LP, Golano P, Fariñas O, Cerezal L, Hidalgo C. The radial portal for scaphotrapeziotrapezoid arthroscopy. Arthroscopy. 2003;19:547–53.

60. Viegas SF. Midcarpal arthroscopy: anatomy and portals. Hand Clin. 1994;10:577–87.

61. Bettinger PC, Cooney WP III, Berger RA. Arthroscopic anatomy of the wrist. Orthop Clin North Am. 1995;26:707–19.

62. Viegas SF, Wagner K, Patterson R, Peterson P. Medial (hamate) facet of the lunate. J Hand Surg Am. 1990;15:564–71.

63. Garcia-Elias M, An KN, Cooney WP III, Linscheid RL, Chao EY. Stability of the transverse carpal arch: an experimental study. J Hand Surg Am. 1989;14:277–82.

64. Whipple TL. Arthroscopy of the distal radioulnar joint. Indications, portals, and anatomy. Hand Clin. 1994;10:589–92.

65. Bowers WH, Whipple TL. Arthrosopic anatomy of the wrist. In: McGinty J, editor. Operative arthroscopy. New York: Raven Press; 1991. p. 613–23.

66. Atzei A, Rizzo A, Luchetti R, Fairplay T. Arthroscopic foveal repair of triangular fibrocartilage complex peripheral lesion with distal radioulnar joint instability. Tech Hand Up Extrem Surg. 2008;12:226 35.

Evaluation of the Painful Wrist

2

Enrique Pereira

Introduction

The human wrist connects the forearm to the hand. Under healthy conditions, the wrist is capable of precise hand positioning in space due to a wide range of motion (flexion/extension, pronation/supination, and radio/ulnar deviation). Such freedom of wrist movement and position is necessary to perform highly complex and delicate movements of the thumb and fingers.

Following the notion that *function follows anatomy*, wrist's ample range of motion is the product of the complex interplay of a sophisticated arrangement of bony and ligamentous structures added to normal function of the five carpal joints (radioulnar, the radiocarpal, midcarpal, intercarpal, and carpometacarpal joints) [1, 2].

After evaluating 52 standardized tasks of activities of daily living, Palmer et al. [3] showed that the wrist *normal functional range of motion* allows 5° of flexion, 30° of extension, 10° of radial deviation, and 15° of ulnar deviation. On the other hand, according to the *ideal range of motion* for activities of daily living described by Ryu et al. [4], the wrist should reach 54° of flexion, 60° of extension, 17° of radial deviation, and 40° of ulnar deviation.

The presence of wrist pain may lead to functional impairment of the entire upper extremity, and thus, greatly impacting the patient's quality of life. In view of the fact that there is a wide range of etiologies for wrist pain, the treating physician should keep a high index of suspicion during patient's history and physical examination. Collected findings during patient examination (along with auxiliary studies) are intended to generate the most likely diagnosis. As expected, further comprehension of the underlying anatomic abnormalities is pivotal for a precise diagnosis.

A brief discussion of some core anatomic concepts of the wrist is necessary though before addressing patient assessment. Considering that there are no muscles or tendons attached to the carpus, the stability of each carpal bone is only dependent on bone surface anatomy and ligament attachments.

There are two main ligament systems in the wrist:

1. Extrinsic system capsular (extra-articular) ligaments that extend from the radius or metacarpals to the carpal bones.
2. Intrinsic system: interosseous (intra-articular) ligaments that take origin from and insert on adjacent carpal bones.

The triangular fibrocartilage complex (TFCC) attaches the distal radius, the lunate, and the triquetrum to the distal ulna. This complex along with the bony architecture provides the stability for the distal radioulnar joint (DRUJ). The vascular pattern and nerve distribution of the pain together with their pathophysiological correlation remain essential when facing a painful wrist. This complexity of the carpus and our incomplete understanding of carpal kinematics makes diagnosis of a painful wrist very difficult.

History

Obtaining a detailed history often helps narrow the differential diagnosis over a number of potential etiologies. Determining the diagnosis is usually a challenge in patients with wrist pain, to some extent due to the large number of structures found in the human wrist (bone, soft tissues, and extra-articular and intra-articular etiologies) as well as their complex biomechanical characteristics (Table 2.1). During the first step in history taking, the patient should be able to express any detail that judges related to the his/her symptomatology. This step creates sympathy toward the patient and a suitable environment during the clinical encounter and enhances the patient's compliance for future diagnostic and therapeutic steps. After that, the physician should direct the history in orderly sequence, collecting facts that have the

E. Pereira (✉)
Department of Hand Surgery, Penta Institute of Traumatology and Rehabilitation, Buenos Aires, Argentina

© Springer Nature Switzerland AG 2022
W. B. Geissler (ed.), *Wrist and Elbow Arthroscopy with Selected Open Procedures*,
https://doi.org/10.1007/978-3-030-78881-0_2

Table 2.1 Most common traumatic and atraumatic etiologies of wrist pain

Wrist pain: outline of most frequent etiologies
Bone
Fractures (distal radius, scaphoid, triquetral, hook of the hamate)
Malunions (distal radius, scaphoid)
Nonunions (scaphoid, hook of the hamate, ulnar styloid)
Impingement (radiocarpal, ulnocarpal / stylocarpal impaction syndrome)
Osteonecrosis (Kienböck's disease, Preiser's disease)
Joint
Synovitis
Loose bodies
Chondral lesions
Posttraumatic arthritis
Degenerative arthritis (radiocarpal, radioulnar, midcarpal, intercarpal)
Crystal arthritis (gout, pseudogout, lupus)
Inflammatory arthritis (rheumatoid arthritis, psoriatic arthritis, Reiter's syndrome)
Ligament
Ligament tear/rupture (TFCC, SLIL, LTIL)
Instability (scapholunate, lunotriquetral, DRUJ, midcarpal, capitolunate, pisotriquetral, STT)
Tendon
Tendonitis and tenosynovitis (De Quervain's)
Tendon tear/subluxation (ECU)
Tendon rupture
Nerve
Trauma/neuroma (superficial branch of radial or ulnar nerve)
Compression (carpal tunnel syndrome, Wartenberg's syndrome, Guyon's canal)
Peripheral neuropathy (diabetes mellitus)
Vascular
Arterial occlusion
Hypothenar hammer syndrome
Tumor
Soft tissue (ganglion cyst, giant cell tumor, fibroma, synovial cell hemangioma)
Bone tumors (primary, metastatic)
Infection
Bacterial arthritis (Staphylococcus, Streptococcus, Lyme disease, tuberculosis, gonorrhea)
Viral arthritis
Other
Complex regional pain syndrome (CRPS)

TFCC triangular fibrocartilage complex, *SLIL* scapholunate interosseous ligament, *LTIL* lunotriquetral interosseous ligament, *DRUJ* distal radioulnar joint, *STT* scaphotrapeziotrapezoid joint, *ECU* extensor carpi ulnaris

greatest clinical relevance like pain characteristics, the presence of other symptoms, and predisposing factors.

Pain

Several pain features are worth recording such as its quality (cramping, dull, aching, sharp, shooting, severe, or diffuse), frequency, duration, intensity, radiation, and movements in conjunction with the activities that may elicit pain. Nerve injury usually manifests as a sharp pain associated to a burning sensation. On the other hand, a deep, constant, boring pain mostly accompanies bone fractures. Pain from a ligamentous injury is often intermittent and elicited upon activity. In addition, location of symptoms can help guide diagnosis. The presence of localized pain may point toward ligamentous disruption, whereas nerve compression (due to carpal tunnel syndrome) is frequently associated with a more diffuse discomfort.

Predisposing Factors

Trauma

The patient should describe thoroughly any recent trauma, as its mechanism of injury may give up the diagnosis. For instance, a fall onto an outstretched hand during practice of contact sports is a common mechanism for fractures of the distal radius or scaphoid, whereas a direct palmar trauma from swinging a baseball bat or golf club could lead to a fracture of the hook of the hamate. Ligament tears may also occur, mainly at the TFCC, scapholunate, and/or lunotriquetral ligaments. Depending on the kinetic energy of the trauma, these ligament injuries could either be partial or complete, isolated or associated with either distal radius fractures or scaphoid fractures. TFCC tears (with or without DRUJ instability) are often seen in gymnastic and racquet sports and may mimic extensor carpi ulnaris (ECU) pathology.

At times, trauma kinetics of a given wrist lesion remains elusive. In these situations, symptom duration may provide a temporal clue related to a vague history of trauma, while the patient refers spontaneous onset of the pain. Sometimes, the examiner faces such challenging scenario in patients with carpal bone nonunion or avascular necrosis, in whom symptoms may manifest several years after the index injury because of ongoing inflammation, leading to arthritis, swelling, pain, and loss of grip strength. The scaphoid is particularly prone to developing nonunions [5]. The latter is due to its vulnerable blood supply that can lead to complete vascular interruption of a bone fragment following wrist trauma. Idiopathic avascular necrosis generally occurs either at the lunate (Kienböck's disease) or at the scaphoid (Preiser's disease).

Patient Occupation or Recreational Activities

Several leisure or labor activities can affect wrist function. For example, long-standing history of typing that involves repetitive motion can trigger wrist pain, while knitting or sewing may lead to compressive neuropathy. Activities requiring forceful grasping with ulnar deviation or repetitive use of the thumb (e.g., caring for a newborn infant) can lead to De Quervain's tenosynovitis with pain and swelling along the first extensor compartment.

Specific details regarding sport activities can be very informative about the mechanism of injury: repetitive stress versus blunt trauma. Contact sports, such as American football or rugby, may lead to blunt trauma, while noncontact sports, such as golf, tennis, or field hockey, involve repetitive stress of the wrist.

The presence of a painful clunking on the ulnar side of the wrist during activities that involve active ulnar deviation indicates midcarpal instability. In patients with symptoms at the ulnar side of the wrist, the examiner should rule out DRUJ arthritis, ulnocarpal, or stylocarpal impaction syndrome.

Medical History

While obtaining a thorough complete medical history, the physician should exclude the presence of systemic inflammatory disorders (lupus, rheumatoid arthritis, and degenerative arthritis) and metabolic diseases (diabetes, gout, and hypothyroidism) in addition to previous surgeries. Pregnancy, hypothyroidism, and diabetes are predisposing risk factors for carpal tunnel syndrome. Rheumatoid arthritis has a tendency to involve the wrist while gouty arthritis and pseudogout can involve the wrist joint, although more commonly they affect the lower extremities.

Patients with septic arthritis typically present with a history of constitutional symptoms or a recent infection and a poorly moveable wrist owing to severe, deep, and unrelenting pain.

Patient's age and sex should also be considered. As example, younger patients are prone to posttraumatic carpal injuries and occult ganglion cysts, whereas older patients are susceptible to systemic diseases and degenerative processes.

Physical Examination

The physician should perform a methodical physical examination, starting with a comprehensive visual inspection of the upper extremity.

Noticeable swelling, ecchymosis, or skin changes at the level wrist can provide major clues to comprehend the mechanism of injury. Gross deformity of the wrist generally indicates an obvious pathologic process that could be due to previous fracture, dislocation, or from soft tissue and/or joint swelling. A malunited distal radius fracture is often the cause of this deformity, presenting radial deviation of the wrist, and the carpus palmary displaced on the radius. Such misalignment of the distal radius may lead to extrinsic carpal

instability and wrist pain. Disruption of the distal radioulnar joint can also produce wrist deformity.

Following inspection, the physician should proceed by palpating the nonpainful areas of the wrist first and then continue to areas of maximal tenderness. This sequence is crucial because once pain/discomfort is elicited, the patient may become apprehensive, preventing further palpation. Anatomical knowledge, especially surface anatomy, can be of great help during wrist exam.

All wrist structures should be palpated and compared with the contralateral side. A systematic circumferential palpation of the wrist is performed according to patient's history and degree of pain [6]. We routinely start on the dorso-radial corner and progress to the dorso-ulnar side and then to the palmar surface. The site of pain and tenderness suggests the presence of pathology of underlying structures; however, we should take into account the intricate three-dimensional features of the wrist structures (Table 2.2).

Subsequently, active and passive range of motion of the wrist along with grip strength should be tested and compared to the contralateral wrist [7, 8]. As a rule, we measure flexion, extension, radial deviation, ulnar deviation, pronation, and supination with a goniometer. Differences in the range of motion among wrists in addition to the presence of pain at extreme range of motion will carry significant information to narrow the differential diagnosis. Assessing neurovascular status is also important, with special focus on the integrity of the median, radial, and ulnar nerves and dual-hand circulation (Allen test).

Routine palpation may not suffice to reproduce patient's symptoms; therefore, it is often necessary to perform provocative tests to locate the specific anatomic structure(s) that is originating pain. These provocative tests apply an external force that is directed to stress specific anatomic structures, which in turn would provoke an expected clinical response. A positive test correlates closely with a specific wrist pathologic diagnosis. Although the specificity of these maneuvers is not always high, the combination of a positive finding during a provocative maneuver with the remainder of the patient's clinical data (history, rest of the exam, and noninvasive imaging) almost always reach a conclusive diagnosis.

Provocative Tests

- Scaphoid Shift Test [5]: It provides a qualitative assessment of scapholunate stability and periscaphoid synovitits compared to the contralateral asymptomatic wrist.

Table 2.2 Topographic palpation of the wrist

Region	Anatomic structure	Pathology
Dorso radial		
Snuffbox (distal)	STT	Carpometacarpal arthritis/instability
		STT arthritis
Snuffbox (middle)	Floor of the snuffbox	Scaphoid fracture/nonunion
		Scaphoid necrosis (Preiser's disease)
Snuffbox (proximal)	Radial styloid	Radial styloid fracture
		Radioscaphoid arthritis
First extensor compartment	APL/EPB	De Quervain's tenosynovitis
		Intersection syndrome (proximal)
Dorso central		
3–4 dorsal recess	Lister tubercule	Dorsal synovitis
		SLIL instability
		Dorsal wrist ganglion
		Kiënbock's disease
Dorso ulnar		
5–6 dorsal recess	LTIL	LTIL instability/arthritis
DRUJ space	DRUJ	DRUJ instability/arthritis
Ulnar head	ECU	ECU tendinosis/instability
Distal ulna	Ulnar styloid	Ulnocarpal/stylocarpal disorders
Midcarpal		Halt syndrome
Palmar ulnar		
FCU	FCU	FCU tendonitis
Distal ulna	Ulnar styloid	TFCC tears
Pisiform	Pisotriquetral joint	Pisotriquetral arthritis/instability
Hypothenar eminence	Hook of the hamate	Fracture of the hook hamate
	Guyon's canal	Ulnar tunnel syndrome
Palmar central	Median nerve	Median nerve inflammation/entrapment
Palmar radial	Palmaris longus	Palmaris longus tendonitis
	Scaphoid tubercule	Scaphoid fracture (distal pole)

APL abductor pollicis longus, *APB* abductor pollicis brevis, *EPB* extensor pollicis brevis, *FCU* flexor carpi ulnaris

Basically, the test is intended to induce dorsal sublixation of the proximal pole of the scaphoid over the dorsal rim of the radius as the wrist is radially deviated.

This maneuver is done by grabbing the patient's hand from its ulnar aspect and placing the physician's thumb on the palmar surface of the distal pole of the scaphoid.

By moving the wrist from ulnar to radial deviation, the examiner exerts pressure to the distal pole of the scaphoid, which prevents the scaphoid from flexing normally.

In patients with ligamentous laxity or instability, the combined stress of thumb pressure and normal motion of the adjacent carpus may induce the scaphoid to pop out of its fossa and up onto the dorsal rim of the radius. By diminishing the pressure exerted in the thumb, the scaphoid usually returns to its normal position. The presence of

pain associated with unilateral hypermobility of the scaphoid is virtually diagnostic of scapholunate instability.

- Pisotriquetral Shear Test: It offers a qualitative evaluation of the pisotriquetral joint. The examiner's thumb is placed over the pisiform and a dorsal directed pressure is applied along with a circular grinding motion over the triquetrum. Pain elicited by the maneuver is consistent with joint instability and/or degenerative. It is central to perform this test before assessing the lunotriquetral joint, to avoid pain overlapping.

- Lunotriquetral Compression Test [7]: It evaluates the integrity of the lunotriquetral ligament. As its overall diagnostic accuracy is considered superior to other lunotriquetral tests, the compression test represents our current first choice. By supporting the wrist and pushing the triquetrum from an ulnar to a radial direction against the lunate, the test is considered positive if elicits pain. A positive test may indicate lunotriquetral ligament tear or instability.

- Lunotriquetral Ballottement Test [9]: It detects lunotriquetral ligament injuries. While holding the lunate with the thumb and the index of one hand, the triquetrum and pisiform are simultaneously displaced dorsally and palmary with the thumb and index of the other hand. Pain and excessive displaceability of the joint will suggest lunotriquetral ligament tear.

- Ulnocarpal Stress Test [10]: It is considered as a screening test for intra-articular ulnocarpal disorders. The test is performed by applying axial stress to the wrist during passive supination-pronation with the wrist in maximum ulnar deviation.

- Piano-Key Test [11]: It examines the stability of the distal radioulnar joint and often reveals instability that cannot be detected even by imaging studies. The piano-key sign is demonstrated by depressing the ulnar head over and under the distal sigmoid notch while supporting the wrist in pronation. The result of this maneuver will be positive whenever the ulnar head returns to its normal position after the applying force is removed from the distal ulna, simulating as a piano key springing up.

- TFCC Compression Test: It helps identify TFCC lesions. Under axial loading and ulnar deviation of the wrist, the test is positive when elicits a painful response and reproduces patient symptoms.

- Ulnar Fovea Test: It identifies foveal disruptions of the TFCC (also ulnotriquetral ligament tears). The examiner pressed his/her thumb into the ulnar fovea, between the flexor carpi ulnaris tendon and ulnar styloid between the volar surface of the ulnar head and pisiform with the forearm in neutral rotation. The test is considered positive when reproduces the patient's symptoms. Clinically, TFCC disruptions can be differentiated from ulnotriquetral ligament tears by assessing DRUJ stability, since in TFCC disruptions the DRUJ is unstable, whereas ulnotriquetral ligament tears have stable DRUJ.

- Midcarpal Shift Test [12]: It confirms midcarpal instability. In this maneuver, the examiner applies an axial load to the wrist while on pronation and mild flexion. In this setting, axial load generates radial to ulnar deviation. This maneuver normally reproduces a characteristic painful "clunk." This finding is based on the loss of the smooth transition from proximal row flexion to extension as the unit moves from radial to ulnar deviation. Based on how much resistance is necessary to maintain the wrist palmary subluxed while in ulnar deviation, wrists are classified into five grades of instability.
- Ice Cream Scoop Test [13]: It exacerbates extensor carpi ulnaris subluxation. The wrist is first positioned in full pronation, ulnar deviation, and extension, and then is slowly moved into supination while maintaining ulnar deviation against resistance with the other hand of the examiner ("as the ice cream is scooped"). The test is considered positive if symptoms are reproduced and snapping of the extensor carpi ulnaris tendon over the distal ulna is visualized, heard, or palpated.

Radiographic Evaluation

Initially, routine X-ray examination (posteroanterior, oblique, and lateral views) may suffice for the detection of gross wrist abnormalities. However, specialized X-ray views such as a scaphoid view (posteroanterior view in ulnar deviation), 45-degree semipronated oblique, and a true lateral may result instrumental for the identification of more subtle problems. We should probably include these specialized X-ray views in the initial imaging assessment [14]. X-ray imaging provides significant information regarding bone integrity, structure, and alignment along with the joint space dimension and symmetry.

A specialized posteroanterior view with the elbow on 90° of flexion (at shoulder height) and the forearm in neutral position is convenient to define ulnar variance (plus, neutral, negative) and constitutes a suitable view to analyze breaks in Gilula's lines. The Gilula's lines represent the arcs formed by the proximal and distal articular surfaces of the proximal row of carpal bones and the proximal articular surfaces of the distal row of carpal bones. A wide carpal joint space or a break in Gilula's lines suggests carpal instability.

In the neutral posteroanterior view, the lunate remains in a trapezoidal shape. A true lateral must be done though (elbow adducted to the patient's side and the wrist in neutral rotation) to allow the pisiform locate between the palmar

Table 2.3 Radiographic examination of the wrist: complementary views

View	Area of interest/pathologic finding
PA with radial deviation	Lunotriquetral interval/lunotriquetral instability
PA with ulnar deviation	Scapholunate interval/scapholunate instability
PA clenched fist view	Scapholunate interval/scapholunate instability
Oblique view pronated 20°	Dorsal triquetrum avulsion
	Distal pole waist scaphoid fractures
	Fourth and fifth CMC joint fracture dislocation
Oblique view pronated 60°	Scaphoid fractures
Oblique view supinated 30°	Pisotriquetral joint status
	Hook of the hamate fractures
	Second and third CMC joint fracture dislocation
Carpal tunnel view	Trapezium, scaphoid tuberosity, capitate, hook of the hamate, triquetrum, and the entire pisiform

surface of the distal scaphoid tuberosity and the capitate head. This view is particularly helpful for assessing carpal alignment. Carpal alignment has historically been determined using specific distances and measuring various angles on PA and lateral X-ray views. Several angles (capitolunate, scapholunate, and radiolunate) and indexes (carpal height, capitate-radius, and ulnar translocation) have been used showing modest (at best) diagnostic accuracy. Nonetheless, a scapholunate angle greater than 60° suggests scapholunate instability, whereas a small angle (less than 30°) points toward ulnar-sided wrist instability. Other measures can confirm this diagnosis: a radioscaphoid angle greater than 60° and a radiolunate angle greater than 15°. In case of suspecting carpal collapse secondary to Kienböck's disease, carpal height can be compared with the length of the third metacarpal. Several specialized views are sometimes required to narrow the diagnosis. The most frequently used are listed in Table 2.3.

Computed Tomography

Computed tomography (CT) constitutes an excellent imaging modality to assess bone and articular lesions as well as bone healing pattern after fracture or surgery. This technique can also detect with great precision cysts and tumors. The ability to perform multiple plane images and three-dimensional reconstruction proves particularly useful for the evaluation of bone with oblique axis like the scaphoid. Furthermore, CT may represent the imaging method of choice for detecting DRUJ instability. This technique is also valuable in certain situations in which performing a magnetic resonance imaging (MRI) is impractical (e.g., evaluation of the hook of the hamate).

Magnetic Resonance Imaging

MRI is very useful for the assessment of the integrity of soft tissues of the wrist and the vascular status of the carpal bones [15]. Nonetheless, accurate reading of MRI requires considerable anatomical knowledge and radiologist's experience. T1-weighted images provide optimal resolution for the assessment of anatomy while T2-weighted images are more suitable for the detection fluid, cysts, and tumors. This modality can evaluate the quality of carpal bone blood perfusion, including the lunate, the scaphoid, and the capitate [16]. MRI is particularly accurate to gage lunate perfusion and is superior to bone scanning when assessing Kienböck's disease [17]. Even minimal changes in bone perfusion (e.g., ulnar abutment syndrome) can be identified by MRI.

MRI enables optimal visualization of occult ganglions, soft tissue tumors, tendinitis, and joint fluid collection [18]. In addition, this imaging technique may detect subtle bone abnormalities such as bone bruises and micro fractures [19]. Consequently, this imaging modality is very reliable for diagnosing occult scaphoid fractures [20].

MRI constitutes an excellent study for the evaluation of intrinsic carpal ligaments and TFCC. State-of-the-art MRI technology (with 3.0 Tesla) have an improved ability for the detection of TFCC tears compared to MRIs with 1.5 Tesla. These lesions appear as linear hyperintense defects on coronal gradient-echo or T2-weighted pulse sequences. The assessment of the scapholunate and lunatotriquetral ligaments is somewhat more challenging, but it is also feasible with reasonable accuracy (71% sensitivity and 88% specificity), especially with addition of arthrographic contrast. Although 1.5 Tesla MRIs are capable of diagnosing scapholunate tear, 3.0 Tesla MRIs are more precise (89% sensitivity and 100% specificity) and thus represents the imaging modality of choice for evaluating the status of the scapholunate ligament.

MRI identifies lesion of the extrinsic carpal ligaments; however, their role in these lesions is still unclear since the information acquired by MRI rarely changes their management.

In patients with carpal tunnel syndrome, axial imaging with T2 weighting can clearly display masses within the confines of the carpal tunnel, as well as edema and swelling of the median nerve. However, this advanced imaging modality is often unnecessary when suspecting carpal tunnel syndrome, since this syndrome is usually diagnosed with after a good history and physical exam.

Radionuclide Imaging

Bone scans have high sensitivity for detection of wrist lesions (particularly in patients with chronic wrist pain) but low specificity. Thus, bone scans are quite useful as a screening imaging modality chiefly for bone integrity. Osteonecrosis of the scaphoid, lunate, and capitate can be picked with scintigraphy. Bone scanning can also detect occult fractures or the presence of osteoblastic activity (bone turnover). In order to confirm a positive bone scan, CT imaging should then be performed to precise the location and the amount of fracture material. CT imaging can identify fracture subluxations that were overlooked by routine X-ray imaging. Scintigraphy can also be useful for the early detection of complex regional pain syndrome, and evaluating soft tissue lesions. Bone scans are usually abnormal (93%) in cases of complete intrinsic ligament ruptures; however, detection rates diminished substantially in partial lesions. Compared to bone scans, MRIs have equal sensitivity and higher specificity for the detection soft tissue injuries.

Arthroscopy

Arthroscopic examination of the wrist enables direct visualization and palpation of intra-articular structures such as intrinsic ligaments, TFCC, and the articular cartilage. Its diagnostic accuracy is high for the detection of soft tissue injuries or small fractures, and for that reason, at the end of the day, arthroscopy has gradually replaced other diagnostic studies as the gold standard [21–23]. Undoubtedly, the role of wrist arthroscopy has evolved, especially for the detection of associated soft tissue lesions associated to distal radius or scaphoid fractures in active, high-demanding patients. This procedure currently has a well-established role in the evaluation of wrist pain, providing a conclusive diagnosis in most cases. However, a potential pitfall of this procedure is the identification of asymptomatic (incidental) lesions, which in turn could lead to unnecessary treatment.

References

1. Zancolli EA, Cozzi EP. The wrist. In: Zancolli EA, Cozzi EP, editors. Atlas of surgical anatomy of the hand. New York: Churchill Livingstone Inc; 1992.
2. Zancolli EA. Structural and dynamic bases of hand surgery. 2nd ed. Philadelphia: Lippincott; 1979.

3. Palmer AK, Werner FW. Biomechanics of the distal radioulnar joint. Clin Orthop Relat Res. 1984;187:26–35.

4. Ryu JY, Cooney WP 3rd, Askew LJ, An KN, Chao EY. Functional ranges of motion of the wrist joint. J Hand Surg Am. 1991;16:409–19.

5. Watson HK, Dt A, Makhlouf MV. Examination of the scaphoid. J Hand Surg Am. 1988;13:657–60.

6. Nagle DJ. Evaluation of chronic wrist pain. J Am Acad Orthop Surg. 2000;8:45–55.

7. Linscheid RL. Examination of the wrist. In: Nakamura R, Linscheid RL, Miura T, editors. Wrist disorders, current concepts and challenges. Tokyo: Springer Verlag; 1992. p. 13–25.

8. Czitrom AA, Lister GD. Measurement of grip strength in the diagnosis of wrist pain. J Hand Surg Am. 1988;13:16–9.

9. Reagan DS, Linscheid RL, Dobyns JH. Lunotriquetral sprains. J Hand Surg Am. 1984;9:502–14.

10. Nakamura R, Horii E, Imaeda T, Nakao E, Kato H, Watanabe K. The ulnocarpal stress test in the diagnosis of ulnar-sided wrist pain. J Hand Surg Br. 1997;22:719–23.

11. Keiserman LS, Cassandra J, Amis JA. The piano key test: a clinical sign for the identification of subtle tarsometatarsal pathology. Foot Ankle Int. 2003;24:437–8.

12. Feinstein WK, Lichtman DM, Noble PC, Alexander JW, Hipp JA. Quantitative assessment of the midcarpal shift test. J Hand Surg Am. 1999;24:977–83.

13. Ng CY, Hayton MJ. Ice cream scoop test: a novel clinical test to diagnose extensor carpi ulnaris instability. J Hand Surg Eur Vol. 2012;38:569–70.

14. Mann FA, Wilson AJ, Gilula LA. Radiographic evaluation of the wrist: what does the hand surgeon want to know? Radiology. 1992;184:15–24.

15. Cristiani G, Cerofolini E, Squarzina PB, Zanasi S, Leoni A, Romagnoli R, Caroli A. Evaluation of ischaemic necrosis of carpal bones by magnetic resonance imaging. J Hand Surg Br. 1990;15:249–55.

16. Haygood TM, Eisenberg B, Hays MB, Garcia JF, Williamson MR. Avascular necrosis of the capitate demonstrated on a 0.064 T magnet. Magn Reson Imaging. 1989;7:571–3.

17. Imaeda T, Nakamura R, Miura T, Makino N. Magnetic resonance imaging in Kienbock's disease. J Hand Surg Br. 1992;17:12–9.

18. Kettner NW, Pierre-Jerome C. Magnetic resonance imaging of the wrist: occult osseous lesions. J Manip Physiol Ther. 1992;15:599–603.

19. Sferopoulos NK. Bone bruising of the distal forearm and wrist in children. Injury. 2009;40:631–7.

20. Brydie A, Raby N. Early MRI in the management of clinical scaphoid fracture. Br J Radiol. 2003;76:296–300.

21. Weiss AP, Akelman E, Lambiase R. Comparison of the findings of triple-injection cinearthrography of the wrist with those of arthroscopy. J Bone Joint Surg Am. 1996;78:348–56.

22. Schers TJ, van Heusden HA. Evaluation of chronic wrist pain. Arthroscopy superior to arthrography: comparison in 39 patients. Acta Orthop Scand. 1995;66:540–2.

23. Cooney WP. Evaluation of chronic wrist pain by arthrography, arthroscopy, and arthrotomy. J Hand Surg Am. 1993;18:815–22.

Lasers and Electrothermal Devices

3

Daniel J. Nagle

A significant part of arthroscopic wrist surgery includes debridement of the triangular fibrocartilage (TFC), interosseous ligaments, synovium, cartilage, and even bone. Until the mid-1980s, these procedures were carried out using mechanical devices such as mini-banana blades, mini-suction punches, graspers, and motorized cutters and abraders. Good results were achieved with these instruments but with some difficulty because of the small size of the wrist joint. The small joint instruments were limited in variety and efficacy. This problem was first addressed by the holmium YAG (yttrium aluminum garnet) laser and later by radiofrequency (RF) devices, both of which are small, precise cutting, and ablating tools.

Lasers

The bulk of the research on laser/RF-assisted arthroscopy has been on the knee and shoulder. There has been some controversy on the use of lasers in the knee due to the report of four cases of femoral condyle avascular necrosis [1]. Whether the laser played a role in these cases remains to be seen. Avascular necrosis has also been reported after meniscectomy performed using mechanical devices [2]. Janecki et al. reviewed 504 laser-assisted knee arthroscopies and noted no new cases of avascular necrosis of the femur [3].

There was also concern regarding the "sonic shock" produced by the vaporization of the water at the tip of the holmium YAG (Ho:YAG) laser. Gerber and his associates [4] have studied this issue and have concluded that there is no acoustic trauma associated with the use of the Ho:YAG laser.

The CO_2 laser was the first laser to be used in arthroscopy, but it proved difficult to use. The CO_2 laser energy cannot be transmitted through a fiberoptic cable and therefore requires a series of prisms in an articulated arm for delivery.

Furthermore, the joint must be inflated with a gas (CO_2) because water strongly absorbs CO_2 laser light. This inflation often produces subcutaneous emphysema. Finally, the CO_2 laser produces a significant amount of char. The one advantage of the CO_2 laser is that its thermal effect remains very superficial (tissue penetration of ± 50 μm), thus producing very little damage to adjacent tissue.

The shortcomings of the CO_2 laser contributed to the introduction of Ho:YAG laser-assisted arthroscopy. The holmium laser functions (as does the CO_2 laser) in the infrared region of the electromagnetic spectrum at 2.1 nm. In contrast to the CO_2 laser, the Ho:YAG energy can be transmitted through a quartz fiber and functions well underwater. Also, it is well absorbed by cartilage, fibrocartilage, synovial tissue, scar tissue, and hemoglobin. This last point explains the Ho:YAG's hemostatic capabilities.

Other types of lasers have been used in arthroscopy. The neodymium YAG laser has a wavelength of 1.064 nm, which, like the Ho:YAG and CO_2 lasers, is in the infrared region of the electromagnetic spectrum. Like the Ho:YAG laser, it can be used in a liquid medium. However, it has proved difficult to control the depth of penetration of the laser energy, and because of this the neodymium YAG laser is no longer used in arthroscopy.

Erbium lasers have also been used. Like the CO_2 and Ho:YAG lasers, the erbium is an infrared laser. The erbium laser combines the advantages of the Ho:YAG with the reduced collateral tissue injury seen with the CO_2 laser. Its use in the United Sates has been limited.

The excimer laser has also been used in arthroscopy. The wavelength of the excimer laser is in the ultraviolet region of the electromagnetic spectrum. This laser's ablative potential is based on its ability to resonate with and disrupt the covalent bonds of the tissues being ablated. This interaction produces no heat, and therefore thermal collateral injury is eliminated (hence the term *cold laser*). As mentioned, the excimer laser functions in the ultraviolet region of the electromagnetic spectrum; for this reason, there is some concern

D. J. Nagle (✉)
Department of Orthopedics, Northwestern University Feinberg School of Medicine, Chicago, IL, USA

© Springer Nature Switzerland AG 2022
W. B. Geissler (ed.), *Wrist and Elbow Arthroscopy with Selected Open Procedures*,
https://doi.org/10.1007/978-3-030-78881-0_3

it may be mutagenic. Hendrich et al. evaluated the mutagenic effect of ultraviolet light of the same wavelength (308 nm) as that used by the excimer laser and concluded that excimer laser energy is not mutagenic [5]. The excimer laser has not been used widely in arthroscopy, for two reasons. The first is that these lasers are extremely expensive. The second reason is that the fluence, or the amount of energy that can be transmitted through the quartz fiber carrying the laser energy, is barely sufficient to ablate fibrocartilage. Attempts to increase the fluence have resulted in destruction of the fiberoptic delivery system.

The Ho:YAG laser functions by superheating the tissues to be ablated. When the laser fires, it creates a small bubble of water vapor at its tip (the Moses effect). The tissue within this bubble absorbs the majority of the laser energy and is vaporized, leaving a layer of "caramelized" protein behind, but no char. Beyond the vapor bubble, the laser energy is quickly attenuated as it is absorbed by the water in the joint. This drop-off in energy allows the surgeon to titrate the amount of energy transmitted to the tissues in the joint. By "defocusing" the laser (pulling the tip away from the tissue), the tissue is taken out of the Moses bubble and less energy is imparted to the tissue. This allows the "melting" of chondromalacic fronds and capsular shrinkage without injuring adjacent tissues. The water in the joint not only absorbs the laser energy, but it also acts as a large, continually renewed heat sink. The problems of heat buildup and collateral tissue damage are also addressed by pulsing the laser light. The time between pulses allows the tissues outside the ablation zone to transmit the energy they absorb to the heat sink (water) and thus remain protected from thermal injury. Continuously applied laser energy does not permit the flow of heat energy away from the ablation site and results in significant collateral damage. Thus, with appropriate technique, one can modulate the energy imparted to the tissues by changing the laser pulse frequency, by changing the amount of energy per pulse, and finally by focusing or defocusing the laser.

Radiofrequency Devices

Radiofrequency devices, like lasers, ablate/shrink tissue by heating the tissue. The RF devices transmit energy to the tissues via radiofrequency waves in the 100–450 kHz range. This electromagnetic energy causes the electrolytes within the tissue to oscillate very rapidly. This molecular oscillation creates friction within the tissue that, in turn, heats the tissue. The RF energy produces enough friction to either denature the collagen and cause shrinkage or vaporize the tissue. Monopolar and bipolar radiofrequency devices are available. Monopolar units require a grounding pad be attached to the patient, while the bipolar devices do not. The RF devices oscillate the polarity of the active and passive electrodes to

produce the RF energy. The energy of the monopolar devices flows from the active electrode *through* the tissue being treated to the passive, ground electrode. Bipolar devices have both the active and passive electrodes in the tip of the probe. The energy flows from the active electrode back to the passive electrode, passing through the superficial layers of the tissue near the probe tip (Fig. 3.1). The depth of penetration of the monopolar devices is greater than that noted with bipolar devices (4 mm vs. 0.2–0.3 mm). With monopolar devices, the depth of tissue penetration also depends on the impedance of the tissue (Table 3.1). It follows that the energy will penetrate deeper into a ligament than into cartilage. The RF current follows the path of least resistance.

Monopolar and bipolar devices both require a conductive milieu such as normal saline or lactated Ringer's. The tips of the RF probes are available in many shapes and sizes to accommodate the anatomy of the problem being treated.

While the following discussion focuses on the use of the Ho:YAG laser, radiofrequency (RF) devices can be used in

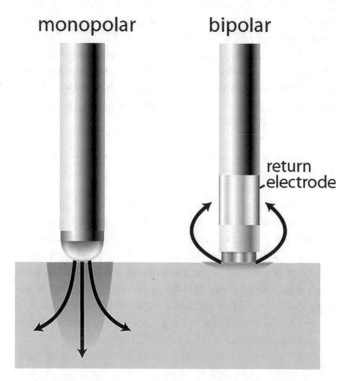

Fig. 3.1 Monopolar: electrical current is conducted into the tissue to the grounding pad. Bipolar: current is conducted away from the tip to the return electrode on the probe shaft

Table 3.1 Tissue impedance

Tissue/substance	Impedance (Ω)
Saline	90–120
Ligaments	100–140
Cartilage	350–500
Bone	1100

Based on data from Refs. [23, 27]

place of the laser [6]. The only exception to this generalization is the ablation of bone, which is more readily accomplished with the laser. The RF probes can be used through the same portals described for the laser probes. Radiofrequency devices can ablate and shrink tissue. However, one must be careful while using RF wands to not overheat the joint or the structures adjacent to the joint. Adequate inflow/outflow is essential while using the RF devices. Prolonged use of the RF probes without an adequate heat sink (fluid flow) can lead to diffuse thermal injury of the joint surfaces and adjacent peri-articular structures. The RF energy penetrates the tissue to a depth of 4 mm or more as compared to the 0.5 mm penetration of the laser. There is therefore a greater potential for injury to adjacent extraarticular structures (nerves) when using the RF probes.

Laser/RF-Assisted TFCC Debridement

Andrew Palmer [7] devised a classification scheme for TFCC tears that divides TFCC tears into traumatic tears (type I) and degenerative tears (type II) [7]. While both types of tears can be treated arthroscopically, types I-A, II-C, and II-D lend themselves to laser-assisted debridement (Fig. 3.2).

Before starting arthroscopic treatment of TFCC tears, the ulnar variance must be evaluated. This is done by taking an X-ray with the shoulder abducted to 90° and the elbow flexed to 90° with the hand flat on the X-ray cassette (the "90 × 90" view of Palmer) [8]. Triangular fibrocartilage debridement in face of an ulnar-plus variance is doomed to fail, as the simple debridement of the TFCC is insufficient to decompress the ulnar side of the wrist. In such cases of ulnar abutment syndrome, an ulnar shortening is needed. The results of TFCC debridement in patients with an ulnar-zero variance can be good, but there lingers the possibility of having to perform an ulnar shortening later. It is recommended that this possibility be discussed with the patient preoperatively. In con-trast to the patient with an ulnar plus variance, the patient who presents with an ulnar minus variance is very likely to respond to simple debridement of the central portion of the triangular fibrocartilage [9, 10].

The technique of laser-assisted triangular fibrocartilage debridement is similar to that of mechanical debridement of the triangular fibrocartilage with the exception that the arthroscope can be left in the 3–4 portal while the laser is kept in the 4–5 portal. The laser is set to 1.4–1.6 J at a frequency of 15 pulses per second. With the help of a side-firing 70-degree laser tip, the triangular fibrocartilage can be very rapidly and precisely debrided. The 70-degree laser tip permits ablation not only of the radial and palmar portions of the TFCC tear, but also the ulnar and dorsal components. There is no need to bring the laser probe in through the 3–4 portal. During the debridement, care must be taken not to injure the ulnar head. This is avoided by firing the laser tangentially to the head of the ulna or passing the probe beneath the triangular fibrocartilage and firing distally. This latter technique presents minimal danger to the lunate or triquetrum, in that the fluid used to expand the joint acts as a heat sink and absorbs the laser energy as it emerges from beneath the triangular fibrocartilage. The central portion of the TFCC is debrided back to stable edges, taking care not to injure the dorsal and palmar radioulnar ligaments.

The arthroscopic treatment of the ulnar abutment syndrome is facilitated by using the Ho:YAG laser [11]. Hyaline cartilage is very efficiently removed with the laser at higher energy settings (2.0 J at 20 pulses per second). Not only are the ulnar head hyaline cartilage and subchondral bone rapidly removed, but, in contrast to burring, they are removed without producing much debris. Once the cancellous bone of the ulnar head is exposed, however, the bur becomes the most effective tool to complete the ulnar shortening. This is because it becomes very time consuming to focus the laser beam on each trabecula. During the ulnar head resection, care must be taken not to injure the sigmoid notch with either

Fig. 3.2 Palmer classification of TFCC tears. (Adapted from Palmer [7]. With permission from Elsevier)

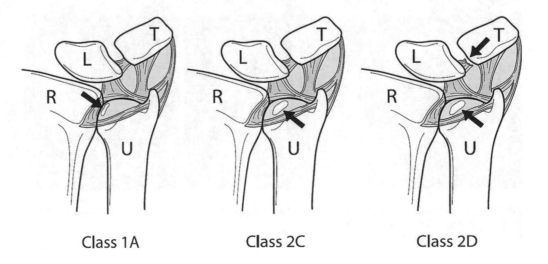

Class 1A   Class 2C   Class 2D

the laser or the bur. Also, care must be taken not to detach the insertion of the triangular fibrocartilage from the fovea at the base of the ulnar styloid. The successful arthroscopic ulnar shortening relies on teamwork. The assistant brings the surfaces of the ulnar head to be resected to the laser being held by the operating surgeon. By progressively supinating and pronating the forearm, an appropriate amount of ulnar head is excised. The goal is to resect sufficient ulna to produce a 2 mm negative ulnar variance. The amount of ulna resected must be verified with intraoperative fluoroscopy. Occasionally, complete visualization of the ulnar head requires that the scope be placed in the 4–5 portal with the laser entering the distal radioulnar joint through the distal radioulnar joint portal. This portal is established just proximal to the 4–5 portal and TFCC.

An effort is made to leave a smooth surface on the remaining distal ulna. The trabeculae of the distal ulna always produce a somewhat rough distal ulna at the completion of the procedure. These irregularities, however, disappear during the months following the surgery (Figs. 3.3 and 3.4). Large irregularities must be avoided, as they can catch on the proximal surface of the residual TFCC during supination and pronation.

The postoperative regimen after TFCC debridement, with or without ulnar shortening, includes providing the patient with a wrist splint to be worn as needed, as well as a home therapy program consisting of active and passive range of motion exercises. The sutures (wounds are closed using subcuticular sutures of 4–0 Prolene) are removed at 2 weeks.

Strengthening exercises can be started at 6 weeks if needed. Premature resumption of heavy lifting or repetitive activities will lead to radiocarpal synovitis. Some patients feel so good after as little as 2 weeks that the surgeon must temper the patient's desire to return to full activity. In the case of an ulnar shortening, the recovery can be as long as 6 months, as suggested by Feldon [12]. However, the majority of patients will be improved long before 6 months.

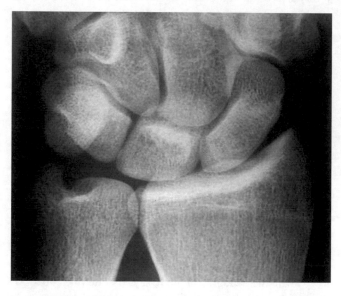

Fig. 3.3 Ulnar abutment

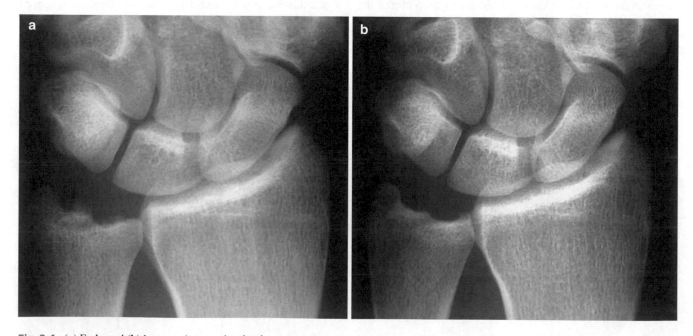

Fig. 3.4 (**a**) Early and (**b**) late post-laser-assisted arthroscopic ulnar shortening demonstrating smoothing of resection site with time. (**a**) 6 weeks postoperative and (**b**) 6 months postoperative

Other Indications for Laser/RF-Assisted Wrist Arthroscopy

Synovectomy

Synovectomy is probably the most frequently performed laser-assisted procedure. This procedure is often needed to permit complete joint visualization, particularly of the lunotriquetral and ulnocarpal joints. The laser, set at 1.2–1.5 J and 15 pulses per second, vaporizes the inflamed synovium and scar tissue quickly and with minimal bleeding due to the hemostatic effect of the laser. The hemoglobin in the inflamed synovium absorbs the laser energy better than the adjacent capsule, thus providing an extra level of safety for the capsule. Scar tissue and synovitis in the radiocarpal, ulnocarpal, and midcarpal joints can be rapidly debrided. When performing a dorsal wrist synovectomy, or for that matter anytime the laser is being used, care should be taken to avoid aiming the laser at the arthroscope, as the laser energy will destroy the scope.

Partial Interosseous Ligament Tears

Partial tears of the scapholunate and lunotriquetral ligaments can be nicely treated with the laser set at 0.2–1.0 J and 15 pulses per second. The ablation of these tears can be done very precisely without scuffing or injuring the adjacent intact articular cartilage.

Chondromalacia

Chondromalacia has been treated with the laser and RF devices. There is, however, evidence that at least in regard to the RF devices, significant injury to the underlying healthy cartilage can occur even when exercising caution and using low power settings [13, 14]. Based on this information, it is difficult to recommend RF treatment of chondromalacia. Chondromalacic fronds can, however, be gingerly vaporized with the laser set at 0.2–0.8 J and 15 pulses per second. The laser beam must be oriented tangentially to the joint surface so that only the fronds of frayed cartilage are treated. Great care must be taken to not injure the underlying healthy cartilage. Because the laser radiation can be directed selectively toward the chondromalacic fronds, sparing the underlying cartilage, it is safer in this situation than are RF devices. However, great care must be exercised. It should be kept in mind that the long-term effectiveness of debridement of chondromalacic fronds has not been established, and the potential for significant injury to healthy cartilage cannot be ignored even with the laser.

Bone Resection

We have seen that the Ho:YAG laser can be used to resect the distal ulna. Similarly, the laser can be used to perform radial styloidectomies, osteophytectomies, and complete resection of the ulnar head. The principles outlined in the section describing the laser-assisted arthroscopic Feldon procedure apply to these procedures as well. The articular cartilage and subchondral bone are vaporized with the laser, while the cancellous bone is removed with a bur.

Radial styloidectomy is performed with the arthroscope in the 4–5 portal and the laser and bur entering through the 1–2 and 3–4 portals. (The 1–2 portal is approached with caution, as the radial artery and branches of the superficial radial nerve course through this area. Only blunt dissection should be used in establishing the 1–2 portal.) A clear junction usually exists between the area of the radial styloid to be debrided (exposed subchondral bone) and the adjacent healthy cartilage. If this is not the case, a K-wire can be placed under both fluoroscopic and arthroscopic control through the radial styloid at the ulnar limit of the proposed bone resection. This provides an intra-articular landmark. The amount of styloid resected should be just enough to solve the problem being addressed, taking care to leave the attachments of the radioscaphocapitate and long radiolunate ligaments intact. Postoperative care after this procedure is similar to that described for a TFCC debridement.

Laser-assisted arthroscopic Darrach procedures and matched ulnar resections are logical extensions of the laser-assisted arthroscopic Feldon procedure. The technique used for these procedures is essentially the same as that used for the laser-assisted arthroscopic Feldon procedure. One would anticipate less morbidity with this technique, though no published series are currently available. The use of the laser to treat grade IV chondromalacia has been successful in our hands in a limited number of cases. Two approaches are used, depending on the clinical presentation. If the joint surfaces involved cannot be unloaded (i.e., the proximal lunate), the laser is used to ablate the detached cartilage and subchondral plate. The laser debridement is extended to expose a healthy cartilage/bone interface. This "crater" margin is "freshened" with the bur. The subchondral bone is burred back to bleeding, cancellous bone. This last step is needed, as laser cauterization slows the fibrous tissue ingrowth necessary for the success of chondroplasty in this setting. Early range of motion is essential. The use of continuous passive motion has proven to be important.

The second approach is that applied to joint surfaces that can be unloaded through limited carpal shortening. A prime example of this is chondromalacia of the proximal pole of the hamate often seen in patients with a type II lunate [15]. In this situation, the goal is not to promote soft tissue ingrowth but rather to unload the lunatohamate joint. This can be accomplished by establishing a viewing portal at the radial midcarpal port and an instrument portal at the ulnar midcarpal port. The

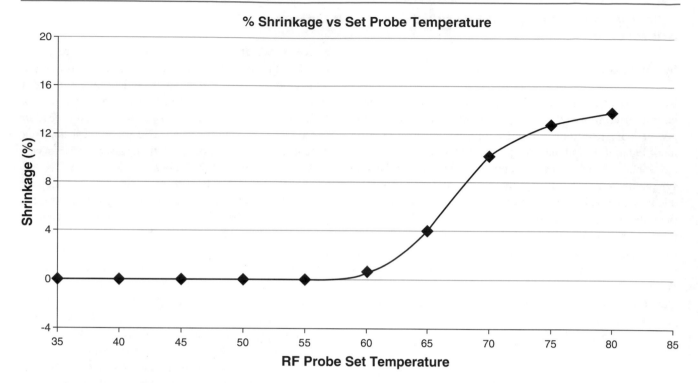

Fig. 3.5 Shrinkage versus RF probe temperature

proximal pole of the hamate is ablated using the laser. The resection is continued until the lunate no longer impinges on the hamate during ulnar deviation. (Care must be exercised not to injure the ulnar limb of the arcuate ligament.) This can be verified by removing the laser and manipulating the wrist while the arthroscope is still in the radial midcarpal joint. In this case, the bur is not used to freshen the hamate defect, as cauterization produced by the laser seems to decrease postoperative discomfort. This effect is attributed to a decrease in postoperative bleeding and inflammation. Though early postoperative range of motion is promoted, continuous passive motion has not been needed. It should be noted that no clinical studies of chondroplasty using the Ho:YAG laser have been published.

Capsular Shrinkage

Wrist capsular shrinkage may offer an attractive alternative to more invasive treatments for subtle forms of carpal instability. It would seem logical to apply to the wrist what has been learned from shoulder capsular shrinkage. The basic science of capsular shrinkage should be the same for both joints. However, the wrist is not the shoulder, and extrapolation of shoulder data to the wrist may not be appropriate.

The biology of capsular shrinkage has been extensively studied in animal models. Capsular shrinkage is a refined "hot poker" technique. The triple helix of collagen unwinds when heated to 60 °C; maximum shrinkage is achieved between 65 and 75 °C (Fig. 3.5). The hydrogen bonds hold-

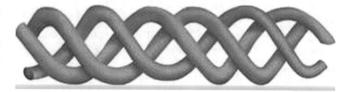

Fig. 3.6 The normal collagen triple helix without shrinkage

ing the type I collagen triple helix together rupture as the collagen is heated beyond 60 °C. As the collagen triple helix unwinds, it shortens (Fig. 3.6). This shortening can reach 50% of the resting length of the untreated collagen. The shortened, denatured collagen acts as scaffolding onto which new collagen is deposited [16]. The new collagen fibers maintain this shortened conformation, thus assuring the long-term maintenance of the shortening.

Biomechanical studies have demonstrated that the tensile strength of heated collagen decreases rapidly and does not return to normal values for 12 weeks [17]. The tensile strength returns to nearly 80% of normal by 6 weeks after heating (Fig. 3.7). This transient loss of tensile strength would suggest that the application of stress to recently heated collagen is contraindicated. Premature loading of the shrunken collagen will lead to a lengthening of the collagen. This has been verified in an animal model [18, 19]. Based on these data, it would seem reasonable to recommend at least 6–8 weeks of joint immobilization after capsular shrinkage. Clearly, heavy loading of the joint should be avoided for 12 weeks.

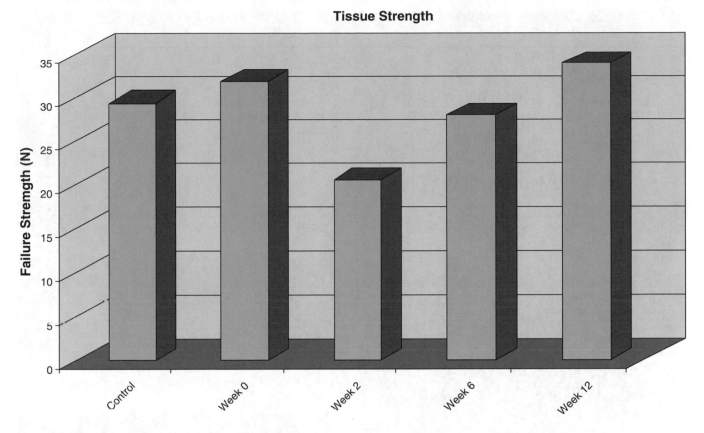

Fig. 3.7 Post-shrinkage tensile strength versus time

Shrinkage requires very low energy settings. The RF devices must be adjusted to heat the tissue to a temperature of between 65 and 75 °C. It is wise to start at low energy and slowly increase the energy output until the desired shrinkage is observed. The laser should be set to very low energy, i.e., 0.2–0.5 J at 15 pulses per second (3–7.5 W). The laser is held away from the target ligament and slowly advanced until the ligament is seen to shrink. Once the shrinkage has stopped, continued laser exposure will only further weaken the ligament without increasing the shrinkage. The color of the ligament changes from white to light yellow during the shrinkage. Lu et al. have suggested that a cross-hatching shrinkage pattern optimizes the ingrowth of healthy tissue and hastens the recovery of the ligament [20]. During the shrinkage, traction on the wrist should be reduced as much as possible to permit optimal shrinkage.

of fibrocartilage, which is not shrinkable (Fig. 3.8). The dorsal and palmar portions of the SL ligament are, however, composed of type I collagen and are shrinkable (Fig. 3.9). Burn et al. [21] have reported excellent long term (minimum 5 year follow up) outcomes in 9 patients with Geissler I, II, and III scapholunate instability treated with shrinkage of the scapholunate ligament.

Capsular shrinkage of the dorsal intercarpal ligament (DIC) could potentially reinforce the stabilizing effect of SL ligament shrinkage. The DIC is attached to the distal dorsal aspect of the scaphoid and the dorsal triquetrum (Fig. 3.10). Shrinkage of this ligament could simulate the tensioning of this ligament noted during open capsulodesis [22]. To accomplish this, the scope and laser would be placed alternately in the radial and ulnar midcarpal portals. Again, no published data are available that support this technique.

Scapholunate Instability

Capsular shrinkage for mild scapholunate (SL) instability could be an attractive alternative to the currently available open procedures. The question is what can or should be shrunk to stabilize the SL axis. The SL interosseous ligament is a heterogeneous structure. Its central portion is composed

Lunotriquetral and Ulnocarpal Instability

Mild forms of lunotriquetral instability can be treated with ulnocarpal ligament shrinkage. I have applied this technique in a limited number of cases with satisfying results. This procedure takes advantage of the anatomy of the ulnotriquetral and ulnolunate ligaments. These ligaments form a V as they

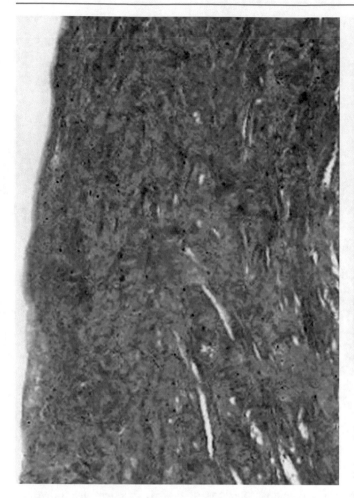

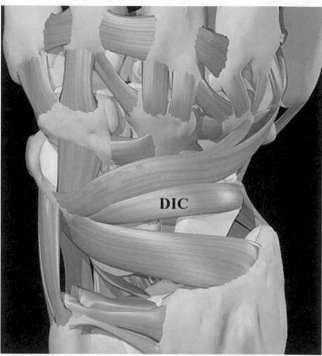

Fig. 3.10 Dorsal intercarpal ligament. (Courtesy of Daniel J. Nagle)

Fig. 3.8 Histology of central fibrocartilaginous portion of the scapholunate ligament. (From Berger [30]; used with permission of Mayo Foundation for Medical Education and Research, all rights reserved

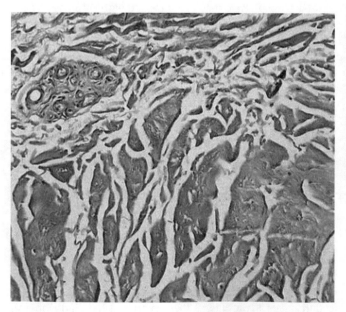

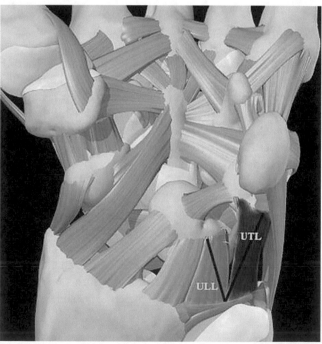

Fig. 3.11 Palmar view of ulnocarpal ligaments demonstrating "V" configuration. (Courtesy of Daniel J. Nagle)

Fig. 3.9 Histology of capsule demonstrating loose collagen (CF) in a fibrous stratum (FS). From Berger [30]; used with permission of Mayo Foundation for Medical Education and Research, all rights reserved

diverge from their origin on the palmar distal radioulnar ligament and insert on the palmar aspect of the lunate or triquetrum (Fig. 3.11). As the ligaments are shrunk, the arms of the V shorten and approximate the lunate to the triquetrum thus stabilizing the LT joint. This stabilization can be further reinforced with the shrinkage of the LT interosseous ligament. The LT ligament histology is similar to that of the SL ligament and can therefore undergo dorsal and palmar but not central shrinkage. Isolated ulnocarpal ligament instability can also be treated with ulnocarpal ligament shrinkage. Ulnocarpal shrinkage is accomplished with the arthroscope in the 3–4 portal and the laser in the 4–5 or 6-U portal.

Midcarpal Instability

It is tempting to apply capsular shrinkage to the treatment of midcarpal instability. Midcarpal instability is associated with attenuation of the ulnar arcuate, triquetrohamate, dorsal intercarpal, ulnocarpal, and radiocarpal ligaments. All of these ligaments can be shrunk. I have had success treating patients with symptomatic chronic mild midcarpal instability and even a patient with significant midcarpal instability due to generalized ligamentous laxity. Mason and Hargreaves have reported excellent short and long term results in 13 patients with palmar midcarpal instability using radio frequency probes to shrink the radioscapholunate ligament, ulnar arcuate ligament, long and short radiolunate ligaments, and accessible areas of the dorsal capsule of the midcarpal and radiocarpal joints [23, 24]. Additional studies of the efficacy of this technique will be long in coming in view of the rarity of this condition and the broad spectrum of pathology associated with midcarpal instability.

Conclusion

Our experience since 1990 with over 350 laser-assisted wrist arthroscopies using the Ho:YAG laser has been excellent. We have encountered no laser-related complications. We have noted no increase in postoperative wrist effusion or pain. These clinical findings echo those found in multiple articles reviewing the use of the Ho:YAG laser in the knee [25] and two articles in the hand/upper extremity literature. Blackwell et al. used the Ho:YAG laser to debride central TFCC tears in 35 patients and noted results similar to those obtained using mechanical debridement [26]. Infanger and Grimm came to the same conclusion after looking at the results of laser-assisted TFCC debridement in 72 patients [27].

The Ho:YAG laser and RF devices should be viewed as additional tools in the wrist surgeon's armamentarium. The advantages of the laser/RF devices include their small size and the efficiency they bring to wrist arthroscopy, as well as their capability to cauterize and to precisely titrate the amount of power delivered to the operative site. The development of aggressive, 2.0 mm mechanical cutting devices has been slow and may be reaching its practical limits. This is not to say, however, that mechanical devices are obsolete.

Certainly, the full-radius cutters and burs continue to be used routinely in wrist arthroscopy.

The future of lasers in wrist and joint surgery in general could be promising if the cost of the lasers decreases. Research is currently being done to evaluate the use of lasers to shrink the wrist capsule to correct subtle forms of carpal instability. Animal and tissue culture research has demonstrated that laser energy of the appropriate frequency can stimulate chonodroblast proliferation and cartilage production [28, 29]. Perhaps one day the laser will help create tissue rather than ablate it.

References

1. Garino JP, Lotke PA, Sapega AA, et al. Osteonecrosis of the knee following laser-assisted arthroscopic surgery: a report of six cases. Arthroscopy. 1995;11:467–774.
2. Johnson TC, Evans JA, Gilley JA, et al. Osteonecrosis of the knee after arthroscopic surgery for meniscal tears and chondral lesions. Arthroscopy. 2000;16(3):254–61.
3. Janecki CJ, Perry MW, Bonati AO, et al. Safe parameters for laser chondroplasty of the knee. Lasers Surg Med. 1998;23:141–50.
4. Gerber BE, Asshauer T, Delacretaz G, et al. Biophysical bases of the effects of holmium laser on articular cartilage and their impact on clinical application technics. Orthopade. 1996;25:21–9.
5. Hendrich C, Werner SE. Mutagenic effects of the excimer laser using a fibroblast transformation assay. Arthroscopy. 1997;13:151–5.
6. Osmond C, Hecht P, Hayashi K, et al. Comparative effects of laser and radiofrequency energy on joint capsule. Clin Orthop. 2000;375:286–94.
7. Palmer AK. Triangular fibrocartilage complex lesions: a classification. J Hand Surg Am. 1989;14:594–606.
8. Palmer AK, Glisson RR, Werner FW. Ulnar variance determination. J Hand Surg Am. 1982;7:376–9.
9. Osterman AL. Arthroscopic debridement of triangular fibrocartilage complex tears. Arthroscopy. 1990;6:120–4.
10. Minami A, Ishikawa J, Suenaga N, et al. Clinical results of treatment of triangular fibrocartilage complex tears by arthroscopic debridement. J Hand Surg Am. 1966;21:406–11.
11. Nagle DJ, Bernstein MA. Laser-assisted arthroscopic ulnar shortening. Arthroscopy. 2002;18(9):1046–51.
12. Feldon P, Terrono AL, Belsky MR. The "wafer" procedure. Partial distal ulnar resection. Clin Orthop. 1992;275:124–9.
13. Edwards RB 3rd, Lu Y, Nho S, et al. Thermal chondroplasty of chondromalacic human cartilage. An ex vivo comparison of bipolar and monopolar radiofrequency devices. Am J Sports Med. 2002;30(1):90–7.
14. Lu Y, Edwards RB 3rd, Cole BJ, et al. Thermal chondroplasty with radiofrequency energy. An in vitro comparison of bipolar and monopolar radiofrequency devices. Am J Sports Med. 2001;29(1):42–9.
15. Nakamura K, Patterson RM, Moritomo H, et al. Type I versus type II lunates: ligament anatomy and presence of arthrosis. J Hand Surg Am. 2001;26(3):428–36.
16. Lopez MJ, Hayashi K, Vanderby R Jr, et al. Effects of monopolar radiofrequency energy on ovine joint capsular mechanical properties. Clin Orthop. 2000;374:286–97.
17. Hecht P, Hayashi K, Lu Y, et al. Monopolar radiofrequency energy effects on joint capsular tissue: potential treatment for joint instability. An in vivo mechanical, morphological, and biochemical study using an ovine model. Am J Sports Med. 1999;27(6):761–71.

18. Naseef GS III, Foster TE, Trauner K, et al. The thermal properties of bovine joint capsule. The basic science of laser- and radiofrequency-induced capsular shrinkage. Am J Sports Med. 1997;25(5):670–4.

19. Hayashi K, Markel MD. Thermal capsulorrhaphy treatment of shoulder instability: basic science. Clin Orthop. 2001;390:59–72.

20. Lu Y, Hayashi K, Edwards RB 3rd, et al. The effect of monopolar radiofrequency treatment pattern on joint capsular healing. In vitro and in vivo studies using an ovine model. Am J Sports Med. 2000;28(5):711–9.

21. Burn MB, Sarkissian EJ, Yao J. Long-Term outcomes for arthroscopic thermal treatment for scapholunate ligament injuries. J Wrist Surgery 2020;9:22–8.

22. Szabo RM, Slater RR Jr, Palumbo CF, et al. Dorsal intercarpal ligament capsulodesis for chronic, static scapholunate dissociation: clinical results. J Hand Surg Am. 2002;27(6):978–84.

23. Mason WTM, Hargreaves DG. Arthroscopic thermal capsulorrhaphy for palmar midcarpal instability. J Hand Surg. 2007;32E:411–6.

24. Hargreaves DG. Long term results of arthroscopic capsular shrinkage for midcarpal instability. Conference proceedings. BSSH Spring meeting, Bath, 2015, pp 30–31.

25. Lubbers C, Siebert WE. Holmium: YAG-laser-assisted arthroscopy versus conventional methods for treatment of the knee. Two-year results of a prospective study. Knee Surg Sports Traumatol Arthrosc. 1997;5(3):168–75.

26. Blackwell RE, Jemison DM, Foy BD. The holmium:yttrium-aluminum-garnet laser in wrist arthroscopy: a five-year experience in the treatment of central triangular fibrocartilage complex tears by partial excision. J Hand Surg Am. 2001;26(1):77–84.

27. Infanger M, Grimm D. Meniscus and discus lesions of triangular fibrocartilage complex (TFCC): treatment by laser-assisted wrist arthroscopy. J Plast Reconstr Aesthet Surg. 2009;62(4):466–71.

28. Torricelli P, Giavaresi G, Fini M, et al. Laser biostimulation of cartilage: in vitro evaluation. Biomed Pharmacother. 2001;55(2):117–20.

29. Morrone G, Guzzardella GA, Tigani D, et al. Biostimulation of human chondrocytes with Ga-Al-as diode laser: 'in vitro' research. Artif Cells Blood Substit Immobil Biotechnol. 2000;28(2):193–201.

30. Berger RA. Chapter 5. In: Cooney WP, Linscheid RL, Dobyns JH, editors. The wrist: diagnosis and operative treatment. St. Louis: Mosby; 1998.

Anatomy of the Triangular Fibrocartilage Complex

4

Jared L. Burkett and William B. Geissler

Introduction

Ulnar-sided wrist pain is a common presenting complaint, so a thorough understanding of the anatomy and biomechanics of the triangular fibrocartilage complex (TFCC) and distal radioulnar joint (DRUJ) is essential for the diagnosis and treatment of these disorders. Over the past 30 years, the knowledge of this complicated structure and its role in the biomechanics of the wrist has increased, leading to improved diagnosis of these injuries and to more effective reconstructive procedures for their treatment [1]. Arthroscopy allows an unparalleled visual examination of the different components of the TFCC, which can aid in differentiating pathologic versus normal anatomy. With this improved ability to see fine details and structures that might go unappreciated in open approaches, the surgeon should possess a comprehensive understanding to guide decision-making and treatment during surgery.

Distal Radioulnar Joint (DRUJ)

DRUJ Anatomy

The DRUJ is a trochoid articulation formed by the sigmoid notch of the distal radius and the seat of the ulnar head. The bony anatomy of this joint is responsible for allowing translation along with pronation and supination of the forearm as the radius rotates around the fixed ulna. Af Ekenstam and Hagert examined the anatomy of the distal radioulnar joint and found that the radius of curvature of the sigmoid notch was 4–7 mm larger than the ulnar head, with the average for the sigmoid notch being 15 mm and the average for the ulnar head being 10 mm (Fig. 4.1) [2]. The articular surface of the ulnar head facing the sigmoid notch, or the seat of the ulna, occupies between 90° and 135° of the circumference of the distal ulna, with a central height of approximately 8 mm [2]. In relation to the ulnar head, the sigmoid notch is relatively flat with an articular surface of between 47° and 80° [2]. This articulation results in rotation of approximately 180°, but also allows for instability of the distal radioulnar joint, allowing palmar translation of the sigmoid notch in pronation and dorsal in supination [1, 2]. Due to this anatomical relationship, the stability of the joint contributed by articular surface contact is approximately 20%, while the remaining stability is imparted by the soft tissue structures [3].

The thin capsule of the DRUJ attaches distally from the sigmoid notch of the radius to the volar and dorsal aspects of

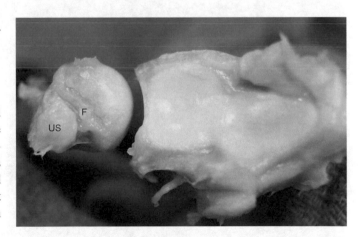

Fig. 4.1 The larger radius of curvature of the sigmoid notch compared to the ulnar head can be seen. With minimal bony restraints, the stability of this joint is dependent on soft tissue structures. The fovea (F) of the ulnar head where the deep portion of the volar and dorsal radioulnar ligaments is seen along with the ulnar styloid (US) where the superficial portions of the radioulnar ligaments attach. Specimens provided by the Anatomical Gifts Program at the University of Mississippi Medical Center

J. L. Burkett
Alabama Orthopaedic Clinic, Mobile, AL, USA

W. B. Geissler (✉)
Division of Hand and Upper Extremity Surgery, Section of Arthroscopic Surgery and Sports Medicine, Department of Orthopedic Surgery and Rehabilitation, University of Mississippi Medical Center, Jackson, MS, USA

© Springer Nature Switzerland AG 2022
W. B. Geissler (ed.), *Wrist and Elbow Arthroscopy with Selected Open Procedures*,
https://doi.org/10.1007/978-3-030-78881-0_4

the radioulnar ligaments of the TFCC before inserting on the base of the ulnar styloid. Due to these attachments, the tip of the ulnar styloid is extra-articular in relation to this joint [4]. Clinically peripheral detachments are more common dorsally, as the volar attachment of the capsule to the TFCC is stronger [5].

During normal forearm supination and pronation, a sliding movement occurs in addition to a rotational movement. In neutral rotation, the principal axis of load bearing of the DRUJ is centrally in the sigmoid notch, with approximately 60% of cartilage surface contact. With pronation, the principal axis of load bearing of the DRUJ moves distally and dorsally in the sigmoid notch, leaving a small portion, approximately 10% of the cartilage surface of the notch, in contact with the ulna. In supination, the reverse is true with the principal axis of load bearing moving proximally and palmarly in the sigmoid notch [2, 6, 7].

To maintain stability of this inherently unstable joint, the function of the DRUJ is intricately related to soft tissue structural support. Both extrinsic and intrinsic structures are present, with the intrinsic stabilizers playing a greater role in

rotational stability [1]. Extrinsic stabilizing structures that will not be described in detail in this chapter include the extensor carpi ulnaris tendon, the sixth dorsal compartment, the pronator quadratus, and the interosseous ligament of the forearm [1, 3]. The TFCC is the primary intrinsic stabilizer of the DRUJ, with the volar and dorsal radioulnar ligaments providing the majority of the support the TFCC imparts to the DRUJ.

Ulnar Variance

As ulnar variance plays a role in TFCC pathology and in the treatment options for ulnar-sided wrist pain, an understanding of the biomechanics of this relationship is needed. As the radius rotates around the fixed ulna, the variance changes with position, being relatively ulnar positive in pronation and ulnar negative in supination (Fig. 4.2a, b). The differences in load transmission through the ulnocarpal joint with differing degrees of ulnar variance or wrist position can be significant. The force transmitted through the ulna has also been found to

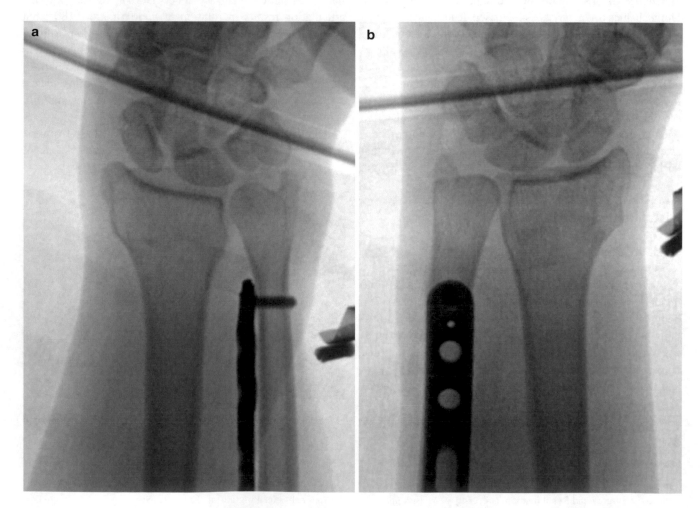

Fig. 4.2 (**a**, **b**) Fluoroscopic images showing the positional changes in ulnar variance with pronation (**a**) and supination (**b**). In pronation, the wrist is found to be significantly ulnar positive, while in supination, the wrist is minimally positive in these images

increase with pronation, extension, and ulnar deviation as this shifts the load medially compared to supination, flexion, and radial deviation [1, 8]. In addition, forced grip has been found to increase ulnar variance an average of 1.95 mm, which will increase load transmission through the TFCC and ulna [9].

In a patient with neutral variance, approximately 80% of the load of the carpus will be transmitted through the radius and 20% through the TFCC and ulna. If the variance increases by 2.5 mm, the load borne by the ulna will increase to approximately 40%, while a decrease in variance of 2.5 mm will decrease the load borne by the ulna to approximately 4% [10]. In addition to the increased load transmitted through the articular disc with increased variance, the space available for the TFCC is diminished, leading to a decreased thickness of the disc [11]. This increased load borne through the TFCC with increased ulnar variance helps explain the association with TFCC injuries, as greater loads and stresses are placed on this structure that already has a decreased thickness [1, 11]. In Palmer and Werner's cadaveric study, they found TFCC perforations in 17% of ulnar minus wrists compared with 73% in ulnar plus or neutral wrists [12].

Radiographic Evaluation

For a complete evaluation of the wrist, an accurate PA and lateral radiograph should be obtained to evaluate carpal and DRUJ pathology, variance, and carpal malalignment. Due to the positional difference in the relationship of the distal radius and ulna, the recommended positioning when taking X-rays to assess for variance is that the forearm be in the zero or neutral rotation position for accurate measurements. A reliable way to obtain this view is with the shoulder abducted 90° and the elbow flexed 90° with the hand flat so that accurate reproducible results can be obtained in subsequent imaging studies [13]. When viewing the radiograph, the ulnar styloid should be at the greatest distance possible from the radius, and if it is not in this position, then the wrist is either pronated or supinated [13]. Another reliable method for obtaining acceptable radiographs is with the arm adducted to the side and the elbow flexed to 90° with the hand in neutral rotation and the thumb toward the ceiling. In this fixed position, the X-ray beam can be rotated 90° to obtain a true PA and lateral radiograph.

Triangular Fibrocartilage Complex

The TFCC is a critical and complex structure that is integral to the normal kinematics and function of the wrist. Palmer and Werner, in their anatomic and biomechanical

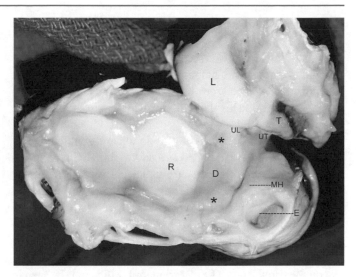

Fig. 4.3 Specimen demonstrating the different components of the ulnar side of the wrist and TFCC. L, lunate; T, triquetrum; R, lunate facet of radius; UT, ulnotriquetral ligament; UL, ulnolunate ligament; D, articular disc, asterisk volar and dorsal radioulnar ligaments; MH, meniscus homologue; E, extensor carpi ulnaris subsheath

testing, described the anatomy of the TFCC as being composed of the articular disc, the meniscus homologue, the ulnar collateral ligament, the sheath of the extensor carpi ulnaris, and the dorsal and volar radioulnar ligaments (Fig. 4.3) [12]. The TFCC originates on the sigmoid notch before inserting on the ulna fovea and styloid, and distally it joins with the ulnar collateral ligament before inserting on the triquetrum, hamate, and base of the fifth metacarpal [12]. While not initially described as part of the TFCC by Palmer, the ulnocarpal wrist ligaments have since been included as components and are important stabilizers of the ulnocarpal joint [14].

These structures forming the TFCC are important in load transmission through the ulnar side of the wrist and are intrinsic stabilizers of the distal radioulnar and the ulnocarpal joints. The TFCC enlarges the contact area between the carpal bones and the ulna and transmits load between these structures. The wide but slim radial attachment is subjected to large amounts of stress during motion and is often a site of tears [15]. The importance of the TFCC in force transmission is demonstrated with resection of the articular disc, which unloads the ulnar column and decreases the load transferred through the ulna from 18% to approximately 6% [16]. The ulnocarpal ligament components of the TFCC contribute very little to DRUJ stability, but are significant in their contribution to ulnocarpal stability. Due to the very limited inherent bony stability of the DRUJ, the major stabilizer of this joint is the TFCC, with the palmar and dorsal radioulnar ligaments playing the most vital role in this process.

Ulnocarpal Ligaments

The ulnocarpal ligaments serve an important role in stabilizing the ulnar carpus and helping prevent supination and volar translocation of the carpus on the distal radius and ulna [17]. Stuart et al. found in their biomechanical study testing the relative contributions to stability of the DRUJ that the ulnocarpal ligament complex was not a significant contributor [3]. Although not always included as a part of the TFCC, the ulnocapitate ligament originates from the palmar aspect of the fovea, where it blends with the palmar radioulnar ligament and then runs superficial to the other ulnocarpal ligaments before inserting onto the capitate [18]. The ulnotriquetral ligament arises from the palmar aspect of the fovea and the meniscus homologue and the palmar radioulnar ligament before inserting on the triquetrum. The pisotriquetral orifice may be seen in the distal aspect of this ligament during arthroscopy. The ulnolunate ligament originates from the palmar aspect of the fovea and the articular disc, with a few fibers from the radius, and is intertwined with the palmar radioulnar ligament before inserting distally on the lunate (Fig. 4.4) [14, 19].

Moritomo et al. found that the length of the ulnotriquetral and ulnocapitate ligaments increased the greatest amount with wrist radial extension, whereas the ulnolunate increased the most with wrist extension, while the palmar radioulnar ligament had minimal change in length with any motion. This stress imparted through the ligaments might explain how a fall on an outstretched hand could lead to a foveal tear of the TFCC from excessive traction imparted through the ulnocarpal ligaments. Morimoto goes on to say, however, that pure wrist hyper-radial extension or hyperextension would not be adequate by itself to cause these injuries and that additional forces would be required to initiate a tear [19].

Meniscus Homologue

The meniscus homologue is a C-shaped vascular tissue located between the superficial portion of the radioulnar ligaments, the capsule, and the triquetrum in the ulnar aspect of the radiocarpal joint. Some debates have occurred over whether this is a true component of the TFCC, as it differs histologically by being composed of loose connective tissue instead of dense collagen and also by being lined by synovial cells on its inner surface [18]. Ishii et al. found in their study that the meniscus homologue, which they classified into three types as related to the prestyloid recess, was not identifiable as the separate structure that was previously described by Bowers and Taleisnik [14, 20, 21].

Prestyloid Recess

The prestyloid recess is a pouch often found anterior to the ulnar styloid where the meniscus homologue does not cover the ulnar styloid, and should not be confused with a tear of the TFCC [18]. It can be found at the apex of radioulnar ligaments and is typically lined with synovial villi (Fig. 4.5) [22]. Ishii described three different variations in the presty-

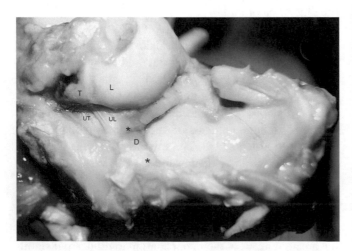

Fig. 4.4 The ulnolunate and ulnotriquetral ligament can be seen arising from the volar distal radioulnar ligament before inserting distally on the lunate and ulna, respectively. The ulnocapitate ligament is not seen as it runs volar to the other ulnar carpal ligaments. The volar and dorsal radioulnar ligaments appear as thickenings of the peripheral articular disc. L, lunate; T, triquetrum; UT, ulnotriquetral ligament; UL, ulnolunate ligament; D, articular disc, asterisk volar and dorsal radioulnar ligaments

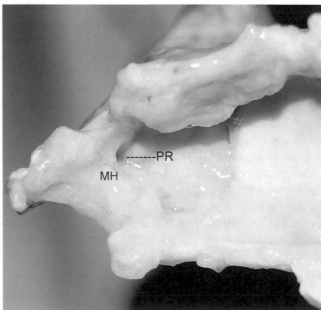

Fig. 4.5 The prestyloid recess is seen and is often found anterior to the ulnar styloid and is the area where the styloid is not covered by the meniscus homologue. The meniscus homologue (MH) composed of loose connective tissue located in the ulnar aspect of the radiocarpal joint and is seen to the *left* and *inferior* to the prestyloid recess (PR) in this image

loid recess: narrow, wide, and no opening types [14]. The narrow opening type was found in 74% of specimens and consisted of the meniscus homologue being attached to the ulnar styloid proximal to its radial, dorsal, and palmar aspects and distal to the ulnar styloid tip circumferential surface [14]. The prestyloid recess was found to communicate with the ulnocarpal space by a long narrow tunnel from the palmar aspect of the styloid [14]. The wide opening type was found in 11% and consisted of the attachments similar to the narrow opening, but without attachment to the tip of the styloid [14]. A short, wide opening was found between the prestyloid recess and the ulnocarpal space [14]. The no opening type was found in 15% of patients, and the prestyloid recess was found to come from the radial aspect of the styloid and to communicate with the distal radioulnar joint instead of the ulnocarpal space [14]. The ligamentum subcruentum, as it was originally described, was not found in this type but was identified in the narrow and wide opening variations [14].

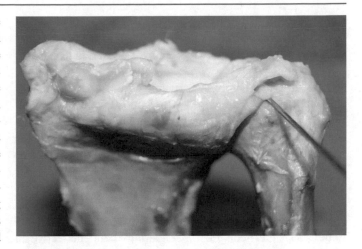

Fig. 4.6 Specimen demonstrating both the superficial and deep volar radioulnar ligaments. The superficial ligament can be seen inserting on the styloid, and the deep ligament (located *superior* to the needle) can be seen inserting into the fovea

Radioulnar Ligaments

The dorsal and palmar radioulnar ligaments are intracapsular intrinsic stabilizers that measure 4–5 mm in thickness and impart the majority of stability to the DRUJ in pronation and supination as translational motion occurs [1–3, 12]. The histologic makeup of these ligaments demonstrates longitudinally oriented parallel fibers, which suggest a tissue that experiences tensile loads, a premise which supports their role as stabilizing structures [23]. The palmar radioulnar ligament forms the proximal attachment of the ulnocarpal ligaments, while the dorsal radioulnar ligament splits ulnarly to form the subretinacular sheath of the extensor carpi ulnaris [15]. These ligaments have both a superficial and deep portion with the insertions on the ulnar styloid and fovea, respectively (Fig. 4.6) [1, 24]. At their broad radial attachment at the distal rim of the sigmoid notch, the radioulnar ligaments are conjoined, but then split prior to reaching the ulnar styloid or fovea into a superficial and a deep portion (Fig. 4.7) [2, 14]. The insertion of the deep portion, commonly called the ligamentum subcruentum, is more lateral and proximal into the fovea compared to the more central and distal insertion of the superficial ligament. The palmar and dorsal portions of the deep ligament converge and intertwine as they insert into the fovea (Fig. 4.8) [15]. The original description of the ligamentum subcruentum was of a vascularized space separating the proximal deep and distal superficial portions of the TFCC, but this term has changed over time to describe the insertion of the deep component of the ligaments [1, 24]. Ishii, in a cadaveric study, found that the deep portion inserts on the fovea, but that there was not a clearly distinct insertion site of the superficial ligament on the styloid [14].

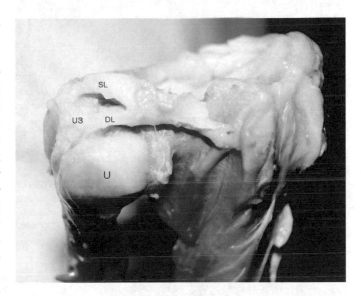

Fig. 4.7 The conjoined deep (DL) and superficial (SL) dorsal radioulnar ligament can be seen prior to splitting and inserting into their respective sites onto the fovea and the ulnar styloid (US). U, ulnar head

The insertion of the deep component of the ligament provides a better mechanical advantage for controlling rotation as its angle of insertion is less acute than that of the superficial ligament [1]. To demonstrate this concept, Kleinman uses the analogy of a team of horses, a buckboard, and a driver, in which the radius is the team of horses, the ulna is the buckboard, and the different angles of the reins going to the driver represent the deep and superficial ligaments [1]. This analogy shows how the less-acute angle of the reins, which represents the deep ligament, is more advantageous in controlling the rotation of the horses, which represents the radius [1]. The radioulnar ligaments have a spiral configuration as they insert onto the ulnar head, and this rotational insertion, along with the differing locations of insertion of the deep and superficial ligaments, allows continuous shifts in tension and compression and is the core of DRUJ stability [7].

The superficial radioulnar ligaments also provide stability to the DRUJ, but their action is the opposite of the deep ligaments, with the dorsal fibers giving stability in pronation and the palmar fibers providing stability in supination. While the superficial fibers do provide stability, they have a more acute angle of insertion and thus less mechanical advantage for rotational control. The second reason the superficial ligaments play a lesser role is that in maximum pronation or supination, the majority of the ulna has escaped out from under the superficial fibers, rendering them ineffective in

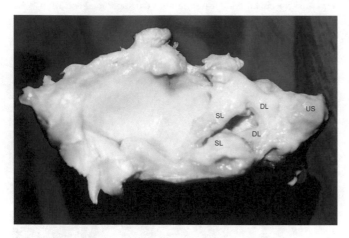

Fig. 4.8 A specimen showing the deep portion of the volar and dorsal radioulnar ligaments (DL) converging prior to inserting into the fovea. The articular disc has been resected and the superficial radioulnar ligaments (SL) have been released from the ulnar styloid (US) and retracted

these extremes of motion (Fig. 4.9a, b). In this position, the deep portion of the radioulnar ligament provides stability by providing a tethering action, thus preventing dislocation of the DRUJ [1, 2].

The Ulnar Collateral Ligament and Extensor Carpi Ulnaris Subsheath

The ulnar collateral ligament and the extensor carpi ulnaris (ECU) subsheath play an important role in the function of the TFCC. The ulnar collateral ligament is found originating on the ulnar styloid before dividing and inserting distally on the triquetrum and pisiform and contributes to ulnocarpal stability. The ECU subsheath is formed from the deep lamina of the antebrachial fascia and is directly adjacent to the articular disc (Fig. 4.10) [4]. The subsheath plays an important role in stabilizing the extensor carpi ulnaris tendon in the ulnar groove in pronation and supination (Fig. 4.11). The role of the extensor carpi ulnaris subsheath in DRUJ stability is somewhat controversial. Iida et al. found that the ECU dynamically stabilized the DRUJ and ulnocarpal joint in supination and neutral rotation after sectioning of the TFCC, and that the ECU subsheath assisted the ECU with stabilization on the ulnar side of the wrist. In contrast, Stuart et al., in their biomechanical study, did not find that the ECU subsheath was a significant contributor to DRUJ stability [3, 25]. Tang did find an increase in excursion of the ECU tendon of 30% during 60° of wrist extension after release of the TFCC from the distal ulna in a Palmar 1B-type lesion, suggesting that the TFCC is an important part of the pulley system for the ulnar wrist extensor [26]. This might suggest that the

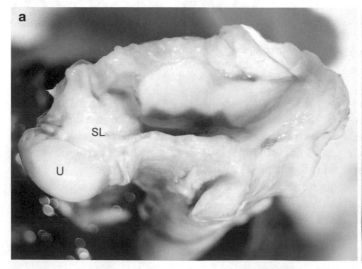
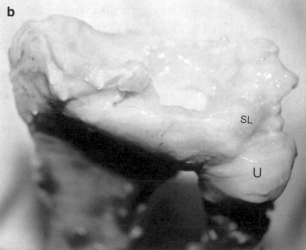

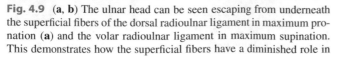

Fig. 4.9 (**a, b**) The ulnar head can be seen escaping from underneath the superficial fibers of the dorsal radioulnar ligament in maximum pronation (**a**) and the volar radioulnar ligament in maximum supination. This demonstrates how the superficial fibers have a diminished role in

the stability of the DRUJ in the extremes of motion, and the majority of the stability is provided by the tethering role of the deep portion of the radioulnar ligaments. SL, superficial portion of the radioulnar ligament; U, ulnar head

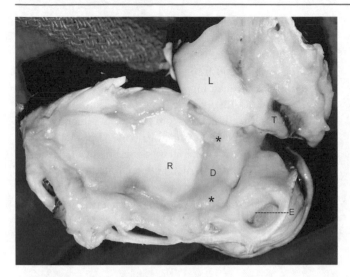

Fig. 4.10 The extensor carpi ulnaris subsheath (E) can be seen directly adjacent to the dorsal portion of the radioulnar ligaments (asterisk) and the articular disc (D). This tissue can provide a stout repair for peripheral tears in this location

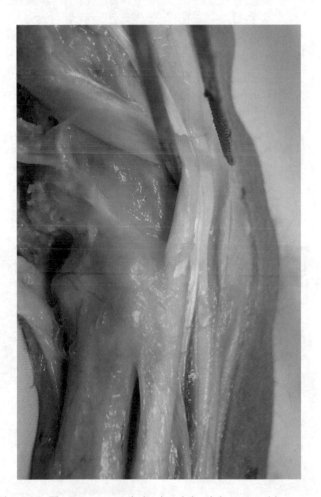

Fig. 4.11 The extensor carpi ulnaris subsheath is seen and is responsible for stabilizing the tendon in the ulnar groove during pronation and supination

TFCC plays a more significant role as part of the ulnar wrist extensor pulley system than the ECU subsheath does as a stabilizer of the DRUJ.

The Articular Disc

The articular disc forms the radial and central aspect of the TFCC and extends from the radius and covers the ulnar head before reaching the meniscus homologue and capsule. It does not attach directly to the ulnar head and is bounded on its palmar and dorsal aspect by the radioulnar ligaments, which are the main supporting structures of the DRUJ. These ligaments cannot be distinctly distinguished from the disc during arthroscopy and appear as thickenings on the periphery. The disc appears wedge-shaped in the coronal plane, being thinner on the radial aspect and then thickening ulnarly. The disc is also found to be thicker on the peripheral aspects and thinner in the central region. It should be noted that the disc is thicker in people with negative ulnar variance and thinner in people with positive or neutral variance [4]. The collagen of the disc is composed of interweaving sheets of collagen fibers, which is consistent with a structure experiencing multidirectional stresses [23]. An important finding regarding surgical treatment showed that resection of the central two-thirds of the disc with maintenance of the radioulnar ligaments and the ulnocarpal ligaments had no significant effect on axial load transmission [27, 28]. Adams also found that resection of two-thirds of the disc with preservation of the peripheral 2 mm had no significant effect on the normal kinematics [29]. With resection of greater than two-thirds of the disc and resection of the peripheral 2 mm, the ulnar column is unloaded, transferring the load to the distal radius in addition to possibly destabilizing the DRUJ [27–29].

Blood Supply

Work done by Thiru et al. demonstrated that the central 80–85% of the disc is relatively avascular, and the blood supply to the peripheral 15–20% is supplied from contributions from the ulnar artery through the palmar and dorsal radiocarpal branches and also from the anterior interosseous artery through the palmar and dorsal branches [30]. Works by Bednar et al. and Chidgey expanded on this knowledge by showing that the vessels enter the TFCC from the palmar, dorsal, and ulnar attachments of the capsule, but that there is limited vascularity at the radial attachment [23, 31]. These anatomical studies suggest that due to the avascular nature of the central TFCC, repair would not be possible in this region, and Bednar and colleagues further expanded this to include tears along the radial attachment. While Bednar suggested from anatomical studies that radial-sided tears might not be amenable to repair, several clinical studies have shown good results with radial-sided repairs despite the poor blood supply in this region [15, 31–33]. An interesting finding was reported by Tatebe et al. with second look arthroscopic surgery in patients who had previously undergone arthroscopic surgery with or without debridement of central TFCC tear followed by an ulnar shortening osteotomy [34]. They found that 16 out of 32 patients had healed their previous central tear with fibrous connective tissue and fibrocartilaginous components with no infiltration of inflammatory cells or vascular invasion seen in the regenerated tissues [34]. Their findings showed that rounded and more ulnarly located tears had a higher tendency to heal compared with linear and radial-central tears [34].

Innervation

The innervation of the TFCC is fairly consistent with contributions from the posterior interosseous nerve in the dorsal aspect, the ulnar nerve in the volar aspect, and the dorsal sensory branch in the ulnar region [7, 35]. Cavalcante et al. found increased free nerve endings in the dorsal and ulnar aspects of the TFCC, which correlate with Ohmori et al.'s findings of more free nerve endings in the region of the meniscus homologue and the collagen fiber area of the ulnar peripheral portion of the articular disc [36, 37]. Gupta et al. suggested the possible entry site for sensory nerves is the internal portion of the TFCC; located deep in the styloid recess, it has the highest density of neural elements and free nerve endings and might be a source of ulnar-sided pain [38]. Mechanoreceptors have been identified in different regions, suggesting a proprioceptive role of the TFCC [7, 36, 37]. Cavalcante et al. found a higher density of Pacini corpuscles in the dorsal and radial aspects, suggesting that this area is responsible for detecting the onset or cessation of movement; they also found an even distribution of Ruffini corpuscles throughout the TFCC [37].

TFCC Injuries

Injuries of the TFCC are not uncommon, with the most common mechanism being a fall onto an outstretched hand, resulting in extension and pronation of an axially loaded carpus [39, 40]. Other common injury mechanisms of the TFCC include a rapid twisting and loading of the ulnar side of the wrist, often occurring on the athletic field or in the workplace, and a distractive force along the ulnar aspect of the wrist [27, 40]. Palmer described a classification of lesions of the TFCC which describes both traumatic (Type 1) and

degenerative lesions (Type 2) (Table 4.1) [39]. An understanding of these lesions and the various treatment options of each should be familiar to the surgeon; however, this discussion will be brief and limited to traumatic lesions and will not go into detail regarding the treatment options.

Type 1A tears involve the central avascular portion of the disc several millimeters from the radial attachment and are usually oriented from dorsal to volar (Fig. 4.12). Type 1B lesions represent a peripheral detachment of the insertion of the TFCC onto the distal ulna. Clinically this type of injury is important, as it involves detachment of the radioulnar ligaments from the ulna either from a fracture or from a pure avulsion-type injury, and can lead to DRUJ instability. Type 1C lesions represent an ulnocarpal ligament avul-

Table 4.1 Classification of tears of the triangular fibrocartilage complex

Class I traumatic injuries	
Subtype	Characteristics
IA	Tears or perforations of the horizontal portion of the triangular fibrocartilage complex (TFCC) Usually 1–2 mm wide Dorsal palmar slit located 2–3 mm medial to the radial attachment of the sigmoid notch
IB	Traumatic avulsion of TFCC from insertion into the distal ulna May be accompanied by a fracture of the ulnar styloid at its base Usually associated with distal radiocarpal joint instability
IC	Tears of TFCC that result in ulnocarpal instability, such as avulsion of the TFCC from the distal attachment of the lunate or triquetrum
ID	Traumatic avulsions of the TFCC from the attachment at the distal sigmoid notch

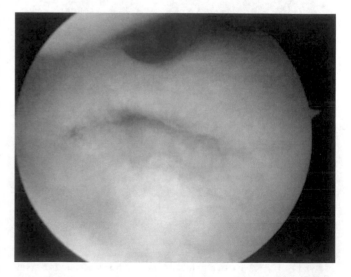

Fig. 4.12 An arthroscopic image showing a Palmer 1A tear of the *central portion* of the disc. The radioulnar ligaments are not involved, and this tear is oriented from volar to dorsal in the usual manner. The ulnar head is visible from the radiocarpal space through this full-thickness tear

sion and can result in ulnocarpal instability with volar translocation of the carpus [27, 39]. Type 1D tears represent an avulsion of the TFCC from its wide but thin radial attachment to the sigmoid notch and are more rare than central and peripheral tears [39].

Arthroscopic Anatomy of the TFCC

Arthroscopy allows better visualization of the different components of the TFCC than can often be obtained with open approaches. With this improved ability to see fine details and structures, the surgeon must possess a comprehensive understanding of the anatomy to help differentiate normal anatomical variants from a pathologic process. The TFCC can be visualized from both the radiocarpal and the DRUJ spaces, and different aspects of the complex can be examined. MRI has been shown to be a valuable resource in the detection of these injuries, with Tanaka et al. finding that high-resolution MRI has improved the detection of central and radial-sided lesions when compared to arthroscopy with findings of 100% sensitivity and specificity [41]. Unfortunately, MRI was not as accurate regarding injuries to the ulnar attachment of the TFCC, DRUL, PRUL, and ulnolunate ligaments with a higher false positive rate and lower specificity [41]. Due to the remaining limitations of MRI, arthroscopy still remains a valuable technique not only for the treatment, but also for the diagnosis of these injuries.

Radiocarpal Space

From the radiocarpal space, the TFCC can first be visualized as the scope is moved ulnarly along the lunate facet of the radius, exposing the broad insertion of the TFCC onto the ulnar border of the radius. The appearance of the TFCC is that of a broad white ligamentous sheet and can be very similar in appearance to the articular cartilage of the lunate facet (Fig. 4.13) [22]. This junction between the medial border of the radius and the TFCC may be clear, but it may be very subtle in some patients [22]. If difficulty is encountered in differentiating where the radius ends and the TFCC begins, a probe can be utilized for help with identification, as the firm border of the radius gives way to the softer disc [42, 43]. The articular disc lies in between the dorsal and palmar radioulnar ligaments and extends from the sigmoid notch toward the ulnar styloid and meniscus homologue. The ulnar head should not be seen from the radiocarpal space with an intact TFCC, but may be visualized with a full-thickness tear [42].

The dorsal and palmar radioulnar ligaments appear as thickenings of the peripheral aspect of the disc where it joins the capsule, but they are not seen as distinct, separate structures. The insertion of the deep portion of these ligaments

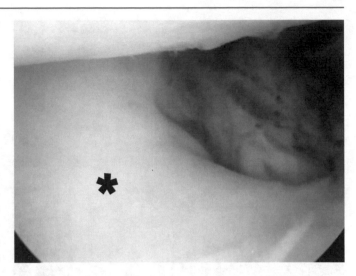

Fig. 4.13 An arthroscopic image showing the taut, white sheet-like appearance of the TFCC (*asterisk*). The volar and dorsal radioulnar ligaments cannot be seen as distinct structures arthroscopically and appear as thickenings where the TFCC meets the capsule

cannot be visualized from the radiocarpal space, but can still be evaluated. The hook test, as described by Ruch, can be used to determine if there is a foveal detachment of the deep portion of the radioulnar ligaments representing a Palmer 1B-type lesion [44]. This is performed by inserting a probe in the 4–5 or 6-R portal and pulling traction to the most ulnar aspect of the TFCC. This test is positive for a tear of the foveal attachment if the ulnar aspect of the TFCC is able to be pulled radially and distally [45]. The probe can further be used to palpate the disc and perform the trampoline test by compressing the TFCC. An intact TFCC will be taut with the tension maintained, whereas with a significant tear, the disc will be soft and pliable (Fig. 4.14) [17, 42]. The central disc and the periphery should be thoroughly inspected and probed to determine the integrity of the TFCC and to ensure that there are no subtle tears present [42].

In the dorsal ulnar aspect, the TFCC can be seen attached to the floor of the subsheath of the extensor carpi ulnaris tendon. This tissue provides good fixation of the disc back to the sheath when a peripheral tear occurs in this area [40]. The ECU subsheath and the dorsal ulnotriquetral ligament should be visualized and probed after removing the covering synovium if an injury is suspected in this region [40]. The prestyloid recess can be visualized, ulnar to the short radiolunate ligament and palmar to the styloid, but should not be mistaken for a TFCC tear, as this is a normal finding. This opening can have a variable appearance and is usually lined with synovial villi and capillaries (Fig. 4.15) [15].

The ulnolunate and ulnotriquetral ligaments can be seen passing from the palmar aspect of the radioulnar ligament before attaching to the volar aspect of the lunate and the triquetrum (Fig. 4.16). The ulnolunate ligament can be seen originating from the palmar radioulnar ligament before

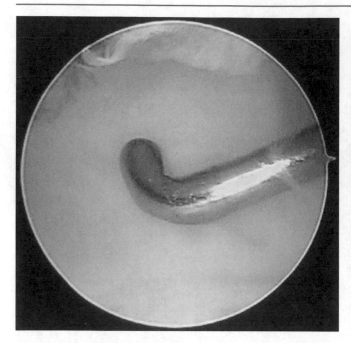

Fig. 4.14 The "Trampoline" test is performed by compressing the TFCC with a probe and assessing the tension. An intact disc will be taut, and a tear should be suspected if the disc is found to be soft and pliable

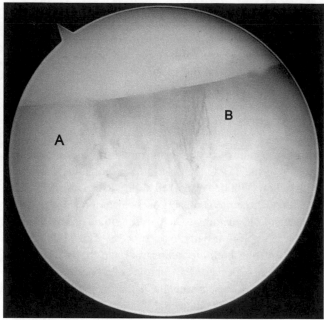

Fig. 4.16 Arthroscopic image showing the ulnolunate (**a**) and the ulnotriquetral (**b**) ligament passing from the palmar aspect of the volar radioulnar ligament to their insertions on the lunate and triquetrum, respectively

seen between these ligaments [22]. Moving ulnarly, the ulnotriquetral ligament can be visualized originating from the palmar radioulnar ligament and inserting distally on the palmar aspect of the triquetrum. The pisotriquetral orifice may be seen as a small defect in the distal aspect of the ulnotriquetral ligament and is a communication between the ulnocarpal and pisotriquetral joints (Fig. 4.17). This is best seen using the 4–5 or 6-R portal, and through this opening, the dorsal surface of the pisiform may be visualized along with the insertion of the flexor carpi ulnaris [22]. Both of these ligaments should be inspected and probed to test their integrity, as they limit wrist extension and radial deviation and can be a source of pain when injured, even though they do not contribute significantly to DRUJ stability. The lunotriquetral interosseous ligament can be located in the interval of these ligaments by following them distally (Fig. 4.18) [42]. The ulnocapitate ligament is not normally visible during radiocarpal arthroscopy as it is superficial to the ulnolunate and ulnotriquetral ligaments [22].

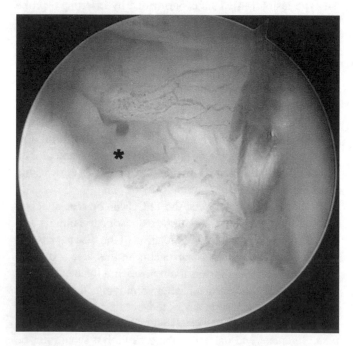

Fig. 4.15 Arthroscopic image showing the prestyloid recess (*asterisk*) with the synovial villi lined opening, along with the surrounding loose tissue of the meniscus homologue. This structure can have a variable appearance and should not be mistaken for a TFCC tear

inserting distally on the lunate just ulnar to the short radiolunate ligament. Depending on the tension of the proximal radioulnar ligament during forearm rotation, a fold may be

DRUJ Space

Although arthroscopy of the DRUJ is not as commonly performed as that of the radiocarpal space, it can provide important diagnostic information. The DRUJ can be entered using either a 2.7-mm or a 1.9-mm arthroscope for visualizing the sigmoid notch, distal ulna, undersurface of the TFCC, and

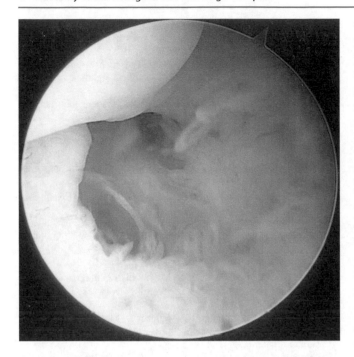

Fig. 4.17 An arthroscopic image taken from the 6R portal demonstrating the pisotriquetral orifice. This communication between the ulnocarpal and pisotriquetral joints can be located by following the ulnotriquetral ligament distally. The dorsal surface of the pisiform is not visible in this image, but it may be seen along with insertion of the flexor carpi ulnaris

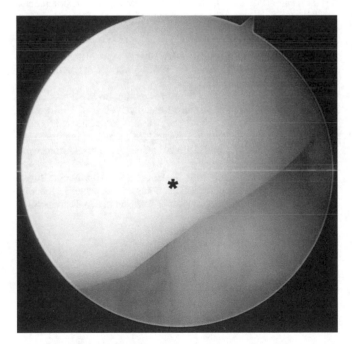

Fig. 4.18 The ulnotriquetral interval (*asterisk*) is seen in this arthroscopic image and may be identified in the interval of the ulnolunate and ulnotriquetral ligaments by following them distally

the deep portion of the palmar and dorsal radioulnar ligaments along with their attachment into the fovea. Arthroscopy of this joint takes advantage of the mismatch of the radius of

curvature of the ulnar head and the sigmoid notch to allow passage of the scope [22]. With the scope in the dorsal DRUJ portal, the sigmoid notch and the ulnar head can be visualized as the scope is directed distally. The ulnocapitate ligament can be seen inserting on the most radial aspect of the fovea with the radioulnar ligaments converging and inserting ulnarly on the fovea. From the volar DRUJ portal, the undersurface of the TFCC can again be seen attaching to the ulnar border of the radius. A probe can be placed from the dorsal portal allowing this broad attachment to be evaluated. As the scope is directed ulnarly, the ulnar head and the undersurface of the articular disc come into view and can be inspected. Directing the scope more ulnarly toward the fovea exposes the deep portions of the radioulnar ligaments, which can be seen converging and inserting onto the fovea. These ligaments can then be probed to check for tears of their insertion into the fovea.

Conclusion

A thorough understanding of the anatomy and biomechanics of the TFCC is invaluable in treating patients with ulnar-sided wrist pain. While instructional texts and videos can provide a basic foundation of knowledge, the arthroscopic anatomy of the TFCC and wrist in general may best be learned through cadaveric training initially. This knowledge can then be further enhanced through clinical practice, as often the intraoperative findings may be subtle or not as classically described. Once the surgeon has mastered this sometimes-difficult anatomy, pathologic findings can be identified and the proper surgical treatment may be performed.

References

1. Kleinman WB. Stability of the distal radioulnar joint: biomechanics, pathophysiology, physical diagnosis, and restoration of function what we have learned in 25 years. J Hand Surg Am. 2007;32A:1086–106.
2. Af Ekensam F, Hagert CG. Anatomical studies on the geometry and stability of the distal radio ulnar joint. Scand J Plast Reconstr Surg. 1985;19:17–25.
3. Stuart PR, Berger RA, Linscheid RL, An KN. The dorsopalmar stability of the distal radioulnar joint. J Hand Surg Am. 2000;25A:689–99.
4. Berger RA. Wrist anatomy. In: Cooney WP, editor. The wrist. 2nd ed. Philadelphia: Lippincott Williams & Wilkins; 2010. p. 25–76.
5. Whipple TL. Arthroscopy of the distal radioulnar joint-indications, portals, and anatomy. Hand Clin. 1994;10(4):589–92.
6. Hagert CG. The distal radioulnar joint. Hand Clin. 1987;3(1):41–50.
7. Hagert E, Hagert CG. Understanding stability of the distal radioulnar joint through an understanding of its anatomy. Hand Clin. 2010;26(4):459–66.
8. Ekenstam FW, Palmer AK, Glisson RR. The load on the radius and ulna in different positions of the wrist and forearm. Acta Orthop Scand. 1984;55:363–5.

9. Friedman SL, Palmer AK, Short WH, et al. The change in ulnar variance with grip. J Hand Surg Am. 1993;18:713–6.

10. Palmer AK, Werner FW. Biomechanics of the distal radioulnar joint. Clin Orthop Relat Res. 1984;187:26–35.

11. Palmer AK, Glisson RR, Werner FW. Relationship between ulnar variance and TFCC thickness. J Hand Surg Am. 1984;9:681–3.

12. Palmer AK, Werner FW. The triangular fibrocartilage complex of the wrist anatomy and function. J Hand Surg Am. 1981;6:153–62.

13. Michalko K, Allen S, Akelman E. Evaluation of the painful wrist. In: Geissler WB, editor. Wrist arthroscopy. New York: Springer; 2005. p. 15–21.

14. Ishii S, Palmer AK, Werner FW, Short WH, Fortino MD. An anatomic study of the ligamentous structure of the triangular fibrocartilage complex. J Hand Surg Am. 1998;23A:977–85.

15. Jantea CL, Baltzer A, Ruther W. Arthroscopic repair of radial-sided lesions of the fibrocartilage complex. Hand Clin. 1995;11(1):31–6.

16. Werner FW, Glisson RR, Murphy DJ, et al. Force transmission through the distal radioulnar carpal joint: effect of ulnar lengthening and shortening. Handchirurgie. 1986;18:304–8.

17. Osterman AL, Terrill RG. Arthroscopic treatment of TFCC lesions. Hand Clin. 1991;7:277–81.

18. Moritomo H, Kataoka T. Anatomy of the ulnocarpal compartment. In: Piñal FD, Mathoulin C, Nakamura T, editors. Arthroscopic management of ulnar pain. Berlin; New York: Springer; 2012. p. 1–14.

19. Moritomo H, Murase T, Arimitsu S, Oka K, Yoshikawa K, Sugamoto K. Change in the length of the ulnocarpal ligaments during radiocarpal motion: possible impact on triangular fibrocartilage complex foveal tears. J Hand Surg Am. 2008;33A:1278–86.

20. Bowers WH. The distal radioulnar joint. In: Green DP, editor. Operative hand surgery, vol. vol. 1. 3rd ed. New York: Churchill Livingstone; 1993. p. 973–1019.

21. Taleisnik J. The ligaments of the wrist. In: Taleisnik J, editor. The wrist. New York: Churchill Livingstone; 1985. p. 13–38.

22. Berger RA. Arthroscopic anatomy of the wrist and distal radioulnar joint. Hand Clin. 1999;15(3):393–413.

23. Chidgey LK. Histologic anatomy of the triangular fibrocartilage. Hand Clin. 1991;7(2):249–62.

24. Kauer JMG. The articular disc of the hand. Acta Anat. 1975;93:590–605.

25. Iida A, Omokawa S, Moritomo H, Aoki M, Wada T, Kataoka T, Tanaka Y. Biomechanical study of the extensor Carpi ulnaris as a dynamic wrist stabilizer. J Hand Surg Am. 2012;37A:2456–61.

26. Tang JB, Ryu J, Kish V. The triangular fibrocartilage complex: an important component of the pulley for the ulnar wrist extensor. J Hand Surg Am. 1998;23A:986–91.

27. Bednar JM. Arthroscopic treatment of triangular fibrocartilage tears. Hand Clin. 1999;15(3):479–88.

28. Palmer AK, Werner FW, Glisson RR, et al. Partial excision of the triangular fibrocartilage complex. J Hand Surg Am. 1988;13:391–4.

29. Adams BD. Partial excision of the triangular fibrocartilage complex articular disc: a biomechanical study. J Hand Surg Am. 1993;18:334–40.

30. Thiru RG, Ferlic DC, Clayton ML, McClure DC. Arterial anatomy of the triangular fibrocartilage of the wrist and its surgical significance. J Hand Surgery Am. 1986;11:258–63.

31. Bednar MS, Arnoczky SP, Weiland AJ. The microvasculature of the triangular fibrocartilage complex: its clinical significance. J Hand Surg Am. 1991;16:1101–5.

32. Trumble TE, Gilbert M, Vedder N. Isolated tears of the triangular fibrocartilage: management by early arthroscopic repair. J Hand Surg Am. 1997;22:57–65.

33. Sagerman SD, Short W. Arthroscopic repair of radial-sided triangular fibrocartilage complex tears. Arthroscopy. 1996;12:339–42.

34. Tatebe M, Horii E, Nakao E, Shinohara T, Imaeda T, Nakamura R, Hirata H. Repair of the triangular fibrocartilage complex after ulnar-shortening osteotomy: second-look arthroscopy. J Hand Surg Am. 2007;32(4):445–9.

35. Shigemitsu T, Tobe M, Mizutani K, Murakami K, Ishikawa Y, Sato F. Innervation of the triangular fibrocartilage complex of the human wrist: quantitative immunohistochemical study. Anat Sci Int. 2007;82(3):127–32.

36. Ohmori M, Azuma H. Morphology and distribution of nerve endings in the human triangular fibrocartilage complex. J Hand Surg Br. 1998;23(4):522–55.

37. Cavalcante ML, Rodrigues CJ, Mattar R Jr. Mechanoreceptors and nerve endings of the triangular fibrocartilage in the human wrist. J Hand Surg Am. 2004;29(3):432–5.

38. Gupta R, Nelson SD, Baker J, Jones NF, Meals RA. The innervation of the triangular fibrocartilage complex: nitric acid maceration rediscovered. Plast Reconstr Surg. 2001;107(1):135–9.

39. Palmer AK. Triangular fibrocartilage complex lesions: a classification. J Hand Surg Am. 1989;14:594–606.

40. Geissler WB. Arthroscopic knotless peripheral ulnar-sided TFCC repair. Hand Clin. 2011;27(4):273–9.

41. Tanaka T, Yoshioka H, Ueno T, Shindo M, Ochiai N. Comparison between high-resolution MRI with a microscopy coil and arthroscopy in triangular fibrocarilage complex injury. J Hand Surg Am. 2006;31(8):77–84.

42. Lee JH, Taylor NL, Beekman RA, Rosenwasser MP. Arthroscopic wrist anatomy. In: Geissler WB, editor. Wrist arthroscopy. New York: Springer; 2005. p. 7–13.

43. Whipple LT. Arthroscopic surgery: the wrist. Philadelphia: Lippincott Williams & Wilkins; 1992. p. 55–60.

44. Ruch DS, Yang CC, Smith BP. Results of acute arthroscopically repaired triangular fibrocartilage complex injuries associated with intra-articular distal radius fractures. Arthroscopy. 2003;19(5):511–6.

45. Atzei A, Rizzo A, Luchetti R, Fairplay T. Arthroscopic foveal repair of triangular fibrocartilage complex peripheral lesion with distal radioulnar joint instability. Tech Hand Up Extrem Surg. 2008;12:226–35.

Management of Type 1A TFCC Tears

Laith Al-Shihabi, Robert W. Wysocki, and David S. Ruch

History and Physical Examination

Triangular fibrocartilage complex (TFCC) injuries are among the most common causes of ulnar sided wrist pain and can result from both acute and chronic mechanisms of injury. Acute injuries are typically traumatic and result from compression or shear of the TFCC between the distal ulna and the proximal carpus, while chronic injuries are degenerative and occur in the setting of positive ulnar variance and ulnocarpal impaction syndrome [1]. The most common mechanism of acute injury to the TFCC is via a fall onto outstretched hands. With the wrist in pronation, as is often the case when bracing for a fall forward, the ulna is brought into relative positivity versus the radius and a greater portion of the load is applied across the ulnocarpal joint and TFCC than would be experienced with the forearm in neutral or supination. Ulnar deviation of the wrist also increases compression through the TFCC, and extremes of pronation or supination tighten the dorsal and volar radioulnar ligaments [2–5], respectively, and may expose them to injury.

Patients will typically present with complaints of ulnar-sided wrist pain that is exacerbated by motions that stress or load the TFCC. Symptomatic weakness, mechanical catching or crepitus, and distal radioulnar joint (DRUJ) instability may also be present. Detailed inquiry should be directed toward onset and duration of symptoms, exacerbating factors, history of trauma or fracture, and any previous treatment. The physical exam is centered around identifying points of tenderness, response to provocative tests, and stability of the DRUJ. Understanding surface anatomy is key to distinguishing pain from an injured TFCC versus other causes of ulnar-sided pain such as lunotriquetral (LT) ligament injury, hamate hook fracture, ulnar artery thrombosis, piso-triquetral arthritis, or extensor carpi ulnaris tendinitis. The TFCC is palpated in the soft spot bordered by the distal ulna proximally, pisiform distally, ulnar styloid dorsally, and flexor carpi ulnaris tendon volarly. Pain in this area is considered a positive ulnar fovea sign, and has been found to have a 95.2% sensitivity and 86.5% specificity for ulnotriquetral ligament tears or foveal avulsion of the TFCC [6]. The ulnocarpal stress test is performed by axially loading an ulnarly deviated and extended wrist in neutral, supination, or pronation. Nakamura arthroscopically examined 45 patients with persistent ulnar-sided pain and a positive ulnocarpal stress test, and in all instances identified a source of pathology. Injuries identified included signs of ulnocarpal abutment syndrome, TFCC tears, LT ligament tears, and degenerative arthritis among others, suggesting it is a sensitive but not specific examination maneuver [7]. To test the DRUJ, the ulna is stabilized while the radius is manually translated dorsally and volarly in neutral, pronation, and supination. Increased excursion compared to the unaffected side is a positive result. Alternatively, the piano key test can be used to assess the DRUJ by having the patient place both palms flat onto the examination table. The patient either actively pushes their ulna down toward the table or the examiner applies a volar-directed force on the ulna 4 cm proximal to the DRUJ; pain at the DRUJ with stress is indicative of TFCC pathology, while increased ulnar motion relative to the unaffected side suggests a tear which has destabilized the DRUJ [8].

Supplementary Information The online version of this chapter (https://doi.org/10.1007/978-3-030-78881-0_5) contains supplementary material, which is available to authorized users.

L. Al-Shihabi
Department of Orthopaedic Surgery, Rush University Medical Center, Chicago, IL, USA

R. W. Wysocki (✉)
Department of Orthopedic Surgery, Rush University, Chicago, IL, USA

D. S. Ruch
Department of Orthopaedic Surgery, Duke University Medical Center, Durham, NC, USA

© Springer Nature Switzerland AG 2022
W. B. Geissler (ed.), *Wrist and Elbow Arthroscopy with Selected Open Procedures*,
https://doi.org/10.1007/978-3-030-78881-0_5

Triangular Fibrocartilage Complex Tear Classification

The distinction between acute and traumatic vs. chronic and degenerative injuries to the TFCC forms the basis of the Palmer classification into Type I and Type II tears, respectively [1]. Further subclassifications are defined based on tear location and associated pathology. Type 1A tears are the most common [8] and occur within the central substance fibrocartilaginous disc, typically sagittally oriented and 2–3 mm ulnar to the radial border of the TFCC. This area corresponds to the region and orientation of maximal strain through the fibrocartilage when the forearm is pronated [9]. As both the bony attachments of the TFCC on the radius and ulna and the dorsal and volar radioulnar ligaments are left intact, stability of the distal radioulnar joint (DRUJ) is not compromised. Central tears are unlikely to heal either spontaneously or with repair as only the periphery of the TFCC is vascularized, while the central 80–85% that includes the disc is avascular (Fig. 5.1) [10–12]. Pain is likely not from the tear proper, as the central disc is similarly poorly innervated [13], but rather traction on the peripheral TFCC from catching of unstable tear flaps during wrist motion. Simple debridement of the loose fibrocartilaginous flaps of Type 1A tears does not alter TFCC or DRUJ biomechanics [14], and is the preferred surgical treatment.

Type 1B tears involve avulsion of the TFCC from the ulnar fovea or an avulsion fracture through the base of the ulnar styloid, and the fibrocartilaginous disc may also be torn from the dorsal wrist capsule. DRUJ instability is often, but not always, associated. Tears in which the disc pulls away from the ulnar capsule with intact deep insertional fibers to the ulna are seen with ulnar sided wrist pain in the absence of DRUJ instability [15]. As 1B tears are through the vascularized periphery and may heal, surgical repair is preferred

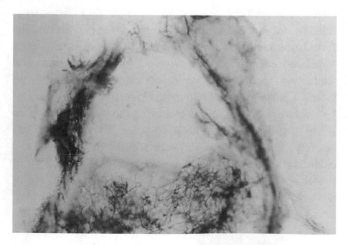

Fig. 5.1 The periphery of the TFCC is well vascularized, and thus capable of healing. The central disc is avascular and thus has poor healing potential. (Courtesy of Michael Bednar, MD)

either directly to bone or to the ulnar capsule depending on whether DRUJ instability is or is not present, respectively [15–20]. Type 1C tears occur along the volar margin and are associated with disruption of the ulnolunate, ulnotriquetral, or ulnocapitate ligaments of the wrist. These are typically high-energy injuries, often associated with ulnocarpal instability and volar translation of the ulnar carpus. Open repair is the most common surgical treatment to restore stability [21]. Type 1D lesions result from detachment of the TFCC from the ulnar radius, either via rupture of the radioulnar ligaments or an avulsion fracture of the radius at the sigmoid notch. If the radius and radioulnar ligaments are intact, the lesion is treated as a Type 1A tear and can be debrided [9, 22]. If DRUJ instability is present or the origin of one or more radioulnar ligaments disrupted, repair is preferred [23–25].

Type II lesions represent degeneration of the TFCC and surrounding structures due to chronic ulnar positive variance and consequent ulnocarpal impaction syndrome. Even small changes in ulnar variance can dramatically affect load-sharing, with 2.5 mm of ulnar positivity causing 42% of load to be borne through the ulnocarpal joint vs. 18% in an ulnar-neutral wrist [26]. In contrast to Type I tears, which represent distinct traumatic injuries, Type II lesions represent a spectrum of progressive pathology. Type 2A lesions involve wear of the proximal side of the TFCC only, without perforation or associated pathology. Type 2B lesions demonstrate the same degree of TFCC wear but in association with chondromalacia of the lunate or ulnar head. Type 2C lesions involve a perforation of the fibrocartilaginous disc, but unlike Type 1A tears they are typically ovoid in shape and more ulnar within the substance of the disc. Type 2D lesions involve both the TFCC perforations, lunate and ulnar head chondromalacia, and lunotriquetral ligament disruption. Finally, Type 2E lesions show frank degenerative arthritis of the ulnocarpal joint, lunotriquetral ligament disruption, and may also be associated with ulnar lunate collapse or DRUJ arthritis [1, 27]. Treatment for Type II TFCC lesions centers around correcting positive ulnar variance, with ulnar shortening osteotomy or arthroscopic debridement and ulna wafer resection being the most common treatments [28, 29]. For advanced pathology or failed primary surgery, either a distal ulna resection or Sauve-Kapandji procedure along with lunotriquetral pinning may be necessary.

Imaging

Standard posterior–anterior (PA), lateral, and oblique radiographs are the first-line imaging study to assess the TFCC, DRUJ, and wrist joint. Acute injury to the TFCC can be inferred by examining the integrity and alignment of the distal radius and ulna relative to the carpal bones. Widening of the DRUJ on a PA radiograph or anterior/posterior displacement of the ulna on a lateral radiograph suggests injury and instability; however, given anatomic variability it is important to compare to the unaffected extremity. Soft tissue Type 1B, 1C, and 1D injuries may still be associated with instability, however, and the presence of normal radiographs cannot exclude injury [30]. Ulnar variance should also be assessed on radiographs, including a power-grip PA in pronation if dynamic ulnocarpal impaction is suspected. Computed tomography (CT) can also be used to further clarify bony anatomy, and can compare DRUJ alignment side to side in positions of neutral, supination, and pronation to help detect subtle instability. CT scan is also more sensitive for detecting degenerative change within the DRUJ, distal ulna, or carpus associated with chronic pathology [8].

Magnetic resonance imaging (MRI) and arthrography (MRA) have largely replaced traditional arthrography as imaging modalities of choice, given the poor correlation of traditional arthrography with arthroscopic findings [31, 32]. To improve diagnostic accuracy, MRI should ideally be performed with the use of a microscopy wrist coil and at least a 1.5-T magnet [33]; newer 3.0-T magnets are significantly more accurate at imaging the TFCC, but are also more costly and less widely available [34]. Golimbu has also recommended imaging with 3 mm-thick sections and with the wrist in radial deviation to stretch ulnar tissues as techniques to improve accuracy, but no comparative studies have been performed regarding the effect of wrist position [35]. Systematic review of MRA vs. MRI by Smith demonstrated MRA to be superior to MRI for the detection of TFCC pathology, with pooled sensitivity of 84% and specificity of 95% for MRA vs. 75% and 81% for noncontrast MRI [36]. Given these findings, they concluded that MRA should be the study of choice for evaluating ulnar-sided wrist pain despite the invasiveness of the procedure. Diagnostic accuracy may vary depending on location of the TFCC injury, however, as some authors report superior results at detection of central and radial tears versus those involving the radioulnar ligaments [33]. MRI or MRA findings should always be considered in the context of the history and physical exam, however, as the rate of TFCC abnormalities on MRI in asymptomatic adults has been reported as 33.7% in those under 50, 62.5% in those 50–59, and 100% in those over 60 [37].

Treatment of Type 1A TFCC Tears

In the absence of DRUJ instability most acute TFCC injuries can initially be managed nonoperatively, with up to 57% of patients symptom-free after 1 month [38]. Temporary splinting or casting of the wrist for up to 2–6 weeks along with oral analgesics and anti-inflammatory medications relieves pain and may allow peripheral tears to heal without surgery.

While Type IA tears do not have a good intrinsic ability to heal, they are typically not structurally significant for wrist biomechanics and corticosteroid injections to the ulnocarpal joint can eliminate inflammation surrounding the tear, thus eliminating pain and avoiding surgical intervention in many cases [22]. Cortisone injection should not be undertaken within the first 6 weeks after symptom onset so as not to interfere with the normal biologic processes of healing. Patients with persistent pain despite nonoperative treatment or with instability of the DRUJ are indicated for surgery. High-performance athletes with confirmed TFCC tears on imaging can also be considered for early operative intervention [39, 40]. Arthroscopy is considered the gold-standard diagnostic modality to evaluate the TFCC, and the majority of tears can be treated with this approach.

Arthroscopic Evaluation

The patient's wrist is positioned, traction applied, and arthroscopic access established as described in Chapter 1. Initial evaluation is typically performed with the arthroscope placed in the 3,4 portal and instrumentation in the 6-R portal. Inflow pressure should be minimized in order to allow the TFCC to assume a more normal position within the ulnocarpal joint and minimize blanching, which allows for easier identification of inflamed soft tissue. Visual examination for obvious signs of injury or tears is performed, and associated synovitis or chondromalacia is also noted (Fig. 5.2a). Pronation and supination may aid in visualization of the entire TFCC, and stability of the DRUJ can be assessed with manual stress testing. If necessary, the arthroscope may also be moved to the 6-R portal to better view the radial and ulnar attachments of the disc. A probe is used to assess the integrity of the fibrocartilage by palpating the disc for intrasubstance tears, and when depressed it should readily spring back into its normal position (Fig. 5.2b). Loss of this so-called trampoline effect can indicate either peripheral or foveal detachment [41]. The hook and drag tests use the probe to apply traction along the periphery of the TFCC, and displacement vertically or in the direction of traction similarly indicates either a peripheral tear or foveal injury [6]. If a reparable tear is identified, its full extension must be explored in order to determine whether the repair should be to the subsheath only or, in the case of deep fiber involvement, directly to the ulna [15].

Arthroscopic Debridement of Type 1A Tears

Once the diagnosis of a Type 1A tear is made, arthroscopic debridement is the treatment of choice given the central disc's poor vascularity and inability to heal. Detailed man-

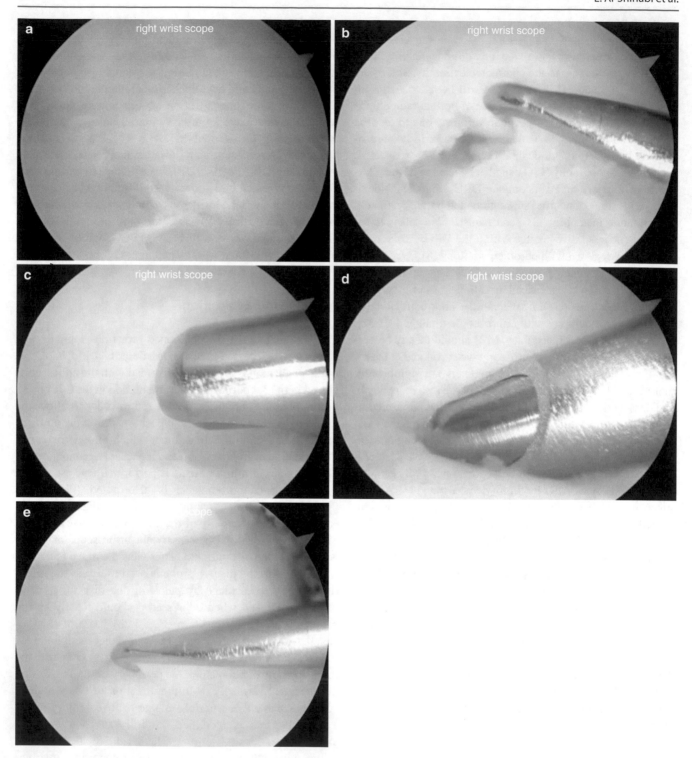

Fig. 5.2 (**a**) The arthroscopic appearance of a Type 1A TFCC tear, the extent and margins of which are defined with the aid of a probe (**b**). An arthroscopic shaver or other instrument is used to debride the unstable flaps of the tear back to stable edges, taking care to avoid the volar and dorsal radioulnar ligaments (**c**, **d**). The margins are then rechecked with the probe to confirm the adequacy of resection (**e**)

agement of tears amenable to repair will be covered in subsequent chapters. The goal of the procedure is to debride unstable flaps of the central fibrocartilage that are likely to catch on surrounding tissue back to a stable rim.

Biomechanical studies demonstrate that up to 2/3 of the central region can safely be resected without destabilizing the DRUJ; more important is to avoid damage to the peripheral 2 mm of the TFCC as this tissue contains the dorsal and volar radioulnar ligaments [14, 42] (Video 5.1). Debridement techniques have been described with multiple instruments including scalpels, banana blades, shavers, radiofrequency probes, and lasers [43–45]. Each has its own advantages and disadvantages, and the ideal instrument is ultimately the surgeon's preference. Ours is to use a banana blade or arthroscopic shaver to perform the bulk of resection followed by radiofrequency ablation, if necessary, to stabilize the borders of the resection (Fig. 5.2c, d). As with arthroscopic evaluation, debridement is started with the arthroscope in the 3,4 portal and instrumentation is introduced via the 6-R portal. The radial side of the torn fibrocartilaginous disc is outlined and resected with the blade, then removed with an arthroscopic grasper. The arthroscope is then moved to the 6-R portal, and with instrumentation through the 3,4 portal the same procedure is performed on the ulnar side of the tear. The TFCC is then reexamined to ensure the absence of any further unstable tissue and the integrity of the peripheral ligaments (Fig. 5.2e). The LT ligament and articular surfaces should also be examined and repair or debridement performed as indicated. In most cases, acute IA tears should not have significant carpal chondromalacia or LT ligament insufficiency as these are more often seen with chronic Type II patterns.

In the case of a patient with a Type 1A tear and concomitant positive ulnar variance, most authors argue for the addition of a primary ulnocarpal decompression along with TFCC debridement [8, 22, 28, 29, 46, 47]. The ulnar-shortening osteotomy [46] and ulnar wafer procedure [47] have both been proposed as treatment options that can be combined with arthroscopic debridement. In an early report of arthroscopic TFCC debridement Osterman noted some patients with positive ulnar variance to have degenerative chondromalacia of the ulnar head despite traumatic mechanisms, suggesting some tears may be acute-on-chronic injuries [48]. Minami subsequently reported that patients with positive ulnar variance have inferior outcomes compared to those with neutral or negative variance after debridement alone, and argued for primary ulnar-shortening osteotomy for these patients [46, 49]. Ulnar-shortening osteotomy is also a successful secondary procedure for persistent pain after primary debridement regardless of preoperative ulnar variance [50], suggesting dynamic positive ulnar variance may contribute to failure even if routine X-rays are normal [51]. In comparing primary ulnar wafer resection to ulnar-shortening osteotomy, when combined with debridement both show equivalent postoperative pain relief and function. Higher rates of tendinitis and reoperation (for hardware removal) have been reported with ulnar-shortening osteotomy, however [28, 52].

As previously discussed, if only the central region of the TFCC is debrided and the periphery remains intact, the biomechanics and stability of the wrist will not be affected. Further, as there is no repair to protect, postoperative immobilization is unnecessary and patients are able to begin rehabilitation immediately, including unrestricted active and passive motion and light progressive strengthening once pain is diminished [42]. If an ulnar-shortening osteotomy or ulnar wafer resection is performed a splint is used for 6 weeks to protect the osteotomy or allow a clot (and subsequently fibrocartilage) to form over the distal ulna, respectively. Strengthening exercises are delayed until the osteotomy is healed radiographically in the setting of an ulnar shortening (typically 6–8 weeks).

Results

Arthroscopic debridement has become the treatment of choice and standard of care for Type 1A TFCC tears, offering superior visualization of the TFCC with a less invasive approach and superior outcomes when compared to open procedures. In separate studies, Osterman and Roth both described the initial technique of arthroscopic TFCC debridement [48, 53]. Osterman also reported on 52 patients prospectively followed after arthroscopic debridement with either a motorized shaver or pituitary rongeur for traumatic or degenerative TFCC tears. At an average follow-up of 23 months, 73% were pain-free and 12% further were improved; among the five patients who failed treatment no relationship to ulnar variance was identified [48]. Subsequent studies have found similar results. Comparing arthroscopic debridement in 11 posttraumatic vs. 5 degenerative cases, Minami found a posttraumatic etiology to be associated in all cases with an excellent recovery based on superior patient satisfaction, pain relief, and function [49]. Using Minami's criteria, Miwa also found good or excellent results in 9/10 patients undergoing debridement for Type 1A tears [54]. Using the modified Mayo Wrist Score, Husby and Haugstvedt reviewed 32 patients at a median of 39 months after arthroscopic debridement and found 27 good or excellent results vs. 4 fair and 1 poor result; all but 2 patients in their study would have had surgery performed again [55].

Among patients failing debridement alone, Hulsizer found a subsequent ulnar shortening osteotomy resulted in complete relief of pain for 12/13 patients regardless of preoperative ulnar variance [50]. In cases of positive ulnar variance, failure rates of up to 25% have been described for debridement alone [49], and primary procedures to decompress the ulnocarpal joint should be considered in addition. Outcomes after debridement with ulnar-shortening osteotomy or an ulnar wafer procedure are equal or superior to those published for debridement alone. However, rates of reoperation, most commonly removal of osteotomy hardware, as well as ulnar-sided tendinitis are higher with ulnar-shortening osteotomy, leading some authors to favor the wafer procedure [28, 52]. Animal models also suggest that the clot formed by bleeding from the distal ulna may allow for fibrous reconstitution of the debrided central TFCC, but this has yet to be shown in humans [56].

Complications

Arthroscopic TFCC debridement is a minimally invasive, safe technique for the treatment of persistent ulnar-sided wrist pain due to traumatic tears of the central fibrocartilage. It is not without risk, however. The general risks of wrist arthroscopy are well known and well described, the most common being tendon and nerve injuries, local infections, cyst formation, and postoperative edema and stiffness [57–59]. Specific to TFCC debridement surgeons should be aware of the risks associated with their chosen instruments, such as laceration of surrounding tissues with a banana blade or burns and thermal injury with a radiofrequency device [60]. Surgeons should also develop a comprehensive, systematic preoperative workup to avoid diagnostic pitfalls, as coexistent DRUJ instability, lunotriquetral ligament injury, or ulnocarpal impaction left untreated will lead to a poor outcome and the need for additional surgery. If the correct diagnosis is made and treated, however, arthroscopic debridement yields excellent outcomes and a high degree of patient satisfaction.

References

1. Palmer AK. Triangular fibrocartilage complex lesions: a classification. J Hand Surg Am. 1989;14(4):594–606.
2. Ward LD, Ambrose CG, Masson MV, Levaro F. The role of the distal radioulnar ligaments, interosseous membrane, and joint capsule in distal radioulnar joint stability. J Hand Surg Am. 2000;25(2):341–51.
3. DiTano O, Trumble TE, Tencer AF. Biomechanical function of the distal radioulnar and ulnocarpal wrist ligaments. J Hand Surg Am. 2003;28(4):622–7.
4. Schuind F, An KN, Berglund L, Rey R, Cooney WP, Linscheid RL, Chao E. The distal radioulnar ligaments: a biomechanical study. J Hand Surg Am. 1991;16(6):1106–14.
5. Xu J, Tang JB. In vivo changes in lengths of the ligaments stabilizing the distal radioulnar joint. J Hand Surg Am. 2009;34(1):40–5.
6. Tay SC, Tomita K, Berger RA. The "ulnar fovea sign" for defining ulnar wrist pain: an analysis of sensitivity and specificity. J Hand Surg Am. 2007;32(4):438–44.
7. Nakamura R, Horii E, Imaeda T, Nakao E, Kato H, Watanabe K. The ulnocarpal stress test in the diagnosis of ulnar-sided wrist pain. J Hand Surg Br. 1997;22(6):719–23.
8. Sachar K. Ulnar-sided wrist pain: evaluation and treatment of triangular fibrocartilage complex tears, ulnocarpal impaction syndrome, and lunotriquetral ligament tears. J Hand Surg Am. 2012;37(7):1489–500.
9. Adams BD, Holley KA. Strains in the articular disk of the triangular fibrocartilage complex: a biomechanical study. J Hand Surg Am. 1993;18(5):919–25.
10. Thiru RG, Ferlic DC, Clayton ML, McClure DC. Arterial anatomy of the triangular fibrocartilage of the wrist and its surgical significance. J Hand Surg Am. 1986;11(2):258–63.
11. Mikić Z. The blood supply of the human distal radioulnar joint and the microvasculature of its articular disk. Clin Orthop Relat Res. 1992;275:19–28.
12. Bednar MS, Arnoczky SP, Weiland AJ. The microvasculature of the triangular fibrocartilage complex: its clinical significance. J Hand Surg Am. 1991;16(6):1101–5.
13. Gupta R, Nelson SD, Baker J, Jones NF, Meals RA. The innervation of the triangular fibrocartilage complex: nitric acid maceration rediscovered. Plast Reconstr Surg. 2001;107(1):135–9.
14. Adams BD. Partial excision of the triangular fibrocartilage complex articular disk: a biomechanical study. J Hand Surg Am. 1993;18(2):334–40.
15. Wysocki RW, Richard MJ, Crowe MM, Leversedge FJ, Ruch DS. Arthroscopic treatment of peripheral triangular fibrocartilage complex tears with the deep fibers intact. J Hand Surg Am. 2012;37(3):509–16.
16. Hauck RM, Skahen J, Palmer AK. Classification and treatment of ulnar styloid nonunion. J Hand Surg Am. 1996;21(3):418–22.
17. Wolf MB, Haas A, Dragu A, Leclère FM, Dreyhaupt J, Hahn P, Unglaub F. Arthroscopic repair of ulnar-sided triangular fibrocartilage complex (palmer type 1B) tears: a comparison between short- and midterm results. J Hand Surg Am. 2012;37(11):2325–30.
18. Reiter A, Wolf MB, Schmid U, Frigge A, Dreyhaupt J, Hahn P, Unglaub F. Arthroscopic repair of palmer 1B triangular fibrocartilage complex tears. Arthroscopy. 2008;24(11):1244–50.
19. Moritomo H, Masatomi T, Murase T, Miyake J, Okada K, Yoshikawa H. Open repair of foveal avulsion of the triangular fibrocartilage complex and comparison by types of injury mechanism. J Hand Surg Am. 2010;35(12):1955–63.
20. Chou KH, Sarris IK, Sotereanos DG. Suture anchor repair of ulnar-sided triangular fibrocartilage complex tears. J Hand Surg Br. 2003;28(6):546–50.
21. Mikic ZD. Treatment of acute injuries of the triangular fibrocartilage complex associated with distal radioulnar joint instability. J Hand Surg Am. 1995;20(2):319–23.
22. Henry MH. Management of acute triangular fibrocartilage complex injury of the wrist. J Am Acad Orthop Surg. 2008;16(6):320–9.
23. Sagerman SD, Short W. Arthroscopic repair of radial-sided triangular fibrocartilage complex tears. Arthroscopy. 1996;12(3):339–42.
24. Cho CH, Lee YK, Sin HK. Arthroscopic direct repair for radial tear of the triangular fibrocartilage complex. Hand Surg. 2012;17(3):429–32.
25. Jantea CL, Baltzer A, Rüther W. Arthroscopic repair of radial-sided lesions of the triangular fibrocartilage complex. Hand Clin. 1995;11(1):31–6.
26. Palmer AK. The distal radioulnar joint. Anatomy, biomechanics, and triangular fibrocartilage complex abnormalities. Hand Clin. 1987;3(1):31–40.
27. Palmer AK. Triangular fibrocartilage disorders: injury patterns and treatment. Arthroscopy. 1990;6(2):125–32.
28. Bernstein MA, Nagle DJ, Martinez A, Stogin JM, Wiedrich TA. A comparison of combined arthroscopic triangular fibrocartilage complex debridement and arthroscopic wafer distal ulna resection versus arthroscopic triangular fibrocartilage complex debridement and ulnar shortening osteotomy for ulnocarpal abutment syndrome. Arthroscopy. 2004;20(4):392–401.
29. Tomaino MM, Elfar J. Ulnar impaction syndrome. Hand Clin. 2005;21(4):567.
30. Lindau T, Adlercreutz C, Aspenberg P. Peripheral tears of the triangular fibrocartilage complex cause distal radioulnar joint instability after distal radial fractures. J Hand Surg Am. 2000;25(3):464–8.

31. Chung KC, Zimmerman NB, Travis MT. Wrist arthrography versus arthroscopy: a comparative study of 150 cases. J Hand Surg Am. 1996;21(4):591–4.
32. Weiss AP, Akelman E, Lambiase R. Comparison of the findings of triple-injection cinearthrography of the wrist with those of arthroscopy. J Bone Joint Surg Am. 1996;78(3):348–56.
33. Tanaka T, Yoshioka H, Ueno T, Shindo M, Ochiai N. Comparison between high-resolution MRI with a microscopy coil and arthroscopy in triangular fibrocartilage complex injury. J Hand Surg Am. 2006;31(8):1308–14.
34. Saupe N, Prüssmann KP, Luechinger R, Bösiger P, Marincek B, Weishaupt D. MR imaging of the wrist: comparison between 1.5- and 3-T MR imaging—preliminary experience. Radiology. 2005;234(1):256–64.
35. Golimbu CN, Firooznia H, Melone CP, Rafii M, Weinreb J, Leber C. Tears of the triangular fibrocartilage of the wrist: MR imaging. Radiology. 1989;173(3):731–3.
36. Smith TO, Drew B, Toms AP, Jerosch-Herold C, Chojnowski AJ. Diagnostic accuracy of magnetic resonance imaging and magnetic resonance arthrography for triangular fibrocartilaginous complex injury: a systematic review and meta-analysis. J Bone Joint Surg Am. 2012;94(9):824–32.
37. Iordache SD, Rowan R, Garvin GJ, Osman S, Grewal R, Faber KJ. Prevalence of triangular fibrocartilage complex abnormalities on MRI scans of asymptomatic wrists. J Hand Surg Am. 2012;37(1):98–103.
38. Park MJ, Jagadish A, Yao J. The rate of triangular fibrocartilage injuries requiring surgical intervention. Orthopedics. 2010;33(11):806.
39. Dailey SW, Palmer AK. The role of arthroscopy in the evaluation and treatment of triangular fibrocartilage complex injuries in athletes. Hand Clin. 2000;16(3):461–76.
40. Whipple TL. The role of arthroscopy in the treatment of wrist injuries in the athlete. Clin Sports Med. 1998;17(3):623–34.
41. Hermansdorfer JD, Kleinman WB. Management of chronic peripheral tears of the triangular fibrocartilage complex. J Hand Surg Am. 1991;16(2):340–6.
42. Palmer AK, Werner FW, Glisson RR, Murphy DJ. Partial excision of the triangular fibrocartilage complex. J Hand Surg Am. 1988;13(3):391–4.
43. Nagle DJ. Laser-assisted wrist arthroscopy. Hand Clin. 1999;15(3):495–9. ix.
44. Infanger M, Grimm D. Meniscus and discus lesions of triangular fibrocartilage complex (TFCC): treatment by laser-assisted wrist arthroscopy. J Plast Reconstr Aesthet Surg. 2009;62(4):466–71.
45. Darlis NA, Weiser RW, Sotereanos DG. Arthroscopic triangular fibrocartilage complex debridement using radiofrequency probes. J Hand Surg Br. 2005;30(6):638–42.
46. Minami A, Kato H. Ulnar shortening for triangular fibrocartilage complex tears associated with ulnar positive variance. J Hand Surg Am. 1998;23(5):904–8.
47. Tomaino MM, Weiser RW. Combined arthroscopic TFCC debridement and wafer resection of the distal ulna in wrists with triangular fibrocartilage complex tears and positive ulnar variance. J Hand Surg Am. 2001;26(6):1047–52.
48. Osterman AL. Arthroscopic debridement of triangular fibrocartilage complex tears. Arthroscopy. 1990;6(2):120–4.
49. Minami A, Ishikawa J, Suenaga N, Kasashima T. Clinical results of treatment of triangular fibrocartilage complex tears by arthroscopic debridement. J Hand Surg Am. 1996;21(3):406–11.
50. Hulsizer D, Weiss AP, Akelman E. Ulna-shortening osteotomy after failed arthroscopic debridement of the triangular fibrocartilage complex. J Hand Surg Am. 1997;22(4):694–8.
51. Tomaino MM. The importance of the pronated grip X-ray view in evaluating ulnar variance. J Hand Surg Am. 2000;25(2):352–7.
52. Constantine KJ, Tomaino MM, Herndon JH, Sotereanos DG. Comparison of ulnar shortening osteotomy and the wafer resection procedure as treatment for ulnar impaction syndrome. J Hand Surg Am. 2000;25(1):55–60.
53. Roth JH, Poehling GG. Arthroscopic "-ectomy" surgery of the wrist. Arthroscopy. 1990;6(2):141–7.
54. Miwa H, Hashizume H, Fujiwara K, Nishida K, Inoue H. Arthroscopic surgery for traumatic triangular fibrocartilage complex injury. J Ortho Sci. 2004;9(4):354–9.
55. Husby T, Haugstvedt JR. Long-term results after arthroscopic resection of lesions of the triangular fibrocartilage complex. Scand J Plast Reconstr Surg Hand Surg. 2001;35(1):79–83.
56. Whatley JS, Dejardin LM, Arnoczky SP. The effect of an exogenous fibrin clot on the regeneration of the triangular fibrocartilage complex: an in vivo experimental study in dogs. Arthroscopy. 2000;16(2):127–36.
57. Warhold LG, Ruth RM. Complications of wrist arthroscopy and how to prevent them. Hand Clin. 1995;11(1):81–9.
58. Culp RW. Complications of wrist arthroscopy. Hand Clin. 1999;15(3):529–35.
59. Ahsan ZS, Yao J. Complications of wrist arthroscopy. Arthroscopy. 2012;28(6):855–9.
60. Pell RF, Uhl RL. Complications of thermal ablation in wrist arthroscopy. Arthroscopy. 2004;20(Suppl 2):84–6.

Arthroscopic Management of Peripheral Ulnar Tears of the TFCC

William B. Geissler

Introduction

The wrist is a complex labyrinth of eight carpal bones, multiple articular surfaces combined with intrinsic and extrinsic ligaments, including the triangular fibrocartilage complex (TFCC) all within a 5 cm interval. This perplexing joint continues to challenge clinicians with no array of potential diagnoses and treatments. Arthroscopy has continued to revolutionize the practice of orthopedic surgery by providing the surgeon the capability to examine and treat multiple intraarticular abnormalities. Wrist arthroscopy allows for direct visualization of the cartilage surfaces, ligaments, and the components of the triangular fibrocartilage complex under bright light and magnified conditions.

The triangular fibrocartilage complex is a complex soft tissue support system whose purpose is to stabilize the ulnar side of the wrist [1]. It acts as an extension of the articular surface of the radius to support the proximal carpal row and to stabilize the distal radial ulnar joint. Palmer classically described the components of the triangular fibrocartilage complex being the fibrocartilage articular disk, the volar and dorsal radial ulnar ligaments, and the floor of the extensor carpi ulnaris tendon sheath. The central disk is wedge-shaped in the coronal section and radially inserted on the articular surface of the radius by merging with the hyaline cartilage of the sigmoid notch and lunate facet. Chigley evaluated the collagen structure of the TFCC in an attempt to correlate its biomechanical function [2]. They found that the radial side of articular disk fibrocartilage has thick collagen fibers pro-

jecting 1–2 mm into the disk. The central portion of the articular disk has an oblique wave pattern for strength, tension, and compression. The ulnar aspect of the articular disk has two main bundles. One bundle is directed to the ulnar styloid and the second bundle to the fovea. Proximal limbs of the palmar and dorsal radial ulnar ligaments conjoin and insert onto the fovea just medial to the pole of the distal ulna. These structures have previously been referred to as the ligamentum subcruetum. However, Benjamin et al. have used this same term to describe the vascularized tissue between the fovea ligaments and the ulnar styloid. The exact function of the superficial deep components of the volar and dorsal radial ulnar ligaments is controversial. The distal superficial portions of the volar and dorsal radial ligament insert directly into the base of the ulnar styloid and are independent of the function of the ligamentum subcruetum insertion.

This chapter reviews the indication for wrist arthroscopy and the management of peripheral ulnar-sided tears of the articular disk involving the triangular fibrocartilage complex. Several techniques for outside-in or inside-out repair of peripheral ulnar-sided tears of the triangular fibrocartilage complex have been previously described in the literature. In addition, a new technique allows arthroscopic-assisted fixation of the articular disk back down to bone with a knotless suture anchor technique has recently been described.

Palmer and Warner defined the articular disk of the triangular fibrocartilage complex to be an axial loadbearing structure [1]. They found that in the static state 82% of the axial compressive load of power grasp was transmitted from the forearm through the radial carpal joint. The remainder 18% was supported by the articular disk on the ulnar side of the wrist. The peripheral attachment of the articular disk is approximately 5 mm thick and becomes thinner near its radial insertion, narrowing to less than 2 mm. It is the central portion of the disk that accepts the majority of the compressive loads transmitted from the carpus to the ulna. The thickness of the articular disk varies from individual to individual with an inverse relationship between the thickness of the

Supplementary Information The online version of this chapter (https://doi.org/10.1007/978-3-030-78881-0_6) contains supplementary material, which is available to authorized users.

W. B. Geissler (✉)
Division of Hand and Upper Extremity Surgery, Section of Arthroscopic Surgery and Sports Medicine, Department of Orthopedic Surgery and Rehabilitation, University of Mississippi Medical Center, Jackson, MS, USA

articular disk and ulnar variance. Adams demonstrated that when the disk is excised, loadbearing by the ulna drops to approximately 5% of the total load [3].

Dorsally, the triangular fibrocartilage complex has attachments to the ulna carpus and to the sheath of the extensor carpi ulnaris. This is a frequent area of peripheral detachment of the articular disk. The floor of the sheath of the extensor carpi ulnaris is quite stout and thick. This stout, fibrous tissue allows for firm fixation of the articular disk back to the floor of the extensor carpi ulnaris utilizing outside-in arthroscopic-assisted technique. The remaining component of the triangular fibrocartilage complex is classically described by Palmer as the ulnar carpal meniscus homolog. This is a quite controversial structure as to its function and even existence. It is a layer of fibrous connective tissue with variable thickness. The prestyloid recess typically presents between the bony ulnar styloid and a thickening of the ulnar soft tissues known as the meniscus homolog. It is vital to understand that the prestyloid recess is a normal fovea and it should not be mistaken for a peripheral tear of the articular disk. The prestyloid recess is the site of the 6-U portal which is frequently used for inflow.

Although not classically described as part of the triangular fibrocartilage complex, the ulna carpal ligaments are composed of the ulna lunate and ulna triquetral ligaments. These are primarily stabilizers of the ulna and the palmar carpus. The origin has been shown by cadaver studies to be along the palmar margin of the triangular fibrocartilage complex. They insert independently on the triquetrum and lunate with additional insertion into the lunotriquetral interosseous ligament.

Thiru et al. evaluated the arterial blood supply of the triangular fibrocartilage complex in 12 cadaver specimens with latex injections [4]. They determined there were three main arterial supplies to the triangular fibrocartilage complex. The ulnar artery supplies the majority of the blood to the triangular fibrocartilage complex supporting the ulna portion to the dorsal palmar radial carpal branches. Thiru documented a complex of vessels which filled with latex dye in the peripheral 15–20% of the ulnar articular disk. Bednar et al. similarly examined ten cadavers with an ink injection study and found penetration of the vessels into the peripheral 10–40% of the articular disk [5]. These studies are very significant regarding procedures for arthroscopic repair of peripheral tears to the articular disk. They confirm an intact blood supply to the peripheral articular disk, and theoretically, peripheral tears of the articular disk should be able to heal following repair with this vascular blood supply.

Classification of TFCC Tears

In 1989, Palmer proposed a classification system for tears of the triangular fibrocartilage complex [1]. He divided the injuries into two basic categories. Class I are traumatic and Class II are degenerative (Tables 6.1 and 6.2).

Class I injuries are true traumatic tears and are subdivided into four basic types based on the pattern of injury. Type IA lesions involve the central avascular portion of the articular disk and are not suitable for suture repair. Arthroscopic management includes the debridement of a central tear to remove any symptomatic flaps. Type IB (ulnar avulsion) injuries occur when the ulnar side of the articular disk is avulsed from its insertion. These injuries may or may not be associated with a fracture to the ulnar styloid. Because these tears occur over in the region of a documented vascular supply, they are very amenable to arthroscopic repair by a number of techniques. Type IC injuries involve rupture of the volar attachment of the triangular fibrocartilage complex over the ulnar carpal ligaments. Type ID involves a tear of the radial

Table 6.1 Classification of traumatic injuries class I

Class IA	Tears or perforations of the horizontal portion of the triangular fibrocartilage complex (TFCC)
	Usually 1–2 mm wide
	Dorsal palmar slit located 2–3 mm medial to the radial attachment of the sigmoid notch
Class IB	Traumatic avulsion of TFCC from insertion into the distal ulna
	May be accompanied by a fracture of the ulnar styloid at its base
	Usually associated with distal radiocarpal joint instability
Class IC	Tears of TFCC that result in ulnocarpal instability, such as avulsion of the TFCC from the distal attachment of the lunate or triquetrum
Class ID	Traumatic avulsions of the TFCC from the attachment at the distal sigmoid notch

Table 6.2 Classifications of degenerative lesions class II

Class IIA	Wear of the horizontal portion of the TFCC distally, proximally, or both; with no perforation
	Possible ulnar plus syndrome
Class IIB	Wear of the horizontal portion of the TFCC and chondromalacia of lunate and/or ulna
Class IIC	TFCC perforation and chondromalacia of the lunate and/or ulna
Class IID	TFCC perforation and chondromalacia of the lunate and/or ulna
	Perforation of the lunotriquetrum ligament
Class IIE	TFCC perforation and chondromalacia of the lunate and/or ulna
	Perforation of the lunotriquetrum ligament
	Ulnocarpal arthritis

attachment of the articular disk as well as the radioulnar ligament separate from the radius with or without a fracture of the radial sigmoid notch.

Class II lesions are considered degenerative tears of the triangular fibrocartilage complex and involve a central portion of the articular disk. These are stage A through E depending on the presence or absence of perforation to the triangular fibrocartilage complex, ulnar head and lunate chondromalacia, perforation of the lunotriquetral interosseous ligament, and degenerative arthritis of the radial ulnar joint. These lesions generally arise from ulna impaction and surgical management mostly consists of a variety of procedures to decrease the load across the ulnar side of the wrist, either arthroscopic or open management.

Diagnosis

Injuries to the triangular fibrocartilage complex commonly occur with extension and pronation of an axially loaded carpus. The most common mechanism occurs with a fall on an outstretched hand. Peripheral tears of the articular disk are frequently common athletic injuries, which occur in sports and require rapid twisting and loading of the ulnar side of the wrist such as golf or racket sports. Peripheral ulnar-sided tears of the articular disk may also be a common work injury. Patients often describe a mechanism of traction and torsion of the forearm which may occur with the use of a drill motor when the drill bit suddenly binds resulting in a twisting injury to the wrist.

Patients with symptoms of peripheral tears of the triangular fibrocartilage complex complain of a deep diffused aching across the ulnar side of the wrist. They may complain of pain with firm gripping as well as a clicking sensation with rotation of the forearm. They frequently complain of pain with resistance to forearm rotation such as twisting lids off jars or twisting a doorknob. Frequently, they may complain of generalized wrist weakness.

Patients with an ulnar-sided peripheral tear of the articular disk frequently describe point tenderness right at the prestyloid recess and point to that location. This pain may be accentuated by hypo-pronation or supination of the forearm. This pain may be further aggravated by passive anterior/posterior translation of the ulna in relation to the radius with the wrist in pronation and supination. Dorsal subluxation of the ulnar head in relation to the radius may be seen particularly if a large peripheral tear is present involving both the superficial and deep layers of the articular disk.

Several tests have been described that are used for the diagnosis of ulnar-sided wrist pain. The TFCC compression test is considered positive with axial loading of the articular disk with the wrist in ulnar deviation and results in signifi-

cant pain. Araujo described the ulna impaction test which is considered to be positive when the wrist is positioned in ulnar deviation, hyperextension and axial load reproduces the ulnar-sided wrist pain. The piano key sign is frequently described for instability of the distal radioulnar joint, which can be seen with a peripheral tear of the articular disk. The test is positive if the distal ulna can be pressed volarly by dorsal thumb pressure in a pronated wrist as compared to the opposite side. In general, patients with a central tear of the articular disk hurt more over the ulnar head while patients with a peripheral tear present complaining about the prestyloid recess region.

Diagnostic Modalities

Patients who present with acute or chronic ulnar-sided wrist pain should be evaluated initially with standard anterior/posterior, lateral, and oblique radiographs of the wrist. It is important in the AP view to take the radiograph in neutral position to evaluate for ulnar variance. It is frequently helpful to take a fist compression view to evaluate for possible ulnar impaction which should be in the differential diagnosis. Radiographic signs of ulnar impaction include cystic changes on the medial side of the lunate (kissing lesion). These changes are indicated by excessive loading to the ulnar side of the wrist, which may require an ulnar shortening procedure. The distal radioulnar joint should also be evaluated for signs of radioulnar impingement, which must be differentiated from pain related to the triangular fibrocartilage complex. In addition, signs of acute or chronic injury to the ulnar styloid may be assessed on plain radiographs. Plain radiographs also are helpful to evaluate for signs of ulnar styloid abutment.

Triple injection arthrography was the gold standard in the past in diagnosing pathology of the triangular fibrocartilage complex [6]. However, ulnar-sided peripheral tears of the articular disk may be frequently missed by arthrography particularly in the chronic setting. This is secondary to chronic synovitis that develops over the peripheral tear blocking the flow of dye between the radial carpal and distal radial ulnar joint.

Several studies have evaluated the use of magnetic resonance imaging in diagnosing TFCC injuries [7–9]. Golimbu et al. and Skahen et al. both reported that the use of magnetic resonance imaging for detection of central and radial detachment of the articular disk with an accuracy of 95% [7, 8]. Corso et al. in their study of ulnar-sided tears of the triangular fibrocartilage complex found sensitivity in only 76% with magnetic resonance imaging [9]. Bednar reported his results of MR imaging and noted the sensitivity was 44% with specificity set at 5% for TFCC tears [5]. Fulcher and Poehling recommended the use of arthroscopy for definitive diagnosis and felt that MRI overstates some injuries of the TFCC while understating other TFCC pathology [10].

Studies comparing wrist arthroscopy with arthrography confirm that arthroscopy is the gold standard in detecting injuries to the triangular fibrocartilage complex [9]. Pederzini et al. compared MRI, arthrography, and arthroscopy on 11 patients with tears to the triangular fibrocartilage complex [9]. Utilizing arthroscopy as the gold standard, he reported 1% sensitivity with MRI and arthrography and 80% sensitivity for arthrography and 82% sensitivity for MRI evaluation alone. Arthroscopy has a clear advantage of visualization of the articular disk under bright light and magnified conditions. The tension of the disk may be assessed by palpation with a probe. In most instances, a loss of tension will be detected to the articular disk when a peripheral tear is present. Frequently, synovitis has formed over the peripheral ulnar tear marking the site of pathology. Once the synovitis is debrided, the peripheral tear would be well visualized. Wrist arthroscopy is a useful adjunct and not only has the advantage of being sensitive and accurate to make the diagnosis but at the same sitting proceeding with definitive management.

Management

Indications

Patients who present with acute ulnar-sided wrist pain with normal radiographs and tenderness over the periphery of the TFCC, initial immobilization is a rule of thumb. Potentially small ulnar peripheral tears of the articular disk may heal from immobilization due to the vascular blood supply. Further diagnostic modalities are initiated after 2 or 3 months of immobilization when patients continue to be symptomatic or when an early diagnosis is important to the patient (professional athlete). MRI evaluation is certainly a common option, but the author prefers to proceed directly to wrist arthroscopy when the history and physical examination are classic for an injury to the triangular fibrocartilage complex and the patient does not improve with immobilization.

Indications for surgical intervention include persistent ulnar-sided wrist pain not relieved by conservative management for at least 3 months. Additional indications include symptomatic distal radial ulnar joint instability not improved by immobilization. It is also felt that a subluxation to the extensor carpi ulnaris tendon is usually associated with a peripheral tear to the articular disk.

Contraindications for surgical management are in those patients who are minimally symptomatic despite radiographic findings and patients with low physical demand who are medically not healthy enough for surgery. In addition, patients with significant degenerative changes either to the radial carpal or radial ulnar joint may be better managed by addressing the arthritic symptoms rather than an arthroscopic procedure.

Arthroscopic Technique

The wrist is suspended with 10 lb. of traction in a traction tower (Fig. 6.1). The volar forearm and arm are well padded with towels so the skin does not come into contact with the tower itself. This will help prevent any potential burns from heat of the tower if it has been recently sterilized. The skin is incised with the tip of an 11 blade at the 3–4 portal and blunt dissection is continued with a hemostat to the level of the joint capsule. The arthroscope with a blunt trocar is introduced into the 3–4 portal and a working portal is made in the standard 6-R portal. Inflow may be provided through the 1–2 portal if a tear of the triangular fibrocartilage complex is suspected. In this manner, the inflow is out of the way during the arthroscopic repair to the TFCC complex. Alternatively, inflow may be provided through the arthroscope itself or through the needle in the 6-U portal.

It is always important to identify the exact location of the 6-R portal just distal to the articular disk with an 18-gauge needle inserted into the radial carpal space. The needle is viewed arthroscopically as it is being inserted. If ideal placement is confirmed, then the skin is incised and the 6-R portal is made. In this manner, there is no potential damage to the articular disk when making the 6-R portal. Cooney described the trampoline test in which there should be good tension to the articular disk when palpated with a probe inserted through the 6-R portal [11]. The articular disk will be lax to

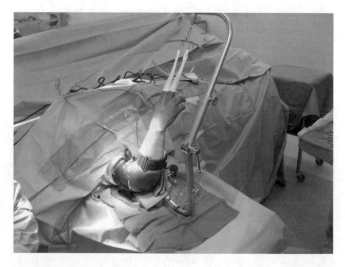

Fig. 6.1 The wrist is suspended in a wrist traction tower (Acumed, Hillsboro, OR). The wrist is suspended in approximately 10–20° of flexion to allow easier entry of instrumentation into the radiocarpal space

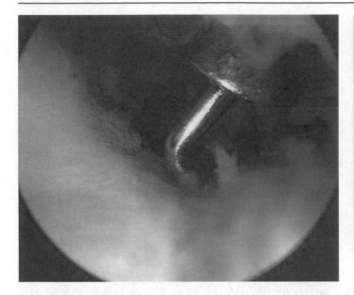

Fig. 6.2 Arthroscopic view with the arthroscope in the 3–4 portal showing a peripheral tear to the articular disk of the TFC in a right wrist. Note the proliferative synovitis about the tear

palpation and has a sunken appearance when a peripheral ulnar tear of the articular disk is present. Synovitis is frequently present marking the location of the peripheral tear which is debrided out to further expose the injury (Fig. 6.2).

There are several arthroscopic techniques for repair of peripheral ulnar-sided tears of the articular disk. Indications for which type of repair vary from author to author. Each technique has its advantages and disadvantages. It is thought when a greater degree of instability of the distal radioulnar joint is present, arthroscopic repair back to bone will provide greater stability as compared to soft tissue repair alone.

Whipple Technique

Whipple et al. described the outside-in technique to reattach the articular disk back to the floor of the sixth compartment [12]. This is ideal for peripheral tears of the articular disk that arise dorsally. The advantage of this technique is that it is relatively simple and does not require any special instrumentation. It is particularly indicated in those patients that are point tender about the prestyloid recess area and have a minimal amount of instability to the distal radioulnar joint. The disadvantage of this procedure is that it does require an incision around the extensor carpi ulnaris tendon sheath, which has to be closed after the procedure. Potentially, there would be a risk for subluxation or instability to the extensor carpi ulnaris if the sheath is not fully closed or does not heal. In addition, patients may complain about irritation of the ECU tendon secondary to the suture knots.

In this technique, the arthroscope is introduced in the standard 3–4 portal. The 6-R portal is elongated approxi-

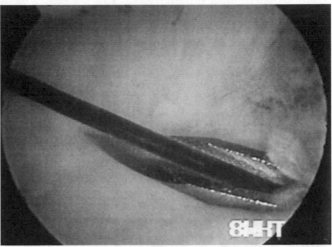

Fig. 6.3 Arthroscopic view with the arthroscope in the 3–4 portal showing an 18-gauge needle perforating through the articular disk with a stitch of monofilament suture being passed through the cannula

mately 12–15 mm in length along the radial border of the extensor carpi ulnaris tendon. The extensor retinaculum is sharply released along its radial side and the extensor carpi ulnaris tendon is retracted volarly. It is important to protect the articular branch of the dorsal sensory branch of the ulnar nerve as it crosses the incision in an attempt to decrease the risk of sympathetic dystrophy. A curved or straight 18-gauge needle is inserted through the floor of the extensor carpi ulnaris tendon sheath through the peripheral tear as visualized with the arthroscope in the radiocarpal space. Once the needle is identified, it is pulled back and then perforates through the articular disk (Fig. 6.3). It is important to insert the needle as perpendicular as possible to the articular disk. The suture may potentially pull through or shred the disk if it is placed too horizontal or shallow. A 2.0 monofilament suture is placed through the needle into the joint (Fig. 6.4). One trick to help get the suture started into the needle is to cut the plastic off the needle as close as possible. This makes it easier to thread the suture into the needle and into the joint. It is sometimes frustrating to fight the pressure of the fluid being injected through the needle as one is trying to insert the suture. Following insertion of the suture through the needle into the joint, a suture retriever is inserted through the floor of the extensor carpi ulnaris tendon sheath distal to the articular disk to grab the suture (Fig. 6.5). If a suture retriever is not available, a standard wrist arthroscopy grasper may work. Two or three sutures are placed in vertical fashion to close the tear (Figs. 6.6 and 6.7). The wrist is then taken out of traction, and the sutures are tied with the wrist in neutral position. A trick is to tie an arthroscopic slip knot to help slide the suture down against the tendon sheath of the extensor carpi ulnaris with tension. It is frequently difficult to slide the knot with the surgeon's finger down into such a small hole and maintain good tension to the repair. It is very impor-

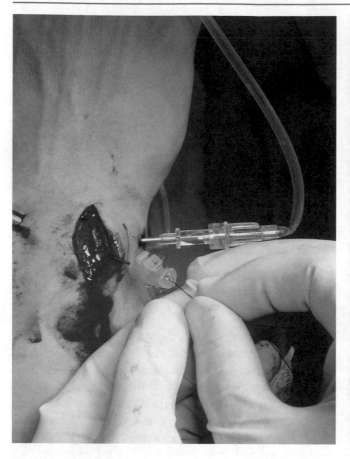

Fig. 6.4 Outside view showing an incision of the extensor carpi ulnaris tendon sheath. The extensor carpi ulnaris is retracted volarly and an 18-gauge needle is passed through the floor of the sheath of the extensor carpi ulnaris into the radiocarpal space and a monofilament suture is being inserted

tant to use dissolvable sutures so the knots of the sutures do not continue to irritate the tendon of the extensor carpi ulnaris. It is important to close the sheath of the extensor carpi ulnaris to limit the risk of instability to the tendon.

Occasionally, a second surgery is required to remove the irritating suture knot.

Tuohy Needle Technique

Poehling et al. described this inside-out technique [13]. The advantage of this technique is that it utilizes a smaller outside incision where the sutures are to be tied down. The Tuohy needle technique allows for a horizontal mattress stitch to be placed across the peripheral tear. It allows for excellent visualization as the needle and the suture are being placed. The disadvantage of this particular technique is that sometimes it is difficult to help control the needle across the radiocarpal joint to pierce the articular disk. Another disadvantage of this technique is that it primarily repairs the superficial layer of the articular disk and does not involve the deeper layers of

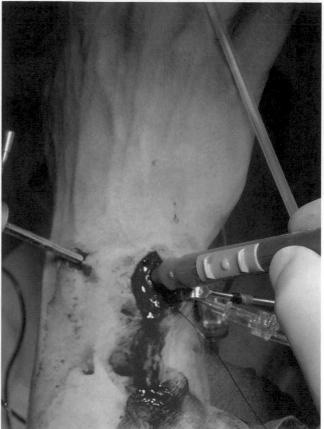

Fig. 6.5 Outside view showing a suture grasper being placed through the incision distal to the articular disk to retrieve the suture

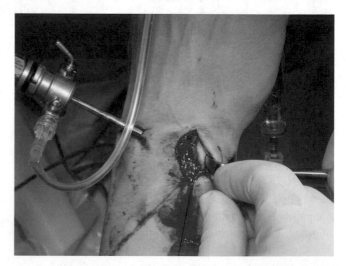

Fig. 6.6 Outside view showing the first suture passed. Note the good tissue on the floor of the extensor carpi ulnaris tendon sheath to which the suture will be tied securing the repair

the ligamentum subcruetum. In addition, it is very important to dissect down to the capsule as the suture is being tied so that it does not encompass a branch of the dorsal sensory branch of the ulnar nerve.

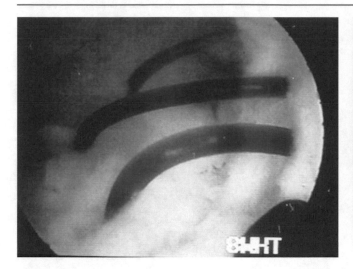

Fig. 6.7 Arthroscopic view with the arthroscope in the 3–4 portal showing three simple sutures passed through the disk securing the tear back to the capsule

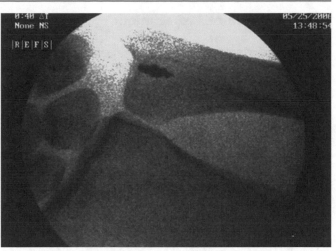

Fig. 6.8 Radiographic view showing a suture anchor placed at the base of the fovea of the ulna reattaching the articular disk back down to bone

The Tuohy needle is a needle used in the practice of anesthesia. The needle is blunt tipped and will not cut a suture as it exits the end of the needle.

In this technique, the arthroscope is placed in the 4–5 portal and a 20-gauge Tuohy needle is inserted into the radiocarpal joint through the 1–2 or 3–4 portals. Under direct visualization, the needle is placed through the torn edge of the triangular fibrocartilage complex and exits the skin. A 2.0 absorbable suture is threaded through the needle and exits along the ulnar side of the wrist. The suture is anchored at each end with a hemostat. The needle is then pulled back into the joint and passed back through the free edge of the peripheral tear in a horizontal mattress fashion. The needle is again advanced out through the tear and out the skin where the loop of suture is retrieved. Multiple sutures may be placed with this technique. Blunt dissection is carried down under direct visualization and the suture is tied directly on the capsule.

Suture Anchor Technique

Sutures may be placed in an arthroscopic-assisted fashion utilizing a suture anchor inserted at the base of the fovea to the ulna (Fig. 6.8). The advantage of this technique is that it allows for repair of the articular disk back down to bone with permanent suture. This technique may be indicated for greater instability to the distal radioulnar joint as determined clinically as it provides fixation of the deep layers of the articular disk back down to bone rather than the superficial fibers alone.

Another advantage of this technique is that it allows the use of a softer braided suture which may be less irritating to the surrounding soft tissues as compared to a monofilament suture. In addition, the extensor carpi ulnaris tendon sheath is not opened decreasing the risk of instability to the extensor carpi ulnaris tendon sheath and irritation from suture knots. The disadvantage of the technique is that it does require an open incision and dissection proximal to the articular disk for insertion of the anchor.

In this technique, the arthroscope is initially placed in the 3–4 portal and the working 6-R portal is made. The 6-R portal is then elongated and the fifth dorsal compartment is then opened releasing the extensor digiti minimi tendon once the tear is identified. The 6-R portal marks the distal portion of the articular disk. Blunt dissection is then continued proximal to the 6-R portal over the head of the ulna. The dorsal aspect of the ulnar head is identified through this small incision. A small burr can then be used to debride any bone to facilitate soft tissue reattach and vascularization. A small anchor with braided suture may be inserted at the base of the ulnar styloid under direct visualization.

The suture is then inserted into the sharp-pointed end of an 18-gauge needle. This loaded 18-gauge needle is then placed perpendicular to the articular disk and inserted through the disk into the joint as viewed with the arthroscope in the 3–4 portal. The tip of the needle is identified arthroscopically and pulled back. As the needle is pulled back, this leaves a loop of braided suture through the articular disk in the radiocarpal space. A suture retriever is then brought in distal to the articular disk to retrieve the suture. The process is repeated with a second limb of the braided suture so that a horizontal mattress suture has been placed. The wrist is then taken out of traction and the suture is tied over the dorsal extensor retinaculum being careful not to entrap the tendon of the extensor digiti minimi.

Arthroscope Knotless Technique

Geissler described the all arthroscopic knotless technique (Bad to the Bone) [14] (Video 6.1). The advantage of the all arthroscopic knotless technique is that it allows for repair of both the superficial and deep layers of the articular disk back down to bone with no knots all arthroscopically. Another advantage of this technique is that it can be done rather quickly compared to the other techniques. It is the author's opinion that patients with this technique hurt less as compared to the previously described techniques and can be moved sooner. Also, since both layers of the articular disk are repaired back down to bone, this technique may be indicated in those patients who have greater instability to the distal radioulnar joint. It is important to remember that in patients with gross instability to the distal radial ulnar joint, peripheral TFCC repair alone may not provide enough stability. The disadvantage of this technique is that there is a significant learning curve. It involves passage of sutures back and forth between portals, and there is always concern of soft tissue entrapment around the suture. Also, the anchors will be inserted blindly into the previously drilled hole in the ulna.

In this technique, the standard 3–4 and 6-R portals are made (Fig. 6.9). An accessory 6-R portal is made approximately one-half centimeters distal in line with the 6-R portal. It is important to have the wrist flexed in the traction tower about 20–30° when making this portal. The portal is located by utilizing an 18-gauge needle inserted through the skin aimed at the fovea of the ulna head (Fig. 6.10). The base of the ulna can be palpated with the needle. It is important that

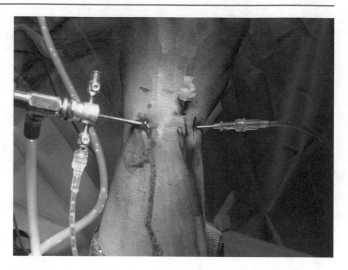

Fig. 6.10 A standard 3–4 outside view showing the standard 3–4 and 6-R portals have been made. An 18-gauge needle is being used to identify the most ideal location for the more distal accessory 6-R portal

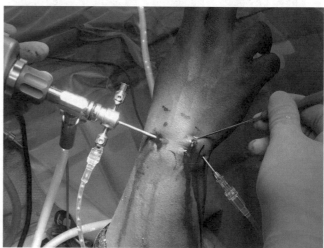

Fig. 6.11 Outside view showing a suture lasso (Arthrex, Naples, FL) being passed through the accessory 6-R portal through the articular disk

the needle is close to being parallel to the dorsum of the hand so that with eventual drilling of the bone, the drill does not slide off the volar aspect of the ulna. Once ideal placement of the accessory 6-R portal has been identified, a portal is made.

A suture lasso (Arthrex, Naples, FL) is then placed through the accessory 6-R portal into the joint as viewed arthroscopically (Fig. 6.11). The curved lasso is then placed through the tear in a proximal to distal direction and it pierces through the disk. The lasso is just gently twisted between the thumb and index finger to allow it to more easily perforate through the articular disk. A suture passing wire is then inserted through the lasso and with a crochet grasper inserted through the 6-R portal is retrieved (Fig. 6.12). A 2.0 fiber wire suture (Arthrex, Naples, FL) is then placed through the suture retriever wire and is pulled through the lasso and out

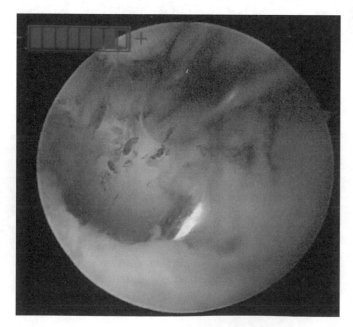

Fig. 6.9 Arthroscopic view with the arthroscope in the 3–4 portal demonstrating a peripheral tear to the articular disk in a right wrist

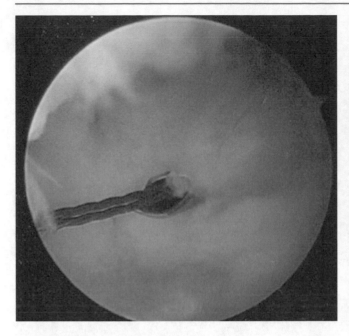

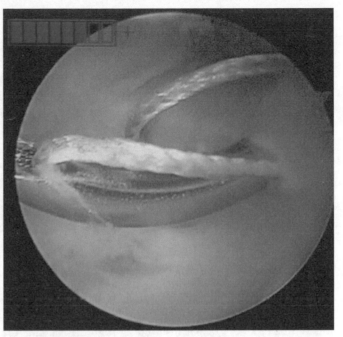

Fig. 6.12 Arthroscopic view showing the suture lasso being perforated through the articular disk with a wire retriever passed through the lasso to retrieve the suture

Fig. 6.14 The suture lasso then re-perforates through the articular disk leaving a loop of suture as view arthroscopically

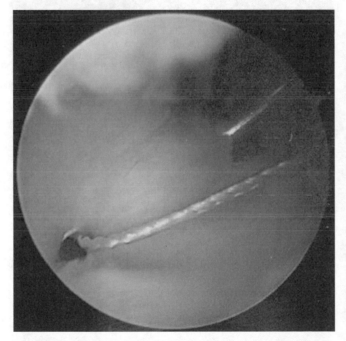

Fig. 6.13 The wire retriever is retrieving the suture through the suture lasso out distally

Fig. 6.15 Arthroscopic view showing the crochet hook grabbing the loop of suture retrieving both limbs out the standard 6-R portal

distally through the handle (Fig. 6.13). The lasso is then pulled back from the disk but still kept in the radiocarpal space. The lasso is then reinserted through the articular disk and a loop of suture is formed at the end of the lasso (Fig. 6.14). This loop of suture is pulled out through the 6-R portal with the crochet grasper (Fig. 6.15).

A horizontal mattress stitch with permanent braided suture is now been formed through both layers of the articular disk and both suture limbs are exiting the 6-R portal. The arthroscopic cannula developed for this technique has a serrated end and a smooth end. The smooth end of the cannula with a trocar is then inserted through the accessory 6-R por-

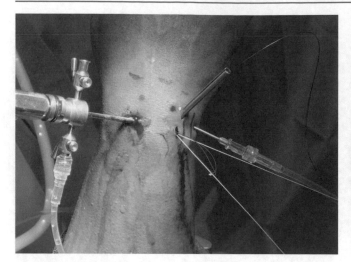

Fig. 6.16 Outside view showing the suture wire retriever pulling both limbs of the suture through the 6-R portal out through the accessory 6-R portal in the cannula

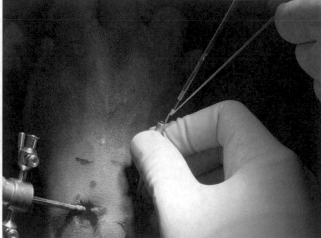

Fig. 6.17 Outside view showing the sutures being passed through a mini push lock anchor (Arthrex, Naples, FL) being inserted through the cannula securing the repair of the articular disk back to bone with a knotless technique

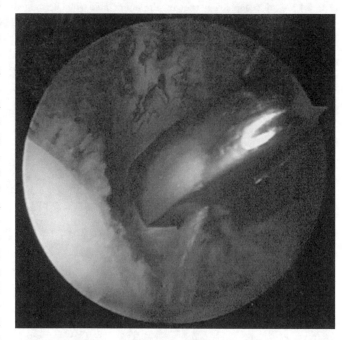

Fig. 6.18 Arthroscopic view showing the two fiber wire suture limbs being cut

tal. With a crochet grasper inserted through the cannula, the two suture limbs are pulled back from the 6-R portal through the cannula exiting the accessory 6-R portal (Fig. 6.16). The two suture limbs are then pulled through the slot in the cannula so they will not be entangled with the drill. The cannula is held firmly against the ulna head and the drill is placed. The drill is cannulated, so if the surgeon wants to place a K-wire to confirm the ideal placement into the base of the ulna, that option is available. The wire is placed and can be visualized under fluoroscopy. Once ideal placement is found, the drill is inserted through the cannula over the guide wire and the base of the ulna is drilled. Alternatively, when no guide wire is used, the drill is inserted through the cannula alone and the base of the ulna is drilled, which is recommended. Once the head of the ulna has been drilled, the cannula is not moved. The two suture limbs are then inserted into the mini push lock anchor (Arthrex, Naples, FL) and the anchor is slid down the cannula and inserted into the drill hole (Fig. 6.17). As the anchor is being passed down the cannula, it is important that the suture limbs are pulled back through the slot so they can be advanced into the bone of the ulna. As the anchor is inserted into the previously drilled hole, the sutures are then tensioned and the articular disk is evaluated arthroscopically. Once ideal tension has been confirmed, the push lock anchor is advanced into the head of the ulna. Following insertion of the anchor into the bone, the anchor is gently pulled on the handle to insure that the anchor has a good purchase into the bone of the ulna. Once confirmed, the sutures are cut (Fig. 6.18). This technique repairs the articular disk back down to bone with the all arthroscopic knotless technique (Fig. 6.19).

Rehabilitation

Postoperative management of peripheral TFCC repair is controversial with multiple techniques being suggested. In the author's practice, the patient is immobilized in slight supination in an above elbow splint for 3–4 weeks. A removable

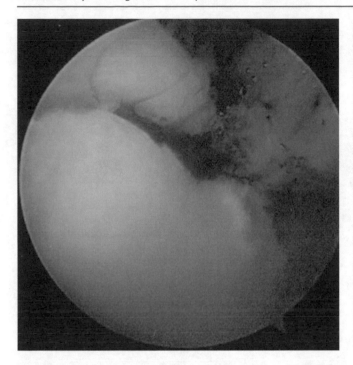

Fig. 6.19 Arthroscopic view with the arthroscope in the 3–4 portal showing repair of the articular disk back down to bone with an all-arthroscopic knotless technique. Note the good tension to the articular disk

wrist splint is then used for an additional 3 weeks. Digital range of motion exercises are started immediately. Range of motion and strengthening exercises of the forearm and wrist are initiated at approximately 7 weeks.

Discussion

It is controversial whether a repair of a peripheral tear of the triangular fibrocartilage complex should be repaired back to bone or if a soft tissue repair to the capsule satisfactorily restores stability. Ruch et al., in a biomechanical study, compared TFCC repairs of the articular disk back to the extensor carpi ulnaris subsheath (Whipple technique) as compared to open transosseous repair in six matched pairs of fresh frozen cadavers [15]. He reported that in both groups distal radioulnar joint stability was restored and there was no statistical biomechanical difference.

Corso et al. reported their results in a multicenter study of patients who underwent an outside-in Whipple technique [9]. Patients were contributed to the study by Drs. Geissler, Savoie, and Whipple. They found 41 of 45 patients had a good or excellent result utilizing the Mayo modified wrist score and returned to normal activity by 3 months. Fulcher reported his results with the Tuohy needle technique. He reported a 70% satisfaction rate at 16–24 months follow-up in 17 patients.

Estrella et al. reviewed their results in 35 patients repaired by either the Whipple or Tuohy needle technique [16]. They found that 74% of their patients had good or excellent results utilizing the Mayo modified wrist score. They found that the patients had significant increased grip strength and pain relief, and in addition, had increased capacity to perform daily activities.

Ruch and Papadonikolakis reported their results in 35 patients who had a repair of a peripheral ulnar tear utilizing the disabilities of the arm, shoulder, and hand (DASH score) as statistical analysis to identifying factors [17]. They found that positive ulnar variance and increased age correlated with a poorer outcome. They also noted that patients who had loss of wrist rotation and grip strength reported poorer outcomes.

It is controversial in a patient with a peripheral ulnar tear in an ulnar positive patient should the ulna be shortened at the time of the repair. In the author's experience, sutures are initially placed arthroscopically, an ulnar shortening osteotomy is performed, and then the sutures are tied. It is the author's experience that in patients who are ulnar positive, an ulnar shortening osteotomy improves the patient's pain relief in addition to the repair of the articular disk.

A peripheral ulnar-sided tear of the articular disk may be the first stage of a complex multifactorial ligamentous injury (Figs. 6.20 and 6.21). Trauma to the ulnar side of the wrist

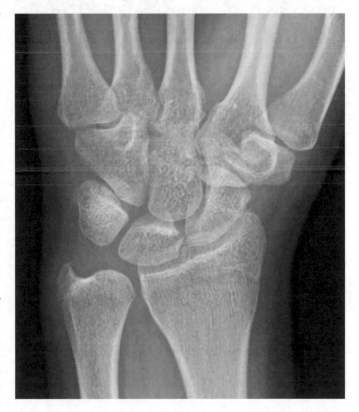

Fig. 6.20 AP radiograph of a young female who sustained a severe ulnar-sided perilunate injury

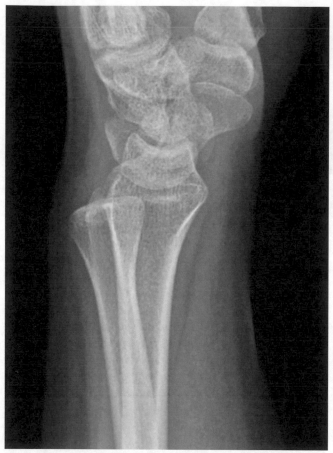

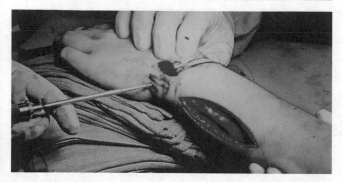

Fig. 6.22 The patient underwent arthroscopic evaluation which showed a complete tear, Geissler Grade IV, to the lunotriquetral interosseous ligament as well as a large peripheral tear to the articular disk. The patient underwent arthroscopic stabilization of the peripheral tear utilizing the Whipple technique without tying the sutures. The patient then underwent placement of a SLIC screw (Acumed, Hillsboro, OR) across the LT interval for the complete tear to the interosseous ligament. The patient then underwent an open ulnar shortening osteotomy with the ulnar shortening plate (Acumed, Hillsboro, OR) to further tighten the instability of the distal radioulnar joint

Fig. 6.21 Lateral radiograph of the same patient with a severe ulnar-sided perilunate injury with subluxation of the distal radioulnar joint

usually involves a spectrum of injury. Wrist arthroscopy is a useful adjunct in the management of these complex injuries to the triangular fibrocartilage complex (Figs. 6.22, 6.23, and 6.24) Current arthroscopic techniques for repair of peripheral ulnar-sided tears of the articular disk have produced good and excellent results as documented in the literature. Potential further refinements such as the newer all arthroscopic knotless technique described in this chapter may further enhance the treatment of these injuries and improve patient's satisfaction and outcomes.

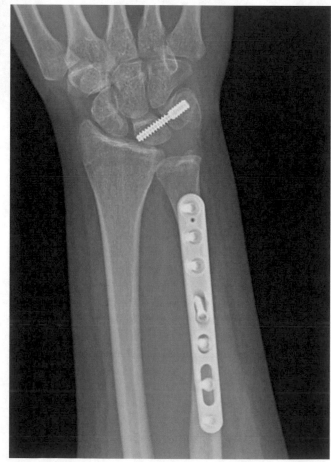

Fig. 6.23 PA radiograph following stabilization of the peripheral tear of the TFC, LT interval, and open ulnar shortening osteotomy

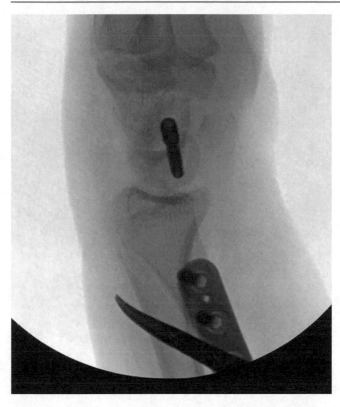

Fig. 6.24 Lateral radiograph following stabilization. The lateral radiograph demonstrates reduction to the distal radioulnar joint as compared to preoperative radiographs

References

1. Palmar AK. Triangular fibrocartilage complex lesions: a classification. J Hand Surg. 1989;14:594–606.
2. Chidgey LK, Dell PC, Bittar ES, et al. Histologic anatomy of the triangular fibrocartilage. J Hand Surg. 1991;16:1084–100.
3. Adams B. Partial excision of the triangular fibrocartilage complex articular disk, a biomechanical study. J Hand Surg. 1993;184:334–40.
4. Thiru RG, Ferlic DC, Clayton MI, et al. Arterial anatomy of the triangular fibrocartilage of the wrist and its surgical significance. J Hand Surg. 1986;11:258–63.
5. Bednar MS, Arnoczky SP, Weiland AJ. The microvasculature of the triangular fibrocartilage complex: its clinical significance. J Hand Surg. 1991;16:1101–5.
6. Weiss A, Akelman E, Lambiase R. Comparison of the findings of triple-injection cinearthrography of the wrist with those of arthroscopy. J Bone Joint Surg Am. 1996;78A:348–56.
7. Golimbu C, Firooznia H, Melone CJ, et al. Tears of the triangular fibrocartilage of the wrist: MR imaging. Radiology. 1989;173:731–3.
8. Skahen JI, Palmer A, Levinsohn E, et al. Magnetic resonance imaging of the triangular fibrocartilage complex. J Hand Surg. 1990;15A:552–7.
9. Pederzini L, Luchetti R, Soragni O, et al. Evaluation of the triangular fibrocartilage complex by arthroscopy, arthrography, and magnetic resonance imaging. Arthroscopy. 1992;8:191–7.
10. Fulcher S, Poehling G. The role of operative arthroscopy for the diagnosis and treatment of lesions about the distal ulna. Hand Clin. 1998;14:285–96.
11. Cooney WP, Linscheid RL, Dobyns JH. Triangular fibrocartilage tears. J Hand Surg. 1994;19:143–54.
12. Whipple T, Geissler W. Arthroscopic management of wrist triangular fibrocartilage complex injuries in the athlete. Orthopedics. 1993;16(9):1061–7.
13. de Araujo W, Poehling G, Kuzma G. New Tuohy needle technique for triangular fibrocartilage complex repair: preliminary studies. Arthroscopy. 1996;12:699–703.
14. Geissler W. Arthroscopic knotless peripheral triangular fibrocartilage repair. J Hand Surg Am. 2012;37(2):350–5.
15. Ruch DS, Anderson SR, Ritter MR. Biomechanical comparison of transosseous and capsular repair of peripheral triangular fibrocartilage tears. Arthroscopy. 2003;19(4):391–6.
16. Estrella EP, Hung LK, Ho PC, Tse WL. Arthroscopic repair of triangular fibrocartilage complex tears. Arthroscopy. 2007;23(7):729–37.
17. Ruch DS, Papadonikolakis A. Arthroscopically assisted repair of peripheral triangular fibrocartilage complex tears: factors affecting outcome. Arthroscopy. 2005;21(9):1126–30.

Arthroscopic TFCC Peripheral Repair Through Bone Tunnel

7

Christopher G. Larsen and Andrew S. Greenberg

Introduction

The triangular fibrocartilage complex (TFCC) is a structure based on the ulnar side of the wrist that consists of an articular disc, a meniscus homologue, the ulnar collateral ligament (UCL), the dorsal and volar radioulnar ligaments, the ulnocarpal ligaments, and the sheath of the extensor carpi ulnaris (ECU) (Fig. 7.1) [1]. The complex originates from the ulnar aspect of the lunate fossa of the ulnar styloid and courses ulnarly to an insertion onto the base of the ulnar styloid. Distal to the ulnar styloid insertion, the TFCC becomes thickened as it is joined by fibers of the UCL and the meniscus homologue before again inserting distally onto the triquetrum, hamate, and base of the fifth metacarpal. It serves as the main stabilizer of the distal radioulnar joint (DRUJ), as the typically shallow sigmoid notch offers little bony constraint [1]. Tears of the TFCC are a common cause of ulnar-sided wrist pain and have historically been grouped into two categories: acute and chronic, or type 1 and type 2 injuries, respectively [2]. In his landmark paper, Palmer further classified acute tears into subtypes 1A–D based on location of the tear, with 1A representing central perforations, 1B representing avulsions of the TFCC from its insertion on the ulna, 1C representing tears involving the volar ulnar extrinsic ligaments, and 1D representing avulsions from the distal radius (Fig. 7.2) [2]. First-line treatment for these injuries has typically consisted of nonoperative management, including, but not limited to, activity modification, immobilization, anti-inflammatory medications, and corticosteroid injections. However, for patients who fail conservative treatment, surgery may be beneficial [3]. Much like the meniscus of the knee, it has been demonstrated that the periphery of the

TFCC has an adequate vascular supply to support surgical repairs (Fig. 7.3) [4]. As such, there is literature that indicates that type 1B injuries respond well to surgical repair, as well as some data showing that the more rare type 1C and 1D injuries also can be repaired surgically [3, 5, 6]. Due to the poor blood supply of the TFCC centrally, surgical treatment of 1A injuries is generally limited to arthroscopic debridement of the central unstable portions of the articular disc as, as well as performing a limited synovectomy [3, 4]. One of the causes for failure of nonoperative treatment is DRUJ instability as a result of the TFCC tear, which can be seen with type 1B tears because of a disruption of the attachment to the ulnar fovea [3, 7, 8]. Type 1B tears are the main focus of the literature on TFCC repairs and they were even subclassified by Atzei and Luchetti in 2011 to predict DRUJ stability and guide treatment of these tears [8] (Fig. 7.4). In this classification, foveal tears are described as involving the distal component (dc-TFCC), which consists of the UCL and distal hammock structure, and/or the proximal component (pc-TFCC), which consists of the proximal triangular ligament and dorsal and ulnar radioulnar ligaments [8]. As they explain, the portion of the TFCC that is visualized from the radiocarpal/ulnocarpal joint is just one portion of the TFCC, more specifically the dc-TFCC. There is much more below the surface that needs to be explored, which they describe as the "Iceberg Concept" [8] (Fig. 7.5). The pc-TFCC, which is a part of the iceberg below the surface, contains the radioulnar ligaments making it important for DRUJ stability and tears there are more clinically relevant than the dc-TFCC. When performing a radiocarpal and ulnocarpal arthroscopy, the most easily visualized portion of the TFCC is the articular disc. A common mistake many surgeons make is to mistake the articular disc for the TFCC itself. As has been previously stated, the TFCC is in fact a complex and focusing repairs on the visualized articular disc alone could lead to poor surgical outcomes.

Surgical repairs were initially all performed open, but since the mid-1990s many studies have been published

C. G. Larsen (✉)
Department of Orthopaedic Surgery, Northwell Health, North Shore University Hospital/Long Island Jewish Medical Center, New Hyde Park, NY, USA

A. S. Greenberg
Orthopaedic Associates of Manhasset, P.C., Great Neck, NY, USA

© Springer Nature Switzerland AG 2022
W. B. Geissler (ed.), *Wrist and Elbow Arthroscopy with Selected Open Procedures*,
https://doi.org/10.1007/978-3-030-78881-0_7

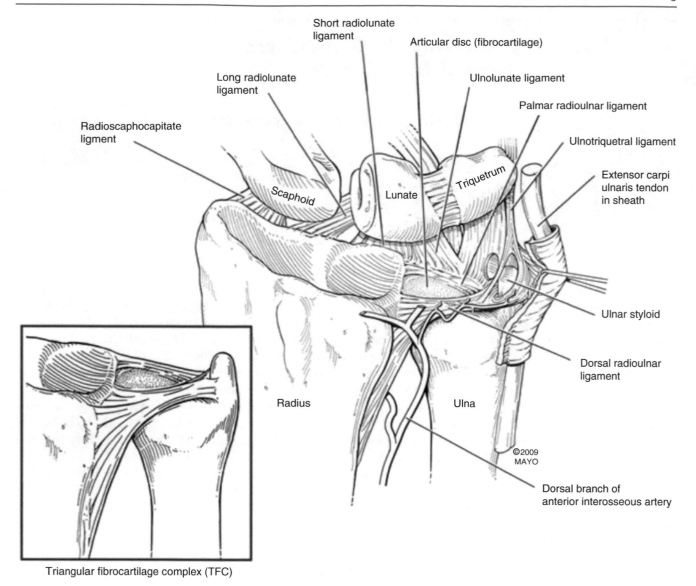

Short radiolunate ligament
Articular disc (fibrocartilage)
Long radiolunate ligament
Ulnolunate ligament
Palmar radioulnar ligament
Radioscaphocapitate ligment
Ulnotriquetral ligament
Scaphoid
Lunate
Triquetrum
Extensor carpi ulnaris tendon in sheath
Ulnar styloid
Dorsal radioulnar ligament
Radius
Ulna
©2009 MAYO
Dorsal branch of anterior interosseous artery

Triangular fibrocartilage complex (TFC)

Fig. 7.1 A detailed illustration showing the complex anatomy of the TFCC. The inset (bottom left) highlights the insertion of the TFCC onto the ulnar fovea which is integral to the stability of the distal radioulnar junction. (Reprinted from Carlsen et al. [32], Copyright 2009, with permission from Elsevier)

showing that there are no significant differences in outcomes and postoperative DRUJ stability between open and arthroscopic repair techniques. However, there is still a lack of high-quality evidence in support of either repair technique [9–13]. Most early arthroscopic repair techniques involved repair of the TFCC to the ulnar side of the capsule through either and inside-out or outside-in technique. However, recent literature supports that a more anatomic approach of repairing the TFCC to the ulnar fovea for type 1B tears is biomechanically more similar to the native TFCC [14, 15]. Furthermore, positive results have been reported for arthroscopic foveal repair through a transosseous bone tunnel both with regard to biomechanics and clinical outcomes [16–19]. Ma et al. demonstrated in cadavers that arthroscopic

transosseous foveal TFCC repair has biomechanically superior strength compared to foveal TFCC repair using a suture anchor [16]. Abe et al. compared clinical outcomes of 21 patients who underwent arthroscopic TFCC repair compared to 8 patients who underwent open repair, all of which were repaired to the ulnar fovea in a transosseous fashion, and reported that there were no significant differences in outcomes with a significantly shorter operative time in the arthroscopic group [17]. A series of 16 patients receiving arthroscopic transosseous foveal TFCC repair by Park et al. demonstrated improvement in postoperative outcome measures and DRUJ stability, and successful return to work in all patients [18]. In a study of 24 arthroscopic transosseous foveal repairs compared to 66 open transosseous foveal

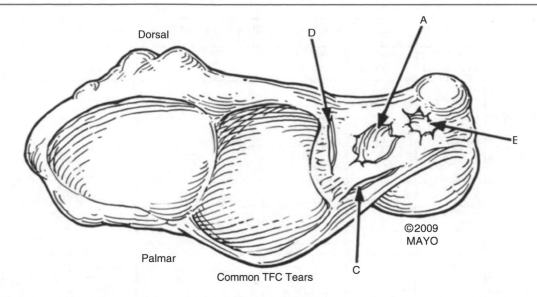

Fig. 7.2 Illustration showing the different types of acute TFCC tears that are included in the Palmer classification (1A–D). A: central perforations; B: avulsions of the TFCC from its insertion on the ulna; C: avulsion of the TFCC from the volar ulnar extrinsic ligaments; D: avulsions from the distal radius. (Reprinted from Carlsen et al. [32], Copyright 2009, with permission from Elsevier)

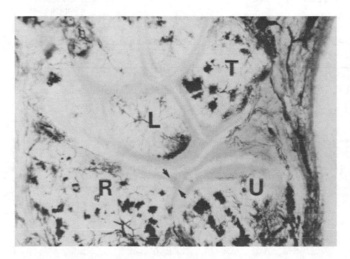

Fig. 7.3 Coronal section of a wrist showing blood vessels from the peripheral soft tissues (joint capsule and synovium) that penetrate the TFCC. There are no blood vessels supplying the radial attachment of the TFCC (black arrows). R: radius; U: ulna; T: triquetrum; L: lunate. (Reprinted from Bednar et al. [4], Copyright 1991, with permission from Elsevier)

repairs, Nakamura et al. showed no significant differences in clinical outcomes; however, patients with the best outcomes following arthroscopic repair had surgery within 7 months of their injury and had neutral or negative ulnar variance [19]. Additionally, there is some evidence to support ulnar shortening osteotomy (USO) in conjunction with TFCC repair in those patients who have foveal tears with DRUJ instability and positive ulnar variance to reduce ulnar impaction on the repaired TFCC and allow for healing [10, 18–20]. In 1996, Trumble et al. anecdotally reported that patients with ulnar positive variance had poor outcomes and frequent re-tearing

following TFCC repair [10]. Similarly, in 2011, Nakamura et al. reported in their series of 24 transosseous arthroscopic TFCC repairs, that in 5 patients with +2 mm positive ulnar variance their outcomes were graded as 1 excellent, 2 fair, and 2 poor compared to the other 19 patients with neutral or negative ulnar variance who had outcomes graded as 12 excellent, 3 good, 2 fair, and 2 poor [19]. In 2016, Seo et al. showed that transosseous arthroscopic TFCC repair performed along with USO is a viable operative combination and that patients receiving both procedures had better outcome scores than patients that received USO with TFCC debridement alone [20].

Indications

For patients with ulnar-sided wrist pain, a careful clinical examination is the key to guiding further workup and management. The "fovea sign," which is positive when there is tenderness to palpation in the soft spot between the ulnar head and the pisiform distally and dorsal to the flexor carpi ulnaris tendon, is 95.2% sensitive and 86.5% specific for detecting either foveal or ulnocarpal tears (type 1B and 1C) of the TFCC [21]. DRUJ stability can be assessed by a number of provocative examination maneuvers; some of the most commonly cited tests are the ulnocarpal stress test, DRUJ ballottement test, and the piano-key test with the ballottement test being cited as the most reliable test [22]. To perform the ballottement test, the examiner grasps the radius and radiocarpal bones firmly and with the other hand assesses the anterior and posterior translation of the ulnar head with the forearm in neutral, supinated, and pronated. The results

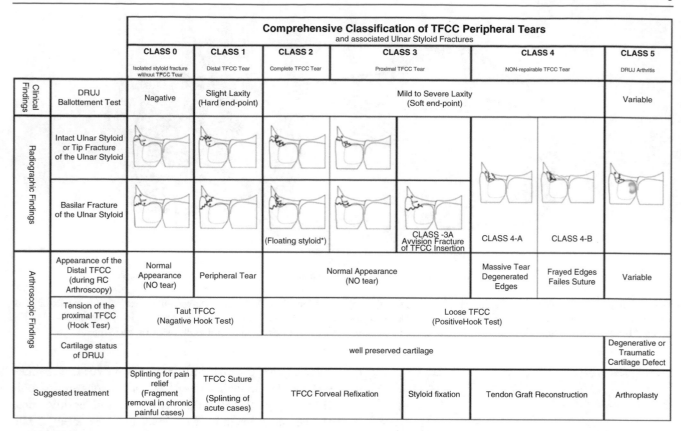

		CLASS 0	CLASS 1	CLASS 2	CLASS 3		CLASS 4		CLASS 5
		Isolated styloid fracture without TFCC Tear	Distal TFCC Tear	Complete TFCC Tear	Proximal TFCC Tear		NON-repairable TFCC Tear		DRUJ Arthritis
Clinical Findings	DRUJ Ballottement Test	Nagative	Slight Laxity (Hard end-point)	Mild to Severe Laxity (Soft end-point)					Variable
Radiographic Findings	Intact Ulnar Styloid or Tip Fracture of the Ulnar Styloid								
	Basilar Fracture of the Ulnar Styloid		(Floating styloid*)		CLASS -3A Avvision Fracture of TFCC Insertion		CLASS 4-A	CLASS 4-B	
Arthroscopic Findings	Appearance of the Distal TFCC (during RC Arthroscopy)	Normal Appearance (NO tear)	Peripheral Tear	Normal Appearance (NO tear)			Massive Tear Degenerated Edges	Frayed Edges Failes Suture	Variable
	Tension of the proximal TFCC (Hook Tesr)	Taut TFCC (Nagative Hook Test)		Loose TFCC (PositiveHook Test)					
	Cartilage status of DRUJ	well preserved cartilage							Degenerative or Traumatic Cartilage Defect
	Suggested treatment	Splinting for pain relief (Fragment removal in chronic painful cases)	TFCC Suture (Splinting of acute cases)	TFCC Forveal Refixation	Styloid fixation		Tendon Graft Reconstruction		Arthroplasty

Comprehensive Classification of TFCC Peripheral Tears and associated Ulnar Styloid Fractures

Fig. 7.4 Classification of TFCC peripheral tears that considers clinical, radiographic, and arthroscopic findings. (Reprinted from Atzei and Luchetti [8], Copyright 2011, with permission from Elsevier)

Fig. 7.5 "The Iceberg Concept" describes how the distal-most part of the TFCC is what is immediately viewable from the radiocarpal/ulnocarpal joint; however, the more proximal portion of the TFCC contains the attachment to the ulnar fovea and has a larger role in the stability of the DRUJ. (Reprinted from Atzei and Luchetti [8], Copyright 2011, with permission from Elsevier)

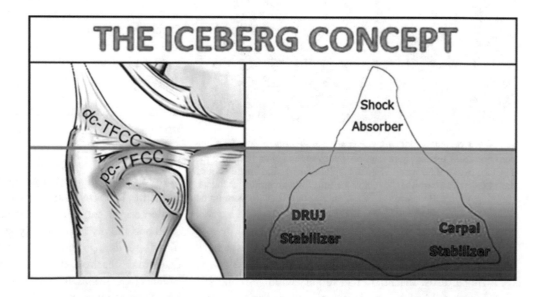

of the test are graded on a scale of 0–3: 0 is equal to the contralateral side, 1 indicates increased laxity with a firm end point in all forearm positions, 2 indicates increased laxity with a firm endpoint in at least one forearm position, and 3 indicates increased laxity without a firm endpoint [18].

Plain radiographs can be helpful for identifying patients with ulnar positive variance or fractures, as these can impact

the treatment plan. Further workup can consist of magnetic resonance imaging (MRI), in which gradient echo sequence T2 weighted and fat-suppressed T1 weighted images provide a good resolution view of the TFCC, or either computed tomography arthrography (CTA) or magnetic resonance arthrography (MRA). Diagnostic arthroscopy is still ultimately considered the gold standard for diagnosis of TFCC tears [19, 23, 24]. It has been shown that there is a high false positive rate for MRI, with more than 50% of all patients over the age of 70 having signal abnormalities in the TFCC despite 90% of those patients presenting with a low clinical suspicion for TFCC pathology [25]. Compared to diagnostic arthroscopy, a recent meta-analysis showed sensitivities of 0.76, 0.78, and 0.89 for MRI, MRA, and CTA, respectively [26]. Despite the slight superiority of arthrography to conventional MRI for diagnostic accuracy, it should be noted that arthrography is an invasive procedure with additional risks and costs [27]. We routinely send our patients for an MRI preoperatively, and find it valuable not only to support the diagnosis of a TFCC tear, but to assist in determining the morphology of the tear, which can be helpful for surgical planning.

For patients with suspected TFCC tear and intact DRUJ stability, a trial of nonoperative treatment with 4 weeks of immobilization, restricting forearm rotation and wrist range of motion in either a cast, brace, or Munster splint, is the first line of treatment.

Corticosteroid injections can be used for pain relief and can provide important diagnostic information when the source of a patient's ulnar-sided wrist pain is in question. Patients who fail conservative treatment or have TFCC tears with gross DRUJ instability on physical exam should be indicated for surgery.

Diagnostic arthroscopy can be performed in isolation or as part of a larger planned arthroscopic procedure. Most of the TFCC and the entirety of the articular disc can be viewed through the 3–4 and 4–5 portals, using various additional working portals, making arthroscopy the gold standard in diagnosis of TFCC tears [8] (Fig. 7.6). A trampoline test should be performed, which is positive when the TFCC is soft and compliant under a compressive load from the probe and indicates a tear of the distal portion of the TFCC [28] (Fig. 7.7). TFCC tears that do not disrupt to foveal attachment, and therefore are not associated with DRUJ instability, can be managed with simple suture repair for those patients who fail non-operative treatment. A hook test should also be performed to indirectly assess the foveal insertion of the TFCC and is performed by hooking the ulnar-most aspect of the TFCC and attempting to displace the TFCC toward the center of the radiocarpal joint; this test is positive if the TFCC can be displaced centrally and indicates that the underlying foveal attachment is disrupted [29]. Additionally, in the setting of a foveal TFCC avulsion, the diagnosis can be made by placing a probe beneath the TFCC from the 6-U portal. The ability to pass beneath the articular disc and probe the fovea is essentially diagnostic for a foveal avulsion of the TFCC. Some surgeons prefer to directly visualize the deep portion of the TFCC via DRUJ arthroscopy; however, this is not something that we do routinely. When desired, DRUJ arthroscopy can be accomplished using a smaller

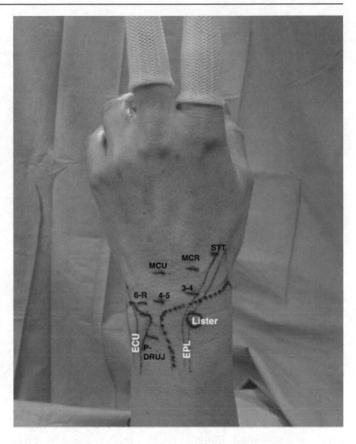

Fig. 7.6 A wrist positioned for arthroscopy with commonly used portals marked on the dorsal surface. Of relevance to our procedure are the 6-R, 4–5, and 3–4 portals. Other portals marked here are: distal radioulnar joint (DRUJ), mid-carpal ulnar (MCU), mid-carpal radial (MCR), and scaphotrapeziotrapezoid (STT). Other landmarks: extensor carpi ulnaris (ECU), extensor pollicis longus (EPL), and Lister's tubercle (Lister). (Reprinted with permission from Badur et al. [33])

(<2 mm) arthroscope. Disruption of the foveal attachment of the TFCC, which can be diagnosed by use of a hook test, probing the fovea from the 6-U portal, or by direct visualization through DRUJ arthroscopy, is indicative of DRUJ instability and should be repaired surgically except for when the tear is degenerative in nature and cannot hold sutures, or if there is preexisting DRUJ arthritis (see Fig. 7.4). Arthroscopic transosseous foveal repair is a validated technique for surgical repair of these aforementioned tears and is the focus of this chapter.

Contraindications

Contraindications to the arthroscopic transosseous foveal TFCC repair technique include the following: degenerated TFCC tissue that is not suitable to hold sutures and advanced arthritis of the DRUJ or ulnocarpal joint [8]. Avulsion fractures of the ulnar styloid with an attached TFCC can undergo internal fixation to restore DRUJ stability, and therefore do

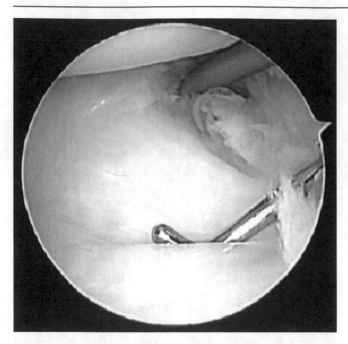

Fig. 7.7 Arthroscopic view of a positive trampoline test

not need TFCC repair [8]. Any prior hardware in the ulna that would prevent drilling of the bone tunnels is also a relative contraindication, unless a removal of hardware procedure is considered clinically appropriate. Ulnar positive variance and ulnar abutment is not a contraindication to this technique, as we have found good results when performed along with USO in patients with signs of chronic abutment or significant ulnar positive variance. This is consistent with the limited data published to support USO and arthroscopic transosseous foveal TFCC repair performed in tandem [18, 20]. It should be noted, however, that previously asymptomatic ulnar positive variance without signs of ulnar carpal impaction (lunate chondromalacia, chronic central articular disc perforation, cystic carpal changes) does not routinely have to be addressed with an osteotomy and may be left to the surgeon's discretion. Lastly, less optimal results have been reported when using the arthroscopic technique for patients with subacute or chronic injuries [19].

Technique

Diagnostic Arthroscopy

Wrist arthroscopy can be performed under either regional or general anesthesia depending on surgeon and anesthesiologist preference and comfort. The patient is placed in supine position with the arm extended onto a hand table. This surgeon's preference is to perform arthroscopy with the use of a well-padded upper arm, non-sterile tourniquet, applied before draping. The arm is prepped and draped below the

tourniquet, just above the elbow. The arm is suspended from a wrist traction tower using finger traps. The traps and suspension can be placed on all of the fingers, or the radial or ulnar digits in isolation, depending on whether or not wrist deviation is desired. Ten pounds of traction is applied to the wrist and the tourniquet is inflated to 250 mm of Mercury (mmHg) following exsanguination of the limb with an Esmarch bandage. Insufflation of the joint with saline prior to establishing the first portal can make it easier to identify the wrist joint. First, a standard 3–4 viewing portal is established carefully by incising the skin with a #11 blade followed by blunt dissection with a hemostat just distal to Lister's tubercle between the tendons of the 3rd and 4th dorsal compartments. If insufflation was successful, perforation of the capsule should be followed by a rush of fluid. Next, a 2.7 millimeter (mm), 30-degree arthroscope with a blunt trocar is introduced. Inflow is established, and after a diagnostic radiocarpal arthroscopy has been performed, the view may be directed ulnarly toward the articular disc and the rest of the visualized TFCC. At this point, a 4–5 and/or 6-R portal needs to be established as both a working portal and an additional viewing portal. Establishing the 4–5 portal (between the tendons of the 4th and 5th compartments) can be assisted by triangulating with a 25-gauge needle. The needle tip can be swept carefully across the joint to make sure that the portal can access all points necessary for TFCC viewing and repair. Once the needle trajectory and placement are deemed appropriate, the portal is created in the identical manner as that previously described for the 3–4 portal. The 6-R and 6-U portals can be established just radial to the ECU tendon in a similar fashion if considered by the surgeon to be necessary for the procedure. It should be noted that these portals can be used for outflow and provide excellent working angles for suture passing as will be described.

Once a working portal has been established, a probe is introduced and the trampoline test and hook test are performed as described previously. Often synovectomy will be required to improve visualization of the ulnar side of the wrist. A positive hook test indicates TFCC detachment from its foveal insertion, and if the tissue can hold a suture, these patients are good candidates for a transosseous foveal repair. When a tear is not repairable, such as when there is a massive tear with retraction of the ligamentous remnants not allowing for approximation, or in more chronic tears where the tissue may be degenerative, surgical options include debridement and in cases of instability, ligamentous reconstruction.

Bone Tunnel Creation

In order to perform a transosseous foveal TFCC repair, an incision will need to be made along the mid-axial line of the ulna, beginning roughly 1–1.5 cm proximal to the ulnar styloid. Care must be taken to keep this incision mid-axial to avoid injury to the sensory branches of the ulnar nerve, and we recommend blunt dissection and identification of this nerve whenever possible. With blunt retractors placed, the guidewire for the 3.0 cannulated drill (Arthrex, Naples, FL, USA) is driven obliquely through the fovea and into the visualized portion of the torn TFCC. This is usually performed with basic triangulation technique, but can be assisted with a C-ring aiming guide to align and drill the bone tunnel (AR-8826) and/or with the use of fluoroscopy. If using a guide, its distal end is placed through the 6-R portal and the tip is wedged onto the fovea, which is assessable given the detached TFCC. The angle of the tunnel should be approximately 45 degrees from a line perpendicular to the long axis of the forearm, but can vary based on patient size and anatomy. The aiming guide is removed leaving the K-wire in place. Care should be taken no to drive the wire into the more distal carpus to prevent unnecessary cartilage damage. Next the K-wire is over-drilled with a 3-mm cannulated drill. It is important not to bend the wire when drilling, as it is possible to break the guidewire and risk drilling a faulty path or leaving a buried portion of the wire in the patient. One must also take care when drilling through the ulnar fovea, not to damage the tissue of the TFCC. Only the wire is visible in the joint at this point. Once the foveal bone is about to be breached, the wire will begin to spin, providing a visual feedback for the surgeon to apply a bit less force. This will help prevent a plunge of the drill bit through the foveal cortex. The drill and K-wire are now removed from the bone tunnel.

Suture Passing

After the bone tunnel has been created, the next step is to pass the sutures used for the TFCC repair. An Arthrex 2-0 FiberStick suture (AR-7222) is loaded onto an Arthrex straight Micro SutureLasso (AR-8703) and about 0.5 cm of the stiffened end of the FiberStick is bent over the blunt end of the metal tip of the SutureLasso, so that it will not back out upon insertion. This waxed suture will maintain its position when this step is perfomed. The Micro SutureLasso is then inserted through the bone tunnel and is advanced through the TFCC on the radial side of the tear. The SutureLasso is twisted in a clockwise manner. The SutureLasso is then slowly backed out from the bone tunnel, leaving a spiral portion of the suture in the wrist distal to the TFCC that it was just passed through (Fig. 7.8). Holding the SutureLasso in between the surgeon's index finger and thumb and performing a rapid pill-rolling motion, while slowly reversing the SutureLasso, should keep the suture from binding the instrument, thus leaving it visible in the joint. The SutureLasso is then reloaded with a black nitinol

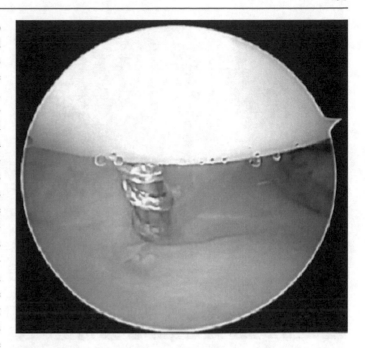

Fig. 7.8 Arthroscopic view of passing of FiberStick from the transosseous ulnar tunnel through the TFCC

wire suture passer and is advanced back through the bone tunnel. This time the SutureLasso is advanced through the TFCC on the ulnar side of the tear, preferably at least 4 mm from where the suture previously penetrated the TFCC. This can be challenging as the same 3 mm tunnel is being used. One technique is to place a slight bend at the tip of the SutureLasso. This angle will allow additional reach and prevent perforating the same region of the TFCC. Additionally, providing a slight volar or dorsal shuck on the ulna will translate the tunnel and alter the point of perforation. Next, an arthroscopic suture retriever can be inserted through the 4–5 portal and is used to retrieve the suture and the nitinol wire and they are pulled out through the 4–5 portal. The two limbs (both suture and wire) must be grabbed by the retriever at the same time. There is no cannula being used in this case, and if they are grabbed separately, a tissue bridge may be created and prevent suture passage. The FiberStick is then threaded through the nitinol wire and both are pulled back into the wrist and then out through the bone tunnel creating a mattress stitch through the torn TFCC (Fig. 7.9). If additional mattress stitches are desired, these steps can be repeated; however, it is recommended that all passes of the suture through the TFCC are at least 4 mm apart from each other to reduce the chances of the sutures pulling through the tissue.

An alternative method for passing the mattress suture is to use an Arthrex Knee Scorpion suture passer (AR-12990) through a 6-U or 6-R working portal [30]. These portals are located just ulnar or radial to the ECU tendon respectively, and a needle should be used to establish either of these portals

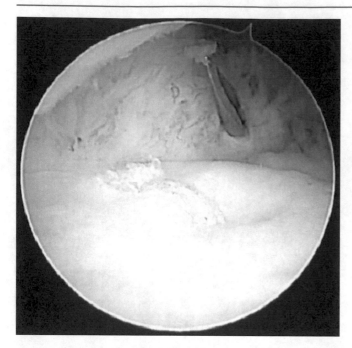

Fig. 7.9 Arthroscopic picture of a completed TFCC repair. The final construct is in a horizontal mattress configuration and was performed using a transosseous technique through an ulnar bone tunnel

under direct visualization from inside the joint to assure that the instrument will have access to the desired portions of the TFCC (see Fig. 7.6). A 2-0 FiberWire (AR-7221) is loaded into the Scorpion and the jaws are closed as the instrument is inserted into the 6-U or 6-R portal. The jaws are opened once the Scorpion is visualized and the instrument is situated to pass the FiberWire from proximal to distal through the TFCC. This is only possible if the TFCC is torn peripherally and from the fovea, as the jaws must go both above and below the articular disc. The Scorpion is deployed and the passed end of the FiberWire is pulled back out through the portal with the Scorpion. The FiberWire end is then reloaded onto the Scorpion and the instrument is re-inserted through the same working portal; however, this time with the instrument flipped 180 degrees such that when the bite is taken with the Scorpion it passes the suture from distal to proximal through the TFCC. This will create a mattress suture with both limbs aiming into the tunnel. An arthroscopic grasper or suture retriever inserted through the bone tunnel is then used to retrieve both the passed end of the FiberWire from the underside of the TFCC and the opposite end that is still exiting the portal. Visualization for suture retrieval can be difficult and may be assisted by viewing through the 4–5 portal.

Suture Anchor Fixation

To complete the repair, the sutures will be secured to the lateral ulna using a suture anchor. The anchor should be placed approximately 1 cm proximal to the bone tunnel along the subcutaneous surface of the ulna. If necessary, the ulnar incision should be extended proximally to accommodate anchor placement at this point. A hole is drilled with either a 1.8- or 2.0-mm drill for placement of a mini-PushLock anchor. This hole is drilled 1 cm proximal to the bone tunnel and at a 45-degree angle in relation to the ulna so that the trajectory of the bone tunnel and the hole for the suture anchor are just divergent from parallel. Alternatively, a punch could be used to complete the prior step if desired.

The suture ends exiting the bone tunnel are loaded into a 2.5-mm Arthrex PushLock anchor (AR-8825). At this point, tension on the sutures should be adjusted as desired by the surgeon by pulling on the suture ends, and then when satisfied with the amount of tension, the anchor is inserted into the hole until flush with the bone. The authors of this chapter recommend performing this step under arthroscopic visualization. If too much tension is applied, the sutures may tear through the tissue, regardless of the distance between the limbs. It should also be stated that placement of the anchor into the bone further tensions the sutures, so less tension is required than may otherwise be expected. Under arthroscopic visualization, the surgeon will clearly notice the dimpling created by the suture tension and the recreation of the trampoline effect, tested with a probe. At this point, the tension is appropriate and the anchor can be seated without tensioning further. The suture ends are cut flush at the edge of the bone to complete this knotless repair without leaving any uncomfortable prominences along the subcutaneous border of the ulna. If a second mattress stitch is desired at this point, a second suture anchor would have to be used to secure those suture ends. Caution must be taken not to damage previously placed sutures while in the bone tunnel.

Repair Assessment and Final Steps

After completion of the TFCC repair, direct visualization should again be performed arthroscopically. Gentle trampoline and hook tests should also be performed to assess the functional stability of the repair; however, care should be exercised not to disrupt the repair with overly aggressive maneuvers (Fig. 7.10). If satisfied with the repair, the arthroscopic inflow is turned off and outflow is opened to drain excess fluid from the joint. The arthroscope is removed and all skin incisions are closed in subcuticular fashion with interrupted buried 4-0 monocryl sutures. Skin adhesive is applied, and then steri strips for added wound closure security. A sterile dressing is applied and then the patient is placed in an above elbow sugartong splint with the wrist in neutral.

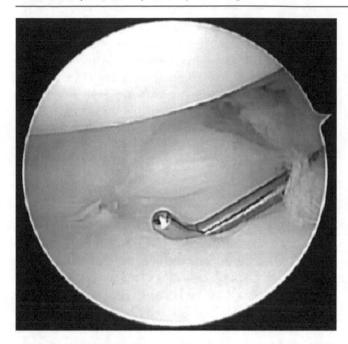

Fig. 7.10 Arthroscopic view of a negative trampoline test following repair of the TFCC

Postoperative Protocol

One of the most important aspects of this surgery, much like other ligament or tendon repairs, is successful completion of a postoperative protocol that protects the integrity of the repair. As discussed above, the patient leaves the operating room in a sugartong splint and remains in this splint until a 1-week postoperative follow-up visit. At this first follow up appointment, the splint is taken off and the patient is placed into a hinged elbow brace that allows for full elbow flexion and extension, but does not allow for pronation or supination. It has been shown that the radioulnar ligaments of the TFCC experience the greatest amounts of force at full pronation and supination, so keeping the forearm neutral during the recovery period maintains a low stress environment on the healing TFCC [31]. The patient will remain in this brace until the 6-week mark and should wear it at all times. The patient is allowed to remove the brace for bathing and dressing, but they are carefully instructed as to which motions to avoid, as certain positions may jeopardize the repair.

Patients after their first visit are prescribed hand therapy, with an initial focus on elbow flexion and extension, as well as finger range of motion to prevent stiffness during these early weeks. At 6 weeks, the brace is removed and active and passive motion of the wrist is permitted. Hand therapy is now advanced to include grip strengthening, as well as active and passive wrist and elbow range of motion. No resistance is applied at this point, and no axial weight bearing is allowed yet. At 10 postoperative weeks, wrist strengthening exercises are begun and weight bearing is progressed. Full weight bearing and return to athletics is not advised until 4 months postoperative.

Tips and Tricks

Performing an arthroscopic TFCC repair can be a challenging procedure, as it requires an advanced level of both arthroscopic skill as well as knowledge of anatomy. The wrist is a very confined space and efforts must be made to utilize this space without crowding. Portal placement is done in the standard fashion, but the use of 25-gauge small needles can be very helpful. They can assist in triangulation, but additionally a gentle sweep with the needle under arthroscopic visualization (to make sure no damage is caused) can confirm that all regions that need treatment can be accessed. Correct portal placement also may require a synovectomy and debridement. The authors of this chapter strongly recommend performing this step as it will improve initial visibility and prevent water-infused synovium from crowding the joint and limiting both the surgeon's sight and the working space. Additional tips are as follows:

Tunnel Drilling

The orientation of the bone tunnel through the ulna is one of the most crucial parts of the operation and correct execution of this step makes sure that the sutures can be passed appropriately through the TFCC to perform the repair. Creating a tunnel that is too vertical could cause the sutures to be passed too ulnar through the TFCC, and similarly a tunnel that is too horizontal could cause the sutures to penetrate the TFCC too radially. Likewise, a tunnel that penetrates the ulnar fovea close to the volar or dorsal sides of the ulnar head could cause sutures to be passed volar or dorsal to the midsubstance of the TFCC, which is the ideal place for suture placement due to the highest quality of tissue being located there. The use of a C-ring guide (Arthrex, Naples, FL, USA) can be helpful when it is available. The angle can be set by placing the tip of the ring onto the fovea and the wire entry against the ulna. However, this guide is not always available and thus triangulation is required to aim the wire. We would recommend the use of a mini-C-arm. This can help confirm the angle and assure the surgeon that the wire is headed toward the correct anatomic location. However, recall that simply breaching the fovea is not the only concern. As noted above, the angle at which the fovea is breached determines the portion of the TFCC that is accessible.

When a C-ring guide is not used, the wire may slide during placement. To avoid this skiving during the initial drilling of the K wire into the ulna, it can be helpful to create a small trough for the wire that is centered on the subcutaneous border and approximately 1–1.5 cm proximal to the ulnar styloid. It is also advisable to be diligent in confirming correct trajectory of the K-wire at multiple points by using fluoroscopy, confirming the direction of the bone tunnel and then also checking while drilling the bone tunnel over the K-wire.

Suture Management

When working with sutures in a closed space, it is critical that they are kept in an area that is accessible, while at the same time, not in contact with other sutures. It is very easy to get sutures tangled, and if that occurs in the radiocarpal or ulnocarpal joints, it is very difficult to deal with. It is therefore important that only one suture is passed at a time in cases where more than one mattress suture is desired.

The other portion of suture management that can be a hindrance in these cases is the formation of a soft tissue bridge. This occurs in situations where no cannula is being used, and thus, small difference in soft tissue pathways can happen when multiple passes are made through the same portal. For example, grasping the twirled limb of the FiberStick suture, and then going back in through the same portal to grasp the SutureLasso. It is possible, though not definite, to wind up with a tissue bridge that will prevent complete passage of the suture through the tunnel. The key to preventing this is to leave the coiled end of the FiberStick in place during passage of the SutureLasso. Once the second bite of tissue is created with the SutureLasso, both limbs (the nitinol wire and the FiberStick) can be grabbed by the retriever at the same time. The suture is then threaded through the lasso and passed with ease.

Portal Usage

The described technique for this procedure is to view the TFCC through the 3–4 portal and to work through the 4–5 portal. We would encourage any surgeon attempting this procedure to not confine themselves to these portals. There are times when visibility through the 3–4 portal can be hindered by instruments placed through the 4–5 portal. A solution to this can be to use the 6-R or 6-U portal to work and shuttle sutures, to view the TFCC through the 4–5 portal, or both. One benefit of viewing through the 4–5 portal is visibility of the lunotriquetral (LT) ligament, tears of which may be a concomitant injury and the cause of persistent ulnar-sided wrist pain.

Forearm Position

The forearm should be positioned in neutral, or midsupination/pronation, so that the thumb is pointing in the same direction as the humerus. This position should be maintained for tunnel drilling, suture passing, suture tensioning, and splinting postoperatively. Changing the forearm rotation between any of these steps could cause the TFCC to move either volar or dorsal with regard to the repair footprint on the ulnar fovea and can throw off the tensioning that was established during suture anchor placement since the length of the TFCC changes based on the position of the forearm.

Suture Tying

Once it is time to tension the sutures and place the anchor, we want to make sure that the tension established is the final tension and that it is appropriately holding the DRUJ reduced. Therefore, before final tensioning of the sutures, an assistant should be holding the ulnar head in a reduced position with regard to the DRUJ. This again can be assisted by fluoroscopy. Additionally, wrist traction should be removed. As was mentioned previously, forearm rotation is also important and should be checked again to make sure that it is maintained in neutral prior to the final tensioning.

It was also discussed above during the description of this technique that we recommend viewing the TFCC when placing tension on the sutures. This tissue can be friable in certain cases and too much tension may tear through the tissue. The goal is approximation of the TFCC to the fovea, which can be seen through dimpling in the tissue and recreation of the trampoline, as well as probing though the 6-R or 6-U portals to confirm the tissue is down. Recall the ability to place a probe beneath the TFCC confirmed its avulsion from the fovea. Loss of this ability helps verify its repair. Lastly, when placing the anchor, additional tension will be added to the sutures as the eyelet of the anchor, loaded with the suture, is driven further into the bone.

Conclusion

TFCC tears present with many different morphologies and while classifications exist to differentiate between these tears, the clinically important factor is if the insertion onto the fovea of the ulna is intact. Loss off the foveal attachment of the TFCC leads to instability of the DRUJ, and while many TFCC tears can be treated with nonoperative measures, persistent pain may warrant surgical intervention, and foveal tears resulting in DRUJ instability are a known cause of failure of conservative management. The data show that restoring the integrity of the TFCC to its ulnar attachment on the fovea successfully eliminates instability at the DRUJ that can be a source of chronic pain in patients with TFCC tears. Historically, TFCC repairs were repaired with open surgery. However, as arthroscopy techniques have improved, many surgeons are now choosing to perform repairs arthroscopically, with studies reporting equivalent outcomes. Initially arthroscopic repair techniques focused on repairing the TFCC to the peripheral wrist capsule in either an outside-in or inside-out method, but now the focus is on performing a more anatomic repair of the TFCC to its normal attachment site on the ulnar fovea. Arthroscopic peripheral TFCC repair through an ulnar bone tunnel is an effective and reproducible method for repairing the TFCC to its anatomic footprint on the ulnar fovea. Workup and diagnosis of peripheral TFCC tears that are indicated for repair is of paramount importance prior to consideration of this technique, and we have discussed this in detail in this chapter. We describe in simple, easy-to-follow steps, how to perform a diagnostic arthroscopy followed by ulnar bone tunnel drilling, suture passing through the torn tissue, and fixation of the sutures with an anchor to complete the repair. Equally important to the repair itself is the postoperative protocol and restriction of forearm rotation to avoid stress on the repair. Our hope is that this detailed technique guide will allow readers to add this repair method to their repertoire for the management of peripheral TFCC tears.

References

1. Palmer AK, Werner FW. The triangular fibrocartilage complex of the wrist--anatomy and function. J Hand Surg Am. 1981;6(2):153–62.
2. Palmer AK. Triangular fibrocartilage complex lesions: a classification. J Hand Surg Am. 1989;14(4):594–606.
3. Kovachevich R, Elhassan BT. Arthroscopic and open repair of the TFCC. Hand Clin. 2010;26(4):485–94.
4. Bednar MS, Arnoczky SP, Weiland AJ. The microvasculature of the triangular fibrocartilage complex: its clinical significance. J Hand Surg Am. 1991;16(6):1101–5.
5. Cooney WP, Linscheid RL, Dobyns JH. Triangular fibrocartilage tears. J Hand Surg Am. 1994;19(1):143–54.
6. Trumble TE, Gilbert M, Vedder N. Isolated tears of the triangular fibrocartilage: management by early arthroscopic repair. J Hand Surg Am. 1997;22(1):57–65.
7. Nakamura T, Yabe Y, Horiuchi Y. Functional anatomy of the triangular fibrocartilage complex. J Hand Surg Br. 1996;21(5):581–6.
8. Atzei A, Luchetti R. Foveal TFCC tear classification and treatment. Hand Clin. 2011;27(3):263–72.
9. Dunn JC, Polmear MM, Nesti LJ. Surgical repair of acute TFCC injury. Hand (N Y). 2019:1558944719828007.
10. Trumble TE, Gilbert M, Vedder N. Arthroscopic repair of the triangular fibrocartilage complex. Arthroscopy. 1996;12(5):588–97.
11. Robba V, Fowler A, Karantana A, Grindlay D, Lindau T. Open versus arthroscopic repair of 1B ulnar-sided triangular fibrocartilage complex tears: a systematic review. Hand (N Y). 2019:1558944718815244.
12. Andersson JK, Åhlén M, Andernord D. Open versus arthroscopic repair of the triangular fibrocartilage complex: a systematic review. J Exp Orthop. 2018;5(1):6.
13. Corso SJ, Savoie FH, Geissler WB, Whipple TL, Jiminez W, Jenkins N. Arthroscopic repair of peripheral avulsions of the triangular fibrocartilage complex of the wrist: a multicenter study. Arthroscopy. 1997;13(1):78–84.
14. Johnson JC, Pfeiffer FM, Jouret JE, Brogan DM. Biomechanical analysis of capsular repair versus arthrex TFCC ulnar tunnel repair for triangular fibrocartilage complex tears. Hand (N Y). 2019;14(4):547–53.
15. Chen WJ. Arthroscopically assisted transosseous foveal repair of triangular fibrocartilage complex. Arthrosc Tech. 2017;6(1):e57–64.
16. Ma CH, Lin TS, Wu CH, Li DY, Yang SC, Tu YK. Biomechanical comparison of open and arthroscopic transosseous repair of triangular fibrocartilage complex foveal tears: a cadaveric study. Arthroscopy. 2017;33(2):297–304.
17. Abe Y, Fujii K, Fujisawa T. Midterm results after open versus arthroscopic transosseous repair for foveal tears of the triangular fibrocartilage complex. J Wrist Surg. 2018;7(4):292–7.
18. Park JH, Kim D, Park JW. Arthroscopic one-tunnel transosseous foveal repair for triangular fibrocartilage complex (TFCC) peripheral tear. Arch Orthop Trauma Surg. 2018;138(1):131–8.
19. Nakamura T, Sato K, Okazaki M, Toyama Y, Ikegami H. Repair of foveal detachment of the triangular fibrocartilage complex: open and arthroscopic transosseous techniques. Hand Clin. 2011;27(3):281–90.
20. Seo JB, Kim JP, Yi HS, Park KH. The outcomes of arthroscopic repair versus debridement for chronic unstable triangular fibrocartilage complex tears in patients undergoing ulnar-shortening osteotomy. J Hand Surg Am. 2016;41(5):615–23.
21. Tay SC, Tomita K, Berger RA. The "ulnar fovea sign" for defining ulnar wrist pain: an analysis of sensitivity and specificity. J Hand Surg Am. 2007;32(4):438–44.
22. Moriya T, Aoki M, Iba K, Ozasa Y, Wada T, Yamashita T. Effect of triangular ligament tears on distal radioulnar joint instability and evaluation of three clinical tests: a biomechanical study. J Hand Surg Eur Vol. 2009;34(2):219–23.
23. Nakamura T, Yabe Y, Horiuchi Y. Fat suppression magnetic resonance imaging of the triangular fibrocartilage complex. Comparison with spin echo, gradient echo pulse sequences and histology. J Hand Surg Br. 1999;24(1):22–6.
24. Tanaka T, Yoshioka H, Ueno T, Shindo M, Ochiai N. Comparison between high-resolution MRI with a microscopy coil and arthroscopy in triangular fibrocartilage complex injury. J Hand Surg Am. 2006;31(8):1308–14.
25. Bendre IIII, Oflazoglu K, van Leeuwen WF, Rakhorst H, Ring D, Chen NC. The prevalence of triangular fibrocartilage complex signal abnormalities on magnetic resonance imaging relative to clinical suspicion of pathology. J Hand Surg Am. 2018;43(9):819 26.e1.
26. Treiser MD, Crawford K, Iorio ML. TFCC injuries: meta-analysis and comparison of diagnostic imaging modalities. J Wrist Surg. 2018;7(3):267–72.
27. Boer BC, Vestering M, van Raak SM, van Kooten EO, Huis In't Veld R, Vochteloo AJH. MR arthrography is slightly more accurate than conventional MRI in detecting TFCC lesions of the wrist. Eur J Orthop Surg Traumatol. 2018;28(8):1549–53.
28. Hermansdorfer JD, Kleinman WB. Management of chronic peripheral tears of the triangular fibrocartilage complex. J Hand Surg Am. 1991;16(2):340–6.
29. Atzei A. New trends in arthroscopic management of type 1-B TFCC injuries with DRUJ instability. J Hand Surg Eur Vol. 2009;34(5):582–91.
30. Birdsong E. TFCC repair to fovea using knee scorpion suture passer: Arthrex; 2016. Available from: https://www.arthrex.com/resources/video/x_H6sELFPCUmJoAFT7XuiBA/tfcc-repair-to-fovea-using-knee-scorpion-suture-passer.
31. Af Ekenstam F, Hagert CG. Anatomical studies on the geometry and stability of the distal radio ulnar joint. Scand J Plast Reconstr Surg. 1985;19(1):17–25.
32. Carlsen BT, Rizzo M, Moran SL. Soft-tissue injuries associated with distal radius fractures. Oper Tech Orthop. 2009;19:107–18.
33. Badur N, Luchetti R, Atzei A. Arthroscopic wrist anatomy and setup. In: Wrist and elbow arthroscopy: a practical surgical guide to techniques. 2nd ed. New York: Springer Science; 2015.

UT Ligament Split Tears

Nicholas Munaretto and Sanjeev Kakar

Introduction

The anatomy comprising the ulnar side of the wrist has a layered complexity that makes diagnosis and treatment very challenging. This has often contributed to the ulnar side of the wrist being referred to as the "black box" or the "low back pain" of the wrist [1–5]. However, ulnar-sided wrist pain is common and can frequently be debilitating to patients. Therefore, it is important to have a detailed anatomic understanding and to be adept at the diagnosis and treatment of this difficult area of the wrist.

Although the UT ligament is a small ligament located on the ulnar side of the wrist, it can be a significant source of pain and disability. UT ligament split tear can be diagnosed and treated with a combination of anatomic knowledge, a detailed history, physical exam, imaging, and wrist arthroscopy. Although there is limited literature on outcomes of UT ligament split tear treatment, newer studies have highlighted that its treatment has potential favorable outcomes and can make a significant difference in patient pain and function [2].

Anatomy

TFCC Anatomy

PRU and DRU Ligaments

Having an understanding of the palmar radioulnar (PRU) and dorsal radioulnar (DRU) ligaments is imperative (Fig. 8.1). The PRU and DRU ligaments are the primary stabilizers of the distal radioulnar joint. Each originates from their respective sides of the sigmoid notch and converges on the ulnar fovea [3, 6–10]. Additionally, some fibers insert on the ulnar

styloid as well. The PRU ligament and DRU ligaments leave an opening between them centrally that is named the triangular fibrocartilage. The PRU ligament, DRU ligament, and triangular fibrocartilage collectively make up the triangular fibrocartilage complex (TFCC) [3, 6–10].

PRU as Proximal Attachment of UL and UT

The palmar radioulnar ligament is of particular interest in this chapter as it makes up the proximal attachment of the UT ligament and ulnolunate (UL) ligament (see Fig. 8.1). Although these two ligaments have similar origins, the only way to distinguish them is by their insertions, as there is no clearly discernable demarcation seen arthroscopically [3]. The UT ligament lies ulnar to the UL ligament proximally and inserts at the palmar and ulnar aspect of the triquetrum. It inserts dorsal to the palmar lunotriquetral ligament (LT), which is the distal portion of the palmar radiotriquetral ligament [11]. Conversely, the UL ligament inserts on the palmar aspect of the lunate, allowing for distinction from the UT ligament.

UT Ligament

Although the UT ligament is described as one ligament, arthroscopically, it often contains two perforations. The prestyloid recess (PR) perforation is found just ulnar to the union between the proximal radioulnar ligament and the UT ligament. The pisotriquetral orifice is anterior to the proximal articular surface of the triquetrum and just distal to the prestyloid recess [3, 6–10].

UC Ligament

Another ligament that is important to understand when diagnosing UT ligament split tears is the ulnocapitate (UC) ligament, given its proximity. The UC ligament does not arise from the PRU ligament but instead arises from the fovea of the ulna superficially [3]. The UC ligament then travels distally, palmar to the UT and UL ligaments where it reinforces the palmar LT. Distal to this, it continues and eventually

N. Munaretto · S. Kakar (✉)
Department of Orthopedic Surgery, Mayo Clinic,
Rochester, MN, USA
e-mail: kakar.sanjeev@mayo.edu

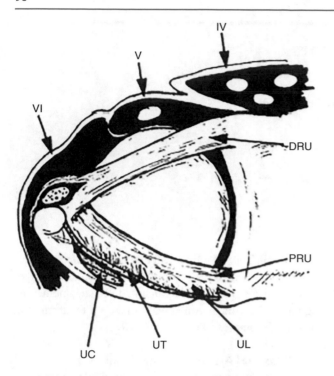

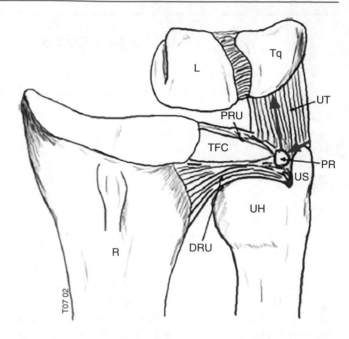

Fig. 8.1 As seen from a distal perspective, the DRU ligament splits to form the ECU subsheath, which is deep to the sixth extensor compartment (VI). The PRU ligament provides the origin for the ulnolunate (UL) and ulnotriquetral (UT) ligaments. The ulnocapitate (UC) ligament, however, is more superficial and has a direct bony attachment to the fovea of the ulnar head. (Reprinted from Tay et al. [3], Fig. 1. With permission from Elsevier)

Fig. 8.2 A representative image showing the likely mechanism for UT split tear propagation. The ulnar styloid fibers likely detach first (horizontal red arrow) and then the ligament injury propagates along the path of weakness between the PR and pisotriquetral orifice (vertical red arrow). (Reprinted from Tay et al. [3], Fig. 3. With permission from Elsevier)

becomes confluent with the radioscaphocapitate ligament at the midcarpal joint [3].

Ligament Biomechanics and Injury Mechanism

Biomechanical studies of the UT ligament by Moritomo and DiTano et al. suggest that the UT ligament is at maximal stretch and tension when the wrist is in maximal extension, radial deviation, and supination [12, 13]. Additionally, the authors concluded that an axial load or forearm rotation applied to the wrist when it is in this position can cause a UT ligament split tear. This biomechanical study was consistent with a retrospective study by Berger that showed that 96% of patients that reported a history of trauma with a UT ligament split tear reported that the wrist was in wrist extension and forearm supination during the inciting trauma [3]. Berger hypothesized that the UT ligament may tear in a split fashion due to a proposed longitudinal zone of weakness between the two perforations of the ligament. Additionally, Berger felt that the ulnar styloid attachment may fail before the foveal attachment, causing a split tear in the ligament (Fig. 8.2).

Diagnosis

Introduction

Split tears of the UT ligament can be difficult to diagnose. A combination of history, physical examination, imaging, and, in some situations, diagnostic arthroscopy should be utilized to diagnose this injury effectively. Brogan et al. and Kakar and Garcia-Elias noted the importance of recognizing the myriad of pathologies that need to be considered when managing ulnar wrist pain as these tend not to be mutually exclusive. These include but are not exhaustive of foveal avulsions of the TFCC, peripheral tears of the TFCC, extensor carpi ulnaris subsheath tears, lunotriquetral ligament injuries, UT ligament injuries, and ulnar styloid impaction [1–3, 14–18].

History

Patient Profile/Demographics

In a retrospective review of 96 patients by Clark et al. studying patients with UT ligament inter-substance split tears, the average patient age was 38 years old at time of injury. The dominant extremity was involved in 51% of cases, and 28% of patients had previous surgery for their ulnar-sided wrist pain [2].

Although a UT ligament split tear can be an isolated diagnosis in patients, it often can be associated with other ulnar-sided pathologies. Clark et al. noted that UT ligament split tear was the lone diagnosis in 74 out of 96 wrists. However, UT ligament tear and TFCC tear was observed in 10 wrists, UT ligament tear and ECU pathology in 5 wrists, UT ligament tear and ganglion cyst in 3 wrists, UT ligament tear and scapholunate (SL) ligament tear in 3 wrists, and 1 wrist also had ulnar impaction. Additionally, 48% reported a traumatic event leading to diagnosis of UT split tear [2].

Berger et al. showed that all patients with a UT split tear had a chief complaint of ulnar-sided wrist pain with average duration of symptoms being 14.9 months. All patients reported worsening of pain with gripping and most (80%) had worsening with pronosupination of the forearm [3].

Physical Exam

Given the myriad of possible diagnoses when evaluating a patient with ulnar-sided wrist pain as a chief complaint, a complete wrist examination should be completed [5]. The senior author begins by evaluating the specific site of ulnar-sided wrist pain by asking the patient to use a finger to point to the area of maximal tenderness. Next, the wrist is palpated by the examiner. This is a deliberate and thorough process where the myriad of disorders that can cause ulnar wrist pain are ruled in or out. Range of motion should be recorded in wrist flexion, extension, radial and ulnar deviation, and pronation and supination. Grip strength should be recorded as well. Berger et al. noted that wrist range of motion should be normal in isolated UT ligament split tears and if motion is found to be abnormal, another diagnosis may be more likely, such as DRUJ pathology [3, 19].

Aside from a comprehensive wrist examination, the most important physical exam test for diagnosing split tears of the UT ligament is the "ulnar fovea sign," described and validated by Tay and colleagues [3, 19]. Performing the ulnar fovea sign requires knowledge of the surface anatomy of the ulnar side of the wrist. First, the examiner should palpate the ulnar styloid process with the forearm in neutral rotation and next palpate the flexor carpi ulnaris (FCU). The ulnar fovea lies between the ulnar styloid and the FCU. Proximally, this space is bordered by the ulnar head and distally is bordered by the pisiform bone.

In order to elicit the presence or absence of tenderness in the ulnar fovea, the examiner must properly position the patient. The examiner should sit opposite of the patient's elbow, supporting the patient's hand with the elbow relaxed and in 90° of flexion with the wrist in neutral rotation. While supporting the wrist, the examiner presses his/her thumb tip into the fovea as described above (Fig. 8.3). The ulnar fovea sign is positive when there is tenderness compared to the

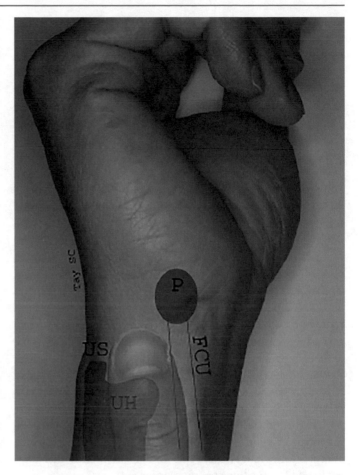

Fig. 8.3 With the forearm in neutral rotation, the fovea region is bound dorsally by the ulnar styloid, proximally by the curved surface of the ulnar head (UH), volarly by the flexor carpi ulnaris (FCU) tendon, and distally by the pisiform (P). The semitransparent thumb tip of the examiner is shown pressing into the fovea region. (Reprinted from Tay et al. [3], Fig. 4. With permission from Elsevier)

opposite side and should replicate the patients' ulnar-sided wrist pain [3, 19]. Additionally, the sign is less useful in patients with global wrist pain, as this then becomes nonspecific.

Once a positive ulnar fovea sign is elicited, it is critical to determine DRUJ stability. If the DRUJ is stable, split tear of the UT ligament is suspected. If the DRUJ is unstable, a foveal avulsion of the TFCC may be more likely [3, 19].

A validation study by Tay et al. showed that the ulnar fovea sign has a sensitivity of 95.2% and specificity of 87% for detecting foveal disruptions and/or UT ligament injuries. The ulnar fovea sign was 90% sensitive and 88% specific for UT split tears in patients with a stable DRUJ [3, 19].

Imaging

Although X-rays are often used when evaluating patients for UT split tears, they are generally used to exclude underlying bony pathology.

MRI is often useful in the diagnosis of underlying pathology associated with ulnar-sided wrist pain, such as with tears of the TFCC. However, the utility of MRI in diagnosing split tears of the UT ligament is debatable. One study demonstrated that signal change consistent with fluid accumulation in the UT ligament substance, the foveal insertion of the TFCC or in both structures may represent a UT split tear. However, this study failed to find any specific MRI findings to be used to definitively diagnose UT split tears [20].

In a study by Ringler et al., 40 patients with arthroscopically proven longitudinal UT ligament tears and 20 patients with intact UT ligaments were retrospectively evaluated in a blinded fashion for preoperative 3T MRI findings [21]. The authors utilized two musculoskeletal radiologists who were blinded to the surgical results and clinical information to review MRIs for UT split tears along with other pathologies. The overall sensitivity for definitive UT split tear detection on MRI was 58% for the first radiologist and 30% for the second radiologist. Specificity was 60% for both. There were no statistically significant discriminatory findings. Therefore, the authors concluded that 3T MRI had poor sensitivity and specificity for detecting split tears of the UT ligament. They felt that MRI may be more helpful for excluding other potential diagnoses [21]. See Fig. 8.4 for an MRI image of a UT split tear.

Ultrasound (US) may be a possible alternative to MRI in diagnosis of split tears of the UT ligament. However, to the author's knowledge, there are no specific studies that have evaluated US for this specific purpose.

Arthroscopy

Wrist arthroscopy remains the gold standard for diagnosis of split tears of the UT ligament. In order to diagnose UT split tears using wrist arthroscopy, an arthroscope is placed in the 3–4 viewing portal. The area between the prestyloid recess

and the pisotriquetral joint is examined. Proliferative synovial villi will often be observed in this space. After debridement of these villi, the UT ligament will be visible, allowing diagnosis of UT ligament longitudinal split tears. The intact fibers of the UT ligament will be observed on either side of the longitudinal tear. External pressure at the ulnar fovea, as in the ulnar fovea sign, can help to confirm correct location of the injury [3]. See Figs. 8.5 and 8.6.

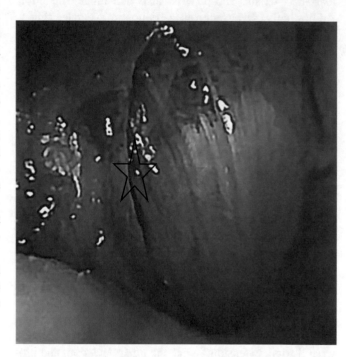

Fig. 8.5 Arthroscopic image demonstrating a UT split tear (asterisk)

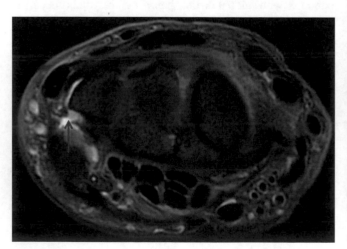

Fig. 8.4 Axial image of a right wrist showing a UT split tear (arrow) with associated edema

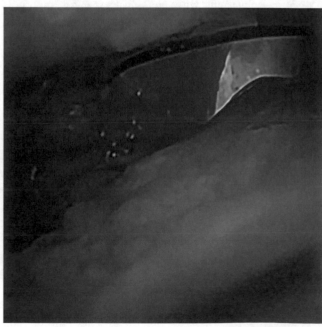

Fig. 8.6 Arthroscopic image showing placement of a PDS suture

Indications

- Treatment of a UT ligament split tear is indicated in a symptomatic patient who demonstrates a history, physical exam, and/or imaging that is consistent with this as a pain generator.
- A patient with ulnar-sided wrist pain who has a positive foveal sign on exam and a stable DRUJ should have a UT ligament split tear on the differential. Next, advanced imaging can be used to rule out other pathologies but can be unreliable for definitive diagnosis. Diagnostic arthroscopy is the gold standard and next step for definitive diagnosis.
- Furthermore, if there is a patient with a positive foveal sign and unstable DRUJ, UT split tear cannot be fully ruled out, as the patient may have concomitant TFCC disruption and UT split tear. As such, multiple pathologies can make definitive UT ligament split tear diagnosis difficult. Nonetheless, if a UT split tear is diagnosed during arthroscopy at the time of treatment of another ulnar-sided pathology, the authors advocate for UT ligament split tear repair given the low morbidity and promising clinical results of the procedure [2, 3]. Of note, clinical outcomes of UT split tear repair in all patients versus UT split tear repair with concomitant other pathology treatment did not show any significant difference [2].

Contraindications

- If the patient's history, pain location, exam, and imaging are not consistent with UT ligament split tear, other pathologies must be considered.
- The physician needs to decipher between a UT ligament split tear versus an avulsion of the UT ligament off the triquetrum, as the latter is treated by a different approach.
- Other generic contraindications to surgery include an active infection, medical comorbidities precluding surgery, etc.

Technique

The patient is positioned supine on a normal operating room table and hand table under general or regional anesthesia. Non-sterile tourniquet can be utilized intraoperatively for hemostasis. The hand is suspended in a well-padded arthroscopy tower and wrist arthroscopy can be performed using either a 1.9-mm or 2.7-mm arthroscope using the 3–4 and 6R portals. Midcarpal portals can be used if treating other concomitant pathologies such as carpal instabilities [2, 3]. We tend to perform dry wrist arthroscopy using the automated washout technique [22–24].

As part of the standard diagnostic arthroscopy, the integrity of the TFCC should be assessed centrally with a probe and assessment of the trampoline sign [25]. The TFCC foveal attachments (DRU and PRU) are evaluated by hooking the TFCC with a probe at the prestyloid recess and looking for distal laxity/displacement [26, 27]. The "suction test" is also performed to evaluate the tension of the TFCC [28]. Additionally, any synovitis overlying the UT ligament should be debrided to determine if an underlying UT ligament split tear exists. The UT ligament can be repaired using the following "outside inside technique" [2, 3].

A 3-cm longitudinal incision is made from ulnar styloid to the hamate, just anterior to the ECU tendon. The dorsal sensory branches of the ulnar nerve are identified and protected using a vessel loop. The UT ligament split tear is identified and repaired using 2-0 polydioxanone suture (PDS) placed in a horizontal mattress fashion. This is completed with the help of the Meniscus Mender II suture system in a standard outside-to-inside technique. Once the traction has been released, the sutures are pulled tight and tied, thereby repairing the split tear. At the conclusion of the procedure, the arthroscopic instruments are removed, excess fluid expressed, and wounds closed [2, 3].

Tips and Tricks

It is critical to rule out associated DRUJ instability at the time of surgery by performing an examination under anesthesia if this is clinically suspected.

The above technique applies when there is a longitudinal split tear of the UT ligament as compared to when the UT ligament avulses of the triquetrum which may require an open approach and anchor repair.

Postoperative Care

After operative intervention, the patient is placed in a sugar tong splint in neutral rotation. Typically, 2 weeks later, sutures are removed and the patient is placed into a Muenster cast in neutral forearm rotation for an additional 4 weeks. After this, the cast is removed and a Muenster splint is fabricated by hand therapy and worn for an additional 6 weeks in combination with a formalized UT split tear hand therapy program.

The formalized hand therapy program is as follows:

Conservative Management: Therapy

0–6 Weeks

- A Muenster orthosis is fabricated with the elbow at 90° of flexion and forearm in neutral. They are encouraged to work on scapulothoracic strengthening and conditioning exercises with their hand therapist.

6–12 Weeks

- The patient comes out of the Muenster splint and starts working on active pronation and supination. When the patient is able to achieve 45/45 of active supination/pronation in a consistent, pain-free arc, they are transitioned to a removable wrist support.
- Assuming the patient is relatively pain-free, progressive strengthening and dynamic proprioceptive exercises to the hand and wrist can be initiated while incorporating scapulothoracic, arm, and forearm strengthening and conditioning.

Surgical Management: Therapy

6 Weeks Postoperative

- Postoperative cast is removed and fabrication of a Muenster orthosis: elbow at 90°, wrist included, and forearm in a neutral position.

Therapy with a certified hand therapist is initiated at 6 weeks following surgery with the following exercises:

- Scar massage: 2–3 minutes, 3×/day.
- Passive and active motion of the elbow.
- Scapulothoracic and arm strengthening and conditioning exercises are initiated with the hand therapist.
- Active range of motion of the wrist and forearm: wrist flexion/extension/RD/UD/supination/ pronation.
- Exercises completed 10 repetitions, 3–5×/day.
- Patients are also taught wrist proprioceptive exercises.
  - Able to discharge the Muenster orthosis and wean to a volar wrist support when the patient is able to complete 45° of active supination and 45° of active pronation comfortably (typically will take 3–6 weeks.) If the patient does not achieve 45° of pronation and supination 10 weeks after surgery, may transition to a volar wrist support.
  - If the patient already has 45/45° active range of motion pronation/supination, the patient should wear the Muenster orthosis for a minimum of 2 weeks.
  - Patient can begin passive motion to the wrist and forearm approximately 10–12 weeks following surgery assuming they are pain-free. Typically, we let the patients advance as they tolerate rather than working on passive range of motion assuming they are not too stiff.
  - Begin strengthening once 90% of ROM returns.
  - Once 90% of motion has returned and 80% grip strength, patients are started on a sports-specific rehabilitation program.

Overall Therapy Note While the patient is immobilized in a sugar tong splint and then a Muenster cast/orthosis, they work with therapy on scapulothoracic stabilization, strengthening, and postural control. In addition, strengthening and conditioning exercises are performed on the shoulder and arm as tolerated.

Clinical Outcomes

Clinical outcomes after UT split tear repair have shown excellent outcomes in recent series. Clark et al. demonstrated a significant improvement in grip strength, pain scores, and Mayo wrist scores postoperatively compared to before surgery [2]. Forty-nine percent of patients had complete pain resolution and 87% experienced pain relief. Range of motion was unaffected postoperatively in the study. Clinical outcomes for short-term (6 months to 2 years) vs mid-term (>2 years) follow-up showed no statistically significant difference.

Surgical complications associated with UT split tear repair occurred in 8% of cases (8 of 96 wrists) [2]. Of these, recurrent pain was found in 3% (3 of 96), dysesthesia of the dorsal sensory branch of the ulnar nerve in 4% (4 of 96), and superficial infection in one case. All cases of dorsal sensory ulnar nerve dysesthesia fully resolved without further intervention in this series [2]. Finally, in the cohort, 5% (5 of 96 wrists) underwent revision operations that included revision for recurrent tear (2), ulnar shortening osteotomy (1), scar revision (1), and prominent suture removal (1).

Conclusion

UT ligament split tear diagnosis and treatment can be difficult given the complex and overlapping anatomy associated with ulnar-sided wrist pain. However, utilizing a combination of history, physical examination, and imaging in a systematic fashion can lead to a successful outcome.

In any patient with a positive ulnar fovea test, the stability of the DRUJ should be tested. If the DRUJ is unstable, a foveal tear of the TFCC should be suspected.

Although UT ligament split tear can be difficult to diagnose on MRI, this is the most useful adjunct (besides diagnostic arthroscopy) to rule out other pathologies and diagnose UT split tear.

If UT ligament split tear is highly suspected, and the patient failed nonoperative treatment, diagnostic arthroscopy is the gold standard for diagnosis and repair, if indicated.

As evidenced by recent studies, arthroscopic UT split tear repair can reliably improve pain and function for patients with ulnar-sided wrist pain with low complication and reoperation rate [2].

References

1. Shin AY, Deitch MA, Sachar K, Boyer MI. Ulnar-sided wrist pain: diagnosis and treatment. Instr Course Lect. 2005;54:115–28.
2. Clark NJ, Munaretto N, Ivanov D, Berger RA, Kakar S. Outcomes of ulnotriquetral split tear repair: a report of 96 patients. J Hand Surg Eur Vol. 2019:1753193419876066.
3. Tay SC, Berger RA, Parker WL. Longitudinal split tears of the ulnotriquetral ligament. Hand Clin. 2010;26(4):495–501.
4. Brogan DM, Berger RA, Kakar S. Ulnar-sided wrist pain: a critical analysis review. JBJS Rev. 2019;7(5):e1.
5. Kakar S, Garcia-Elias M. The "four-leaf clover" treatment algorithm: a practical approach to manage disorders of the distal radioulnar joint. J Hand Surg. 2016;41(4):551–64.
6. Berger RA. The ligaments of the wrist. A current overview of anatomy with considerations of their potential functions. Hand Clin. 1997;13(1):63–82.
7. Berger RA. The anatomy of the ligaments of the wrist and distal radioulnar joints. Clin Orthop Relat Res. 2001;383:32–40.
8. Haugstvedt JR, Berger RA, Nakamura T, Neale P, Berglund L, An KN. Relative contributions of the ulnar attachments of the triangular fibrocartilage complex to the dynamic stability of the distal radioulnar joint. J Hand Surg. 2006;31(3):445–51.
9. Haugstvedt JR, Langer MF, Berger RA. Distal radioulnar joint: functional anatomy, including pathomechanics. J Hand Surg Eur Vol. 2017;42(4):338–45.
10. Nakamura T, Yabe Y. Histological anatomy of the triangular fibrocartilage complex of the human wrist. Ann Anat = Anat Anz. 2000;182(6):567–72.
11. Ishii S, Palmer AK, Werner FW, Short WH, Fortino MD. An anatomic study of the ligamentous structure of the triangular fibrocartilage complex. J Hand Surg. 1998;23(6):977–85.
12. Moritomo H, Murase T, Arimitsu S, Oka K, Yoshikawa H, Sugamoto K. Change in the length of the ulnocarpal ligaments during radiocarpal motion: possible impact on triangular fibrocartilage complex foveal tears. J Hand Surg. 2008;33(8):1278–86.
13. DiTano O, Trumble TE, Tencer AF. Biomechanical function of the distal radioulnar and ulnocarpal wrist ligaments. J Hand Surg. 2003;28(4):622–7.
14. Rhee PC, Sauve PS, Lindau T, Shin AY. Examination of the wrist: ulnar-sided wrist pain due to ligamentous injury. J Hand Surg. 2014;39(9):1859–62.
15. Sachar K. Ulnar-sided wrist pain: evaluation and treatment of triangular fibrocartilage complex tears, ulnocarpal impaction syndrome, and lunotriquetral ligament tears. J Hand Surg. 2012;37(7):1489–500.
16. Yamabe E, Nakamura T, Pham P, Yoshioka H. The athlete's wrist: ulnar-sided pain. Semin Musculoskeletal Radiol. 2012;16(4):331–7.
17. Nakamura R. Diagnosis of ulnar wrist pain. Nagoya J Med Sci. 2001;64(3–4):81–91.
18. Tang CQY, Lai SWH, Leow G, Tay SC. Patient-reported outcome following ulnotriquetral ligament Split tear repair. J Hand Surg Asian Pacific Vol. 2017;22(4):445–51.
19. Tay SC, Tomita K, Berger RA. The "ulnar fovea sign" for defining ulnar wrist pain: an analysis of sensitivity and specificity. J Hand Surg. 2007;32(4):438–44.
20. Anderson ML, Skinner JA, Felmlee JP, Berger RA, Amrami KK. Diagnostic comparison of 1.5 Tesla and 3.0 Tesla preoperative MRI of the wrist in patients with ulnar-sided wrist pain. J Hand Surg. 2008;33(7):1153–9.
21. Ringler MD, Howe BM, Amrami KK, Hagen CE, Berger RA. Utility of magnetic resonance imaging for detection of longitudinal split tear of the ulnotriquetral ligament. J Hand Surg. 2013;38(9):1723–7.
22. Atzei A, Luchetti R, Sgarbossa A, Carita E, Llusa M. Set-up, portals and normal exploration in wrist arthroscopy. Chir Main. 2006;25(Suppl 1):S131–44.
23. del Pinal F, Garcia-Bernal FJ, Pisani D, Regalado J, Ayala H, Studer A. Dry arthroscopy of the wrist: surgical technique. J Hand Surg. 2007;32(1):119–23.
24. Kakar S, Burnier M, Atzei A, Ho PC, Herzberg G, Del Pinal F. Dry wrist arthroscopy for radial-sided wrist disorders. J Hand Surg. 2020;45(4):341–53.
25. Hermansdorfer JD, Kleinman WB. Management of chronic peripheral tears of the triangular fibrocartilage complex. J Hand Surg. 1991;16(2):340–6.
26. Atzei A, Luchetti R. Foveal TFCC tear classification and treatment. Hand Clin. 2011;27(3):263–72.
27. Ruch DS, Yang CC, Smith BP. Results of acute arthroscopically repaired triangular fibrocartilage complex injuries associated with intra-articular distal radius fractures. Arthroscopy. 2003;19(5):511–6.
28. Greene RM, Kakar S. The suction test: a novel technique to identify and verify successful repair of peripheral triangular fibrocartilage complex tears. J Wrist Surg. 2017;6(4):334–5.

Management of Type 1D Tears

Fernando Corella, Miguel Del Cerro,
and Montserrat Ocampos

Anatomy of the TFCC

The so-called triangular fibrocartilage complex (TFCC) is an anatomical structure which is fundamental for the stability of the distal radioulnar joint (DRUJ). It is denominated "complex" as it is not a single anatomical structure, but various. The first author to define the term was Palmer in the year 1989 [1]. Since then, it has been understood that the TFCC is formed by an articular disk, the radioulnar ligaments (RUL) dorsal (DRUL) and volar (VRUL), the meniscus homologue, the ulnar collateral ligament, the ulnocarpal ligaments, and the tendon sheath of the extensor carpi ulnaris tendon (ECU) (Fig. 9.1).

The articular disk is a triangular meniscus-shaped structure. It is thinner in its central portion and widens out in the more dorsal and palmar part, where it becomes to dorsal and volar radioulnar ligaments. Histologically speaking, in the union with the radius there exists a reinforcement of short collagenous fibers, oriented radially, with an extension of 1–2 mm, while the fibers of the rest of the disk have a greater tendency toward intertwining and are less organized. The area of the union of the short fibers with the rest of the articular disk is where the type 1D tear commonly takes place [2].

The radioulnar ligaments stabilize the DRUJ joint. Ishii, in his anatomical study [3], shows how they have both a superficial and deep layer. The deep portion, called subcruentum ligament, is inserted in the fovea of the ulna, whereas the superficial part envelops the articular disk and becomes united to it in the more ulnar part. Nowadays it is known that the deeper part has greater importance in maintaining the stability of the distal radioulnar joint [4, 5].

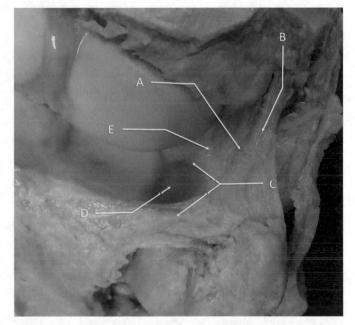

Fig. 9.1 (A) Meniscus homologue. (B) Ulnar collateral ligament. (C) Radioulnar ligaments. (D) Articular disk. (E) Ulnocarpal ligaments

The so-called meniscus homologue refers to the tissue, which is to be found between the superficial insertion of the radioulnar ligaments and the articular capsule [3]. In a certain anatomical study, it has been postulated that it consists of the remains of a large apophysis of the ulnar styloid which, in primates, is joined to the pisiform and pyramidal [6].

The ulnar collateral ligament is a thick structure, which is inserted proximally into the base of the ulnar styloid and distally in the pisiform and triquetrum. It is in close contact with the ECU and distally its fibers converge with the meniscus homologue [7].

The last structure that forms the TFCC is the tendon sheath of the ECU. It is connected to the head of the ulna and the ulnar fovea by means of Sharpey fibers.

From a didactic viewpoint, the TFCC has been compared to a tridimensional structure with two walls and a floor. The

F. Corella (✉) · M. Ocampos
Orthopedic and Trauma Department, Hospital Universitario Infanta Leonor, Madrid, Spain

Hand Surgery Unit, Hospital Universitario Quironsalud Madrid, Madrid, Spain

M. Del Cerro
Hand Surgery Unit, Hospital Beata María Ana, Madrid, Spain

© Springer Nature Switzerland AG 2022
W. B. Geissler (ed.), *Wrist and Elbow Arthroscopy with Selected Open Procedures*,
https://doi.org/10.1007/978-3-030-78881-0_9

floor of this structure would be the articular disk and the volar and dorsal radioulnar ligaments; the palmar wall would be formed by the ulnocarpal ligaments; and the dorsal wall would be formed by the tendon sheath of the ECU.

The integrity of the TFCC is fundamental for two functions. The first of these maintains the stability of the distal radioulnar joint that, as has already been commented, is carried out fundamentally by the radioulnar ligament [4, 5, 8]. The second function refers to the correct transmission of the load. It is known that approximately 20% of the wrist load is transferred through its ulnar border, that is to say, through the TFCC, so that any lesion may alter it [1].

Vascularization of the TFCC

The ulnar artery is that which gives greater blood supply to the TFCC, above all in its ulnar portion. The more radial part is irrigated by means of volar and dorsal branches of the anterior interosseous artery.

In histological studies, such as those carried out by Bednar [9] and Thiru [10], it has been seen that the blood vessels penetrate the TFCC from the periphery and can be observed only in an external 10–40% of their size. These vessels may be observed above all in the dorsal, ulnar, and palmar area of the TFCC. Thus, the "radial and central portion" is relatively avascular, unlike the volar radial and dorsal radial, that is to say, the radioulnar ligaments.

It has been considered that the central area, as it has lesser vascular supply, it lacks a healing capacity. But Cooney [11] in a series of 23 patients with peripheral tears of the radial margin treated by open surgery obtained good or excellent results in 80% of the cases. By the same token, he verified that 2 years after surgery, there still existed continuity of the reparation in four out of five patients.

That is, the fact that in histological studies the central area of the radial portion of the TFCC should not have a large number of vessels does not mean that the radioulnar ligaments do not have them and neither does it mean that the healing may not be obtained after a correct bone bed preparation for the anchoring. In the same way that a meniscal lesion of the knee is not sutured in the white–white area, in the TFCC, healing is not attained by suturing a tear of the most central part (1A lesion), but the healing can be attained of the "central radial" portion with the radius (this would be a red–white area) or of the radioulnar ligaments with the radius (it would be a red–red area).

Diagnosis

Physical Examination

Patients with a radial lesion usually recall a traumatic precedent, above all in a fall with the wrist in hyperextension and ulnar deviation or also a sharp twist of the wrist.

The patient complains of pain and swelling in the ulnar area of the wrist and discomfort with the movements of ulnar deviation and pronosupination. If the lesion is a significant one and involves radioulnar instability, the dorsal prominence of the ulna may be observed, but it should always be compared with the contralateral wrist in order not to confuse it with a hypermobile wrist.

There exist several exploration tests of the TFCC, but in our view, the most useful ones are the three following ones (Fig. 9.2).

Ulnar fovea sign [12]: With the elbow of the patient in a state of flexion, the thumb palpates the depression formed by the flexor carpi ulnaris, the ulnar styloid, the head of the ulna, and the pisiform. It may be regarded as positive when pain appears compared with the contralateral. It is one of the most

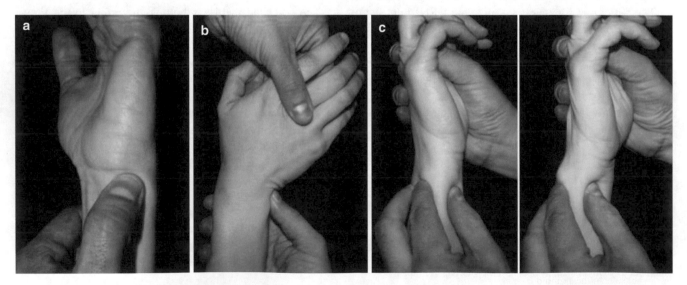

Fig. 9.2 (**a**) Ulnar fovea sign. (**b**) Ulnocarpal stress test. (**c**) Radioulnar instability exploration

important signs in this kind of pathology, as it has a very high sensitivity and specificity (95% and 87%, respectively).

Ulnocarpal stress test [13]: is carried out by the application of axial loading to the wrist in a state of maximal ulnar deviation while a movement of pronation and supination is applied. It is a very sensitive sign but not a very specific one as it can be positive in a number of pathologies that affect the ulnar region of the wrist.

Radioulnar instability [5]: In order to evaluate the stability of the distal radioulnar joint, the ulna is displaced with respect to the radius in an anteroposterior plane with the wrist in a neutral position, in supination and pronation. These maneuvers should be carried out in both the affected side and the contralateral one, because instability should not be confused with articular laxness.

Diagnostic Modalities

Tears in the TFCC are not detected by simple radiographic examination, but they can reveal indirect data, which may indicate the possibility of a lesion. Thus, lateral and oblique and AP projections are useful to diagnose the presence of fractures-avulsions of the sigmoid notch and DRUJ instability as, with a complete radial desinsertion, the space of this joint will increase.

Tricompartmental arthrography has been the standard method used for the diagnosis of lesions of the intra-articular ligaments of the wrist [14]. It consists of a contrast injection under radiological control in the radiocarpal joint, midcarpal, and DRUJ. In the presence of a radial tear, there appears an extravasation of the contrast.

With the development of new technical advances in magnetic resonance imaging (MRI), improvement has been achieved in the resolution and diagnosis of TFCC lesions; the former being the preferential technique of several authors [15, 16]. Arthro-MRI may add further information to the study and is shown to be superior to the standard MRI for the detection of complete tears of the TFCC [17].

The carrying out of helical computerized axial tomography (CT) together with arthrography combines the advantages of both techniques; the intra-articular structures and compartments remain distinctly defined in multiple planes. Thanks to this, the location of the tear may be determined with greater precision [18] and may be regarded as an alternative technique to that of arthro-MRI [19].

But without any shade of doubt, the "gold standard" in the diagnosis of 1D-type lesions of the TFCC is still arthroscopy of the wrist, as it allows a direct visualization of the tear, determines the location and lesion type, and detects other associated lesions.

Classification

In 1989, Palmer classified TFCC lesions into two large groups [1]. The first of these included traumatic lesions and he denominated them class 1, and the degenerative lesions class 2. Likewise, the traumatic lesions are subdivided according to their location, a central slit as 1A, ulnar tear as 1B, distal tear as 1C, and radial tear as 1D.

Radial tears are avulsions of the TFCC from the radial sigmoid notch and may or may not include bone fragments.

Although controversy exists as to what a 1D tear is and what it is not, one of the best classifications which define them is that of Nakamura [20] who subdivided the radial lesions of the TFCC into six groups (Fig. 9.3).

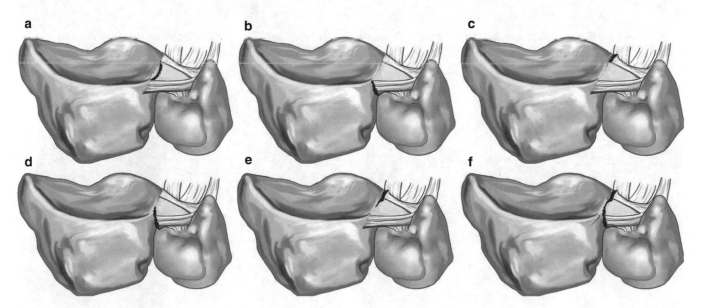

Fig. 9.3 (**a**) Fibrocartilage tear between the hyaline cartilage of the sigmoid notch of the radius and TFCC. (**b**) Dorsal edge tear between the dorsal edge of the sigmoid notch of the radius and dorsal portion of the radioulnar ligament. (**c**) Palmar edge tear between the palmar edge of the sigmoid notch of the radius and palmar portion of the radioulnar ligament. (**d**) Combination of (**a**) + (**b**). (**e**) Combination of (**a**) + (**c**). (**f**) Complete detachment of the TFCC from the sigmoid notch of the radius

(a) Fibrocartilage tear between the hyaline cartilage of the sigmoid notch of the radius and TFCC

(b) Dorsal edge tear between the dorsal edge of the sigmoid notch of the radius and dorsal portion of the radioulnar ligament

(c) Palmar edge tear between the palmar edge of the sigmoid notch of the radius and palmar portion of the radio-ulnar ligament

(d) Combination of (a) + (b)

(e) Combination of (a) + (c)

(f) Complete detachment of the TFCC from the sigmoid notch of the radius

As has already been seen, the stability of the DRUJ depends on the integrity of the radioulnar ligaments, and thus a type 1D-a may not be associated with DRUJ instability, whereas a type 1D-b–f can induce DRUJ instability.

Further doubt may exist with regard to differentiating a 1D-a lesion (radial lesion) from a 1A lesion (central lesion), as the only difference is a few millimeters of fibrocartilage tissue. In our view, the most important thing is to determine the treatment to be carried out rather than an evaluation as to whether a fibrocartilage tissue exists or not between the tear and the radius.

We would advocate a debridement of the portion of the fibrocartilage united to the radius and an evaluation as to whether the articular disk can be approximated to the radius without tension. If this is the case, the reattaching of the lesion would be carried out and we would denominate it 1D-a. If the disk cannot be approximated without tension, only the debridement would be carried out and the lesion would be classified as 1A (Fig. 9.4).

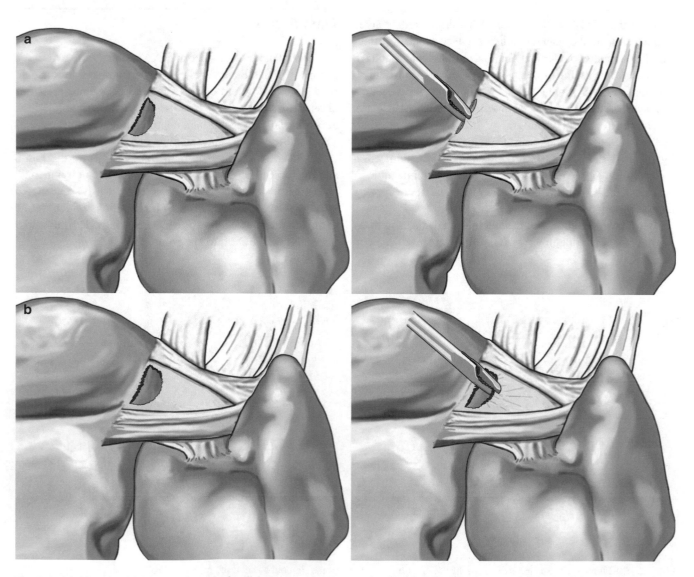

Fig. 9.4 (**a**) After the debridement the articular disk can be approximated without tension to the radius sigmoid notch. We would classify the lesion as 1D-a and the reattachment back down to the bone could be made. (**b**) After the debridement the articular disk cannot majorly be approximated without tension to the radius sigmoid notch. We would classify the lesion as 1A and only a debridement would be carried out

Treatment

Conservative Treatment

Treatment in the acute phase of lesions of the TFCC, not associated with clinical instability, includes immobilization for 3–4 weeks, nonsteroid anti-inflammatories, steroid injections, and physiotherapy.

Indication of Surgical Treatment

Both the failure of a conservative treatment, without improvement after 3 months, and the existence of associated distal radioulnar instability indicate the need for surgical treatment.

Surgical Treatment

Many classical papers advocate the treatment of most of the lesions of the TFCC by means of debridement or excision [21, 22]. This practice has been supported by a study, which concludes that the resectioning of at least two thirds of the articular disk does not influence in the DRUJ biomechanics [23]. However, in this study the peripheral margins of the TFCC were respected, that is to say, the radioulnar ligaments. More recent studies have highlighted the importance of the integrity of these ligaments in order to maintain DRUJ stability [4, 5]. This has increased the interest of many authors to repair the TFCC instead of a debridement.

In the case of radial side tears, there exists greater agreement on carrying out a repair when the radioulnar ligaments are affected. As we have seen supra, these ligaments are vascularized structures with potential healing. Greater doubt exists with regard to the repair of a central radial tear without affecting the radioulnar ligaments, but, as we have already mentioned, our view is that, if after the debridement the articular disk can be approximated without tension, we would advocate its repair back to the bone. With this reparation we believe that there may be avoided a possible progression toward the radioulnar ligaments.

One of the first open techniques described for the repair of the radial edge of the TFCC was described in 1994 by Clooney [11] who obtained good or excellent results in 80% of his patients. Since that time numerous arthroscopic techniques have been described:

Trumble [24, 25] used a meniscal suture system with two preloaded needles; the suture was knotted on the radial side of the radius. He obtained improvement in the range of motion up to 89% and grip strength up to 95% with respect to the contralateral side.

Sagerman and Short [26] described a similar technique, whose difference was based on the carrying out of three bone tunnels through which there passed the meniscal suture systems. The results were good or excellent in 8 out of 12 patients.

Plancher [27] described a technique in which a suture was also carried out by passing it through the radius. With the usage of an external guide, he managed to make two tunnels in the radius with a single outward opening in the sigmoid notch. A suture passer was used in an outside-inside way, and the threads were knotted on the radial side of the radius.

Fellinger [28] described the repair of tears of the radial side using the T-Fix Device® (Acufix). A single bone tunnel was made through which this system was passed in an outside-to-inside manner. Once the TFCC had been traversed, the "T" form anchorage was established, maintaining united the TFCC to its insertion zone.

Jantea [29] also used an external guide to create the tunnels. In one of them a spinal needle loaded with an absorbable monofilament was passed and in the other a suture retriever. The sutures were knotted on the dorsal side of the radius. Good results were obtained in 11 out of 12 patients.

Geissler [30] developed a new anchorage system with technology similar to the system of meniscal suture RAPIDLOC® (De Puy Mitek). Through two bone tunnels the system is introduced, the fibrocartilage is perforated, and the topHat is extended. It slides toward the radial region of the radius where the TFCC remains fixed.

All of these techniques require the use of bone tunnels which pierce the radius and through which the sutures are passed. With the development of new implants and instruments nowadays, the reattachment can be carried out arthroscopically without the necessity of carrying out bone tunnels or knots. The following explains the technique of making it.

Arthroscopic Knotless Radial-Side TFCC Repair

The portals that this technique requires are the dorsal 3/4, 6R, and 4/5 radiocarpal portals. The wrist is placed in the traction tower, applying 10 lb of traction. Firstly the 3/4 radiocarpal portal is performed, it is marked with an 18-gauge needle, the tip of a number 11 scalpel is introduced, and the portal is widened with a blunt dissector. Through this portal the arthroscope is introduced, the whole of the radiocarpal joint is inspected, and the TFCC is visualized.

The second portal that should be made is the 6R. As well as in the case of the 3/4 portal, an 18-gauge needle is introduced; on this occasion it is verified under arthroscopic control that it is located just above the TFCC, afterward the tip of the scalpel is introduced, and finally the portal is widened with a blunt dissector. By carrying out the portal under direct

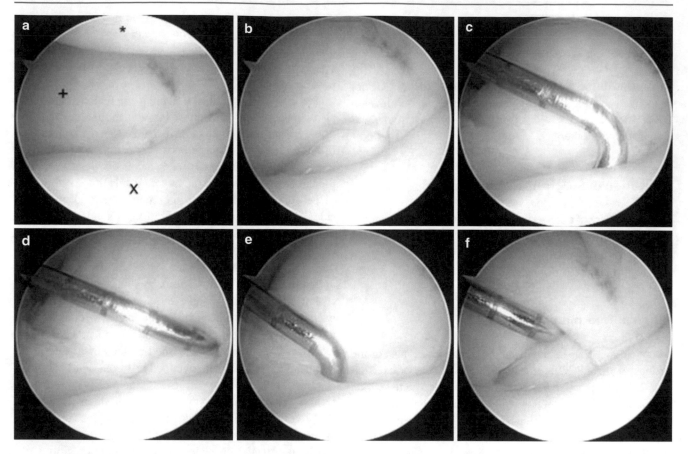

Fig. 9.5 (a) Ulnar compartment seen from the 3/4 portal (*Lunate, ⁺TFCC, ˣRadius). (b) Radial lesion of the TFCC. (c) Probe in the sigmoid notch. (d) The tear extends to the volar radioulnar ligament. (e) Integrity of the dorsal radioulnar ligament. (f) The ulnar head is seen under the radial lesion of the TFCC

visualization, it is not probable to cause lesion of the TFCC or the articular cartilage.

The probe is inserted through the 6-R portal, and the location and extension of the radial tear in the TFCC is evaluated. In order to be able to classify this type of lesion correctly, particular attention should be paid to its dorsal or palmar extension, that is to say, the injury of the dorsal and palmar radioulnar ligaments (Fig. 9.5).

If the lesion extends to the radioulnar ligaments, or if it is a central tear but as has already been commented, approximation to the sigmoid notch can be made without tension, the repair of the TFCC back down to the bone can be performed as follows.

In the same way as the reattached of a peripheral ulnar tear [31], this technique requires one visualization portal (the 3/4 portal) and two working portals. Instead of carrying out a 6R accessory portal as it is made in an ulnar tear, a 4/5 portal is performed. Given the radial location of the lesion, this portal will greatly facilitate the technique. The 4/5 portal may be made also under arthroscopic control, first it is located with an 18-gauge needle (Fig. 9.6), afterward incised with the scalpel, and finally dilation is made. In a cadaver study published by the authors of this chapter [32], it has been found that while performing the 4/5 portal, an injury of

the fifth extensor tendon could happen, and thus special care should be taken with it.

The TFCC SutureLasso 70°® (Arthrex, Naples, FL, USA) is introduced through the 6R portal. Its tip is situated just above the articular disk, penetrating from distally to proximally, coming out just below the tear. In order to penetrate easily the TFCC, a probe may be used to make counterpressure from the inferior side. The whole thickness of the TFCC is pierced through, and it can be verified how the tip of the SutureLasso appears between the inferior side of the disk and the ulnar head (Fig. 9.7).

The SutureLasso is loaded with a Fiber-Stick Suture® (Arthrex, Naples, FL, USA), which is a 2/0 Fiberwire suture with a more rigid end which facilitates its insertion in the passer. It is recovered with a Mini Suture Hook® (Naples, FL, USA) or a grasper through the 4/5 portal (Fig. 9.8).

Following this, the SutureLasso is withdrawn and, without removing it from the radiocarpal joint, it is reinserted a few millimeters from the first point and in the same distal and to proximal direction until it comes out below the TFCC. As the SutureLasso is still loaded with the Fiber-Stick, the suture is retrieved again through the 4/5 portal, and thus the horizontal mattress-type suture is complete (Fig. 9.9).

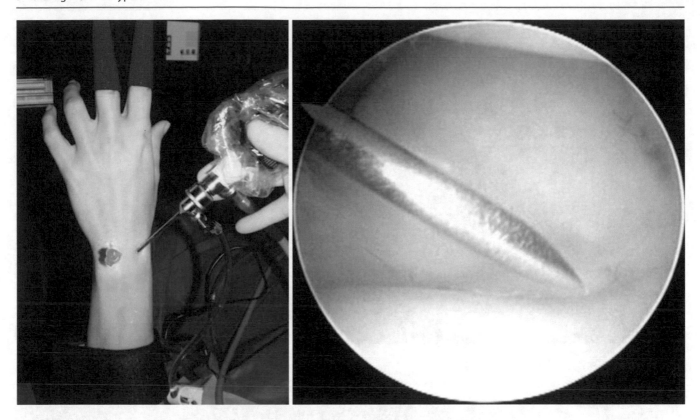

Fig. 9.6 Establishment of the working accessory portal; in this technique it would be the 4/5 portal

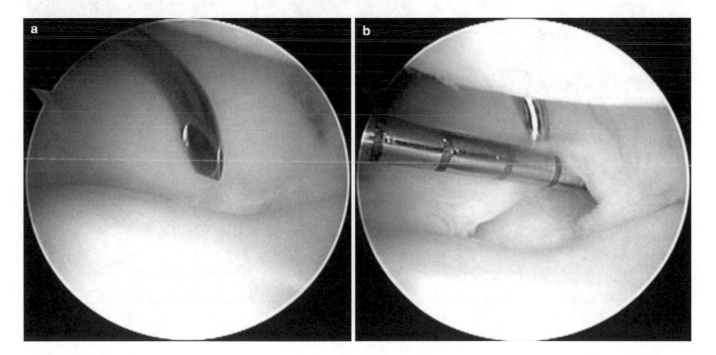

Fig. 9.7 (a) The TFCC SutureLasso 70° (Arthrex, Naples, FL, USA) is introduced through the 6R portal. (b, c) With the help of the probe, the whole thickness of the TFCC is pierced through. (d) The tip of the SutureLasso appears between the inferior side of the TFCC and the ulnar head

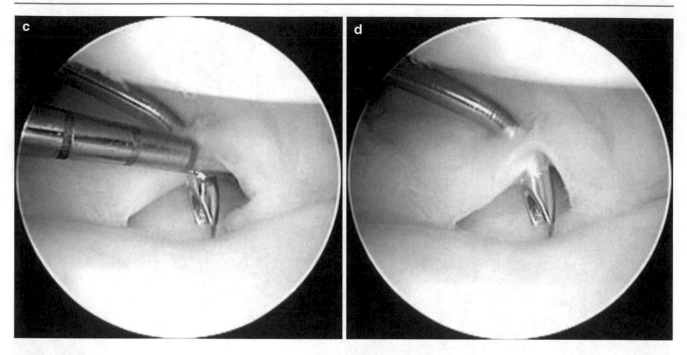

Fig. 9.7 (continued)

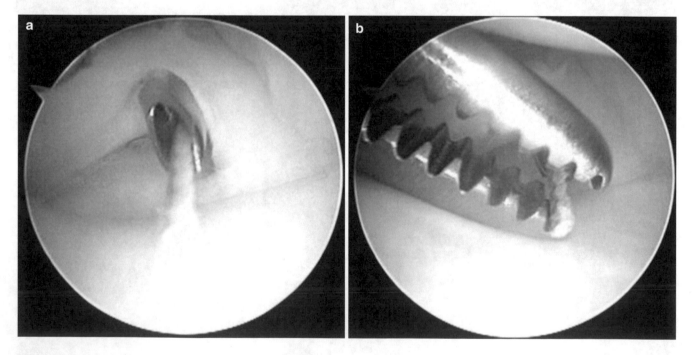

Fig. 9.8 (**a**) The SutureLasso is loaded with a Fiber-Stick suture (Arthrex, Naples, FL, USA). (**b–d**) It is retrieved to the 4/5 portal

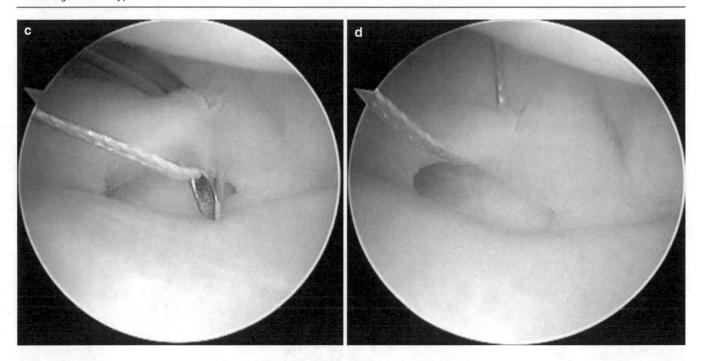

Fig. 9.8 (continued)

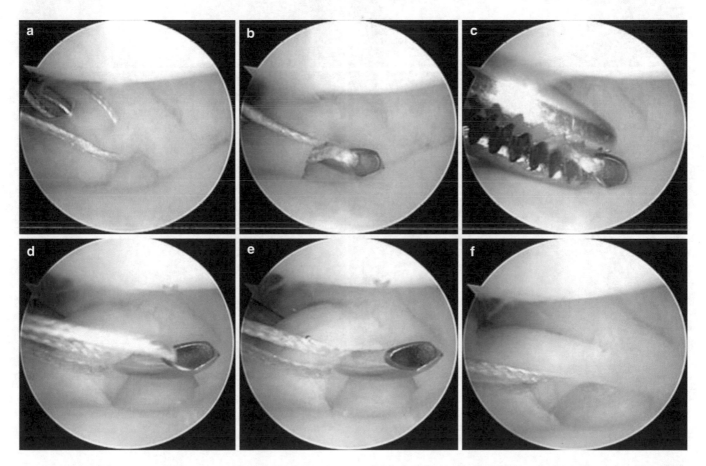

Fig. 9.9 (**a**) The SutureLasso is reinserted a few millimeters from the first point and in the same distal and to proximal direction. (**b**) It comes out again below the TFCC. (**c–e**) The Fiber-Stick suture is retrieved again to the 4/5 portal. (**f**) In this way, the horizontal mattress-type suture is complete, with the sutures coming out through the 4/5 portal

The SutureLasso is withdrawn, and the slotted cannula together with the obturator of the TFCC instrument Kit® (Arthrex, Naples, FL, USA) is inserted through the 6R portal, the obturator is withdrawn from the cannula, and the Mini Suture Hook is inserted to retrieve the two sutures from the 4/5 portal to the 6R portal (Fig. 9.10).

The threads are passed outside of the cannula through the slot in order that the drilling afterward should not break them. The obturator is then inserted into the cannula and is placed at the desire point of reattachment in the sigmoid notch of the radius. Through the obturator the guidewire of the kit is inserted into the radius. At this point it is useful to

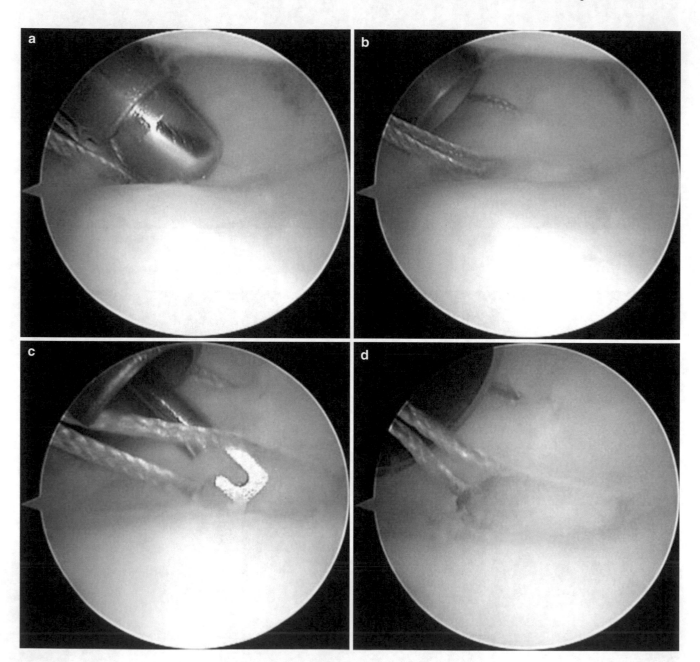

Fig. 9.10 (**a**) The slotted cannula together with the obturator of the TFCC instrument Kit (Arthrex, Naples, FL, USA) is inserted through the 6R portal. (**b**) The obturator is withdrawn from the cannula. (**c**) The Mini Suture Hook is inserted to recover the two sutures from the 4/5 portal to the 6R portal. (**d**) The two wires are retrieved from the cannula through the slot

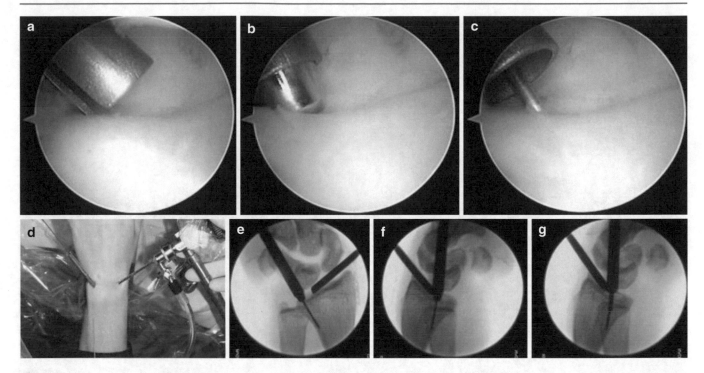

Fig. 9.11 (**a–d**) The Kirschner guidewire is placed through the obturator and inserted into the radius. (**e–g**) Fluoroscopy control to check the correct position of the guidewire and the drill

check under fluoroscopy in order to ascertain that the position is correct. The obturator is removed and the cannulated drill bit from the TFCC kit can be placed over the guidewire and drilled until the positive stop of the drill meets the cannula (Fig. 9.11).

On retrieving the cannulated drill and the guidewire, it is of paramount importance that the surgeon should maintain the cannula in the same direction in order not to lose the location of the tunnel. In order to do this, it is useful for one surgeon to hold only the arthroscope and the cannula and for the other one to carry out the fixation with a 2.5-mm PushLock Anchor® (Arthrex, Naples, FL, USA). The PushLock tip is positioned in the predrilled hole, and the suture tails can be tensioned by pulling on the suture and holding the PushLock anchor in place. The laser line of the PushLock should be advanced until flush with the bone, locking the anchor and suture in the predrilled hole (Fig. 9.12).

The sutures are cut and the tension is verified again (Fig. 9.13).

Conclusion

Two factors have conditioned the fact that many surgeons advocate the debridement of the radial lesions of the TFCC. The first one is considering the radial side of the TFCC as an avascular zone and the second one is the fact that the arthroscopic fixation techniques were very complex.

Nowadays, we know that the more dorsal and volar portion of the TFCC, that is to say, the radioulnar ligaments, are essential for maintaining adequate radioulnar stability. It is also known that these ligaments have an adequate blood supply, which allows its healing. For such motives, its repair back to bone is indicated. We also know that the more central and avascular portion can heal if a correct cruentation of the radius is performed and forms an adequate bed for the reattaching. For these reasons, we advocate the reinsertion of radial lesions (including the central ones) always provided that a correct tension can be attained.

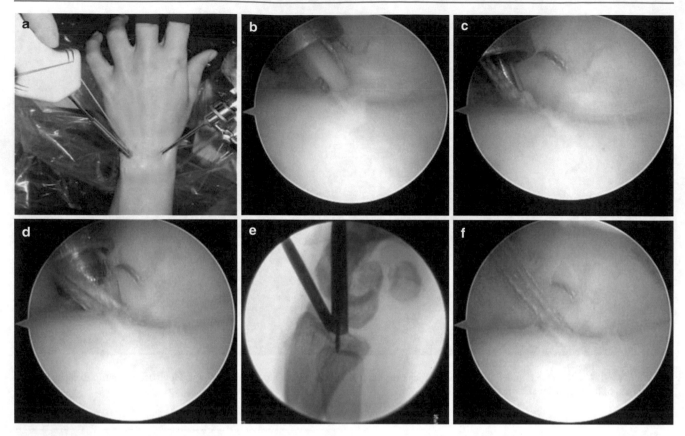

Fig. 9.12 (**a**) The 2.5-mm PushLock Anchor (Arthrex, Naples, FL, USA) and sutures are fed into the slotted cannula. (**b–d**) The 2.5-mm PushLock Anchor is introduced into the predrill hole in the sigmoid notch. (**e**) Fluoroscopy control. (**f**) The radial peripheral tear is repaired back to bone. The suture tails can now be cut flush with the disk

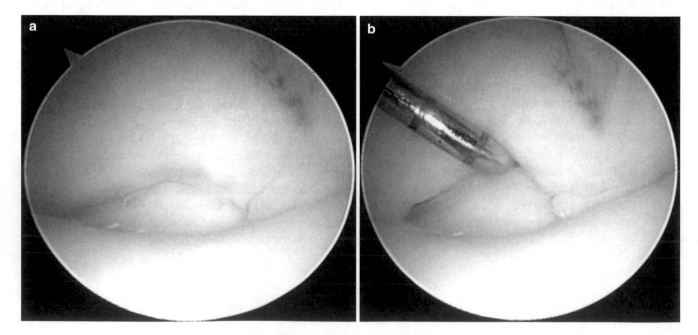

Fig. 9.13 (**a, b**) Initial aspect of the radial tear. (**c, d**) TFCC reattached to the sigmoid notch

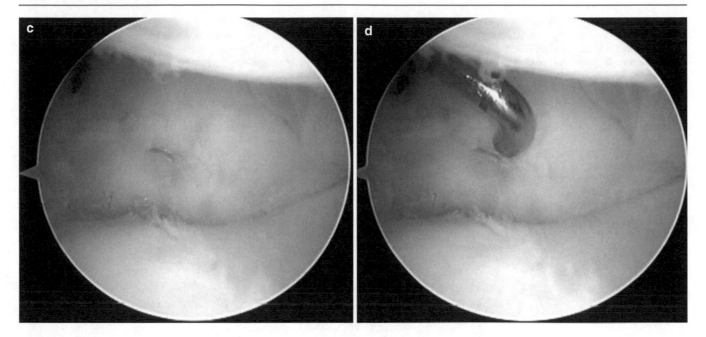

Fig. 9.13 (continued)

Advances in the development of surgical instruments have resulted in the technique for the reattaching of radial lesions presented in this chapter being simple to carry out through the 6R and 4/5 portals without the need of knots or bone tunnels through the radius.

References

1. Palmer AK. Triangular fibrocartilage complex lesions: a classification. J Hand Surg Am. 1989;14(4):594–606.
2. Chidgey LK, Dell PC, Bittar ES, Spanier SS. Histologic anatomy of the triangular fibrocartilage. J Hand Surg Am. 1991;16(6):1084–100.
3. Ishii S, Palmer AK, Werner FW, Short WH, Fortino MD. An anatomic study of the ligamentous structure of the triangular fibrocartilage complex. J Hand Surg Am. 1998;23(6):977–85.
4. Hagert E, Hagert CG. Understanding stability of the distal radioulnar joint through an understanding of its anatomy. Hand Clin. 2010;26(4):459–66.
5. Kleinman WB. Stability of the distal radioulna joint: biomechanics, pathophysiology, physical diagnosis, and restoration of function what we have learned in 25 years. J Hand Surg Am. 2007;32(7):1086–106.
6. Lewis OJ, Hamshere RJ, Bucknill TM. The anatomy of the wrist joint. J Anat. 1970;106(Pt 3):539–52.
7. Zancolli E, Cozzi EP. Atlas de anatomía quirúrgica de la mano. Médica Panamericana; 1993.
8. Haugstvedt JR, Berger RA, Berglund LJ, Neale PG, Sabick MB. An analysis of the constraint properties of the distal radioulnar ligament attachments to the ulna. J Hand Surg Am. 2002;27(1):61–7.
9. Bednar MS, Arnoczky SP, Weiland AJ. The microvasculature of the triangular fibrocartilage complex: its clinical significance. J Hand Surg Am. 1991;16(6):1101–5.
10. Thiru RG, Ferlic DC, Clayton ML, McClure DC. Arterial anatomy of the triangular fibrocartilage of the wrist and its surgical significance. J Hand Surg Am. 1986;11(2):258–63.
11. Cooney WP, Linscheid RL, Dobyns JH. Triangular fibrocartilage tears. J Hand Surg Am. 1994;19(1):143–54.
12. Tay SC, Tomita K, Berger RA. The "ulnar fovea sign" for defining ulnar wrist pain: an analysis of sensitivity and specificity. J Hand Surg Am. 2007;32(4):438–44.
13. Nakamura R, Horii E, Imaeda T, Nakao E, Kato H, Watanabe K. The ulnocarpal stress test in the diagnosis of ulnar-sided wrist pain. J Hand Surg Br. 1997;22(6):719–23.
14. Weiss AP, Akelman E, Lambiase R. Comparison of the findings of triple-injection cinearthrography of the wrist with those of arthroscopy. J Bone Joint Surg Am. 1996;78(3):348–56.
15. Anderson ML, Skinner JA, Felmlee JP, Berger RA, Amrami KK. Diagnostic comparison of 1.5 Tesla and 3.0 Tesla preoperative MRI of the wrist in patients with ulnar-sided wrist pain. J Hand Surg Am. 2008;33(7):1153–9.
16. Schweitzer ME, Brahme SK, Hodler J, Hanker GJ, Lynch TP, Flannigan BD, et al. Chronic wrist pain: spin-echo and short tau inversion recovery MR imaging and conventional and MR arthrography. Radiology. 1992;182(1):205–11.
17. Smith TO, Drew B, Toms AP, Jerosch-Herold C, Chojnowski AJ. Diagnostic accuracy of magnetic resonance imaging and magnetic resonance arthrography for triangular fibrocartilaginous complex injury: a systematic review and meta-analysis. J Bone Joint Surg Am. 2012;94(9):824–32.
18. Theumann N, Favarger N, Schnyder P, Meuli R. Wrist ligament injuries: value of post-arthrography computed tomography. Skelet Radiol. 2001;30(2):88–93.

19. Moser T, Khoury V, Harris PG, Bureau NJ, Cardinal E, Dosch JC. MDCT arthrography or MR arthrography for imaging the wrist joint? Semin Musculoskelet Radiol. 2009;13(1):39–54.

20. Nakamura T. Radial side tear of the triangular fibrocartilage complex. Arthroscopic management of distal radius fractures. Berlin, Heidelberg: Springer-Verlag; 2010.

21. Roth JH, Poehling GG, Whipple TL. Arthroscopic surgery of the wrist. Instr Course Lect. 1988;37:183–94.

22. Osterman AL. Arthroscopic debridement of triangular fibrocartilage complex tears. Arthroscopy. 1990;6(2):120–4.

23. Adams BD. Partial excision of the triangular fibrocartilage complex articular disk: a biomechanical study. J Hand Surg Am. 1993;18(2):334–40.

24. Trumble T. Radial side (1D) tears. Hand Clin. 2011;27(3):243–54.

25. Trumble TE, Gilbert M, Vedder N. Isolated tears of the triangular fibrocartilage: management by early arthroscopic repair. J Hand Surg Am. 1997;22(1):57–65.

26. Sagerman SD, Short W. Arthroscopic repair of radial-sided triangular fibrocartilage complex tears. Arthroscopy. 1996;12(3):339–42.

27. Plancher KD, Faber KJ. Arthroscopic repair of radial-sided triangular fibrocartilage complex lesions. Tech Hand Up Extrem Surg. 1999;3(1):44–51.

28. Fellinger M, Peicha G, Seibert FJ, Grechenig W. Radial avulsion of the triangular fibrocartilage complex in acute wrist trauma: a new technique for arthroscopic repair. Arthroscopy. 1997;13(3):370–4.

29. Jantea CL, Baltzer A, Ruther W. Arthroscopic repair of radial-sided lesions of the triangular fibrocartilage complex. Hand Clin. 1995;11(1):31–6.

30. Geissler W. Repair of peripheral radial TFCC tears. In: Wrist arthroscopy. New York: Springer; 2005. p. xiv, 201 p.

31. Geissler WB. Arthroscopic knotless peripheral ulnar-sided TFCC repair. Hand Clin. 2011;27(3):273–9.

32. Corella F, Ocampos M, Del Cerro M. Are extensor tendons safe on your first wrist arthroscopy? J Hand Surg Eur. 2011;36(9):817–8.

Management of Ulnar Impaction

10

Megan Anne Meislin and Randy Bindra

Introduction

The ulnocarpal joint bears a fifth of the loads transmitted across the wrist. Ulnocarpal impaction or ulnar abutment is chronic overloading of the distal ulnar head against the triangular fibrocartilage and the proximal lunate and proximal triquetrum. The condition is usually associated with positive ulnar variance; this dynamic or static overloading leads to degeneration of the central aspect of the TFCC, chondromalacia of the proximal lunate, proximal triquetrum and distal ulnar head, perforation of the lunotriquetral ligament, and ultimately ulnocarpal arthritis.

Pathogenesis

The triangular fibrocartilagenous complex (TFCC) consists of the articular disk, palmar radioulnar ligament, dorsal radioulnar ligament, extensor carpi ulnaris and its subsheath, ulnar capsule, ulnolunate, and ulnotriquetral ligaments. Ulnar abutment is caused by increased loading through the TFCC creating a central perforation through the avascular articular disk that advances to degenerative changes to bony and ligamentous connections of the ulnocarpal joint. While ulnar abutment can occur in neutral and negative ulnar variance, it is more commonly attributed to wrists with positive ulnar variance. This may be a congenital anomaly or can result from injury or other pathologic processes that cause relative shortening of the radius. In patients with neutral variance, positive ulnar variance may be a dynamic phenomenon seen with forceful gripping. The increase in ulnar length facilitates a shift in load transfer through the wrist. Palmer showed that with neutral variance, the load across the wrist joint is born 82% by the radius and 18% by the ulna [1]. However, if the ulnar variance is increased by 2.5 mm, the ulnocarpal loading is increased by 42% [1]. A cadaveric study showed 73% of ulnar-positive wrists had TFCC perforations while only 17% of ulnar negative had perforations [2]. In addition, ulnar positive wrists have been shown to have thinner articular disks creating less mitigation of ulnocarpal loading when compared to an ulnar neutral or negative wrist [3]. There is a strong association between age and degenerative tears with only 7% seen by the third decade and 53% by age 60 suggesting that relationship of the radius and ulna changes with age [4].

Ulnar variance can be congenital or acquired. Isolated congenital positive ulnar variance from birth is frequently seen; however, it is important to get a detailed history so that clues of acquired positive ulnar variance can be identified. Previous injuries like distal radius fractures with malunion, radial shortening, Essex-Lopresti injury, an acute or chronic physeal injury to the radius, and developmental conditions such as Madelung's deformity can cause positive ulnar variance [5]. Besides shortening of the distal radius, change in dorsal tilt of the distal radius can also dramatically increase the ulnar loads from 20% to as much as 65% with dorsal tilt of 40° [6].

Ulnar variance is a dynamic phenomenon. As the axis of forearm rotation runs obliquely from the radial head to the ulnar fovea, there is a relative lengthening of the ulna as it rotates about the radius. Additionally, loading the wrist by gripping can further narrow the ulnocarpal relationship.

Stages

Ulnar abutment is chronic overloading of the ulnocarpal joint that leads to a predictable pattern of degeneration of the ulnocarpal joint. Initially the central horizontal portion of the

M. A. Meislin (✉)
Department of Orthopaedic Surgery, Loyola University Medical Center, Maywood, IL, USA

R. Bindra
Department of Orthopaedic Surgery, Griffith University School of Medicine, Gold Coast University Hospital, Southport, QLD, Australia

© Springer Nature Switzerland AG 2022
W. B. Geissler (ed.), *Wrist and Elbow Arthroscopy with Selected Open Procedures*,
https://doi.org/10.1007/978-3-030-78881-0_10

Fig. 10.1 Palmer's classification of TFCC injuries based on arthroscopic findings

I: Traumatic

A: central TFCC tear

II: Degenerative

A: TFCC wear

B: TFCC wear, lunate +/- ulnar head chondromalacia

C: TFCC perforation, lunate +/- ulnar head chondromalacia

D: TFCC perforation, lunate +/- ulnar head chondromalacia, lunotriquetral ligament perforation

E: TFCC perforation, lunate +/- ulnar head chondromalacia, lunotriquetral ligament perforation, ulnocarpal arthritis

fibrocartilagenous disk, an avascular zone responsible for force transfer, starts to wear and demonstrates fibrillation. This wear causes increased stress on the ulnar head, lunate, and triquetrum resulting in chondromalacia of their opposing articular surfaces. Eventually the central disk will perforate causing the ulnar head and ulnar carpus to be exposed and able to directly articulate [7]. This leads to lunotriquetral ligament attenuation and rupture with eventual inevitable ulnocarpal arthritis [7].

In 1989, Palmer described a classification of TFCC injuries based on arthroscopic findings (Fig. 10.1). TFCC changes are broadly subdivided into two groups, traumatic (I) or degenerative (II). Degenerative perforations of the TFCC are subclassified by progressive involvement of the ulnocarpal joint. Type A is TFCC wear, type B has additional lunate and/or ulnar head chondromalacia. In type C lesions, the TFCC is perforated in the center. Type D lesions additionally demonstrate lunotriquetral ligament perforation with type E lesions signifying ulnocarpal arthritis [8].

Clinical Features

Clinical features vary with severity of the disease; the usual presenting symptom is chronic ulnar-sided wrist pain. The onset is usually insidious and progressive without any history of trauma. In early stages, pain is brought on or exacerbated with activity. Specifically, pain is exacerbated with movements that include power grip, ulnar deviation of the wrist, and pronation and/or supination of the forearm. Some patients will complain of swelling over the ulnar side of the wrist, and in advanced cases, the pain is persistent and associated with decreased motion of the forearm and wrist.

Ulnar-sided tenderness to palpation can be elicited especially around the volar and dorsal aspects of the ulnar head, the lunate, and triquetrum. A positive ulnar impaction test produces pain with passive full ulnar deviation of wrist. In order to differentiate ulnar impaction from other causes of ulnar-sided wrist pain, it is necessary to provoke symptoms with physical maneuvers. Nakamura et al. described the ulnocarpal stress test in which the wrist is placed in maximal ulnar deviation, axially loaded and then the forearm is pas-

sively rotated through supination to pronation. If this causes pain, then the test is positive [9]. Another test is the "press test" in which pain is reproduced by asking a seated patient to push off a chair using the affected wrist [10]. To test the lunatotriquetral ligament, the Reagan shuck test or the Kleinman shear test should be performed [11].

Differential Diagnosis

It is important to differentiate ulnar abutment from other possible conditions. Pathology of the distal radioulnar joint such as arthritis or instability can be identified with pain on forearm rotation. Careful palpation and radiographic assessment are also needed to rule out other bony conditions such as pisotriquetral arthritis or hamate hook nonunions; soft tissue conditions like extensor carpi ulnar wrist tendonitis or subluxation, carpal ligamentous tears, and traumatic TFCC tears also need to be taken into consideration. Finally nerve pathology like neuritis of the dorsal cutaneous branch of the ulnar nerve must also be excluded.

Imaging

Standard posteroanterior (PA) and lateral radiographs of the wrist should be obtained. The shoulder should be abducted to 90°, the elbow flexed to 90° with the forearm pronated to obtain a neutral rotation wrist film. The PA of the wrist will show static positive ulnar variance if present. If standard films are negative, dynamic positive ulnar variance can be demonstrated with a pronated grip PA view of the wrist. A study of 22 patients with ulnar-sided wrist pain showed increase of ulnar variance of an average 2.5 mm with a pronated grip view [12]. In advanced cases, subchondral sclerosis and cystic changes are visualized within the ulnar side of the lunate, the triquetrum, and the ulnar head. Radiographs must also be examined for widening of the lunotriquetral joint, carpal collapse, and degenerative changes of the ulnocarpal or distal radioulnar joint.

Advanced imaging techniques may be helpful in some cases. Triple injection arthrogram is preferred over single injection to assess both the TFCC and lunatotriquetral ligaments. MR imaging with or without an arthrogram is beneficial for demonstrating integrity of the lunotriquetral ligament and TFCC. MR is particularly helpful in demonstration of early stages of the disease with bony edema, cyst formation, and chondromalacia in the ulnocarpal joint [13].

Role of Arthroscopy

Arthroscopy allows confirmation of the diagnosis, staging of the disease, and the option to proceed with therapeutic procedures such as debridement or ulnar recession. Patients with a positive history, clinical exam, and imaging that have failed nonoperative treatment of activity modification, NSAIDs, splinting, and injection are candidates for intervention. Weiss et al. compared the effectiveness of triple injection arthrogram versus arthroscopy. They found that arthrography was 83% specific, 56% sensitive, and 60% accurate when compared to arthroscopy [14]. Wrist arthroscopy has been shown to be more accurate in assessing the ligaments, articular surfaces, and TFCC than arthrography [15].

Management of Ulnar Abutment

The goal of management is relief of symptoms and prevention of progression of ulnocarpal degeneration. Debridement of a degenerate TFCC will be helpful in the short term, but in the presence of uncorrected ulnocarpal, loading is not likely to produce long-lasting relief [16]. Relieving the increased ulnar pressure is the essence of management and can be achieved by either shortening the ulna or recession of the distal articular surface of the ulna. The latter can be achieved arthroscopically. Debridement of the central portion of the TFCC and the resection of the distal ulna to subchondral bone can result in significant unloading of the ulnocarpal joint in a cadaver model [17].

Treatment of TFCC Wear and Perforation

In early stages of ulnar abutment, pathology is confined to the central avascular portion of the TFCC [18]. These lesions have no healing potential and should be treated with arthroscopic debridement rather than attempt to repair [19].

When debriding the TFCC, the defect should be enlarged until fresh borders of the tear are created. It is imperative to leave the dorsal and volar radioulnar ligaments intact. If not, this will alter the load bearing at the distal radioulnar joint and the stabilizing effect at the TFCC [20]. The precise mechanism of symptomatic relief achieved by enlarging the

tear is not clear and is likely by prevention of entrapment of flaps of the TFCC during impaction loading of the ulnocarpal joint.

Arthroscopic Technique

The 3–4 and 6R arthroscopic portals are utilized for management of ulnocarpal impaction. The wrist is placed in traction with finger traps applied through the index and middle finger using an overhead boom or specialized traction device. The wrist joint is then insufflated with fluid. A routine diagnostic scope should be performed using the 3–4 portal with outflow through the 6R portal (Fig. 10.2). A probe is introduced by developing the 6R portal in order to probe the TFCC and determine the location and extent of the tear. It is not uncommon to encounter significant synovitis on the ulnar side of the joint requiring initial debridement with an arthroscopic shaver prior to examination with the probe. The articular surfaces of the lunate and triquetrum are examined carefully for any loose chondral flaps that should be debrided. The presence of a TFCC central tear with signs of chondromalacia of the lunate and possibly the ulnar head and triquetrum is classified as a Palmar IIC. If there is LTIL laxity with a TFCC tear, this transitions the diagnosis to a Palmar IID or IIE.

Radial and ulnar midcarpal portals are then used to assess the stability of the lunotriquetral ligament. A shuck test should be used intraoperatively to test the lunatotriquetral laxity.

Once the disease has been staged, attention is turned to debridement of the ulnocarpal joint. Large flaps of the TFCC can be debrided with a curved punch, and the edges of the tear are debrided and smoothened with a toothed powered resector inserted through the 6R portal.

Care is taken to leave the dorsal and palmar radioulnar ligament and the foveal attachment of the TFCC intact. Debridement of the central portion of the TFCC can provide temporary symptomatic relief but does not address the underlying problems of ulnocarpal abutment. Decompression of the ulnocarpal joint in the presence of ulnar positive variance is also of benefit in the management of acute traumatic TFCC tears (Palmer, type IA) as debridement alone in this scenario is associated with poorer results [21]. It is our recommendation that isolated debridement should be reserved for patients with Palmer IA tears without positive ulnar variance. It has been shown that TFCC defects, both acute and chronic, that are addressed with debridement and arthroscopic wafer were satisfied with their outcome [16]. Also, Palmar reported a favorable result at 2-year follow-up with the arthroscopic wafer procedure performed in patients with Palmar IIC TFCC pathology [18].

The wafer procedure was first presented as an alternative to ulnar shortening osteotomy by Feldon in 1992 [22]. The

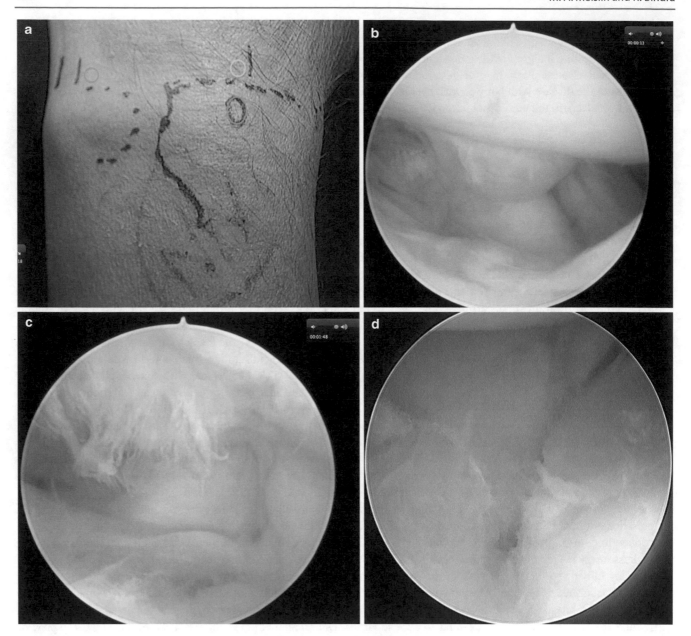

Fig. 10.2 Arthroscopic wafer procedure. (**a**) Portal placement for the wafer procedure mainly uses the 6R portal (*blue circle*) and 3–4 portal (*green oval*) with Lister's tubercle denoted with a *purple oval*. (**b**) Once the scope has been introduced and a routine scope has been performed, the radial side of the wrist will be normal without any signs of pathology pertaining to ulnar abutment. (**c**) The ulnar side of the radiocarpal joint shows a central tear and chondromalacia of the ulnar half of the lunate. (**d**) Midcarpal view shows lunotriquetral instability

main goal is to decrease loading across the ulnar side of the wrist. The wafer procedure is intended to resect the distal most part of ulnar head while still preserving the ulnar styloid and the attachments of the ulnocarpal ligaments and horizontal portion of the TFCC. The DRUJ is also left undisturbed by limiting the amount of resection to 2–4 mm [23]. It has been shown that shortening the ulnar head by 3 mm decreases the force transmitted across ulnar head by 50%; however, more resection did little to decrease forces transmitted [17].

In a retrospective comparative study, combined arthroscopic TFCC debridement and arthroscopic wafer procedure provided similar pain relief and restoration of function with fewer secondary procedures when compared with arthroscopic TFCC debridement and open ulnar shortening osteotomy [24]. Unlike ulnar shortening osteotomy, the wafer procedure bypasses complications such as delayed union or nonunion and late hardware problems that can occur with diaphyseal shortening of the ulna [24].

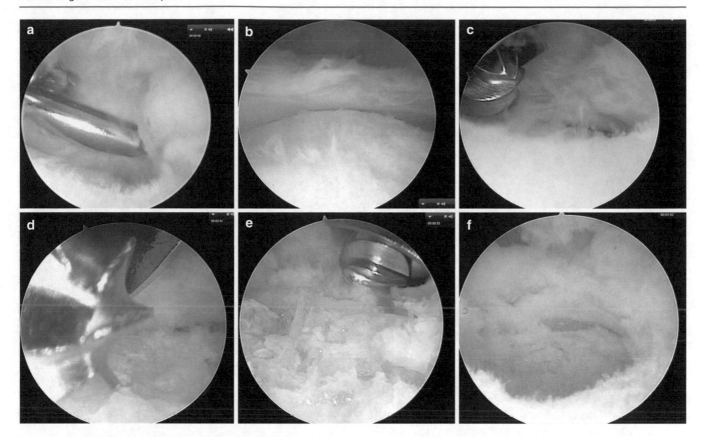

Fig. 10.3 Once finishing the diagnostic scope, (**a**) the shaver is introduced through the 6R portal to enlarge the central tear. (**b**) Debridement with the shaver allows appropriate visualization of the ulnar head. (**c**) The burr is then introduced through the 6R portal and the height of the burr is used to create the depth of resection of the ulnar head. (**d**) A more aggressive burr is then brought into the 6R portal to level off the resection to the depth of the burr and (**e**) is switched into the 3–4 portal to obtain an even resection. (**f**) After resection is completed, the forearm should be pronated and supinated to check for an even resection

Ulnar Wafer

Arthroscopic wafer procedure involves appropriate resection of the dome of the ulnar head accessed through the central perforation in the TFCC (Fig. 10.3). Typically, 2–3 mm of ulnar head removal is sufficient to remove the protuberance of the ulnar head through the TFCC tear. The initial debridement is performed using a 2.9-mm round burr that is gently seated into the distal ulna to its full depth to achieve a 3-mm shortening. A larger oval burr may then be introduced and carefully oscillated from side to side to evenly resect the distal ulna. By rotating the forearm, different parts of the distal ulna are brought into view through the central TFCC tear. In particularly sclerotic bone, a straight narrow osteotome may be introduced into the 6R portal to initiate bone resection. Upon completion, the scope is introduced into the 6R portal to confirm that there is no protruding bone spike. Intraoperative fluoroscopy is important to confirm that an appropriate amount of ulnar head has been removed evenly and that the distal radial articular surface of the distal ulna is not violated (Fig. 10.4).

Management of LT Instability

In patients with lunotriquetral instability (Palmer IID or IIE) debridement of the tear is performed. In cases with significant LT instability additional stabilization may be necessary [21]. In the setting of LT instability, diaphyseal ulnar shortening osteotomy has been advocated because it tensions the extrinsic ulnocarpal ligaments, which help stabilize lunotriquetral joint [11, 23, 25]. In milder cases of attenuation and stretching of the LT ligament, thermal shrinkage may be effective [26]. A bipolar radiofrequency probe is applied to the entire area of the arthroscopically accessible portion of the LT intercarpal ligament, beginning at the distal end (dorsal and palmar parts) of the ligament and moving proximally to the membranous part. Changes in color and consistency of the ligament tissue are visually confirmed. The radiofrequency probe is applied intermittently for a few seconds at a time, and continuous irrigation is ensured throughout the entire procedure to prevent heat injury to articular cartilage and periarticular soft tissues. In cases with an LT step-off visualized from the midcarpal joint, supplemental pinning is

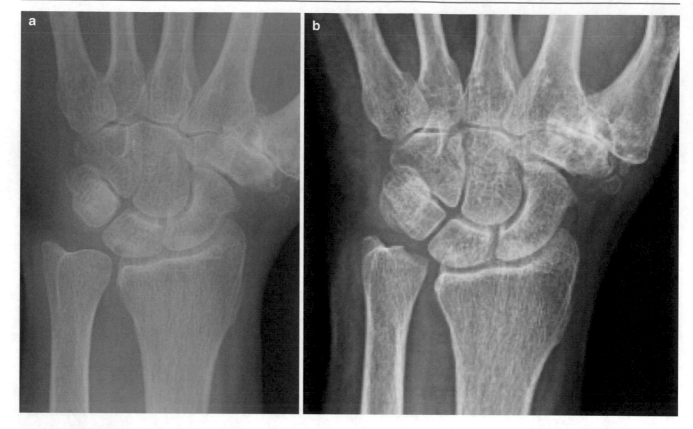

Fig. 10.4 PA X-rays of the wrist showing (**a**) ulnar positive variance with cystic changes of the lunate. (**b**) Shows the same wrist after undergoing the wafer procedure

performed. Two 1.2-mm K-wires are introduced into the lunate though an incision on the ulnar side of the wrist and then the triquetrum is reduced under vision by using the wires as a joystick while the other is driven into the lunate. The K-wires are retained for about 6 weeks.

Postoperative Management

The wrist is immobilized in a splint immediately postoperatively. Early range of motion is encouraged within the first week after surgery. The patient uses a splint for comfort as needed. Strengthening is commenced by about 6 weeks when the patient has regained preoperative motion of the wrist.

Results

In a retrospective series, 9 of 12 patients were very satisfied and 3 of 12 were satisfied after arthroscopic wafer resection. Only four patients reported minimal symptoms. Additionally, 11 of 12 patients returned to work by 8 weeks, with maximum benefit noted at a mean of 6.5 weeks [16]. Contrasting these authors, in a separate report of a large series of 42

patients, less encouraging results were reported with only 40% of patients satisfied, 30% were dissatisfied, and 30% undecided [27].

Summary

The cornerstone of ulnar abutment syndrome is unloading the ulnocarpal joint by recession of the distal ulna. In the presence of a central perforation of the TFCC, it is possible to perform the recession arthroscopically. Arthroscopic wafer resection allows quicker recovery and avoids the morbidity and complications of ulnar shortening. Wafer resection, however, is limited to cases where only a few millimeters of ulna shortening is needed. Additionally, in the presence of advanced LT instability, diaphyseal shortening of the ulna may be preferable.

References

1. Palmer AK, Werner FW. Biomechanics of the distal radioulnar joint. Clin Orthop Relat Res. 1984;187:26–35.
2. Palmer AK, Werner FW, et al. The triangular fibrocartilage complex of the wrist-anatomy and function. J Hand Surg [Am]. 1981;6:153–62.

3. Palmer AK, Glisson RR, et al. Relationship between ulnar variance and triangular fibrocartilage complex thickness. J Hand Surg [Am]. 1984;9:681–2.

4. Mikic ZD. Age changes in the triangular fibrocartilage of the wrist joint. J Anat. 1978;126(Pt 2):367–84.

5. Tolat AR, Sanderson PL, et al. The gymnast's wrist: acquired positive ulnar variance following chronic epiphyseal injury. J Hand Surg [Br]. 1992;17:678–81.

6. Palmer AK. Fractures of the distal radius. In: Green DP, editor. Operative hand surgery. 3rd ed. New York: Churchill Livingstone; 1993. p. 861–928.

7. Bickel KD. Arthroscopic treatment of ulnar impaction syndrome. J Hand Surg [Am]. 2008;33(8):1420–3.

8. Palmer AK. Triangular fibrocartilage complex lesions: a classification. J Hand Surg [Am]. 1989;14(4):594–606.

9. Nakamura R, Horil E, Imaeda T, et al. The ulnocarpal stress test in the diagnosis of ulnar-sided wrist pain. J Hand Surg (Br). 1997;22(6):719–23.

10. Lester B, Halbrecht J, Levy IM, et al. "Press Test" for office diagnosis of triangular fibrocartilage complex tears of the wrist. Ann Plast Surg. 1995;35:41–5.

11. Sammer DM, Rizzo M. Ulnar impaction. Hand Clin. 2010;26:549–57.

12. Tomaino MM. The importance of the pronated grip x-ray view in evaluating ulnar variance. J Hand Surg [Am]. 2000;25:352–7.

13. Imaeda T, Nakamura R, Shionoya K, et al. Ulnar impaction syndrome: MR imaging findings. Radiology. 1996;201(2):495–500.

14. Weiss A-PC, Akelman E, Lambiase R. Comparison of the findings of triple-injection cinearthrography of the wrist with those of arthroscopy. J Bone Joint Surg Am. 1996;78:348–56.

15. North ER, Meyer S. Wrist injuries: correlation of clinical and arthroscopic findings. J Hand Surg. 1990;15A:915–20.

16. Tomaino MM, Weiser RW. Combined arthroscopic TFCC debridement and wafer resection of the distal ulna in wrists with triangular fibrocartilage complex tears and positive ulnar variance. J Hand Surg [Am]. 2001;26(6):1047–52.

17. Wnorowski DC, Palmer AK, Werner FW, et al. Anatomic and biomechanical analysis of the arthroscopic wafer procedure. Arthroscopy. 1992;8(2):204–12.

18. Palmar AK. Triangular fibrocartilage disorders: injury patterns and treatment. Arthroscopy. 1990;6:125–32.

19. Pomerance J. Arthroscopic debridement and/or ulnar shortening osteotomy for TFCC tears. J Hand Surg [Am]. 2002;2(2):95–101.

20. Palmer AK, Werner FW, Glisson RR, et al. Partial excision of the triangular fibrocartilage complex: an experimental study. J Hand Surg [Am]. 1988;13A:391–4.

21. Minami A. Clinical results of treatment of triangular fibrocartilage complex tears by arthroscopic debridement. J Hand Surg [Am]. 1996;21(3):406–11.

22. Feldon P, Terrono AL, Belsky MR. Wafer distal ulna resection for triangular fibrocartilage tears and/or ulna impaction syndrome. J Hand Surg [Am]. 1992;17:731–7.

23. Deitch MA, Stern SJ. Ulnocarpal abutment: treatment options. Hand Clin. 1998;14(2):251–63.

24. Bernstein MA, Nagel DJ, Martinez A, et al. A comparison of combined arthroscopic triangular fibrocartilage complex debridement and arthroscopic wafer distal ulna resection versus arthroscopic triangular fibrocartilage complex debridement and ulnar shortening osteotomy for ulnocarpal abutment syndrome. Arthroscopy. 2004;20(4):392–401.

25. Nagel DJ. Arthroscopic treatment of degenerative tears of the triangular fibrocartilage. Hand Clin. 1994;10:615–24.

26. Lee J, Nha KW, Lee GY, et al. Long-term outcomes of arthroscopic debridement and thermal shrinkage for isolated partial intercarpal ligament tears. Orthopedics. 2012;35(8):1204–9.

27. DeSmet L, DeFerm A, Steenwerckx A, et al. Arthroscopic treatment of triangular fibrocartilage complex lesions of the wrist. Acta Orthop Belg. 1996;62:8–13.

DRUJ Tendon Allograft Arthroplasty

Loukia K. Papatheodorou and Dean G. Sotereanos

Introduction

Despite the many modifications of the distal ulnar resection, Darrach procedure, the reported failure rate remains between 7% and 40% [1–7]. The most common causes of failure of distal ulnar resection procedures are distal radioulnar instability and radioulnar convergence. The patient with a symptomatic failed distal ulnar resection presents with wrist pain especially with forearm rotation and grip weakness (Fig. 11.1a). Painful grinding and mechanical limitations to forearm rotation result in upper extremity disuse.

Many techniques have been described for the management of the failed distal ulnar resection with varying success to prevent recurrent distal radioulnar impingement [1, 3, 8–15]. In an effort to eliminate the symptoms associated with painful radioulnar convergence and instability and to avoid metallic implant failure, the senior author (D.G.S.) developed an interpositional technique using Achilles tendon allograft between the distal radius and the resected distal ulna [16–19].

Indications–Contraindications

The interpositional arthroplasty using Achilles tendon allograft can be used for the management of painful distal radioulnar convergence following a distal ulna resection. Patients with incapacitating pain and instability of the distal stump of the ulna after distal ulnar resection should be assessed with careful physical examination for ballottement of the distal ulna in dorsal and palmar directions, and with

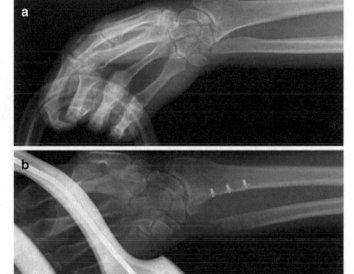

Fig. 11.1 Gripping "weight-bearing" PA radiograph. (**a**) Preoperative radiograph showing impingement between the distal ulnar stump and the distal radius after failed Darrach procedure. (**b**) Three-year postoperative radiograph after tendon allograft interposition showing maintenance of a wide space without impingement between the distal ulna and radius

direct compression of the ulna into the radius. The interpositional arthroplasty is especially useful for young, active patients who may not be candidates for implant arthroplasty.

The cost of the tendon allograft may be considered a relative contraindication. Disadvantages of all allografts include cost, availability, and immunologic reaction. Nonetheless, they are currently widely used in orthopedic surgery. Thus far, there have been no reports on immune reactions or infections with this technique.

L. K. Papatheodorou
Department of Orthopaedic Surgery, University of Pittsburgh School of Medicine, Pittsburgh, PA, USA

D. G. Sotereanos (✉)
Department of Orthopaedic Surgery, University of Pittsburgh School of Medicine, Pittsburgh, PA, USA

University of Pittsburgh Medical Center, Pittsburgh, PA, USA

Surgical Technique

The interpositional arthroplasty using Achilles tendon allograft can be performed under regional or general anesthesia with tourniquet control. The patient is positioned supine with the affected extremity on a hand-table extension. If possible, the previous skin surgical incisions are incorporated into the approach with extension dorsally to the fifth dorsal compartment. Dissection through the fifth dorsal compartment provides access to the resected distal ulna and to the medial cortex of the distal radius. Attention must be paid to preserve the dorsal cutaneous branch of the ulnar nerve. Then subperiosteal exposure of the distal ulna is performed approximately 4–6 cm proximal to the distal stump. A smooth surface of the distal ulna is created by removing any prominent bone that have been developed around the ulnar stump. To expose the medial cortex of the radius, the ulna is retracted volarly using Hohmann retractors over the ulna and under the radius (Fig. 11.2). Three or four mini unicortical suture anchors are placed into the medial cortex of the distal radius, proximal to the sigmoid notch at the site of the impingement (Fig. 11.3). These anchors should extend 3–4 cm along the medial cortex of the radius. Along the distal ulna (2–3 cm) three or four drill holes are made in a medial-to-lateral direction and then sutures are passed through each of the holes for later fixation of the allograft between the two bones (Fig. 11.4).

An Achilles tendon allograft is prepared for implantation. The calcaneal remnant is removed from the allograft and then the allograft is rolled onto itself creating a large interpositional "pillow" (usually size, 5 cm × 3 cm) (Fig. 11.5). The

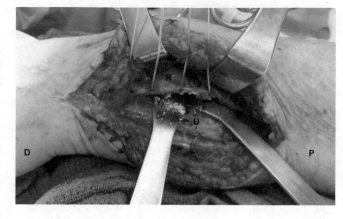

Fig. 11.3 Intraoperative view. Suture anchors are placed into the medial cortex of the distal radius. D, distal; P, proximal; R, radius; U, ulna

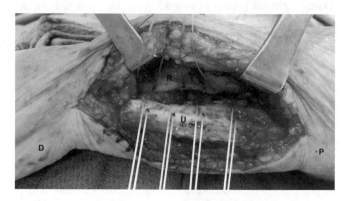

Fig. 11.4 Intraoperative view. Drill holes are made in the distal ulna and sutures are passed through each of the holes. D, distal; P, proximal; R, radius; U, ulna

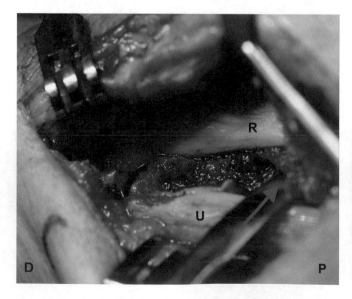

Fig. 11.2 Intraoperative view. Exposure of the medial cortex of the distal radius using Hohmann retractors (blue arrow) over ulna and under radius. D, distal; P, proximal; R, radius; U, ulna

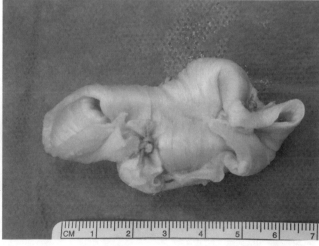

Fig. 11.5 Achilles tendon allograft. The calcaneal remnant has been removed and the allograft is rolled onto itself creating a large interposition "pillow"

allograft is interposed between the distal radius and ulna to act as a soft tissue buffer between the two bones to prevent radioulnar impingement. To secure the allograft between both forearm bones sutures from the anchors to radius are passed through the "graft pillow" and sutures from the drill holes to ulna are passed through the "graft pillow" as well (Fig. 11.6). With final allograft placement there should be significant padding between the distal radius and the ulna to prevent any palpable crepitus or impingement during forearm rotation under compression (Figs. 11.7 and 11.8). If crepitus is noted, the size of the allograft pillow is increased until no further crepitus occurs with passive forearm rotation. Generally, the entire soft tissue allograft is utilized. No other tissues are used to stabilize the ulnar stump. Standard capsular and soft tissue closures are completed over the allograft and the retinaculum is closed followed by routine skin closure.

The wrist is placed in a well-padded, long-arm splint in neutral rotation and flexion. The long-arm splint is converted to a long-arm cast at the initial postoperative follow-up, usu-

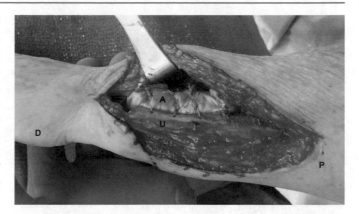

Fig. 11.8 Intraoperative view. Final placement of the allograft between the distal radius and ulnar stump. D, distal; P, proximal; A, allograft; U, ulna

ally in 10 days. The cast is removed after 6 weeks and a removable long-arm splint is used. At this time, the patient begins a rehabilitation program, initially consisting of active and active-assisted range of motion exercises with appropriate progression to strengthening exercises. Protected range of motion and interval splinting is continued until 12 weeks postoperative.

Outcomes

Since the original clinical series, consistently good-to-excellent results with the interpositional arthroplasty using Achilles tendon allograft have been noted in more than 40 patients with failed distal ulnar resection in the senior author's (D.G.S.) personal series. Marked alleviation of pain and improvement of forearm rotation and grip strength have been demonstrated. Maintenance of space between the distal radius and ulna was also demonstrated radiographically at 2–14 years after surgery (see Fig. 11.1b) [16, 19]. Radiographic evaluation revealed ulnar scalloping in three patients (2–3 years postoperative), although the patients remain asymptomatic.

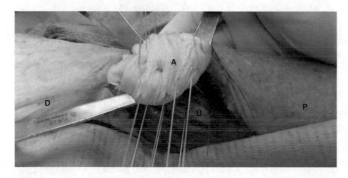

Fig. 11.6 Sutures from the anchors to distal radius are passed through the "graft pillow" and sutures from the drill holes to distal ulna are passed through the "graft pillow". D, distal; P, proximal; A, allograft; U, ulna

Tips and Tricks

- The size of the allograft "pillow" must be given great attention. For sufficient size of allograft bulk, obtain as much as necessary – increase allograft size if crepitus is palpated. The allograft "pillow" should prevent the ulnar stump from contacting the radius during pronation and supination under compression.
- Allograft dislodgement can occur if the graft is not sutured to radius and ulna or if the graft is not large enough to prevent impingement.

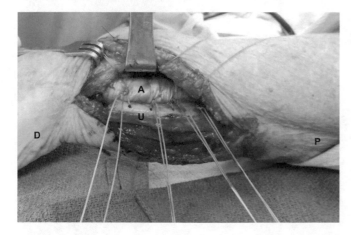

Fig. 11.7 Intraoperative view. The allograft is placed and sutured between the distal radius and ulnar stump (using sutures from anchors to radius and drill holes to ulna). D, distal; P, proximal; A, allograft; U, ulna

- Use mini unicortical suture anchors into the medial cortex of the radius for graft fixation to avoid radial shaft fracture.
- Immobilize the wrist in long-arm splint in neutral position for 10 days and convert to cast for 6 weeks.
- Physical therapy can be started after 6 weeks to advance motion and strength.

Conclusion

Although the Achilles allograft interposition does not restore normal biomechanics of the DRUJ, it can prevent impingement, crepitus, and painful distal radioulnar convergence following distal ulnar resection. The interpositional arthroplasty with the Achilles tendon allograft is an attractive alternative especially for young, active patients, in which an implant or alternative procedure may not be appropriate.

References

1. Garcia-Elias M. Failed ulnar head resection: prevention and treatment. J Hand Surg Br. 2002;27(5):470–80.
2. Sauerbier M, Berger RA, Fujita M, Hahn ME. Radioulnar convergence after distal ulnar resection: mechanical performance of two commonly used soft tissue stabilizing procedures. Acta Orthop Scand. 2003;74(4):420–8.
3. Adams BD. Distal radioulnar joint instability. In: Wolfe SW, Hotchkiss RN, Pederson WC, Kozin SH, editors. Green's operative hand surgery. 6th ed. Philadelphia: Churchill Livingstone Elsevier; 2011. p. 523–60.
4. Greenberg JA. Reconstruction of the distal ulna: instability, impaction, impingement, and arthrosis. J Hand Surg Am. 2009;34(2):351–6.
5. Minami A, Iwasaki N, Ishikawa J, Suenaga N, Yasuda K, Kato H. Treatments of osteoarthritis of the distal radioulnar joint: long-term results of three procedures. Hand Surg. 2005;10(2–3):243–8.
6. Bieber EJ, Linscheid RL, Dobyns JH, Beckenbaugh RD. Failed distal ulna resections. J Hand Surg Am. 1988;13(2):193–200.
7. McKee MD, Richards RR. Dynamic radio-ulnar convergence after the Darrach procedure. J Bone Joint Surg Br. 1996;78(3):413–8.
8. Kleinman WB. Salvage procedures for the distal end of the ulna: there is no magic. Am J Orthop (Belle Mead NJ). 2009;38(4):172–80.
9. Jupiter JB. Tendon stabilization of the distal ulna. J Hand Surg Am. 2008;33(7):1196–200.
10. Minami A, Iwasaki N, Ishikawa J, Suenaga N, Kato H. Stabilization of the proximal ulnar stump in the Sauvé-Kapandji procedure by using the extensor carpi ulnaris tendon: long-term follow-up studies. J Hand Surg Am. 2006;31(3):440–4.
11. Axelsson P, Sollerman C, Kärrholm J. Ulnar head replacement: 21 cases; mean follow-up, 7.5 years. J Hand Surg Am. 2015;40(9):1731–8.
12. van Schoonhoven J, Mühldorfer-Fodor M, Fernandez DL, Herbert TJ. Salvage of failed resection arthroplasties of the distal radioulnar joint using an ulnar head prosthesis: long-term results. J Hand Surg Am. 2012;37(7):1372–80.
13. Kakar S, Swann RP, Perry KI, Wood-Wentz CM, Shin AY, Moran SL. Functional and radiographic outcomes following distal ulna implant arthroplasty. J Hand Surg Am. 2012;37(7):1364–71.
14. Scheker LR. Implant arthroplasty for the distal radioulnar joint. J Hand Surg Am. 2008;33(9):1639–44.
15. Bellevue KD, Thayer MK, Pouliot M, Huang JI, Hanel DP. Complications of semiconstrained distal radioulnar joint arthroplasty. J Hand Surg Am. 2018;43(6):566.e1–9.
16. Sotereanos DG, Papatheodorou LK, Williams BG. Tendon allograft interposition for failed distal ulnar resection: 2- to 14-year follow-up. J Hand Surg Am. 2014;39(3):443–448.e1.
17. Papatheodorou LK, Rubright JH, Kokkalis ZT, Sotereanos DG. Resection interposition arthroplasty for failed distal ulna resections. J Wrist Surg. 2013;2(1):13–8.
18. Greenberg JA, Sotereanos D. Achilles allograft interposition for failed Darrach distal ulna resections. Tech Hand Up Extrem Surg. 2008;12(2):121–5.
19. Sotereanos DG, Gobel F, Vardakas DG, Sarris I. An allograft salvage technique for failure of the Darrach procedure: a report of four cases. J Hand Surg Br. 2002;27(4):317–21.

Alan E. Freeland and William B. Geissler

Introduction

Although the wrist is commonly thought to move in flexion and extension in the anatomic sagittal plane and radial and ulnar deviation in the anatomic frontal (coronal) plane, it is actually a universal joint that is capable of multidirectional or global motion. Although full wrist motion may allow peak performance, most important daily functions are performed in the midrange and along the coupled dart thrower's "out-of-plane" pathway [1–9]. The dart thrower's motion (DTM) takes place primarily at the midcarpal joint, and follows a plane or corridor 30–45° obliquely to the anatomic sagittal and coronal planes, extending from approximately 60° of wrist extension and 20° of radial deviation, through the neutral zone, to 60° of wrist flexion and 40° of ulnar deviation and back. The radioscaphocapitate ligament (RSCL), long radiolunate (LRLL), short radiolunate (SRLL), and dorsal radiolunotriquetral ligament (DRLTL) are aligned parallel, or nearly parallel, to the dart thrower's pathway.

Motion at the radiocarpal joint (RCJ) is the primary source of global wrist flexion, whereas motion at the midcarpal joint (MCJ) is the primary source of wrist extension [2–9]. The proximal carpal row (PCR) does not function as a single unit during normal global wrist motion. The scaphoid, lunate, and triquetrum each have a unique arc of motion. Scapholunate motion approaches zero during the DTM. The

primary motion of the scaphoid and lunate is in the flexion-extension arc regardless of the direction of wrist motion. The scaphoid and lunate flex and the capitate extends during radial deviation. The scaphoid and lunate extend and the capitate flexes during ulnar deviation.

The wrist is comprised of eight carpal bones, seven of which act synchronously and synergistically within the confines of the wrist to allow normal wrist motion. The scaphoid, lunate, triquetrum, trapezium, trapezoid, capitate, and hamate are guided and constrained by a complex system of viscoelastic intrinsic and extrinsic ligaments. A total of 24 muscles cross or insert on the carpal bones, move the wrist and hand, and assist in providing wrist stability. No tendons insert into the bones of the intercalated PCR. The pisiform articulates with the palmar surface of the triquetrum, but acts primarily as a fulcrum to enhance flexor carpi ulnaris strength and power during wrist flexion and ulnar deviation, especially during the DTM, rather than to intrinsically influence wrist kinematics or stability.

Historical Perspective

Early investigations applied planar concepts that attempted to correlate carpal structure and function. Johnston reported in 1907 that carpal motion was initiated at the midcarpal joint and occurred largely between the carpal rows [10]. In 1943, Guilford et al. promoted the row concept of wrist motion, envisioning three "links" (rows): the distal radius, the PCR, and the distal carpal row (DCR). He described the scaphoid as a rod "linking" the carpal "rows" [11]. In 1972, Linscheid et al. refined the "link" concept of carpal motion to propose the "slider crank" analogy, in which the scaphoid acts as a mobile bridge between the two carpal rows, much as the slider crank controls motion between a piston and drive shaft [12] (Fig. 12.1). In 1977, Sarrafian et al. noted that radiocarpal motion comprised 40% and midcarpal motion 60% of maximum wrist flexion, while motion was 66.5%

Supplementary Information The online version of this chapter (https://doi.org/10.1007/978-3-030-78881-0_12) contains supplementary material, which is available to authorized users.

A. E. Freeland (Deceased)
Department of Orthopaedic Surgery and Rehabilitation, University of Mississippi Medical Center, Brandon, MS, USA

W. B. Geissler (✉)
Division of Hand and Upper Extremity Surgery, Section of Arthroscopic Surgery and Sports Medicine, Department of Orthopedic Surgery and Rehabilitation, University of Mississippi Medical Center, Jackson, MS, USA

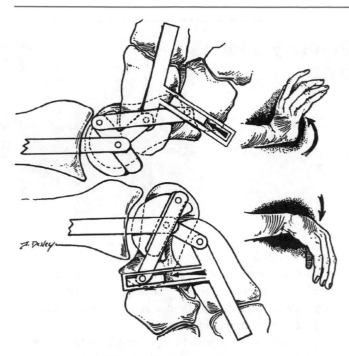

Fig. 12.1 The "slider crank" concept of wrist flexion and extension. (Reprinted from Linscheid et al. [12])

radiocarpal and 33.5% midcarpal during maximum extension [13]. These researchers theorized that the scaphoid functioned with the PCR during flexion and with the distal carpal row (DCR) during extension.

Although most investigators had long believed that the center of rotation (COR) of the wrist was confined solely within the head of the capitate, Wright reported in 1935 that the COR of the wrist joint resided in the head of the capitate during wrist flexion and shifted to the intercarpal joint during extension [14]. The distal carpal row DCR rotates about a fixed axis within the head of the capitate throughout radioulnar deviation [15, 16]. The distance between the base of the third metacarpal and the distal radial articular surface (carpal height index [CHI] − normal C/MC = 0.56) on a neutrally positioned anteroposterior image is constant throughout radioulnar motion.

CHI can be used to measure carpal collapse [15, 16]. The perpendicular distance from the distally projected longitudinal axis of the ulna to the axis of rotation for radioulnar deviation on a neutrally positioned anteroposterior image is used to measure carpal translation. Three-dimensional analysis of the instantaneous screw axes (ISA) calibrated for the position of the third metacarpal base with respect to the distal radius revealed that the COR of wrist motion is not fixed or limited to the capitate during global motion [3]. ISA data also demonstrated that translational motion in the normal wrist may account for the difference between this study and previous reports.

In 1921, Navarro conceptualized a columnar wrist model to better explain the sophisticated and multidirectional movements of the wrist [17]. He theorized that three inter-dependent columns best correlated carpal anatomy with function. The lateral column (scaphoid, trapezium, and trapezoid) supported the thumb and transferred load between the other two carpal columns. The central column (lunate, capitate, and hamate) flexed and extended the wrist. Rotation was controlled by the medial column (triquetrum and pisiform). In 1978, Taleisnik modified the column theory to exclude the pisiform, recognizing that it played no integral role in intercarpal motion [18]. He also determined that the bones of the normal DCR are securely fixed together by stout ligaments, have very little intercarpal motion, and act as a unit. He therefore included the trapezium and trapezoid, along with the capitate, hamate, and lunate, as parts of the central column. The DCR is also rigidly secured to the bases of the second and third metacarpals and, consequently, moves with the hand (Fig. 12.2). Weber took a slightly different view of the columnar theory [19]. He divided the carpus into two columns: the load-bearing radial column composed of the scaphoid, lunate, trapezium, trapezoid, and capitate and the ulnar control column, consisting of the triquetrum and hamate. He viewed the helicoid triquetrohamate joint as the key to wrist position during rotation and load changes.

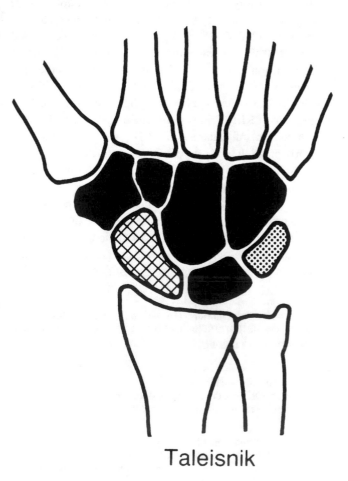

Taleisnik

Fig. 12.2 Taleisnik's columnar concept

Lichtman et al. formulated the next step toward a better understanding of three-dimensional wrist motion with their "oval-ring" theory [20] (Fig. 12.3). Their theory perceived the wrist as four interdependent segments: the DCR, scaphoid, lunate, and triquetrum. Ligamentous links connect each segment to its two adjacent elements. The scaphotrapezial (radial link) and triquetrohamate (ulnar link) joints form two reciprocal physiologic links. Radial deviation creates an unbalanced flexion moment at the radial link inducing proximal row flexion and palmar capitate and hamate subluxation (physiologic VISI). An unbalanced extension moment at the ulnar link causes the triquetrum to extend against the hamate with the PCR following and the capitate and hamate transitioning dorsally (physiologic DISI). Continuity of the ligaments assures synchronous synergistic carpal motion within the moving wrist. Disruption of any link(s) results in dysfunction. Craigen and Stanley pointed out that certain elements of both the column and row theories, although sometimes contradictory, are useful in our understanding of multidimensional wrist motion [21].

During wrist flexion-extension, the motion of the capitate closely follows that of the third metacarpal, while the lunate motion is approximately 50% of the total motion, the triquetrum 65%, and the scaphoid 90% [2, 22]. Similar differences in motion for these carpal bones occur during radioulnar deviation, circumduction, and the DTM. This suggests that the scaphoid, lunate, and triquetrum do not normally function as a single unit, but that each bone has a unique arc of motion during global wrist motion. This three-dimensional study of carpal rotational behavior supported a row concept of wrist motion as opposed to a carpal column model [2, 22].

Perhaps, at this point in time, we can conclude that the forearm, wrist, hand, and articular contact position at the moment of impact; point of impact; columns; rows; individual carpal bones; amount, direction, and rate of the applied and resistance forces; individual bone and articular cartilage morphology and containment; and viscoelastic ligament properties and relative strengths, especially in the PCR, interact to provide various multiplanar global wrist motions and play a role in injury susceptibility. Each of these parameters allows some measure of integral static and continuous dynamic quantification for biometric analysis, comparisons, communication, and management of these injuries as we unravel the comprehensive three-dimensional geometrics of normal and abnormal carpal motion with and without loading.

Normal Carpal Kinematics

The PCR is intercalated between the radius and ulna proximally and the DCR distally [23]. The scaphoid pivots over the radioscaphocapitate ligamentous fulcrum at its waist. The distal pole of scaphoid flexes as the trapezium and radial styloid close over it during wrist flexion and/or radial deviation. The scaphoid extends as the distance between the trapezium and radial styloid widens during wrist extension and/or ulnar deviation. The scaphoid and lunate flex and pronate during wrist flexion and/or radial deviation, while extending and supinating during wrist extension and/or ulnar deviation. Scaphoid flexion, extension, and rotation exceed that of the lunate [2, 22]. During full wrist flexion in the sagittal anatomic plane, the scaphoid flexes 35° more than the lunate and pronates three times as much. Lunate radioulnar and dorsopalmar translation in its radial fossa is minimal, but exceeds that of the scaphoid. The distal pole of the scaphoid has relatively more motion than has the proximal dorsal pole. The scaphoid moves somewhat as a rotating triplanar pendulum [2, 22]. The palmar SLIL fibers lengthen and the dorsal fibers shorten with wrist flexion [24]. The opposite occurs with wrist extension.

Radial and ulnar deviations primarily occur in the midcarpal joint. Midcarpal motion accounts for 60% of radial deviation and 86% of ulnar deviation [25]. The radiocarpal and scapholunate joints remain relatively stable. In radial deviation, the PCR flexes and the capitate moves slightly radiodorsally relative to the lunate. The scaphoid flexes and

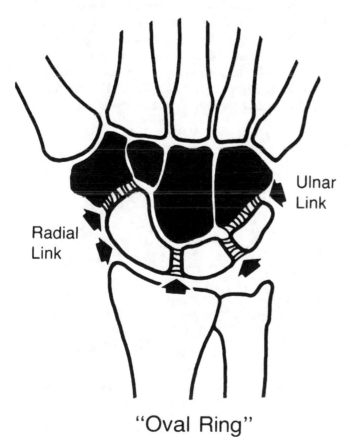

Fig. 12.3 Lichtman's oval ring. Redrawn from Lichtman et al. [72]. (With permission from Elsevier)

radially deviates. In ulnar deviation, the PCR extends and the capitate moves slightly ulnopalmarly on the lunate. Midcarpal motion relative to the capitate rotates in a plane from dorsoradial to ulnopalmar, similar to the DTM [2–9, 25, 26].

The PCR translocates radiopalmarly and rotates dorsally during ulnar deviation as the triquetrum pronates and shifts palmarly, distally, and ulnarly on the hamate's helicoid articular slope [16, 19]. The midcarpal joint slightly flexes. Conversely, the PCR translocates dorsoulnarly and rotates palmarly during radial deviation as the triquetrum supinates and shifts dorsally, proximally, and radially. The lunate geometry accommodates the rotational shifts within the PCR, maintaining a constant carpal height throughout radioulnar wrist motion in the frontal plane [15, 16]. The scaphotrapeziotrapezoidal ligament complex (STTL) and the lateral portion of the RSCL support the distal scaphoid throughout extension and ulnar deviation.

The SLIL has three anatomic regions [27, 28]. The dorsal SLIL (dSLIL) is thick and composed of short, transversely oriented collagen fibers. The palmar SLIL (pSLIL) is thin and contains obliquely oriented collagen fascicles. The proximal midregion of the SLIL (mSLIL) is composed of fibrocartilage, with a few superficial, longitudinally oriented collagen fibers and extends distally into the scapholunate joint (SLJ) space, resembling a meniscus. The mesentericlike radioscapholunate ligament (RSLL) separates the mSLIL and pSLIL, and spreads distally over the proximal scaphoid, SLIL, and lunate. The RSLL encloses small caliber neurovascular elements to and from the scaphoid, lunate, and SLIL. The yield strength of the dSLIL component is 260 ± 118 N, the mSLIL 63 ± 32 N, and the pSLIL 118 ± 21 N. The RSLL provides little, if any, structural support and depends on its elasticity and neighboring structures for protection.

There is no dorsal radioscaphoid ligament (DRSL) [29–31]. Such a ligament would require an elastic coefficient three times its resting length. This prerequisite exceeds the inherent physical capacity of ligaments. The dorsal radiolunotriquetral (DRLTL) and dorsal intercarpal (DICL) ligaments form a V-shaped configuration on the dorsum of the wrist with its converging apex on the ulnar side. The DRLTL originates from the dorsal lip of the distal radius, passes over the proximal pole of the scaphoid, extends obliquely, attaching to the distal dorsal ulnar lunate, dorsal ulnar lunate ligament (DULL), and dorsal LTIL, and inserts onto the dorsal tubercle of the triquetrum. The DRLTL lends support to the midcarpal joint and passively pronates the attached carpus during forearm pronation. The DICL has a thick proximal and a thinner distal transverse band. The DICL originates from the dorsal triquetrum and hamate, extends radially, attaches to the dorsal lip of the lunate, and inserts its thickest

attachment into the dorsal groove of the scaphoid where its anterior fibers blend imperceptibly with the strong dorsal fibers of the dSLIL before fanning onto the dorsal trapezium and proximal trapezoid.

The DVL substitutes for some of the function that a DRSL might provide throughout normal carpal kinematics by maintaining an indirect stabilizing effect on the proximal pole of the scaphoid by threefold narrowing and widening of the distance between the DRLTL origin and the scaphoid insertion of the DICL during maximum wrist extension and flexion, respectively. The STTL, RSCL, DRLTL, and DICL individually and conjointly are secondary stabilizers of the scapholunate joint (SLJ) [29–32].

The normal relationship of the scaphoid, lunate, and their related ligaments is illustrated in Fig. 12.4. The normal SLIL has an inverted V appearance with the apex of the V distally ("Tushy sign"), as visualized from the radiocarpal (3–4) arthroscopic portal. From the radial midcarpal portal, the normal SLJ is congruently aligned and immobile (Fig. 12.5). The scaphoid is flexed approximately 47° relative to the third metacarpal-capitate-lunate-radial longitudinal axis in the lateral X-ray view. The SLJ space is stable, congruent, and does not exceed 2 mm on the AP X-ray.

The triquetrum is the fulcrum for wrist rotation and motion in the radioulnar plane. The helicoid geometry of the triquetrohamate joint is instrumental in accommodating this screw-like movement [20]. The tensile strengths of dLTIL and pLTIL are the obverse or reciprocal of the dSLIL and pSLIL. The dLTIL yield strength 121 ± 42 N, the mLTIL 64 ± 14 N, and the pLTIL (pLTIL) 301 ± 36 N [33]. Although the pLTIL is stronger than the dLTIL, it is less flexible.

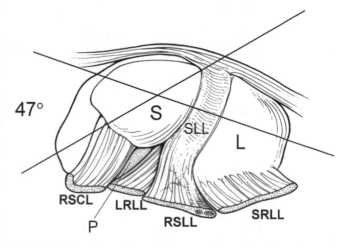

Fig. 12.4 Normal scapholunate alignment. S scaphoid, SLL scapholunate ligament, L lunate, RSCL radioscaphocapitate ligament, P interligamentous sulcus leading to the space of Poirier, LRLL long radiolunate ligament, RSLL radioscapholunate ligament, SRLL short radiolunate ligament

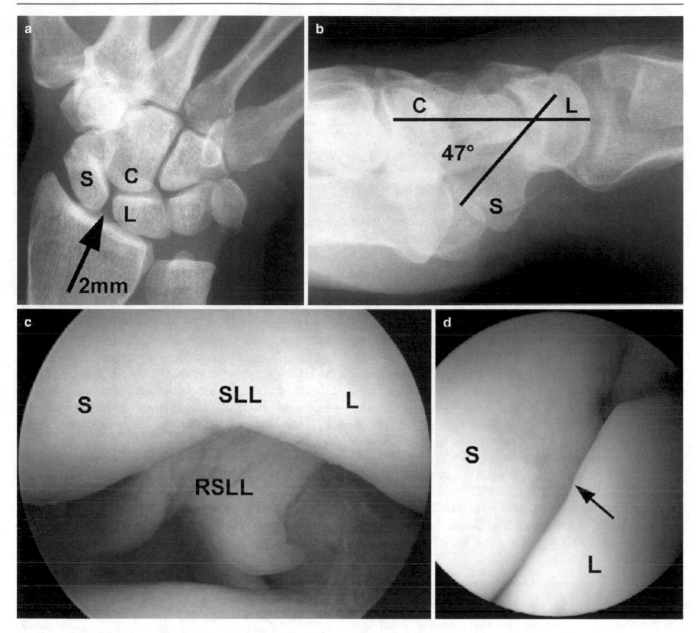

Fig. 12.5 Normal scapholunate alignment. (**a**) Normal AP X-ray (*arrow* points to the scapholunate joint). (**b**) Normal lateral X-ray and scapholunate angle. (**c**) Radiocarpal (3–4 portal) arthroscopic image demonstrating a normal SLL and RSLL. (**d**) Midcarpal arthroscopic view with normal scapholunate alignment

Classification of Carpal Instabilities

Although there is probably no single uncontested, comprehensive, or perfect classification for carpal instabilities, several parameters allow some measure of quantification that is useful for analysis, comparison, communication, and management of these injuries [34]. These parameters include chronicity, constancy, etiology, location, direction, and pattern.

Chronicity

Classification by chronicity relates to the time interval between injury and diagnosis. This categorization is based on the capacity for carpal reduction and, especially, on the intrinsic capability for ligament healing after treatment. Acute carpal instabilities are those diagnosed and treated within 1 week of injury. These instabilities are reducible and have the highest potential for ligament healing. Subacute tears are those diagnosed and treated between 1 and 6 weeks after injury. Although they are reducible, the capacity for primary ligament healing is diminished. Injuries seen after longer than 6 weeks from the time of injury are considered chronic, have little capacity for ligament healing, and may occasionally be irreducible.

Constancy

Carpal instability and symptoms may be apparent immediately in some cases; in others, they may take an initially indeterminate amount of time to appear as the carpi settle or the tear(s) extend. Ligaments that tear beyond the axis connecting the centers of rotation of two bones often have carpal malalignment that may be seen on standard wrist X-rays with the wrist at rest. This type of carpal collapse is termed static carpal instability. This category may be further divided into reducible and irreducible injuries.

Patients with lesser ligament injuries often have normal standard X-rays, yet carpal malalignment and symptoms occur during motion and loading. This type of carpal collapse is termed dynamic carpal instability. The diagnosis of dynamic instability may require stress X-rays, such as an anteroposterior (AP) distraction X-ray with digital traction, manual stress X-rays, a six-view AP (radial deviation, neutral, and ulnar deviation), and lateral (extension, neutral, and flexion) X-ray with a tightly gripped fist; fluoroscopic cineradiography; enhanced gap-free MRI; and/or arthroscopic evaluation. Attenuation and partial ligament tears may propagate over a period of time and use. Carpal collapse, correlative symptoms, and classification may advance accordingly.

Etiology

Trauma and synovitis are the principal causes of carpal ligament disruption. The former is more common. The healing capacity of traumatic ligament injuries is limited and unreliable, owing to a disrupted and/or meager blood supply and technical difficulties in achieving successful repair by suturing. Synovitis erodes ligaments and renders them irreparable.

Location

Location refers to the specific ligament(s) injured, fracture(s), and carpal bones and joints involved.

Direction

Direction is primarily determined by evaluating a true lateral X-ray in the sagittal plane with the resting wrist in a neutral

position. The axial and tangential methods of radiographic measurement are equally accurate in assessing carpal angles [35–37] (Fig. 12.6). The scaphoid tubercle and pisiform must be maximally superimposed to assure a true lateral (sagittal plane) wrist X-ray or image and to eliminate or minimize observer variability [38, 39]. The normal scapholunate angle on lateral X-ray views increases from an average of 35° of flexion in full wrist extension to 76° in full flexion. With the normal wrist in a neutral position, the scaphoid is flexed at about 47° (the angle of Alexander).

The doubly intercalated lunate is a prime radiographic sentinel for both normal and pathophysiologic carpal kinematics [23]. First, the lunate is intercalated *between* the scaphoid and the triquetrum. Lunate flexion and extension occur with the PCR and wrist during normal motion. The lunate is collinear with the capitate in a true lateral (sagittal plane) X-ray or imaging study in the normal resting wrist. The lunate is normally balanced between the scaphoid, which independently tends to flex, and the triquetrum, which intrinsically tends to extend.

In scapholunate dissociation, the lunate dorsiflexes and the lunocapitate and scapholunate angles increase [23]. In lunotriquetral dissociation, the lunate palmar flexes and the lunocapitate angle increases in the direction opposite to that of scapholunate dissociation. The lunotriquetral angle increases.

Second, the lunate is intercalated *within* the proximal row [23]. In midcarpal instability (MCI), when the lunate dorsiflexes and subluxes under the head of the capitate, the injury is termed a dorsal intercalary segment instability (DISI). When the lunate palmar (volar) flexes and subluxes over the

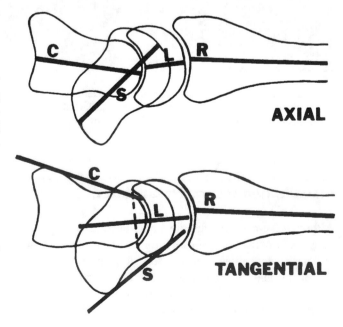

Fig. 12.6 Axial (*above*) and tangential (*below*) methods of measuring carpal angles. C capitate, S scaphoid, L lunate, R radius. (Reprinted from Garcia-Elias et al. [37]. With permission from Elsevier)

head of the capitate, the injury is termed a volar intercalary segment instability (VISI). Knowledge of the lunate as a marker helps to sort out midcarpal, adaptive, and combined or complex carpal instabilities.

Pattern

Four intrinsic carpal instability patterns are recognized. When the ligaments restraining the scaphoid and triquetrum to the lunate are intact, the PCR flexes and extends as a unit. Scapholunate or lunotriquetral ligament injuries cause dissociative and reciprocally opposite rotation of the scaphoid and the triquetrum, respectively, within the PCR. These injuries are therefore defined as carpal instability dissociative (CID). Displaced transtriquetral, and especially transscaphoid, fractures may result in similar patterns. In displaced scaphoid fractures, the proximal scaphoid fragment extends with the lunotriquetral unit and the distal fragment flexes owing to opposing forces. Ligament injuries between the radius and/or ulna and the PCR (the radiocarpal and/or ulnocarpal joints) or between the PCR and DCR (the midcarpal joint) are labeled carpal instability nondissociative (CIND). Carpal instability adaptive (CIA) refers to MCI (*CIND*) from a skeletal injury adjacent to, but not directly involving, the carpal bones and their connecting ligaments. Extra-articular distal radial fractures and malunions with loss of dorsal inclination and dorsal second and third carpometacarpal dislocations or fracture dislocations may cause *CIA* [40, 41]. If *CIA* is corrected with reduction of the causative skeletal deformity, the carpal bones usually realign in a normal or nearly normal posture. Coexisting *CID* and *CIND* are classified as carpal instability combined or complex (CIC).

Pathophysiology

Patients with ulnar negative variance are at increased risk of SLIL injury [42]. Patients with ulnar negative variance and a lunate fossa with an increased radioulnar slope on anteroposterior images are at increased risk of MCI [43]. Larger and deeper scaphoid fossae and greater palmar tilt of the distal radius and greater proximal articular curvatures may shield the wrist from incurring SLIL injury or developing instability after SLIL injury [44]. Wrists with a *Type II* lunate tend to be less susceptible to SLIL injury and progressive perilunar instability (PPI) than patients with a *Type I* lunate; however, they have an increased risk of developing lunohamate arthrosis [45, 46].

Ligament injury is one of degree and may be divided into attenuation or stretch injuries (in which the elastic coefficient of the ligament is exceeded without tearing), partial tears, and complete tears [47]. Attenuation may occasionally be associated with predynamic instability that is unapparent even with joint loading or stress. Attenuation and partial ligament tears are frequently associated with dynamic instability that is apparent only with joint loading or stress. Complete ligament tears, and in some instances specific isolated ligament sectioning, are associated with static instability, owing to some degree of adjacent external secondary ligament injury or division. Bone avulsion may occur in concert with ligament tears and sometimes helps to locate and identify these injuries.

Vertical Carpal Instabilities

Scapholunate Instability (SLI) and Progressive Perilunar Injury (PPI)

PPI results from sequential ligamentous injuries due to wrist extension, ulnar deviation, and supination in relation to a stable forearm during a fall or force on the outstretched hand (FOOSH) [48]. The sequence continues until the energy from the force is completely expended. These forces may also disrupt the wrist ligaments when they occur during other wrist injuries, particularly radial styloid fractures and intra-articular, or even extra-articular, distal radial fractures [48, 49]. Injuries to the SLIL and/or LTIL ligaments are classified as lesser arc injuries [50]. Transscaphoid, transcapitate, and transtriquetral fractures are greater arc lesions (Fig. 12.7). Fractures, in these instances, are more easily treated and heal

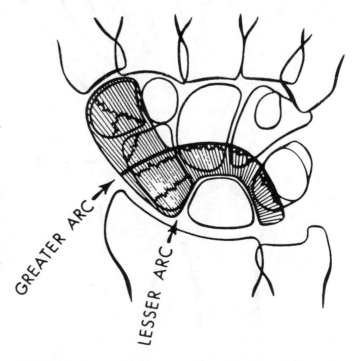

Fig. 12.7 The lesser and greater carpal arcs. (Reproduced with permission from Blazar and Lawton [50])

more reliably than ligament injuries. Concurrent proximal pole fractures of the scaphoid and SLIL tears have been reported and are challenging both to diagnose and treat [51–53].

Mayfield et al. have reported four progressive, representative, integral *stages* within the *spectrum* of PPI [48] (Fig. 12.8). Stage I injuries are characterized by disruption of the SLIL and adjacent ligaments. The SLIL is the primary stabilizer of the scapholunate joint [54–56]. The RSCL and STTL are secondary stabilizers. The SLIL usually tears from its attachment to the scaphoid. Stage I PPI injuries attenuate or tear the space of Poirier palmarly and distally and progressively extend proximally to disrupt the pSLIL until there is scapholunate diastasis with disruption of the RSCL or radial styloid fracture and tearing of the dSLIL and scaphoid insertion of the DICL. Complete scapholunate instability (SLI) occurs when the DICL attachment to lunate is disrupted. Attenuation and partial SLIL tears anterior to the scapholunate axis between the

centers of rotation of the scaphoid and the lunate usually result in dynamic scapholunate instability. Partial SLIL tears dorsal to the scapholunate axis between the centers of rotation of the scaphoid and the lunate and complete SLIL tears result in static scapholunate instability.

Laboratory studies have demonstrated that in vitro complete sectioning of the SLIL alone does not cause scapholunate widening or carpal instability in the resting wrist [54–56]. In vitro sectioning of the SLIL caused mild scapholunate instability during wrist flexion and extension, but only minimal scapholunate instability throughout radioulnar deviation. Loading causes slight abnormal motion between the scaphoid and the lunate that may account for predynamic or mild dynamic instability. Although laboratory sectioning of the entire SLIL causes minimal SLI, traumatic clinical SLIL disruption can cause marked static scapholunate diastasis and instability, owing to involvement of adjacent extra-articular ligaments.

The computation of the total hysteresis area from the hysteresis effect is a sensitive technique that can determine the subtle onset of abnormal carpal motion [57]. Whereas the sectioning of the SLIL, RSCL, and STTL is required to produce changes in the hysteresis area in flexion-extension curves, in vitro sectioning of the SLIL alone increases the total hysteresis area during wrist radioulnar deviation. This subtle finding may identify the onset of dynamic SLI. The total hysteresis area of the lunate may increase as well; however, a paradoxical decrease of the total hysteresis effect of the lunate with hypermobile (lax) wrists may explain why some patients with SSI do not develop DISI deformities.

Further in vitro sectioning of the DICL causes scapholunate widening without static carpal collapse [31, 58]. Additional sectioning of the DICL attachments to the lunate causes greater scapholunate widening. The scaphoid flexes and dissociates from the extending lunotriquetral unit causing static carpal collapse. The proximal pole of the scaphoid subluxes dorsoradially in the scaphoid fossa of the distal radius [59]. Conversely, the lunate subluxes palmarly and ulnarly within the lunate fossa of the distal radius. Abnormal widening of the scapholunate and lunocapitate angles results.

In the intact wrist, scapholunate motion is greater in circumduction than in the DTM, where motion is, in fact, minimal [2–9, 54–56]. Following in vitro sectioning of the RSCL, STTL, and SLIL, the scaphoid flexes more and the lunate extends more during both circumduction and the DTM. Both before and after sectioning, scaphoid motion is greater than that of the lunate. Overall, after in vitro sectioning of the RSCL, STTL, and SLIL, scaphoid motion substantially increased, while lunate motion decreased. This helps to explain the observation that after SLIL tears with associated secondary restrain involvement and continuous motion, arthritic changes occur in the radioscaphoid fossa, but not in the radiolunate joint [60, 61].

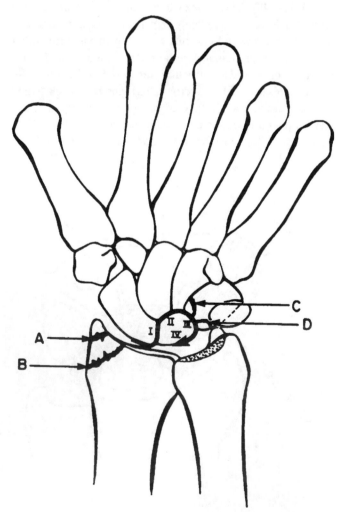

Fig. 12.8 Mayfield's stages of progressive perilunate dislocation. (Reprinted from Mayfield et al. [48]. With permission from Elsevier)

Geissler et al. combined radiocarpal and midcarpal diagnostic arthroscopic evaluation to classify the progressive *spectrum* of SLIL injuries that occur in Mayfield Stage I PPI injuries into four integral arthroscopic *grades* [62] (Video 12.1).

Mayfield Stage I PPI, Geissler SLIL Grade I Injuries

Arthroscopic Grade I SLIL injuries start palmarly and distally and progress proximally and are confined to attenuation or tear in the space of Poirier between the RSCL and LRLL and SLIL attenuation without tear (Fig. 12.9). The attenuation is visualized from the radiocarpal (3–4) portal. From the radial midcarpal portal, the normal SLJ remains congruently aligned and immobile or may have very slight widening palmarly. No abnormality is seen on plain X-rays

(Fig. 12.10). Arthroscopic Grade I lesions create predynamic or dynamic instabilities.

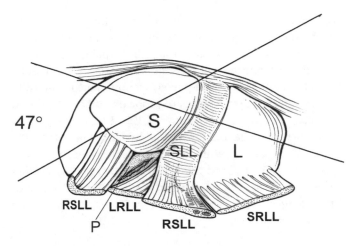

Fig. 12.9 Grade I scapholunate ligament tear

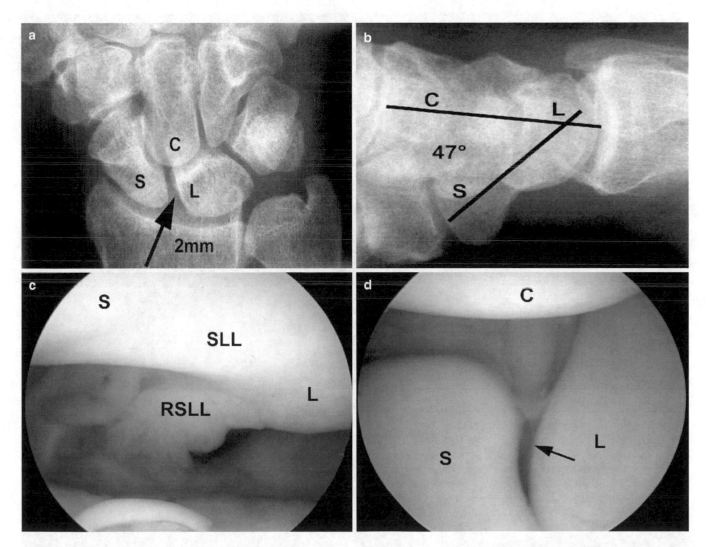

Fig. 12.10 Grade I scapholunate ligament tear. (a) Normal AP X-ray (*arrow* points to the scapholunate joint). (b) Normal lateral X-ray and scapholunate angle. (c) Radiocarpal (3–4 portal) arthroscopic image demonstrating attenuation of the SLL and RSLL. (d) Midcarpal arthroscopic view with opening of the volar portion of the scapholunate interval

Mayfield Stage I PPI, Geissler Grade II SLIL Injuries

Avulsion of the palmer radial corner of the SLIL from the scaphoid or tears of the pSLIL anterior to the scapholunate axis of rotation as seen from the radiocarpal (3–4) portal is classified as arthroscopic Grade II lesions (Fig. 12.11). From the radial midcarpal portal, scapholunate incongruity may be apparent, but a standard probe cannot be introduced between the two bones (Fig. 12.12). Slight multiplanar instability may be demonstrated by stressing either the scaphoid or lunate with the probe or by manual stress applied to the scaphoid tubercle. Usually, there is no discernible abnormality on standard resting X-rays. Stress or MRI images may reveal the lesion. These lesions create dynamic instability.

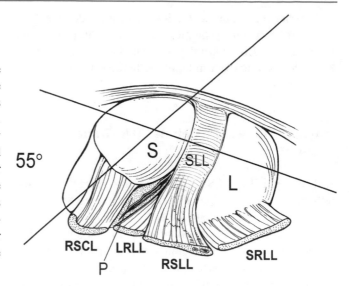

Fig. 12.11 Grade II scapholunate ligament tear

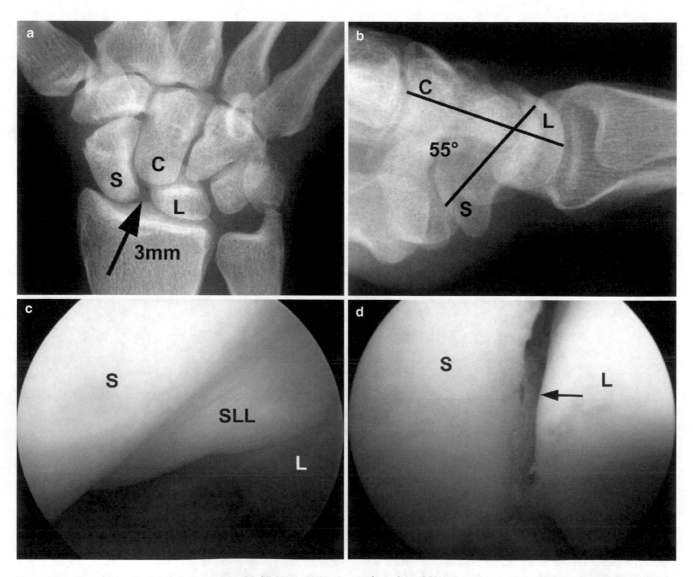

Fig. 12.12 Grade II scapholunate ligament tear. (**a**) Slight diastasis of the scapholunate joint on AP X-ray (*arrow* points to the scapholunate joint). (**b**) Slight flexion of the scaphoid and increase of the scapholunate angle on lateral X-ray. (**c**) Radiocarpal (3–4 portal) arthroscopic image demonstrating attenuation of the SLL. (**d**) Midcarpal arthroscopic view with a uniform opening (1.0–1.5 mm) of the scapholunate interval

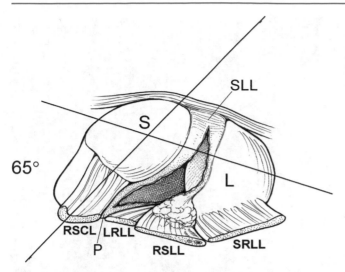

Fig. 12.13 Grade III scapholunate ligament tear

Mayfield Stage I PPI, Geissler Grade III SLIL Injury

Arthroscopic Grade III lesions extend throughout the membranous midportion of the SLIL, but do not involve or only attenuate or partially involve the dSLIL, leaving it as a soft tissue hinge (Fig. 12.13). Some arthroscopic Grade II SLIL lesions and all Grade III involve the mesenteric RSLL. The SLIL tear may be seen from both the 3–4 radiocarpal and the midcarpal portals and a probe (but not the 2.7-mm arthroscope) may be introduced between the scaphoid and the lunate (Fig. 12.14). Multiplanar instability is present and is easily demonstrated with the probe or by digital compression of the scaphoid tubercle. There is definite static instability. Slight scapholunate diastasis (3–4 mm) is seen on AP X-ray, and slight scaphoid flexion and lunate extension are seen on lateral resting X-ray.

Mayfield Stage I PPI, Geissler Grade IV SLIL Injuries

Arthroscopic Grade IV lesions avulse or tear the dorsal segment of the SLIL and then the insertion of the DICL from the scaphoid. The dorsal SLIL and the DICL insertion blend are difficult to distinguish at their interface (Fig. 12.15). The DICL attachment to the lunate may also be torn. The 2.7-mm arthroscope may be passed into the interval between the scaphoid and the lunate. Geissler termed this the "drive-through sign." The head of the capitate may be visualized from the 3–4 radiocarpal portal

(Fig. 12.16). Multiplanar instability between the scaphoid and lunate within the midcarpal portal is readily apparent or easily demonstrated with manual stress testing. The scaphoid is foreshortened by carpal collapse, creating a scapholunate advanced collapsed (SLAC) wrist [60, 61]. On AP X-ray, there is a wide scapholunate gap (4–5 mm or more), and the scaphoid tubercle appears circular creating a "signet ring sign." On the lateral X-ray view, the scaphoid is vertical, or nearly so, and if the DICL attachment to the lunate is torn, the lunate is extended.

Progressive correlative scaphoid flexion, lunotriquetral unit extension, and scapholunate gap widening may be seen on standard resting images as the tear propagates through the arthroscopic grades of classification.

Mayfield Stage II PPI

Scapholunate diastasis and further separation of the space of Poirier is followed by sequential or simultaneous attenuation and/or partial or complete failure of the capitate insertion of the RSCL, the dorsal scaphocapitate segment of the DICL, dorsal capitohamate ligament/capsule, DRLTL, distal insertions of the ulnar limb of the anterior arcuate ulnolunocapitate ligament (triquetrocapitate, triquetrohamate, capitohamate ligaments/capsule), dLTIL, and/or mLTIL, causing capitolunate dissociation [48]. The midcarpal joint becomes unstable and may sublux and/or angulate (see Fig. 12.8).

Mayfield Stage III PPI

Mayfield Stage III lesions are subclassified into Type A (without perilunate dislocation) and Type B (with perilunate dislocation) [48] (see Fig. 12.8). In Type III A, there is failure of the DRLTL between the lunate and triquetrum and separation between the lunate and the triquetrum, indicating at least attenuation or partial tear of the LTIL, creating lunotriquetral instability. The head of the capital remains contained, albeit sometimes dorsally subluxed in the lunate concavity so as to create a DISI deformity. The radiolunate portion of the DRLTL may remain intact, whereas the lunotriquetral segment may be torn. In Type III B, the capitate is dorsally dislocated on top of the lunate (perilunate dislocation), indicating a complete tear of the SLIL, LTIL, and both the radiolunate and lunotriquetral segments of the DRLTL. When both the SLIL and LTIL are torn, the lunate may appear neutral or be flexed or extended on lateral imaging, but the scaphoid will be abnormally flexed.

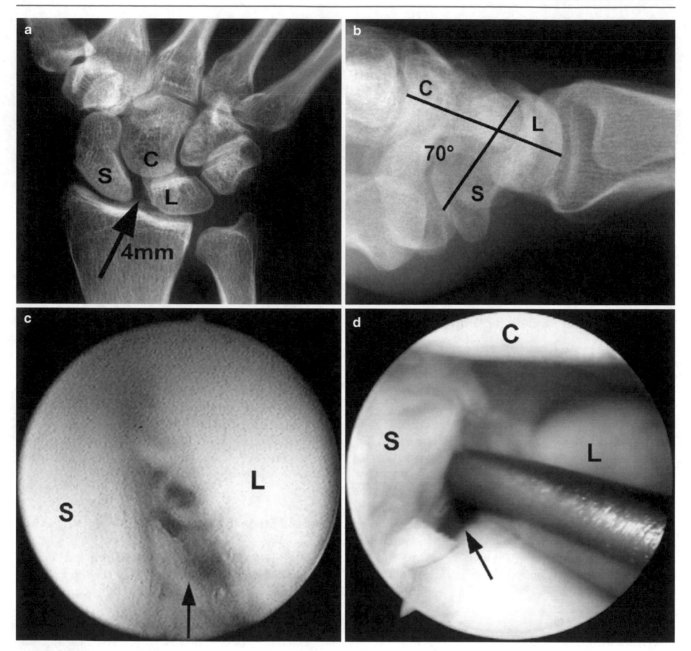

Fig. 12.14 Grade III scapholunate ligament tear. (**a**) Four-millimeter diastasis of the scapholunate joint on AP X-ray (*arrow* points to the scapholunate joint). (**b**) Moderate flexion of the scaphoid and increase of the scapholunate angle to 70° on lateral X-ray. There is slight extension of the lunate in relation to the head of the capitate, a sign of early DISI pattern. (**c**) Radiocarpal (3–4 portal) arthroscopic image demon- strating a complete tear of the volar portion and midsubstance of the SLL. The dorsal scapholunate segment remains intact. (**d**) Midcarpal arthroscopic view demonstrating increased widening and instability of the scapholunate joint sufficient to allow the introduction of a metallic probe

Mayfield Stage IV PPI

Palmar lunate dislocation identifies Stage IV PPI [48]. The SLIL and LTIL are completely ruptured. The lunate attach- ments of the DRLTL and DICL are torn (see Fig. 12.8). Palmar dislocation of the lunate occurs through the space of Poirier (between the RSCL and LRLL). Palmar ligament/ capsular structures may remain sufficiently intact and act as a hinge on the palmer pole of the lunate. There is a wide gap between the scaphoid and the triquetrum. The capitate migrates proximally.

The DCR migrates proximally in terminal Stage I and in Stages II, III, and IV lesions. Consequently, we believe that these injuries should be considered CIC lesions.

Fig. 12.15 Stage II (Grade IV) scapholunate ligament tears

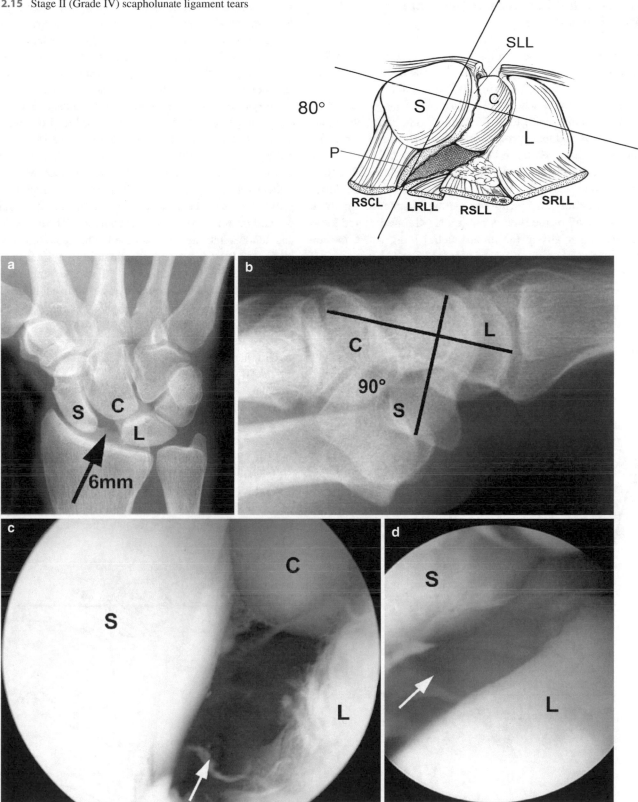

Fig. 12.16 Stage II (Grade IV) scapholunate ligament tear. (**a**) Six-millimeter diastasis of the scapholunate joint on AP X-ray (*arrow* points to the scapholunate joint). (**b**) Severe flexion of the scaphoid and increase of the scapholunate angle to 90° on lateral X-ray. The lunate is extended and subluxed in relation to the head of the capitate, a sign of an established DISI pattern. (**c**) Radiocarpal (3–4 portal) arthroscopic image demonstrating a complete tear of the entire SLL. The head of the capitate can be visualized in the widened interval between the scaphoid and the lunate. (**d**) A midcarpal arthroscopic view demonstrating severe widening and instability of the scapholunate joint sufficient to allow the introduction of the arthroscope

Ulnar-Sided Progressive Perilunar Instability (UPPI)

Lunotriquetral dissociation is substantially less frequent than its dissociative counterpart at the SLJ. The LTIL usually tears from the triquetrum. UPPI results from a fall or a force on the hypothenar eminence of the outstretched hand positioned in radial deviation with PCR pronation. Ulnar-sided perilunate attenuation and tears progress through a spectrum of severity similar to that of SLIL and PPI diastasis [63–68] (Fig. 12.17).

Horii et al. experimentally sectioned the entire LTIL [64]. In a second stage, they additionally sectioned both the dorsal radiotriquetral and scaphotriquetral ligaments. In both instances, all of the intercarpal joints exhibited altered kinematics, especially at the lunotriquetral joint, where motion was increased in all phases of wrist motion. Only in Stage II did a VISI deformity occur.

Viegas et al. have identified three successive stages of ulnar-sided perilunate instability in the laboratory [65]. Similar to the SLIL, partial or complete laboratory partial sectioning of the LTIL alone (Stage I) allowed very slight divergent motion between the lunate and triquetrum, without static deformity. There was no significant difference in the load distribution between a normal wrist and a Stage I lesion. With complete division of the LTIL (Stage II), the scapholunate complex flexed and subluxed dorsally and radially and the triquetrum extended away from the lunate. The lunotriquetral angel increased from a normal value of 14° as lunotriquetral dissociation progressed [66] (Fig. 12.18). Complete sectioning of the LTIL and the lunotriquetrohamate complex of the DRLTL (Stage III) caused ulnar-sided MCI. Static VISI deformity occurred. The head of the capitate migrated proximally from the metacarpal-radial midaxis and subluxed palmarly against the palmar flexed lunate. The lunotriquetral and lunocapitate angles increased. The scaphoid flexed in relation to the capitate while maintaining a normal scapholunate angle. The lunate again acted as a sentinel signaling intrinsic PCR and midcarpal intercarpal instabilities. Wrist extension or ulnar deviation beyond 25° caused a "catch-up clunk" as the PCR and VISI deformities were reduced.

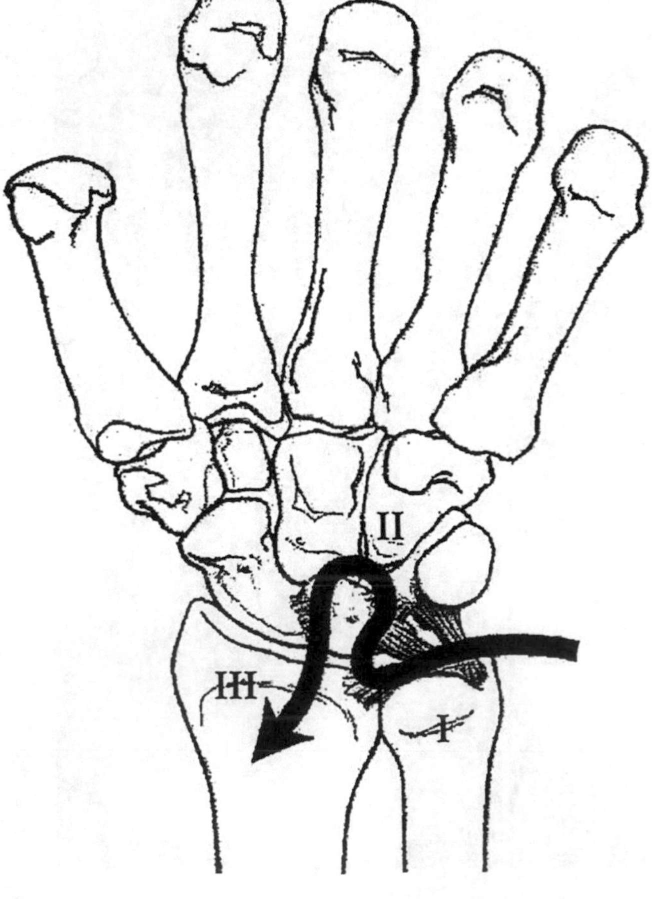

Ritt et al. demonstrated that sectioning of the mLTIL and dLTILL had little effect on carpal kinematics, but sectioning of the mLTIL and pLTIL resulted in flexion of the scapholunate complex and triquetrum extension, producing a VISI deformity [67]. The triquetrum supinated away from the lunate after complete sectioning of the LTIL. VISI deformity increased after additional sectioning of the adjacent components, the DRLTL and DICL. Cycling increased the instability.

Taleisnik identified two clinical *types* of ulnar carpal instability, lunotriquetral and triquetrohamate [68]. Lunotriquetral instability is a Viegas Stage III manifestation of UPPI and has a loss of the dorsiflexion influence of the

Fig. 12.17 The direction, pattern, and stages of progressive lunotriquetral tear leading to perilunate involvement. A Stage I injury has disruption of the ulnolunate and lunotriquetral (ulnar leash) ligament complex. The lunotriquetral ligament is involved in a Stage II injury. In Stage III, the lesion progresses through the midcarpal joint and the scapholunate ligament is disrupted. (Reprinted from Reagan et al. [66]. With permission from Elsevier)

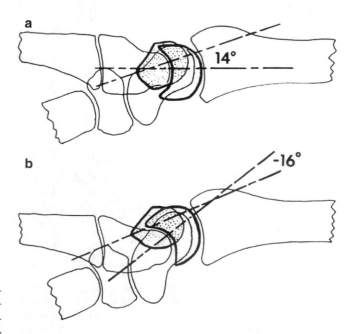

Fig. 12.18 Normal lunotriquetral angle (**a**) and the loss of this relationship with lunotriquetral tear (**b**). (Reprinted from Garcia-Elias et al. [69]. With permission from Elsevier)

triquetrum on the lunate causing static VISI collapse. Triquetrohamate instability will be discussed under MCIs.

Axial Carpal Instability (ACI)

Axial carpal instability (ACI) refers to vertical splits between metacarpal bases and bones in both carpal rows [69, 70]. Crush or blast injuries are frequent precursors. Axial wrist dislocations are not purely intrinsic and extrinsic carpal ligamentous injuries and can be complicated by a variety of other adjacent hand and wrist bone, joint, and/or soft tissue injuries. Open wounds, intrinsic compartment syndromes, and median and ulnar nerve compression, especially of the ulnar motor branch, are frequently seen.

A longitudinal split of the carpus and metacarpal bases characterizes axial dislocations of the carpus (Fig. 12.19). Both the proximal (carpal) and distal (metacarpal) trans-

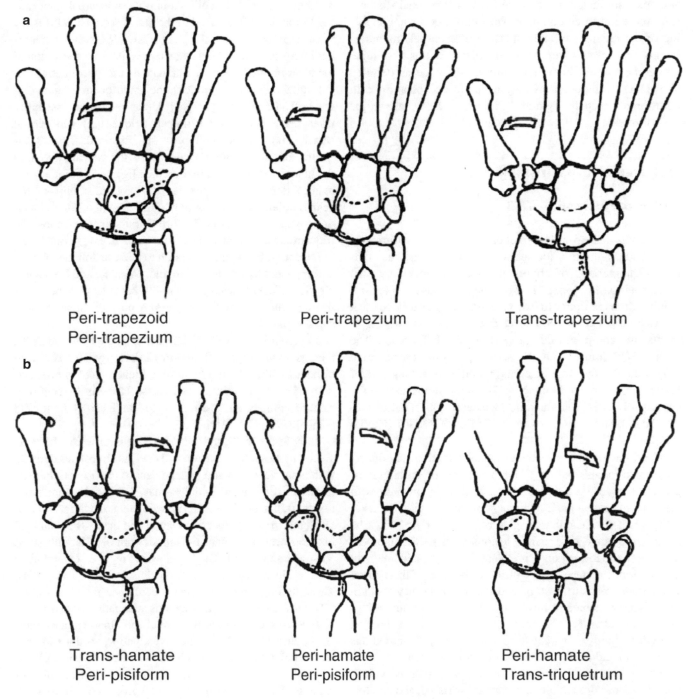

Peri-trapezoid
Peri-trapezium

Peri-trapezium

Trans-trapezium

Trans-hamate
Peri-pisiform

Peri-hamate
Peri-pisiform

Peri-hamate
Trans-triquetrum

Fig. 12.19 Some of the more common patterns of (**a**) axial-radial dislocation and (**b**) axial-ulnar dislocation patterns. (Reprinted from Garcia-Elias et al. [69]. With permission from Elsevier)

verse arches are disrupted. There are three types of axial wrist dislocations: radial, ulnar, and combined radioulnar [69, 70]. In radial and ulnar axial carpal dislocations, the carpus splits into two columns. In radial axial dislocations, the ulnar column maintains a normal and stable relationship with the distal radius and ulna, whereas the radial column separates proximally and radially and may pronate. In ulnar axial dislocations, the radial column maintains a normal and stable relationship with the distal radius and ulna, whereas the ulnar column separates proximally and ulnarly and may supinate. In combined radioulnar axial dislocation, there are three columns. The central column, consisting of the lunate, capitate, and third metacarpal, maintains its normal relationship with the distal radius and ulna, while the radial and ulnar columns displace as detailed above. Axial dislocations may occur in combination with additional carpal ligament injuries and intercarpal deformities.

Transverse Carpal Instabilities

Midcarpal Instability (MCI)

MCI represents several distinct clinical entities, differing in cause and direction of the subluxation, but sharing the common characteristic of abnormal force transmission at the midcarpal joint [64–68, 71]. MCI may be caused by various combinations of injury to extrinsic ligaments as they connect the two carpal rows. Whenever one or more of these ligaments are compromised, proportionate MCI occurs. The radius, PCR (lunate), DCR (capitate), and third metacarpal longitudinal axes no longer have collinear resting and/or load midaxes on lateral imaging. The longitudinal axis of the capitate diverges from the third metacarpal-distal radius longitudinal axis. Dynamic or static VISI or DISI MCI (CIND) follows.

Here, once more, the lunate acts as a sentinel, signifying the direction and extent of MCI. Lunocapitate angles of greater than 15° on a resting, true lateral X-ray or image with the wrist in neutral position highly correlate with static instability [12]. Lunocapitate angles of less than 15° may be static, suggestive of dynamic lesions with partial ligament tears or, in the lower range, predynamic or dynamic ligament attenuation. Palmar sagging of the ulnar side of the neutral wrist, midcarpal shift testing, and stress images may assist in identifying evidence of instability. Fluoroscopic cineradiography can identify MCI and its related ulnarly directed reduction "jump" or "catch-up clunk" [72]. Ligamentous attenuation and/or laxity may be difficult to define.

There are a number of subtypes of MCI: palmar (volar), dorsal, palmar/dorsal, ulnar, radial, ulnar/radial, and capitolunate; often with overlapping features [71]. Distal radial malunions, scaphoid malunions, ulnar negative variance, second and third carpometacarpal dislocation or fracture dislocation, advanced Kienbock's disease, and rheumatoid arthritis account for additional etiologies of MCI. A specific consistent anatomic source(s) has not been verified for many of the MCI patterns published and their direction as they have been difficult to ascertain on diagnostic studies and at the time of operative intervention. We have consequently been left to informed conjecture and speculation.

MCI instability can result from extension of scapholunate and lunotriquetral instabilities into the midcarpal joint during PPI and UPPI as noted in the above sections. VISI is the most commonly reported type of MCI. VISI malalignment is not injury specific. VISI frequently results from disruption of the ulnar limb of the palmar arcuate ligament (triquetrohamatocapitate ligament complex), the lunotriquetral segment of the DRLTL, or both [71, 72]. Ulnar midcarpal instability takes place between the medial (triquetrum) and central (lunate and hamate) columns [68]. Taleisnik Type 2 triquetrohamate instability occurs across the midcarpal joint in the ulnar limb of the palmar arcuate ligaments (triquetrohamatocapitate ligament complex) with loss of stability of the central column presenting only during radial or ulnar deviation (dynamic VISI) [68, 71–73]. During ulnar deviation, the triquetrohamate joint and PCR undergo an exaggerated shift or relocation from palmar flexion to dorsiflexion that may be accompanied by an uncomfortable, palpable, and even audible clunk. Lunotriquetral instability has a loss of the dorsiflexion influence of the triquetrum on the lunate causing static VISI collapse.

In pure primary MCI (CIND) *between* the PCR and DCR, there is no intrinsic SLIL and/or LTIL injury or dissociation of bones within the proximal row. Rather, there is dissociation between the two carpal rows. There is a reciprocal smaller compensatory effect at the radiocarpal joint [71] (Figs. 12.20 and 12.21).

In both the VISI and DISI directions of MCI, the PCR always moves into extension and the DCR translates dorsally with ulnar deviation and engagement of the triquetrohamate joint. In VISI, it is the initial palmar PCR translocation (subluxation) in neutral that reduces with ulnar deviation [71]. In DISI, the wrist is reduced in neutral and the PCR dorsal subluxation occurs in ulnar deviation. Some MCIs with static VISI demonstrated DISI behavior of the capitolunate joint ± the radiolunate joint on dorsal stress testing [74]. These findings may represent a combined radial and ulnar MCI and/or increased ligamentous attenuation or laxity.

In vitro sectioning of the dorsal and ulnar triquetrohamate ligament/capsule in one investigation produced slight midcarpal laxity, but no clunk, whereas division of the stout ulnar limb of the palmar arcuate (triquetrohamatocapitate) ligament caused MCI and produced a clunk [72]. Ensuing studies have shown that sectioning either the pal-

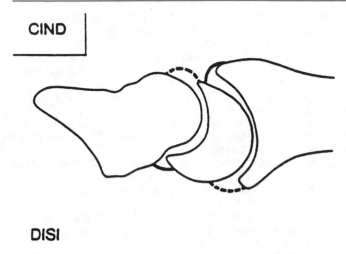

Fig. 12.20 A DISI pattern of deformity occurs with CIND owing to attenuation or tear of the palmar radiocarpal or dorsal midcarpal ligaments or of both. (Reprinted from Amadio [23], pp. 1–12. With permission from John Wiley & Sons, Inc)

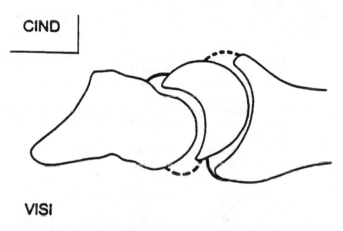

Fig. 12.21 A VISI pattern of deformity occurs with CIND owing to attenuation or tear of the dorsal radiocarpal or volar midcarpal ligaments or of both. (Reprinted from Amadio [23], pp. 1–12. With permission from John Wiley & Sons, Inc)

mar arm of the arcuate ligament or the DRLTL produces a VISI deformity and pathomechanics characteristic of ulnar VISI MCI [75].

In capitolunate instability pattern (CLIP) and chronic capitolunate instability (CCI), the head of the capitate progressively subluxes dorsally on the lunate, especially during ulnar deviation. The entire PCR dorsiflexes. A static or dynamic DISI deformity occurs. Louis et al. and Johnson and Carrera implicated both palmar and dorsal ligamentous/capsular structures attaching to the capitate, including the scaphocapitate segment of the RSCL and the radiolunate ligaments [76, 77]. Traumatic separation and/or extension of the space of Poirier should also be considered.

Hankin et al. postulated two types of radial MCI with rotatory subluxation of the scaphoid. They postulated that one type was due to STTL laxity and the other, to RSCL

disruption. Conceivably, a combination of the two could occur. STTL complex disruption causes a radial-sided MCI with a VISI deformity [78].

Adaptive MCI has also been reported with progressive loss of lateral inclination of the radius in distal radius fractures and malunions [12, 40]. The lunate migrates and angulates dorsally in a DISI configuration to compensate for the loss of lateral angulation of the distal radius. The capitate remains collinear with the lunate, but dorsal to the longitudinal loadline of the distal radius. In these instances, the primary problem occurs at the radiocarpal joint and the reciprocal compensatory response occurs at the midcarpal joint. This type of external MCI has been attributed to repetitive loading and attenuation of the dorsal carpal ligaments and/or acquired laxity of the palmar carpal ligaments attaching to the DCR [40, 71]. Similarly, second and third carpometacarpal dislocation or fracture dislocation can cause a secondary VISI midcarpal malalignment [41]. Patients with ulnar negative variance and a lunate fossa with an increased radioulnar slope on anteroposterior images are at increased risk of MCI [43].

Radiocarpal Instability (RCI)

Posttraumatic ulnar radiocarpal translocation is a rare type of instability, often subtle, highly unstable, and potentially devastating manifestation of severe "inferior arc" injury at the radiocarpal and ulnocarpal joints [79–82]. RCI is a common sequela of radiocarpal dislocation. Shearing axial force is involved. Dorsal radiocarpal dislocation with reciprocal wrist supination and forearm pronation is more common than its palmar counterpart with concomitant wrist pronation and forearm supination. Combined radial and ulnar styloid fractures may herald "inferior arc" injuries. Excessive removal of bone during radial styloidectomy can cause TCI [83].

A spectrum of instabilities occurs, as the following structures are fractured, avulsed, attenuated, or partially or completely disrupted in a radial to ulnar sequence: radial styloid fracture, RSCL or SLIL disruption, LRLL and SRLL disruption, DRLTL disruption, palmar ulnolunate ligament (PULL) disruption, palmar ulnotriquetral ligament (PUTL) and dorsal ulnotriquetral ligament (DUTL) disruption, and ulnar styloid fracture [79–82]. The elements of injury and resistance forces determine the extent of injury until the energy is expended. Distal radioulnate joint (DRUJ) disruption frequently accompanies this injury, as do dorsal and or palmar distal radial lip fractures. Palmar and dorsal Barton's fractures are subsets of RCI. A slice fracture of the distal radius occasionally occurs. RCI may be obscure following radiocarpal reduction and may only be identified by initial distraction X-rays or, later, after the wrist settles into deformity.

The lateral radiocarpal ligament (LRCL) is thin and narrow; it offers little resistance to transverse forces. Siegel et al. demonstrated the importance of the integrity of the RSCL and the radiolunate ligaments in preventing ulnar radiocarpal translocation [83]. There are two configurations of this lesion [84]. Type I RCI involves ulnar translocation of the proximal carpal row as a unit owing to extrinsic radiocarpal ligament injuries with or without radial and/or ulnar styloid fractures. The less common Type II RCI has a dissociative lesion of the SLIL. The sulcus between the radial styloid (Type I injuries) and the scaphoid or between the scaphoid and lunate (Type II injuries) widens in proportion to the injury severity. In Type I RCI with radial styloid fractures and Type II injuries, the RSCL may remain intact. The lunate subluxes or dislocates ulnarly. The proximal pole of the scaphoid subluxes onto or beyond the scapholunate ridge of the distal radius. This constellation of injuries may present dynamic or static patterns and may be accompanied by dorsal or palmar carpal subluxation. Attenuation or tear of the RSCL and/or LRLL may only cause marginal radiocarpal palmar subluxation and dynamic instability [79–81]. Attenuation, or tear, of the SRLL and DRLTL leads to more severe dynamic instability or mild static instability, whereas disruption of the ulnocarpal ligaments accounts for severe static ulnar shift and multidirectional instability. Commensurate progressive radioscaphoid or scapholunate diastasis occurs. Static radiocarpal shifts of this nature may be identified on neutral AP and/or PA and lateral X-rays using standardized measurements of carpal position in relation to the longitudinal midaxis of the radius and third metacarpal [15].

References

1. Palmer AK, Werner FW, Murphy D, et al. Functional wrist motion: a biomechanical study. J Hand Surg Am. 1985;10A:39–46.
2. Werner FW, Short WH, Fortino MD. The relative contribution of selected carpal bones to global wrist motion during simulated planar and out-of-plane motion. J Hand Surg Am. 1997;22A:708–13.
3. Patterson RM, Nicodemus CL, Viegas SF, et al. High speed, three-dimensional kinematic analysis of the normal wrists. J Hand Surg Am. 1998;23A:446–53.
4. Werner FW, Green JK, Short WH, et al. Scaphoid and lunate motion during a wrist dart throw motion. J Hand Surg Am. 2004;29A:418–22.
5. Moritomo H, Murase T, Goto A, et al. Capitate-based kinematics of the midcarpal joint during wrist radioulnar deviation: an in vivo three-dimensional motion analysis. J Hand Surg Am. 2004;29A:668–75.
6. Crisco JJ, Coburn JC, Moore DC, et al. In vivo radiocarpal kinematics and the dart thrower's motion. J Bone Joint Surg. 2005;87A:2729–40.
7. Moritomo H, Apergis EP, Herzberg G, et al. 2007 IFSSH committee report of wrist biomechanics committee: biomechanics of the so-called dart-throwing motion of the wrist. J Hand Surg Am. 2007;32A(32A):1447–53.
8. Calfee RP, Leventhal EL, Wilkerson J, et al. Simulated radioscapholunate fusion alters carpal kinematics while preserving dart-thrower's motion. J Hand Surg Am. 2008;33A:503–10.
9. Crisco JJ, Heard WM, Rich RR, et al. The mechanical axes of the wrist are oriented obliquely to the anatomical axes. J Bone Joint Surg. 2011;93A:169–77.
10. Johnston HM. Varying positions of the carpal bones in the different movements at the wrist. Part I. Extension, ulnar, and radial flexion. J Anat Physiol. 1907;41:109–22.
11. Guilford W, Boltan R, Lambrinudi C. The mechanism of the wrist joint. Guys Hosp Rep. 1943;92:52–9.
12. Linscheid RL, Dobyns JH, Beabout JW, et al. Traumatic instability of the wrist: diagnosis, classification, and pathomechanics. J Bone Joint Surg. 1972;54A:1612–32.
13. Sarrafian SK, Malamed JL, Goshgarian GM. Study of wrist motion in flexion and extension. Clin Orthop. 1977;126:153–9.
14. Wright DR. A detailed study of the movement of the wrist joint. J Anat. 1935;70:137–43.
15. Youm Y, McMurty RY, Flatt AE, et al. Kinematics of the wrist. I. An experimental study of radio-ulnar deviation and flexion-extension. J Bone Joint Surg. 1978;60A:423–31.
16. Wolfe SW, Gupta A, Cristo JJ. Kinematics of the scaphoid shift test. J Hand Surg. 1997;22A:801–6.
17. Navarro A. Luxaciones del carpo. Anal Fac Med Montevideo. 1921;6:113–41.
18. Taleisnik J. Wrist anatomy, function, and injury. AAOS Instr Course Lect. St. Louis: Mosby; 1978. p. 61–87.
19. Weber ER. Concepts governing the rotational shift of the intercalated segment of the carpus. Orthop Clin North Am. 1984;15:193–207.
20. Lichtman DM, Schneider JR, Swafford AR, et al. Ulnar midcarpal instability. J Hand Surg Am. 1981;6:515–23.
21. Craigen MA, Stanley JK. Wrist kinematics. Row, column or both? J Hand Surg Am. 1995;20B:165–70.
22. Berger RA, Crowninshield RD, Flatt AE. The three-dimensional rotational behavior of the carpal bones. Clin Orthop. 1982;167:303–10.
23. Amadio PC. Carpal kinematics and instability: a clinical and anatomic primer. Clin Anat. 1991;4:456–68.
24. Upal MA, Crisco JJ, Moore DC, et al. In vivo elongation of the palmar and dorsal scapholunate interosseous ligament. J Hand Surg Am. 2006;31A:1326–32.
25. Moojen TM, Snel JG, Ritt MJ, et al. In vivo analysis of carpal kinematics and comparative review of the literature. J Hand Surg Am. 2003;28A:81–7.
26. Kaufmann R, Pfaeffle J, Blankenhorn B, et al. Kinematics of the midcarpal and radiocarpal joints in radioulnar deviation: an in vitro study. J Hand Surg Am. 2005;30A:937–42.
27. Berger RA. The gross and histologic anatomy of the scapholunate ligament. J Hand Surg Am. 1996;21A:170–8.
28. Berger RA, Imeada T, Bergland L, et al. Constraint and material properties of the subregions of the scapholunate interosseous ligament. J Hand Surg Am. 1999;24A:953–62.
29. Viegas SF, Yamaguchi S, Boyd NL, et al. The dorsal ligaments of the wrist: anatomy, mechanical properties, and function. J Hand Surg Am. 1999;24A:456–68.
30. Viegas SF. The dorsal ligaments of the wrist. Hand Clin. 2001;17:65–75.
31. Mitsuyasu H, Patterson RM, Shah MA, et al. The role of the dorsal intercarpal ligament in dynamic and static scapholunate instability. J Hand Surg Am. 2004;29A:279–88.
32. Werner FW, Short WH, Green JK. Changes in patterns of scaphoid and lunate motion during functional arcs of wrist motion induced by ligament division. J Hand Surg Am. 2005;30A:1156–60.
33. Ritt MJ, Bishop AT, Berger RA, et al. Lunotriquetral ligament properties: a comparison of three anatomic subregions. J Hand Surg Am. 1998;23A:425–31.
34. Larsen CF, Amadio PC, Gilula LA, et al. Analysis of carpal instability. I. Description of the scheme. J Hand Surg Am. 1995;20A:757–64.

35. Schuind FA, Leroy B, Comtet J-J. Biodynamics of the wrist: radiologic approach to scapholunate instability. J Hand Surg Am. 1985;10A:1006–8.

36. Nakamura R, Hori M, Imamura T, et al. Method for measurement and evaluation of carpal bone angles. J Hand Surg Am. 1989;14A:412–6.

37. Garcia-Elias M, An KN, Amadio PC, et al. Reliability of carpal angle determination. J Hand Surg Am. 1989;14A:1017–21.

38. Yang Z, Mann FA, Gilula LA, et al. Scaphopisocapitate alignment: criteria to establish a neutral lateral view of the wrist. Radiology. 1997;205:865–9.

39. Larsen CF, Stigsby B, Lindequist S, et al. Observer variability in measurements of carpal bone angles on lateral wrist radiographs. J Hand Surg Am. 1992;16A:893–8.

40. Taleisnik J, Watson HK. Midcarpal instability caused by mal-united fractures of the distal radius. J Hand Surg Am. 1984;9A:350–7.

41. Freeland AE, McAuliffe JA. Dorsal carpal metacarpal fracture dislocation associated with nondissociative segmental instability. Orthopedics. 2002;25:753–5.

42. Czitrom AA, Dobyns JH, Linscheid RL. Ulnar variance in carpal instability. J Hand Surg Am. 1987;12A:205–8.

43. Wright TW, Dobyns J, Linscheid RL, et al. Carpal instability non-dissociative. J Hand Surg Am. 1994;19B:763–73.

44. Werner FW, Short WH, Green JK, et al. Severity of scapholunate instability is related to joint anatomy and congruency. J Hand Surg Am. 2007;32A:55–60.

45. Rhee PC, Moran SL, Shin AY. Association between lunate morphology and carpal collapse in cases of scapholunate dissociation. J Hand Surg Am. 2009;34A:1633–9.

46. Nakamura K, Patterson RM, Viegas SF. Type I versus type II lunates: ligament anatomy and presence of arthrosis. J Hand Surg Am. 2001;26A:428–36.

47. Watson HK, Weinzweig J, Zeppierri J. The natural progression of scaphoid instability. Hand Clin. 1997;13:39–49.

48. Mayfield JK, Johnson RP, Kilcoyne RK. Carpal dislocations: pathomechanics and progressive perilunar instability. J Hand Surg Am. 1980;5:226–41.

49. Mudgal CS, Jones WA. Scapho-lunate diastasis: a component of fractures of the distal radius. J Hand Surg Am. 1990;15B:503–5.

50. Blazar PE, Lawton JN. Diagnosis of carpal ligament injuries. In: Trumble TE, editor. Carpal fracture-dislocations. Rosewood: American Academy of Orthopaedic Surgery; 2002. p. 21.

51. Black DM, Watson HK, Vender MI. Scapholunate gap with scaphoid nonunion. Clin Orthop. 1987;224:205–9.

52. Monsivais JJ, Nitz PA, Scully TJ. The role of carpal instability in scaphoid nonunion: casual or causal? J Hand Surg Am. 1986;11B:201–6.

53. Vender MI, Watson HK, Black DM, et al. Acute scaphoid fracture with scapholunate gap. J Hand Surg Am. 1989;14:1004–7.

54. Short WH, Werner FW, Green JK, et al. Biomechanical evaluation of ligamentous stabilizers of the scaphoid and lunate. J Hand Surg Am. 2002;27A:991–1002.

55. Short WH, Werner FW, Green JK, et al. Biomechanical evaluation of the ligamentous stabilizers of the scaphoid and lunate. Part II. J Hand Surg. 2005;30A:24–34.

56. Short WH, Werner FW, Green JK, et al. Biomechanical evaluation of the ligamentous stabilizers of the scaphoid and lunate. Part III. J Hand Surg Am. 2007;32A:297–309.

57. Berdia S, Short WH, Werner FW, et al. The hysteresis effect in carpal kinematics. J Hand Surg Am. 2006;31:594–600.

58. Elsaidi GA, Ruch DS, Kuzma GR, et al. Dorsal wrist ligament insertions stabilize the scapholunate interval: cadaver study. Clin Orthop Relat Res. 2004;425:152–7.

59. Blevens AD, Light TR, Jablonsky WS, et al. Radiocarpal articular contact characteristics with scaphoid instability. J Hand Surg Am. 1989;14A:781–90.

60. Watson HK, Ballet FL. The SLAC wrist. Scapholunate advanced collapse pattern of degenerative arthritis. J Hand Surg Am. 1984;9A:356–65.

61. Watson HK, Ryu J. Evolution of arthritis of the wrist. Clin Orthop. 1986;202:57–67.

62. Geissler WB, Freeland AE, Savoie FH, et al. Intracarpal soft tissue lesions associated with intra-articular fracture of the distal end of the radius. J Bone Joint Surg. 1996;78A:357–65.

63. Shin AY, Murray PM. Biomechanical studies of wrist ligament injuries. In: Trumble TE, editor. Carpal fracture-dislocations. Rosewood: American Academy of Orthopaedic Surgery; 2002. p. 14.

64. Horii E, Garcia-Elias M, An KN, et al. A kinematic study of lunotriquetral dissociations. J Hand Surg Am. 1991;16A:355–62.

65. Viegas SF, Patterson RM, Peterson PD, et al. Ulnar sided perilunate instability: an anatomic and biomechanical study. J Hand Surg Am. 1990;15A:268–77.

66. Reagan DS, Linscheid RL, Dobyns JH. Lunotriquetral sprains. J Hand Surg Am. 1984;9:502–14.

67. Ritt MJ, Linscheid RL, Cooney WP, et al. Lunotriquetral ligament properties: the lunotriquetral joint: kinematic effects of sequential ligament sectioning, ligament repair, and arthrodesis. J Hand Surg Am. 1998;23A:432–45.

68. Taleisnik J. Triquetrohamate and triquetrolunate instabilities (medial carpal instability). Ann Chir Main. 1984;3:331–43.

69. Garcia-Elias M, Dobyns JH, Cooney WP, et al. Traumatic axial dislocations of the carpus. J Hand Surg Am. 1989;14A:446–57.

70. Freeland AE, Rojas SL. Traumatic combined radial and ulnar axial wrist dislocation. Orthopedics. 2002;245:1161–3.

71. Lichtman DM. Understanding midcarpal instability. J Hand Surg Am. 2006;31A:491–8.

72. Lichtman DM, Schneider JR, Swatford AR, et al. Ulnar midcarpal instability – clinical and laboratory analysis. J Hand Surg Am. 1981;6A:515–23.

73. Garth WP Jr, Hoffamann DY, Rooks MD. Volar intercalated instability secondary to medial carpal ligament laxity. Clin Orthop. 1985;201:94–105.

74. Aspergis EP. The unstable capitolunate and radiolunate joints as a source of wrist pain in young women. J Hand Surg Am. 1996;21B:501–6.

75. Trimble T, Bour CT, Smith RJ, et al. Kinematics of ulnar carpus related to the volar intercalated segment instability pattern. J Hand Surg Am. 1990;15A:384–92.

76. Louis DS, Hankin FM, Greene TL. Chronic capitolunate instability. J Bone Joint Surg. 1987;69A:950–1.

77. Johnson RP, Carrera GF. Chronic capitolunate instability. J Bone Joint Surg. 1986;68A:1164–76.

78. Hankin FM, Amadio PC, Wojtys EM, et al. Carpal instability with volar flexion of the proximal row associated with injury to the scapho-trapezial ligament: report of two cases. J Hand Surg Am. 1988;13B:298–302.

79. Graham TJ. The inferior arc injury: an addition to the family of complex carpal fracture-dislocation patterns. Am J Orthop (Belle Mead NJ). 2003;32(9 Suppl):1–19.

80. Rayhack JM, Linscheid RL, Dobyns JH, Smith JH. Posttraumatic ulnar translocation of the carpals. J Hand Surg Am. 1987;12A:180–9.

81. Allieu Y, Garcia-Elias M. Dynamic radial translation instability of the carpus. J Hand Surg Am. 2000;25B:33–7.

82. Freeland AE, Ferguson CA, McCraney WO. Palmar radiocarpal dislocation resulting in ulnar radiocarpal translocation and multidirectional instability. Orthopedics. 2006;29:604–8.

83. Siegel DB, Gelberman RH. Radial styloidectomy: an anatomic study with special reference to radiocarpal intracapsular ligamentous morphology. J Hand Surg Am. 1991;16A:40–4.

84. Moneim MS, Bolger JT, Omer GE. Radiocarpal dislocation-classification and rationale for management. Clin Orthop. 1995;192:199–209.

Management of Scapholunate Ligament Pathology

13

Mark Ross, William B. Geissler, Jeremy Loveridge, and Gregory Couzens

Introduction

Management of pathology involving the scapholunate ligament complex presents a number of unique challenges. These challenges are derived not only from difficulty in defining the temporal, structural, and biomechanical nature of such pathology, but also from the lack of uniformly good outcomes from a wide variety of existing surgical treatments.

Initially, arthroscopy offered the capacity to directly visualize interosseous ligaments within the wrist and even a dynamic evaluation of some intercarpal relationships. A partial tear of the scaphulonate interosseous ligament (SLIL) may be difficult to detect with imaging studies, but is identifiable arthroscopically. In addition, arthroscopy allows the assessment of the status of articular cartilage, with greater accuracy than imaging techniques, for planning therapeutic intervention. It continues to remain the gold standard for diagnosis [1, 2]. Improvements in resolution and scanning protocols have seen improved diagnostic utility from magnetic resonance imaging (MRI).

Nevertheless, the utility of wrist arthroscopy has been extended to facilitate treatment options for SLL ligament pathology beyond diagnosis.

The indications for wrist arthroscopy continue to expand from Whipple's original description [3] as new techniques and instrumentation develop. Further advances in instrumentation, such as electrothermal shrinkage and pathology-specific arthroscopic drill guides, will continue to play a role in the management of pathology of the SLIL.

Anatomy

Improved understanding of the biomechanics of the carpus and their dynamic relationships has altered the conceptualization of the SLL interface. We have moved from considering the SLL in isolation to considering it one component of the "SLL complex" (SLLC) that involves both intrinsic and extrinsic ligamentous components [4]. The intrinsic portion of the SLLC includes the palmar, central membranous, and dorsal portions. The dorsal portion appears to be the primary biomechanical functioning component of the interosseous ligament. It is composed of stout transverse fibers to resist rotation. The volar portion of the interosseous ligament is comprised of longer oblique fibers that allow for sagittal rotation. The central membranous portion of the ligament frequently demonstrates perforations, which increase in frequency with age [4, 5].

The extrinsic components include the volar radio-scapho-capitate, long radiolunate, and short radiolunate ligaments on the volar aspect [6]. Further secondary stabilizers of the SLL interval include the capsule of the scapho-trapezio-trapezoid (STT) joint and the dorsal intercarpal (DIC) ligament [7, 8].

M. Ross
Brisbane Hand and Upper Limb Research Institute, Brisbane, QLD, Australia

Orthopaedic Department, Princess Alexandra Hospital, Woolloongabba, QLD, Australia

The University of Queensland, St. Lucia, QLD, Australia

W. B. Geissler (✉)
Division of Hand and Upper Extremity Surgery, Section of Arthroscopic Surgery and Sports Medicine, Department of Orthopedic Surgery and Rehabilitation, University of Mississippi Medical Center, Jackson, MS, USA

J. Loveridge
Brisbane Hand and Upper Limb Research Institute, Brisbane, QLD, Australia

G. Couzens
Orthopaedic Department, Princess Alexandra Hospital, Woolloongabba, QLD, Australia

Brisbane Hand and Upper Limb Research Institute, Brisbane Private Hospital, Brisbane, QLD, Australia

Institute of Health and Biomedical Innovation, Queensland University of Technology, Brisbane, QLD, Australia

© Springer Nature Switzerland AG 2022
W. B. Geissler (ed.), *Wrist and Elbow Arthroscopy with Selected Open Procedures*,
https://doi.org/10.1007/978-3-030-78881-0_13

Radiographic abnormalities may not be seen initially until attenuation or failure of the extrinsic stabilizers occurs. This may result in delayed detection of SLL pathology on plain radiographs.

Pathomechanics/Mechanism of Injury

Injury is usually caused by a fall onto the outstretched wrist resulting in a dorsiflexion injury. Wrist extension and carpal supination are the primary mechanisms of injury to the SLL. Similar to other ligamentous injuries in the body, the interosseous ligament may stretch and eventually tear. The SLL may double in length prior to failure. Mayfield has shown the percent elongation to failure to be up to 225% [9]. A spectrum of injury is seen to the SLL itself. An isolated injury to the SLL may not yield SL disassociation or widening on plain radiographs. However, a combined injury to both the intrinsic and extrinsic ligaments will usually cause SL diastasis [10]. The difficulty is that there is a paucity of natural history studies that define the evolution of either acute or chronic SL pathology. Although some patients present with the typical history of a hyperextension injury to the wrist, other patients may not recall an acute injury in a fall, but rather a "popping" or giving way sensation on heavy lifting, or even no history of injury at all. Many patients who present with an established scapholunate advanced collapse (SLAC) wrist do not recall any history of acute injury. It is clear that there is a complex interplay between acute traumatic disruptions, serial lesser injuries, and attenuation over time from subclinical events.

Assessment

History

A history of acute dorsiflexion injury should raise concern about injury to the SLLC. Patients may present with dorsal wrist pain and giving way or mechanical symptoms without a history of serious acute injury.

Examination

Physical examination reveals localized tenderness directly over the dorsum of the SL interval. The principal provocative maneuver to assess the SL instability is the "scaphoid shift test" [7]. This test evaluates motion of the scaphoid during radial deviation and wrist flexion, while pressure is applied to the tubercle of the scaphoid in a volar to dorsal direction. Partial tears to the SLL may produce pain directly over the dorsum of the SL interval with no palpable click. Pain over

the scaphoid tubercle when palpated is not clinically significant. A complete tear of the SLL results in subluxation of the proximal pole of the scaphoid over the dorsal lip of the distal radius. When this occurs, a palpable shift or click is felt. Both the injured and noninjured wrists should be assessed with the scaphoid shift test to evaluate for inherent laxity, particularly in individuals with a classified generalized ligamentous laxity [11]. The radiocarpal joint may be injected with local anesthetic to evaluate for potential shift if pain prevents performance of the test.

Imaging

Plain Radiographs

Radiographs are essential at the initial evaluation to assess the SL articulation. It should be stressed from the outset that all radiographic views may only be definitely interpreted when compared with the opposite side. Standard radiographic views include the posteroanterior (PA) view in ulnar deviation; an oblique, true lateral; and clenched-fist views.

In the PA view, three smooth radiographic arcs may be drawn to define normal carpal relationships [12]. A step-off in the continuity of any of these arcs indicates an intercarpal instability at the site where the arc is broken. Any overlap between the carpal bones or any joint width exceeding 4 mm strongly suggests carpal ligamentous injury. A standardized clenched-fist view in 30° ulna deviation has been shown to yield the widest diastasis in ruptured SLL injuries [13].

A "Terry-Thomas" sign is considered present when the space between the scaphoid and lunate appears abnormally wide as compared to the opposite wrist [14]. The SL interval should be measured in the middle of the flat medial facet of the scaphoid. Less than 3 mm is considered normal, 3–5 mm is suspicious, and any asymmetric SL gap greater than 5 mm is said to be diagnostic of SL dissociation [15]. The scaphoid ring sign occurs when the scaphoid has collapsed into flexion and has a foreshortened appearance on a PA radiograph. The ring sign is present in all causes of scaphoid flexion, regardless of the etiology [16]. Therefore, the presence of a scaphoid ring sign does not necessarily indicate instability of the SL interval.

In lateral radiographs, the SL angle is defined by a line tangential to the two proximal and distal convexities of the palmar aspect of the scaphoid. The angle formed by this line and a line through the central axis of the lunate determines the SL angle. Normal values range between 30° and 60°, with an average of 47°. Angles greater than 80° are strongly indicative of SL instability [16]. Assessment of the radiolunate and capitolunate angles may also give an assessment of the degree of intercalated segment instability.

On the lateral radiograph, concentricity between the arc of the proximal pole of the scaphoid and the scaphoid facet of the radius is usually seen. When there is carpal instability, dorsal translation of the proximal pole is seen with loss of this concentric relationship. Subtle manifestation of this altered relationship may be identified on sagittal plane high-resolution MRI scanning before plain radiographic abnormality is identified.

Assessing the contralateral side radiographically for comparison is useful. In addition, the sensitivity of plain radiographs may be increased by performing so-called "dynamic views." There are a variety of views described. Although not truly dynamic, these static stress views look at changes in carpal alignment with specific wrist positioning and with load from grip. Flexion and extension lateral views and radial/ulnar deviation PA views are most frequently suggested and a standardized clenched-fist pencil view in 30° ulna deviation has been shown to yield the widest diastasis in ruptured SLIL injuries [13, 17].

Fluoroscopy

True dynamic assessment of carpal motion and intercarpal relationships can be achieved with the use of fluoroscopy.

Ultrasound

Ultrasound has been used for the assessment of SLL injury. It offers the possibility to assess the pathology dynamically in real time. The SLL and proximal pole of the scaphoid are identified and ultrasound is performed in the transverse and longitudinal planes. The wrist is scanned in ulnar and radial deviation, the clenched-fist view, and resisted extension. Ultrasound scans can show osteophytes, a joint effusion, bulging of the SLL, and a degenerate capsule. The technique and the interpretation of the findings can be difficult, especially due to the variations in anatomy and kinetics. Its main role is probably to complement clinical examination and other imaging studies. It has the potential to show subtle rotatory instability of the scaphoid [18].

Dao et al. in 2004 reported on the efficacy of ultrasound for evaluating dynamic SLL instability and compared it to arthroscopy [18]. Of the 64 wrists analyzed, ultrasound had a low sensitivity of 46.2%, a high specificity of 100%, and an accuracy of 89.1%. The authors recommended its use as an adjunct to other diagnostic modalities for this purpose [18].

Taljanovic et al. in 2008 described the use of ultrasound for the assessment of SLLs and its correlation with magnetic resonance (MR) and magnetic resonance angiography (MRA). For the SLL, the results were concordant for all imaging modalities in 15, partially concordant in 3 (18.75%), and discordant in 1 (6.25%). The arthroscopic and imaging findings were concordant for three SLLs [19].

The preliminary results are encouraging. Sonography may be used at least as a screening imaging modality in evaluation of the SLL.

MRI

Patients who are suspected clinically of having a SLL injury, but whose radiographs are normal should undergo MRI scanning of the injured wrist with interpretation by an experienced radiologist. The SLL can be challenging to assess on MRI.

High-resolution MRI using 3.0 T magnetic strength is optimal for definitively demonstrating the three components of the SLL (dorsal, volar, and membranous components) and their integrity [20].

High-resolution MRI of the SLL is best performed on a 3 T magnet with a dedicated 8ch or 16ch wrist coil. It is also accepted that interpretation of the MRI should be completed by a radiologist with expertise in wrist imaging [20]. In the unit of two of the senior authors (MR, GC), high-resolution noncontrast MRI is performed on a Siemens 3 T Verio platform using the in vivo 8ch wrist coil. The patients are positioned with the arm above their head while lying prone in the scanner, that is, "Superman position" [20]. The reason for this is that this position is at the isocenter of the magnet providing the best signal-to-noise ratio possible. Two-millimeter slice axial views are performed from the proximal radius and ulna to distal to the capitate. Direct coronal views of the wrist are obtained with the slice orientation parallel to the anterior border of the distal radius and ulna. Sagittal views are obtained with the slice orientation perpendicular to the wrist joint. Proton density scans with fat suppression are used. A T1 coronal sequence with 2-mm slices and a three-dimensional (3D) axial gradient echo sequence with 0.5-mm slices are also performed.

High-resolution coronal and axial images delineate whether the dorsal or volar fibers are intact. The intact dorsal band is well demonstrated on the most dorsal of the coronal plane slices that show scaphoid and lunate, with dark linear fibers being visible. Secondary signs of SLL rupture are seen with dorsal scaphoid translation in relation to the scaphoid facet of the radius and cartilage loss, which are best seen on the sagittal views (Fig. 13.1). Widening of the SL interval should not be an exclusive indication that the SLL has been ruptured, as it could still be intact, but redundant. Ganglia are often present with SLL tears, and visualization is best seen on T2-weighted scans with uniform fat suppression.

Computed Tomography

Recently, Kakar described a novel imaging technique for 4D CT (computed tomography) imaging (3D + time), which has promising clinical utility in accurately diagnosing SL instability [21]. The 4D CT allows dynamic image data (4D movies) to be recorded while the patient moves their wrist

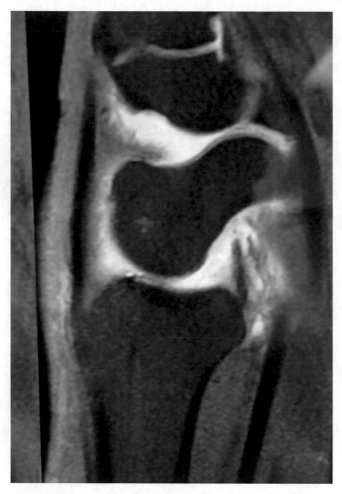

Fig. 13.1 Dorsal scaphoid translation and cartilage loss on proximal scaphoid on sagittal plane MRI

through various movements including radial-ulnar deviation, flexion-extension, and dart thrower's motion.

Classification of SLL Pathology

This table summarizes the various methods of classifying SLL pathology and identifies what level of pathology each type of assessment can ascertain (Table 13.1). Various systems for classifying SLL pathology have been described, both temporally and structurally.

Temporal Classification

There is no clear consensus on what constitutes acute, subacute, and chronic injuries. Whichever criteria are used, the principal aim is to define the potential for healing of the native ligament.

Larsen et al. classified *carpal instability* in a temporal way. Acute was defined as less than a week old, subacute was defined as between 1 and 6 weeks, and chronic was described as more than 6 weeks old [22].

Geissler and Haley defined an acute injury as up to 3–4 weeks old. Subacute was defined as an injury more than 3–4 weeks old and up to 6 months old. A chronic injury was defined as symptoms present greater than 6 months [23].

The current trend has been to consider injuries as "chronic" at an earlier time point due to the observed poorer outcomes in terms of radiographic maintenance of SL gap after direct ligament repair, at relatively early intervals after the apparent index injury.

Table 13.1 Classification of SLL pathology

Classification type	Description		
Temporal	Acute		
	Subacute		
	Chronic		
Structural	Imaging	Radiographs	Static radiographs—complete static dissociation
			Dynamic radiographs/fluoroscopy—complete dynamic dissociation
		MRI	Incomplete and partial
			Dorsal band
			Membranous
			Volar band
			Complete—dynamic or static
	Arthroscopic	Geissler classification	See Table 13.2 for detail
	Operative	Incomplete	
		Complete	Dynamic
			Static
			Reducible
			Irreducible

This lack of consensus as to what constitutes an acute injury means that algorithms for management based on temporal classification remain inconsistent.

Clinical Examination Classification Systems

Clinically, we can define four types of instability: (1) predynamic instability, (2) dynamic instability, (3) reducible static instability, and (4) nonreducible instability [24]. Predynamic instability was initially termed by Kirk Watson [7] and applies to instability that may be observed clinically on physical examination but not by radiographic studies, and corresponds to a Geissler Grade I or II instability [23]. Dynamic SL instability is applied to a complete SLL tear, but the secondary scaphoid stabilizers remain intact [25]. SL instability can be observed radiographically under loaded conditions or in specific wrist positions, "clenched fist" or loading the wrist in ulnar deviation. Static reducible SL dissociation occurs when the ligament tear is chronic and irreparable; the secondary stabilizers are insufficient and a dorsal intercalated segment instability (DISI) deformity results; carpal subluxation is reducible [24].

Structural Classification

A structural classification can be based on imaging studies, or arthroscopic or open operative evaluation. Imaging studies may be static X-ray films, stress/positional radiographs, fluoroscopy, ultrasound, or MRI.

Arthroscopic Structural Classification

The key to treatment of SLL complex pathology is recognition of what is normal and what is pathological anatomy. Both the radiocarpal and midcarpal spaces must be evaluated arthroscopically when carpal instability is suspected. Wrist arthroscopy is usually not considered complete if the midcarpal space has not been evaluated, particularly with a suspected diagnosis of carpal instability.

The SLL is best visualized with the arthroscope in the 3–4 portal. It should have a concave appearance as viewed from the radiocarpal space (Fig. 13.2). In the midcarpal space, the SL interval should be tight and congruent without any step-off (Fig. 13.3). This is in contrast to the luno-triquetral (LT) interval, in which a 1-mm step-off occasionally is seen, which is considered normal and slight motion is seen between the lunate and triquetrum. When it tears, the SLIL hangs down and blocks visualization with the arthroscope in the radiocarpal space from the 3–4 portal. The normal concave appearance between the carpal bones becomes convex.

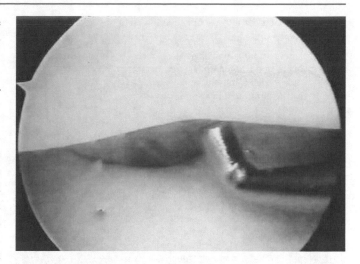

Fig. 13.2 Arthroscopic view of the normal concave appearance of the SLIL as seen from the 3–4 portal in the radiocarpal space

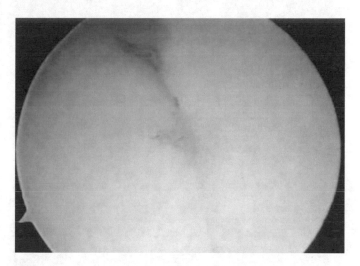

Fig. 13.3 Arthroscopic view of the normal, tight, congruent SL interval as seen from the midcarpal space

However, the degree of rotation of the carpal bones and any abnormal motion or separation are best appreciated from the unobstructed view available in the midcarpal space.

A spectrum of injury to either the SL or LT interosseous ligament is possible. The interosseous ligament appears to attenuate and then tear from volar to dorsal. Geissler devised an arthroscopic classification of carpal instability and suggested management of acute lesions to the interosseous ligament (Table 13.2) [23, 25]. The management options as listed from this original article have evolved as the understanding of the compromise of ligament healing potential over time has changed.

In *Grade I* injuries, there is loss of the normal concave appearance of the scaphoid and lunate as the interosseous ligament bulges with the convex appearance (Fig. 13.4). Evaluation of the SL interval from the midcarpal space shows the SL interval still to be tight and congruent. These

Table 13.2 Geissler arthroscopic classification of carpal instability

Grade	Description	Management
I	Attenuation/hemorrhage of interosseous ligament as seen from the radiocarpal joint. No incongruency of carpal alignment in the midcarpal space	Immobilization
II	Attenuation/hemorrhage of interosseous ligament as seen from the radiocarpal joint. Incongruency/step-off as seen from the midcarpal space. A slight gap (less than width of probe) between carpals may be present	Arthroscopic reduction and pinning
III	Incongruency/step-off of carpal alignment is seen in both the radiocarpal and midcarpal spaces. The probe may be passed through the gap between carpals	Arthroscopic/open reduction and pinning
IV	Incongruency/step-off of carpal alignment is seen in both the radiocarpal and midcarpal spaces. Gross instability with manipulation is noted. A 2.7-mm arthroscope may be passed through the gap between carpals	Open reduction and repair

Based on data from Ref. [25]

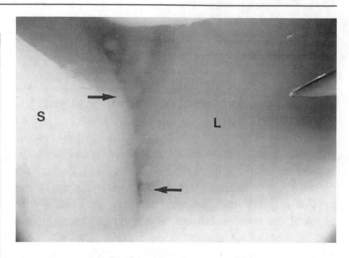

Fig. 13.5 Arthroscopic view of a Type II SLIL injury as seen from the radial midcarpal space. The dorsal lip of the scaphoid is no longer congruent with the lunate as it is palmar flexed (S scaphoid, L lunate)

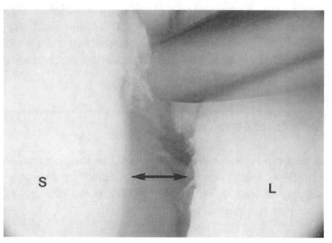

Fig. 13.6 Arthroscopic view of a Type III SLIL tear as seen from the radial midcarpal space. Note the gap between the scaphoid and lunate (S scaphoid, L lunate)

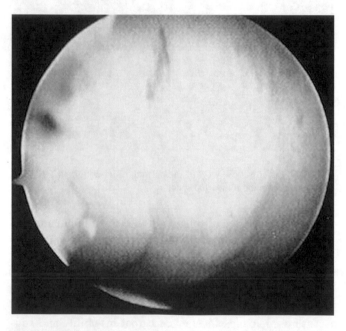

Fig. 13.4 Arthroscopic view of a Grade I interosseous ligament injury to the SLIL as seen from the 3–4 portal in the radiocarpal space. Note that the normal concave appearance at the SL interval has now become convex

mild *Grade I* injuries usually resolve with simple immobilization.

In *Grade II* injuries, the interosseous ligament bulges similarly to *Grade I* injuries as seen from the radiocarpal space. In the midcarpal space, the SL interval is no longer congruent. The scaphoid flexes and its dorsal lip is rotated distal to

the lunate (Fig. 13.5). This can be better appreciated with the arthroscope placed in the ulnar midcarpal portal looking across the wrist to assess the wrist to assess the amount of flexion to the scaphoid. This is analogous to the dorsal translation of the proximal pole of the scaphoid that can be identified on sagittal plane MRI imaging (see Fig. 13.1).

In *Grade III* injuries, the interossesous ligament starts to separate, and a gap is seen between the scaphoid and lunate from both the radiocarpal and midcarpal spaces. A 1-mm probe may be passed through the gap and twisted between the scaphoid and lunate from both the radiocarpal and midcarpal spaces (Fig. 13.6). Sometimes the gap between the scaphoid and lunate is not visible until the probe is used to push the scaphoid away from the lunate. A portion of the dorsal SLIL may still be attached.

In *Grade IV* injuries, the interosseous is completely torn, and a 2.7-mm arthroscope may be passed freely from the

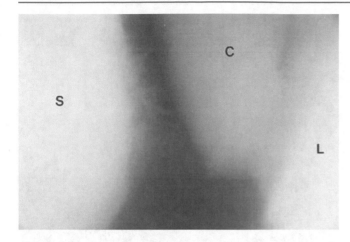

Fig. 13.7 Arthroscopic view of a Type IV SLIL tear. The scaphoid and lunate are completely separated, and the arthroscope may pass freely between the radiocarpal and midcarpal spaces. The capitate is seen between the SL intervals (S scaphoid, L lunate; C, capitate)

midcarpal space to the radiocarpal space between the scaphoid and lunate (the drive-through sign) (Fig. 13.7). This corresponds to the widened SL gap seen on plain radiographs with a complete SL dissociation.

Radiographic Structural Classification

Incomplete/Partial Rupture: Dorsal, Membranous, Volar Band

Partial rupture—usually only the palmar band of ligament is ruptured or occasionally only the dorsal segment is ruptured.

Static and dynamic radiographs are usually normal. Chronicity of the injury and partial healing may also be identified with high-resolution MRI scanning. Dorsal translation of the proximal pole relative to the facet of the radius may be identified on sagittal plane MRI images in spite of normal static plain radiographic alignment and may be an early indicator of functionally more significant partial injury. Early chondral loss on the proximal pole may also be identified on MRI before plain radiographic abnormality.

Complete Rupture: Static Versus Dynamic

Static versus dynamic dissociation is best identified by comparing static versus stress radiographs, or by fluoroscopy.

1. Complete rupture—dynamic—All components of SLIL are ruptured but the extrinsic ligaments/secondary stabilizers are usually intact. Static plain radiographs may be normal but there is disruption of normal relationships on stress radiographs.
2. Complete rupture—static—Complete SLL rupture and extrinsics also injured and static plain radiographs dem-

onstrate widened SL interval on PA radiographs and increased SL angle on the lateral radiographs (modified by Watson) [26].

Static Reducible Versus Static Irreducible

This is determined intraoperatively. Static deformity is present on resting plain radiographs. It may be easily reducible during surgery to repair or reconstruct the SLIL. When deformity is not reducible intraoperatively, salvage options should be utilized. This usually follows a temporal relationship with the more chronic ruptures leading to a static deformity, which may then become irreducible.

Treatment

Correct classification of the injury can assist in the selection of appropriate treatment options. Nonetheless, the greatest challenge is that there is no consensus on which surgical treatment option should be undertaken. Various options exist including pinning, repair, capsulodesis, and reconstruction and each has been applied to virtually all grades of injury. Moreover, surgical interventions can be either open or arthroscopic.

The authors have defined a unified classification system for treatment options of SLL complex pathology (Table 13.3).

Closed Pinning: Image Intensifier or Arthroscopically Guided

This surgery may be appropriate for acute lower grade injuries.

The wrist is evaluated arthroscopically for direct visualization of SLL injury and indirect evidence of disordered intercarpal mechanics. Arthroscopic assessment is achieved through the preferred means of arthroscopy and traction. The wrist may be suspended at approximately 10 lbs of traction in a traction tower [27, 28]. Alternately, traction may be applied with the forearm horizontal using a variety of traction devices [28, 29]. The 3–4 portal is the most ideal viewing portal for visualization of the SLL. A working 4–5 or 6-R portal is also used. The wrist is systematically evaluated from radial to ulnar. The SL interval is probed. The degree of injury may not be fully appreciated until the tear is palpated with a probe (Fig. 13.8). Torn fibers of the SLL, if present, are then debrided with the arthroscope in the 6-R portal, and a shaver inserted into the 3–4 portal. A probe is inserted into the SL interval to note particularly any gap between the scaphoid and lunate. Following arthroscopic debridement of a torn SLL from the radiocarpal space, the midcarpal space

Table 13.3 Classification system for treatment options for SL pathology

Treatment options		
Closed pinning	Fluoroscopic guided	
	Arthroscopic guided	
Open repair and pinning		
Capsulodesis, capsulorrhaphy, and partial repair	Arthroscopic— volar or dorsal	"Abrasion" capsulorrhaphy
		Shrinkage
		Suture
	Open	Dorsal—Blatt/ reverse Blatt (often adjunct to open repair or reconstruction)
Reconstruction: defined as an attempt to reestablish a soft tissue relationship between scaphoid and lunate ± stabilization through other soft tissue augmentation)	Local tissue	Dorsal intercarpal ligament
	RASL (arthroscopic or open)	
	Free tissue grafts—"Bone– Tissue–Bone"	Bone– Retinaculum–Bone
		Hand/wrist graft options
		Foot/tarsal graft options
		Other tissue
	Tendon grafts	Brunelli
		Three ligament tenodesis
		Scapholunate axis method
		Scapho-luno-triquetral tenodesis
Salvage	Proximal row carpectomy (PRC) [59]	
	Partial fusion (arthroscopic or open)	Four-corner fusion ±e/o scaphoid
		Radio-scapho-lunate fusion
		Capitolunate fusion
		STT fusion
	Total wrist fusion	

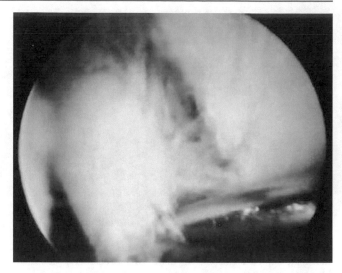

Fig. 13.8 Arthroscopic view of a Type II SLIL tear as seen from the 3–4 portal in the radiocarpal space. A probe is used to palpate the interosseous ligament and the separation, which was not initially noted, is identified

is then evaluated. The arthroscope is initially placed in the radial midcarpal space. Close attention is paid to any rotational displacement of the scaphoid with the dorsal lip being rotated distal to that of the lunate. This may be best visualized with the arthroscope placed in the ulnar midcarpal portal. Also, any gap where the probe or arthroscope itself can be passed between the scaphoid and lunate is identified. If this is achieved easily, then there are serious doubts as to whether closed pinning is appropriate [28].

Patients with a Grade II lesion may be most ideally suited for arthroscopic-assisted reduction and pinning, although efficacy of this treatment must be interpreted in the context of the interval since injury, which will affect the healing potential. Alternate treatment options with arthroscopic capsular abrasion or shrinkage have also been advocated for

Grade II pathology, particularly in more chronic injury, and will be discussed later. The use of closed pinning for Grade III injuries is difficult to justify based on current literature.

For arthroscopic pinning, the arthroscope is placed in the 3–4 portal, after the midcarpal space has been evaluated in patients who have an acute or perhaps subacute Grade II SLIL injury. A 0.045 Kirschner wire (K-wire) is inserted through a soft tissue protector or through a 14-G needle placed dorsally in the anatomic snuff box to the scaphoid. A soft tissue protector may be used in order to avoid injury to the sensory branches of the radial nerve. A small incision is made, and blunt dissection is continued down with a hemostat; a soft tissue protector may be placed directly on the scaphoid.

The K-wire can then be seen as it enters the scaphoid with the surgeon looking down the radial gutter with the arthroscope. In an easier alternative technique, the wrist is taken out of traction and the K-wires can be positioned under fluoroscopic control. If there is concern regarding the reduction, then placing the arthroscope in the ulnar midcarpal portal during stabilization allows the surgeon to look across the wrist to better judge the rotation of the scaphoid in relation to the lunate.

Additionally, a probe may be inserted through the radial midcarpal space to control the palmar flexion of the scaphoid. The wrist may be extended and ulnar deviated to help further reduce the palmar flexion of the scaphoid. After the first wire is placed controlling the reduction, an additional wire may be placed in the SL interval. Placement of wires between scaphoid and capitate remains controversial. A scapho-capitate wire gives excellent control of scaphoid rotation but some authors have questioned the advisability of violating the uninjured scapho-capitate articulation. In addition, immobilization of the midcarpal joint through scapho-capitate wires may be considered undesirable in the context of renewed interest in the "dart throwing" plane of motion.

The K-wires are best buried under the skin as this avoids secondary infection and need for premature removal. The wrist is immobilized in a below elbow thermoplastic splint. Gentle inner range radiocarpal flexion-extension range of motion exercise is usually possible, as restricted by the wires. The K-wires are then removed in theater after 6–8 weeks. Grip strength exercises for the wrist are initiated at 3 months.

Treatment for patients with Grade III and Grade IV injuries to the SLL, either acute, subacute, or chronic, remains unclear. Results of closed treatment for higher-grade injuries have largely been unsatisfactory [30] and the dichotomy between repair and reconstruction has remained difficult to clarify. There has undoubtedly been a trend toward earlier adoption of reconstruction for higher-grade injuries.

Whipple reviewed the results of arthroscopic management of SL instability, utilizing the previously described techniques in patients who were followed for 1–3 years [31]. In his series, patients were classified into two distinct groups of 40 patients each, according to the duration of symptoms and the radiographic SL gap. Thirty-three patients (83%) who had a history of instability for 3 months or less and had less than 3 mm side-to-side difference in the SL gap had maintenance of the reduction and symptomatic relief. When symptoms were present for greater than 3 months and there was more than a 3-mm side-to-side SL gap, only 21 patients (53%) had symptomatic relief following arthroscopic reduction and pinning. Patients with less than 3 months symptoms duration and 3-mm side-to-side SL gap were followed for 2–7 years. Whipple found that 85% continued to maintain their stability and comfort in his series. This report emphasized the need for early diagnosis and intervention prior to the onset of fixed carpal alignment and diminished capacity for ligamentous healing.

Open Repair and Pinning

Patients with acute Grade III and Grade IV injuries to the SLIL are best treated with open repair or reconstruction. The efficacy of direct repair remains controversial; however, there is little doubt that the trend is toward earlier adoption of reconstructive techniques rather than direct repair due to the strong impression that complete ruptures lose the capacity for primary healing very soon after injury. The critical interval has not been defined and indeed it may be that once a complete rupture of the SLIL has occurred, the potential for healing may be compromised. Furthermore, the tear morphology may influence the healing potential. When the ligament is avulsed from either the scaphoid or lunate, it may

have a greater capacity to heal than a midsubstance rupture. Prior to arthrotomy, the wrist is evaluated arthroscopically for any additional injuries, including potential cartilaginous loose bodies, triangular fibrocartilage complex tears, and possible injury to the LT interosseous ligament. Open repair is undertaken through a dorsal 3–4 extensor compartment approach. A Berger ligament sparing arthrotomy [32] is preferred by the authors. It is essential that an intraoperative assessment is made as to the healing potential of the residual ligament and alternate reconstructive or salvage procedures undertaken if the residual ligament is of poor quality or there is concern regarding the cartilage surfaces of the carpus and radius.

Capsulodesis, Capsulorrhaphy, and Partial Repair

Restraint of scaphoid flexion has long been identified as a desirable intervention in the treatment of SL pathology [33–35]. The dorsal subluxation of the proximal scaphoid and loss of congruence of the distal pole in relation to the radial styloid have long been considered the principal initial biomechanical abnormalities requiring intervention. Procedures that restrict scaphoid flexion have been advocated as an alternative to repair or reconstruction. There is no consensus as to when such alternate stabilizing procedures should be undertaken in preference to repair or other reconstructive options.

Arthroscopic Techniques for Capsulodesis, Capsulorrhaphy, and Partial Repair

Abrasion Capsulodesis

Although not previously reported in the literature, a new surgical technique receiving attention is abrasion capsulodesis. Although alternative arthroscopic capsular tightening has been reported with thermal shrinkage, there are some concerns given the adverse experience of thermal techniques in the shoulder. Although there have not been reports of similar problems in the wrist, abrasion of the dorsoradial capsule has been considered as a safer alternative. In lower grade injuries, this may improve stability by inciting a scar reaction with an increase in the extrinsic restraint to scaphoid flexion. The dorsoradial capsule is abraided with a chondrotome blade to stimulate a scar reaction. Consideration may be given to temporary K-wire pinning (either SL or scaphocapitate) to prevent scaphoid flexion, and flexion is usually restricted for 4–6 weeks with a thermoplastic splint. This technique is currently being studied in a prospective cohort by Ross and colleagues in Brisbane.

Arthroscopic Dorsal Capsular Thermal Shrinkage

Thermal capsular shrinkage using a thermal probe has been suggested in the treatment of Grade II injuries [36]. Although this technique demonstrated a number of unsatisfactory results in the treatment of anterior shoulder instability, it has been argued that the wrist capsule behaves differently and that it is easier to immobilize the wrist and allow adequate healing.

In Geissler Grade I and II SL instability, Danoff et al. in a small series have used arthroscopic thermal capsular shrinkage [37]. Using the fact that collagen shrinks with heat, nonablative thermal energy was also applied to the palmar SLIL in predynamic instability to effectively tighten up the ligament. Seven of eight patients had improved pain and preserved mobility, while one patient failed this treatment and progressed to fusion.

Darlis et al. performed arthroscopic debridement and capsular shrinkage on 16 patients with 14 reported good to excellent results (8 of those pain free) and 2 failures [38]. Similarly, Hirsh et al. reported on a cohort of 10 patients with 90% pain free at an average follow-up of 28 months [39]. In contrast, Geissler reported on his findings in the management of 19 patients with chronic partial tears of the SLL (Geissler Grade II or III) or LT tears [36]. He reported variable results from poor to excellent using the Mayo wrist score at 6–22 months postoperation. Grade II tears appeared to have better results than Grade III injuries. However, as these are preliminary studies with small samples, no firm conclusions can be drawn.

Arthroscopic Suture Capsulorrhaphy, Capsulodesis, or Partial Repair

In the circumstance where complex open reconstruction is considered undesirable, then arthroscopic reconstruction of chronic tears may be considered.

Mathoulin et al. describe an arthroscopic dorsal capsule-ligamentous repair for chronic reducible SLL tears [40, 41]. The technique involves passing a 3/0 PDS suture through a needle visualized arthroscopically and passed into the remnants of ligament and capsule between the scaphoid and lunate at the distal capsular reflection of the SLL and then tied to form a capsuloplasty. In his series of 36 patients with a mean 13-month follow-up, the results of the technique were generally excellent. The main advantage of the technique appeared to be the reduction in postoperative stiffness related to minimizing the dorsal capsular dissection needed during conventional surgical exposure with open techniques and hence the minimizing of scar tissue. Patient's pain scores were generally excellent, they regained 96% grip strength compared to the contralateral side, and seven of the sports persons were able to return to the same level of sport postoperatively.

Del Pinal et al. [42] describe an all-inside technique for arthroscopic suturing of the volar SLL. This technique used sutures introduced volarly via a Tuohy needle to plicate the volar ligament remnants and the long radiolunate ligament. Although this appears to be a favorable procedure, the technique had been applied to four patients with minimal follow-up reported, hence no meaningful conclusions for this technique can be made.

Recently, van Kampen and Moran reported on a new technique of a volar capsulodesis used to reconstruct the volar SLL using a portion of the long radiolunate ligament [43]. Although only results from a preliminary cadaveric study are published, they found that this approach allowed a strong repair with no compromise on the vascularity of the scaphoid or lunate.

Open Capsulodesis

Blatt's original description [33] in 1987 used a dorsoradial flap of wrist capsule to differentially restrict scaphoid flexion. He left the flap of capsule attached to the radius and advanced it dorsally on the scaphoid. In his original series of 12 patients of late rotatory subluxation, he reported excellent recovery of range of movement, average grip strength recovered to 80%, and the majority returning to the preinjury work. Later, Muermans and colleagues reported on 17 cases (11 cases of preradiographic instability; 3 dynamic; 3 static) with an average age of 30 years [44]. Patients had previously undergone conservative management and were on average 23 months postinjury at the time of surgery. On blinded examination, they reported ten patients with excellent to good outcomes (pain and activities of daily living (ADL)) and six had fair to poor results. Sixteen patients had a negative Watson test. However, X-rays failed to reveal any significant improvement in SL gap or angle.

The reverse Blatt procedure leaves the capsule attached to the scaphoid and advances it proximally on the dorsal radius. It has been employed as an adjunct to various other open repairs and reconstructions [32]. Megerle et al. followed up 59 patients for an average of 8 years following dorsal capsulodesis [45]. A Berger flap was performed and a slip of the proximal aspect of the dorsal intercarpal ligament left attached distally onto the scaphoid and either sutured to the lunate (36 untethered cases) or distal radius (16 tethered cases) periosteum or attached with an anchor. K-wires were used to transfix the reduced SL interval while the capsulodesis healed. The K-wires were removed at 12 weeks. Carpal reduction was not maintained over time and 78% went on to have radiographic evidence of arthritis and an average SL angle of 70°.

Reconstruction

We have defined this as an attempt to reestablish a soft tissue connection between scaphoid and lunate that may be augmented by other secondary stabilizing soft tissues to provide additional stability.

The various techniques described use local tissue or tendons as grafts, such as flexor carpi radialis (FCR), the majority of which are still left attached to the wrist distally, and others use autologous free tissue grafts as a bone–tissue–bone construct.

Local Tissue: Dorsal Intercarpal Ligament

Dobyns et al. [13] described the early technique for reconstruction in 1974. The Mayo capsulodesis in 1982 [2] used half of the dorsal intercarpal ligament left attached to the distal pole of the scaphoid but detached from its ulna side and reattached to the dorsal lunate with suture anchors and to the dorsal radiocarpal ligament. Moran and colleagues reported on an update of results of 14 patients who had a Mayo capsulodesis and compared them to 15 patients who had a modified Brunelli tenodesis procedure [46]. They reported similar wrist range of movement (63% and 64% of the unaffected side, respectively) and grip strength (91% and 87% of the unaffected side, respectively) in both groups. No failures were reported in the capsulodesis group.

More recently, Gajendra et al. reported on the long-term outcomes of dorsal intercarpal ligament capsulodesis (DILC) for chronic SL dissociation [47]. The DILC was followed up in 16 patients for on average 84 months, and despite a 58% satisfaction rate thus far, radiographic signs of arthrosis were present in 50%. Despite this, it is still advocated by the authors for the treatment of reducible static SL dissociation.

Local Tissue: RASL

This technique is difficult to classify and may be considered a variation in repair. Nevertheless, we consider it more analogous to a reconstruction, particularly where the cartilage between the scaphoid and lunate is removed to encourage fibrous tissue growth between the two surfaces. The "Reduction and Association of the Scaphoid and Lunate" (RASL) procedure reported by Rosenwaser et al. involves open reduction of the SL diastasis and holding the reduction with a headless compression screw [48]. Thirty-two patients with an average follow-up of 6.2 years results have now been reported. Range of motion was maintained at 80% of the unaffected side and grip strength at 90%. Radiographic reduction parameters were well maintained at follow-up with two failures resulting in SL advanced collapse and salvage.

The RASL procedure has also been described as an arthroscopic technique and a modified articulated screw (scapholunate intercarpal (SLIC) screw) has been proposed by Geissler to decrease problems with screw breakage.

Free Tissue Grafts: Bone–Tissue–Bone

These techniques harvest ligament or ligament-like tissue as free grafts with their bony origins from sacrificeable locations elsewhere in the body.

Bone–Retinaculum–Bone

Weiss et al. described the bone–retinaculum–bone autograft technique of reconstruction in 1997 [49]. The graft was harvested from Lister's tubercle between second and third compartments and the overlying retinacular tissue, and the bone plugs were inserted into the scaphoid and lunate. This technique was initially advocated in dynamic instability but not in static cases.

The long-term follow-up at an average of 11.9 years has now been reported [49–51].

Clinical and radiographic outcomes deteriorated moderately from the initial report. There were three failures, resulting in one proximal row carpectomy and two total wrist arthrodeses. Findings at repeat surgery in the failed group included an intact graft without any apparent abnormalities, a partially ruptured graft (after a subsequent reinjury), and a completely resorbed graft.

This bone–retinaculum–bone reconstruction may be a viable treatment option for dynamic SL instability in which the scaphoid and lunate can be reduced. Results may deteriorate but are similar to those reported previously from other techniques. Problems with graft strength or stiffness may necessitate further surgery.

Bone–Tissue–Bone: Hand/Wrist Options

Harvey and Hanel [52, 53] tested the SLL in cadavers against bone–tissue–bone grafts taken from cadaveric second metacarpal–trapezoid ligaments, third metacarpal–capitate ligaments, and the dorsal retinaculum. The third metacarpal–carpal bone–tissue–bone technique in a clinical series was published in 2002 [54]. Although used in chronic SLL injuries, with numbers of cases not included in the report, the results were documented to be best when there was a shorter period between injury and reconstruction and when there was a dynamic deformity with a radiolunate angle no more than 30°. The complications were related to bone fragmentation at the screw site acutely or at a later date secondary to trauma.

Harvey et al. later described the lack of healing with graft pullout and graft stretching as complications from his non-vascularized bone–tissue–bone reconstructions and developed the third metacarpal–carpal vascularized pedicle graft from the radial sided intermetacarpal artery to address these shortcomings [55].

Capitohamate autografts were advocated by Ritt and colleagues in 1996 [56].

Bone–Tissue–Bone: Tarsal Options

Svoboda et al. [57] in 1995 tested bone–ligament–bone grafts from cadavers as potential ligament complex grafts to reconstruct the SLL using the dorsal ligament of the fourth and fifth metatarsals, a dorsal tarso-metatarsal ligament graft, and a dorsal calcaneo-cuboid graft. The tarso-metatarsal ligament graft produced in vitro results closest to the SLL.

Davis et al. in 1998 described a bone–ligament–bone graft harvested and biomechanically tested from the cadaveric foot [58]. They used the dorso-medial portion of the navicular–first cunieform ligament.

Free Tissue Grafts: Tendon

Four Bone Technique

Almquist et al. described a four bone technique of SLL reconstruction in 1991 using a graft harvested from extensor carpi radialis brevis (ECRB) [59]. The ECRB tendon remained attached distally. Tunnels in the capitate, scaphoid, lunate, and distal radius allowed passage of the tendon graft from its attachment distally to its reattachment proximally on the radius. The graft is passed first from dorsal to volar through the capitate tunnel. It is then passed through the scaphoid tunnel from volar to dorsal. In this way, it allows the tendon graft to pass between the dorsal scaphoid and dorsal lunate before passing through the lunate tunnel exiting on the volar aspect of the lunate. Finally, the graft passes from here onto the volar aspect of the distal radius or through a tunnel into the volar distal radius to be tensioned and finally anchored in the tunnel or to suture anchors. The SL interval is also stabilized with a wire loop.

The results of this technique have been published for the first 36 patients with an average age of 34 years at an average of 4.8 years' follow-up. Average flexion was 37° and average extension was 52°. Grip strength remained on average 73% of the contralateral side. A return to preinjury levels was noted in 86% with no evidence of advancing arthritic changes in X-ray.

Brunelli Technique

In 1995, Brunelli and Brunelli described a technique using the local tissue for a tenodesis effect with a partial FCR tendon graft [34, 60]. It was left attached distally and passed through a tunnel in the scaphoid from volar to dorsal and then sutured to the dorsal capsule of the radius. This aims to address the rotary subluxation of the scaphoid with scaphoid flexion and proximal pole subluxation dorsally. Although this does not attempt to anatomically reconstruct the SLL, we mention it in the reconstructive tendon graft section because it introduced the concept of harvesting a portion of the FCR left attached distally and passing the tendon volar to the STT joint and through to the dorsal aspect of the wrist via a transosseous tunnel in the scaphoid. This has formed the basis of many of the subsequent successful techniques for reconstruction.

Three Ligament Tenodesis

The "modification" of the Brunelli technique popularized by Garcia-Elias and Stanley in 2006 as the three ligament tenodesis (3LT) eliminates the tether to the radius [61]. It reinforces the volar capsule of the STT joint to add restraint to scaphoid flexion, in keeping with the Brunelli technique, while reconstructing the dorsal band of the SLL and reinforcing the dorsal intercarpal ligament. They published a series of 38 patients with an average age of 31 years with symptomatic SL dissociation (21 wrists stage 3; 8 stage 4; 9 stage 5). The majority had dynamic instability (79%). At an average follow-up of 46 months (7–98 months), satisfactory pain relief was achieved in 28 patients. Twenty-nine resumed normal preinjury work. Acceptable range of movement was achieved (mean flexion 51°; mean extension 52°). Average grip strength was 65% of the contralateral side. Progression of carpal collapse was noted in two wrists.

Nienstedt published his 10-year results with a small series using a modified Brunelli procedure using a strip of FCR tendon as a ligament substitute for static SL instability [62], based on the technique originally described by Van Den Abbeele and colleagues [63]. The FCR tendon was passed through the scaphoid tunnel and fixed to the dorsal lunate with an anchor. The mean follow-up was 13.8 years in a cohort of eight patients. The reduction of the SL gap from 5.1 mm preoperatively and obtained intraoperatively to 2.4 mm was maintained at 2.8 mm long term. Average disabilities of the arm, shoulder and hand (DASH) score was 9, and six out of eight patients were pain free. One case had occasional slight pain and the other had chronic pain. With small numbers, valid conclusions are difficult but the follow-up interval is significant and maintaining radiographic parameters with only one case developing arthritis might suggest a successful procedure.

Scapholunate Axis Method (SLAM)

In 2012, Lee et al. described the scaphulonate (SL) axis method (SLAM), which involves drilling a tunnel between the scaphoid and lunate and anchoring a free tendon graft in the lunate with an intraosseous bullet anchor and in the scaphoid with an interference screw [64]. This was compared to the modified Brunelli and Blatt capsulodesis in 12 cadavers and in this, experimental data were deemed a more anatomical and less restrictive reconstruction.

Cable Augmented Quad Ligament Tenodesis

Bain et al. in 2013 described a small series using tensionable suture anchors and an FCR tendon graft combination [65]. The technique was adapted from the modified Brunelli and has the theoretical advantage of maintaining SL reduction with a cable during the healing phase. Initial clinical results were promising but longer-term follow-up is needed.

Scapho-Luno-Triquetral Tenodesis (SLT)

The open reconstruction technique favored by Ross, Couzens, and colleagues has been developed for the treatment of dynamic or intraoperatively reducible static SL instability where other forms of SL reconstruction may previously have been considered [66]. It may also offer an augmentation for acute and semi-acute repairs of the SLL. It has also been successfully used in acute reconstruction/repair following perilunate dislocations where both the SLL and LT ligaments are damaged. Since the development of this technique in 2009, Ross and colleagues have performed this operation on over 60 patients with Grade III or IV SLL injuries [66]. They have reported preliminary results on the first 11 consecutive patients who received this technique and were prospectively reviewed over a 12- to 24-month period [66]. At an average follow-up of 14 months (12–24 months) postoperation, they reported good early radiological and clinical outcomes. When comparing the preoperative clinical results with their most recent follow-up, the cohort demonstrated pain relief with normal activities, improved Patient-Rated Wrist Evaluation, quick disabilities of arm, shoulder and hand (QuickDASH), range of movement, and grip strength scores. Radiological outcomes (SL angle and SL gap) were improved.

The technique involves the passage of a distally based partial FCR graft across the volar STT joint and through a scaphoid tunnel. The graft exits the scaphoid between the scaphoid and lunate and is then passed through a second tunnel in the lunate and triquetrum (Fig. 13.9). It is tensioned and anchored with an interference screw in the ulnar aspect of the triquetrum and then passed back across the midcarpal joint to reinforce the dorsal intercarpal ligament. It can also be used to augment acute and semi-acute repairs of the SLL. By reconstructing the SLL and LT ligaments, it is also suitable for the treatment of perilunate dislocations.

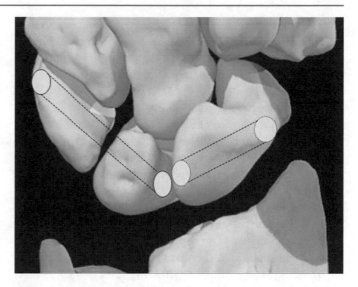

Fig. 13.9 Scapho-luno-triquetral tenodesis transosseous tunnel placement

This technique may be suitable for adaption to arthroscopic, or arthroscopic-assisted techniques, particularly with the development of procedure-specific targeting jigs and instruments. The authors are undertaking this development currently.

This technique is contraindicated in SL advanced collapse (SLAC) or irreducible static instability intraoperatively. The authors believe that this technique combines a large number of desirable features from previous procedures and addresses many of the potential facets of SL pathology to achieve a stable reconstruction of carpal stability. The features include:

1. In keeping with the initial intent of Brunelli's original description [60], the procedure provides a volar restraint to flexion of the distal pole of the scaphoid and a reinforcement of the volar capsule of the STT joint.
2. There is no tethering of the dorsal carpus to the scaphoid. Therefore, there is no absolute restraint to radio carpal flexion.
3. The tunnels are positioned at, or close to, the isometric point of rotation between the scaphoid and the lunate. As a consequence, the potential for the normal sagittal plane rotation between the scaphoid and the lunate is not restricted. In addition, as the graft is tensioned, there is uniform apposition of the scaphoid and the lunate facets. This avoids excessive tensioning dorsally, with consequent opening on the volar aspect, or vice versa, as may occur with volar or dorsal reconstruction or capsulodesis techniques.
4. As the graft is tensioned, there is an automatic reduction in the major aspects of pathology, including the rotary dorsal subluxation of the proximal scaphoid, and closure of the gap between the scaphoid and the lunate.

5. The transosseous passage of the graft avoids soft tissue bulk or formation of dorsal scar tissue, as occurs when a tendon graft is passed dorsally in the region of the dorsal band of the SLL and anchored to the lunate dorsally.

6. The central positioning of the graft between the scaphoid and lunate does not compromise the possibility of repairing any residual native SLIL that may remain.

7. The triquetrum is ideally suited for anchoring of a tendon using an interference screw, and this anchoring in the triquetrum avoids excessive instrumentation or anchor placement in the lunate or scaphoid.

8. Passage of the graft across the LT interval allows additional stabilization of the LT interval. Many of these injuries are part of a spectrum of perilunate injury, and as a consequence, there may be subtle recognized or unrecognized pathology affecting the LT ligament. As a consequence, this reconstruction is particularly suitable for the reconstruction of complete perilunate injuries.

9. The secondary passage of the tendon graft across the dorsal aspect of the midcarpal joint back to the scaphoid reinforces and reconstructs the dorsal intercarpal ligament, which may also be secondarily involved in these patterns of injury. This secondary reconstruction also provides an additional reinforcement to the relationships of the proximal row of the carpus in the coronal plane.

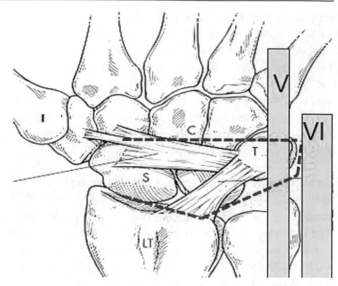

Fig. 13.10 Modified Berger flap exposure for the scapho-luno-triquetral tenodesis technique

Scapho-Luno-Triquetral Tenodesis (SLT): Surgical Technique

Exposure

A standard midline approach over the central dorsal aspect of the wrist is utilized.

A ligament sparing Berger capsular flap [44] is developed further to the ulnar side than is usual, to gain access to the ulnar border of the triquetrum immediately radial to the extensor carpi ulnaris (ECU) subsheath, which is not opened (Fig. 13.10). In addition to the usual elevation of the third and fourth compartments, division of the septum between fourth and fifth compartment and elevation of the extensor digiti minimi tendon is required (Fig. 13.11).

Exposure of the ulnar aspect of the triquetrum, drilling the LT tunnel, and graft tensioning can be facilitated by placing a small Hohmann retractor in the vicinity of the pisotriquetral joint. If there is a perilunate dissociation, the lunate and triquetrum should be reduced anatomically and pinned with a K-wire before drilling the LT tunnel. Elevate the flap, stopping over the dorsal ridge of the scaphoid. This preserves the capsular attachments to the dorsum of the scaphoid that carry the blood supply.

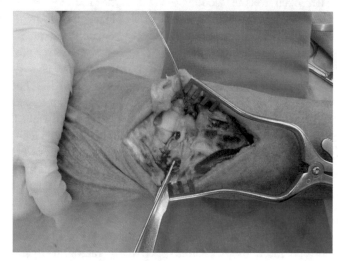

Fig. 13.11 Exposure for scapho-luno-triquetral tenodesis

Alternate Exposure

Once a degree of familiarity is achieved with the technique using the large dorsal exposure described above, it may be possible to decrease the dorsal exposure by accessing the ulnar border of the triquetrum through a separate direct ulnar approach. This allows a limited dorsal exposure. The fifth compartment does not need to be elevated and the capsulotomy is more limited incorporating only a portion of the typical Berger flap, without the need to extend the flap past the triquetrum.

Expose the ulnar side of the triquetrum through a separate small direct ulnar incision approximately 2 cm long just volar to the ECU. Care should be taken to protect dorsal branches of the ulnar nerve which have variable anatomy in this region. The LT tunnel can be drilled via this approach. Use of fluoroscopy to check cannulated drill guide wire positioning is recommended before drilling the definitive tunnel.

After it has been tensioned and secured with the interference screw through the ulnar incision, the graft can be passed subperiosteally under the sixth and fifth compartments back toward the central dorsal exposure of the scaphoid and lunate, using a fine hemostat. Prior to this passage back to the dorsal incision, the graft may also be secondarily secured with sutures to the soft tissues over the ulnar triquetrum in the floor of the "ulnar snuff box." The remainder of the attachment of the graft to the dorsal scaphoid is the same as described with the more extensive dorsal exposure.

Harvesting the Graft and Preparation

Volar exposure of the scaphoid is similar to the volar approach for scaphoid fixation and grafting described by Russe [67]. Expose the tubercle and the distal half of the scaphoid. Minimize the division of the radio-scapho-capitate ligament at this point. Harvest approximately 40% of the FCR tendon using a technique allowing the tendon to be stripped from proximal to distal, leaving it attached distally. Tendon graft thickness should correspond to the transosseous tunnel diameter, which is usually 3 mm. Once the portion of tendon is harvested, mobilize it until it is distal to the ST joint.

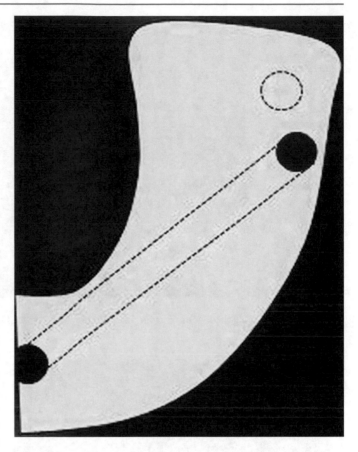

Fig. 13.12 Scaphoid tunnel placement for the scapho-luno-triquetral tenodesis technique

Preparing the Scaphoid Tunnel

Drill a hole using a 3-mm cannulated drill bit, in a process similar to a traditional style Brunelli reconstruction [34, 60], except that the entry point dorsally is on the articular facet of the scaphoid for the lunate (not at the dorsal insertion of the SLL). The tunnel should be just dorsal to the center point of lunate facet of the scaphoid. The exit point on the volar side of the scaphoid is a few millimeters proximal and radial to the normal point that would be used for a traditional dorsal band reconstruction (Fig. 13.12). The position of the tunnel exit on the volar side needs to be accurate, so that the tunnel can enter on the lunate facet of the scaphoid without violating the scapho-capitate joint. The point on the scaphoid facet should be just dorsal to the midpoint of the articular surface for the lunate. The reason for this is that if the corresponding point on the facet of the lunate is volar to the midpoint, the tendon graft will be traveling obliquely, from dorsal on the scaphoid, to volar on the lunate. This causes the graft to naturally reduce the rotary subluxation between the scaphoid and the lunate, and correct the dorsal subluxation of the proximal pole of the scaphoid, as it is tensioned.

Preparing the Luno-Triquetral Tunnel

The LT tunnel is drilled from the ulnar side of the triquetrum, across the LT joint to exit on the lunate just volar to the midpoint of the articular facet. Care is taken not to make the entry point on the ulnar aspect of the triquetrum too dorsal to avoid the risk of fracturing the tunnel when the interference screw is inserted. Care must also be taken not to enter too proximal on the triquetrum as the medial-lateral dimension of the triquetrum decreases significantly in its more proximal portion, and the tunnel needs to be long enough to accommodate the 8-mm length of the interference screw without it protruding across the LT joint.

Passing the Graft

The graft is then passed sequentially through the scaphoid from volar to dorsal then across the LT tunnel. The tendon needs to be approximately of the same dimension as the tunnel, so that the interference screw fit is tight. Ensure there is no slack in the graft between the FCR insertion and the volar entry to the tunnel before tensioning dorsally (Fig. 13.13).

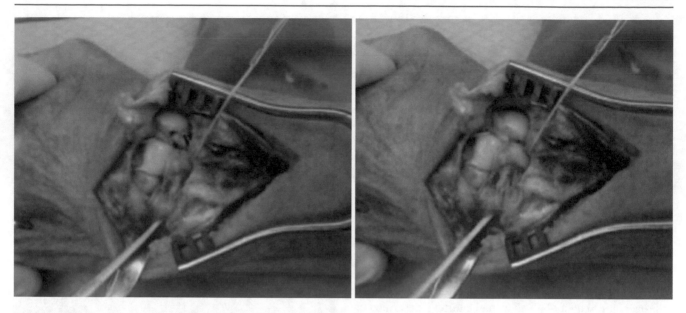

Fig. 13.13 Tensioning the tendon to reduce the SL interval for the scapho-luno-triquetral tenodesis

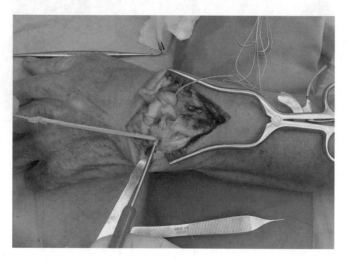

Fig. 13.14 Inserting the interference screw for the scapho-luno-triquetral tenodesis

Reducing the Joint

Pull on the tendon as it exits the triquetrum. The dorsal subluxation of the scaphoid will reduce and close the SL interval. Insert the interference screw (e.g., 3 × 8 mm PEEK screw, Arthrex Inc.) into the triquetrum volar to the tendon (Fig. 13.14). We have found that it is best to tension the graft with the wrist in ulnar deviation to ensure maximum tension. A similar biocomposite (e.g., tricalcium phosphate (TCP)) screw would be preferable. We are reluctant to use a polylactic acid (PLA) screw due to probable cyst formation in small carpal bones.

Once the graft is secured if there is any residual SLL tissue, it may be repaired using the surgeon's preferred technique. The graft is then passed across the dorsum of the midcarpal joint. The goal is to augment (or reconstruct) the dorsal intercarpal ligament. Place a small absorbable anchor with 2° suture in the waist of the scaphoid, being careful to avoid the tunnel containing the FCR graft. Suture the graft to the waist of the scaphoid. This is also the base of the Berger flap, so use either an artery forceps (hemostat) or tendon braiding forceps to pass the graft through the base of the Berger flap.

Closure

To protect the reconstruction, a single 1.1-mm wire is placed between the distal pole of the scaphoid and the capitate, or between the scaphoid and lunate, being careful not to perforate the graft. Surgeon preference may be to use two wires. The K-wire is left in situ for 6–8 weeks.

Rehabilitation

Postoperatively, the patient is allowed to mobilize the wrist to 30° of flexion and 30° of extension. If only one SL wire is used, oblique axis (dart throwing) motion can be commenced early with the wire in situ. Custom-made thermoplastic wrist splint is worn at all other times, until the K-wire is removed (i.e., 6–8 weeks). After the wire is removed, wrist mobilization exercises are upgraded to include orthogonal flexion/extension exercises and oblique dart throwing type exercises, which focus on the midcarpal joint.

SLT Case Presentation

A 40-year-old male right-hand dominant cane farmer presents with an acute SL dissociation (with static deformity) and simultaneous distal radius fracture of his left wrist. Preoperative X-ray is depicted in Fig. 13.15. Surgery for internal fixation of distal radius and SL reconstruction using the scapho-luno-triquetral tenodesis technique was performed at 10 days postinjury. At 7 months postsurgery, he had good radiological outcome (Fig. 13.16). He had returned to normal work and function, and had achieved a good clinical outcome (Fig. 13.17).

Salvage

Wrist arthroscopy can be used to evaluate the degree and extent of articular cartilage degeneration in patients with SLL pathology. The status of the articular cartilage, as determined arthroscopically, helps to determine whether a reconstructive procedure, such as ligament reconstruction or capsulodesis versus a salvage procedure (e.g., a four-corner fusion or proximal row carpectomy), is indicated [68, 69]. Arthroscopic evaluation of the status of the articular cartilage of the head of the capitate is extremely useful in determining the indications for four-corner fusion versus proximal

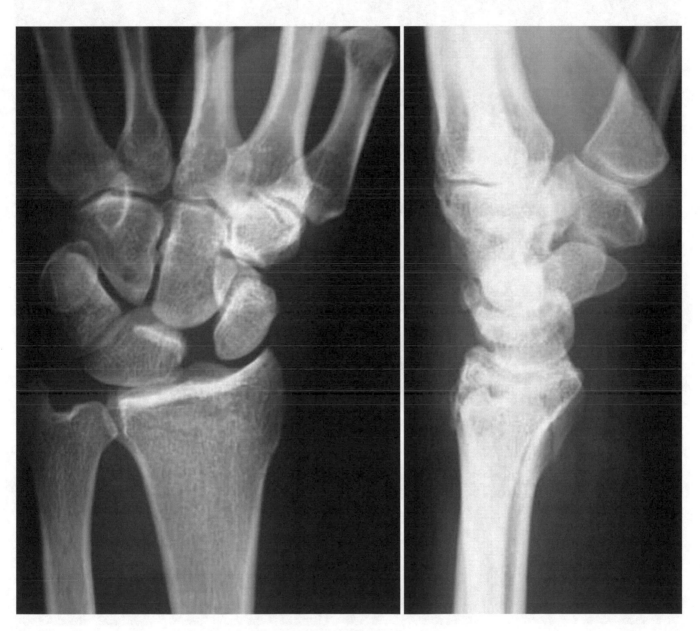

Fig. 13.15 Preoperative X-ray depicting SL dissociation and undisplaced distal radius fracture

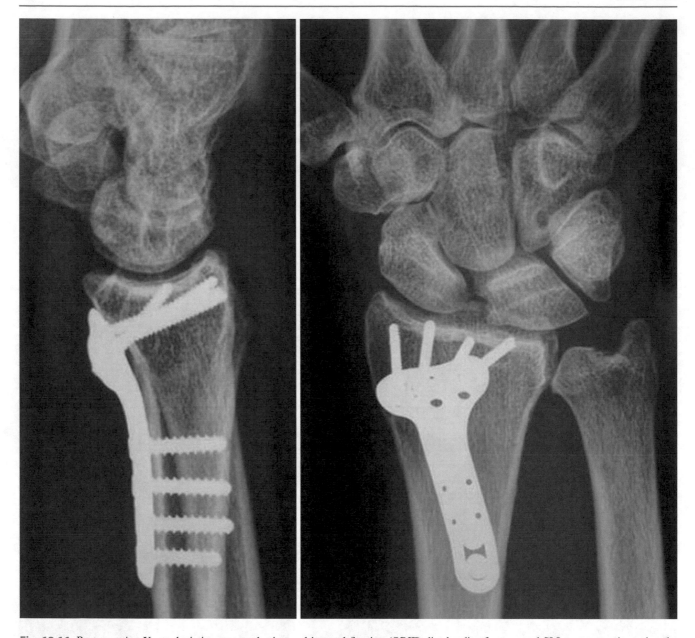

Fig. 13.16 Postoperative X-ray depicting open reduction and internal fixation (ORIF) distal radius fracture and SLL reconstruction using the authors' technique

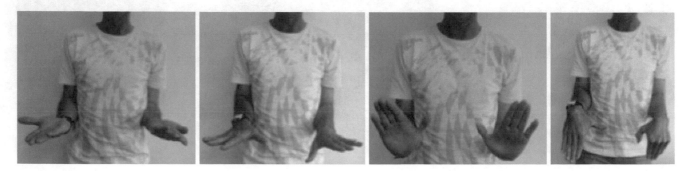

Fig. 13.17 Range of movement at 7 months postsurgery

row carpectomy. In selecting individuals with early SLAC wrist who desire only minimal arthroscopic intervention, debridement and radial styloidectomy may be an option. This is further described in a later chapter.

The hitherto unpredictable results of soft tissue reconstructions have led some authors to consider bony procedures preferentially [68, 69]. The chronicity of the injury and the difficulty in reducing the SL relationship will influence this decision.

Proximal Row Carpectomy

Proximal row carpectomy is a motion-preserving salvage procedure not reliant on bony union. It allows earlier mobilization than four-corner fusion and is technically less demanding [69].

Fusion

Partial Intercarpal Fusions

Limited carpal fusions may be a suitable salvage for some patients [70].

STT Joint Fusion

There is a paucity of recent literature on the use of STT joint fusion as a salvage technique since Kirk Watson and colleagues described this initially in 1991 [35].

Scapho-Capitate Fusion

The concern with scapho-capitate fusion is the alteration in carpal mechanics with loss of midcarpal oblique plane motion and increased contact stresses between the scaphoid and radius. Deletang et al. in 2011 reported on 31 scapho-capitate fusions for chronic scapholunate instability which were followed for an average of 5 years [71]. The conclusion was that capsulodesis and ligament reconstruction provide the same functional results as SC fusion, but with slightly less stiffening.

Luegmair et al. in 2013 reported on scapho-capitate arthrodesis for SL instability in manual workers [72]. This high-demand group of 20 patients with an average follow-up of 10 years had a significant reduction in pain symptoms and maintained an average 87° flex-extension arc and 41° radioulnar deviation arc. Grip strength was 60% of the opposite wrist. All patients united, 90% of patients returned to work but 30% had radiocarpal arthritis at last follow-up.

Four-Corner Fusion ± Excision of Scaphoid

Four-corner fusion and proximal row carpectomy are often compared and contrasted as salvage procedures. Cadaveric work by DeBottis et al. in 2013 showed a reduced range of motion compared to normal wrists with either procedure [73]. Wrist flexion was reduced similarly in both by 12–13°. Extension was decreased by 20° in the four-corner fusion and 12° in the PRC.

Radio-Scapholunate Fusion

Radioscapholunate ligament (RSL) arthrodesis is technically challenging, although improved implants including memory staples and specific internal fixation implants have helped to improve union rates. It remains important to respect the three-dimensional relationship of the scaphoid and lunate to preserve the shape of the articulation with the proximal capitate.

Bain et al. described RSL arthrodesis with distal pole of scaphoid excision and triquetral excision for isolated radiocarpal arthritis secondary to a variety of pathologies [74]. The midcarpal joint must be normal for this limited arthrodesis to be justified. Resection of the distal scaphoid and triquetrum was shown to increase range of motion in prior cadaveric studies [75].

Mühldorfer-Fodor et al. report on the results of RSL arthrodesis for posttraumatic arthritis with or without distal pole of scaphoid excision [76]. The distal pole excision group had not only better radial deviation but better union rates too. Although this procedure is suitable for salvage in failed SLL reconstruction, in this cohort of 35 patients with follow-up, however, only two cases were due to SL pathology, while the majority of cases were arthritis secondary to intraarticular distal radial fractures.

Capitolunate Fusion

Wang et al. report on capitolunate and triquetrohamate fusions for scapholunate advanced collapse and scaphoid nonunion advanced collapse salvage [77]. In a consecutive series of 27 patients, there was a 96% union rate. Postoperative results showed a 21% reduction in mean flexion-extension arc compared to preoperatively. There was no change in radio-ulnar deviation. The mean grip strength postoperatively increased by 27%.

Total Wrist Fusion

Total wrist fusion is best reserved for the salvage of pancarpal arthritis or failed limited carpal arthrodesis or other motion-preserving procedures [78]. The overwhelming challenge of all treatments for SL pathology is avoidance of the need for total wrist fusion.

Summary of Treatment Options

Partial Tears

Acute partial tears may heal without treatment or may benefit from simple immobilization. There may also be a role for closed pinning, with or without arthroscopic assistance.

Symptomatic chronic partial tears are less likely to be suitable for closed pinning; however, the residual ligament function may be too good for major reconstruction. In these cases, capsulodesis (arthroscopic or open) or capsulorrhaphy (abrasion, thermal, suture) may be appropriate.

Complete Tears: Dynamic

In acute dynamic tears, most authors would favor primary repair over reconstructive techniques. This still requires a pragmatic assessment of ligament quality intraoperatively before proceeding to repair. In chronic dynamic tears, the balance shifts toward reconstruction over repair. The challenge is in establishing the interval that defines a chronic tear.

Complete Tears: Static

When these tears are reducible at operation the preference may be for reconstruction or capsulodesis, although there are some authors who consider this pathology beyond the limit of soft tissue reconstruction to achieve stability and prefer partial fusion. Consideration may also be given to less invasive arthroscopic capsulodesis or capsulorrhaphy techniques.

In a static irreducible dissociation, the only predictable options are partial or total fusion.

Conclusion

The management of SLL injury is continuing to evolve with both arthroscopic and more anatomical open reconstruction techniques being developed. The biggest dilemma facing the surgeon is when to apply repair versus reconstructive versus salvage techniques. This challenge is complicated by the difficulty in defining chronicity of the injury, the poor results of open primary repair in many series, and the lack of good natural history studies for both partial and complete ligament tears. In addition, it remains difficult to make direct outcome comparisons with other techniques in the published literature. There is currently no standard for reporting preoperative and postoperative outcome data in relation to either clinical or radiographic results for SLIL pathology.

Acknowledgments We would like to acknowledge Dr. Nick Daunt, Radiologist, QLD Xray, for his assistance with the "Imaging" section of the chapter. We would also like to acknowledge Susan Peters, Senior Research Coordinator and Hand Therapist, Brisbane Hand and Upper Limb Research Institute, for assistance with manuscript preparation.

References

1. Walsh JJ, Berger RA, Cooney WP. Current status of scapholumate interosseous ligament injuries. J Am Acad Orthop Surg. 2002;10:32–42.
2. Cooney WP. Evaluation of chronic wrist pain by arthrography, arthroscopy and arthrotomy. J Hand Surg. 1993;18:815–22.
3. Whipple TL, Marotta JJ, Powell JH. Techniques of wrist arthroscopy. Arthroscopy. 1986;2:244–53.
4. Berger RA. The anatomy of the ligaments of the wrist and distal radioulnar joints. Clin Orth Rel Res. 2001;383:32–40.
5. Berger RA, Landsmeer JMF. The palmar radiocarpal ligaments: a study of adult and fetal wrist joints. J Hand Surg Am. 1990;15:847–54.
6. Chung KC, Zimmerman NB, Travis MT. Wrist arthrography versus atthroscopy: a comparative study of 150 cases. J Hand Surg Am. 1995;27:591–4.
7. Watson HK, Ashmead D, Makhlouf MV. Examination of the scaphoid. J Hand Surg Am. 1988;13:657–60.
8. Lk R, An KN, Linschield RL. The effect of scapholunate ligament section on scapholunate motion. J Hand Surg Am. 1996;12:767–71.
9. Mayfield JK, Williams WJ, Erdman AG, et al. Biochemical properties of human carpal ligaments. Orthop Trans. 1979;3:143.
10. Mead TD, Schneider LH, Cherry K. Radiographic analysis of selective ligament sectioning of the carpal scaphoid: a cadaver study. J Hand Surg Am. 1990;15:855–62.
11. Wynne-Davies R. Heritable disorders in orthopaedic practice. Oxford: Blackwell Scientific; 1973. p. 138.
12. Gilula LA. Carpal injuries: analytic approach and case exercises. Am J Roentgenol. 1979;133:503–17.
13. Dobyns JH, Linscheid RL, Chao EYS, et al. Traumatic instability of the wrist. Instr Course Lect. 1975;24:182–99.
14. Frankel VH. The Terry Thomas sign. Clin Orthop Relat Res. 1977;129:321–2.
15. Cautilli GP, Wehbe MA. Scapholunate distance and cortical ring sign. J Hand Surg Am. 1991;16:501–3.
16. Linschied RL, Dobyns JH, Beabout JW, Bryan RS. Traumatic instability of the wrist: diagnosis, classification and pathomechanics. JBJS. 1972;54:1612–32.
17. Lawland A, Foulkes GD. The "clenched pencil" view: a modified clenched fist scapholunate stress view. J Hand Surg. 2003;28:414–8.
18. Dao KD, Solomon DF, Shin AY, Puckett ML. The efficacy of ultrasound in the evaluation of dynamic scapholunate ligamentous instability. JBJS. 2004;86A:1473–8.
19. Taljanovic MS, Sheppard JE, Jones MD, Switlick DN, Hunter TB, Rogers LF. Sonography and sonoarthrography of the scapholunate and lunotriquetral ligaments and triangular fibrocartilage disk: initial experience and correlation with arthrography and magnetic resonance arthrography. J Ultrasound Med. 2008;27:179–91.
20. Ringler MD. MRI of wrist ligaments. J Hand Surg Am. 2013;38:2034–46.
21. Kakar S. Use of dynamic 4DCT for the diagnosis of scapholunate instability. J Wrist Surg. 2013;1(S1):520.
22. Larsen CF, Amadio PC, Gilula LA, Hodge JC. Analysis of carpal instability: I description of the scheme. J Hand Surg Am. 1995;20:757–64.
23. Geissler WB, Haley T. Arthroscopic management of scapholunate instability. Atlas Hand Clin. 2001;6:253–74.
24. Luchetti R, Atzei A, Cozzolino R, Hairplay T. Current role of open reconstruction of the scapholunate ligament. J Wrist Surg. 2013;2:116–25.
25. Geissler WB, Freeland AE, Savoie FH, et al. Intracarpal soft tissue lesions associated with intraarticular fracture of the distal end of the radius. J Bone Joint Surg. 1996;78:357–65.

26. Watson HK, Ballet FL. The SLAC wrist: scapholunate advanced collapse pattern of degenerative arthritis. J Hand Surg Am. 1984;9:358–65.
27. Geissler WB, Freeland AE, Weiss APC, Chow JCY. Techniques in wrist arthroscopy. JBJS Am. 1999;81:1184–97.
28. Gupta R, Bozentka DJ, Osterman AL. Wrist arthroscopy: principles and clinical applications. J Am Acad Orthop Surg. 2001;9:200–9.
29. Geissler WB. Arthroscopic management of scapholunate instability. J Wrist Surg. 2013;2:129–35.
30. Tang JB, Shi D, Gu YQ, Zhang QG. Can cast immobilization successfully treat scapholunate dissociation associated with distal radius fractures? J Hand Surg Am. 1996;21:583–90.
31. Whipple TL. The role of arthroscopy in the treatment of scapholunate instability. Hand Clin. 1995;11:37–40.
32. Berger RA, Bishop AT, Bettinger PC. New dorsal capsulotomy for the surgical exposure of the wrist. Ann Plast Surg. 1995;35:54–9.
33. Blatt G. Capsulodesis in reconstructive hand surgery. Dorsal capsulodesis for the unstable scaphoid and volar capsulodesis following excision of the distal ulna. Hand Clin. 1987;3:81–102.
34. Brunelli GA, Brunelli GR. A new technique to correct carpal instability with scaphoid rotary subluxation : a preliminary report. J Hand Surg. 1995;20A:S82–5.
35. Watson HK, Belniak R, Garcia-Elias M. Treatment of scapholunate dissociation: preferred treatments—STT fusion vs. other methods. Orthopedics. 1991;14:365–8.
36. Geissler WB. Electrothermal shrinkage in interosseous ligament tears (SS-29). Arthroscopy. 2002;18:24–5.
37. Danoff JR, Birman MV, Rosenwasser MP. The use of thermal shrinkage for scapholunate instability. Hand Clin. 2011;27:309–17.
38. Darlis NA, Weiser RW, Sotereanos DG. Partial scapholunate ligament injuries treated with arthroscopic debridement and thermal shrinkage. J Hand Surg Am. 2005;30:908–14.
39. Hirsh L, Sodha S, Bozentka D, et al. Arthroscopic electrothermal collagen shrinkage for symptomatic laxity of the scapholunate interosseous ligament. J Hand Surg Br. 2005;30:643–7.
40. Mathoulin CL, Dauphin N, Wahegaonkar AL. Arthroscopic dorsal capsuloplasty in chronic scapho-lunate ligament tears: a new procedure. Hand Clin. 2011;27:563–72.
41. Wahegaonkar AL, Mathoulin CL. Arthroscopic dorsal capsule ligamentous repair in the treatment of chronic scapho-lunate ligament tears. J Wrist Surg. 2013;2:141–8.
42. del Piñal F, Studer A, Thams C, Glasberg A. An all-inside technique for arthroscopic suturing of the volar scapholunate ligament. J Hand Surg Am. 2011;36:2044–6.
43. Van Kampen RJ, Moran SL. A new volar capsulodesis for scapholunate dissociation. J Wrist Surg. 2013;1(2):s16–7.
44. Muermans S, De Smet L, Van Ransbeeck H. Blatt dorsal capsuldesis for scapholunate instability. Acta Orthop Belg. 1999;54:434–8.
45. Megerle K, Bertel D, Germann G, Lehnhardt M, Hellmich S. Long-term results of dorsal intercarpal ligament capsulodesis for the treatment of chronic scapholunate instability. J Bone Joint Surg Br. 2012;94:1660–5.
46. Moran SL, Ford JS, Wulf CA, Cooney WP. Outcomes of dorsal capsulodesis and tenodesis for treatment of scapholunate instability. J Hand Surg Am. 2006;31:1438–46.
47. Gajendran VK, Peterson B, Slater RR Jr, Szabo RM. Long-term outcomes of dorsal intercarpal ligament capsulodesis for chronic scapholunate dissociation. J Hand Surg Am. 2007;32:1323–33.
48. Rosenwasser MP, Miyasajsa KC, Strauch RJ. The RASL procedure: reduction and association of the scaphoid and lunate using the Herbert screw. Tech Hand Up Extrem Surg. 1997;1:263–72.
49. Weiss APC, Sachar K, Glowacki KA. Arthroscopic debridement alone for intercarpal ligament tears. J Hand Surg Am. 1997;22:344–9.
50. Weiss AP, Providenc RI. Scapholunate reconstruction using a bone-retinaculum-bone autograft. J Hand Surg Am. 1998;23:205–15.
51. Soong M, Merrell VA, Orthoman F, Weiss AP. Long-term results of bone-retinaculum-bone autograft for scapholunate instability. J Hand Surg Am. 2013;38:504–8.
52. Harvey E, Hanel D. Autograft replacements for the scapholunate ligament: a biomechanical comparison of hand based autografts. J Hand Surg. 1999;24A:963–7.
53. Harvey E, Hanel D. What is the ideal replacement for the scapholunate ligament in a chronic dissociation? Can J Plast Surg. 2000;8:143–6.
54. Harvey EJ, Hanel DP. Bone—ligament—bone reconstruction for Scapholunate disruption. Tech Hand Upper Extrem Surg. 2002;6:2–5.
55. Harvey EJ, Sen M, Martineau P. A vascularized technique for bone-tissue-bone repair in scapholunate dissociation. Tech Hand Up Extrem Surg. 2006;10(3):166–72.
56. Ritt MJ, Berger RA, Bishop AT, An KN. The capitohamate ligaments. A comparison of biomechanical properties. J Hand Surg Br. 1996;21:451–4.
57. Svoboda S, Eglseder A, Belkoff S. Autografts from the foot for reconstruction of the scapholunate interosseous ligament. J Hand Surg. 1995;20A:980–5.
58. Davis CA, Culp RW, Hume EL, Osterman AL. Reconstruction of the scapholunate ligament in a cadaver model using a bone-ligament-bone autograft from the foot. J Hand Surg Am. 1998;23(5):884–92.
59. Almquist EE, Bach AW, Sack JT, Fuhs SE, Newman DM. Four bone ligament reconstruction for treatment of chronic complete scaholunate separation. J Hand Surg. 1991;16A:322–7.
60. Brunelli GA, Brunelli GR. A new surgical technique for carpal instability with scapho-lunar dislocation (eleven cases) (French). Ann Chir Main Memb Supér. 1995;14:207–13.
61. Garcia-Elias M, Lluch AL, Stanley JK. Three-ligament Tenodesis for the treatment of Scapholunate dissociation: indications and surgical technique. J Hand Surg. 2006;31A:125–34.
62. Nienstadt F. Treatment of static scapholunate instability with modified Brunelli tenodesis: results over 10 years. J Hand Surg Am. 2013;38:887–92.
63. Van Den Abbeele KL, Loh YC, Stanley JK, Trail IA. Early results of a modified Brunelli procedure for scapholunate instability. J Hand Surg Br. 1998;23:258–61.
64. Lee SK, Zlotolow DA, Sapienza A, Karia R, Yao J. The scapholunate axis method: a new technique for scapholunate ligament reconstruction. J Wrist Surg. 2013;1:S17.
65. Bain GI, Watts AC, McLean J, Lee YC, Eng K. Cable-augmented, quad ligament tenodesis scapholunate reconstruction: rationale, surgical technique, and preliminary results. Tech Hand Up Extrem Surg. 2013;17:13–9.
66. Ross M, Loveridge J, Cutbush K, Couzens G. Scapholunate ligament reconstruction. J Wrist Surg. 2013;2:110–5.
67. Russe O. Fracture of the carpal navicular: diagnosis, non-operative treatment, and operative treatment. JBJS Am. 1960;42:759–68.
68. Strauch RJ. Scapholunate advanced collapse and scaphoid non-union advanced collapse arthritis—update of evaluation and treatment. J Hand Surg Am. 2011;36:729–35.
69. Wall LB, Stern PJ. Proximal row carpectomy. Hand Clin. 2013;29:69–78.
70. Mulford JS, Ceulemans LJ, Nam D, Axelrod TS. Proximal row carpectomy vs. four corner fusion for scapholunate (SLAC) or scaphoid nonunion advanced collapse (SNAC) wrists: a systematic review of outcomes. J Hand Surg Eur. 2009;34(2):256–63.
71. Deletang F, Segreta J, Dapb F, Daute G. Chronic scapholunate instability treated by scaphocapitate fusion: a midterm outcome perspective. Orthop Traumatol Surg Res. 2011;97:164–71.
72. Luegmair M, Saffar P. Scaphocapitate arthrodesis for treatment of scapholunate instability in manual workers. J Hand Surg. 2013;38:878–86.

73. Debottis DP, Werner FW, Sutton LG, Harley BJ. 4-corner arthrodesis and proximal row carpectomy: a biomechanical comparison of wrist motion and tendon forces. J Hand Surg Am. 2013;38:893–8.

74. Bain GI, Ondimu P, Hallam P, Ashwood N. Radioscapholunate arthrodesis—a prospective study. Hand Surg. 2009;14(2–3):73–82.

75. McCombe D, Ireland DCR, McNab I. Distal scaphoid excision after radioscaphoid arthrodesis. J Hand Surg Am. 2001;26(5):877–82.

76. Muhldorfer-Fodor M, Phan Ha H, Hohendorff B, Low S. Results after radioscapholunate arthrodesis with or without resection of the distal scaphoid pole. J Hand Surg Am. 2012;37:2233–9.

77. Wang ML, Bednar JM. Lunatocapitate and triquetrohamage arthrodesis for degenerative arthritis of the wrist. J Hand Surg Am. 2012;37:1136–41.

78. Hayden RJ, Jebson PJ. Wrist arthrodesis. Hand Clin. 2005;21:631–40.

New Concepts in Carpal Instability

Senthooran Raja, Daniel Williams, Scott W. Wolfe, Gregory Couzens, and Mark Ross

Introduction

Our understanding of carpal anatomy and kinematics continues to evolve through continued research and clinical experience. Conventional thinking has supported the belief that the intrinsic ligaments are the main stabilisers of the proximal carpal row with extrinsic structures acting as secondary stabilisers.

The intrinsic ligaments originate and insert onto carpal bones whereas the extrinsics are capsuloligamentous structures that cross the radiocarpal and ulnocarpal joints. The intrinsic ligaments given most importance are the scapholunate interosseous ligament (SLIL) and the lunotriquetral interosseous ligament (LTIL). These are considered primary stabilisers of the proximal carpal row whereas the extrinsics are conventionally thought of as secondary stabilisers. There

S. Raja · D. Williams
Brisbane Hand and Upper Limb Research Institute, Brisbane, QLD, Australia

Orthopaedic Department, Princess Alexandra Hospital, Woolloongabba, QLD, Australia

S. W. Wolfe
Hand and Upper Extremity Service, Department of Orthopedic Surgery, The Hospital for Special Surgery, New York, NY, USA

G. Couzens
Brisbane Hand and Upper Limb Research Institute, Brisbane Private Hospital, Brisbane, QLD, Australia

Orthopaedic Department, Princess Alexandra Hospital, Woolloongabba, QLD, Australia

Institute of Health and Biomedical Innovation, Queensland University of Technology, Brisbane, QLD, Australia

M. Ross (✉)
Brisbane Hand and Upper Limb Research Institute, Brisbane, QLD, Australia

Orthopaedic Department, Princess Alexandra Hospital, Woolloongabba, QLD, Australia

The University of Queensland, St. Lucia, QLD, Australia
e-mail: research@upperlimb.com

remains debate as to whether ligaments that span across multiple carpal bones without origin on the radius or ulna are intrinsic or extrinsic ligaments, although the distinction is less important than recognising their critical stabilising function.

The extrinsic' ligaments include the radioscaphocapitate (RSC), long radiolunate (LRL), short radiolunate (SRL), dorsal radiocarpal (DRC), ulnolunate, ulnotriquetral, and ulnocapitate ligaments. The dorsal intercarpal (DIC) and dorsal scaphotriquetral (DST) ligaments are robust intrinsic ligaments that stabilize the proximal row.

The distinct notion of intrinsic ligaments acting as primary stabilisers and thus treatment being directed at either repairing or reconstructing these structures alone is not entirely supported by the current literature. Viegas et al. demonstrated through cadaveric dissection and load testing that the dorsal extrinsic ligaments play a greater and more important role in carpal kinematics and stability [1].

This chapter discusses new concepts in carpal stability as briefly outlined above exploring in particular the 'extrinsic' critical stabilisers with particular focus on dorsal radiocarpal and dorsal intercarpal ligaments and their broad insertions onto the dorsal lunate non-articular surface which we have termed the 'bare area'. In doing so we offer an algorithm-based approach to investigation, treatment and how best to approach the dorsal carpus without worsening instability iatrogenically.

Dorsal Ligament Complex

A number of studies have helped improve our understanding of dorsal carpal anatomy and in particular that of the DRC and DIC ligaments [1–6].

The work carried out by Berger, Bishop and Bettinger in 1995 culminated in their dorsal ligament-sparing, fibre-splitting capsulotomy. It was suggested as an optimal exposure of the dorsal wrist while preserving the integrity of the dorsal extrinsic ligaments and is widely used [7, 8]. In ratio-

W. B. Geissler (ed.), *Wrist and Elbow Arthroscopy with Selected Open Procedures*,
https://doi.org/10.1007/978-3-030-78881-0_14

nalising the capsulotomy, they revisited the dorsal extrinsic anatomy. Here, they described the DRC proximal origin being distal and ulnar to Lister's tubercle, also being broader at its origin spanning Lister's tubercle to the dorsal rim of the sigmoid notch. The capsulotomy is continued along the DRC as it narrows to its insertion of the dorsal cortex of the triquetrum. It is often fused to the septum between the fourth and fifth extensor compartments at the triquetrum. In the same plane, the incision is made from the proximal origin of the DIC and continued along its length to its insertion onto the scaphoid waist and trapezium. The DIC was described as passing superficially to the midcarpal joint on its way to the trapezium [7].

The original description of Berger's dorsal capsulotomy was in part based on an understanding that the DIC had no noticeable attachment onto the lunate which is evident in the illustration provided in the same publication (Fig. 14.1). They were also unclear in the original text as to any distinct insertion of the DRC to the lunate along its course.

However, in 1999, Viegas et al. undertook a cadaveric study of 90 wrists and identified a 100% consistent attachment of the DRC onto the dorsal ulna aspect of the lunate.

Naturally, there are anatomical variations between individuals and Viegas et al. reported the common types they had encountered. Four types of DRC were observed with the commonest being a single ligament widest at its origin on the distal radius, attaching to the dorsal horn of the lunate and proceeding onto the triquetrum. The other types involved an accessory band with varying configurations and insertions (Fig. 14.2).

The DIC was also found to have, in 90% of the wrist specimens, an attachment onto the lunate at its dorsal distal aspect [1]. It also attached to the SLIL and LTIL along its route to the proximal rim of the trapezium (Fig. 14.3).

Three anatomical variants of the DIC were seen. The commonest (Type A—44%) had two thick bands with the proximal one extending from the triquetrum to the scaphoid and then distally to the trapezium. A single thick band was found in 30% of wrists (Type B) followed by multiple bands (Type C—26%) [1].

Berger later modified his illustration of the dorsal carpus to show the dorsal coverage of the lunate passing over the SLIL and LTIL (Fig. 14.4). In the illustration shown, a Viegas type A DIC is seen with proximal limb extending to the distal pole of scaphoid and a distal limb to the trapezium [8].

These findings were further corroborated by Nagao et al. in 2005. This cadaveric study utilised three-dimensional imaging to define attachment sites and dimensions of the ligaments to the volar and dorsal aspects of the carpal bones. Like Viegas, they observed a consistent attachment of the DIC to the dorsal pole of the lunate (Fig. 14.5). The DIC was also attached to the scaphoid proximally and at its waist, the triquetrum, the trapezium and to the dorsal SLIL and LTIL. The largest attachment was to the scaphoid and when considering the insertions onto the lunate and triquetrum, they concluded that the DIC is a major stabiliser of the proximal carpal row [5].

Dorsal Scaphotriquetral Ligament

The literature is not clear as to whether the dorsal scaphotriquetral ligament (DST) is truly a ligament or rather a fibrocartilaginous labral-like acetabular roof for the midcarpal joint.

Berger first described the DST as a distinct dorsal carpal structure of varying widths closely related to the DIC [2, 3]. It arose proximal to the DIC, merging with the dorsal SLIL. Interestingly, Berger remarked that the DST often appeared as an integral part of the DIC and a point of discussion was whether it is indeed a distinct structure at all or merely the deep proximal band of the DIC (Figs. 14.6 and 14.7).

Based on the inconsistent description in the literature and lack of consensus, Wessel et al. undertook a cadaveric study of 17 specimens and demonstrated that the DST represented an inseparable deep subsection of the DIC [10]. It had consistent attachments to the lunate (65.0 ± 28.3 mm^2) and scaphoid ridge (67.4 ± 26.8 mm^2) as did the DIC and DRC,

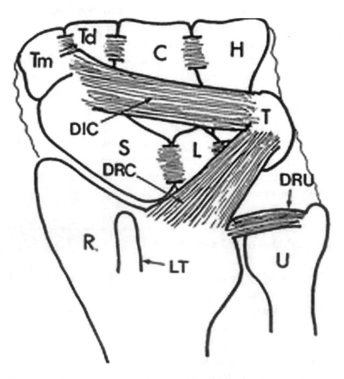

Fig. 14.1 Image appears to show the DIC having no clear attachment to the dorsal lunate [7]. (Reproduced with permission from Berger et al. [7])

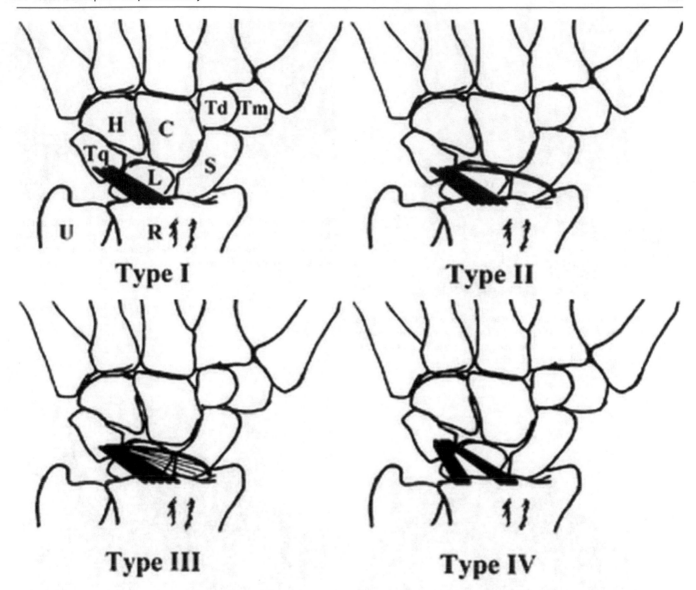

Fig. 14.2 Four anatomical variants of the DRC ligament. (Reproduced with permission from Viegas et al. [1]. With permission from Elsevier)

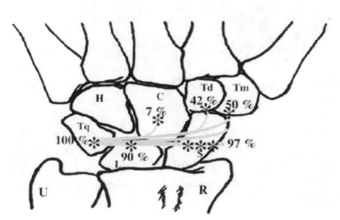

Fig. 14.3 Variable course of the DIC and its insertions. (Reproduced with permission from Viegas et al. [1]. With permission from Elsevier)

creating a labral-like covering for the dorsal capitate (see Fig. 14.7).

They concluded that the DST constituted a stout deep subsection of the DIC that spanned the entire proximal row and recommended it being renamed the dorsal scapholu-notriquetral (DSLT) ligament.

The midcarpal acetabulum is completed by the palmar scaphotriquetral ligament (PST) whose structure and function were clarified by Sennwald et al. in 1994 [11]. This collagenous structure is found deep to the radioscaphocapitate ligament and lies on the palmar surface of the capitate head. The PST has a thin fan-shaped attachment to the scaphoid extending transversely to the triquetrum with a robust 2 mm thick attachment. It has no attachment to the capitate itself but is embedded within the capsule which in turn has con-

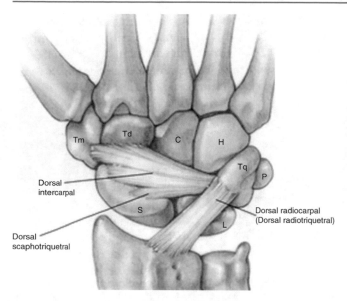

Fig. 14.4 Updated Berger carpal anatomy drawing with coverage of lunate and type A Viegas DIC [9]. (Republished with permission of Wolters Kluwer Health, Inc., from Berger et al. [9]. Permission conveyed through Copyright Clearance Center, Inc)

Fig. 14.5 Three-dimensional image. Dorsal carpal ligament attachments (dSLIO, dorsal scapholunate interosseous; pSLIO, proximal scapholunate interosseous) [5]. (Reproduced from Nagao et al. [5]. With permission from Elsevier)

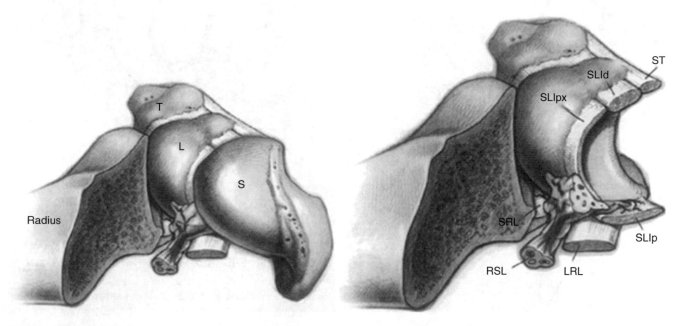

Fig. 14.6 The dorsal scaphotriquetral ligament [2]. (Reproduced from Ritt et al. [2]. With permission from Elsevier)

nections to the lunate proximally and capitate distally. It forms a palmar labral-like structure like the DSLT. In wrist dorsiflexion, the PST is taught preventing palmar translation of the capitate head.

This notion of a midcarpal acetabulum gives rise to the concept of a ball and socket articulation with the capitate head and emphasises the role of the DSLT in preventing dorsal translation of the capitate with associated extension of the lunate.

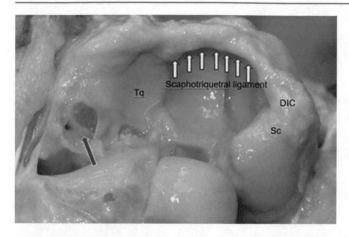

Fig. 14.7 Cadaveric specimen demonstrating labral-like dorsal acetabular roof comprised of the DSLT and DSLIL

The Dorsal Capsulo-Scapholunate Septum (DCSS)

The DCSS is a confluence of the dorsal capsule, DIC and SLIL. It is a fibrous structure arising from the dorsal capsule as two transverse arches and one longitudinal inserting onto the scaphoid and lunate at the bone-ligament interface and into the SLIL itself [12] (Fig. 14.8).

Overstraeten et al. found the DCSS to be a well-defined reproducible structure and proceeded to assess its contribution to scapholunate stability [13]. Arthroscopic sectioning of the DCSS notably increased the European Wrist Arthroscopy Society (EWAS) classification grading with increased gapping visualised. However, there was no change in radiographic markers of instability. With or without load,

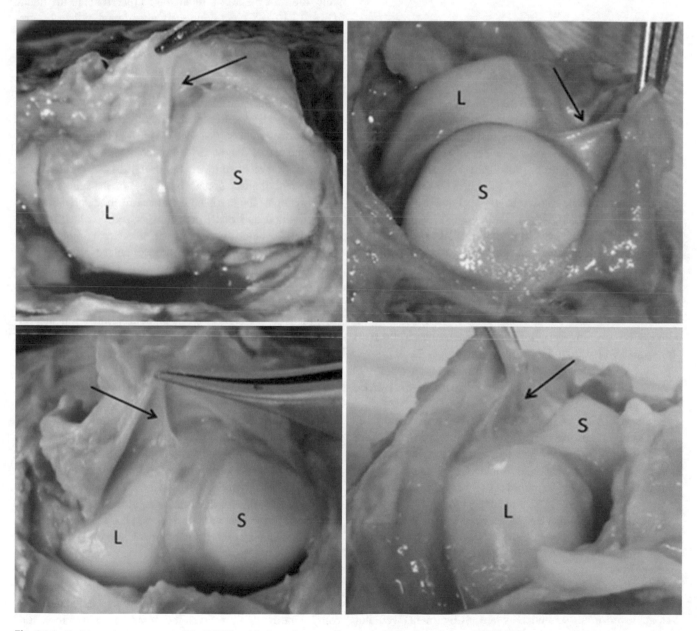

Fig. 14.8 Gothic-arch appearance of the DCSS and its insertion onto the scaphoid, lunate and dorsal SLIL [12]

there was no increase in static scapholunate gapping, scapholunate angle, or radiolunate angle [13].

Its significance was reinforced by Binder et al. who noticed a degree of SL instability (Geissler Grade 2) in individuals with an arthroscopically diagnosed DCSS detachment from the SLIL [14]. Subsequent arthroscopic repair of the DCSS to the DSLIL appeared to be a successful treatment option with excellent postoperative results.

We postulate that a significant part of the benefit of the DCSS repair is that by virtue of the route of suture passage through the stump of the SLL/DCSS into the midcarpal joint, it re-establishes contact between the DICL and the dorsal lunate and scaphoid. This may even be more significant than the side-to-side closing effect between the scaphoid and lunate.

Critical Stabilisers

As mentioned earlier, the proximal row intrinsic ligaments have been largely thought of as the primary stabilisers of the carpus with the extrinsics having a secondary function.

Instability and deformity typically attributed to isolated injury to the SLIL range from scapholunate gapping and scaphoid rotatory subluxation or dorsal translation to dorsal intercalated segment instability (DISI) and ulna translation.

However, multiple cadaveric studies have used sequential sectioning of carpal ligaments and cyclical loading to demonstrate that complete division of the SLIL alone does not result in a significant change in static carpal posture nor does it cause a DISI deformity [4, 15–19].

Equally, in surgical practice, the repair or reconstruction of the SLIL following traumatic injury achieves at best 80–85% functional outcomes and radiological recurrence of gapping between the scaphoid and lunate is frequently seen, sometimes worse than the original deformity [20, 21].

This experience suggests an incomplete understanding of carpal stability with perhaps excessive focus on the interosseous ligaments.

A change in carpal posture and stability arises only when extrinsic ligaments are sectioned in addition to the SLIL. A combination of injury to the SLIL and any of the following extrinsic ligaments leads to significant carpal instability; DIC at its insertion onto the scaphoid (DIC^S) or lunate (DIC^L), scaphotrapeziotrapezoid (STT) and LRL [1, 4, 6, 17].

Perez et al. randomised cadaveric specimens to five varied sequences of intrinsic and extrinsic ligament sectioning all commencing with the SLIL first [17]. They used a radiolunate angle of 15 degrees or more to define the presence of a DISI deformity, as well as looking at SL gapping, lunate extension and dorsal scaphoid translation. DISI deformity was achieved in all sequences when all ligaments were cut;

however, when either the DIC^L or volar STT (vSTT) was cut alongside the SLIL, a DISI resulted (Fig. 14.9).

Based on these findings and those of other investigators, we propose that the extrinsic ligaments are in fact 'critical stabilisers' of the proximal carpal row. The term secondary stabilisers should be dispensed with. The DIC$^{L(lunate\ attachment)}$ and vSTT have a particularly critical role to play in carpal posture and stability.

The various manifestations of dissociative carpal instability would now appear to result from a combination of injury to the SLIL and either acute injury to one or more critical stabilisers such as the DIC^L and vSTT or late attenuation to the LRL [22, 23].

Using diagnostic measures such as magnetic resonance imaging (MRI), with or without an arthrogram (MRA), one may look for the dorsal ligamentous insertions to the lunate (Fig. 14.10). We had previously abandoned MR arthrography as it did not seem to add to the assessment of the intrinsic ligaments. More recently, we have revisited the use of intra-articular gadolinium. It may increase the identification of the dorsal lunate 'bare area' representing the loss of attachment of DIC/DRC to the lunate; however, other details may be compromised, so currently we are utilising a combination of non-contrast and contrast scans (Fig. 14.11).

In the use of diagnostic arthroscopy, one needs to ensure visualisation of the critical stabilisers. It is essential to look for the pathological dorsal 'bare area' of the lunate created by avulsion of the extrinsic ligaments from the area between the proximal and distal articular surfaces. This inspection should take place from both the midcarpal joint and the radiocarpal joint. It may be more difficult to visualise from the 3–4 portal, so utilisation of the 6R or 1–2 portal is recommended.

In identifying which critical stabilisers are injured or attenuated one can then devise an appropriate surgical strategy. An early algorithm touching on the idea of matching treatment to the overall kinematic problem was published by Kuo and Wolfe [23].

Once a surgical strategy has been committed to, it is worthwhile considering if the surgical exposure taken to carry out the treatment is likely to cause further injury and worsen instability. Based on the evidence supporting critical stabilisers, a ligament-splitting, radial-based capsulotomy flap otherwise known as a fibre-splitting capsulotomy (FSC) is perhaps not the optimal approach [7, 8]. It does provide an excellent exposure of the dorsal carpal bones and intrinsics, but this is at the cost of the robust and broad insertion of the critical stabilisers on the dorsal lunate, namely the DRC and DIC^L.

Where arthroscopic intervention is not possible, a solution to the dorsal capsulotomy is the 'window' approach. This approach creates a radiocarpal and midcarpal capsulotomy window that preserves the broad and robust insertions

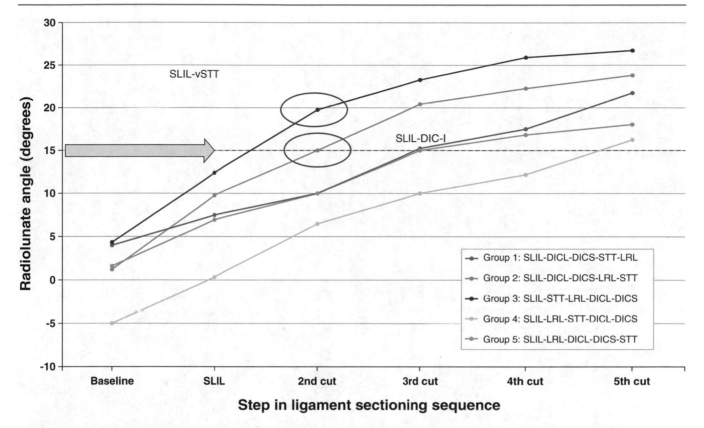

Fig. 14.9 Graph demonstrating increases in radiolunate angle with subsequent sectioning of extrinsic ligaments after SLIL initially [17]. Sectioning of the SLIL with either the DIC^L or vSTT leads to a DISI deformity (circled in red). (Reproduced with permission from Pérez et al. [17])

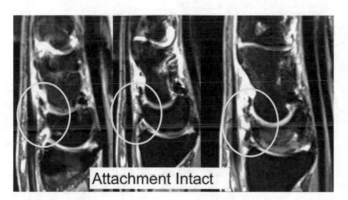

Fig. 14.10 MR arthrogram demonstration of DRC and DIC attachments to the dorsal lunate

of the DRC, DSLT and DIC^L critical stabilisers onto the lunate (Fig. 14.12).

Loisel et al. compared the FSC and 'window' approaches [24]. Following capsulotomy, increases in S-L gap, RLA and dorsal scaphoid translation were observed during the FSC causing iatrogenic proximal row instability (Figs. 14.13 and 14.14). The 'window' approach, however, did not cause instability while allowing good exposure of the dorsal carpus.

Closure of the FSC does restore some stability but not to baseline and this was only seen when secure closure was obtained using anchor fixation into the dorsal carpus. Simple suturing together of the split ligament fibres did not restore stability [24].

Carpal Instability, Non-dissociative, Traumatic (CINDT)

Aside from the classical dissociative types of carpal instability discussed in this chapter so far, there is a spectrum of non-dissociative instability known as CIND. This spectrum may include a traumatic mechanism with primary disruption of extrinsic ligamentous stabilisers. Consideration of the pathomechanics involved in a pathological sagittal plane rotation of the entire proximal row has helped to evolve our understanding of the critical stabilisers in both dissociative and non-dissociative instability.

Non-dissociative instability arises at both the radiocarpal and midcarpal joints. It differs from dissociative carpal instability (CID) as there is no disruption of ligaments between carpal bones within the same row. Pathologic flexion or extension of the entire non-dissociated proximal row has

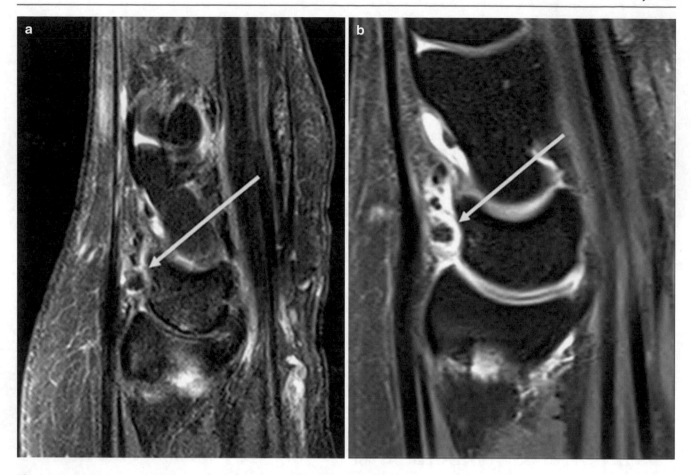

Fig. 14.11 (**a**) Non-contrast proton density fat-saturated MRI indeterminate for bare area. (**b**) T1 fat-saturated MRI with intra-articular gadolinium demonstrating loss of dorsal ligament insertion to lunate

been observed following traumatic episodes. A common misnomer for this traumatic non-dissociative instability is 'midcarpal instability'; however, we prefer CINDT as it is in fact instability of the proximal row with malalignment at both the midcarpal and radiocarpal joints. Indeed, an argument could be made to replace the term midcarpal instability with proximal row instability.

CINDT may present much like traditional 'midcarpal instability' with a dynamic and pathological rotation of the entire proximal row under load combined with radio-ulnar deviation. However, we and others have observed progressive static deformities following a traumatic event including distal radius fractures and undisplaced scaphoid fractures [25, 26].

In normal wrist kinematics, the proximal carpal row is flexed with the wrist radially deviated and extended. The flexion of the proximal row is due in part to the compressive forces of the trapezium and trapezoid directed on the distal pole of the scaphoid [27, 28]. As the wrist flexes and ulnarly deviates, the proximal row extends and this is thought to occur as the helicoidally shaped triquetro-hamate-capitate joint engages and drives the triquetrum into extension and in turn the proximal row [28, 29]. This motion is reliant on intact palmar and dorsal critical stabilisers such as the STT, the ulnar component of the palmar arcuate ligament (triquetro-hamate-capitate or THC) becoming taut, further pulling the proximal row into extension. The combined effort of the extensor and flexor carpi ulnaris tendons completes the complex interplay of static and dynamic structures in achieving the 'dart-throwers' motion of the wrist [30].

Traumatic injury to the critical stabilisers can lead to CINDT.

Four types have been described under the umbrella of CIND: Palmar (or VISI), dorsal (or DISI), combined and adaptive. Some have queried the application of the terms VISI and DISI to this pathological sagittal plane rotation of the entire proximal row. It may be more descriptive to describe it as flexion or extension deformity of the proximal row.

Palmar is by far the commonest form of CIND. In the traditional dynamic type, there is volar translation of the capitate as the proximal row does not extend as usual during ulnar deviation and the proximal row remains flexed. At maximum ulnar deviation, the triquetro-hamate joint engages causing sudden extension of the proximal row and a palpable

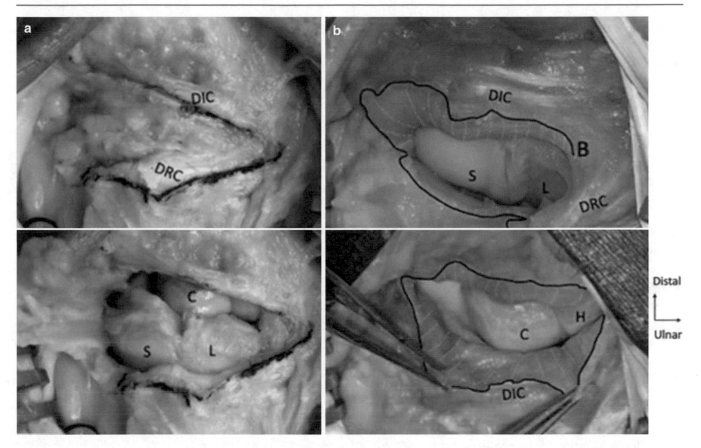

Fig. 14.12 Cadaveric dissection demonstrating the classical fibre-splitting capsulotomy (**a**) and the recommended window approach (**b**). The window approach maintains the broad and robust insertion of the DRC and DIC while the fibre-splitting approach detaches them from the proximal carpal row

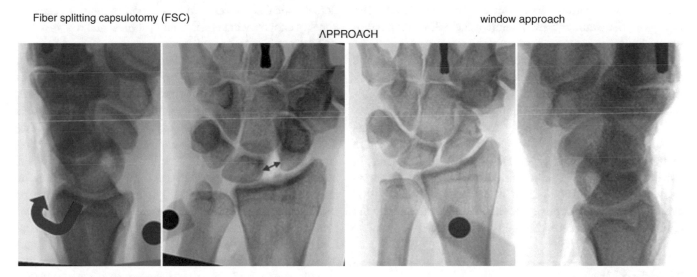

Fig. 14.13 Stress radiographs in normal uninjured cadaveric specimens following FSC on left and window approach on right. The FSC caused proximal row instability as highlighted by the red arrows. The window approach did not affect carpal instability

clunk. In CINDT (flexion), we have observed a more static and progressive pathologic flexion of the proximal row with abnormal capitolunate and radiolunate angles. In this setting, we have observed injury to the volar STT ligaments, volar arcuate ligament complex and the dorsal insertion of the DRC to the lunate.

Dorsal CINDT (proximal row extension) is thought to result from injury to the dorsal insertion of the DIC to the

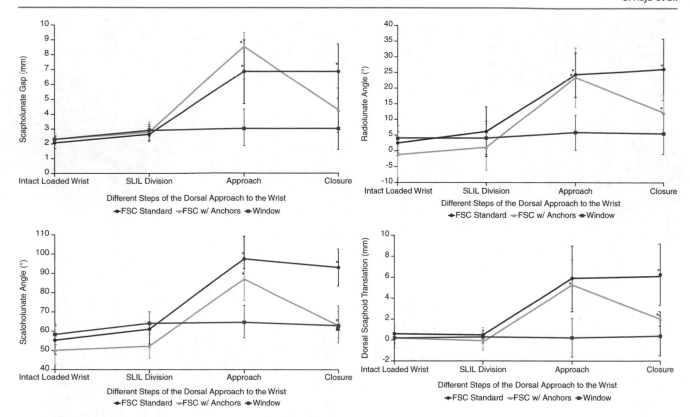

Fig. 14.14 Graphs illustrating the development of proximal row instability following FSA (black line), whereas the window approach (red
line) does not. There is some improvement in stability following closure
of the FSA using anchors to reattach the critical stabilisers (blue line)
but less so without (black line)

lunate (including the deep DSLT ligament fibres that form
the labral-like restraint to dorsal capitate translation) and
injury or post-traumatic attenuation of the palmar long radiolunate ligament.

We have not observed combined CIND in a post-traumatic
setting although a traumatic worsening of known instability
should prompt a careful investigation for traumatic compromise of the relevant critical stabilisers.

Adaptive CIND is typically secondary to distal radius
malunion. The changes in tilt, height and inclination result in
alterations in distances traversed by the carpal ligaments, in
particular the palmar stabilisers. Usually these are successfully treated with the correction of the bony deformity; however, in severe cases, consideration of additional injury to the
extrinsic ligaments should be considered [30].

Mooring Lines

A proposed explanation of the kinematics of proximal row
instability as manifested in both CID and CINDT is based
on the concept of 'mooring lines'. Mooring in boating terminology involves securing the position of a boat or ship on
a body of water by means of secure lines or anchors to the
sea floor.

Using the lunate to represent our boat and our palmar and
dorsal critical stabilisers acting as mooring lines, we can rea-
sonably explain what is necessary for proximal row instability to occur.

In this concept, our mooring lines are the DIC^L, DRC,
LRL and STT. The specific pattern of injury to these ligaments will determine the behaviour of the proximal row.
There are restraints on the dorsal and volar aspects of both
the midcarpal and radiocarpal joint. In order for the proximal
row or lunate to rotate in the sagittal plane, there would be
expected to be compromise of a dorsal midcarpal and volar
radiocarpal restraint, or vice versa. For instance, injury or
attenuation of the DRC and STT ligaments will remove the
restraint to a flexion (VISI) deformity of the proximal row.
Similarly, an extension (DISI) deformity of the proximal row
results from injury to the DIC^L and LRL (Figs. 14.15 and
14.16).

This concept of the critical impact of these stabilising
structures on the sagittal plane rotational stability of the
proximal row and particularly the lunate aligns well with the
stable central column theory proposed by Sandow et al.
(2014) [31].

Although much of carpal instability, both dissociative and
non-dissociative, can be managed non-operatively, early recognition and treatment of injury to these mooring lines leads

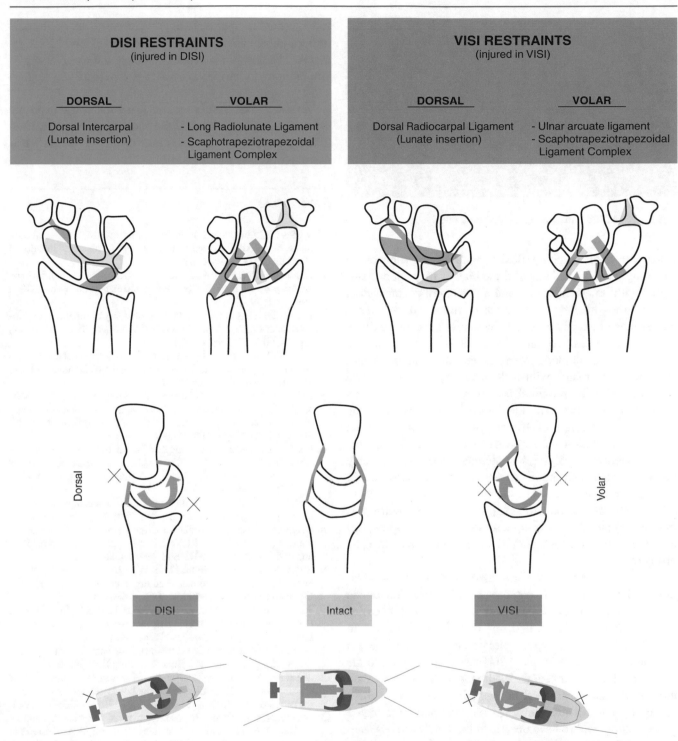

Fig. 14.15 Mooring lines concept of proximal row instability. VISI restraints (orange) and DISI restraints (blue) centred around the lunate

to better restoration of carpal alignment and stability compared to delayed treatment.

Implications for Treatment Choice

There have been many different procedures proposed for the management of carpal instability. For SL dissociation alone, the options are myriad. One of the trends has been a tendency to recommend an author's preferred method for all manifestations of SLD. However, a careful examination of presentations reveals a number of varied kinematic problems, associated with different ligamentous injury patterns, and perhaps requiring differing surgical approaches informed by the kinematic problem.

As an example, significant SLD (Geissler 3/4 or EWAS III/IV) may be manifested by SL gapping, scaphoid pronation, scaphoid flexion without dorsal subluxation (pivoting

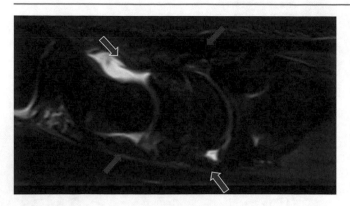

Fig. 14.16 MRI demonstrating the 'mooring lines'

proximally), or scaphoid flexion with dorsal subluxation (pivoting distally) and any of these may or may not be associated with lunate extension and dorsal capitate translation. Clearly, they all have a complete disruption of the SLIL; however, the individual altered kinematics depends on which critical stabilisers are injured or secondarily attenuated. Purely as an example, gapping alone, albeit quite uncommon, may be treated with a dorsal reconstruction. Dorsal subluxation of the proximal pole may be suited to an axis method such as the SLT tenodesis which reconstructs the volar STT, central axis of SLL and particularly targets dorsal scaphoid translation and reconstructs the DICL [32]. Severe lunate extension implying late attenuation of the LRL may be best treated with the ANAFAB reconstruction which, in addition to reconstruction of the volar STT and dorsal SLL, specifically targets the LRL [33]. The important concept is that one should not see every case of SLD as the same, and the reconstructive choice should be tailored to the kinematic problem.

Another observation we have made relates to the association of lower grade SL pathology with disruption of the extrinsic ligament attachment to the dorsal lunate. Many of these patients can be treated non-operatively; however, in refractory cases requiring operative management, if there is such a disruption, attention to this lesion in addition to the SLIL may improve outcome. Dealing with the 'bare area' on the dorsal lunate can assist in managing lower grade SLIL pathology and in augmenting other treatments for higher grade pathology. We have described the repair and augmentation of the DIC^L (RADICL), which will be discussed in greater detail in the next chapter.

Conclusion

This chapter outlines newer concepts in carpal stability and the implications this has on current practice. While our understanding of carpal instability will continue to improve,

it is essential to appreciate the role of the critical stabilisers of the carpus, namely, the DIC^L, DRC, vSTT and LRL ligaments. The specific kinematic problem and associated pattern of injury to the critical stabilisers should inform surgical choices.

We should be careful to ensure that our surgical exposure does not further compromise the integrity of the critical stabilisers, particularly the insertions on to the non-articular dorsal portion of the lunate.

References

1. Viegas SF, Yamaguchi S, Boyd NL, Patterson RM. The dorsal ligaments of the wrist: anatomy, mechanical properties, and function. J Hand Surg. 1999;24:456–68.
2. Ritt MJPF, Berger RA, Kauer JMG. The gross and histologic anatomy of the ligaments of the capitohamate joint. J Hand Surg. 1996;21:1022–8.
3. Berger RA, Garcia-Elias M. General anatomy of the wrist. In: biomechanics of the wrist joint. New York: Springer; 1991. https://doi.org/10.1007/978-1-4612-3208-7_1.
4. Short WH, Werner FW, Green JK, Masaoka S. Biomechanical evaluation of ligamentous stabilizers of the scaphoid and lunate. J Hand Surg Am. 2007 Mar;32(3):297–309.
5. Nagao S, Patterson RM, Buford WL, Andersen CR, Shah MA, Viegas SF. Three-dimensional description of ligamentous attachments around the lunate. J Hand Surg. 2005;30(4):685–92. https://doi.org/10.1016/j.jhsa.2005.03.002.
6. Elsaidi GA, Ruch DS, Kuzma GR, Smith BP. Dorsal wrist ligament insertions stabilize the scapholunate interval: Cadaver study. Clin Orthop Relat Res. 2004; https://doi.org/10.1097/01.blo.0000136836.78049.45.
7. Berger RA, Bishop AT, Bettinger PC. New dorsal capsulotomy for the surgical exposure of the wrist. Ann Plast Surg. 1995;35:54–9.
8. Berger RA, Bishop AT. A fiber-splitting capsulotomy technique for dorsal exposure of the wrist. Tech Hand Upper Extrem Surg. 1997; https://doi.org/10.1097/00130911-199703000-00002.
9. Berger RA, Doyle JR, Botte MJ. Section II: regional anatomy. In: Surgical anatomy of the hand and upper extremity. Philadelphia: Lippincott Williams & Wilkins; 2003. p. 486–531.
10. Wessel LE, Kim J, Morse KW, Loisel F, Koff MF, Breighner R, Doty S, Wolfe SW. The dorsal ligament complex: a cadaveric, histology and imaging study. J Hand Surg. 2021. [in press]
11. Sennwald GR, Zdravkovic V, Oberlin C. The anatomy of the palmar scaphotriquetral ligament. J Bone Joint Surg B. 1994;76:147–9.
12. de Sambuy MT, Burgess TM, Cambon-Binder A, Mathoulin CL. The anatomy of the dorsal capsulo-scapholunate septum: a cadaveric study. J Wrist Surg. 2017; https://doi.org/10.1055/s-0036-1597922.
13. Overstraeten L, Camus E, Wahegaonkar A, Messina J, Tandara A, Binder A, Mathoulin C. Anatomical description of the dorsal capsulo-scapholunate septum (DCSS)—arthroscopic staging of scapholunate instability after DCSS sectioning. J Wrist Surg. 2013;02:149–54.
14. Binder A, Kerfant N, Wahegaonkar A, Tandara A, Mathoulin C. Dorsal wrist capsular tears in association with scapholunate instability: results of an arthroscopic dorsal capsuloplasty. J Wrist Surg. 2013; https://doi.org/10.1055/s-0032-1333426.
15. Lee SK, Desai H, Silver B, Dhaliwal G, Paksima N. Comparison of radiographic stress views for scapholunate dynamic instability in a cadaver model. J Hand Surg. 2011; https://doi.org/10.1016/j.jhsa.2011.05.009.

16. Meade TD, Schneider LH, Cherry K. Radiographic analysis of selective ligament sectioning at the carpal scaphoid: a cadaver study. J Hand Surg. 1990; https://doi.org/10.1016/0363-5023(90)90003-A.

17. Pérez AJ, Jethanandani RG, Vutescu ES, Meyers KN, Lee SK, Wolfe SW. Role of ligament stabilizers of the proximal carpal row in preventing dorsal intercalated segment instability: a cadaveric study. J Bone Joint Surg Am. 2019;101(15):1388–96. https://doi.org/10.2106/JBJS.18.01419.

18. Ruby LK, An KN, Linscheid RL, Cooney WP. The effect of scapholunate ligament section on scapholunate motion. J Hand Surg Am. 1987;12(5 Pt 1):767–71.

19. Mitsuyasu H, Patterson RM, Shah M. The role of the dorsal intercarpal ligament in dynamic and static scapholunate instability. J Hand Surg Am. 2004;29(2):279–88.

20. Rohman EM, Agel J, Putnam MD, Adams JE. Scapholunate interosseous ligament injuries: a retrospective review of treatment and outcomes in 82 wrists. J Hand Surg. 2014; https://doi.org/10.1016/j.jhsa.2014.06.139.

21. Daly LT, Daly MC, Mohamadi A, Chen N. Chronic scapholunate interosseous ligament disruption: a systematic review and meta-analysis of surgical treatments. Hand. 2020;15:27–34.

22. Wolfe SW, Katz LD, Crisco JJ. Radiographic progression to dorsal intercalated segment instability. Orthopedics. 1996; https://doi.org/10.3928/0147-7447-19960801-18.

23. Kuo CE, Wolfe SW. Scapholunate instability: current concepts in diagnosis and management. J Hand Surg. 2008; https://doi.org/10.1016/j.jhsa.2008.04.027.

24. Loisel F, Wessel LE, Morse KW, Victoria C, Meyers K, Wolfe SW. Is the dorsal fiber-splitting approach to the wrist safe? A kinematic analysis and introduction of the window approach. J Hand Surg. 2021. [in press]

25. Fok MWM, Fernandez DL, Maniglio M. Carpal instability non-dissociative following acute wrist fractures. J Hand Surg. 2020; https://doi.org/10.1016/j.jhsa.2019.11.018.

26. Loisel F, Orr S, Ross M, Couzens G, Leo AJ, Wolfe SW. Traumatic non-dissociative carpal instability: a case series. J Hand Surg Am. 2021 Jun 24:S0363-5023(21)00248-3. https://doi.org/10.1016/j.jhsa.2021.04.024.

27. Moritomo H, Murase T, Goto A, Oka K, Sugamoto K, Yoshikawa H. Capitate-based kinematics of the midcarpal joint during wrist radioulnar deviation: an in vivo three-dimensional motion analysis. J Hand Surg. 2004; https://doi.org/10.1016/j.jhsa.2004.04.010.

28. Garcia-Elias M. The non-dissociative clunking wrist: a personal view. J Hand Surg Eur Vol. 2008; https://doi.org/10.1177/1753193408090148.

29. Weber ER. Concepts governing the rotational shift of the intercalated segment of the carpus. Orthop Clin N Am. 1984 Apr;15(2):193–207.

30. Wolfe SW, Garcia-Elias M, Kitay A. Carpal instability nondissociative. J Am Acad Orthop Surg. 2012; https://doi.org/10.5435/JAAOS-20-09-575.

31. Sandow MJ, Fisher TJ, Howard CQ, Papas S. Unifying model of carpal mechanics based on computationally derived isometric constraints and rules-based motion – the stable central column theory. J Hand Surg Eur Vol. 2014; https://doi.org/10.1177/1753193413505407.

32. Ross M, Loveridge J, Cutbush K, Couzens G. Scapholunate ligament reconstruction. J Wrist Surg. 2013; https://doi.org/10.1055/s-0033-1341962.

33. Sandow M, Fisher T. Anatomical anterior and posterior reconstruction for scapholunate dissociation: preliminary outcome in ten patients. J Hand Surg Eur Vol. 2020; https://doi.org/10.1177/1753193419886536.

Arthroscopic-Assisted Combined Dorsal and Volar Scapholunate Ligament Reconstruction with Tendon Graft for Chronic SL Instability

15

Siu-cheong Jeffrey Justin Koo and Pak-cheong Ho

Introduction

Scapholunate (SL) dissociation is the most common carpal instability [1]. As described by Mayfield et al., the injury is often due to a fall on the hypothenar area with the wrist in extension and ulnar deviation resulting in intercarpal supination. This leads to progressive failure of carpal osteoligamentous architecture, traveling from radial to ulnar around the lunate [2]. The scapholunate joint stability depends on two systems of ligament: intrinsic scapholunate interosseous ligament (SLIL) and secondary extrinsic stabilizers such as dorsal radiocarpal (DRC) ligament, dorsal intercarpal (DIC) ligament, scaphotrapezial (ST) ligament, and radioscaphocapitate (RSC) ligament. Each has a distinct role, but they work in concert to form the scapholunate ligament complex (SLLC) [3].

Numerous surgical techniques have been described to restore or improve the stability of the SL joint and to retard or prevent the progression to arthritis [4–29]. Among those focused on SLIL reconstruction, most methods provide only dorsal and uniplanar reconstructions, and the importance of the SLIL volar component is often underrated [11, 12, 20, 21, 26]. The volar component has an important role in rotational constraint of SL joint and will create shear stress between the scaphoid and lunate when sectioned [30, 31].

Based on the results of biomechanical studies, it is more logical and ideal to restore both the dorsal and volar components of the SL ligament. Yi et al. used a palmaris longus tendon to pass through drill holes in the anteroposterior plane of the scaphoid and the lunate. The SL diastasis was effectively reduced to normal, and the scaphoid and lunate contact pressure on the radius and the scaphoid-to-lunate contact ratio were significantly improved after the reconstruction [32]. Zdero used bovine tendons passing through double bone tunnels of the scaphoid and lunate in 19 cadaveric wrists and found no difference in the mechanical property from the normal wrists [33].

Dobyns used a portion of tendon to pass through anteroposterior bone tunnels in the proximal pole of the scaphoid and lunate to reconstruct the SL linkage. Stability was obtained by tightly looping the tendon graft across the scaphoid and lunate [34]. However, creating drill holes across poorly vascularized areas of bone in an open fashion severely compromised their blood supply and resulted in fractures and avascular necrosis.

In 2002, the senior author (PC Ho) developed an arthroscopic-assisted technique to reconstruct both the dorsal and volar SL ligament simultaneously using a free tendon graft in a box-like structure without violating the major blood supply to the scaphoid and soft tissue envelope [35] (Fig. 15.1).

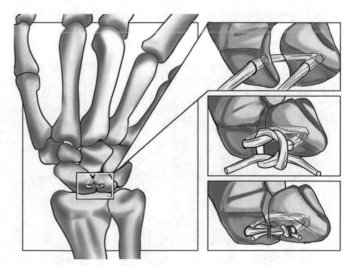

Fig. 15.1 Simultaneous reconstruction of the dorsal and palmar SL ligaments anatomically with the use of tendon graft in a box-like manner (Courtesy of Mr. Joey Lau Chun Yin)

S.-c. J. J. Koo

Department of Orthopaedics and Traumatology, Alice Ho Miu Ling Nethersole Hospital, Hong Kong, China

P.-c. Ho (✉)

Department of Orthopaedics and Traumatology, Prince of Wales Hospital, Hong Kong, China
e-mail: pcho@cuhk.edu.hk

© Springer Nature Switzerland AG 2022

W. B. Geissler (ed.), *Wrist and Elbow Arthroscopy with Selected Open Procedures*,
https://doi.org/10.1007/978-3-030-78881-0_15

Indications

The indication is subacute and chronic SL dissociation of 6 weeks or beyond with reducible SL diastasis and dorsal intercalated segmental instability (DISI) deformity confirmed arthroscopically and radiologically.

Contraindications

Contraindications include SL advanced collapse (SLAC) wrist beyond stage I and chronic non-reducible SL dissociation after adequate intra-articular fibrosis and capsular contracture release.

Operative Techniques

We advise to perform diagnostic wrist arthroscopy under portal site local anesthesia prior to the definitive surgery for complete diagnostic purpose, especially if the SL dissociation cannot fully account for the wrist pain [36]. This helps to evaluate the cause of the chronic wrist pain, confirm the status of the SL ligaments, evaluate the reducibility of the SL diastasis and rotation malalignment, and assess any cartilage or SLAC changes. Also, arthroscopic lysis performed at this stage can help to improve the SL joint reducibility. If not, then we will need to consider alternative treatment methods.

Patient Preparation and Positioning

After anesthesia and before the patient is subjected to surgery, a thorough fluoroscopic assessment of the SL joint sta-

bility and reducibility is conducted. The amount of SL joint diastasis, DISI deformity, and dorsal scaphoid translation is noted. Reducibility can be evaluated by doing a passive radial deviation of the wrist to observe for apposition of the SL gap (Fig. 15.2). Reduction of the DISI deformity can be assessed by applying a volarly directed pushing force to the dorsal scaphoid (Fig. 15.3). Easily reducible SL dissociation will constitute a good indication for the captioned technique.

The surgery is performed under general anesthesia or regional block with the patient in a supine position and the operated arm in 90° shoulder abduction resting on a hand table. The elbow joint is flexed to 90° and the affected hand is subjected to 10–13 lb of traction force through the plastic finger traps applying to the middle three digits by using a sterilizable Wrist Traction Tower (ConMed Linvatec Corp., Goleta, CA, USA). The well-padded arm is strapped to the base plate of the tower to provide countertraction.

The arm tourniquet is not inflated initially. Two percent lignocaine with 1:200,000 adrenaline was injected into the portal sites to reduce bleeding. Continuous saline irrigation of the joint was achieved with a bag of 3 L of normal saline hung up at about 1.5 meters instilled under gravity.

Exploration of Radiocarpal Joint and Midcarpal Joint

A 1.9-mm or 2.7-mm arthroscope is used. Small transverse skin crease incisions are made on the portal sites. Radiocarpal joint arthroscopy is performed initially through the 3–4 and 4–5 portals with 6U as the outflow portal, followed by midcarpal joint arthroscopy through the midcarpal radial (MCR) and midcarpal ulnar (MCU) portals. SL joint gapping, drive-through sign, articular step-off, status of the torn SL liga-

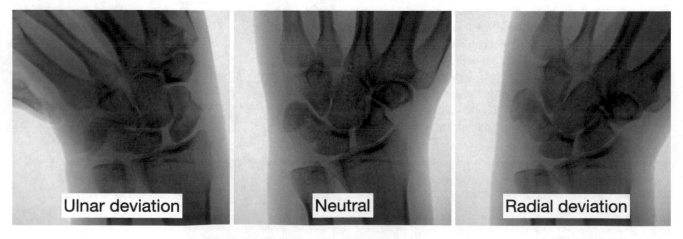

Fig. 15.2 Reducibility of SL joint can be assessed under fluoroscopy, where radial deviation reduces the SL gap, while ulnar deviation widens the gap

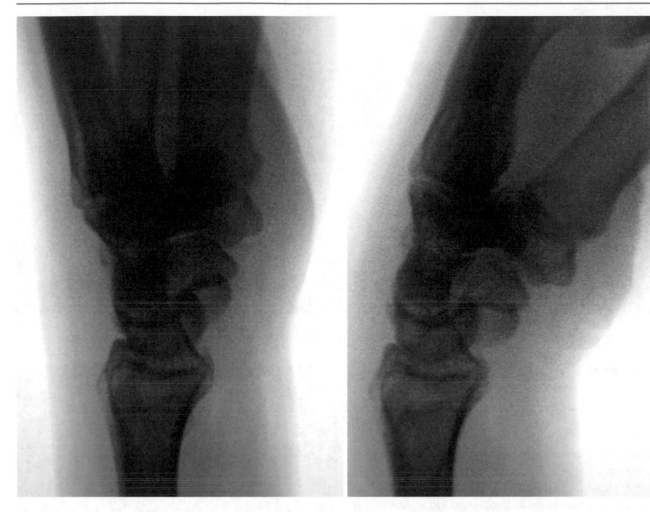

Fig. 15.3 By applying wrist flexion force, reducibility of lunate in DISI deformity can be observed under fluoroscope

ment remnant, associated chondral lesions, and changes in the extrinsic ligaments can be observed. Synovectomy and radial styloidectomy can be performed at the same time, if necessary, using a 2-mm shaver, small radiofrequency ablation probe, and 2.9-mm burr.

Taking Down of Intra-articular Fibrosis

In chronic SL dissociation with significant diastasis and DISI deformity, intra-articular fibrosis and capsular contracture are often found. Bundle of scar tissue interposed at the SL joint interval can prevent its adequate reduction (Fig. 15.4). Fibrosis and scar tissue are resected with a shaver to improve the capsular elasticity and to facilitate subsequent reduction of the SL gap, malalignment, and DISI deformity. The carpal bones in the proximal carpal row can be squeezed manually under a reduced traction force to assess the reduction of the SL gap (Fig. 15.5). Reducibility of scaphoid and lunate should also be confirmed by fluoroscopy before proceeding to next stage.

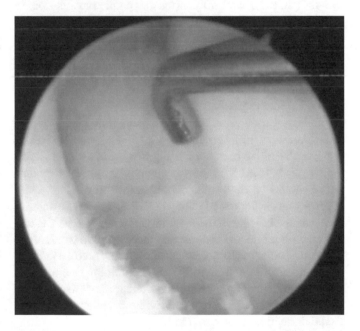

Fig. 15.4 A view from MCR portal looking into the midcarpal joint showing the dense scar tissue interposed between SL interval, which would hinder subsequent reduction

Before reduction

After reduction

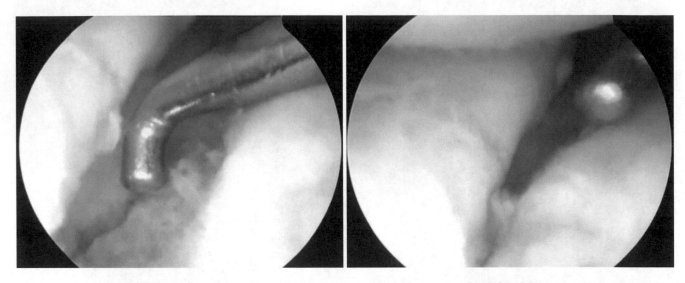

Fig. 15.5 By removing the scar tissue in between SL interval, the gap can be reduced with squeezing proximal carpal bone externally

Preparation of Scaphoid and Lunate Bone Tunnels

The operated arm is taken off the traction tower and put on the hand table. The arm tourniquet is then inflated after the hand and forearm are exsanguinated. A 2-cm transverse incision is centered at the 3–4 portal and extended 1 cm radially and 1 cm ulnarly toward the 4–5 portal (Fig. 15.6). The extensor retinaculum is split along its oblique fibers. The extensor digitorum communis (EDC), extensor carpi radialis brevis (ECRB), and the extensor carpi radialis longus (ECRL) tendons are identified. Lunate can be exposed by retracting the EDC tendons ulnarward or more preferably by passing between the EDC tendons. The ideal scaphoid tunnel position can be spotted between ECRB and ECRL tendons (Fig. 15.7). The tendons are being slung with cotton tapes for protection and retraction.

Volarly, a transverse incision is made along the proximal wrist crease from the radial border of the palmaris longus (PL) to the ulnar border of the flexor carpi radialis (FCR) tendon (Fig. 15.8). The palmar cutaneous branch of median nerve should be dissected out and safeguarded (Fig. 15.9). PL free graft is harvested with a tendon stripper. The anterior forearm fascia is incised. The interval between the FCR tendon, the finger flexor tendons, and median nerve is entered to reach the volar wrist joint capsule (Fig. 15.10). Both the volar and dorsal wrist joint capsules containing the important extrinsic ligaments and, hence, secondary stabilizers of the SL joint are carefully preserved without violation. The soft tissue dissection is kept to a minimum.

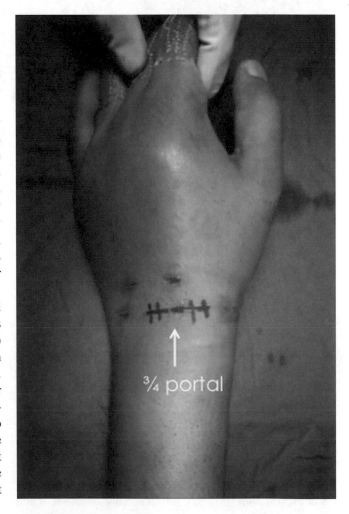

Fig. 15.6 Planning of dorsal skin incision. Using the 3–4 portal as the center, skin incision is extended 1 cm radially and 1 cm ulnarly

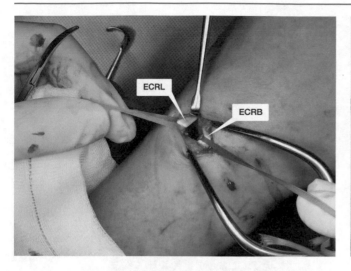

Fig. 15.7 By retracting the ECRB and ECRL, the "sweet" spot for placing the scaphoid bone tunnel can be located

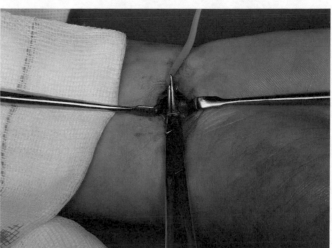

Fig. 15.9 The palmar cutaneous branch of median nerve should be dissected out and safeguarded, which is often found on radial side of skin incision

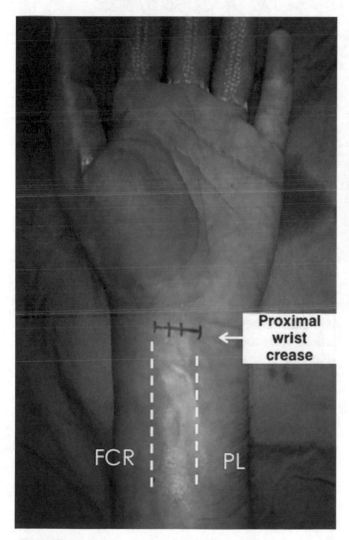

Fig. 15.8 Placement of volar skin incision. Transverse incision is made along the proximal wrist crease from the radial border of the palmaris longus (PL) to the ulnar border of the flexor carpi radialis (FCR) tendon

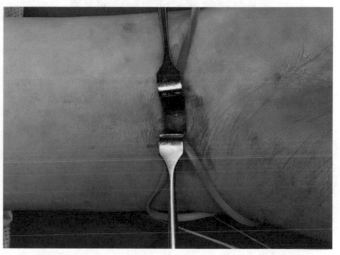

Fig. 15.10 The volar joint capsule can be visualized by retracting FCR and palmar cutaneous branch of median nerve radially while median nerve and finger flexor tendons retract ulnarly

Correction of DISI Deformity

DISI deformity needs to be corrected before drilling the bone tunnel. The hand is examined under the fluoroscope. The extended lunate can be corrected by the Linscheid maneuver with wrist flexion to realign the lunate with radius. The lunate position can be maintained by transfixing the RL joint with a 1.6-mm K-wire, which is inserted percutaneously through the dorsum of distal radius. The RL pin should be aimed at the ulnar half of the lunate to avoid conflict with the lunate bone tunnel (Fig. 15.11). The wrist is now ready for bone tunnel preparation.

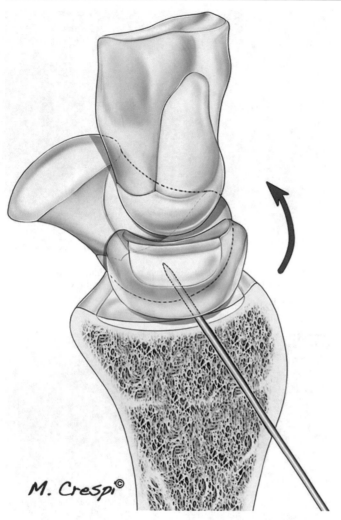

Fig. 15.11 The lunate reduction by the Linscheid maneuver. The radiolunate joint is transfixed with a 1.6-mm K-wire with the lunate in a neutral position. (Reprinted with permission from Mathoulin [40])

Preparation of Lunate Bone Tunnel

Lunate bone tunnel is created through the dorsal incision. Either by retracting the tendons ulnarly or more preferably passing through the EDC tendons, the dorsal portion of lunate can be reached. A 1.1-mm guide pin is inserted into the lunate perpendicular to the long axis of the lunate, that is, parallel to the line joining the tip of the volar and dorsal lips of the lunate, through the capsule under fluoroscopic guidance. The guide pin should aim at the center of lunate to avoid iatrogenic blow-out fracture. For cases with mild DISI deformity, RL pinning may not be necessary. If the lunate is not being transfixed to the radius, manual traction of the wrist can help bring the lunate to a more distal position to uncover the lunate from the dorsal rim of the distal radius and hence facilitating the pinning process. Over the volar side, an assistant helps to gently retract and protect the flexor

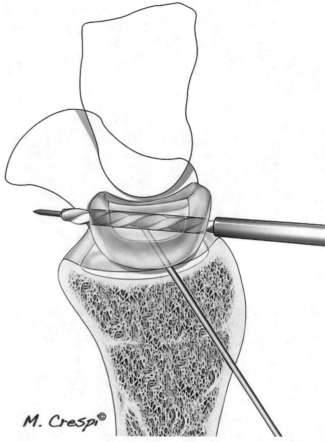

Fig. 15.12 The preparation of lunate bone tunnel. 1.1-mm guide pin is inserted into the lunate perpendicular to the long axis of the lunate under fluoroscopic guidance. The guide pin should aim at the center of lunate and not too close to the articular margin to avoid iatrogenic blow-out fracture. Then the bone tunnel is prepared with cannulated drill form dorsal to volar direction. Using a 4.5-mm drill sleeve to protect the soft tissue from the K-wire and cannulated drill is often useful to avoid iatrogenic damage to flexors and median nerve. (Reprinted with permission from Mathoulin [40])

tendons and median nerve ulnarward. The surgeon advances the lunate tunnel guide pin to perforate the volar cortex of the lunate, volar capsule, and exit through the volar wound (Fig. 15.12).

Preparation of Scaphoid Bone Tunnel

Another guide pin is inserted through the dorsal wound onto the scaphoid in the interval between the ECRB and ECRL tendons. The guide pin aims at the proximal scaphoid at least 2–3 mm from the surrounding articular margin to avoid iatrogenic fracture both in coronal and sagittal planes. It provides counterrotational force on the scaphoid to correct the flexion pronation deformity when the guide pin trajectory is slightly directed proximally and volarly (Figs. 15.13 and

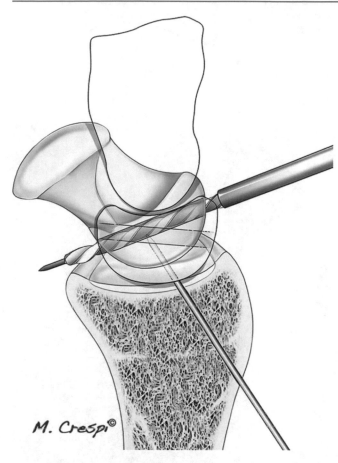

Fig. 15.13 The preparation of scaphoid bone tunnel. Again, guide pin should be 2–3 mm away from articular margin to avoid blow-out. Guide pin trajectory is preferably slightly directed proximally and volarly to correct the flexion pronation deformity when the tendon graft is tightened. (Reprinted with permission from Mathoulin [40])

15.14). With the FCR tendon retracted radially, the scaphoid guide pin exited through the volar wound. Both the lunate and scaphoid bone tunnels are subsequently enlarged using 2.0-mm and 2.4-mm cannulated drill bits. It must be borne in mind that the bone tunnels should not be too large, because there is risk of iatrogenic fracture or inducing bone ischemia. If the tunnel size is too small, it may cause jamming of tendon graft inside the tunnel, causing graft attrition or even avulsion when being pulled through the tunnel. It is mandatory to use protection sheaths of adequate size on both the dorsal and volar sides to protect the soft tissue during the pinning and drilling processes under fluoroscopic control.

Passing the Palmaris Longus Tendon Graft through the Scaphoid and Lunate Bone Tunnel

The free PL tendon graft is delivered through the capsular vents and the bone tunnels with a 2-mm arthroscopic grasper, from the volar side of the scaphoid to dorsal, and from the

volar aspect of the lunate to dorsal (Fig. 15.15). It is critically important to be sure that the grasper is passing through inside the tunnels instead of slipping through the surface of the carpal bones. The tendon graft is passed outside the capsule to cross the SL interval so that the reconstruction also helps to tighten the capsule and the extrinsic ligaments, which confer added stability to the SL joint (Fig. 15.16). It is mandatory to check that the volar loop of the tendon graft does not trap on any of the flexor tendons and the median nerve before the tendon should be tied.

Assessment through Midcarpal Joint Arthroscopy and Scapholunate Interval Reduction with Palmaris Longus Tendon Graft

The hand is put on the traction tower again. The MCJ is inspected through the MCR portal. The RL pin is then withdrawn from the lunate so that the lunate becomes mobile. Traction should be reduced to minimum. When the two ends of the tendon graft are pulled manually, any SL gapping and step-off is corrected and can be visualized under arthroscopic and fluoroscopic surveillance. Any interposing soft tissue at the SL joint can be removed arthroscopically. Quality of reduction can be reassured. If necessary, the reduction can be facilitated by using a large bone reduction clamp placed between the scaphoid and triquetrum percutaneously. Once adequate reduction is confirmed by tensioning the tendon graft, the hand is put back on the hand table. The two ends of the tendon graft are passed underneath all the extensor tendons to meet each other at the SL joint. The tendon graft is maximally tensioned and tied in a shoelace manner over the dorsal capsule and secured with 2–0 nonabsorbable braided sutures on a non-cutting needle (Fig. 15.17). Additional sutures can be stitched through the adjacent capsular structure to augment the repair strength. SL reduction and stability are confirmed arthroscopically and fluoroscopically. If the reduction and stability is suboptimal, the suturing can be revised after further tensioning until reduction is satisfactory. The tendon graft is then tied once more and sutured securely. Two knots of the tendon graft suffice as further knotting may produce an unacceptable bump at the back of the wrist. Two 1.1-mm K-wires are inserted through a small incision in the anatomic snuffbox region to transfix the scaphocapitate (SC) joint to unload the SL joint and hence protect the reconstructed ligament during the healing process (Fig. 15.18). The pins are cut short and buried underneath the skin for later removal. We advised against pinning of the SL joint as this may risk the injury and weakening of the tendon graft at the bone tunnels. Additional suture anchors can be placed next to the dorsal bone tunnels over the scaphoid and lunate and tied for additional repair

a

b

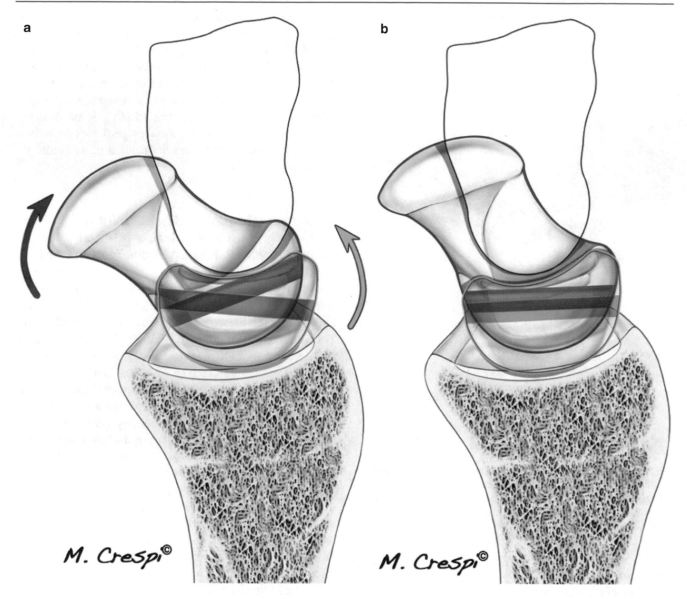

Fig. 15.14 (**a**) The position of tunnels before passage of tendon graft and before reduction. (**b**) The reduction of both tunnels after tensioning of the PL graft. (Reprinted with permission from Mathoulin [40])

strength. The RL pin is then advanced to maintain the lunate reduction if necessary. If the reconstruction is considered solid and stable, the protective pinning can be omitted. The extensor tendons are repositioned and the extensor retinaculum repaired.

Closure and Postoperative Care

The wound is closed with absorbable subcuticular sutures. Bulky dressing and scaphoid plaster slab are applied with wrist in a neutral position and the thumb in neutral palmar abduction.

The wrist is immobilized in a short arm thumb spica cast for 6 weeks. The RL pin is removed at the beginning of the third week. The cast is then changed to a thumb spica splint for an additional 2 weeks, at which time gentle active wrist mobilization exercise is allowed out of the splint. The SC pins are removed at the beginning of the 9th week under local anesthesia. The splint is worn at nighttime for another 4–6 weeks. Gradual wrist range of motion exercises under physiotherapist supervision is started after the pin removal. Passive motion exercise can be commenced at the beginning of the 11th week and gradual strengthening exercises at 13th week after surgery. The SL reduction should be monitored at interval with radiological examination.

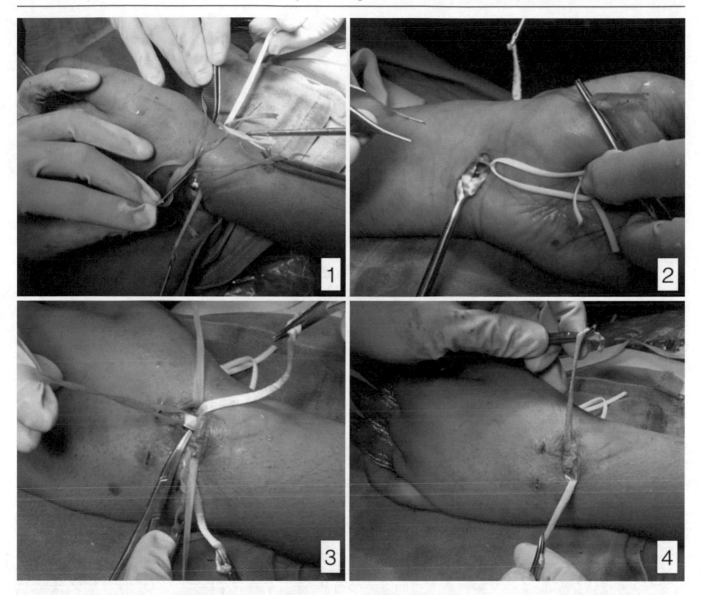

Fig. 15.15 Operative view of PL tendon graft delivered through the wrist capsule and the bone tunnels. (1) Passing the 2 mm arthroscopic grasper from dorsal side to volar side to grab the PL tendon graft end and deliver through the bone tunnel to dorsal side. (2) Careful retraction helps to prevent trapping of flexor tendons and median nerve by the tendon graft. (3) Passing of PL tendon graft underneath the extensors to avoid iatrogenic entrapment of extensors. (4) After checking of no soft tissue entrapment, it is ready for reduction and tightening of tendon graft

Clinical Outcome

In our series of the first 17 patients with chronic SL instability operated between October 2002 and June 2012, there were 3 Geissler grade 3 and 14 grade 4 instability cases. The average preoperative SL interval was 4.9 mm (range 3–9 mm). DISI deformity was present in 13 patients. Six patients had stage 1 SLAC wrist change radiologically. Concomitant procedures were performed in four patients.

The average follow-up was 48.3 months (range 11–132 months). Thirteen returned to their preinjury job level. Eleven patients had no wrist pain, and six had some pain on either maximum exertion or at the extreme of motion. The average extension range compared to pre-op improved for 13%, flexion range 16%, radial deviation 13%, and ulnar deviation 27%. Mean grip strength was 32.8 kg (120% of the preoperative status, 84% of the contralateral side). The average SL interval after reconstruction was 2.9 mm (range 1.6–

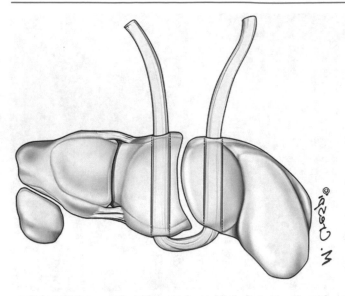

Fig. 15.16 The passage of PL tendon graft from scaphoid, volar to the volar capsule and through the lunate before final tightening and suture. (Reprinted with permission from Mathoulin [40])

5.5 mm). Recurrence of a DISI deformity was noted in four patients but remained asymptomatic. No case reported progressive SLAC wrist change. Ischemic change of proximal scaphoid was noted in one case without symptom or progression. It is likely due to the creation of large bore bone tunnel of 3.5 mm at the initial period of the surgery development. There was no neurovascular or tendon complication. All patients were satisfied with the procedure and outcome.

Naqui et al. had reviewed the 1191 papers related to the management of chronic non-arthritic scapholunate dissociation, of which 17 papers were valid for analysis. From his paper, our method had better pain reduction than others (63% in our study vs. 50% in capsulodesis vs. 52% in tenodesis). This would probably be related to minimal soft tissue disturbance, as our technique is performed with very little soft tissue dissection under arthroscopic guidance. Flexion-extension arc has improved for 15% in our series while tenodesis and capsulodesis have reduction in flexion-extension range for 32% and 22%, respectively. The greater loss of motion in tenodesis and capsulodesis can be

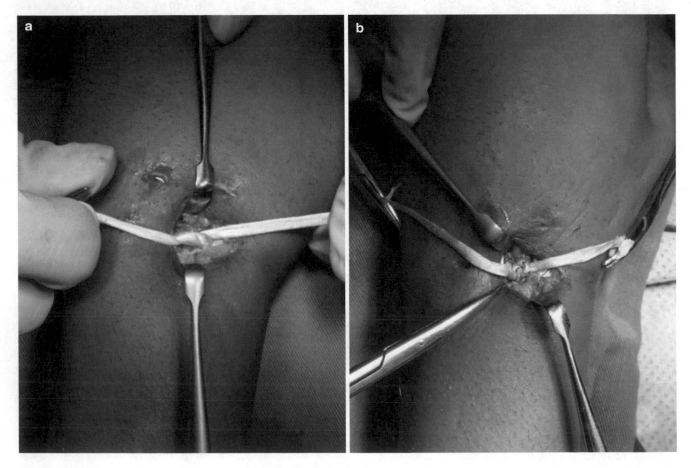

Fig. 15.17 (a) The tendon graft is knotted and (b) sutured under maximal tension on the dorsal surface of the SL joint extracapsularly in the shoelace manner

explained by the fact that tenodesis crosses radiocarpal and midcarpal joint, whereas in capsulodesis the reinforcement of the dorsal SLIL repair through the capsular flap will limit the radiocarpal joint motion [37]. Our technique involves tendon graft spanning over scaphoid and lunate only can minimize the restaining effect to other carpal bones motion. Also, as the tendon graft is placed at extracapular level, it helps to reinforce the extrinsic secondary stabilizers when the graft is tied in its maximal tension. Moreover, another potential advantage is that, since there is no need to open the joint capsule to expose the scapholunate interval, this leaves the innervation pathways intact, thus improving the scapholunate stabilizing effect further [38, 39].

The following case illustrates the clinical result of one of our cases with chronic SL dissociation. The patient had right wrist injury 1 year before during tennis playing. He felt pain over right wrist during backhand serve and had persistent weakness of grip and painful clicks during movement since then for 1 year. Physical examination showed tenderness at anatomical snuffbox, proximal scaphoid, and SL interval region. Watson test was positive with a painful clunk. Radiologically, a widely open SL interval, marked DISI deformity, and mild dorsal scaphoid translation were noted (see Fig. 15.18). With the SL ligament complex reconstructed by PL graft, SL interval, DISI deformity, and dorsal translation were well reduced. The construct was stabilized by the RL pin and SC joint pinning. The reconstruction remained stable with well-maintained SL angle and SL interval after 9.5 years (Fig. 15.19). He had no pain (VAS 0) with reasonable range of wrist motion (extension 77.8%, flexion 60%), grip strength (107% compared with contralateral side), and good outcome in functional score (DASH score 0.83/100, PWRE 5/100).

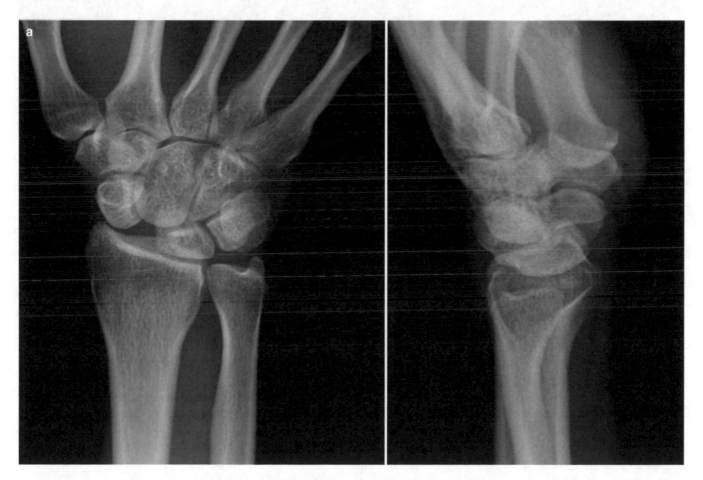

Fig. 15.18 (a) Preoperative X-ray of PA and lateral view for right wrist showing widening of SL interval and developing mild DISI. (b) Immediate postoperative X-ray showing the SL interval gap was reduced compared to preoperative X-ray. DISI deformity is also reduced and stabilized with PL pinning and the construct is further stabilized by SC pinning

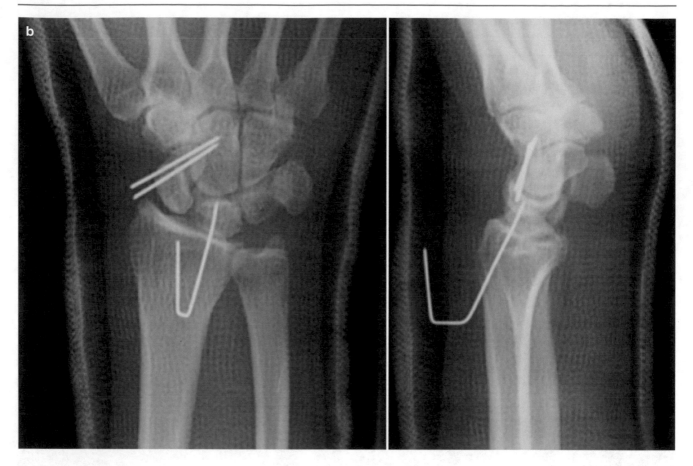

Fig. 15.18 (continued)

Tips and Tricks

- *Reducibility of scaphoid and lunate*. Intra-articular fibrosis is often found in radiocarpal joint interposed at the region between dorsal joint capsule and the region of previous ligament. The fibrosis and scar tissue need to be shaved away to restore the reducibility of scaphoid and lunate, which facilitates subsequent reduction of SL malalignment. Fluoroscopic assessment is required to assess whether DISI deformity can be reduced or not before proceeding to tendon harvesting and bone tunnel creation.

- *Protecting the palmar cutaneous branch of median nerve during creation of volar skin incision*. When making skin incision for volar incision, palmar cutaneous branch of median nerve should be identified and protected; otherwise, the nerve will be injured in subsequent procedure.

- *K-wire pinning of the RL joint should be aimed at ulnar half of lunate*. When transfixing the RL joint, the 1.6-mm pin is inserted percutaneously through the dorsum of dis-

tal radius. Blunt dissection is required to avoid iatrogenic injury to the extensor tendons. The RL pin should be aimed at the ulnar half of the lunate to avoid conflict with the lunate bone tunnel.

- *Precise bone tunnel position should be confirmed with fluoroscopy to avoid blow out fracture*. The lunate bone tunnel should be perpendicular to the long axis of the lunate, that is, parallel to the line joining the tip of the volar and dorsal lips of the lunate. The pin should aim at the center of lunate to avoid iatrogenic blow-out fracture.

  In a more severe case of DISI deformity, using the Linscheid maneuver helps to reduce the deformity. In a mild case of DISI, however, the lunate pin can be inserted slightly obliquely from dorsal proximal to volar distal direction to increase the correction force on the dorsal rotation of the lunate.

  The scaphoid bone tunnel aims at the proximal scaphoid at least 2–3 mm from the surrounding articular margin to avoid iatrogenic fracture. The guide pin trajectory is slightly directed proximally and volarly so that it provides

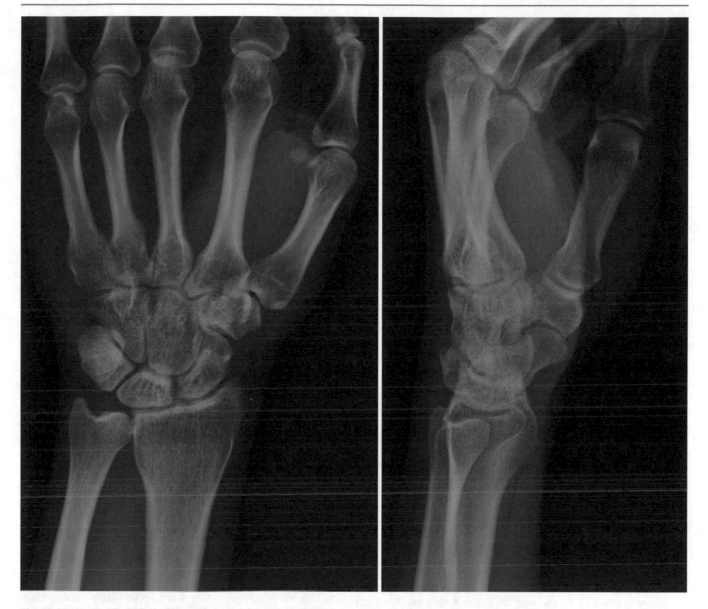

Fig. 15.19 X-ray of PA view and lateral view of the same patient taken 9.5 years after the SL reconstruction. There is no reopening up of the SL interval and corrected scapholunate angle maintained

counterrotational force on the scaphoid to correct the flexion pronation deformity when tendon graft is passed and tightened.

Under fluoroscopic guidance, we can assess guide pin placement inside scaphoid and lunate before proceed to bone tunnel drilling.

- *Pay attention to bone tunnel size, and soft tissue protection is needed when passing K-wire and cannulated drill.* The bone tunnels should not be too large, because there is risk of iatrogenic fracture or inducing bone ischemia. Tunnel size of about 2.5 mm is appropriate. Too small the tunnel size may cause jamming of tendon graft inside the tunnel, causing graft attrition or even avulsion when being

pulled through the tunnel. The tunnels should not be closed to the articular surfaces.

The flexor tendons and median nerve have to be gently retracted and protected when the guide pins and cannulated drills are passing out from the volar side of scaphoid and lunate. A large soft tissue protection sheath is essential when using the cannulated drills.

The assistant surgeon working on the volar side should preferably be a knowledgeable and reliable partner because it is hard for the arthroscopic surgeon to visualize both the dorsal and palmar sides at the same time. There should be good lighting and loupe magnification to avoid complications.

- *Use non-absorbable round-bodied suture when securing the tied tendon graft.* Make sure the suture has equipped with round-bodied suture needle; otherwise, it can create iatrogenic injury and lacerate the tendon graft.
- *Avoid inserting K-wire for pinning the SL joint.* It may injure and weaken the tendon graft inside the scaphoid and lunate bone tunnels.

Conclusion

Different methods have been described to reconstruct scapholunate ligament in chronic scapholunate dissociation over the past 50 years. It is logical and more preferable to reconstruct both the dorsal and volar components and to augment the extrinsic ligaments as secondary joint stabilizer. Our study demonstrated that it could be performed in arthroscopic-assisted manner. The ideal indication for this technique is a non-reparable complete scapholunate ligament injury with dissociation. The presence of DISI deformity does not preclude this method, as long as the deformity is reducible. While arthroscopic shaving of intra-articular fibrosis and lysis of capsular scar helps to convert non-reducible DISI into a reducible one, the DISI deformity can further be corrected and stabilized with the RL pinning.

References

1. Daniels JM II, Zook EG, Lynch JM. Hand and wrist injuries: part I. Nonemergent evaluation. Am Fam Phys. 2004;69(8):1941–8.
2. Mayfield JK, Johnson RP, Kilcoyne RK. Carpal dislocations: pathomechanics and progressive perilunar instability. J Hand Surg Am. 1980;5(3):226–41.
3. Short WH, Werner FW, Green JK, Sutton LG, Brutus JP. Biomechanical evaluation of the ligamentous stabilizers of the scaphoid and lunate: part III. J Hand Surg Am. 2007;32:297–309.
4. Peterson HA, Lipscomb PR. Intercarpal arthrodesis. Arch Surg. 1967;95:127–34.
5. Palmer AK, Dobyns JH, Linscheid RL. Management of post-traumatic instability of the wrist secondary to ligament rupture. J Hand Surg Am. 1978;3:507–32.
6. Uematsu A. Intercarpal fusion for treatment of carpal instability: a preliminary report. Clin Orthop Relat Res. 1979;144:159–65.
7. Watson HK. Limited wrist arthrodesis. Clin Orthop Relat Res. 1980;149:126–36.
8. Glickel SZ, Millender LH. Ligamentous reconstruction for chronic intercarpal instability. J Hand Surg Am. 1984;9:514–27.
9. Hastings DE, Silver RL. Intercarpal arthrodesis in the management of chronic carpal instability after trauma. J Hand Surg Am. 1984;9:834–40.
10. Blatt G. Capsulodesis in reconstructive hand surgery. Dorsal capsulodesis for the unstable scaphoid and volar capsulodesis following excision of the distal ulna. Hand Clin. 1987;3:81–102.
11. Conyers DJ. Scapholunate interosseous reconstruction and imbrication of palmar ligaments. J Hand Surg Am. 1990;15:690–700.
12. Almquist EE, Bach AW, Sack JT, Fuhs SE, Newman DM. Four-bone ligament reconstruction for treatment of chronic complete scapholunate separation. J Hand Surg Am. 1991;16:322–7.
13. Pisano SM, Peimer CA, Wheeler DR, Sherwin F. Scaphocapitate intercarpal arthrodesis. J Hand Surg Am. 1991;16:328–33.
14. Rotman MB, Manske PR, Pruitt DL, Szerzinski J. Scaphocapitolunate arthrodesis. J Hand Surg Am. 1993;18:26–33.
15. Brunelli GA, Brunelli GR. A new surgical technique for carpal instability with scapho-lunar dislocation. (Eleven cases). Ann Chir Main Memb Super. 1995;14:207–13.
16. Wintman BI, Gelberman RH, Katz JN. Dynamic scapholunate instability: results of operative treatment with dorsal capsulodesis. J Hand Surg Am. 1995;20:971–9.
17. Rosenwasser MP, Miyasajsa KC, Strauch RJ. The RASL procedure: reduction and association of the scaphoid and lunate using the Herbert screw. Tech Hand Up Extrem Surg. 1997;1:263–72.
18. Uhl RL, Williamson SC, Bowman MW, Sotereanos DG, Osterman AL. Dorsal capsulodesis using suture anchors. Am J Orthop. 1997;26:547–8.
19. Van Den Abbeele KL, Loh YC, Stanley JK, Trail IA. Early results of a modified Brunelli procedure for scapholunate instability. J Hand Surg Br. 1998;23:258–61.
20. Weiss AP. Scapholunate ligament reconstruction using a bone-retinaculum-bone autograft. J Hand Surg Am. 1998;23:205–15.
21. Harvey EJ, Hanel DP. Bone-ligament-bone reconstruction for scapholunate disruption. Tech Hand Up Extrem Surg. 2002;6:2–5.
22. Moran SL, Ford KS, Wulf CA, Cooney WP. Outcomes of dorsal capsulodesis and tenodesis for treatment of scapholunate instability. J Hand Surg Am. 2006;31(9):1438–46.
23. Darlis NA, Kaufmann RA, Giannoulis F, Sotereanos DG. Arthroscopic debridement and closed pinning for chronic dynamic scapholunate instability. J Hand Surg Am. 2006;31:418–24.
24. Garcia-Elias M, Lluch AL, Stanley JK. Three-ligament tenodesis for the treatment of scapholunate dissociation: indications and surgical technique. J Hand Surg Am. 2006;31:125–34.
25. Aviles AJ, Lee SK, Hausman MR. Arthroscopic reduction-association of the scapholunate. Arthroscopy. 2007;23:105.e1–5.
26. Papadogeorgou E, Mathoulin C. Extensor carpi radialis brevis ligamentoplasty and dorsal capsulodesis for the treatment of chronic post-traumatic scapholunate instability. Chir Main. 2010;29:172–9.
27. Mathoulin CL, Dauphin N, Wahegaonkar AL. Arthroscopic dorsal capsuloligamentous repair in chronic scapholunate ligament tears. Hand Clin. 2011;27:563–72.
28. Camus EJ, Van Overstraeten L. Dorsal scapholunate stabilization using Viegas' capsulodesis: 25 cases with 26 months-follow-up. Chir Main. 2013;32:393–402.
29. Ross M, Couzens G. A new technique for scapholunate ligament reconstruction utilizing FCR and interference screw fixation. J Hand Surg Am. 2013;38(Suppl):e51.
30. Berger RA, Imeada T, Berglund L, An KN. Constraint and material properties of the subregions of the scapholunate interosseous ligament. J Hand Surg Am. 1999;24:953–62.
31. Berger RA. The ligaments of the wrist. A current overview of anatomy with considerations of their potential functions. Hand Clin. 1997;13:63–82.
32. Yi IS, Firoozbakhsh K, Racca J, Umeda Y, Moneim M. Treatment of scapholunate dissociation with palmaris longus tendon graft: a biomechanical study. Univ Pennsylvania Orthop J. 2000;13:53–9.
33. Zdero R, Olsen M, Elfatori S, Skrinskas T, Nourhosseini H, Whyne C, et al. Linear and torsional mechanical characteristics of intact and reconstructed scapholunate ligaments. J Biomech Eng. 2009;131(4):41009.
34. Dobyns JH, Linscheid RL, EYS C, Weber ER, Swanson GE. Traumatic instability of the wrist In Instructional Course Lectures, The American Academy of Orthopaedic Surgeons, vol. 24. St. Louis: C. V. Mosby; 1975. p. 182–99.
35. Ho PC, Wong WYC, Tse WL. Arthroscopic-assisted combined dorsal and volar scapholunate ligament reconstruction with tendon graft for chronic SL instability. J Wrist Surg. 2015;4(4):252–63.

36. Koo SC, Ho PC. Wrist arthroscopy under portal site local anesthesia without tourniquet and sedation. Hand Clin. 2017;33(4):585–91.

37. Naqui Z, Khor WS, Mishra A, Lees V, Muir L. The management of chronic non-arthritic scapholunate dissociation: a systematic review. J Hand Surg Eur Vol. 2018;43(4):394–401.

38. Salva-Coll G, Garcia-Elias M, Hagert E. Scapholunate instability: proprioception and neuromuscular control. J Wrist Surg. 2013;2(2):136–40.

39. Hagert E, Lluch A, Rein S. The role of proprioception and neuromuscular stability in carpal instabilities. J Hand Surg Eur Vol. 2016;41(1):94–101.

40. Koo SC, Ho PC. Arthroscopic-assisted Box Reconstruction of scapho-lunate ligament with tendon graft. In Mathoulin C, Ed. Wrist Arthroscopy Techniques. Stuttgart, Germany; 2019:87–92.

Internal Brace for Carpal Instability

Robert M. Zbeda and Steven J. Lee

Introduction

Scapholunate (SL) instability is the most frequent cause of carpal instability [1]. SL instability represents a spectrum of injuries that ranges from dynamic instability to static instability. If left untreated, these injuries can progress and result in abnormal wrist mechanics and degenerative changes. For patients with SL instability, this ultimately leads to wrist dysfunction, lost time from work, and interference with daily activities.

The goals of treatment include restoring ligamentous continuity and normalizing carpal kinematics to ultimately preserve wrist function. A multitude of non-operative and operative treatment options exist for treating SL instability. Surgical techniques include thermal shrinkage, dorsal capsulodesis, and tendon reconstructions [2–7]. Indicating the proper surgical procedure is based on the patient's demands, whether the scapholunate interosseous ligament (SLIL) is repairable, and whether there is any pre-existing arthritis.

Surgical treatment methods have largely been able to improve pain but at the cost of reduced range of motion and grip strength. Long-term, SL gapping and carpal malalignment can occur despite an adequate repair or reconstruction [1]. Despite an abundance of procedures described to date, no surgical technique has demonstrated the ability to consistently provide long-term carpal stability in this challenging patient cohort.

In this chapter, we aim to describe novel techniques for treating SL instability with internal bracing. Although long-term data for internal bracing is pending, we believe that it is an attractive alternative to existing techniques due to its ability to add biomechanical strength to repairs and reconstructions while restoring carpal anatomy and kinematics.

Anatomy

A thorough understanding of the anatomy and biomechanics of the scapholunate joint is essential in guiding potential treatment strategies. The carpus consists of the distal radio-ulnar joint, radiocarpal joint, midcarpal joint, and carpometacarpal joints. The distal carpal row (trapezium, trapezoid, capitate, and hamate) is tightly connected via strong ligaments. Rigid ligamentous attachments exist between the second and third metacarpal bases with the trapezoid and capitate. The distal carpal bones have minimal motion and function as a single unit. In contrast, the scaphoid, lunate, and triquetrum of the proximal carpal row are without tendinous insertions and function as an intercalated segment. The motion of the proximal carpal row is largely dependent on its surrounding articulations [1, 8].

The scapholunate interosseous ligament (SLIL) is the primary stabilizer of the SL joint. The SLIL is C-shaped and attaches along the dorsal, proximal, and volar aspects of the articular surfaces of the scaphoid and lunate. The dorsal component is the thickest, strongest, and most critical portion that provides a restraint to not only distraction but also rotational and translational moments. The volar component is thinner and has some contributions to rotational stability. The proximal portion is a fibrocartilaginous structure with minor contributions to SL stability [1]. Berger et al. noted that the dorsal and volar SL ligaments have a yield strength of approximately 300 N and 120 N, respectively [9]. Together, the SLIL and lunotriquetral interosseous ligament (LTIL) are the major stabilizers of the proximal carpal row and carpus.

The secondary stabilizers of the wrist are also important to maintain carpal stability. The key extrinsic ligaments on the

R. M. Zbeda (✉)
Department of Orthopaedic Surgery, Lenox Hill Hospital, New York, NY, USA

S. J. Lee
Surgery of the Hand/Upper Extremity, Lenox Hill Hospital, New York, NY, USA

Nicholas Institute of Sports Medicine and Athletic Trauma, New York, NY, USA

© Springer Nature Switzerland AG 2022
W. B. Geissler (ed.), *Wrist and Elbow Arthroscopy with Selected Open Procedures*,
https://doi.org/10.1007/978-3-030-78881-0_16

volar-radial side of the wrist include the radioscaphocapitate (RSC), long radiolunate (LRL), short radiolunate (SRL), and radioscapholunate ligament (ligament of Testut). On the volar-ulnar side, there are the ulnolunate and ulnotriquetral ligaments. The scaphotrapezial ligament complex is also an important volar secondary stabilizer of the scaphoid. On the dorsal side, there are the dorsal radiotriquetral (or dorsal radiocarpal) and dorsal intercarpal (DIC or scaphotriquetral) ligaments. The V-arrangement of the dorsal radiotriquetral and dorsal intercarpal (DIC) are obliquely oriented to the flexion–extension axis of wrist motion and are key secondary stabilizers of the SL complex [10].

Biomechanics

In a normal wrist, the scaphoid, lunate, and triquetrum rotate together in flexion and extension. Radial deviation drives the scaphoid into flexion and the lunate follows via ligamentotaxis through the SLIL. Ulnar deviation drives the hamate into the triquetrum, which results in extension of the triquetrum and also the lunate via the LTIL.

Compared to the distal carpal row, the proximal carpal row has a greater degree of relative motion between its carpal bones. Scaphoid flexion–extension exceeds lunate flex–extension by approximately 35°. Scaphoid pronation is three times that of the lunate, and lunate ulnar deviation exceeds that of the scaphoid [11].

Pathomechanics

The SLIL is the most frequently injured carpal ligament. SL instability is a spectrum of injuries that includes both dynamic and static instabilities. Rupture of the SLIL alone may not result in a static increase in SL gapping. However, isolated injury to the SLIL can lead to dynamic changes with wrist motion and loading that can result in symptoms of catching, popping, and disabling pain despite normal-appearing radiographs [1].

Concomitant injury or gradual attenuation of volar and/or dorsal secondary ligamentous stabilizers are necessary to produce static changes seen on radiographs. The combination of a SLIL and secondary stabilizer injury will result in dorsal intercalated segment instability (DISI). In DISI, the scaphoid flexes, while the lunate and triquetrum extend. In addition, the capitate will migrate both proximally and dorsally, and the lunate will migrate ulnarly. Eventually, the changes in scaphoid, capitate, and lunate position become irreversible and fixed as secondary ligamentous structures are permanently damaged [1].

Over time, abnormal joint mechanics results in cartilage wear and progressive degenerative changes of the carpus. In scapholunate advanced collapse (SLAC), arthritis follows a stepwise progression that initiates in the radial styloid (Stage I) followed by the proximal radioscaphoid joint (Stage II). As the distal carpal row migrates proximally into the widened SL interval, the capitolunate joint becomes arthritic (Stage III). Although the lunate is extended in SLAC wrist, the radiolunate joint often maintains its congruency and is preserved [12]. There are cases of SLAC pancarpal arthritis, in which the radiolunate joint becomes damaged (Stage IV). The same degenerative changes are also seen in scaphoid non-union advanced collapse (SNAC). The statuses of the articular cartilage in the capitolunate and radiolunate joints are both important considerations when indicating various salvage procedures.

Clinical Signs

The typical mechanism of SLIL injury includes history of a fall onto an outstretched hand with the wrist in extension, ulnar deviation, and supination. SLIL injury can occur in an isolated fashion or in combination with carpal or distal radius fractures.

In the acute setting, patients often have tenderness to palpation that is poorly localized. The acute swelling and pain of the injury will often make special physical exam maneuvers difficult to tolerate. After the acute phase, patients will often develop painful popping and clicking, decreased grip strength, sensations of "instability," and tenderness to palpation over the dorsal SL joint located approximately 1 cm distal to Lister's tubercle.

In the Watson test for SL instability, the examiner applies volar-to-dorsal pressure over the scaphoid tubercle and passively brings the wrist from ulnar deviation and slight extension to radial deviation and slight flexion [13]. Normally, the scaphoid will flex and pronate, but thumb pressure will force the proximal scaphoid to subluxate onto the dorsal rim of the radius. Upon relief of the thumb pressure, the proximal pole will spontaneously reduce with an audible clunk and is thus considered a positive test. A history consistent with SL injury and a painful clunk is suggestive of SL instability. However, the Watson test may be falsely positive in up to one-third of individuals due to underlying ligamentous laxity [14].

Radiographs

Radiographic work-up of SL instability includes posteroanterior (PA), lateral, scaphoid, and anteroposterior (AP) pencil grip views of both wrists. In dynamic SL instability, the clenched pencil grip view has been shown to be most useful. SL gapping >3 mm, a scaphoid "ring sign," scaphoid shortening, and disruption of Gilula lines of the carpus are all radiographic signs of static SL instability.

Obtaining a proper lateral radiograph is important for measuring the scapholunate and radiolunate angles and requires that the radius, capitate, long-finger metacarpal be collinear in the sagittal plane. Measurement of the intercarpal angles is based on external contour of each bone. The scaphoid portion of the scapholunate angle is measured by drawing a tangent to the volar cortex of the scaphoid proximal and distal poles. The lunate portion is measured by drawing a perpendicular line to the tangent of the distal volar and dorsal horns of the lunate. A scapholunate angle >60° is considered abnormal (normal 46°, range 30–60°) and suggestive of a DISI deformity. The radiolunate angle is the angle formed by the same perpendicular of the lunate and the longitudinal axis of the radius. A radiolunate angle of >15° of dorsal deviation is indicative of a DISI deformity [1].

Advanced Imaging and Wrist Arthroscopy

Advanced imaging and wrist arthroscopy are important diagnostic tools in confirming the clinical diagnosis of SL instability based on the patient's symptoms and physical exam. With the advent of high-resolution magnetic resonance imaging (MRI) using 3-T magnets, the sensitivity and specificity of diagnosing SL ligament tears have improved to 89% and 100%, respectively [15]. MRI is also an important tool in evaluating the articular cartilage of the radiocarpal and midcarpal joints as significant degenerative changes are a contraindication to soft tissue repairs or reconstructions.

Despite advances in MRI in the evaluation of SL instability, wrist arthroscopy remains the gold standard for diagnosing and staging SL instability. The Geissler Arthroscopic Grading System is utilized to stage the severity of SL instability. Grade I is partial injury of the SLIL without any midcarpal malalignment. Grade II is partial injury of the SLIL with a slight gap between carpal bones. Grade III includes an SL gap large enough to pass a probe, and Grade IV is gross instability with a gap large enough to pass a 2.7-mm arthroscope [16]. Establishing a midcarpal portal to view and probe the SL joint is necessary to accurately diagnose and stage SL instability. Findings on arthroscopy can also inform treatment decisions. Grades I and II can often be managed with thermal shrinkage, pinning, or capsulodesis. Grades III and IV will often require a SLIL repair or reconstruction with capsulodesis.

Treatment

The goals of managing SLIL instability are to restore ligamentous integrity to the carpus and normalize biomechanics to preserve wrist function. To achieve this end, any treatment strategy must address SLIL instability in multiple dimensions. In the coronal plane, dynamic or static gapping of the SL joint must be treated with a SLIL repair or reconstruction. In the sagittal plane, rotatory subluxation of the scaphoid in flexion and lunate in extension requires the addition of a dorsal capsulodesis [1].

Kitay et al. provided a useful framework to guide treatment options based on which ligaments are injured, radiographs, and stress radiographs [1]. SLIL occult instability (Stage 1) occurs due to a partial SLIL tear without clinical or intra-operative findings of instability. Treatment options include thermal shrinkage with or without percutaneous pinning of the SL and scaphocapitate (SC) joints. At this stage, outcomes are more favorable in patients with partial tears versus complete tears [17–19]. Thermal shrinkage must be performed with some caution, as there is some inherent risk of inducing chondrolysis secondary to excessive heat generated by the radiofrequency ablation probe [5].

In dynamic instability (Stage 2), there is instability in both the coronal and sagittal planes that must be addressed. Requirements for SLIL repair include a scaphoid that is easily correctible, SLIL integrity, and preservation of the articular surface. An open SLIL repair with either bone tunnels or suture anchors is performed to address coronal instability. To address the sagittal plane instability, a dorsal capsulodesis is performed with either the Blatt or modified DIC technique. In the Blatt technique, a portion of the dorsal wrist capsule from the distal radius is inserted on the scaphoid distal to the axis of rotation as a checkrein to scaphoid flexion [2, 20]. In the modified DIC technique, a proximal portion of the DIC is detached from the triquetrum, dissected back to the scaphoid, and then inserted onto the dorsal lunate with the scaphoid reduced [5, 21].

Overall, there is no strong evidence to suggest any difference in outcomes between bone tunnels versus suture anchors and between Blatt and modified DIC for dorsal capsulodesis [4, 22–25]. Outcomes are superior in acute repairs versus chronic repairs and when capsulodesis is performed in addition to SLIL repair. Patients usually experience improvement in pain levels, but a decrease in wrist range of motion. Despite the quality of repair, long-term carpal alignment is not consistently well maintained [1]. In addition, patients with physically demanding jobs had significantly more pain and SL gapping [26].

In SL dissociation (stage 3), static changes are seen on radiographs which implies both a complete rupture of the SLIL and injury to the secondary ligamentous stabilizers. Although multiple techniques have been developed, none have been able to provide long-term carpal stability and re-establish normal wrist biomechanics. If the SLIL is not repairable, reconstructive procedures may be necessary to re-establish the SLIL and some of its secondary stabilizers [1].

The modified Brunelli procedure aims to re-create the scaphotrapezial ligament complex, dorsal radiotriquetral ligament, and SLIL and is also known as a triligament tenodesis. This technique involves passing a slip of the flexor carpi radialis (FCR) tendon through the volar scaphoid tuberosity to the scaphoid dorsal ridge to re-create the scaphotrapezial ligament complex. The tendon slip is then attached to the dorsal lunate and passed through a slit in the radiotriquetral ligament and then sutured back on itself to re-create the dorsal radiotriquetral ligament and SLIL [7]. In 4- to 5-year follow-up, patients undergoing the modified Brunelli procedure had a satisfaction rate of 79%, maintenance of 65–80% of grip strength relative to contralateral side, but average of 30% loss of range of motion [7, 27]. Conceptually, the issue with using tendon for reconstruction is that the elastic moduli of tendon and ligaments are not equivalent. The use of a tendon slip to restrict scaphoid motion requires a significant amount of tension, which ultimately reduces wrist range of motion [8].

Rosenwasser and colleagues developed a technique for SL dissociation called the reduction and association of scaphoid and lunate (RASL) procedure [28]. Before SLIL repair, the SL joint is reduced and fixed with a headless compression screw, which is left in for 12 months or more. Arthroscopic-assisted RASL procedure enables preparation of bony surfaces and reduction under direct visualization [29]. The screw is a rigid construct that does not re-create normal SL joint biomechanics but instead aims to create a fibrous union across the SL joint.

Outcomes on the RASL procedure have been somewhat varied. White et al. reported a series of 31 patients at an average of 6.4 years follow-up with a scapholunate gap and angle of 2.1 mm and 55°, respectively [30]. In a series of eight patients with a mean of 34.6 months follow-up, Caloia et al. reported an improvement in pain, post-op grip strength 78% of the contralateral wrist, average wrist range of motion 20% less than pre-op, and removal of hardware in three patients [31]. Larson et al. reported on eight patients at 38 months follow-up, with five patients having recurrence of deformity or progression of radiographic arthritis [32]. In order to avoid these complications, several surgical alternatives have been developed including the jointed Scapholunate Intercarpal Screw (SLIC, Acumed, Hillsboro, OR, USA) and SL-axis method (SLAM, Arthrex, Naples, FL, USA) [33]. The SLIC has been discontinued, and clinical outcomes of the SLAM technique are pending. Overall, patients with SL dissociation remain a challenging patient cohort as no technique has demonstrated consistent long-term carpal stability.

In the next stage of SL instability, DISI deformity (stage 4), treatment is dependent on patient activity level and chronicity of injury. If the patient has well-preserved grip strength and function, non-operative treatment with activity modification and splint wear may be a reasonable option. Patients may ultimately need a salvage procedure if they develop

arthritis, but the timeline for this is often unpredictable. Surgical treatment options for DISI deformity largely depend on whether the SL joint is reducible and preserved. If the SL is reducible, soft tissue reconstruction may be considered. However, if the DISI deformity is chronic and irreducible, selective intercarpal arthrodesis must be considered. Outcomes may be improved with the addition of an anterior interosseous nerve (AIN) and posterior interosseous nerve (PIN) neurectomy to denervate the wrist joint. Additionally, a radial styloidectomy or arthroscopic debridement may also help decrease pain [1].

After the development of scapholunate advanced collapse (stage 5), patients will often require a wrist salvage procedure as soft tissue reconstruction will likely fail to alleviate pain due to degenerative changes. Salvage procedures include proximal row carpectomy, scaphoid excision four-bone fusion, lunocapitate fusion, wrist arthroplasty, or total wrist arthrodesis [1].

Internal Bracing

The concept of internal bracing was first conceived by Dr. Gordon Mackay from Scotland to augment the repair of the lateral ligament complex in ankle instability using FiberTape (Arthrex, Naples, FL, USA) and two biocomposite SwiveLock anchors (Arthrex, Naples, FL, USA) [34]. The purpose of internal bracing is to add immediate strength to the repair at time zero and to protect the healing ligament while allowing early mobilization. The concept to use strong, synthetic suture as a checkrein for ligament repairs has been applied all over the body. This includes all knee ligaments—anterior cruciate ligament, posterior cruciate ligament, medial collateral ligament, lateral collateral ligament, anterolateral ligament, and patellofemoral ligament [34]. In the upper limb, shoulder acromioclavicular joint ligament augmentation, elbow ulnar collateral ligament, and lateral ulnar collateral ligament repair with internal brace augmentation have also been described [35–40]. FiberTape has excellent biocompatibility with more than 750,000 inserted over 9 years and 0.0008% reported synovial reactions [34].

More recently, the concept of internal brace has been applied to hand and wrist surgery to treat basal joint arthritis, collateral ligament injuries, carpometacarpal dislocations, and midcarpal instability [41]. Thumb ulnar collateral ligament (UCL) repairs with SutureTape (Arthrex, Naples, FL, USA) augmentation have been described. Biomechanical studies have shown a higher load to failure in UCL repair with SutureTape versus repair-only [42]. Moreover, a clinical study using internal bracing for thumb ulnar collateral ligament repairs has shown its efficacy and safety with a

1year minimum follow-up [43]. In addition, the use of the internal brace in UCL repair has obviated the need for K-wires post-operatively and expedited the recovery and rehabilitation process with an earlier return to sport or activity. The quicker recovery time has been particularly impactful in the professional athlete population but also is important for patients in the general population trying to get back to work.

Internal bracing has also been applied to SL instability with three techniques described: all-dorsal SL reconstruction, SL interosseous reconstruction, and SL ligament intrinsic brace 360° tenodesis (SLITT) reconstruction [44]. This chapter will focus on the all-dorsal SL reconstruction and SL interosseous reconstruction.

The all-dorsal and interosseous reconstruction utilizes biologic tendon graft, SutureTape, and the 3.5 mm × 8.5 mm DX SwiveLock SL anchor (Arthrex, Naples, FL, USA). The SwiveLock used in this technique is a knotless, pitchfork-style anchor that can accommodate both tendon graft and SutureTape. This anchor was made shorter than previously developed SwiveLock anchors to better accommodate the smaller bones in the hand and wrist. The 3.5-mm SwiveLock technique involves reconstruction with biologic tendon graft and a strong anchor construct that is reinforced with static, synthetic SutureTape. The SutureTape is a 1.3 mm wide, #2 FiberWire (Arthrex, Naples, FL, USA) braided flat that we prefer over LabralTape (Arthrex, Naples, FL, USA), which is 1.5 mm wide and used in shoulder arthroscopy. The purpose of the internal brace is to prevent SL gapping while the graft incorporates and to increase the overall strength of the reconstruction. The goal of the all-dorsal reconstruction is to address dorsal and central tears of the SLIL. The goal of the interosseous reconstruction is to address complete tears of dorsal, central, and volar portions of the SLIL, especially when there is no ligament to repair.

Biomechanical testing of the SL reconstruction with 3.5-mm SwiveLock, LabralTape, and ECRB tendon graft compared to the native dorsal component of the SLIL showed no significant difference between the reconstruction and native ligament strength [45]. Biomechanical testing of the all-dorsal SL reconstruction with extensor tendon autograft, SutureTape, and 3 × 3.5 mm SwiveLock anchors versus SL repair with 2 × Micro Corkscrew FT with 2-0 FiberWire (Arthrex, Naples, FL, USA) demonstrated that the SL reconstruction had higher load to failure than SL repair (82.0N vs. 41.7N) in vitro. Failure occurred primarily through suture anchor pullout in the reconstruction group and suture pullout in the repair group [46].

The SLITT reconstruction aims to re-create both the dorsal and volar SL ligaments to not only provide restraint to SL gapping in the coronal plane but also address torsional instability in the sagittal plane. Kakar et al. theorized that reconstruction of the dorsal SL ligament in the setting of a combined volar and dorsal SL ligament injury may be a reason why outcomes SL reconstructions are varied and unpredictable [44]. In this procedure, a palmaris longus graft is passed through bone tunnels in the scaphoid and lunate in a continuous loop and then secured with two biotenodesis screws. A SutureTape is then passed from dorsal to volar through the cannulation of the biotenodesis screws and is then tied volarly. Additionally, the volar tail of the tendon graft and SutureTape can be secured to the volar rim of the distal radius to reconstruct the long radiolunate ligament and provide a checkrein to ulnar translocation of the carpus.

In a biomechanical study, Kakar et al. demonstrated a higher load to failure in the 360 tenodesis group with internal brace (283.47 ± 100.25 N) versus the 360 tenodesis group (143.61 ± 90.54 N) [47]. In a case report, Kakar and Greene describe a patient who underwent a SLITT procedure with 4 weeks of post-operative immobilization and no K-wires. At 13 months, the patient was back at work and happy, carpal alignment was maintained, and the patient had 66% of grip strength relative to the contralateral side (46% pre-op) with symmetrical range of motion [47].

Although these techniques have been described, follow-up data are still pending. However, SutureTape augmentation of SL reconstruction is conceptually appealing, because it can prevent ligament attenuation and post-operative carpal malalignment that has been problematic for previous techniques. Long-term results will be needed to determine if techniques involving internal brace lead to better patient outcomes.

Indications

SL reconstruction with internal brace ligament augmentation is recommended for cases of both dynamic and static SL instabilities. This procedure can be performed in acute or chronic SLIL ruptures and partial or complete tears. The SL joint must be reducible in both the coronal and sagittal planes. In addition, the articular surface of the involved carpal bones should be well preserved in order to ensure a pain-free, satisfactory outcome. Prior to the reconstruction, radiographs, MRI, and wrist arthroscopy can be used to further stage and characterize the SL tear. Once the decision is made to perform reconstruction, open exposure of the SL joint can help guide management. If the dorsal portion of the SLIL is torn and the volar portion is intact, an all-dorsal reconstruction can be performed. If the dorsal and volar portions of the SLIL are torn, then the interosseous SL reconstruction is preferable.

Contraindications

SL reconstruction with internal bracing is not recommended in all patients. Patients with degenerative changes (SLAC wrist) and a DISI deformity that is not reducible may be candidates for intercarpal arthrodesis or salvage procedure, but not reconstruction. History of inflammatory arthritis, septic arthritis, or osteomyelitis is also a contraindication. Insertion of anchors should be avoided in pediatric patients with carpal bones that have not yet ossified. Pre-existing hardware and large cystic changes in carpal bones can compromise anchor fixation and lead to reconstruction failure and SL gapping. Patients with unusually small anatomy may not have enough surface area to accommodate the 3.5-mm SwiveLock SL anchor.

Technique

A 4–6″ longitudinal incision is made between the bases of the second and third metacarpals centered over the radiocarpal joint (Fig. 16.1). The length of the incision is necessary in order to harvest the graft safely. Subcutaneous dissection is carried out down to the level of extensor retinaculum. The retinaculum is incised between the third and fourth extensor compartments. An AIN and PIN neurectomy is routinely per-

formed in order to denervate the wrist and provide pain relief. The PIN is found in the radial aspect of the floor of the fourth compartment. The AIN is found just deep to the interosseous membrane proximal to the distal radioulnar joint. Both the AIN and PIN are excised using bipolar electrocautery. The wrist capsule is then exposed, and an inverted T-capsulotomy is made with the transverse portion taken down directly off the distal radius to completely expose the scaphoid and lunate. Alternatively, a ligament-sparing capsulotomy can also be performed if preferred by the surgeon.

Our preference for tendon graft is a 2-mm to 2.5-mm intratendinous slip of the extensor carpi radialis brevis (ECRB) tendon taken at its insertion on the base of the third metacarpal (Fig. 16.2). Alternatively, a slip of the extensor carpi radialis longus (ECRL) tendon or palmaris longus can also be used. The second extensor compartment is opened, and care is taken to not injure the extensor pollicis longus (EPL) crossing over the ECRB. A tendon stripper is used to harvest the graft to achieve a length greater than 10 cm. The tendon should be measured in a tendon sizer to ensure that the graft is not too large in diameter as larger grafts will not fit properly in the pitchfork anchor and drill hole. Once the graft is harvested, a 2-0 FiberLoop suture (Arthrex, Naples, FL, USA) is used to whipstitch both ends of the graft to help secure the tendon graft onto the anchor (Fig. 16.3). The tendon is stretched out to avoid tendon creep during the healing process. In order to reduce the DISI deformity, 0.054" K-wires are inserted into the waist of the scaphoid and the proximal-ulnar aspect of the lunate, and the SL joint is reduced (Fig. 16.4). A needle driver or hemostat is used to clamp the wires and hold the reduction in place. Care should be taken to place the joysticks in a position that avoids planned tunnels.

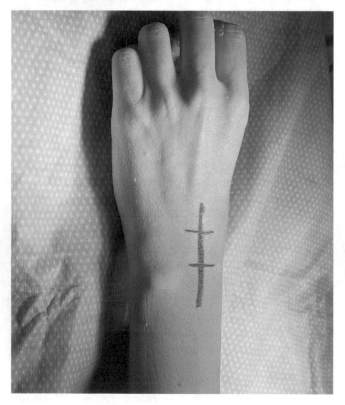

Fig. 16.1 A 4–6″ longitudinal incision is made between the bases of the second and third metacarpals and centered over the radiocarpal joint

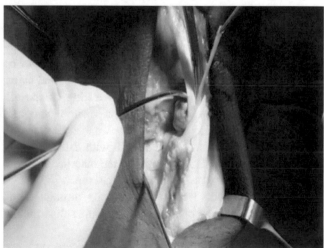

Fig. 16.2 A 2-mm intratendinous slip of the ECRB tendon is taken distally to proximally starting from its insertion on the base of the third metacarpal. Care is taken not to injure the EPL crossing over

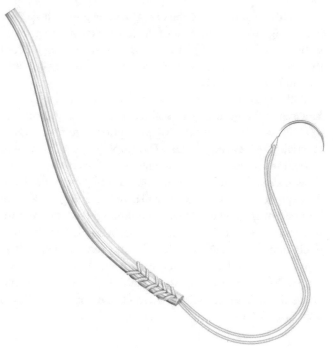

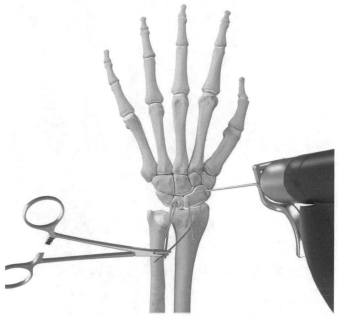

Fig. 16.5 Three additional K-wires are placed in the proximal pole of the scaphoid, central lunate, and distal pole of scaphoid

Fig. 16.3 Both ends of the tendon graft are whipstitched with 2-0 FiberLoop in this configuration

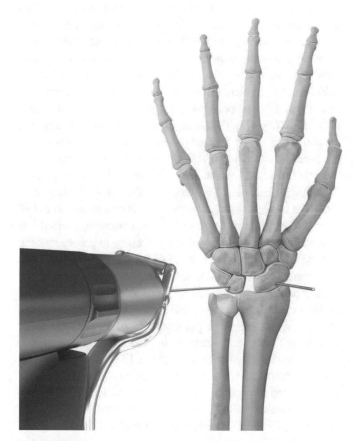

Fig. 16.4 Joystick K-wires are inserted into the waist of the scaphoid and proximal-ulnar aspect of the lunate

All-Dorsal Scapholunate Reconstruction with Internal Brace Ligament Augmentation

Three additional 0.054″ K-wires are placed into the proximal pole of the scaphoid, central lunate, and distal pole of scaphoid (Fig. 16.5). At this point, fluoroscopy is used to confirm that the placement of the guidewires is satisfactory. The 3.5-mm diameter of the cannulated drill for constructs with suture and tendon graft must be taken into account when placing guidewires as breaking out of the cortex will compromise anchor fixation. The proximal pole of scaphoid, central lunate, and distal pole of scaphoid are drilled over the guidewires, and all soft tissue is removed from the drill holes to ease the insertion of the suture and graft construct (Fig. 16.6).

The tendon graft and SutureTape are placed in the pitch-fork eyelet approximately 3 mm from the end (Fig. 16.7). The SutureTape and both limbs of the FiberLoop suture are wrapped around the SwiveLock tab. The SwiveLock and graft/SutureTape construct are inserted into the proximal pole of the scaphoid until the laser line is just below the level of cortical bone (Fig. 16.8a). While inserting the anchor, the tendon graft should be on the ulnar aspect of the drill hole so it is closer to the lunate. The tendon graft construct is then loaded in a second SwiveLock anchor and inserted into the lunate hole (Fig. 16.8b). The remaining limb is then loaded onto the third SwiveLock anchor and inserted into the distal

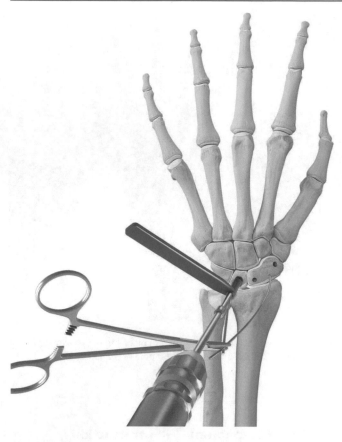

Fig. 16.6 The three K-wires inserted in the proximal pole of scaphoid, central lunate, and distal pole of scaphoid are overdrilled with a 3.5-mm gold cannulated drill

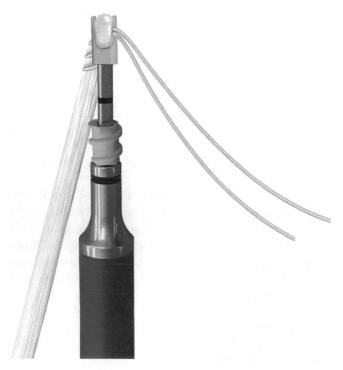

Fig. 16.7 The tendon graft and SutureTape construct are loaded into the pitchfork eyelet approximately 3 mm from the end

pole of the scaphoid, and the excess tendon graft SutureTape is cut (Fig. 16.8c). The goal of the third anchor is to provide stability in the sagittal plane and prevent the scaphoid from flexing and the lunate from extending in a manner similar to the modified DIC technique.

Although internal bracing has obviated the need for K-wires in thumb UCL, we still recommend the insertion of a 0.054″ K-wire across the SC joint prior to removal of the joystick K-wires (Fig. 16.8d). The purpose of the SC K-wire is to allow the secondary ligamentous stabilizers to heal. The K-wire should be inserted from the waist of the scaphoid into the capitate. Care must be taken to avoid inserting the K-wire into one of the anchor holes or binding up the tendon graft. Insertion of an SL K-wire is not recommended as this will likely disrupt the tendon graft and suture reconstruction. The capsule is closed with 0-vicryl (Ethicon, Bridgewater, NJ, USA), the extensor retinaculum with 2-0 vicryl, the subcutaneous tissue is closed with 3-0 vicryl, and the skin is closed with 3-0 prolene.

Interosseous Scapholunate Reconstruction

The exposure to the scaphoid and lunate is the same described in the all-dorsal technique. However, the joystick K-wire must be put into the proximal and ulnar aspect of the lunate so as to avoid the bone tunnels in the lunate. The joystick K-wire is placed in the waste of the scaphoid per usual. Additionally, both ends of the graft are whipstitched with 2-0 fiber loop. After preparation of the graft and insertion of joystick K-wires, the remaining soft tissue in between the scaphoid and lunate is removed so that the two bones can be open-booked. A guidewire is placed along the central axis of the scaphoid and over drilled with the 3.5-mm cannulated drill (Figs. 16.9 and 16.10a). An additional guidewire is placed in the lunate and, this time, a 3.0-mm cannulated drill is used (Fig. 16.10b). Prior to drilling, fluoroscopy should be used to check the position of the guidewire to ensure that the drill will be within the confines of the lunate and scaphoid. Both the 3.5 mm and 3.0 mm have a 1-cm-depth stop.

A separate outside-in tunnel is made in the lunate starting in the dorsal ulnar corner of the lunate and connecting to the central tunnel. Inserting a guidewire into the central tunnel as an aiming target for the outside-in guidewire can be helpful. The guidewire is positioned near the LTIL attachment just distal to the articular surface of the lunate and aimed at a 45° angle toward the central tunnel and overdrilled with the 3.0-mm cannulated drill to create a bone tunnel through the lunate (Fig. 16.10c). Alternatively, a single drill hole can be made from the dorsal ulnar aspect of the lunate through the central axis of the lunate with a 3.0-mm drill bit. Lastly, a final drill hole is made in the distal pole of the scaphoid using a guidewire and the 3.5-mm cannulated drill.

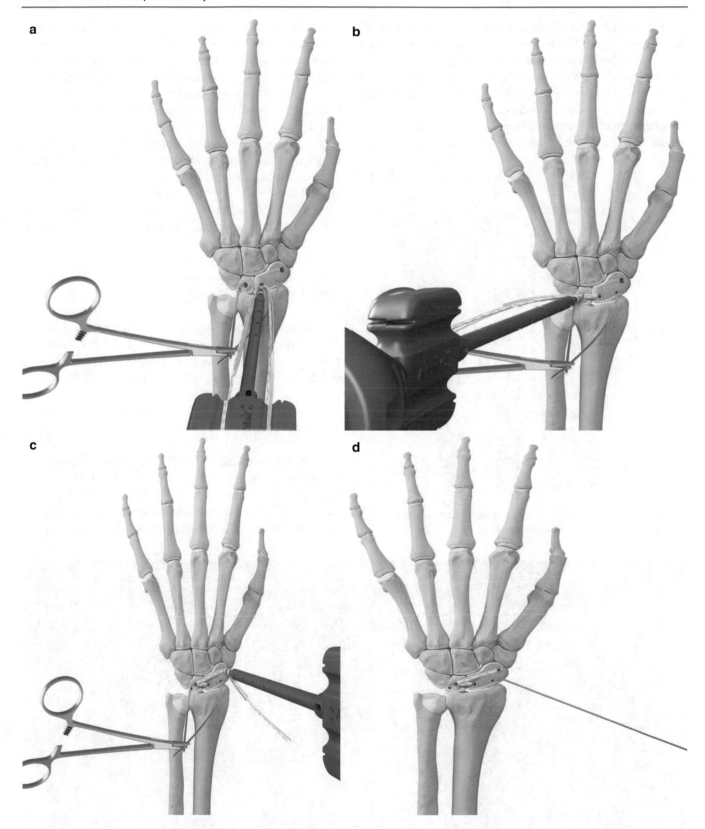

Fig. 16.8 Loaded with tendon graft and SutureTape, the SwiveLock is inserted into the (**a**) proximal pole of scaphoid, (**b**) lunate, (**c**) and distal pole of the scaphoid. (**d**) A K-wire is inserted across the SC joint prior to removal of the joystick K-wires

After preparation of the drill holes in the scaphoid and bone tunnel in the lunate, the graft/SutureTape construct is loaded into the SwiveLock and inserted into the central axis of the scaphoid, and the tendon graft is shuttled through the bone tunnel in the lunate (Fig. 16.11a, b). Using the joystick K-wires the SL joint is reduced, and a 3 mm × 8 mm Tenodesis Screw (Arthrex, Naples, FL, USA) is used to secure the tendon and SutureTape construct in the lunate

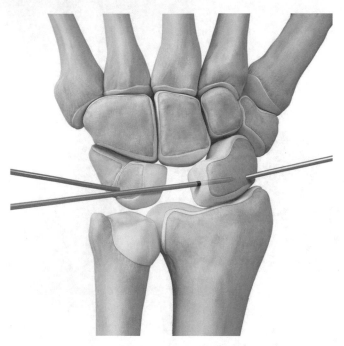

Fig. 16.9 The scaphoid and lunate are open booked, and the K-wire is placed along the central axis of the scaphoid

hole (Fig. 16.11c). Tension must be applied to the tendon graft and SutureTape, while the tenodesis screw is inserted to minimize SL gapping. If the bone tunnel in the lunate is less than 8 mm (length of the biotenodesis screw), the body from the 3.5-mm SwiveLock anchor may be used, but prior to insertion the bone tunnel should be over drilled with a 3.5-mm drill.

The remaining limb of the tendon graft and SutureTape is then loaded onto the SwiveLock and inserted into the distal pole of the scaphoid (Fig. 16.11d). Pressure should be applied to the volar scaphoid while advancing the anchor to correct for scaphoid flexion. The conclusion of the procedure is the same as the all-dorsal reconstruction and includes the SC K-wire.

Post-Operative Course

A forearm-based thumb spica splint is worn for 6–8 weeks. At this point, K-wires are removed and hand therapy is started at this time. A splint is worn for an additional 6 weeks, and the patient can return to full activity at week 12.

Tips and Tricks

Additional K-wires are needed for the joystick reduction and SC fixation. We recommend the use of 0.054″ K-wires. There are two cannulated drill bits that accompany the 3.5-mm DX SwiveLock SL anchor. The silver drill bit is 3.0 mm and is meant for all-suture constructs. The gold drill bit is

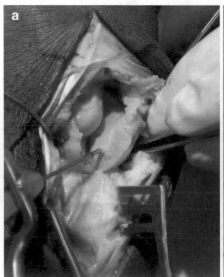
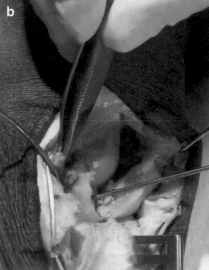
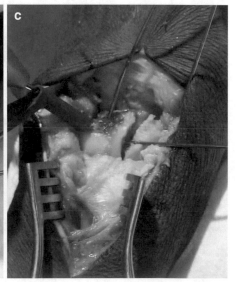

Fig. 16.10 (**a**) A K-wire is placed along the central axis of the scaphoid. (**b**) Another K-wire is placed in the center of the lunate. (**c**) A separate outside-in K-wire starting in the dorsal-ulnar corner of the lunate is inserted. This K-wire is positioned near the LTIL attachment, just distal to the articular surface of the lunate and aimed approximately 45° toward the central tunnel. Note that the K-wire in the central tunnel of the lunate acts as an aiming target

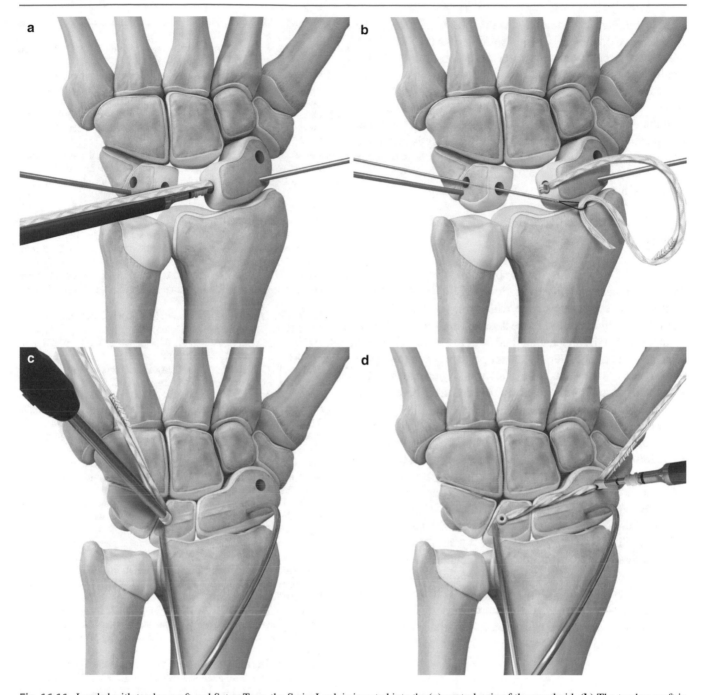

Fig. 16.11 Loaded with tendon graft and SutureTape, the SwiveLock is inserted into the (**a**) central axis of the scaphoid. (**b**) The tendon graft is shuttled through the bone tunnel in the lunate, (**c**) secured with 3 × 8 mm tenodesis screw and then inserted into the distal pole of the scaphoid (**d**)

3.5 mm and is meant for constructs with suture and graft. Any time a drill hole is going to accommodate a 3.5-mm SwiveLock, tendon graft, and suture, and the 3.5-mm drill bit must be used. If a 3-mm biotenodesis screw or 3.5-mm SwiveLock with suture tape only is being used, a 3.0-mm drill bit is preferred. An easy way to remember this is "gold is for graft" and "silver is for suture." The maximum size for any graft taken is 2.5 mm, as any larger graft will lead to issues with graft and anchor fixation.

When drilling, the guidewire must be as perpendicular to the bone as possible. Since the carpal bones have a normal curvature to it, drilling slightly tangential may cause the anchor to be proud. When inserting the SwiveLock anchor, it is important to have the anchor body flush with bone before turning the knob. Additionally, a slight positive pressure should be applied while turning the knob in order to ensure that the threads of the anchor are engaging the bone. In order to properly deploy the SwiveLock, the laser line should be at or below the level of the bone. At this point, there should be a gentle give on the knob, which signifies that the SwiveLock handle has been disengaged from the anchor. If there is difficulty removing the handle from the anchor, the tab can be turned clockwise to release the inserter from the anchor. When inserting a limb of the SutureTape and tendon graft into the SwiveLock, a gentle twist of the construct can aid in completely seating it into the pitchfork. This is important because the graft should be able to freely slide within the pitchfork to allow for self-tensioning of the graft when the anchor is inserted.

Conclusion

SL instability represents a wide spectrum of injuries ranging from dynamic instability to static instability and is associated with wrist pain, lost time from work, and interference with daily activities. Left untreated, SL instability will lead to abnormal wrist mechanics and progressive degenerative changes. The goal of surgical management is to relieve pain and preserve wrist function by restoring ligamentous continuity and normal biomechanics. To date, there have been a multitude of surgical techniques described. However, no technique has been able to consistently prevent SL gapping and the abnormal wrist mechanics due to repair or reconstruction attenuation over time. Internal bracing is a relatively novel concept that uses strong, synthetic suture material as a checkrein for ligament repairs and reconstructions. By applying this concept to hand and wrist surgery, new techniques have been developed for SL reconstruction: all-dorsal SL reconstruction, SL interosseous reconstruction, and SL ligament intrinsic brace 360° tenodesis reconstruction. Although clinical data are still pending, these internal bracing techniques have shown to be biomechanically strong and are promising surgical alternatives to previously described repair and reconstruction techniques and may play a bigger role in the management of SL instability in the future.

References

1. Kitay A, Wolfe SW. Scapholunate instability: current concepts in diagnosis and management. J Hand Surg Am. 2012;37(10):2175–96.
2. Blatt G. Capsulodesis in reconstructive hand surgery. Dorsal capsulodesis for the unstable scaphoid and volar capsulodesis following excision of the distal ulna. Hand Clin. 1987;3(1):81–102.
3. Danoff JR, Karl JW, Birman MV, Rosenwasser MP. The use of thermal shrinkage for scapholunate instability. Hand Clin. 2011;27(3):309–17.
4. Gajendran VK, Peterson B, Slater RR, Szabo RM. Long-term outcomes of dorsal intercarpal ligament capsulodesis for chronic scapholunate dissociation. J Hand Surg Am. 2007;32(9):1323–33.
5. Manuel J, Moran SL. The diagnosis and treatment of scapholunate instability. Hand Clin. 2010;26(1):129–44.
6. Nathan R, Blatt G. Rotary subluxation of the scaphoid. Revisited Hand Clin. 2000;16(3):417–31.
7. Garcia-Elias M, Lluch AL, Stanley JK. Three-ligament tenodesis for the treatment of scapholunate dissociation: indications and surgical technique. J Hand Surg Am. 2006;31(1):125–34.
8. Chim H, Moran SL. Wrist essentials: the diagnosis and management of scapholunate ligament injuries. Plast Reconstr Surg. 2014;134(2):312e–22e.
9. Berger RA. The gross and histologic anatomy of the scapholunate interosseous ligament. J Hand Surg Am. 1996;21(2):170–8.
10. Garcia-Elias M, Lluch AL. Wrist instabilities, misalignments, and dislocations. In: Wolfe SW, Hotchkiss RN, Pederson WC, Kozin SH, Cohen MS, editors. Green's operative hand surgery. 7th ed. Philadelphia: Elsevier; 2017. p. 418–78.
11. Wolfe SW, Neu C, Crisco JJ. In vivo scaphoid, lunate, and capitate kinematics in flexion and in extension. J Hand Surg Am. 2000;25(5):860–9.
12. Watson HK, Ballet FL. The SLAC wrist: scapholunate advanced collapse pattern of degenerative arthritis. J Hand Surg Am. 1984;9(3):358–65.
13. Watson HK, Ashmead D, Makhlouf MV. Examination of the scaphoid. J Hand Surg Am. 1988;13(5):657–60.
14. Wolfe SW, Gupta A, Crisco JJ. Kinematics of the scaphoid shift test. J Hand Surg Am. 1997;22(5):801–6.
15. Magee T. Comparison of 3-T MRI and arthroscopy of intrinsic wrist ligament and TFCC tears. AJR Am J Roentgenol. 2009;192(1):80–5.
16. Geissler WB, Freeland AE, Savoie FH, McIntyre LW, Whipple TL. Intracarpal soft-tissue lesions associated with an intra-articular fracture of the distal end of the radius. J Bone Joint Surg Am. 1996;78(3):357–65.
17. Darlis NA, Weiser RW, Sotereanos DG. Partial scapholunate ligament injuries treated with arthroscopic debridement and thermal shrinkage. J Hand Surg Am. 2005;30(5):908–14.
18. Ruch DS, Poehling GG. Arthroscopic management of partial scapholunate and lunotriquetral injuries of the wrist. J Hand Surg Am. 1996;21(3):412–7.
19. Weiss AP, Sachar K, Glowacki KA. Arthroscopic debridement alone for intercarpal ligament tears. J Hand Surg Am. 1997;22(2):344–9.
20. Kuo CE, Wolfe SW. Scapholunate instability: current concepts in diagnosis and management. J Hand Surg Am. 2008;33(6):998–1013.
21. Slater RR, Szabo RM, Bay BK, Laubach J. Dorsal intercarpal ligament capsulodesis for scapholunate dissociation: biomechanical analysis in a cadaver model. J Hand Surg Am. 1999;24(2):232–9.
22. Bickert B, Sauerbier M, Germann G. Scapholunate ligament repair using the Mitek bone anchor. J Hand Surg Br. 2000;25(2):188–92.
23. Rosati M, Parchi P, Cacianti M, Poggetti A, Lisanti M. Treatment of acute scapholunate ligament injuries with bone anchor. Musculoskelet Surg. 2010;94(1):25–32.
24. Lavernia CJ, Cohen MS, Taleisnik J. Treatment of scapholunate dissociation by ligamentous repair and capsulodesis. J Hand Surg Am. 1992;17(2):354–9.
25. Moran SL, Ford KS, Wulf CA, Cooney WP. Outcomes of dorsal capsulodesis and tenodesis for treatment of scapholunate instability. J Hand Surg Am. 2006;31(9):1438–46.
26. Pomerance J. Outcome after repair of the scapholunate interosseous ligament and dorsal capsulodesis for dynamic scapholunate instability due to trauma. J Hand Surg Am. 2006;31(8):1380–6.
27. Harvey EJ, Hanel D, Knight JB, Tencer AF. Autograft replacements for the scapholunate ligament: a biomechanical comparison of hand-based autografts. J Hand Surg Am. 1999;24(5):963–7.

28. Rosenwasser MP, Miyasajsa KC, Strauch RJ. The RASL procedure: reduction and association of the scaphoid and lunate using the Herbert screw. Tech Hand Up Extrem Surg. 1997;1(4):263–72.

29. Aibinder WR, Izadpanah A, Elhassan BT. Reduction and association of the scaphoid and lunate: a functional and radiographical outcome study. J Wrist Surg. 2019;8(1):37–42.

30. White NJ, Rollick NC. Injuries of the scapholunate interosseous ligament: an update. J Am Acad Orthop Surg. 2015;23(11):691–703.

31. Caloia M, Caloia H, Pereira E. Arthroscopic scapholunate joint reduction. Is an effective treatment for irreparable scapholunate ligament tears? Clin Orthop Relat Res. 2012;470(4):972–8.

32. Larson TB, Stern PJ. Reduction and association of the scaphoid and lunate procedure: short-term clinical and radiographic outcomes. J Hand Surg Am. 2014;39(11):2168–74.

33. Yao J, Zlotolow DA, Lee SK. ScaphoLunate axis method. J Wrist Surg. 2016;5(1):59–66.

34. Mackay GM, Blyth MJ, Anthony I, Hopper GP, Ribbans WJ. A review of ligament augmentation with the InternalBrace: the surgical principle is described for the lateral ankle ligament and ACL repair in particular, and a comprehensive review of other surgical applications and techniques is presented. Surg Technol Int. 2015;26:239–55.

35. Scheiderer B, Imhoff FB, Kia C, Aglio J, Morikawa D, Obopilwe E, et al. LUCL internal bracing restores posterolateral rotatory stability of the elbow. Knee Surg Sports Traumatol Arthrosc. 2019;28(4):1195–201.

36. Byrne PA, Hopper GP, Wilson WT, Mackay GM. Acromioclavicular joint stabilisation using the internal brace principle. Surg Technol Int. 2018;33:294–8.

37. Dugas JR, Looze CA, Capogna B, Walters BL, Jones CM, Rothermich MA, et al. Ulnar collateral ligament repair with collagen-dipped fiber tape augmentation in overhead-throwing athletes. Am J Sports Med. 2019;47(5):1096–102.

38. Dugas JR, Walters BL, Beason DP, Fleisig GS, Chronister JE. Biomechanical comparison of ulnar collateral ligament repair with internal bracing versus modified Jobe reconstruction. Am J Sports Med. 2016;44(3):735–41.

39. Jones CM, Beason DP, Dugas JR. Ulnar collateral ligament reconstruction versus repair with internal bracing: comparison of cyclic fatigue mechanics. Orthop J Sports Med. 2018;6(2):2325967118755991.

40. Bodendorfer BM, Looney AM, Lipkin SL, Nolton EC, Li J, Najarian RG, et al. Biomechanical comparison of ulnar collateral ligament reconstruction with the docking technique versus repair with internal bracing. Am J Sports Med. 2018;46(14):3495–501.

41. De Giacomo AF, Shin SS. Repair of the thumb ulnar collateral ligament with suture tape augmentation. Tech Hand Up Extrem Surg. 2017;21(4):164–6.

42. Shin SS, van Eck CF, Uquillas C. Suture tape augmentation of the thumb ulnar collateral ligament repair: a biomechanical study. J Hand Surg Am. 2018;43(9):868.e1–6.

43. Lee SJ, Rabinovich RV, Kim A. Thumb ulnar collateral ligament repair with suture tape augmentation. J Hand Surg Asian Pac Vol. 2020;25(1):32–8.

44. Kakar S, Greene RM. Scapholunate ligament internal brace 360-degree Tenodesis (SLITT) procedure. J Wrist Surg. 2018;7(4):336–40.

45. Scapholunate reconstruction: a biomechanical analysis of a novel technique. Arthrex research and development invalid date Invalid date.

46. Biomechanical testing of scapholunate reconstruction with internal brace versus scapholunate repair. American academy of orthopaedic surgeons annual meeting new orleans, LA; Invalid date.

47. Kakar S, Greene RM, Denbeigh J, Van Wijnen A. Scapholunate ligament internal brace 360 tenodesis (SLITT) procedure: a biomechanical study. J Wrist Surg. 2019;8(3):250–4.

Geissler "Sling and Cinch" for Carpal Instability

17

William B. Geissler and Kevin F. Purcell

Introduction

There are several ligaments around the lunate providing inherent stability [1, 3, 4]. Perilunate instability can be attributed to complete rupture of the scapholunate (SLIL) and lunotriquetral interosseous (LTIL) ligaments. Perilunate instability can occur in isolation or with associated fractures of scaphoid, capitate, triquetrum, or lunate [5]. If perilunate instability is left untreated, it will eventually progress to chronic misalignment manifesting as volar intercalated segmental instability (VISI) or dorsal intercalated segmental instability (DISI) [2]. These aforementioned chronic deformities are challenging to manage. They are associated with intractable pain, decreased wrist range of motion (ROM)/grip strength, and radiocarpal osteoarthritis secondary to altered joint kinematics [2, 8].

Traditional management of perilunate instability involves an array of different techniques. In addition, temporary Kirschner wires with a period of cast immobilization are usually employed to assist with acute management of SLIL or LTIL repair [2, 9, 10]. Moreover, external fixation can be utilized in conjunction with Kirschner wires for supplemental stability for a tenuous repair [11, 12]. Investigation of Souer et al. discerned that there were no differences in biomechanical stability between temporary screw and Kirschner wire fixation in management of perilunate instability [9]. Scapholunate repair with internal bracing augmentation is a new technique developed to treat perilunate instability [6, 7, 13]. There are few investigations analyzing internal brace augmentation with SLIL repair, but it appears to be more

biomechanically stable than solely SLIL repair or 360-degree tenodesis procedures [6, 7]. In this chapter, we will offer our preferred treatment options for perilunate instability and offer tips and tricks to ameliorate the complexities.

The scapholunate ligament complex consists of both intrinsic and extrinsic components. The intrinsic components include the dorsal, palmar, and fibromembranous portions. Work by Berger and Landsmeer demonstrated that the dorsal portion is composed of stout transverse fibers that contribute the majority of the functional strength to the interosseous ligament [14]. The volar portion consists of longer oblique fibers that play a role in control of rotation between the scaphoid lunates in the sagittal plane. This central fibromembranous portion contributes minimal structural support and frequently develops perforations with age [15].

The scapholunate ligament is capable of stretching up to 225% of its length prior to failure. An isolated injury to the scapholunate interosseous ligament may not demonstrate dissociation or widening on plain radiographs since the secondary stabilizers remain intact [16]. A combined injury to both the intrinsic and extrinsic ligaments will be required to show diastasis of the scapholunate interval [17–19]. A grade of injury is seen to the scapholunate of the interosseous ligament where the ligament stretches, then usually tears from the volar to dorsal direction and then it completely tears. Geissler described "arthroscopic" classification scapholunate instability in Table 17.1.

In Geissler acute or chronic grade III or grade IV injuries, the "sling and cinch" technique would be indicated. The contraindication to the technique would be particularly in chronic injuries with arthritic changes between the radioscaphoid joints present or in fixed static scapholunate instability.

There are many pre-described procedures for scapholunate interosseous ligament reconstruction. These vary from placement of the screw across the interval, multiple tendon reconstructions, and reconstruction with an internal brace. Previously described reconstructions with internal brace

W. B. Geissler (✉)
Division of Hand and Upper Extremity Surgery, Section of Arthroscopic Surgery and Sports Medicine, Department of Orthopedic Surgery and Rehabilitation, University of Mississippi Medical Center, Jackson, MS, USA

K. F. Purcell
Department of Orthopedic Surgery, University of Mississippi Medical Center, Jackson, MS, USA

© Springer Nature Switzerland AG 2022
W. B. Geissler (ed.), *Wrist and Elbow Arthroscopy with Selected Open Procedures*,
https://doi.org/10.1007/978-3-030-78881-0_17

Table 17.1 Geissler arthroscopic classification of interosseous ligament tears

Grade Description
I. Attenuation or hemorrhage of the interosseous ligament as seen from the radiocarpal space. No incongruency of carpal alignment in the midcarpal space.
II. Attenuation or hemorrhage of interosseous ligament as seen from the radiocarpal space. Incongruency or step-off of carpal space. There may be slight gap (less than width of probe) between carpal bones
III. Incongruency or step-off of carpal alignment as seen from both radiocarpal and midcarpal spaces. Probe may be passed through the gap between carpal bones
IV. Incongruency or step-off of carpal alignment as seen from both radiocarpal and midcarpal spaces. There is gross instability with manipulation. A 2.7-mm arthroscope may be passed through the gap between the bones

have included a dorsal only type repair with anchors or an interosseous repair where two holes drilled at 90 degrees perpendicular to each other through the lunate. The concern of this is breakage between the tunnels, or avascular necrosis due to the amount of bone that has been resected which could affect the blood supply. Geissler devised a surgical technique that is interosseous, so it reconstructs both the volar and dorsal aspects of the ligament and passes completely through the lunate and triquetrum. A "locks head" knot is cinched on the radial aspect of the scaphoid which takes the tension off the remaining part of the labral tape as it is inserted into the distal portion of the scaphoid. This makes this part of the procedure easier to perform. The completely transosseous internal brace technique allows for the normal flexibility between the scaphoid and the lunate and completely closes the interval. The patients as they return to clinic have been remarkably pain-free and hard to slow down their return to activities with this reconstruction.

Surgical Technique: Scapholunate and Perilunate Reconstructions

A standard dorsal approach is made to the wrist (Figs. 17.1 and 17.2). The first step is to identify the extensor pollicis longus in the third compartment and release it. The second and fourth dorsal compartments are then opened. A radial-based flap is made to expose the carpus and the interosseous ligament tear or tears. Frequently, wrist arthroscopy is (Mississippi MRI) performed initially to confirm a Geissler grade III or grade IV tear, of the interosseous ligament prior to reconstruction. This can be performed either dry or wet.

Two 0.62 joystick wires are placed in the scaphoid and lunate, respectively, to manipulate the carpal bones and open up the interval. A guidewire is then placed from ulnar to radial in the midline of the scaphoid (Fig. 17.3). The guidewire is angled slightly distally to pass by the radial styloid. By going

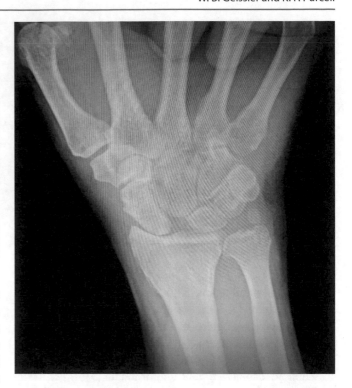

Fig. 17.1 Anterior–posterior radiograph demonstrating a chronic injury to the scapholunate ligament complex. Patient has marked widening between the scaphoid and lunate with minimal degenerative changes at the radioscaphoid articulation

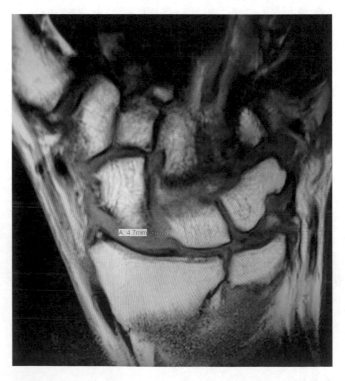

Fig. 17.2 Anterior–posterior MRI evaluation of the same patient demonstrating mark widening between the scaphoid and the lunate with minimal degenerative changes between the scaphoid and the radius

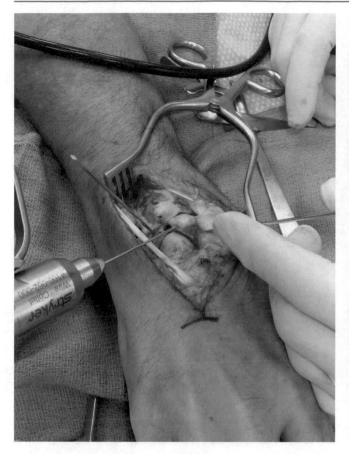

Fig. 17.3 Intraoperative photograph demonstrating placement of the guidewire being placed from ulna to radial in mid-axis of the scaphoid. By placing the guidewire in this manner ensures that the guidewire is inserted in the exact mid-axis of the scaphoid in the anterior–posterior plane

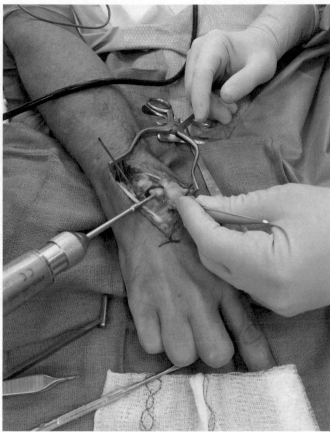

Fig. 17.4 Intraoperative photograph demonstrating drilling of the scaphoid with a cannulated 3-mm drill from ulna to radial

in an ulnar to radial direction ensures that the drill hole will be in the exact center of the scaphoid. The scaphoid is then drilled with a 3-mm cannulated drill (Fig. 17.4). A second guidewire is in place from radial to ulnar through the lunate and exiting the triquetrum (Fig. 17.5). The guidewire is placed slightly volar to the midline to help correct any dorsal rotation of the lunate. The exact position of the guidewire is confirmed under fluoroscopy to make sure the guidewire is passed through both the lunate and triquetrum (Fig. 17.6). The lunate and triquetrum are then drilled with the 3-mm cannulated drill (Fig. 17.7). A Hewson suture passer is then passed through the drill hole through the lunate and triquetrum from radial to ulnar and out the skin along the ulnar aspect of the wrist (Fig. 17.8). The looped end of Arthrex labral tape (Naples, FL) is then passed through the loop of the Hewson suture passer and pulled through the triquetrum and lunate (Fig. 17.9). The suture passer is then passed from radial to ulnar through the scaphoid and pulls the remaining loop portion of the labral tape through the scaphoid (Fig. 17.10). Blunt

dissection is then carried down along the ulnar aspect of triquetrum to find the tails of the labral tape as they exited the triquetrum. The tails are then pulled dorsally across the carpus. A "lark's head" cinch knot is made in the loop end of the labral tape as it exits out the scaphoid (Fig. 17.11). The two tails of the labral tape are then passed through the "lark's head" knot and cinched to close down the carpal interval. Tension is placed on each tail of the labral tape to completely close down the scapholunate interval. Once this has been achieved, a guidewire is placed in the distal aspect of the scaphoid. The remaining joystick in the scaphoid can help dorsiflex the bone to make it easier to visualize the distal pole of the scaphoid. The distal pole of the scaphoid is then drilled with the 3-mm cannulated drill. An Arthrex (Naples, FL) forked anchor is then inserted with the remaining tails of the labral tape which are inserted into the distal pole of the scaphoid (Fig. 17.12). This help maintains dorsiflexion of the scaphoid from the reconstruction. Any remaining portion of the interosseous ligaments can then be repaired with suture anchors in an acute repair. This technique is indicated for both acute and chronic reconstructions (Fig. 17.13).

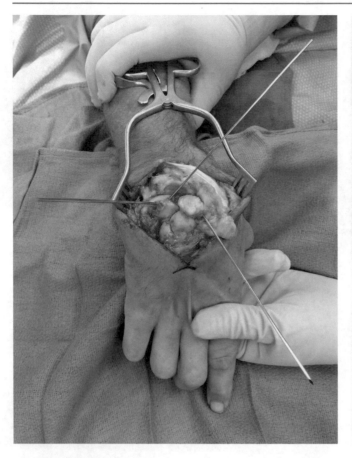

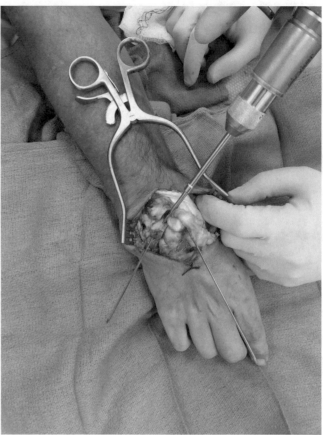

Fig. 17.5 Intraoperative photograph demonstrating placement of the guidewire slightly volar the mid-axis line in the lunate and passing ulnarly through the triquetrum

Fig. 17.7 Intraoperative photograph demonstrating drilling over the guidewire with a 3-mm cannulated drill from the lunate through the triquetrum

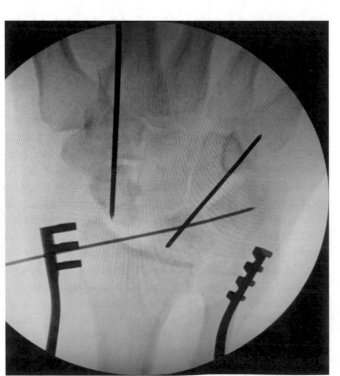

Fig. 17.6 Anterior–posterior fluoroscopy demonstrating ideal placement of the guidewire through the lunate and triquetrum

A dorsal capsulodesis can be performed with this repair as well. Arthrex 1.8-mm anchors are placed in the dorsal aspects of both scaphoid and lunate to facilitate a dorsal capsulodesis. The remaining capsule is closed, but the distal aspect is left open to help improve wrist flexion. The second and fourth dorsal compartments are closed, and the extensor pollicis longus is left free (Figs. 17.14 and 17.15).

Digital range and motion are initiated immediately, and the patient is immobilized for 4 weeks. A removable brace is used for 2 weeks, and then physical therapy for range and motion is then initiated.

The technique is essentially the same for perilunate dislocations (Figs. 17.16 and 17.17). Interosseous drill holes are made in the mid-axis of the scaphoid, reduced lunate, and triquetrum (Fig. 17.18). The labral tape is passed through the carpus (Figs. 17.19 and 17.20). A "lark's head" knot is tied on the looped end of the labral tape (Fig. 17.21).

The remaining suture is passed into the distal pole of the scaphoid (Fig. 17.22). This completes the Geissler "sling and cinch" for the perilunate reconstruction (Fig. 17.23). A dorsal capsulodesis is performed (Figs. 17.24, 17.25, 17.26, and 17.27).

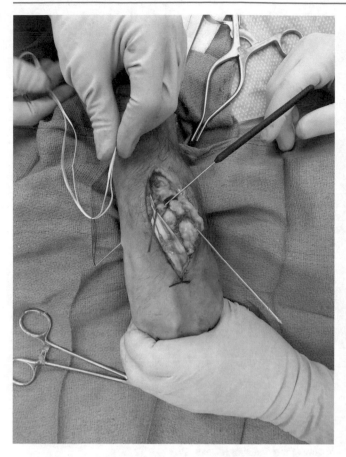

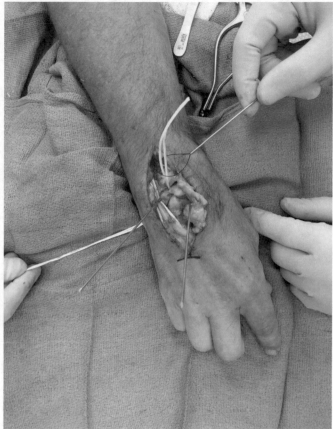

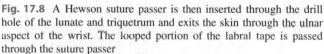

Fig. 17.8 A Hewson suture passer is then inserted through the drill hole of the lunate and triquetrum and exits the skin through the ulnar aspect of the wrist. The looped portion of the labral tape is passed through the suture passer

Fig. 17.9 The labral tape is then pulled through the triquetrum and exited out the lunate

Tips and Tricks

- Joysticks are placed in the scaphoid and lunate to open up the interval. In this way, a guidewire is placed from ulnar to radial through the scaphoid. This allows the guidewire to be exactly in the midline of the scaphoid and avoids any guesswork as compared to going from radial to ulnar.
- The second guidewire is placed from radial to ulnar through the lunate and triquetrum. It is important to place the guidewire slightly volar to the midline to help correct any dorsiflexion rotation of the lunate.
- Confirm the position of the guidewire from the lunate to the triquetrum under fluoroscopy. It is important to ensure

it passes through both carpal bones. The guidewire should be aimed slightly distally to correlate with the distal articulation of the triquetrum to the lunate.
- It is easy to pass the Hewson suture passer through the lunate and triquetrum and through the skin to retrieve the labral tape. It is very difficult to pass the labral tape from the triquetrum across the lunate alone.
- The "lark's head" knot helps to take out the tension from the labral tape after it is cinched across the carpal intervals. It makes it easier to insert the remaining part of the suture into the distal pole of the scaphoid by not fighting the tension of the repair. Any remaining part of the carpal interosseous ligaments is then repaired.

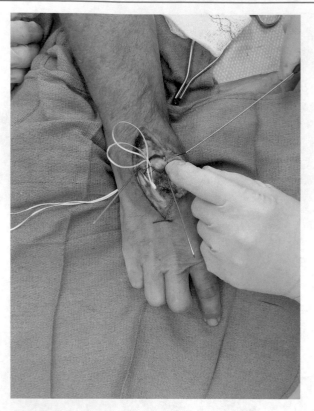

Fig. 17.10 The Hewson suture passer is then passed through the scaphoid from radial to ulnar to retrieve the labral tape

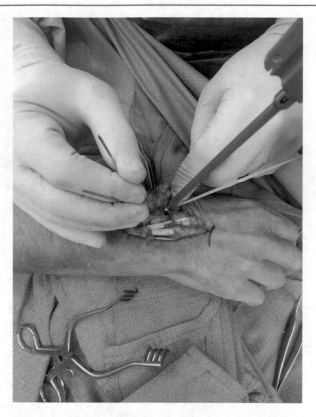

Fig. 17.12 The suture has then been cinched through the "lark's head" knot and then being inserted into the distal pole of the scaphoid with the Arthrex forked anchor (Naples, FL)

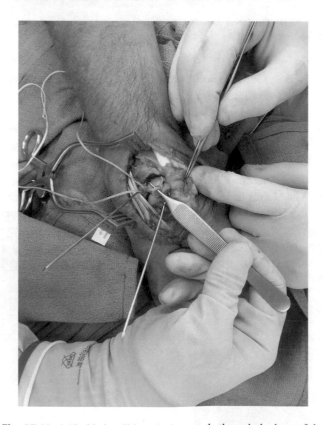

Fig. 17.11 A "lark's head" knot is then made through the loop of the labral tape on the radial aspect of the scaphoid

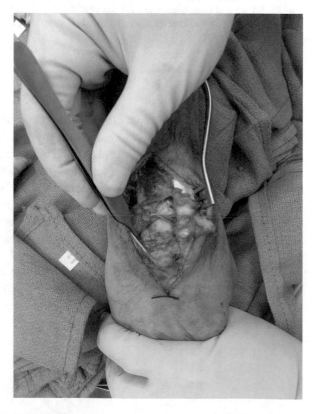

Fig. 17.13 Intraoperative photograph showing the Geissler "Sling and Cinch" complete closure of a chronic tear to the scapholunate interosseous ligament

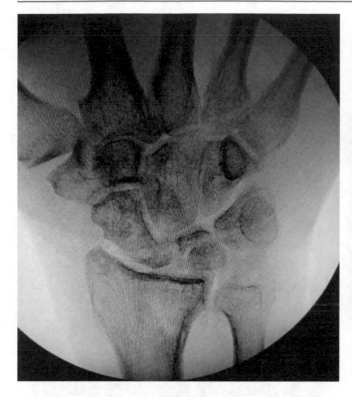

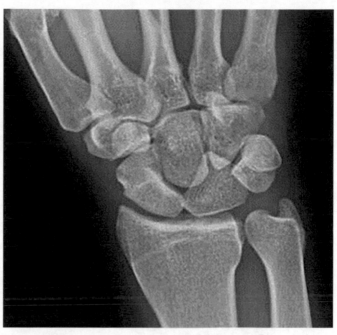

Fig. 17.16 Anterior–posterior radiograph demonstrating the perilunate dislocation

Fig. 17.14 Anterior–posterior fluoroscopy showing complete closure to the scaphoid lunate interval

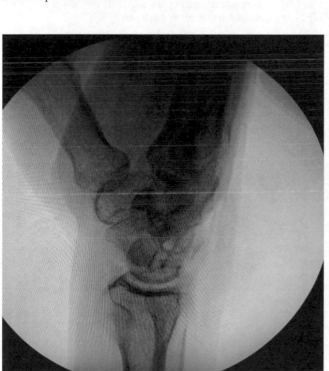

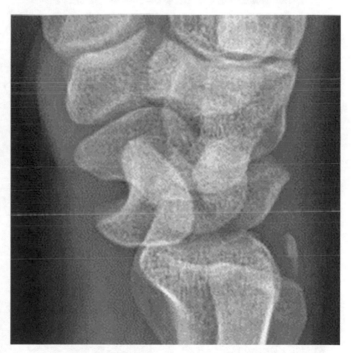

Fig. 17.17 Lateral radiograph demonstrating the anterior dislocation of the lunate

Fig. 17.15 Lateral intraoperative fluoroscopy showing restoration of the normal scapholunate angel. A "lark's head" knot will be tied on the loop portion of the labral tape

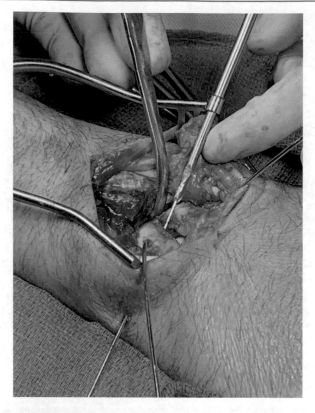

Fig. 17.18 Intraoperative radiograph showing drilling of the cannulated drill through the lunate and triquetrum

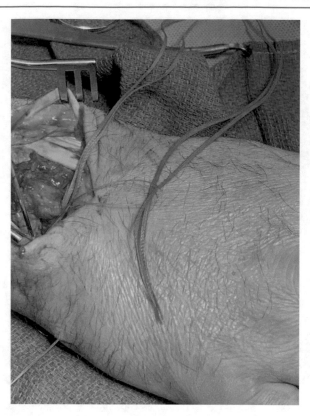

Fig. 17.20 Intraoperative radiograph demonstrating placement of the labral tape through the triquetrum and lunate

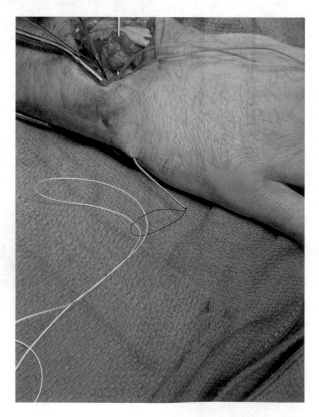

Fig. 17.19 Hewson suture passer is then passed through the drill hole in the scapholunate and triquetrum and out the skin in an ulnar aspect. The labral tape is then passed through the loop of a Hewson suture passer to be passed through the interval of the lunate and triquetrum

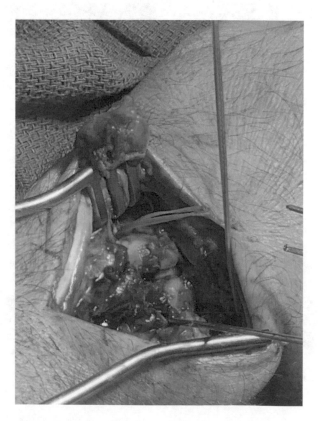

Fig. 17.21 The tails of the labral tape that have been passed through the lunate and triquetrum are then passed through the loop of the labral tape that has been previously passed through the scaphoid

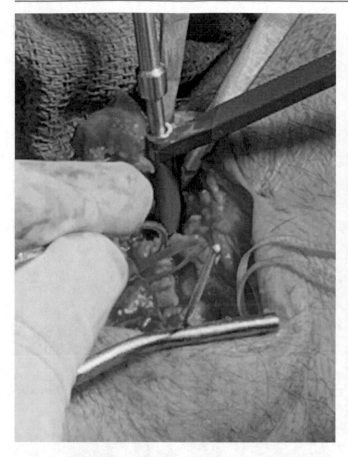

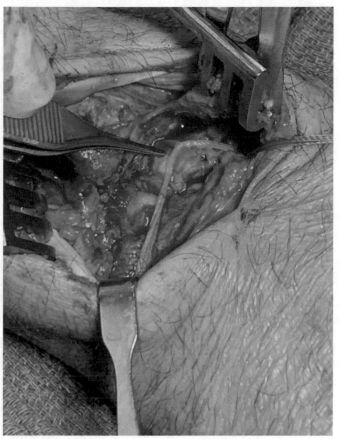

Fig. 17.22 The distal pole of the scaphoid is then drilled for the Arthrex forked anchor (Naples, FL)

Fig. 17.23 The labral tape has been "slinged and cinched" through the loop of the labral tape on the radial aspect of the scaphoid for complete closure to the perilunate dislocation. The labral tape was passed intraosseously for reconstruction of the volar and dorsal portions of the ligament. Note, the labral tape does not impinge on the dorsal aspect of the scaphoid as it is transferred into the distal pole of the scaphoid

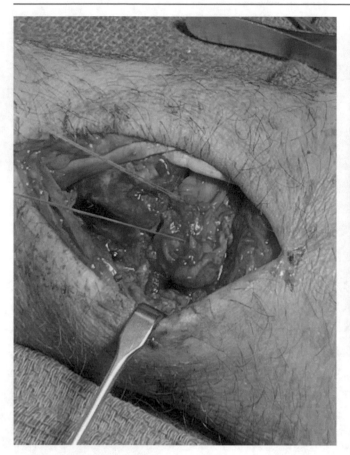

Fig. 17.24 A dorsal capsulodesis is added on top of the perilunate reconstruction

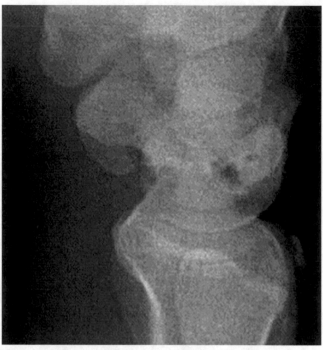

Fig. 17.26 Lateral fluoroscopic views showing complete reduction of the perilunate dislocation with a Geissler "Sling and Cinch" technique

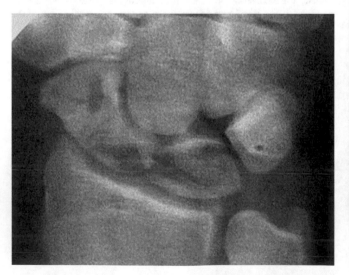

Fig. 17.25 Anterior–posterior fluoroscopic view shows complete closure to the carpus following reconstruction at the perilunate at dislocation

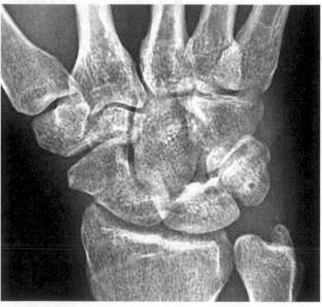

Fig. 17.27 Anterior–posterior radiograph at 8-month follow-up showing complete closure of the perilunate dislocation

Conclusion

Perilunate instability is a complex issue for the hand surgeon. It is important that the hand surgeon has a sound understanding of the different treatment options to manage perilunate instability. It is imperative that these patients undergo surgical intervention early after diagnosis for better outcomes. Traditional techniques have consistently produced good outcomes, but there are newer techniques to manage perilunate instability. Internal bracing augmentation for SLIL repair is a new technique demonstrating promising results. Future studies need to investigate long-term functional outcomes with internal bracing augmentation of perilunate instability.

References

1. Malović M, Pavić R, Milosević M. Treatment of trans-scaphoid perilunate dislocations using a volar approach with scaphoid osteosynthesis and temporary Kirschner wire fixation. Mil Med. 2011;176(9):1077–82.
2. Wolfe SW, Hotchkiss RN, Pederson WC, Kozin SH, Cohen MS. Green's operative hand surgery. Philadelphia: Elsevier; 2016. p. 2060.
3. Jones DB Jr, Kakar S. Perilunate dislocations and fracture dislocations. J Hand Surg Am. 2012;37(10):2168–73. quiz 2174
4. Geissler WB. Arthroscopic management of scapholunate instability. J Wrist Surg. 2013;2(2):129–35.
5. Stanbury SJ, Elfar JC. Perilunate dislocation and perilunate fracture-dislocation. J Am Acad Orthop Surg. 2011;19(9):554–62.
6. Park I-J, Maniglio M, Shin SS, Lim D, MH MG, Lee TQ. Internal bracing augmentation for scapholunate interosseous ligament repair: a cadaveric biomechanical study. J Hand Surg Am. 2020;45(10):985, e1–985.e9. https://doi.org/10.1016/j.jhsa.2020.03.017.
7. Kakar S, Greene RM. Scapholunate ligament internal brace 360-degree tenodesis (SLITT) procedure. J Wrist Surg. 2018;7(4):336–40.
8. Van de Grift TC, Ritt MJPF. Management of lunotriquetral instability: a review of the literature. J Hand Surg Eur Vol. 2016;41(1):72–85.
9. Souer JS, Rutgers M, Andermahr J, Jupiter JB, Ring D. Perilunate fracture-dislocations of the wrist: comparison of temporary screw versus K-wire fixation. J Hand Surg Am. 2007;32(3):318–25.
10. Chou Y-C, Hsu Y-H, Cheng C-Y, Wu C-C. Percutaneous screw and axial Kirschner wire fixation for acute transscaphoid perilunate fracture dislocation. J Hand Surg Am. 2012;37(4):715–20.
11. Savvidou OD, Beltsios M, Sakellariou VI, Papagelopoulos PJ. Perilunate dislocations treated with external fixation and percutaneous pinning. J Wrist Surg. 2015;4(2):76–80.
12. Savvidou OD, Beltsios M, Sakellariou VI, Mavrogenis AF, Christodoulou M, Papagelopoulos PJ. Use of external fixation for perilunate dislocations and fracture dislocations. Strategies Trauma Limb Reconstr. 2014;9(3):141–8.
13. Kakar S, Greene RM, Denbeigh J, Van Wijnen A. Scapholunate ligament internal brace 360 Tenodesis (SLITT) procedure: a biomechanical study. J Wrist Surg. 2019;8(3):250–4.
14. Berger RA, Landsmeer JMF. The palmar radiocarpal ligaments; a study of adult and fetal human wrist joints. J Hand Surg Am. 1990;15(6):847–54.
15. Short WH, Werner FW, Green JK, Masaoka S. Biomechanical evaluation of ligamentous stabilizers of the scaphoid and lunate. J Hand Surg. 2002;27:991–1002.
16. Garcia-Elias M. Carpal instabilities and dislocations. In: Green DP, Hotchkiss RN, Pederson WC, editors. Green's operative hand surgery. 4th ed. New York: Churchill Livingstone; 1999. p. 865–928.
17. Mayfield JK. Wrist ligamentous anatomy and pathogenesis of carpal instability. Orthop Clin North Am. 1984;15(2):209–16.
18. Meade TD, Schneider LH, Cherry K. Radiographic analysis of selective ligament sectioning at the carpal scaphoid: a cadaver study. J Hand Surg Am. 1990;15(6):855–62.
19. Geissler WB, Freeland AE, Savoie FH, McIntyre LW, Whipple TL. Intracarpal soft-tissue lesions associated with an intra-articular fracture of the distal end of the radius. J Bone Joint Surg Am. 1996;78(3):357–65.

The RADICL Procedure: Repair/Augmentation of Dorsal Intercarpal Ligament

Daniel Williams, Senthooran Raja, Mark Ross,
Gregory Couzens, and Scott W. Wolfe

Introduction

The dorsal intercarpal ligament (DIC) and the dorsal radiocarpal ligament (DRC) consistently insert into the dorsal aspect of the lunate [1–3]. Although previously described as secondary stabilisers, the strong insertion of these ligaments into the proximal row, and especially the lunate, has been shown to be pivotal in maintaining normal wrist biomechanics [4]. The dorsal ligaments are perhaps better described as critical stabilisers of the lunate. The detailed kinematic considerations of these ligaments are discussed in the previous chapter.

Disruption to the critical stabilisers can occur in isolation, as part of a larger injury to the dorsal scapholunate complex or as an iatrogenic complication of conventional dorsal approaches to carpus. It is our opinion that there should be a high index of suspicion when investigating dorsal wrist and scapholunate interosseous ligament (SLIL) injuries. When identified through imaging, arthroscopic assessment or during open surgery, injury to the critical stabilisers should be repaired.

Injury to the SLIL complex is the most common cause of symptomatic carpal instability. In 1980, Mayfield suggested a predictable pattern of SLIL injury as a result of extension, ulnar deviation and intercarpal supination, which can eventually lead to scapholunate advanced collapse [5–7]. Sectioning studies have shown that division of the SLIL in isolation does not result in static instability [4, 8]. To reproduce dorsal intercalated segment instability (DISI) in a cadaver, injury need also occur to at least one of the extrinsic ligaments/critical stabilisers [3, 4].

Conventional open approaches for SLIL reconstructions often result in stiffness and can even worsen the gapping at the scapholunate (SL) interval. Wrist arthroscopy has changed how we assess and manage these complex injuries, particularly the initial stages of SLIL disruption. When there is no static malalignment or where carpal re-alignment can be achieved, an arthroscopic procedure to repair and reconstruct the extrinsic ligaments is appealing.

Arthroscopic repair of the dorsal capsular structures has been described [9–14]. The dorsal capsulo-scapholunate septum (DCSS) is dense septum between the DIC and the dorsal fibres of the SLIL [9]. Cadaveric studies have shown that arthroscopic sectioning of the DCSS increases the European Wrist Arthroscopy Society (EWAS) grade for carpal instability. Short-term clinical outcomes of the arthroscopic DCSS repair in 221 patients with a mean follow-up of 39 months have shown a 95.7% satisfaction rate with significant improvement in grip strength (93% of contralateral side) and reduction in DASH score (47 to 9.4), whilst maintaining a good range of motion [10].

Although several classifications exist for the assessment of SLIL injuries, we use both the Geissler and the EWAS classifications to grade SLIL injuries. In discussing the

D. Williams · S. Raja
Brisbane Hand and Upper Limb Research Institute,
Brisbane, QLD, Australia

Orthopaedic Department, Princess Alexandra Hospital,
Woolloongabba, QLD, Australia

M. Ross (✉)
Brisbane Hand and Upper Limb Research Institute,
Brisbane, QLD, Australia

Orthopaedic Department, Princess Alexandra Hospital,
Woolloongabba, QLD, Australia

The University of Queensland, St. Lucia, QLD, Australia
e-mail: research@upperlimb.com

G. Couzens
Brisbane Hand and Upper Limb Research Institute, Brisbane
Private Hospital, Brisbane, QLD, Australia

Orthopaedic Department, Princess Alexandra Hospital,
Woolloongabba, QLD, Australia

Institute of Health and Biomedical Innovation, Queensland
University of Technology, Brisbane, QLD, Australia

S. W. Wolfe
Hand and Upper Extremity Service, Department of Orthopedic
Surgery, The Hospital for Special Surgery, New York, NY, USA

Table 18.1 EWAS stages of scapholunate interosseous instability

Arthroscopic stage (EWAS)	Arthroscopic testing of SLIL from MC joint	AP findings
I	No passage of the probe	
II: Lesion of membranous SLIL	Passage of the tip of the probe in the SL space without widening (stable)	Lesion of proximal/membranous part of SLIL
IIIA: Partial lesion involving the volar SLIL	Volar widening on dynamic testing from MC joint (anterior laxity)	Lesion of anterior and proximal part of SLIL with or without lesion of RSC-LRL
IIIB: Partial lesion involving the dorsal SLIL	Dorsal SL widening on dynamic testing (posterior laxity)	Lesion of proximal and posterior part of SLIL with partial lesion of DIC
IIIC: Complete SLIL tear, joint is reducible	Complete widening of SL space on dynamic testing, reducible with removal of probe	Complete lesion of SLIL (anterior, proximal and posterior), complete lesion of one extrinsic ligament (DIC lesion or RSC/LRL)
IV: Complete SLIL with SL gap	SL gap with passage of the arthroscope from MC to RC joint. No radiographic abnormalities	Complete lesion of SLIL (anterior, proximal and posterior), lesion of extrinsic ligaments (DIC and RSC/LRL)
V	Wide SL gap with passage of the arthroscope through SL joint. Frequent X-ray abnormalities such as increased SL gap, DISI deformity	Complete lesion of SLIL, DIC, LRL, RSC, involvement of one or more ligament (TH, ST and DRC)

Stage	Arthroscopical findings
	Scope through MRC and probe through MCU
Stage I	No passage of the probe in the interosseous scapholunate (SL) space, but synovitis
Stage IIA	Volar passage of the probe in the SL space without the ability to turn the probe (widening less than 1 mm)
Stage IIB	Dorsal passage of the probe in the SL space without the ability to turn the probe (widening less than 1 mm)
Stage IIC	Complete passage of the probe in the SL space without the ability to turn the probe (widening less than 1 mm)
Stage IIIA	Volar widening of the SL space with the ability to turn the probe (widening more than 1 mm, anterior laxity)
Stage IIIB	Dorsal widening of the SL space with the ability to turn the probe (widening more than 1 mm, posterior laxity)
Stage IIIC	Complete widening of the SL space with the ability to turn the probe (widening more than 1 mm, global laxity)
Stage IV	SL gap more than 2.7 mm with passage of the scope from MC to RC joint

Adapted from [7, 8] with permission from Elsevier
Abbreviations: *AP* anatomopathological, *DIC* dorsal intercarpal ligament, *DISI* dorsal intercalated segmental instability, *DRC* dorsoradiocarpal, *EWAS* European Wrist Arthroscopy Society, *MC* midcarpal, *RC* radiocarpal, *RCS* radioscaphocapitate, *LRL* long radiolunate, *SL* scapholunate, *SLIL* scapholunate interosseous ligament, *ST* scaphotrapezial, *TH* triquetrohamate

RADICL repair, we find that the EWAS classification provides more granular detail about partial SLIL injuries (Table 18.1) [15, 16]. As our understanding continues to develop, it is appealing to have a ligament-based approach to SLIL injuries, targeting reconstructions to include DIC, SLIL, volar scaphotrapeziotrapezoid (STT) and long radiolunate ligament (LRL) as required.

As discussed in the previous chapter, a detailed understanding of the anatomy of the dorsal scapholunate complex is vital in the timely and specialised care of these injuries. The RADICL (Repair/Augmentation of Dorsal Intercarpal Ligament) procedure is a technique by which the extrinsic ligaments are re-inserted with arthroscopic or mini-open techniques into dorsal lunate. The same principles and philosophy can be adapted to open procedures where the dorsal capsule should not be dissected off the dorsal lunate and if an avulsion is identified it should be repaired as part of the procedure.

Indications

1. Pain and instability in association with a DIC/DRC avulsion
2. DIC/DRC injury associated with a partial SLIL injury (EWAS 3a, 3b, 3c)
3. In conjunction with SLIL reconstruction (EWAS 3c, 4, 5), lunate/peri-lunate dislocations or complex ligament injuries
4. Following open surgery/iatrogenic injury to the dorsal lunate insertions

We have particularly observed a subset of patients with partial SLIL injury (Geissler 2/EWAS 3a/3b) who have failed non-operative management. At arthroscopy, in addition to the partial SLIL injury, a careful assessment can identify loss of the dorsal ligamentous insertion onto the dorsal lunate. As noted in the previous chapter, the capsular insertions into the lunate should be inspected from the midcarpal joint and from either 1–2 or 6R portals of the radiocarpal joint. Where there is loss of the capsular attachment, we have found good results with arthroscopic or mini-open RADICL repair.

Patient Preparation and Positioning

The procedure is performed as a day case under general or regional anaesthesia. The patient is positioned supine with a tourniquet and the arm resting on an arm board. The senior authors use a horizontal traction system, although vertical traction can also be used.

Diagnostic Arthroscopy

Standard dry arthroscopy techniques are employed [17, 18]. Diagnostic arthroscopy is first performed using the 1–2 or 3–4 portal. The dorsal fibres of the SLIL and the capsular

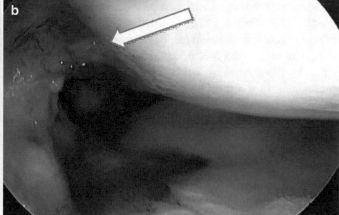

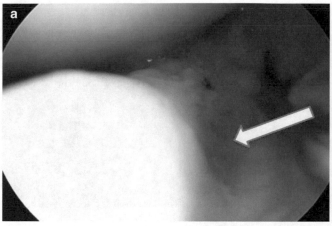

Fig. 18.1 (a) Arthroscopic view from the midcarpal ulnar portal showing the normal capsular insertion of the extrinsic ligaments at the articular cartilage margin. (b) Arthroscopic view from the 1–2 portal showing the normal capsular insertion of the extrinsic ligaments at the articular cartilage margin

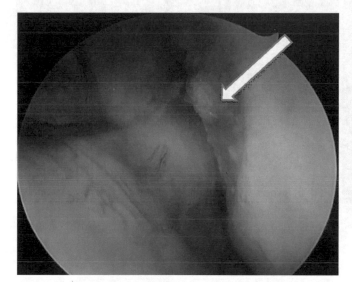

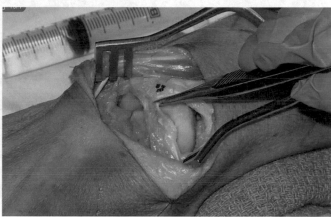

Fig. 18.3 Anatomical dissection demonstrating the firm attachments of the dorsal extrinsic ligaments into the lunate [3]

Fig. 18.2 Arthroscopic view from the 1–2 portal showing the bare area on the dorsal aspect of the lunate following avulsion of the DRC

insertion of the DIC and DRC into the dorsal lunate are best visualised using the 6R, midcarpal ulna (MCU) and 1–2 portal where a clear capsular reflection can be seen in the normal wrist (Fig. 18.1a, b). A shaver is introduced to remove debris and perform a synovectomy. A probe is then inserted to assess the nature of the injury to the SLIL and another intra-articular pathology. Injury to the DRC insertion into the lunate is often best appreciated when viewing from the 6R or 1–2 portal, whereas injury to the DIC insertion into the lunate is best appreciated using the midcarpal portals and moving the scope and probe into the dorsal recess. When an injury to the extrinsic ligaments has occurred, a bare area on the dorsum of the lunate is seen; this is pathognomonic of an injury (Fig. 18.2). In significant injuries, complete disruption of the capsular attachment can be observed. After removal of minor granulation tissue, the probe may be passed between the radiocarpal and midcarpal joints deep to the transverse DIC fibres.

The DIC and DRC are normally firmly attached to the lunate (Fig. 18.3) [3]. In chronic injuries, fibrous bands and scar tissue may form in the dorsal recess. This is not structural and with experience can be clearly differentiated from normal ligamentous insertion. In this situation, a shaver is used to debride and further delineate the bare area of the lunate. At this stage, it is important to prepare the bare area of the lunate for the re-insertion of the DIC.

The RADICL Procedure

In an isolated avulsion of the dorsal critical stabilisers or more commonly in association with lower grade SLIL injuries (EWAS grade 3a, 3b and 3c), it may be possible to perform a RADICL procedure in isolation. Viewing from the 1–2 or MCU portal, the bare area of the lunate is prepared to ensure all of the fibrous scar tissue is removed. The optimum position for the anchor can then be localised with a 21-gage needle. This is often possible utilising the 3–4 portal; however, an accessory incision can be made if required. The incision is made, or the 3–4 portal is extended (approximately 1.5 cm). Care is taken to retract the extensor tendons. An anchor is inserted through the distal edge of the DRC centrally into the bare area of the lunate (Fig. 18.4). The senior author's preference is for an all-suture anchor with a small diameter hole and a 2/0 or 0 non-absorbable suture. One suture strand is then shuttled distally from inside out through the proximal edge of the DIC/dorsal capsule using a fine curved mosquito forceps or the smallest Arthrex Micro SutureLasso with a 70-degree curvature. The sutures are tied extracapsular, taking care not to catch extensor tendons, reinserting the DIC into the bare area of the lunate (Fig. 18.5).

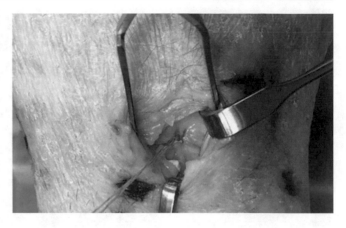

Fig. 18.5 Clinical photograph demonstrating a 2-cm wound with sutures tied over the DIC

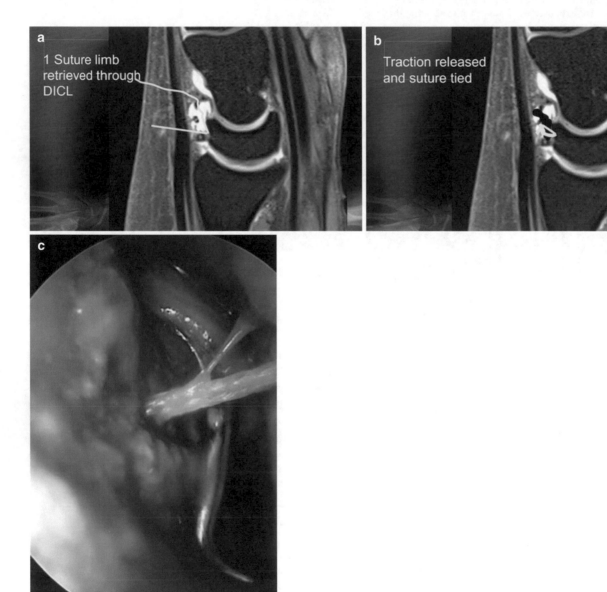

Fig. 18.4 (**a, b**) Diagrammatic representation of RADICL repair. (**c**) Arthroscopic view of anchor placement in dorsal lunate

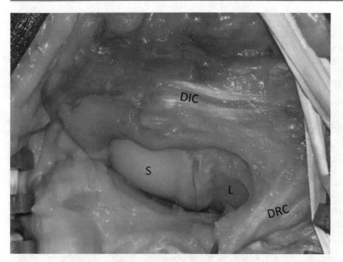

Fig. 18.6 A prosection demonstrating the window approach and the preservation of the DIC and DRC. In clinical practice, all of the tissue does not need to be excised and a transverse capsulotomy alone can be made giving adequate exposure [19]

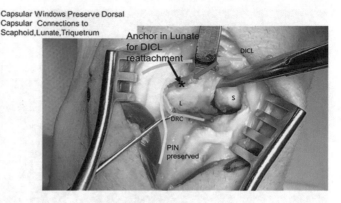

Fig. 18.7 Window approach for open SL reconstruction. Note bare area (blue arrow) on dorsal lunate which was present on opening the capsule (i.e. not iatrogenic). This lesion should be repaired with the RADICL repair at the conclusion of the reconstruction

It is important to release traction and place the wrist in a neutral position when the sutures are tied. The reduction and fixation can then be confirmed arthroscopically. Wounds are irrigated and closed.

The RADICL procedure can also be performed as an open procedure. A 3-cm dorsal incision is made just distal and ulna to Lister's tubercle. Care is taken to protect any rare branches of the superficial radial nerve. The fourth compartment is opened just distal to the extensor retinaculum to expose the dorsal capsule. Release of the distal aspect of the extensor retinaculum may be required to adequately expose the dorsal capsule. A transverse capsulotomy is then made just proximal to the DIC extending from the radius to the DRC. It is important to work in the window between the DRC, DIC and radius to avoid further damaging the extrinsic ligaments (Fig. 18.6) [19]. Through this window, the bare area of the lunate can be prepared and an anchor easily inserted to recreate the attachments of the DRC and DIC. The two suture limbs are then passed, respectively, through the proximal DIC and distal DRC and tied extracapsular.

Post-Operative Care

The wrist is placed in a resting thermoplastic splint, and hand therapy is commenced on day 1 post-op. Therapy focuses on maintaining a full range of finger motion with early active inner range of motion of the wrist from 30° extension to 20° flexion. From 6 weeks, patients work on regaining and full range of motion. Strengthening with a focus on SL protective muscles is commenced between 10 and 12 weeks. The aim is to return to full activity by 16 weeks.

RADICL Procedure In Association with Other Injuries/Surgery

DIC disruption occurs with multiple pathologies, and this chapter is designed to provide a framework to advise when repair/augmentation of the DIC and DRC may be required. When a reduction in carpal malalignment is required as part of the procedure, temporary pinning of the carpus is usually required.

When performing arthroscopic or open surgery for complete SLIL dissociation, it is common to identify the bare area caused by disruption of the dorsal capsular attachments to the lunate. This lesion should not be created or worsened by the surgical approach, and this is best achieved by utilising the window approach. After whatever repair or reconstruction is performed, the dorsal capsule should be re-inserted with a RADICL repair (Fig. 18.7).

The two cases that follow are examples of where the RADICL procedure has been used as part of a complex reconstruction.

Case 1: Trans-styloid Peri-lunate Dislocation (Mayfield 3)

Figure 18.8 demonstrates a trans-styloid lunate dislocation (Fig. 18.8a). In this scenario, the lunate has dissociated from the carpus with injuries to the SLIL and the lunotriquetral interosseous ligament (LTIL). The dorsal attachments of the DRC and DIC were avulsed from the dorsal aspect of the lunate.

An all-arthroscopic reduction and reconstruction of the carpus was performed and held with a combination of percutaneous wires and cannulated screws (Fig. 18.8b). Following this, the RADICL procedure is undertaken to repair the critical stabilisers of the wrist. The red star indicates the location for anchor insertion.

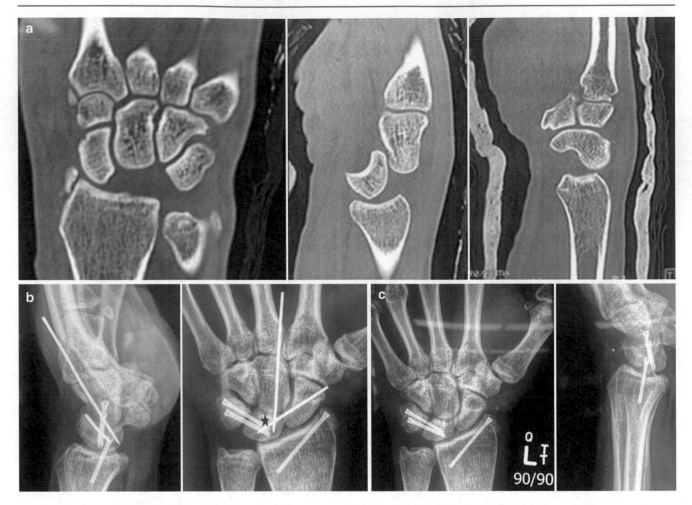

Fig. 18.8 (**a**) Coronal and sagittal computerised tomography images demonstrating a trans-styloid peri-lunate dislocation. (**b**) Following all-arthroscopic reduction, fixation and RADICL procedure. (**c**) 6 months post surgery; 4 months post removal of wires. Lunotriquetral screws were removed at 12 months post surgery

Case 2: Carpal Instability Non-dissociative Traumatic (CINDT)

Figure 18.9a demonstrates a traumatic non-dissociative volar intercalated segment instability (VISI) following a distal radius fracture. In this case, there was an injury to the critical stabilisers of the wrist and attenuation of the volar STT ligaments and volar lunocapitate capsule. Following an arthroscopic dorsal release of pathologic adhesions between the dorsal lunate and the normal bare areas of the capitate, and between the dorsal proximal margin of trapezium/trapezoid and the dorsal ridge of the scaphoid, the fixed deformity was converted to a reducible one. The volar STT was stabilised and volar capsule augmented with flexor carpi radialis tendon graft. The RADICL procedure was then performed as an open procedure through a capsular window created between the DRC, DIC and radius. Figure 18.9b shows the post-operative images with the red star indicating the location for anchor insertion.

Results

Three female and two male patients, average age 40 years, had patient-reported outcome scores collected pre-operatively and at 6 months post RADICL procedure at our institute.

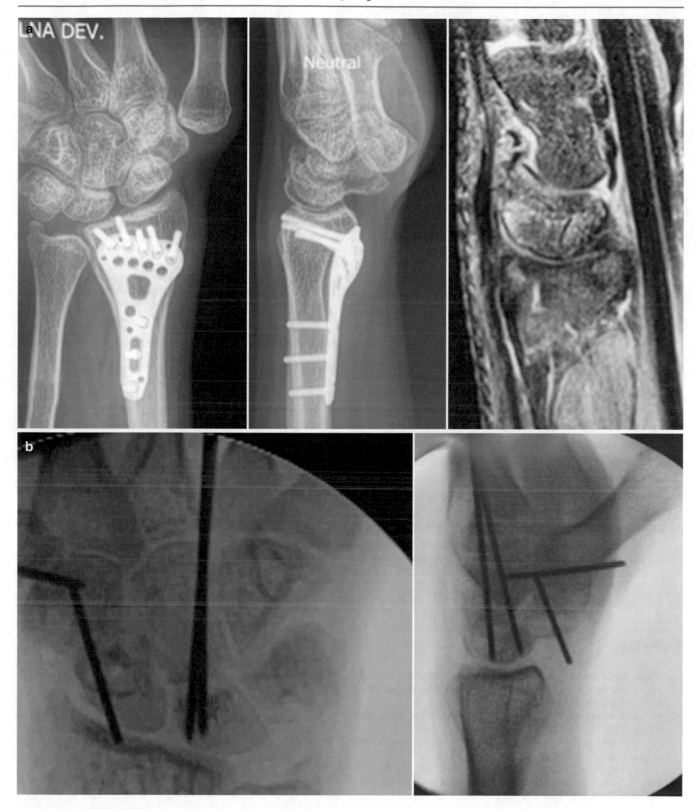

Fig. 18.9 (a) Radiographs and magnetic resonance imaging (following plate removal) demonstrating a non-dissociative traumatic VISI following a distal radius fixation. (b) Radiographs post reconstruction, percutaneous pinning and RADICL procedure. In this case, the patient has also had a first carpometacarpal joint stabilisation

Patient reported pain with normal activities improved from an average of 49.4/100 at pre-operative assessment to 23.8 at 6 months post-surgery. Similarly, Patient-Rated Wrist Evaluation, shortened Disabilities of the Arm, Shoulder and Hand (Quick DASH) and Quick DASH sport scores improved from 65.6, 50.9 and 64 prior to surgery to 27.3, 27.7 and 27.5 at post-op assessment, respectively. Range of motion was maintained after surgery and grip strength improved from an average of 19.6–33.6 kg at 6 months post-surgery.

Conclusion

The importance of the DIC and the DRC as critical stabilisers of the lunate has been underappreciated until relatively recently. The RADICL procedure is a simple and reproducible arthroscopic or open method for recreating this important insertion into the lunate.

Key Points

- The DIC and DRC are critical wrist stabilisers and insert into the dorsal aspect of the lunate.
- Care should be taken to identify and repair injuries to these critical stabilisers.
- The RADICL procedure is the arthroscopic or open repair of the DIC insertion into the lunate.
- These principles should be adopted in open surgery and the insertion of the dorsal capsular ligaments into the lunate should be protected where possible or repaired as part of the procedure.

References

1. Viegas SF, Yamaguchi S, Boyd NL, Patterson RM. The dorsal ligaments of the wrist: anatomy, mechanical properties, and function. J Hand Surg Am. 1999;24:456–68.
2. Nagao S, Patterson RM, Buford WL, Andersen CR, Shah MA, Viegas SF. Three-dimensional description of ligamentous attachments around the lunate. J Hand Surg Am. 2005;30(4):685–92. https://doi.org/10.1016/j.jhsa.2005.03.002.
3. Wessel LE, Kim J, Morse KW, Loisel F, Koff MF, Breighner R, Doty S, Wolfe SW. The dorsal ligament complex: a cadaveric, histology and imaging study. J Hand Surg. 2021. (in press).
4. Pérez AJ, Jethanandani RG, Vutescu ES, Meyers KN, Lee SK, Wolfe SW. Role of ligament stabilizers of the proximal carpal row in preventing dorsal intercalated segment instability: a cadaveric study. J Bone Joint Surg Am. 2019;101(15):1388–96. https://doi.org/10.2106/JBJS.18.01419.
5. Mayfield J. Mechanism of carpal injuries. Clin Orthop Relat Res. 1980;149:45–54.
6. Mayfield JK, Johnson RP, Kilcoyne RK. Carpal dislocations: pathomechanics and progressive perilunar instability. J Hand Surg Am. 1980;5(3):226–41. https://doi.org/10.1016/S0363-5023(80)80007-4.
7. Watson HK, Ballet FL. The SLAC wrist: scapholunate advanced collapse pattern of degenerative arthritis. J Hand Surg Am. 1984;9(3):358–65. https://doi.org/10.1016/S0363-5023(84)80223-3.
8. Mitsuyasu H, Patterson RM, Shah M. The role of the dorsal intercarpal ligament in dynamic and static scapholunate instability. J Hand Surg Am. 2004;29(2):279–88.
9. Overstraeten L, Camus E, Wahegaonkar A, Messina J, Tandara A, Binder A, et al. Anatomical description of the dorsal capsuloscapholunate septum (DCSS)—arthroscopic staging of scapholunate instability after DCSS sectioning. J Wrist Surg. 2013;2:149–54.
10. Mathoulin C. Treatment of dynamic scapholunate instability dissociation: contribution of arthroscopy. Hand Surg Rehabil. 2016;35(6):377–92. https://doi.org/10.1016/j.hansur.2016.09.002.
11. Bednar JM. Acute scapholunate ligament injuries. Hand Clin. 2015;31(3):417–23. https://doi.org/10.1016/j.hcl.2015.04.001.
12. Corella F, del Cerro M, Ocampos M, Larrainzar-Garijo R. Arthroscopic ligamentoplasty of the dorsal and volar portions of the scapholunate ligament. J Hand Surg Am. 2013;38(12):2466–77. https://doi.org/10.1016/j.jhsa.2013.09.021.
13. Carratalá V, Lucas FJ, Miranda I, Prada A, Guisasola E, Miranda FJ. Arthroscopic reinsertion of acute injuries of the scapholunate ligament technique and results. J Wrist Surg. 2020;9(4):328–37. https://doi.org/10.1055/s-0040-1710502.
14. Carratalá V, Lucas FJ, Miranda I, Sánchez Alepuz E, González Jofré C. Arthroscopic scapholunate capsuloligamentous repair: suture with dorsal capsular reinforcement for scapholunate ligament lesion. Arthrosc Tech. 2017;6(1):e113–20. https://doi.org/10.1016/j.eats.2016.09.009.
15. Messina J, van Overstraeten L, Luchetti R, Fairplay T, Mathoulin C. The EWAS classification of scapholunate tears: an anatomical arthroscopic study. J Wrist Surg. 2013;2(2):105–9. https://doi.org/10.1055/s-0033-1345265.
16. Messina J, Dreant N, Luchetti R, Lindau T, Mathoulin C. Scapholunate tears: a new arthroscopic classification. Chir Main. 2009;28:339–40.
17. del Piñal F, García-Bernal FJ, Pisani D, Regalado J, Ayala H, Studer A. Dry arthroscopy of the wrist: surgical technique. J Hand Surg Am. 2007;32(1):119–23. https://doi.org/10.1016/j.jhsa.2006.10.012.
18. del Piñal F. Dry arthroscopy and its applications. Hand Clin. 2011;27(3):335–45. https://doi.org/10.1016/j.hcl.2011.05.011.
19. Loisel F, Wessel LE, Morse KW, Victoria C, Meyers K, Wolfe SW. Is the dorsal fiber-splitting approach to the wrist safe? A kinematic analysis and introduction of the window approach. J Hand Surg. 2021. (in press).

Andrew Y. H. Chin

Introduction

Scapholunate dissociation (SLD) is the most common ligamentous injury of the carpus [1, 2]. The cause is traumatic, most commonly due to a fall on an outstretched hand or sudden overwhelming increase in loading or force across the joint resulting in giving way of the restraining forces of the scapholunate interosseous ligament (SLIL) across the joint, manifested by tear of the ligament. Isolated injury to just the SLIL ligament is uncommon; other secondary restraints (the extrinsic carpal ligaments such as the volar scaphoid–trapezium–trapezoid (STT) ligament, the scaphocapitate (SC) ligament, radioscaphocapitate (RSC) ligament, the dorsal intercarpal ligament (DIC), and the joint capsule) [3, 4] around the region are usually involved to varying degrees. Depending on how much injury to the scapholunate ligament, together with the other secondary stabilizers, will then determine the prognosis and outcome of the patient [3, 5, 6]. If untreated, it will eventually lead to a predictable degenerative pattern known as scapholunate advanced collapse (SLAC) [7, 8].

The SLIL is C-shaped and comprises three parts: the volar, proximal (membranous), and dorsal. Biomechanical studies done showed that the dorsal part is the most important as it is the strongest part of the ligament, resisting substantial torque, translation, and distraction forces generating across the joint during loading and motion [9–12]. It is therefore critical to address the injured dorsal SLIL in patients presenting with SLD.

Hence, SLD is a spectrum where the injury can result in a minor partial tear of the SLIL to a complete tear with loss of functioning secondary stabilizers, which will result in gross carpal instability as evident with carpal malalignment, abnormal kinetics and kinematics, and eventual joint degeneration. Most of the time, such injuries are overlooked as a sprain, and the patient either ignores it or manages the initial phase without consulting a doctor. Only after a period that may range from weeks to months or even years when symptoms of instability such as pain and weakness of grip become intolerable, the patient will seek medical attention. Most often, the SLD would have presented to the hand surgeon in the chronic stage (more than 6 weeks from the time of injury). The natural history of the condition is such that the more acute the presentation and earlier the intervention and treatment, the higher the chance of a possible repair of the SLIL due to the presence of remnant ligaments at either ends of the tear. When the patient presents during chronic stage, the remnant torn ligaments may have already contracted to a degree that primary repair of the ligament is not possible. In such situations, other surgical options comprising soft tissue procedures such as capsular thermal shrinkage [13], SL pinning [14], capsulodesis [15, 16], tenodesis [3, 6, 17–22], and bony ones such as bone–ligament bone grafting [23, 24], Reduction and Association of Scaphoid and Lunate (RASL) procedure [25–27], and intercarpal fusions [28–30] then become relevant in treating such patients. With so many different surgical techniques available, it behooves the treating surgeon to assess the patient carefully and accurately, ensuring correct indications for the most appropriate surgical option are adhered to so as to achieve the best possible outcome for the patient concerned.

Indications

Three-Ligament Tenodesis

Garcia-Elias et al. in 2006 [3] published the SLD treatment algorithm that provides important and relevant questions for the treating surgeon to enquire and assess the patient so that accurate staging of the condition and corresponding treatment options can be offered (Table 19.1).

A. Y. H. Chin (✉)
Singapore General Hospital, Hand and Reconstructive Microsurgery, Singapore, Singapore
e-mail: andrew.chin.y.h@singhealth.com.sg

© Springer Nature Switzerland AG 2022
W. B. Geissler (ed.), *Wrist and Elbow Arthroscopy with Selected Open Procedures*,
https://doi.org/10.1007/978-3-030-78881-0_19

Table 19.1 Staging of scapholunate dissociations

Stage	1	2	3	4	5	6
Is there a partial rupture with a normal dorsal SLIL?	Yes	No	No	No	No	No
If ruptured, can the dorsal SLIL be repaired?	Yes	Yes	No	No	No	No
Is the scaphoid normally aligned (radioscaphoid angle ≤ 45°)?	Yes	Yes	Yes	No	No	No
Is the carpal malalignment easily reducible?	Yes	Yes	Yes	Yes	No	No
Are the cartilages at both RC and MC joints normal?	Yes	Yes	Yes	Yes	Yes	No

Adapted from [3]

Three-ligament tenodesis, or 3LT, procedure [3] is one of the treatment options available to treat patients who have satisfied the stage 4 criteria of the treatment algorithm, which are (1) irreparable complete rupture of the SLIL, in particular, the dorsal aspect, which is biomechanically the most important part of the SLIL [9–12]; (2) normal carpal alignment or, if malaligned, easily reducible; and (3) normal articular cartilage of both radiocarpal and midcarpal joints. This procedure can also be considered in patients with stage 3 of SLD as an alternative to bone–ligament–bone graft procedure [23, 24].

Essentially the procedure involves taking a strip of FCR tendon to achieve the following aims: (1) reinforce the volar–distal connections of the scaphoid, that is, STT ligament; (2) reconstruct the dorsal SLIL; and (3) reduce the ulnar translation of the lunate from the incompetent secondary stabilizers of the SL joint by reinforcing the DRC ligament. As this tenodesis replicates the action of three ligaments (STT, dorsal SLIL, DRC), it is therefore named the three-ligament tenodesis or 3LT procedure [3].

Spiral Tenodesis

Another subset of patients with a more serious injury leading to a complete SLIL rupture and often in the context of a chronic perilunate injury further involving complete lunotriquetral interosseous ligament (LTIL) rupture together with loss of radial sided extrinsic ligamentous restraint.

In such scenario when the SLIL and LTIL are completely torn, the proximal carpal row bones are no longer linked and connected to each other. The scaphoid, based on its anatomy, will inherently go into flexion and pronation and that of the triquetrum, into extension and proximal migration. The distal carpal row will then go into pronation after the scaphoid collapses. In such circumstances, the entire wrist will undergo further passive pronation leading to a dramatic carpal collapse.

Three groups of ligaments have been identified in the prevention of such perilunate pronation instability. They are (1) the volar radiolunotriquetral ligament, including the volar LTIL; (2) the DIC ligament, including the dorsal LTIL and SLIL; and (3) the volar SC ligament. Functionally, these three groups of ligaments act synergistically, preventing intracarpal pronation. This antipronation ligamentous complex confers a spiral configuration around the wrist, with proximal origin at the volar border of the radial styloid, distal insertion at the volar aspect of the capitate, and various attachments along the bones of the proximal carpal row [19].

Hence, on top of the already disrupted or incompetent SLIL and LTIL, prolonged and excessive intercarpal pronation may actually result in further secondary disruption of the long radiolunate (LRL), DIC, DRC, and volar SC ligaments [19, 31]. This presents with inherent carpal instability which may not be immediately obvious, and these patients are usually misdiagnosed at the time of presentation to have just stage 4 SLD. Most of them do undergo the routine 3LT procedure and end up with failure as the LTIL and the loss of radial extrinsic ligament restrain have not been addressed, leading to persistent lunotriquetral dissociation and ulnar translocation.

A high index of suspicion has to be observed especially when the patient presents with a history of being involved in a high-velocity injury with initial paucity of clinical and radiological signs. Therefore, the antipronation spiral tenodesis first described in 2012 [19], aims to deal with patients who present with such a condition by addressing the multiple injuries that lead to a more extensive carpal instability, in this case, a perilunate pronation instability (Fig. 19.1). Another indication will be patients presenting with the Taleisnik type 2 radiocarpal instability involving an SL dissociation with ulnar translocation of the lunate [32].

Contraindications

With such specific indications that demands a careful and accurate assessment of the patients so as to come up with the accurate diagnosis and staging, it is therefore imperative for the treating surgeon to select the correct surgical procedure for the patients. There is no technique that will address the entire spectrum of the SLD entity [31]. More often than not, the inappropriate indications for these surgeries are applied, leading to failures and poor outcomes. Contraindications to both 3LT and spiral tenodesis procedures include patients who already have static, irreducible carpal malalignment and/or established degenerative changes of the radiocarpal and/or midcarpal joints. Patients with milder and more acute

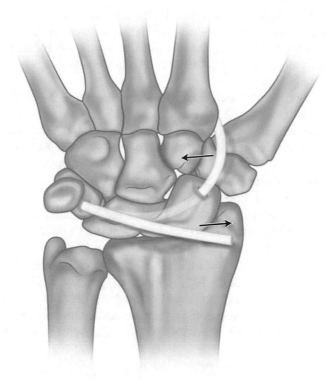

Fig. 19.1 Schematic depiction of the antipronation spiral tenodesis: a strip of flexor carpi radialis tendon passed across the scaphoid from proximal tubercle volarly to the dorsal scaphoid insertion of the dorsal scapholunate ligament dorsally, traversing transversely to the dorsal ridge of triquetrum, and then through a tunnel created through the triquetrum to emerge volarly at the floor of the carpal tunnel just radial to the pisotriquetral joint. The tendon strip is then passed deep to the flexor tendons of the digits and inserted onto the volar aspect of the radial styloid via bone anchor. Blue: Flexor carpi radialis tendon graft traversing the carpal bones to recreate the antipronation tenodesis effect in restoring carpal stability

SLD such as partial tear and reparable SLIL will benefit from direct repair of the SLIL and/or a capsulodesis procedure rather than soft tissue reconstructive procedure such as the 3LT or spiral tenodesis [3, 19, 31].

Three-Ligament Tenodesis (3LT) Technique

Approach

Dorsal longitudinal incision centered over the key landmark, Lister's tubercle. Extend 3 to 4 cm proximally and distally to the landmark. Identify the dorsal cutaneous branches of the superficial radial and ulnar nerves when developing in the incision subcutaneously and protect them. The extensor retinaculum next encountered is divided superficially into the third dorsal extensor compartment where the content, the extensor pollicis longus tendon, is retracted radially. The

retinacular septae between the second to fifth dorsal extensor compartments are then identified and systematically freed, allowing for the II and III compartment tendons to be retracted radially and IV and V compartment tendons ulnarly from the creation of two retinacular flaps. Care has to be taken to cauterize the intraseptal vessels running vertically through the septae.

Exposure of Dorsal Wrist

The terminal branches of the posterior interosseous nerve (PIN) and its branches are located at the floor of the fourth compartment and traced into the dorsal wrist capsule (Figs. 19.2 and 19.3). Visual assessment of the PIN is done, and if it is found to be thickened, irregular, and felt to be hard and cord-like, a neuroma in continuity is most likely and it is recommended for a denervation of the terminal PIN done together with the dorsal capsulotomy described by

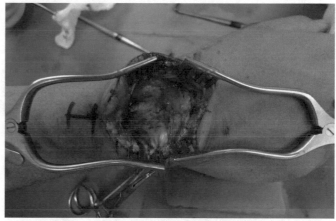

Fig. 19.2 3LT—Dorsal wrist capsule 2 (magnified)

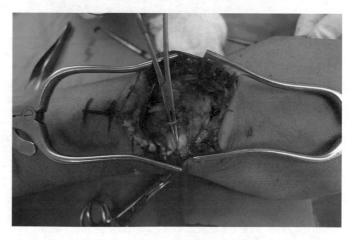

Fig. 19.3 Posterior interosseous nerve (on the forceps)

Berger et al. [33] (Fig. 19.4). However, if the PIN is found to be of normal size and consistency, a nerve-sparing dorsal capsulotomy as described by Hagert et al. [34] is preferred. Also, to preserve as many intact mechanoreceptors on the

dorsal capsule as possible, which is important in the process of proprioceptive feedback for the wrist joint via sensory afferents of the PIN, the superficial fibers of both the SLIL and the LTIL are elevated with the nerve-sparing capsular flap [34, 35].

For the 3LT technique, we will elaborate on the dorsal capsulotomy by Berger et al. [33] (Fig. 19.5a), which is excellent in allowing access to the wrist joint (both radiocarpal and midcarpal joints) and its contents. From radially, the incision commences at the tip of the radial styloid tip and progresses medially along the dorsal rim of the distal radius until the point corresponding to the center of the lunate fossa in a distal-oblique fashion follows the orientation of the fibers of the dorsal radiocarpal ligament (DRC) until its distal insertion onto the dorsal ridge of the triquetrum ulnarly. A second incision is made radially at the level of the scaphoid–trapezium–trapezoid (STT) joint and progresses ulnarly, splitting along the transversely orientated fibers of the dorsal intercarpal ligament (DIC) until its insertion onto the dorsum of the triquetrum. The subsequent longitudinal connection

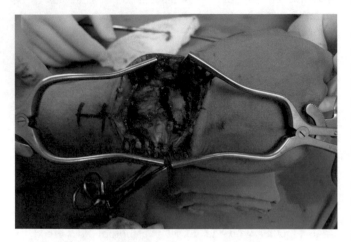

Fig. 19.4 3LT—Berger capsulotomy marking

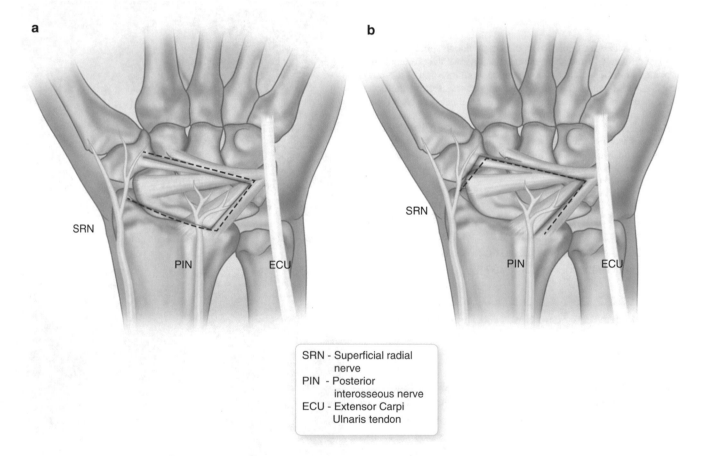

Fig. 19.5 (**a**) Dorsal capsulotomy as described by Berger, Bishop and Bettinger 1996. Note the terminal fibers of the posterior interosseous nerve in the direct path of the incision. (**b**) Nerve-sparing dorsal capsulotomy as described by Hagert, Ferreres and Garcia-Elias 2010. Note the sparing of the terminal branches of the posterior interosseous nerve

when capsulotomy is created. Light blue: dorsal extrinsic ligaments, distal radio-ulnar ligament. Yellow: Superficial radial nerve branches (SBR) and posterior interosseous nerve (PIN). Red: Incisions of the respective dorsal capsulotomies

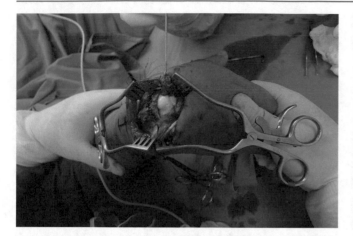

Fig. 19.6 3LT—Carpus exposed after dorsal capsulotomy

between the two incisions on the dorsum of the triquetrum creates a radially based capsular flap which is carefully elevated off the dorsal carpal bones, allowing for a good exposure and access to the dorsal aspect of the wrist (Fig. 19.6).

There should be deliberate planning to leave adequate amount of dorsal radiocarpal ligament attached to the triquetrum to allow for incorporation of the tendon graft through the ligament for tensioning of the tendon reconstruction at later stage of the procedure. Inevitably, by making the proximal transverse capsular incision, the terminal fibers of the posterior interosseous nerve (PIN) will be transected. A painful neuroma may occur post-operatively in patients who have normal PIN pre-operatively which may necessitate a secondary surgery to excise, which is also why the nerve-sparing dorsal capsulotomy is advocated to circumvent this problem [34] (see Fig. 19.5b).

Assessment of Wrist

Once the dorsal wrist is exposed, the SL joint is inspected and the five questions in the treatment algorithm are then answered by visually inspecting and assessing the joint. Visual inspection of the following: of the torn dorsal SLIL proves that the remnant ligament has been severely scarred and retracted or disintegrated beyond repair; all articular cartilage of both the radiocarpal and midcarpal joints are normal. Reducibility of the carpal malalignment is checked by traction or by manipulation with K-wires inserted over the dorsal lunate and scaphoid temporarily as joysticks. In the case of static carpal malalignment, if removal of any interposed fibrosis in the SL joint shows subsequent reduction of the malalignment, then the SLD corresponds to the stage 4 of the algorithm and 3LT procedure is indicated.

Establishing the Scaphoid Tunnel

A 2-cm skin incision is made over the volar radial aspect of the wrist corresponding from the scaphoid tuberosity to the direction of the radial styloid. A 2.7-mm drill hole is made volarly at the scaphoid corresponding to the scaphoid tuberosity, where the sheath of the flexor carpi radialis (FCR) traverses ulnarly, to them through the dorsal scaphoid corresponding to the point of insertion of the scaphoid edge of the dorsal SL ligament, creating a scaphoid tunnel which follows the main axis of the scaphoid. To avoid damage to the surrounding articular surfaces of the scaphoid, it is recommended that a guiding K-wire under direct fluoroscopy control is used to confirm the correct direction and orientation of the proposed scaphoid tunnel before using a cannulated 2.7-mm drill to complete the tunneling process. Drill speed should be slow, sustained, and progressive, and once the tip of the drill is seen to be emerging through the dorsal aspect of the proximal scaphoid incision, the drilling should cease (Figs. 19.7, 19.8 and 19.9).

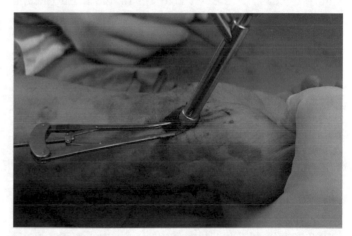

Fig. 19.7 Drilling scaphoid tunnel volar

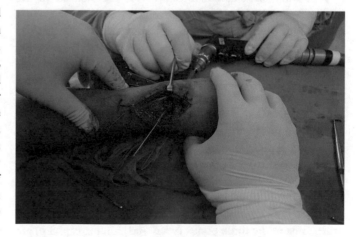

Fig. 19.8 Drilling the scaphoid bone tunnel dorsal

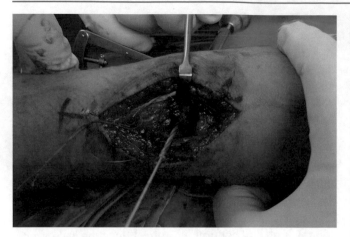

Fig. 19.9 Drilling scaphoid bone tunnel dorsal (magnified)

Harvesting of the FCR Tendon Graft

A distally based strip of FCR tendon is harvested (1/3 thickness and about 12 cm length) through a small transverse incision proximally at distal 1/2 to 1/3 of the radial forearm corresponding to the anatomical course of the FCR tendon. The remnant connections of the FCR tendon sheath and the tendon insertion distal to the trapezium are left intact. This will ensure a correct obliquity of the tendon strip from the volar ridge of the trapezium to the tip of the scaphoid tuberosity, thus mimicking the anatomic disposition of the scaphocapitate ligament. Once at the tuberosity the tendon strip is passed through the scaphoid tunnel using a wire loop or a tendon passer (Figs. 19.10a, b, 19.11a and 19.12).

Dorsal Aspect

Subsequently, turn the wrist dorsally again, create a 3-mm transverse trough deep enough with a burr or ronguer to expose bleeding cancellous bone over the dorsum of the lunate. A small 1.8-mm suture anchor is inserted at the center of the floor of the trough created to hold the tendon graft to the lunate, ensuring close and intimate contact between the two tissues to facilitate the growth of Sharpey's fibers [3] (Figs. 19.10b, 19.13, 19.14 and 19.15). The distal end of the DRC ligament is situated at the proximal and medial to the ulnar corner of the dorsal capsular flap opening. At the most distal level just by the triquetral insertion, a small vertical slit is created in the DRC ligament where the free tendon graft end is passed from deep and out superficially (Figs. 19.10c and 19.16). The slit created acts as a biological pulley from which the free tendon graft end is looped around and pulled toward the radial side of the carpus to tension the tendon graft. Ensure the three bones (scaphoid, lunate, capitate) are reduced and stabilized with two 1.5-mm K-wires across the

SL and scaphocapitate (SC) joints (Fig. 19.10d). The sutures are placed on the tendon graft in the following manner: maintaining the firm tension on the tendon graft at the free end, the anchor suture in the lunate is used to bring the tendon strip in close contact with the trough of cancellous bone at the dorsum of the lunate. The graft end then is sutured back onto itself with 3/0 nonabsorbable sutures (Figs. 19.17 and 19.18). The capsular flap is then reconstituted back to its original position through suturing the split fibers of both the DRC and the DIC ligaments. It is also recommended to place some sutures also from the dorsal capsule to the tendon graft to re-establish the normal capsular attachment to the dorsum of the SL joint. The extensor retinaculum is reconstituted back with sutures, drains are then placed, and skin closure is done.

At End of Surgery

A short-arm thumb spica cast is fashioned and placed on patient, redone on the tenth post-operative day to accommodate removal of stitches, and subsequently maintained for a total of 6 weeks. Supervised rehabilitation with protective removable splint is used for additional 6 weeks. The two stabilizing K-wires across the SL and SC joints are removed at 8 weeks post-surgery. Further supervised rehabilitation should focus especially on strenghtening the supinators of the scaphoids namely the FCR and the ECRB and avoid activating the main pronator of the scaphoid, which is the ECU, as it aggravates the SL distasis. Contact sports and strenuous activities are to be avoided for a total of 6 months post-surgery [31, 36, 37].

Spiral Tenodesis Procedure

Approach

Similar to the 3LT procedure, the initial dorsal approach centered over the key landmark, Lister's tubercle is performed. The incision extends 3–4 cm proximally and distally to the landmark. Alternatively, a transverse 3- to 4-cm incision centered at the Lister's tubercle can also be made as illustrated in Fig. 19.19. The dorsal cutaneous branches of the ulnar nerve and superficial radial nerve are identified and protected. The third dorsal extensor compartment is incised and the content, extensor pollicis longus (EPL), is retracted radially. The retinacular septae between the dorsal extensor compartments II and V are identified and systematically sectioned, raising the two retinacular flaps, one radial and the other ulnar, exposing the second through fifth compartments. The intraseptal vertical blood vessels are carefully identified and cauterized.

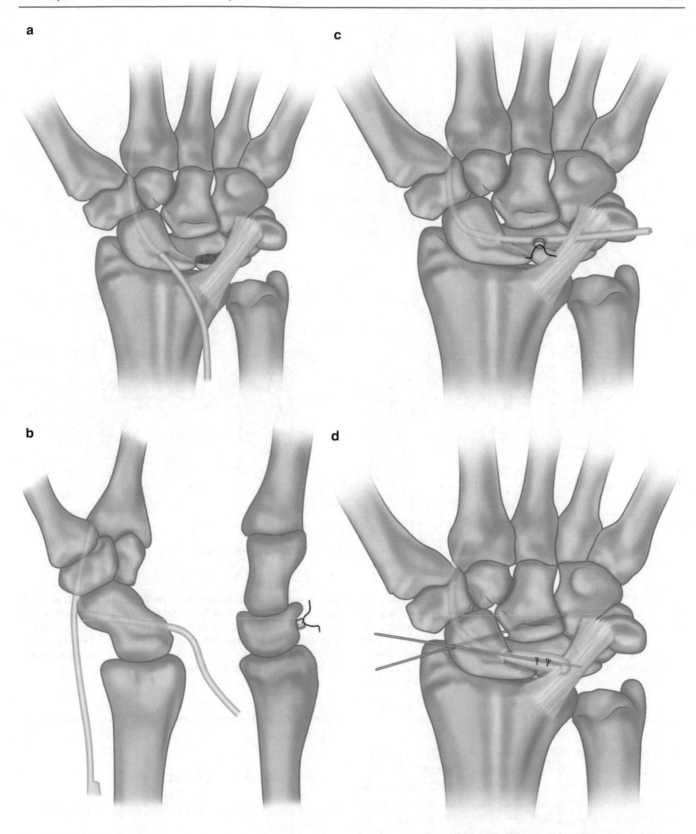

Fig. 19.10 The schematic representation of the three-ligament tenodesis technique. (**a**) A strip of FCR tendon passed from volar scaphoid tuberosity to the dorsal ridge of scaphoid corresponding to the scaphoid insertion of the dorsal scapholunate ligament. (**b**) The FCR tendon graft is set across the SL joint and inset onto the transverse trough created at the dorsal lunate; it is then held in place by a bone anchor inserted in the middle of the trough. (**c**) A slit parallel to the direction of the fibers of the DRC ligament distally at the central portion is created, and the FCR tendon graft is then passed through it and with adequate tensioning. (**d**) The FCR tendon graft is then looped back onto itself and sutured together at the dorsal lunate; two neutralizing K-wires are inserted across the SL and SC joints, respectively. Thus, only the MC joint is immobilized; there is no RC joint immobilization. Blue: Flexor carpi radialis (FCR) tendon graft traversing within the bone tunnel and the opposite far side of the carpus and also parts of the K-wires within carpal bones. Green: Bone anchors and sutures

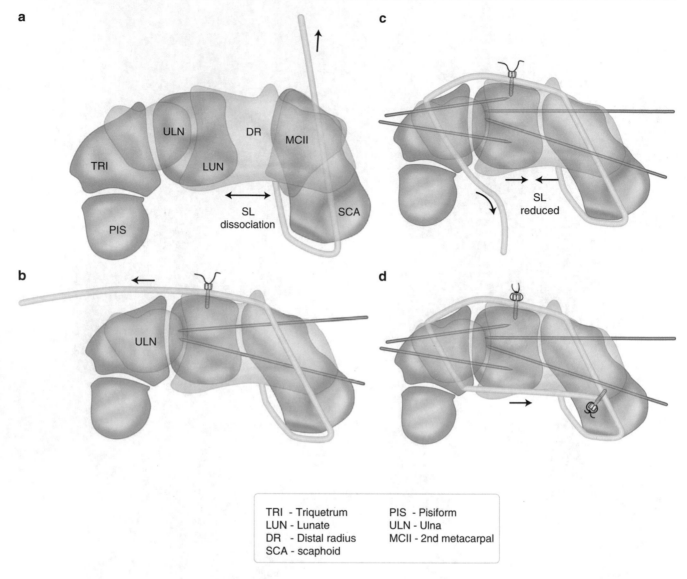

TRI - Triquetrum	PIS - Pisiform
LUN - Lunate	ULN - Ulna
DR - Distal radius	MCII - 2nd metacarpal
SCA - scaphoid	

Fig. 19.11 Schematic representation of the antipronation spiral tenodesis axial perspective. (**a**) FCR tendon strip (distally based) is passed from volar to distal through the scaphoid tunnel created. Note the dissociated SL joint. (**b**) After tensioning of the FCR tendon graft and subsequent reduction of the SL joint, the SL joint is stabilized with two K-wires. The FCR tendon graft traverses the dorsal surface of the lunate, inserted and held firmly onto the dorsal trough created at the dorsal surface with a bone anchor. (**c**) FCR tendon graft is passed through the triquetrum bone tunnel from dorsal to volar aspect, and the LT joint is stabilized with two K-wires. (**d**) FCR tendon graft is then passed deep to the flexor tendons of the digits on the floor of the carpal tunnel and held to the volar surface of the radial styloid by a bone anchor. Green: FCR tendon strip. Blue: K-wires

Assessment of the Wrist

As described in the 3LT procedure previously, the exposure of the dorsal wrist is the same for the spiral tenodesis procedure. Once the carpals are fully exposed after performing the dorsal capsulotomy, a thorough assessment of the articular cartilage status of both the radiocarpal and midcarpal joints as well as the reducibility of any existing carpal collapse or malalignment is made (Fig. 19.20). Likewise, the spiral tenodesis procedure is only recommended if the injured ligaments are irreparable, if the carpal collapse or malalignment is easily reducible and if the articular cartilage is intact.

Establishing the Scaphoid Tunnel

It is the same technique as described in the 3LT procedure.

Harvesting of the FCR Tendon Graft

Again, it is similar to the description for 3LT procedure.

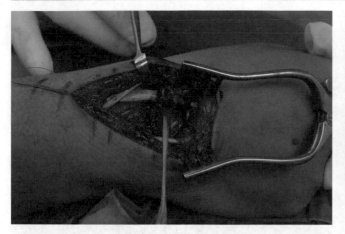

Fig. 19.12 Delivering the FCR graft through scaphoid tunnel

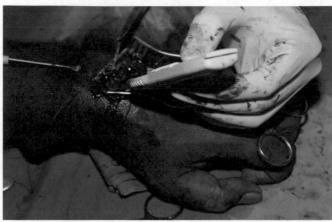

Fig. 19.15 Inserting bone anchor to the dorsum of the lunate

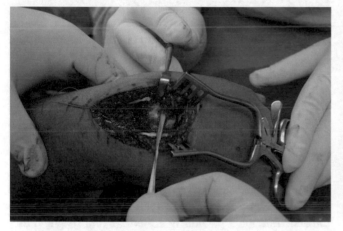

Fig. 19.13 FCR tendon graft across the lunate

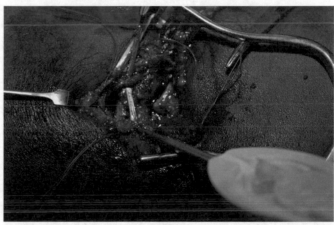

Fig. 19.16 FCR tendon graft placed across the lunate and pierce the DRC ligament

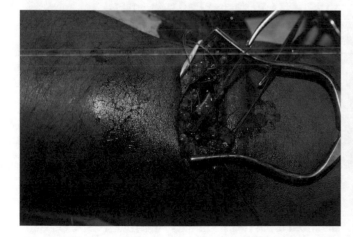

Fig. 19.14 FCR graft as it exits the scaphoid tunnel dorsally

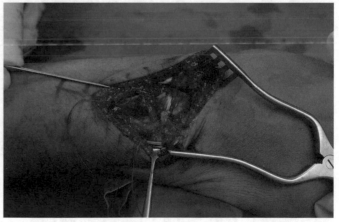

Fig. 19.17 FCR graft looped through the DRC and sutured back onto itself

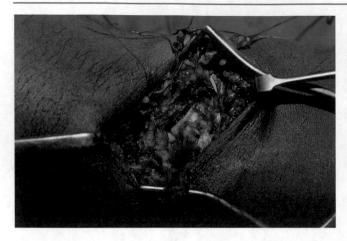

Fig. 19.18 FCR tendon graft folded back to the dorsum of lunate and sutured back down

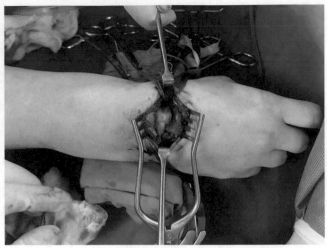

Fig. 19.20 ST—Exposure of dorsal proximal row after capsulotomy

length), the size of that tendon strip of graft is about 2.5 mm in diameter. The distally based strip of ECRL graft is brought from dorsal to volar aspect through the radial aspect of the scapho-trapezial-trapezoid (STT) joint. To aid with this, a small incision can be made over the anterolateral aspect of the scaphoid tuberosity. The capsule overlying the STT joint is pierced volarly and dorsally, and a tendon passer is placed through the capsulotomies created in the STT joint, from volar to dorsal. The distally based strip of the ECRL is then retrieved intracapsularly in a dorsal to volar fashion. Once emerging volarly from the STT joint, the tendon strip is then threaded through a previously drilled 2.7-mm scaphoid tunnel from the scaphoid tuberosity volarly to the dorsal proximal aspect of the scaphoid as previously described in the 3LT procedure (Figs. 19.21, 19.22, 19.23, 19.24, 19.25, 19.26, 19.27, 19.28, 19.29, 19.30 and 19.31).

Dorsal Aspect

A 3-mm transverse trough transversely across the dorsal surface of the lunate is made with a burr or rongeur till bleeding cancellous bone is seen (Fig. 19.32). A 1.8-mm suture anchor inserted into the center of the floor of the trough will be used later to ensure a close and direct contact between the strip of tendon graft and the cancellous bone of the dorsal lunate (Figs. 19.33 and 19.34).

Under fluoroscopic guidance, the SL joint is reduced and stabilized using two 1.5 mm K-wires (Fig. 19.35). One temporary K-wire each to the dorsum of the scaphoid and lunate can be used as joysticks to assist in the reduction process. It is therefore important to note at this point to ascertain if the carpal malalignment is easily reducible. If reduction of the carpal malalignment is difficult, involving a huge struggle, then it is very likely the procedure will not be successful.

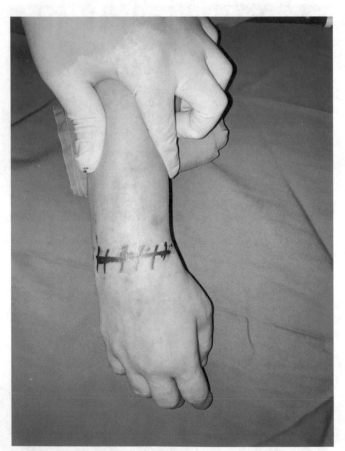

Fig. 19.19 ST—Skin incision—dorsal

Alternatively, Harvesting of the Extensor Carpi Radialis Longus (ECRL) Tendon Graft

A small transverse incision of about 2 cm is made about 15 cm proximal to the dorsum of the wrist overlying the ECRL. Once the ECRL tendon is identified and a distally based radial strip of the tendon is harvested (about 14 cm in

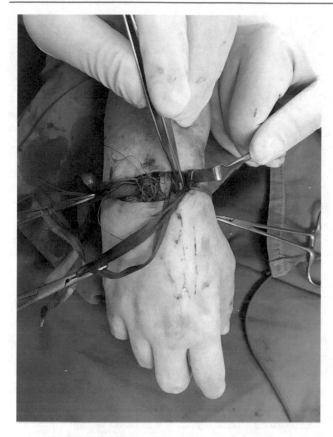

Fig. 19.21 ST—Identifying ECRL tendon

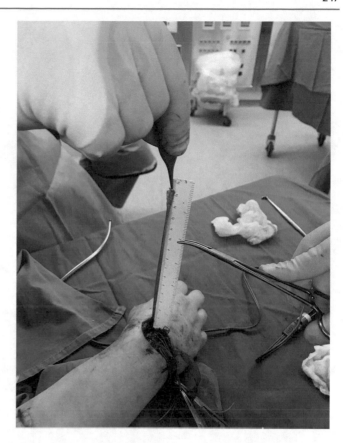

Fig. 19.23 ST—Note the length of ECRL tendon graft

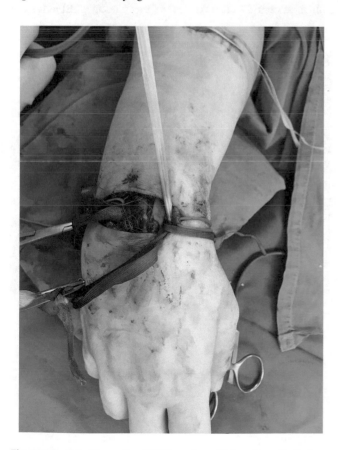

Fig. 19.22 ST—Harvesting ECRL tendon with insertion attached

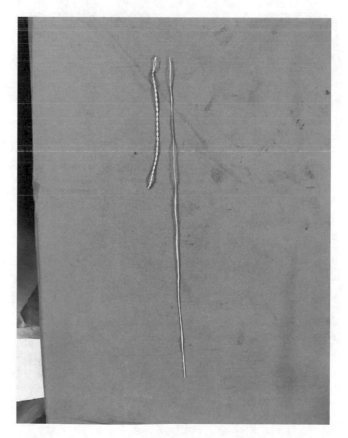

Fig. 19.24 ST—Fashioning the cerclage wire as a tendon passer

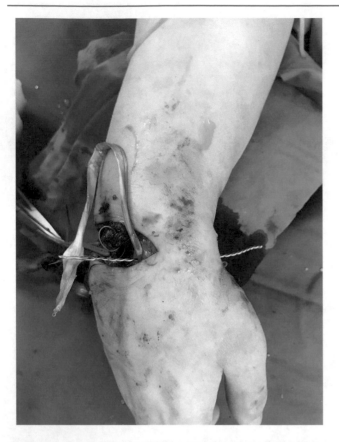

Fig. 19.25 ST—Deliver the ECRL volarly through the STT joint

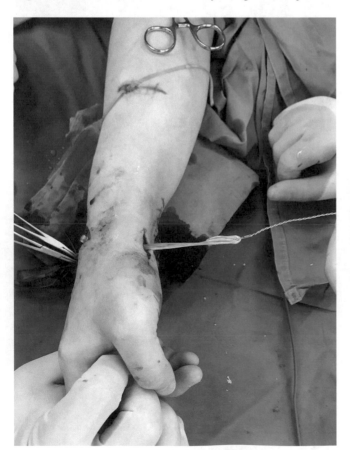

Fig. 19.26 ST—ECRL delivered volarly

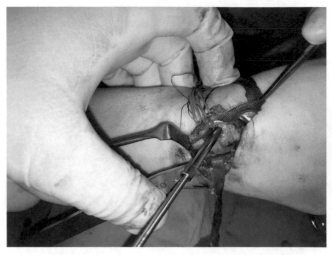

Fig. 19.27 ST—Drilling of scaphoid tunnel

At this critical point, if normal restoration of SL alignment is easily achieved, the spiral tenodesis procedure will proceed further; otherwise, a salvage procedure will have to be considered. It is therefore important to explain this possible situation to the patient during the consent-taking process prior to surgery.

Once the SL joint is properly reduced and stabilized with K-wires, the tendon graft is pulled ulnarly and the pre-set suture anchor is used to secure the tendon graft onto the

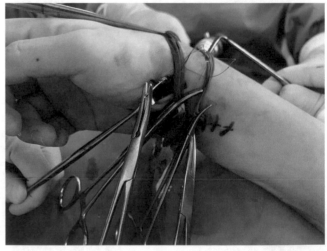

Fig. 19.28 ST—Scaphoid tunnel formed, drill emerging volarly

trough created at the dorsal lunate surface (Fig. 19.11b). This direct contact will promote the growth of Sharpey's fibers as described in the 3LT procedure [3, 19].

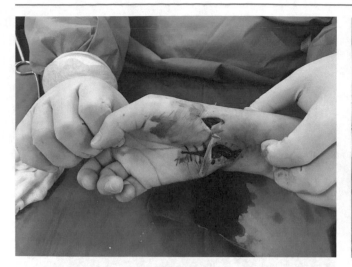

Fig. 19.29 ST—ECRL delivered dorsally through scaphoid tunnel

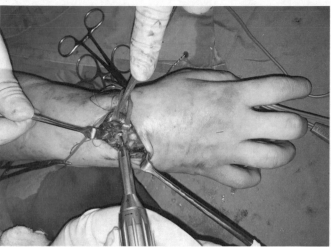

Fig. 19.31 ST—Decorticate dorsal lunate, expose cancellous bone

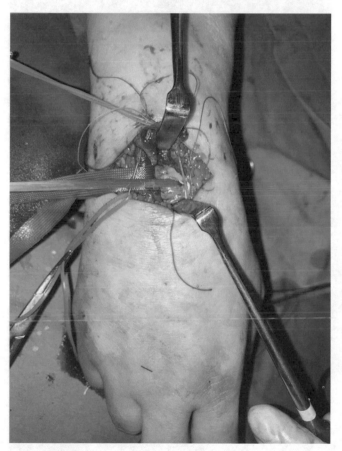

Fig. 19.30 ST—ECRL pass dorsally through scaphoid tunnel

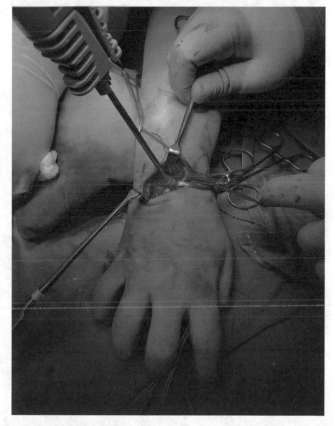

Fig. 19.32 ST—Insertion of bone anchor over dorsal lunate

Volar Aspect

A carpal tunnel incision is then made, following the axis of the ring finger and extending proximally in a zigzag fashion across the palmar wrist crease. The ulnar nerve and artery are identified and protected; the transverse carpal ligament is incised longitudinally exposing the carpal tunnel contents, which are retracted radially (Figs. 19.36 and 19.37). The area of the volar triquetrum just radial to the pisotriquetral (PT) joint is identified, and a guiding K-wire is driven across the bone, toward the dorsal ridge of the triquetrum under fluoroscopic guidance, and once the position and direction of the K-wire are satisfactory, a drill hole is made with a 2.7-mm cannulated drill bit establishing a triquetral

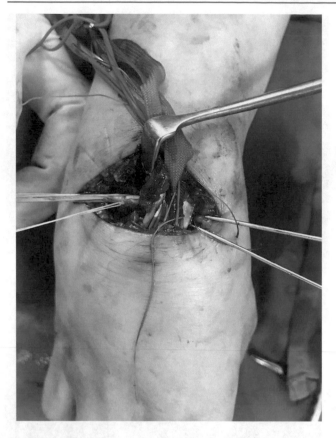

Fig. 19.33 ST—ECRL graft sutured onto the dorsal lunate

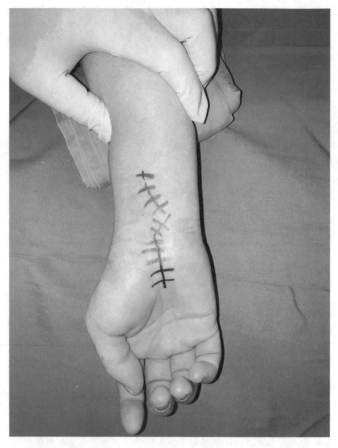

Fig. 19.35 ST—Skin incision marking—volar

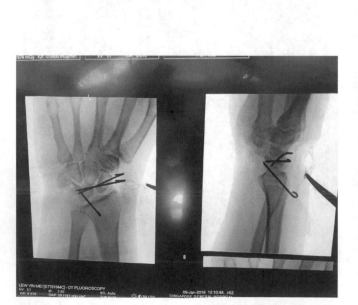

Fig. 19.34 ST—K-wires through SL joint and RL joint if needed

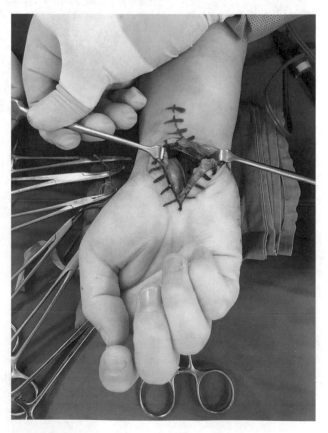

Fig. 19.36 ST—Volar incision and carpal tunnel release

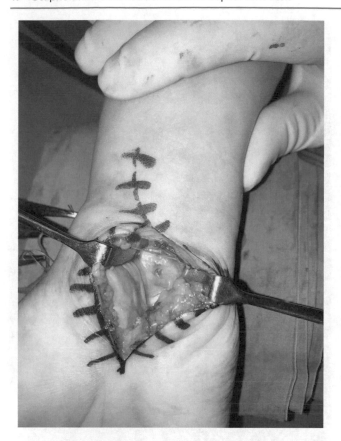

Fig. 19.37 ST—Creation of the triquetral tunnel volarly

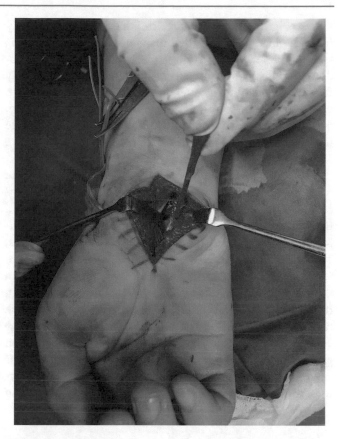

Fig. 19.39 ST—ECRL emerging volarly through triquetral tunnel

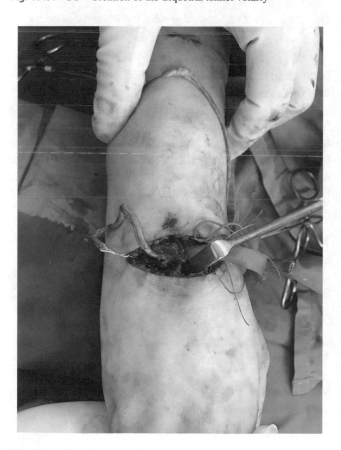

Fig. 19.38 ST—Passage of ECRL from dorsal to volar

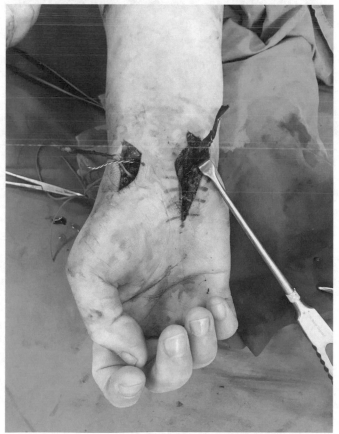

Fig. 19.40 ST—ECRL graft looped through cerclage wire

tunnel (Fig. 19.38). Again, the drilling has to be done slowly in a sustained and controlled manner, also ensuring care is taken to protect the overlying ulnarly situated extensor tendons during this step when the drill bit emerges dorsally from the triquetrum. The tendon strip is then inserted from dorsal to volar through the triquetral tunnel with a wire loop, and the LT joint is then stabilized with two K-wires, while maintaining the tendon strip under tension (Figs. 19.11c, 19.39 and 19.40).

A curved artery forceps clamp is then used to pass the tendon graft from the carpal tunnel incision to the anterolateral incision established earlier in the surgery (scaphoid tuberosity to radial styloid), under the carpal tunnel contents, following the distal edge of the radius (Figs. 19.11d, 19.41 and 19.42). Utmost care is taken to identify and protect the radial artery during this part of the procedure. When the tendon graft is at the volar aspect of the radial styloid, the tendon graft can be attached to the palmar aspect of the radial styloid by means of a suture anchor or an interference screw (Fig. 19.43). Alternatively, if the strip of tendon graft is long enough, it may be threaded through another 2.7-mm oblique bone tunnel, created from volar radial styloid to the dorsum, aiming at the floor of the second

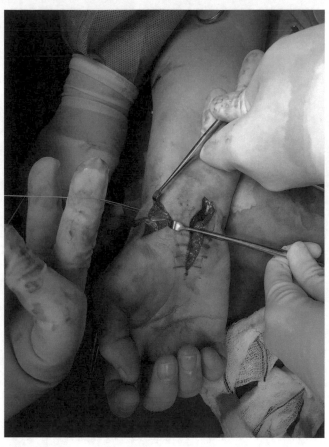

Fig. 19.42 ST—ECRL sutured to radial styloid via suture anchor

compartment, where it is attached firmly to the Lister tubercle with trans-osseous sutures.

The dorsal capsular flap is reconstituted, and the split fibers of the DRC and the DIC ligaments are repaired. Sutures are placed through the capsular flap onto the tendon graft to restore the normal capsular insertion to the dorsum of the SL joint. The extensor retinaculum is reconstituted, drains inserted, and skin closure is done.

At the End of Surgery

It is similar to the 3LT procedure with the only difference is the removal of the stabilizing K-wires across the SL and LT joints, again at 6 weeks post-surgery.

Tips and Tricks

We would like to highlight some important considerations and maneuvers to facilitate smoother and safer surgery. They can be summarized as follows:

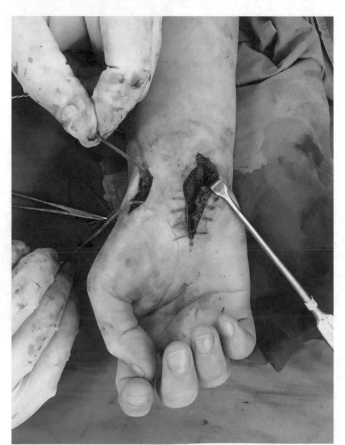

Fig. 19.41 ST—ECRL delivered radially deep to FDP tendons

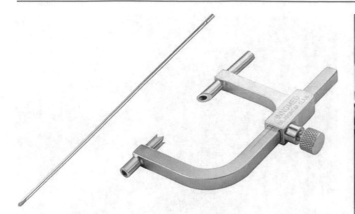

Fig. 19.43 Argintar claw drill guide and wire

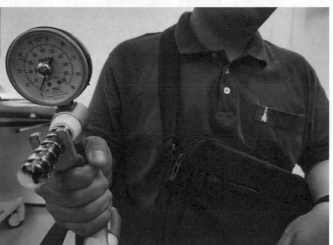

Fig. 19.45 3LT—Grip strength operated side

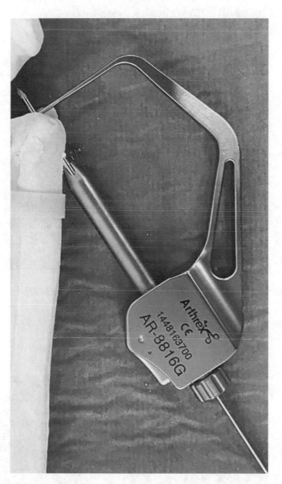

Fig. 19.44 Wrist drill guide and sleeve

Reduction of Carpal Bones Use temporary K-wires drilled perpendicularly at the dorsal proximal row bones to act as joysticks for reduction. Ensure that adequate and sustained tensions are applied onto the tendon graft to facilitate reduc-

tion. Care to not over-tension as it may over-correct the carpal alignment.

Creation of Tunnels There are commercial drill guides and jigs available, such as the Innomed® Argintar Claw Drill Guide (Fig. 19.44) and the Arthrex® Wrist Drill Guide and Sleeve (Fig. 19.45), invented by Dr. Toshiyasu Nakamura, that can be used to facilitate accurate placement for guide wire and subsequent tunnel creation. Such guides are especially useful for minimally invasive adaptation for such procedures.

In the original paper by Garcia-Elias et al. [3], a 3.2-mm drill hole was created for the scaphoid tunnel but subsequently [19, 31], 2.7-mm drill hole has been found to be sufficient for the passage of the tendon graft of about one-third the diameter of the tendon comfortably through the tunnel of that size.

For the creation of triquetral tunnel, it is recommended to drill from volar to dorsal direction so as to visualize the ulnar neurovascular bundle at all times and protect them during the process. Also, the pisiform provides a consistent landmark for placement of the drill hole accurately just radial to the PT joint.

Using Movement to Facilitate Surgery Clean and drape above the elbow to allow unhindered prono-supination of the forearm as the procedures involve both volar and dorsal approaches. Flex the wrist to allow tendon graft to traverse easily along the floor of the carpal tunnel from the triquetral tunnel to the radial styloid for the spiral tenodesis procedure.

Handling of the Drill Adopt slow, sustained, and progressive drill speed to minimize thermal injuries to the bone tunnel and trauma to the overlying soft tissue. Assistant should apply sustained light irrigation to the spinning drill during tunneling to cool the drill bit.

Correct Placement of Drill Hole and Suture Anchors Always confirm with fluoroscopy and ensure that the carpal bones are reduced before commencing the drilling process and the suture anchor placement.

Bear in mind the position of the stabilizing K-wires so as not to interfere or cross path with the drill holes and tunnel position later during surgery.

Ensure that the correct cannulated drill matches and fits the corresponding guide K-wires prior to guide wire placement to the bone.

Avoid creating the scaphoid drill hole too proximally, not to be too close to the SLIL ligament attachment as it may increase the chance of avascularity to the proximal pole [38, 39].

During Harvesting of Graft Sometimes consider additional transverse incisions in distal forearm to deliver the FCR tendon graft especially previous injuries or pre-existing scars seen along the course of the FCR.

Recently, the use of extensor carpi radialis longus (ECRL) as tendon graft has been advocated over FCR for the following reasons: ECRL gives a longer graft length (average of 14 cm versus 11 cm for FCR); through entering the lateral corner of the STT joint, it resists pronation of the scaphoid better [31, 40, 41] and also preserving the FCR, which is an important dynamic stabilizer of the scaphoid [36, 37]. Care has to be taken during the harvesting to avoid injury to the dorsal branches of the superficial radial nerve [31].

Conclusion

SLD presents as a spectrum, and each patient presenting with such a condition should undergo a careful and thorough assessment so as to be corrected diagnosed and staged. Patients with stage 3 or 4 SLD according to the treatment algorithm succinctly thought out and articulated by Gracia-Elias et al. will benefit from the 3 LT procedure [3] (Figs. 19.46, 19.47, 19.48, 19.49, 19.50, 19.51, 19.52, 19.53, 19.54, 19.55 and 19.56). However, there are patients who present with a more severe form of self-reduced chronic peri-

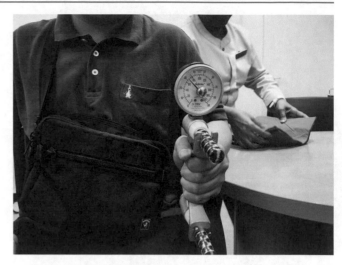

Fig. 19.46 3LT—Grip strength non-operated side

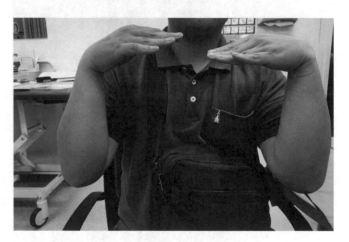

Fig. 19.47 3LT—Wrist flexion (right side operated)

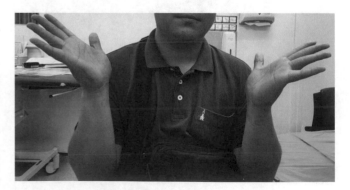

Fig. 19.48 3LT—Wrist extension (right side operated)

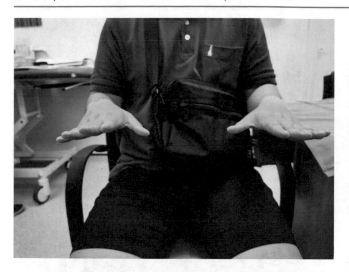

Fig. 19.49 3LT—Pronation

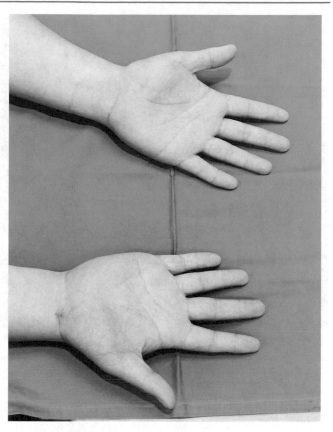

Fig. 19.52 3LT—Volar view

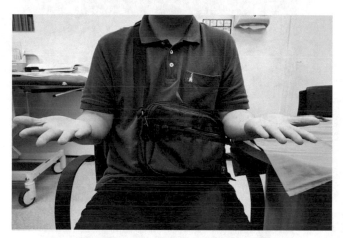

Fig. 19.50 3LT—Supination

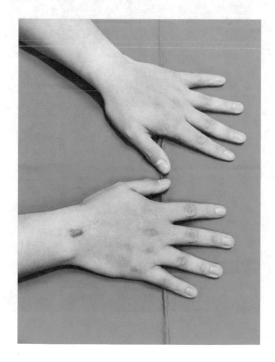

Fig. 19.51 3LT—Dorsal view

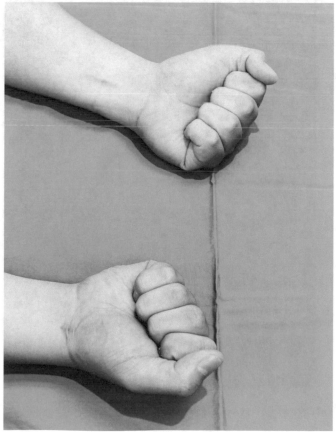

Fig. 19.53 3LT—Fist view

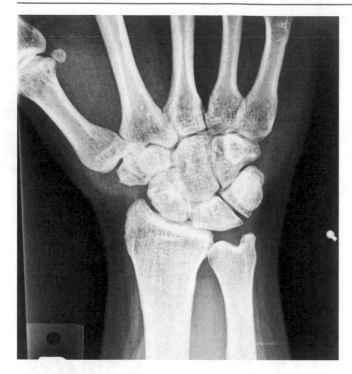

Fig. 19.54 Five years, 11 months post-op X-ray PA view

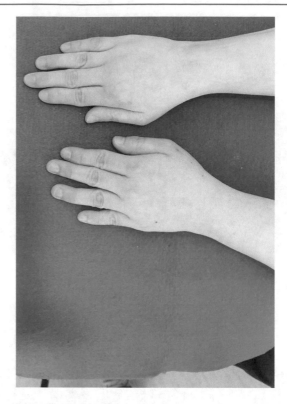

Fig. 19.56 ST—Dorsal view

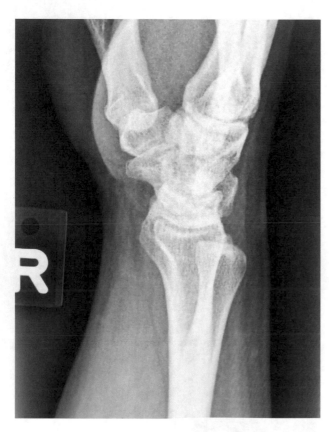

Fig. 19.55 Five years, 11 months post-op lateral view

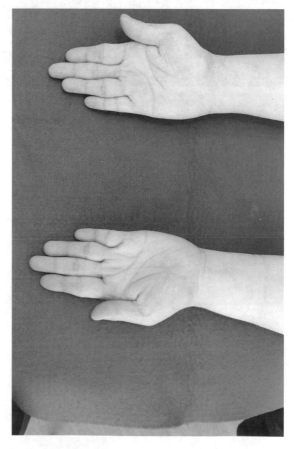

Fig. 19.57 ST—Volar view

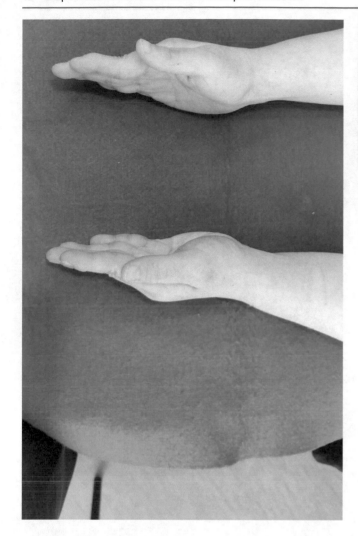

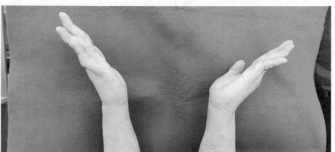

Fig. 19.59 ST—Extension of wrists

Fig. 19.58 ST—Lateral view

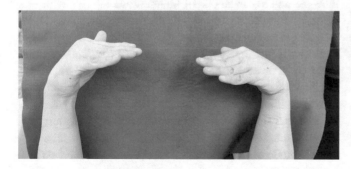

Fig. 19.60 ST—Flexion of wrists

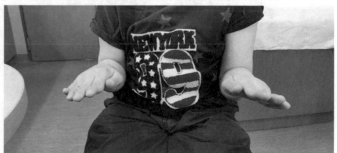

Fig. 19.61 ST—Pronation of the forearms

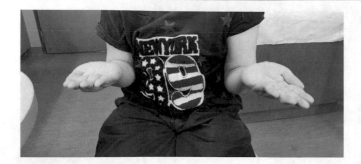

Fig. 19.62 ST—Supination of the forearms

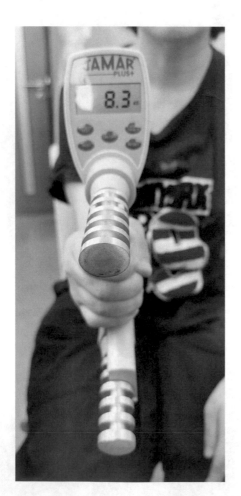

Fig. 19.63 ST—Right grip strength

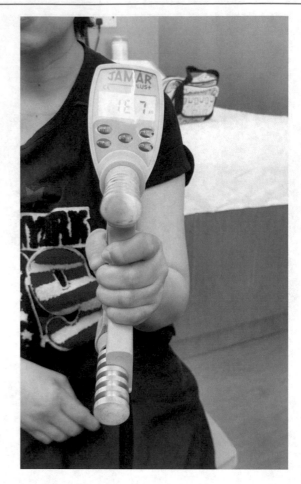

Fig. 19.64 ST—Left grip strength

lunate dislocation with a predominant SL injury component. Such patients may be misdiagnosed as stage 4 SLD and treated inappropriately with 3LT procedure with poor results. Such injuries, usually high velocity in nature, will have both intrinsic and extrinsic carpal ligamentous injuries with loss of functioning secondary stabilizers. Such patients will need to undergo a more extensive spiral tenodesis procedure to address the incompetent ligaments and the secondary stabilizers for a favorable outcome [19, 31] (Figs. 19.57, 19.58, 19.59, 19.60, 19.61, 19.62, 19.63, and 19.64). For both procedures, although there are some commonalities, especially in the initial stages such as the harvesting of the tendon graft and the dorsal exposure, the surgeon still has to be cognizant of the unique differences and nuances between the two procedures to ensure safe and optimal outcomes.

References

1. Kuo CE, Wolfe SW. Scapholunate instability: current concepts in diagnosis and management. J Hand Surg Am. 2008;33:998–1013.

2. Kitay A, Wolfe SW. Scapholunate instability: current concepts in diagnosis and management. J Hand Surg Am. 2012;37(10):2175–96.
3. Garcia-Elias M, Lluch AL, Stanley JK. Three-ligament tenodesis for the treatment of scapholunate dissociation: indications and surgical technique. J Hand Surg Am. 2006;31A:125–34.
4. Short WH, Werner FW, Green JK, Masaoka S. Biomechanical evaluation of ligamentous stabilizers of the scaphoid and lunate. J Hand Surg Am. 2002;27(6):991–1002.
5. Rainbow MJ, Wolff AL, Crisco JJ, Wolfe SW. Functional kinematics of the wrist. J Hand Surg Eur Vol. 2016;41(1):7–21.
6. Pomerance J. Outcome after repair of the scapholunate interosseous ligament and dorsal capsulodesis for dynamic scapholunate instability due to trauma. J Hand Surg Am. 2006;31(8):1380–6.
7. Watson HK, Weinzweig J, Zeppieri J. The natural progression of scaphoid instability. Hand Clin. 1997;13:39–49.
8. Weiss KE, Rodner CM. Osteoarthritis of the wrist. J Hand Surg Am. 2007;32:725–46.
9. Sokolow C, Saffar P. Anatomy and histology of the scapholunate ligament. Hand Clin. 2001;17(1):77–81.
10. Berger RA, Imaeda T, Berglund L, An KN. Constraint and material properties of the subregions of the scapholunate interosseous ligament. J Hand Surg Am. 1999;24A.953–62.
11. Berger RA. The gross and histologic anatomy of the scapholunate interosseous ligament. J Hand Surg Am. 1996;21(2):170–8.
12. Berger RA, Blair WF, Crowninshield RD, Flatt AE. The scapholunate ligament. J Hand Surg Am. 1982;7(1):87–91.
13. Darlis NA, Weiser RW, Sotereanos DG. Partial scapholunate ligament injuries treated with arthroscopic debridement and thermal shrinkage. J Hand Surg Am. 2005;30(5):908–14.
14. Darlis NA, Kaufmann RA, Giannoulis F, Sotereanos DG. Arthroscopic debridement and closed pinning for chronic dynamic scapholunate instability. J Hand Surg Am. 2006;31(3):418–24.
15. Moran SL, Cooney WP, Berger RA, Strickland J. Capsulodesis for the treatment of chronic scapholunate instability. J Hand Surg Am. 2005;30(1):16–23.
16. Szabo RM. Scapholunate ligament repair with capsulodesis reinforcement. J Hand Surg Am. 2008;33(9):1645–54.
17. Brunelli GA, Brunelli GR. A new technique to correct carpal instability with scaphoid rotary subluxation: a preliminary report. J Hand Surg Am. 1995;20(3 Pt 2):S82–5.
18. Henry M. Reconstruction of both volar and dorsal limbs of the scapholunate interosseous ligament. J Hand Surg Am. 2013;38(8):1625–34.
19. Chee KG, Chin AY, Chew EM, Garcia-Elias M. Antipronation spiral tenodesis—a surgical technique for the treatment of perilunate instability. J Hand Surg Am. 2012;37(12):2611–8.
20. Talwalkar SC, Edwards AT, Hayton MJ, Stilwell JH, Trail IA, Stanley JK. Results of tri-ligament tenodesis: a modified Brunelli procedure in the management of scapholunate instability. J Hand Surg. 2006;31B:110–7.

21. Van Den Abbeele KL, Loh YC, Stanley JK, Trail IA. Early results of a modified Brunelli procedure for scapholunate instability. J Hand Surg. 1998;23B:258–61.
22. De Smet L, Van Hoonacker P. Treatment of chronic static scapholunate dissociation with the modified Brunelli technique: preliminary results. Acta Orthop Belg. 2007;73:188–91.
23. Weiss APC. Scapholunate ligament reconstruction using a bone-retinaculum-bone autograft. J Hand Surg Am. 1998;23A:205–15.
24. Harvey EJ, Hanel DP. Bone-ligament-bone reconstruction for scapholunate disruption. Tech Hand Upper Extrem Surg. 2002;6:2–5.
25. Rosenwasser MP, Miyasajsa KC, Strauch RJ. The RASL procedure: reduction and association of the scaphoid and lunate using the Herbert screw. Tech Hand Up Extrem Surg. 1997;1(4):263–72.
26. Aviles AJ, Lee SK, Hausman MR. Arthroscopic reduction-association of the scapholunate. Arthroscopy. 2007;23(1):105. e1–5.
27. Yao J, Zlotolow DA, Lee SK. ScaphoLunate axis method. J Wrist Surg. 2016;5(1):59–66.
28. Watson HK, Ryu J, Akelman E. Limited triscaphoid intercarpal arthrodesis for rotatory subluxation of the scaphoid. J Bone Joint Surg. 1986;68A:345–9.
29. Watson HK, Weinzweig J, Guidera PM, Zeppieri J, Ashmead D. One thousand intercarpal arthrodeses. J Hand Surg. 1999;24B:307–15.
30. Young Szalay MD, Peimer CA. Scaphocapitate arthrodesis. Tech Hand Upper Extrem Surg. 2002;6:56–60.
31. Kakar S, Green RM, Garcia-Elias M. Carpal realignment using a strip of extensor carpi radialis longus tendon. J Hand Surg Am. 2017;42(8):667. e1–8.
32. Taleisnik J. The wrist. New York: Churchill Livingstone; 1985.
33. Berger RA, Bishop AT, Bettinger PC. New dorsal capsulotomy for the surgical exposure of the wrist. Ann Plast Surg. 1995;35:54–9.
34. Hagert E, Ferreres A, Garcia-Elias M. Nerve-sparing dorsal and volar approaches to the radiocarpal joint. J Hand Surg Am. 2010;35A:1070–4.
35. Hagert E, Garcia-Elias M, Forsgren S, Ljung BO. Immunohistochemical analysis of wrist ligament innervation in relation to their structural composition. J Hand Surg Am. 2007;32A:30–6.
36. Salva-Coll G, Garcia-Elias M, Llusa-Perez M, Rodriguez-Baeza A. The role of the flexor carpi radialis muscle in scapholunate instability. J Hand Surg Am. 2011;36A:31–6.
37. Salva-Coll G, Garcia-Elias M, Hagert E. Scapholunate instability: proprioception and neuromuscular control. J Wrist Surg. 2013;2(2):136–40.
38. Taleisnik J, Kelly PJ. The blood supply of scaphoid (carpal navicular). Surg Forum. 1966;17:457–9.
39. Taleisnik J, Kelly PJ. The extraosseous and intraosseous blood supply of the scaphoid bone. J Bone Joint Surg Am. 1966;48(6):1125–37.
40. Petersen SL, Freeland AE. Scapholunate stabilization with dynamic extensor carpi radialis longus tendon transfer. J Hand Surg Am. 2010;35(12):2093–100.
41. Lieber RL, Fazeli BM, Botte MJ. Architecture of selected wrist flexor and extensor muscles. J Hand Surg Am. 1990;15(2):244–50.

RASL Procedure

Seth C. Shoap, Chia H. Wu, Christina E. Freibott,
and Melvin P. Rosenwasser

Introduction

Scapholunate instability is caused by injury to the scapholunate interosseous ligament (SLIL) as well as important secondary intercarpal ligaments such as the dorsal intercarpal, DIC, and the scapho-trapezial, ST, which when incompetent result in this most common type of carpal instability. SLIL injury typically occurs after a fall onto an extended wrist. The combination of axial load, wrist extension, intercarpal supination, and ulnar deviation leads to supraphysiologic loads across the SLIL. Motions of the scaphoid and lunate are linked, such that both bones flex with wrist flexion and radial deviation and extend with wrist extension and ulnar deviation [1]. When disruption of the SLIL occurs, this relative motion between the scaphoid and lunate is no longer linked, causing the scaphoid to flex while the lunate extends [2]. Increased scaphoid flexion creates stress concentration at the radial styloid–scaphoid articulation, leading to scapholunate advanced collapse (SLAC) and osteoarthritis [3]. The extension of the dissociated lunate and scapholunate diastasis is the manifestation of dorsal intercalated segment instability (DISI) and can progress to proximal migration of the capitate and altered kinematics. This can lead to pain, weakness, limitation of wrist motion, and progressive arthritis. Static DISI prior to the onset of osteoarthritis at the capitolunate joint can be corrected with the motion-sparing reduction and association of the scaphoid and lunate (RASL) procedure.

In treating scapholunate dissociation, reconstructions that preserve the motion between the two bones are more physiologic. It has been determined that there are 25 degrees of obligatory physiologic intercarpal rotation between the scaphoid and lunate with wrist flexion and extension, and 10 degrees of rotation with radial and ulnar deviations [4]. Any reconstruction technique must neutralize the forces which result in deformity, while preserving physiologic range of motion. These deforming forces have proven too great for tenodesis weaving techniques even with adjunctive Kirschner wire fixation. The RASL procedure utilizes a headless compression screw with a smooth central shaft in order to stabilize the realigned or re-associated scapholunate articulation. The procedure requires a dechondrification of the scapholunate interface so that a fibrous neoligament may form to provide stability. A few critical technical aspects for achieving favorable functional outcomes when performing the RASL procedure include open radial styloidectomy, and appropriate screw trajectory. Studies have shown that screw trajectory in the RASL procedure is highly predictive of long-term subjective and objective outcomes [5, 6]. The radial styloidectomy is essential regardless of the presence or absence of SLAC 1 radiostyloscaphoid impingement changes. The styloidectomy allows for access to the critical starting point on the carpal scaphoid which is proximal to the dorsolateral ridge. This then allows the trajectory of the screw to be relatively parallel to the radiocarpal inclination and makes targeting in the central to slightly palmar access of the sagittal view of the lunate possible.

Indications

The RASL is primarily indicated for symptomatic subacute to chronic SL dissociation before progression to advanced SLAC arthritis, Grade 3, capitolunate osteoarthritis. Common indications include chronic static DISI deformity, without osteoarthritic involvement of the capitolunate joint. Most of

S. C. Shoap · C. E. Freibott (✉) · M. P. Rosenwasser
Department of Orthopedic Surgery, Columbia University Irving Medical Center, New York, NY, USA
e-mail: scs2217@columbia.edu; cef2141@cumc.columbia.edu; mpr2@cumc.columbia.edu

C. H. Wu
Department of Orthopedic Surgery, Baylor College of Medicine, Houston, TX, USA
e-mail: chia.wu@bcm.edu

© Springer Nature Switzerland AG 2022
W. B. Geissler (ed.), *Wrist and Elbow Arthroscopy with Selected Open Procedures*,
https://doi.org/10.1007/978-3-030-78881-0_20

the injuries on first presentation represent an acute-on-chronic injury pattern leading to the symptomatic DISI deformity. Since the age of the injury can never be assured by the history alone, it cannot be presumed that the integrity and quality of the remnants of scapholunate ligament are reparable by suture or ligament augment techniques [7]. Most patients who present with chronic static SL dissociation cannot recall a specific wrist injury. In reality they have experienced a series of minor wrist sprains, culminating with one final event that exacerbates the symptoms, causing them to seek treatment [8].

Radiographic evaluation is a useful tool in detecting the presence of SLIL injury. In addition to neutral PA, lateral, and oblique views, it is essential to perform PA views in ulnar and radial deviations, as well as a clenched fist PA view in pronation. A scapholunate diastasis that is greater than 3 mm (Fig. 20.1a) may indicate the need for intervention. However, it is crucial to make a comparison to the contralateral side to ensure this is not due to a patient's inherent ligament laxity. It is also important to look for a scaphoid cortical ring sign (see Fig. 20.1a), a scapholunate angle greater than 60 degrees (Figs. 20.1b and 20.2), and a DISI deformity pattern, marked by capitate dorsal translation and decreased carpal height measurements [8]. Plain radiography even with stress views may not uncover the presence of SLIL injury in patients with dynamic instability. Advanced imaging such as MRI with and without contrast and/or arthroscopic evaluation may be necessary.

Physical examinations typically reveal tenderness dorsally, localizing to the scapholunate ligament. Wrist palpation revealing tenderness and pain with end range flexion and extension can correspond to dorsal capsular synovitis, instability, and chondral wear. A corroborating provocative test is the Watson scaphoid shift test, in which a positive test demonstrates dorsal wrist pain with a proximal pole scaphoid reduction clunk that is consistent with SLIL instability. However, it should be noted that a false-positive result may occur in 20% of normal wrists and probably reflects generalized collagen laxity and should be compared to the contralateral wrist [9].

Contraindications

The major contraindication for the RASL procedure is scapholunate advanced collapse (SLAC) osteoarthritis, specifically Stage 3 when the capitolunate articulation is involved. Usually, advanced SLAC is determined by plain X-rays although MRI may be helpful in determining early subchondral edema and cysts indicative of the osteoarthritic process. If there is any question of the integrity of the capitolunate articulation, then a diagnostic arthroscopy can be performed prior or at the same surgical setting as the RASL procedure. Should significant cartilage wear be documented, then alternative salvage procedures should be considered such as a proximal row carpectomy or a limited carpal fusion.

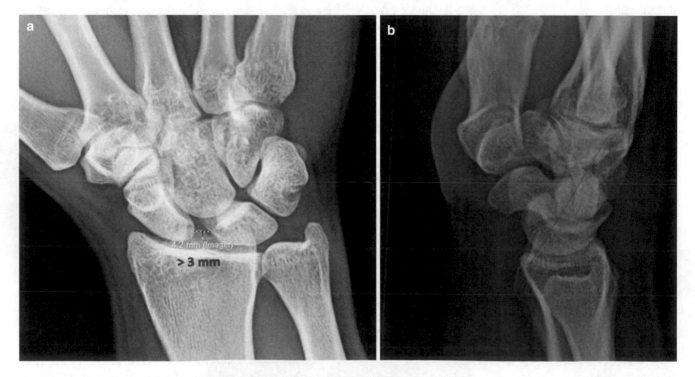

Fig. 20.1 (a) A widened scapholunate interval (>3 mm) and a scaphoid cortical ring sign can be seen on the AP view of the wrist. (b) An obtuse scapholunate angle (>60 degrees) is appreciated on a lateral view of the wrist

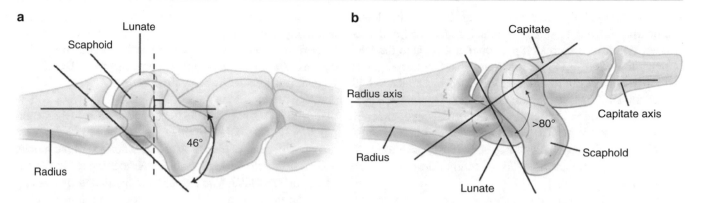

Fig. 20.2 (**a**) The scapholunate angle normally measures 46 degrees with the wrist in neutral position. (**b**) DISI occurs as a result of lunate extension. Consequently, the capitate and distal row migrate proximally and translate dorsally

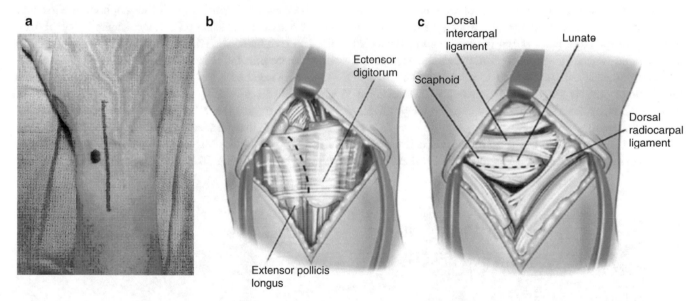

Fig. 20.3 (**a**) A dorsal midline longitudinal incision is made just ulnar to the tubercle of Lister. (**b**) An oblique incision is made through the extensor retinaculum parallel to the EPL tendon. The EPL is retracted radially, and the fourth compartment tendons are retracted ulnarly. (**c**) A transverse incision is made through the dorsal wrist capsule parallel and proximal to the dorsal intercarpal ligament. The DRC ligament is identified and preserved. A second distal window again parallel to the DIC allows inspection of the midcarpal joint

The presence of arthritis at the radial styloid–scaphoid joint, SLAC 1, is not considered a contraindication because a radial styloidectomy is required as part of the RASL procedure. The RASL procedure is for chronic static dorsal intercalated segmented instability patterns, DISI.

Acute injuries may be treated with primary ligament repair and protected with either multiple divergent Kirschner wires of a temporarily placed trans-osseous SL headless bone screw.

Technique in Detail

The procedure is typically performed under either regional or general anesthesia. Patient is in the supine position with the forearm placed pronated with dorsum up on the hand table. Prophylactic antibiotics are administered. Exsanguination with an elastic bandage is followed by inflation of a pneumatic tourniquet on the upper arm. Image intensification is used during the procedure.

For the exposure, a 6-cm longitudinal incision is made on the dorsal wrist, staying just ulnar to the tubercle of Lister (Fig. 20.3a). Soft tissue is bluntly dissected down to the level of the extensor retinaculum, taking care to preserve dorsal veins and cutaneous nerve branches wherever possible. Next, the extensor retinaculum is incised obliquely, parallel to the course of the extensor pollicis longus (EPL) tendon (Fig. 20.3b). The third and fourth extensor compartments are released allowing the EPL to be retracted radially, and the fourth compartment extensor tendons are retracted ulnarly.

A transverse incision through the dorsal wrist capsule is made, with the intention to stay parallel and proximal to the dorsal intercarpal ligament (DIC) (Fig. 20.3c). The dorsal radiocarpal (DRC) ligament should be identified and preserved. Windows are created proximal and distal to the DIC which allow exposure to the radiocarpal and midcarpal joints without the necessity to reflect a V-shaped flap which would detach the DIC. The scapholunate juncture is visualized as is the disruption of the scapholunate interosseous ligaments. Radiocarpal and midcarpal joint surfaces can be inspected for chondral damage. As stated previously, capitolunate arthritis with cartilage wear is a contraindication to the RASL procedure.

Attention is then turned to the midaxial radial wrist to perform a limited radial styloidectomy. A second 5-cm longitudinal incision is made in the midaxial line over the first dorsal compartment (Fig. 20.4a). It starts at 2 cm proximal to the styloid, extending distally to the level of the scapho-trapezial joint. The dorsal branch of the radial artery and the major branches of the superficial radial nerve should be protected and isolated with a vessel loop. A first dorsal compartment retinaculum release is performed to allow for retraction of the abductor pollicis longus and extensor pollicis brevis tendons dorsally. Incise the radiocarpal capsule longitudinally exposing the radial styloid (Fig. 20.4b).

The periosteum overlying the radial styloid is elevated, and an osteotome is used to perform a radial styloidectomy.

Amount of radial styloid removed should be just enough to avoid impingement with radial deviation of the wrist, visualization for proper headless screw starting point, and preservation of the volar radioscaphocapitate ligament. This should be confirmed visually and by fluoroscopy.

Once the carpus is exposed, 2.062 Kirschner wires will be placed as joysticks one in the lunate and another in the scaphoid (Fig. 20.5a). The Kirschner wire is placed in the most proximal portion of the exposed dorsal surface of the lunate, angled from proximal to distal in order to bring the lunate out of extension. This lunate reduction is facilitated by pushing down on the capitate which will derotate the lunate out of extension. A second Kirschner wire may need to be placed, and the above step is repeated if full reduction into neutral of the lunate is not obtained.

To correct the hyperflexion of the scaphoid, a Kirschner wire is placed in the distal pole of the scaphoid angled from distal to proximal. The Kirschner wires must not end up in the ultimate planned axis of the headless bone screw. The scaphoid wire should be distal to this path, and the lunate wire should be proximal.

In order to generate a healing response at the scapholunate interface, it is mandatory to remove the articular cartilage at the interface of the scapholunate joint using a side-cutting burr (Fig. 20.5b), or curettes and the joysticks

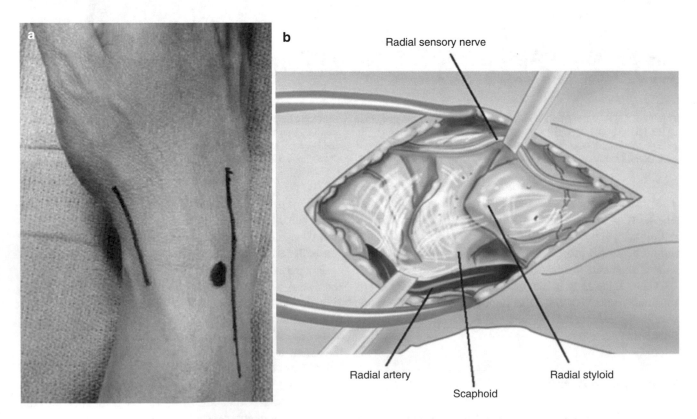

Fig. 20.4 (a) A longitudinal incision is made over the first dorsal extensor compartment. (b) The first compartment is released, and a longitudinal incision is made down to the radial styloid

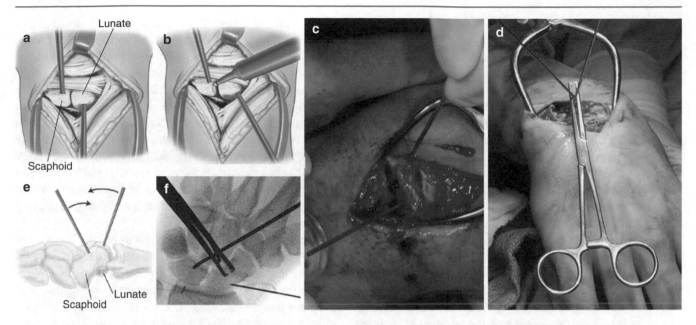

Fig. 20.5 (a) 0.062-inch Kirschner wires are placed in the lunate and scaphoid to serve as joysticks. (b) A side-cutting burr is used to remove the cartilage within the scapholunate joint. (c, e) The joysticks are used to extend the scaphoid and to flex the lunate. (d) A Kocher clamp is used to hold the reduction. (f) The reduction is verified with an image intensifier

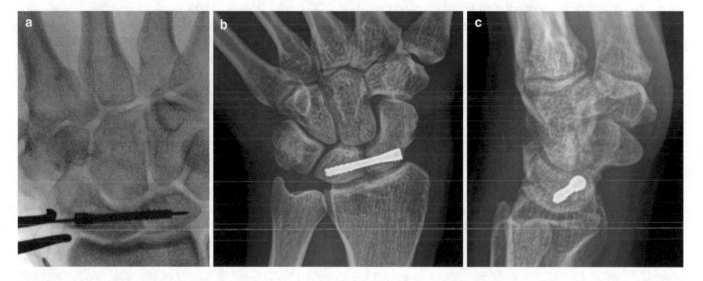

Fig. 20.6 (a) The insertion angle of the headless bone screw should be roughly parallel to the radial inclination of 20 degrees. (b, c) Eight-month follow-up demonstrating stable alignment and ideal screw positioning

can be used to separate the two bones to enhance this process. It is critical to continue to protect the capitate cartilage during this step. Depth of dechondrification should proceed until punctate bleeding in cancellous bone is visualized.

Reduction is performed by derotation of the scaphoid and lunate utilizing the joysticks which are then stabilized by applying a Kocher clamp across the joysticks (Fig. 20.5c, d, e). The reduction can be visually assessed and verified by fluoroscopy (Fig. 20.5f).

Once reduction is achieved, a cannulated headless screw with a smooth central shank is used to secure the reduction,

aiming for the center axis of rotation of the lunate. Continuously threaded variable pitch headless screw is contraindicated. First, start the guidewire through the radial midaxial incision previously made while being careful that the starting point should at or proximal to the dorsal lateral ridge of the scaphoid on PA view of the wrist. The angle of inclination should roughly match the radial inclination of the distal radius (Fig. 20.6a). The termination of the guidewire should aim for medial corner of the reduced lunate. On the sagittal view, the target is center or slightly palmar to center in the lunate. This is critically important to stability of the reduction and implant. The screw must not be placed dorsally in the lunate (Fig. 20.6b, c). Proper trajectory is critical for the restoration of wrist mechanics.

Once guidewire position is confirmed, use a cannulated drill by hand power to prevent binding and possible breakage of the 1-mm wire. As previously mentioned, if the joystick Kirschner wires seem to be impeding the exact placement of the guidewire, then one or both of the joystick wires will have to be repositioned.

Next, measure the screw length with cannulated guide or a second guidewire, and then subtract 4–6 mm for your final screw length so the screw will be completely buried. It is critical that one does not violate the lunotriquetral interosseous ligament. Correct placement should be confirmed by fluoroscopy.

Screw is then inserted by hand and carefully advanced so it is visually confirmed to be below the scaphoid chondral surface. Kocher clamp and the joystick wires can be removed at this point. After the Kocher clamp is released, you will note that the joystick wires do not move signifying stable fixation and alignment. As the screw is now holding the reduction, surgeon should check the stability of the scapholunate reduction while ranging the wrist. It is normal for differential rotation to exist between the scaphoid and lunate.

Once satisfied, tourniquet is released and hemostasis achieved using Bovie or bipolar electrocautery. The dorsal capsular incision is left open. Skin is closed using 5–0 nylon suture and a sterile bulky dressing as well as volar wrist splint applied.

another crucial aspect. Specifically, the axis of the screw should be directed toward the medial corner of the reduced lunate on the coronal view, and central to slightly palmar on the lateral view. If the screw is placed dorsal to the midsagittal line, eccentric screw motion will create excessive wobble or oscillation as the biomechanical axis of rotation was not restored. This will lead to accelerated bone resorption around the screw threads. The screw should also always be placed proximal to or at the dorsal lateral ridge of the scaphoid. It has been shown that screws placed distal to the lateral aspect of the dorsal scaphoid ridge are associated with failure when examined manually, radiographically, and using real-time motion capture [6].

During the procedure, it is critical to bur the interface of the scaphoid and lunate to remove articular cartilage, exposing bleeding cancellous bone to generate a vascular fibroblastic repair response. The resulting neoligamentous structure that forms at the interface is ultimately what provides for the durability of the reconstruction. Screw lucency is expected over time at the lunate end of the screw, but this will not result in scapholunate diastasis due to the soft tissue healing that occurs.

Kirschner wire joysticks must be carefully placed as a reduction tool in consideration of the screw trajectory. If the wires are placed in the center of the scaphoid and lunate, this will block the path of the guidewire and screw. To avoid this, the wires must be placed in the proximal ulnar corner of the lunate and the distal radial corner of the scaphoid, which provides a clear path for the guidewire and screw.

Tips and Tricks

Once the superficial radial sensory nerve branches are identified through the dorsal approach, it is important to avoid self-retaining retractors to prevent a traction neuropraxia. Through the radial approach, the dorsal radial artery must be identified distal to the screw insertion site before the screw is placed. A radial styloidectomy *is mandatory* to access the critical dorsal lateral scaphoid ridge starting point as well as removing radioscaphoid impingement. Sequential osteotomies are performed, one, extra-articular to visualize the scaphoid facet, and the second to titrate the osteotomy to preserve the volar radioscaphocapitate ligaments. It is important that just enough is removed to correct radioscaphoid impingement.

A screw with a smooth central shank is essential to the RASL procedure. The screw maintains reduction during soft tissue healing, while allowing for rotation. A fully threaded screw blocks scapholunate relative motion, which will result in screw breakage with normal rotation of the wrist [10]. In addition to screw type, screw placement especially the dorsal lateral ridge scaphoid starting point is

Conclusion

The RASL procedure is an effective approach to correct static scapholunate instability without midcarpal arthritis. In a clinical outcome's long-term follow-up study conducted by Rosenwasser et al., a cohort of 35 patients reported an average DASH score of 14.96 at 10.89 years of follow-up. The average VAS score was 0.5 out of 10 at rest, and 2.7 out of 10 with activity. The average flexion/extension arc of motion was 102 degrees (std. dev. 28.9, range, 55.0–160.0). This was compared to contralateral arc of motion of 118 degrees (std. dev. 31.9, range, 60.0–170.0), which was not significantly different (p = 0.138). Average radial and ulnar deviations were 19.3 degrees (std. dev. 7.90, range, 10.0–35.0) and 25.2 degrees (std. dev. 10.6, range, 10.0–47.0), respectively. These values were not significantly different from corresponding values on the contralateral uninjured side (p = 0.20 and p = 0.17, respectively). Average grip strength was 66.02 lb (std. dev. 19.6, range, 17.64–68.01), as compared to 79.18 lb (std. dev. 23.28, range, 44.09–123.33) on the contralateral side. This difference was statistically significant (p < 0.005) [9].

In a radiographic assessment of 29 RASL patients with an average follow-up of 6.6 years, we found that 20 patients with screws placed proximal to the dorsal lateral ridge of the scaphoid had an average DASH of 10.89, and 9 patients with the screw through or distal to the ridge had an average DASH of 20.83 [5]. There are a number of studies that have also demonstrated favorable results for this technique and have further highlighted the importance of screw placement [6, 7, 11–14].

Studies by Larson et al. and Aibinder et al. have stated that the RASL procedure is ineffective at providing stability about the SL interval and has a high rate of early failure and reoperation, respectively. However, neither reported performing radial styloidectomies, and both had inconsistent screw placement. Larson et al. had all of their screws inserted distal to the lateral dorsal ridge of the scaphoid, and Aibinder et al. reported that screw placement, "varied significantly in their cohort." Furthermore, Aibinder et al. used four different screws in their cohort of 12 [15, 16].

A critical technical aspect for achieving favorable functional outcomes when performing the RASL procedure is consistent and appropriate screw trajectory—specifically, screw placement in the mid- to slightly volar axis of the reduced lunate, in addition to a starting point proximal to the lateral ridge of the scaphoid. This trajectory, along with a radial styloidectomy for improved visualization, ensures an optimal starting point in the scaphoid. The discrepancies in patient outcomes seen in studies that do not adhere to these criteria further emphasize the importance of screw selection and trajectory in performing the RASL.

References

1. Garcias-Elias MGE. Carpal instability. In: Green DP, Hotchkiss RN, Pederson WC, editors. Green's operative hand surgery. 5th ed. Philadelphia: Elsevier/Churchill Livingstone; 2005.

2. Linscheid RL, Dobyns JH, Beckenbaugh RD, Cooney WP 3rd, Wood MB. Instability patterns of the wrist. J Hand Surg Am. 1983;8:682–6.

3. Watson HK, Ashmead D, Makhlouf MV. Examination of the scaphoid. J Hand Surg Am. 1988;13:657–60.

4. Ruby LK, Cooney WP 3rd, An KN, Linscheid RL, Chao EY. Relative motion of selected carpal bones: a kinematic analysis of the normal wrist. J Hand Surg Am. 1988;13:1–10.

5. Shoap SCNP, Freibott CE, Polzer H, Rosenwasser MP. Radiographic analysis to define optimal screw placement in the reduction and association of the scapholunate (RASL) procedure. New York: Columbia University Department of Orthopaedic Surgery; 2019.

6. Koehler SM, Beck CM, Nasser P, Gluck M, Hausman MR. The effect of screw trajectory for the reduction and association of the scaphoid and lunate (RASL) procedure: a biomechanical analysis. J Hand Surg Eur Vol. 2018;43:635–41.

7. Koehler SM, Guerra SM, Kim JM, Sakamoto S, Lovy AJ, Hausman MR. Outcome of arthroscopic reduction association of the scapholunate joint. J Hand Surg Eur Vol. 2016;41:48–55.

8. Rosenwasser MP, Miyasajsa KC, Strauch RJ. The RASL procedure: reduction and association of the scaphoid and lunate using the Herbert screw. Tech Hand Up Extrem Surg. 1997;1:263–72.

9. Rosenwasser MP, Freibott CE, White NJ, Noback PC, Raskolnikov D, Swart EF. Reduction and association of the scaphoid and lunate (RASL) for chronic static scapholunate instability: 11 year follow-up. [In process of submitting to Journal of Hand Surgery].

10. Geissler WB. Arthroscopic management of scapholunate instability. J Wrist Surg. 2013;2(2):129–35. https://doi.org/10.1055/s-0033-1343354.

11. Aviles A, Lee S, Hausman M. Arthroscopic reduction-association of the scapholunate. Arthroscopy. 2007;23:105.e1–5.

12. Caloia M, Caloia H, Pereira E. Arthroscopic scapholunate joint reduction. Is an effective treatment for irreparable scapholunate ligament tears? Clin Orthop Relat Res. 2012;470:972–8.

13. Lipton CBUO, Sarwahi V. Reduction and association of the scaphoid and lunate for scapholunate ligament injuries (RASL). Atlas Hand Clin. 2003;8:249–60.

14. Fok MW, Fernandez DL. Chronic scapholunate instability treated with temporary screw fixation. J Hand Surg Am. 2015;40:752–8.

15. Larson TB, Stern PJ. Reduction and association of the scaphoid and lunate procedure: short-term clinical and radiographic outcomes. J Hand Surg Am. 2014;39:2168–74.

16. Aibinder WR, Izadpanah A, Elhassan BT. Reduction and association of the scaphoid and lunate: a functional and radiographical outcome study. J Wrist Surg. 2019;8:37–42.

Arthroscopic Management of Lunotriquetral Ligament Tears

Michael J. Moskal and Felix H. Savoie III

Introduction

The diagnosis and treatment of ulnar-sided wrist pain is complex. Arthroscopic evaluation is particularly valuable to examine the anatomy and pathoanatomy of ulnar-sided wrist disorders [1]. Physical examination and radiographs, as well as MRI or arthrography, often do not reveal the full extent of an injury. Wrist arthroscopy facilitates clear characterization of an injury, the quality of the articular surfaces, associated synovitis, as well as treatment based upon an arthroscopic evaluation. Arthroscopic evaluation as well as arthroscopic assessment techniques may allow for specific treatment based upon surgical findings correlated to clinical findings. Arthroscopic treatment needs to be undertaken in the clinical context of history, physical examination, and radiology studies.

Ulnar-sided wrist injuries can be owing to repetitive trauma or to a single traumatic event such as a twisting injury or a fall on an outstretched hand with a pronated forearm in which a dorsally directed force causes the wrist to be extended and radially deviated [2]. Although isolated traumatic lunotriquetral ligament tears are not common, intercarpal pronation causes a disruption of the ulnar ligaments by tearing the lunotriquetral interosseous ligament with associated injury to the disc-triquetral and disc-lunate ligaments tearing leading to greater lunotriquetral instability. It is important to recognize that instability can arise from intrinsic as well as extrinsic ligamentous injury [3–5]. Failure to recognize and treat all the components of a destabilizing injury will lead to a compromised result of treatment.

Lunotriquetral (LT) interosseous ligament tears may be associated with ulnar-sided wrist pain. However, LT ligament tears may not be isolated pathology. Ulnar-sided wrist pain is typically intermittent and associated with forearm rotation with wrist deviation. Pain from a mechanical etiology may be due to impingement of ligament or fibrocartilage tears, instability of the lunotriquetral and or distal radioulnar (DRUJ) joints, and arthritic change. Symptoms of pain and weakness are common and often associated with a give-way sensation.

Clinical scenarios are appropriate for arthroscopic treatment and involve the following anatomical pathology:

1. Isolated lunotriquetral instability.
2. Lunotriquetral instability associated with triangular fibrocartilage cartilage complex (TFFC) tears.
   (a) Traumatic peripheral tears.
   (b) Degenerative radial or central tears.
3. Lunotriquetral instability, degenerative TFFC tears, and ulnar abutment syndrome.

Physical Examination

A comprehensive physical examination is appropriate in the clinical setting. In the context of this chapter, examination focused on ulnar-sided pathology is detailed in brief. Inspection, range of motion in comparison to the opposite side, and palpation are performed. The extensor carpi ulnaris (ECU) is the main anatomic landmark to guide palpation. Radial dorsal and ulnar volar to the ECU is the area of capsular attachment of the peripheral TFC, and both areas should be routinely palpated. Additionally, palpate the area dorsal lunotriquetral joint, extensor carpi ulnaris, the extensor digiti quinti, and flexor carpi ulnaris.

After inspection and palpation, provocative maneuvers for lunotriquetral instability are helpful: lunotriquetral ballottement (compressing the triquetrum against the lunate),

M. J. Moskal (✉)
Orthopaedic Surgery Department, University of Louisville, Sellersburg, IN, USA

F. H. Savoie III
Department of Orthopaedics, Tulane University School of Medicine, New Orleans, LA, USA
e-mail: fsavoie@tulane.edu

W. B. Geissler (ed.), *Wrist and Elbow Arthroscopy with Selected Open Procedures*,
https://doi.org/10.1007/978-3-030-78881-0_21

shuck test as described by Reagan [6], shear test as described by Kleinman [7, 8], distal radioulnar translation (to infer stability) [9, 10]. Localized pain and crepitus may accompany the aforementioned provocative tests.

Ulnar deviation should be performed with the wrist in a flexed, extended, and neutral position. Flexing and extending an ulnar deviated wrist may produce pain associated with crepitus which can be a useful indicator of associated ulnar pathology with LT tears. Ulnar deviation with axial load with the pronated forearm associated with a palpable clunk may be due to lunotriquetral instability but also may be seen in midcarpal instability. Pain and/or weakness-resisted wrist flexion with the forearm in supination increases the suspicion for symptomatic TFC tears.

The radiographic evaluation of a painful wrist should include at least a zero-rotation posteroanterior [11, 12] and a true lateral of the wrist views. Particular attention should be focused toward ulnar variance [13, 14], lunotriquetral interval and the integrity of the subchondral joint surfaces, greater and lesser arc continuity [15], and radiolunate and scapholunate angles which should be recorded. In cases where the physical examination findings are equivocal, an arthrogram or MRI can be obtained.

Ulnar Ligamentous Anatomy

The lunotriquetral interosseous ligament (LT) is thicker both volarly and dorsally [16] with a membranous central portion. Normal lunotriquetral kinematics is imparted from the integrity of the LT interosseous [3], ulnolunate (UL), ulnotriquetral (UT) [3–5], dorsal radiotriquetral (RT), and scaphotriquetral (ST) ligaments [3, 4, 6]. Severe instability (VISI) requires damage to both the dorsal RT and ST ligaments [3, 4, 6]. The TFCC is the primary stabilizer of the distal radioulnar joint via the dorsal and volar radioulnar ligaments [17, 18], helps to stabilize the ulnar carpus, and transmits axial forces to the ulna [9, 19]. TFCC compromise is often a part of more extensive ulnar-sided injuries [20]. The TFCC originates from the ulnar aspect of the lunate fossa of the radius and inserts on the base of the ulnar styloid and distally on the lunate, triquetrum, hamate, and fifth metacarpal base. The volar and dorsal aspects of the lunotriquetral ligament merge with the ulnocarpal extrinsic ligaments volarly and the dorsal radiolunotriquetral ligament dorsally anchoring the triquetrum [21].

The ulnocarpal volar ligaments are composed of the ulnolunate (UL) also known as the disc-lunate, the ulnotriquetral (UT) also known as the disc-triquetral ligaments, and the ulno-capitate. The ulnolunate (UL) and ulnotriquetral (UT) ligaments originate on the volar triangular fibrocartilage complex (TFCC) and insert on the volar lunate and volar triquetrum, respectively, as well as the LT ligament [20, 22, 23]. Just palmar to the disc-carpal ligaments is the ulno-capitate ligament. The ulno-capitate ligament provides a direct attachment from the ulna to the palmar ulnar ligamentous complex. The integrity of the triangular fibrocartilage, volar radiocarpal, as well as dorsal radiocarpal ligaments is visible during arthroscopy. Our approach to LT injuries had evolved from the anatomical concepts of the ulnar ligaments in relationship to the lunotriquetral joint and the TFCC.

Arthroscopic Operative Technique

Chronic isolated lunotriquetral ligament injuries have been treated with ligament repair, ligament reconstruction, and lunotriquetral joint fusion. Compromise of the dorsal extrinsic ligaments (dorsal radiotriquetral and scaphotriquetral) with LT instability producing a VISI deformity is a contraindication to arthroscopic ligament plication. Arthroscopic stabilization of ulnar-sided instability can be used in conjunction with associated pathology such as ulnar abutment syndrome and TFCC tears when associated with an LTIOL tear.

The arthroscopic approach to symptomatic LT instability is a soft tissue procedure reconstruction based upon the contributing factors of the ulnar carpal ligaments to lunotriquetral joint stability. Included in arthroscopic reduction and internal fixation of the lunotriquetral joint, suture plication of the ulnar ligaments serves to shorten the disc-carpal ligaments and augment the palmar capsular tissue.

In the management of capitolunate instability [24], ligament plication of the central portion of the volar radiocapitate ligament was tethered to the radiotriquetral ligament by a volar approach. Ligament plication of the UT–UL ligaments is reminiscent of this technique as was developed by one of us (FHS). Arthroscopic volar ulnar ligament plication allows direct visual assessment of pathology and visual assessment of the plication effect during radiocarpal and midcarpal arthroscopy.

Typical portals used during arthroscopic capsulodesis (ligament plication) and arthroscopic reduction and internal fixation are the 3–4, 6-R, volar 6-U, and the radial and ulnar midcarpal portals. Depending upon each unique case, the addition of a 4–5 portal as either the working or viewing portal can be helpful (Fig. 21.1). The arthroscopic video system should be positioned to allow a clear view of the monitor by the surgeon and assistant. After the limb was exsanguinated, a traction tower is used and eight to ten pounds of traction are applied through finger traps with the arm strapped to the hand table. Diagnostic radiocarpal arthroscopy should include visualization that should also be from the 6-R portal to ensure complete visualization of the lunotriquetral interosseous ligament (LTIOL) from dorsal to palmar. Midcarpal

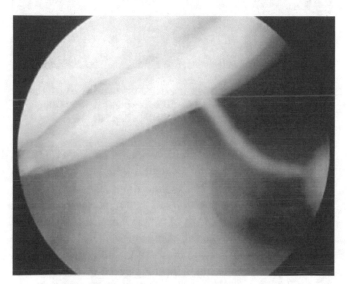

Fig. 21.1 A lunotriquetral ligament tear as seen from the 6-R portal

assessment begins with the arthroscope inserted into the radial midcarpal portal and the ulnar midcarpal portal as the working portal. The lunotriquetral joint is assessed for congruency and laxity of the triquetrum.

1. Congruency
   (a) The lunate and triquetrum should be collinear. If the view of the lunotriquetral joint from the midcarpal radial portal is blocked by a separate lunate facet [25], place the arthroscope in the midcarpal ulnar portal to gain visualization. Under these conditions, the radial articular edge of triquetrum should be aligned with the most ulnar articular edge of the hamate facet of the lunate (Fig. 21.2a, b).
   (b) Although congruent, the LT joint may be unstable due to excessive laxity.
2. Laxity
   (a) Assuming normal, the scapholunate joint can be used as a reference. Laxity should be assessed both upon triquetral rotation and separation from the lunate.
   (b) Upon midcarpal arthroscopic assessment of an unstable LT joint, the dorsal portion of the triquetrum is often rotated such that its articular surface is distal to the lunate (Fig. 21.3). The triquetrum can be translated to a reduced state in which the articular surfaces of the triquetrum and lunate are collinear.
   (c) An unstable LT joint may have collinear articular surfaces; however, the triquetrum can be ulnarly translated so as to "gap open" the LT joint. The normal SL joint can be used as a reference.

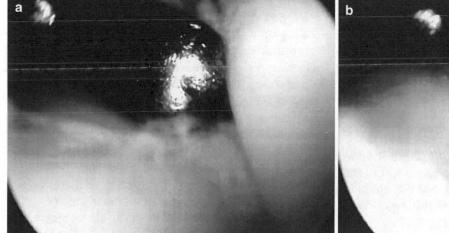 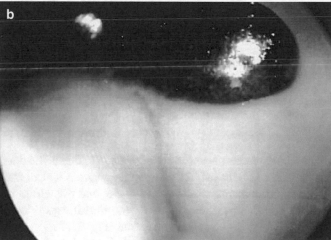

Fig. 21.2 (**a**) An incongruent LT joint as seen from the ulnar midcarpal portal. The probe has been inserted from the radial midcarpal portal. The triquetrum is to the right, and the lunate is to the *left*. (**b**) The triquetrum has been reduced and stabilized with K-wires and now is congruent with the lunate (*left*)

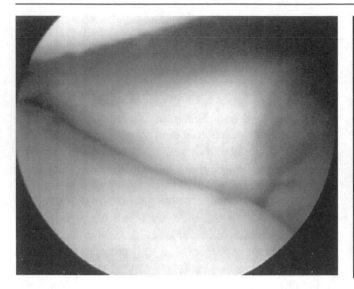

Fig. 21.3 As seen from the radial midcarpal portal, the dorsal portion of the triquetrum is rotated distally with respect to the dorsal portion of the lunate

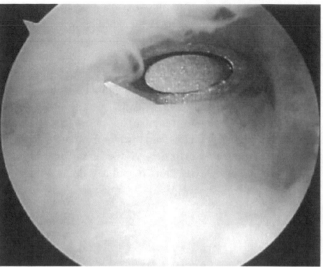

Fig. 21.5 The spinal needle has entered the radiocarpal joint at the level of the ulnar carpal ligaments. Some fraying of the disc-carpal ligaments is seen and is associated with LT ligament injury

The interval between the disc-lunate and disc-triquetral ligament identifies the lunotriquetral joint and interosseous ligament. Debridement of the lunotriquetral ligament, disc-carpal ligaments, and additional pathology is performed. Through the v6-U portal, an 18 G spinal needle is passed just volar to the disc-triquetral, ulno-capitate, and disc-lunate entering the radiocarpal joint at the radial edge of the UL ligament just distal to the articular surface of the radius. A #2–0 PDS suture is placed through the needle into the joint. The suture is retrieved either sequentially through the 6-R and the through the v6-U or directly through the v6-U using a wire loop suture retriever and then and tagged as the first plicating suture (Fig. 21.6a–c). In likewise fashion, a second plicating suture is placed approximately 5 mm distal to the first so that the suture loops are parallel to the lunate and triquetrum and is tagged as the second plicating suture (Fig. 21.7a–c). Tension on the first stitch often facilitates a second needle passage through the ulnolunate and ulnotriquetral ligaments. Adequacy of the plication (tension the stitch) and its effect on LT interval stability should be assessed after each suture passage.

Finally, through the v6-U portal, a spinal needle is passed through the volar aspect of the capsule at the prestyloid recess and then through the peripheral rim of the TFCC. The wire retriever is introduced through the ulnar capsule, and the suture is brought out the v6-U portal to tighten the ulnar capsule (Fig. 21.8a, b). The three sets of sutures are tied at the termination of the procedure after the lunotriquetral joint has been congruently reduced and stabilized with K-wires.

Viewing through the midcarpal radial portal, a midcarpal ulnar (MCU) portal working is created. A spinal needle can be placed from ulnar to radial across the distal aspect of the

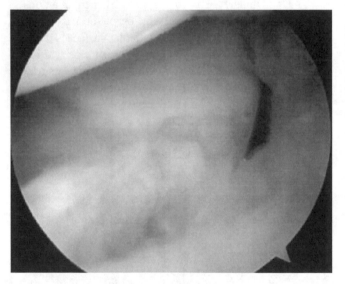

Fig. 21.4 Viewing from the radial midcarpal portal, the dorsal capsuloligamentous structures have been avulsed from their bony attachment

The final midcarpal assessment of the LT joint is the dorsal capsular structures. The dorsal radiocarpal and dorsal intercarpal ligaments attach to the lunate and triquetrum in part. In certain cases, avulsions of the dorsal capsuloligamentous structures have been observed (Fig. 21.4).

The arthroscope is placed in the 3–4 portal during disc-lunate to ulno-capitate to disc-triquetral ligament plication. The volar 6-U (v6-U) is established. The v6-U portal is similar to the normal 6-U portal; however, it is placed just dorsal to the disc-carpal ligaments (Fig. 21.5). Care is taken to avoid injury to the dorsal sensory branches of the ulnar nerve during placement.

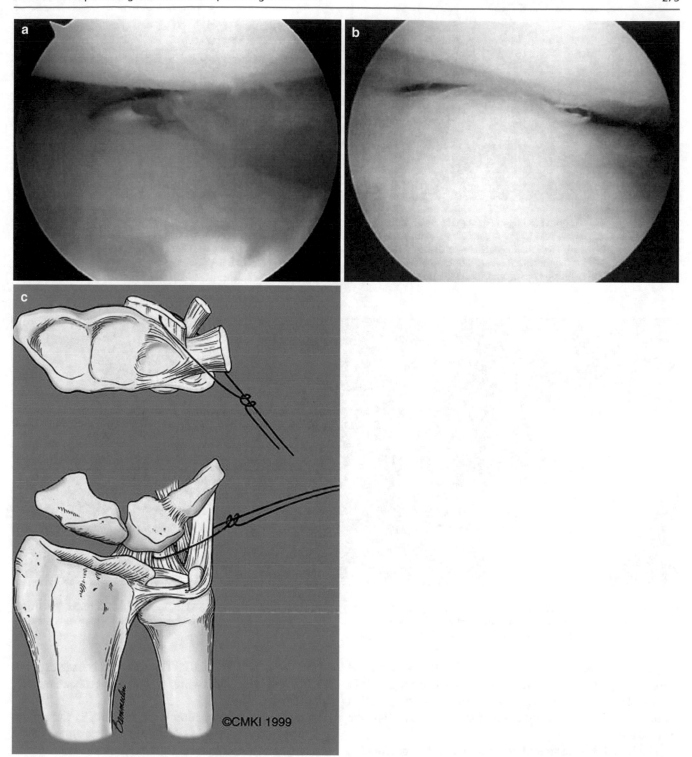

©CMKI 1999

Fig. 21.6 (**a**) The spinal needle has traversed from ulnar to radial just palmar to the ulnar carpal ligaments. The tip of the needle has reentered the radiocarpal joint radial to the disc-carpal ligament. In the photo, the lunate is above and the ulnar border of the distal radius (lunate fossa) is seen obliquely at the level of the spinal needle. (**b**) A 2–0 PDS suture has been passed through the spinal needle and retrieved out the v6-U portal. The disc-carpal ligaments are visualized with the lunate above.

(**c**) The suture passage is diagrammatically represented. The disc-triquetral ligament is to the right. The first 2–0 PDS plication suture is passed from ulnar to radial with a spinal needle through the volar 6-U portal. The disc-triquetral, ulno-capitate, and disc-lunate ligaments are incorporated in the suture. (c) With permission from The Christine M. Kleinert Institute for Hand and Microsurgery, Inc.

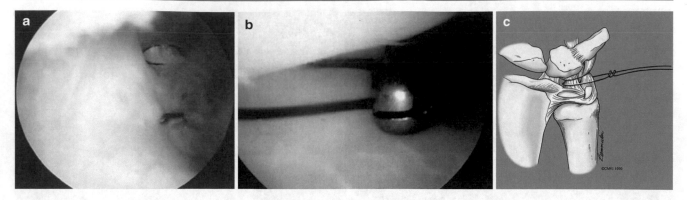

Fig. 21.7 (**a**) The disc-triquetral ligament is to the *left*. The first plicating suture is seen below and to the *right* (ulnar) exiting the ulnarly through the v6-U portal. The spinal needle is seen distal (*above*), as it is ready to be passed for the second plicating suture. (**b**) The second 2–0 PDS plication suture. Tension on the first suture facilitates placement of the second suture, which is placed approximately 5 mm distal to the first suture. (**c**) The plication sutures are represented diagrammatically. ((**c**) With permission from The Christine M. Kleinert Institute for Hand and Microsurgery, Inc)

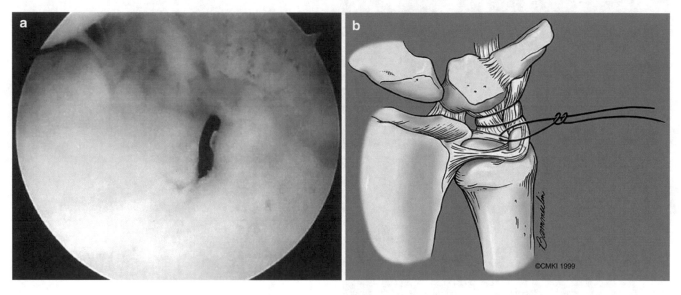

Fig. 21.8 (**a**) The ulnar capsular tension suture is in place. The suture is passed through the ulnar capsule and through the palmar aspect of the peripheral edge of the TFCC. (**b**) Line drawing of the two plication sutures and the prestyloid and TFCC sutures. ((**b**) With permission from The Christine M. Kleinert Institute for Hand and Microsurgery, Inc)

LT joint and used as a guide for percutaneous pin placement into the triquetrum. The triquetrum is reduced congruent to the lunate articular cartilage with traction on the plication sutures and firm pressure on the triquetrum on the triquetrum.

The initial K-wire should be inserted 2–3 mm proximal to the spinal needle. Two 0.045 smooth K-wire are placed percutaneously through the lunotriquetral joint (Fig. 21.9). The first pin is advanced across the lunotriquetral interval from ulnar to radial under fluoroscopic guidance, and the second pin is placed using the first pin as a guide to placement. After satisfactory reduction of the lunotriquetral joint, traction is released, the forearm is held in neutral rotation, and the plication stitches are tied at the 6-U portal with the knots placed below the skin (Fig. 21.10). The peripheral ulnar capsular stitch is retrieved. The K-wires are either cut subcutaneously or bent outside the skin.

If lunotriquetral instability is present with TFCC pathology, ligament plication is not altered and treatment of the traumatic peripheral tears or degenerative tears with or without ulnar abutment syndrome is performed. In degenerative TFCC tears, the central avascular portion is debrided to a stable rim prior to plication. With peripheral traumatic TFCC tears, additional sutures are placed in the dorsal capsule and peripheral TFCC after the initial plication sutures. In the presence of lunotriquetral tears and positive ulnar variance [6, 26, 27], arthroscopic wafer can be added in the presence of ulnar abutment.

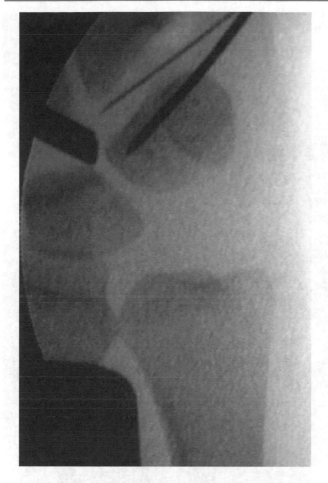

Fig. 21.9 Pin placement. The viewing portal is in the midcarpal space during arthroscopic reduction and pinning of the lunotriquetral joint. A needle has been placed into the midcarpal space to act as a guide to K-wire placement. Two to three K-wires are placed

Postoperative Care

Initially, after surgery the patient is placed in a long arm splint with the elbow flexed at 90°, the forearm in neutral rotation and the wrist in neutral flexion and extension. At approximately 1 week after surgery, a Muenster cast is applied, with the forearm and wrist in neutral rotation and flexion, respectively. At approximately 6 weeks after surgery, the K-wires are removed. A removable Muenster cast is used for an additional 2 weeks to allow daily gentle flexion, extension, pronation, and supination within a painless arc of motion. Eight weeks after surgery, strengthening exercises are instituted and work hardening can begin slowly over 8–24 weeks postoperatively.

Results

In a case series, we looked at a group of 21 patients without ulnar impaction and included seven patients with workman's compensation claims and four patients who sustained injury during sport. All patients complained of ulnar-sided wrist pain, which was invariably increased by use of the wrist, and the mean time between the onset of symptoms and treatment was 2.5 years (range, 1 week to 5.5 years). Seventeen patients recalled a specific injury (hyperextension 12, twisting 2, unknown 3) and four noted a gradual onset of symptoms. Three patients had additional significant injuries to the affected extremity: elbow dislocation, humeral shaft fracture, and anterior shoulder dislocation.

The patients were uniformly tender over the lunotriquetral joint. Provocative tests for lunotriquetral instability were specifically positive in nine and for TFCC in six. Crepitus was produced with pronosupination or ulnar deviation in ten patients. A VISI instability pattern was not present. The average ingo Mayo wrist score was 50 and increased to an outgo score of 88 at a mean of 3.1 years after surgery with 19/21 patients having excellent and good results and two with fair results. The average postoperative score for the nine workman's compensation claimants or litigants was slightly lower than the overall group. Three patients had complications including prolonged tenderness along the extensor carpi ulnaris, and one patient had persistent neuritis of the dorsal branches of the ulnar nerve.

Conclusion

Symptomatic lunotriquetral interosseous ligament tears have been managed in a variety of ways including arthroscopic debridement, ligamentous repair, and intercarpal arthrodesis. Ligamentous repair or grafting requires an extensile approach, and lunotriquetral joint fusion limits flexion and extension and radioulnar deviation by 14% and 25%, respectively [28]. Arthroscopic ulnocarpal ligament plication in addition to LT joint reduction and stabilization is designed to augment the volar aspect of the LT joint.

Arthroscopic evaluation with soft tissue plication with percutaneous lunotriquetral pinning improved comfort and function. Suture plication of the ulnocarpal ligaments which shortens their length to act as a checkrein to excessive lunotriquetral motion and prestyloid recess tightening, which increases tension in the ulnar DRUJ capsule, are goals similar to ulnar shortening procedures.

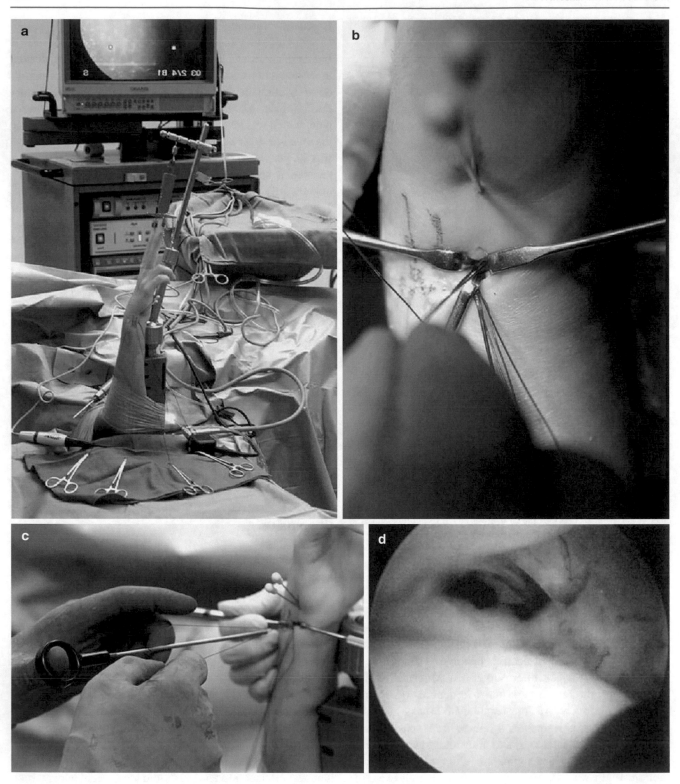

Fig. 21.10 (**a**) The sutures and K-wires are in place. Traction is taken off the wrist, and the forearm is maintained in neutral rotation. (**b**) Retractors can be used to retract soft tissue and protect the ulnar nerve sensory branches. (**c**) A knot passer can be used to pass sequential half hitches. (**d**) The sutures are seen entering the radiocarpal joint. The knot is seen adjacent to the disc-triquetral ligament

References

1. Kulick M, Chen C, Swearingen P. Determining the diagnostic accuracy of wrist arthroscopy. Toronto: Annual meeting of the American Society for Surgery of the Hand; 1990.
2. Palmer C, Murray P, Snearly W. The mechanism of ulnar sided perilunate instability of the wrist. Toronto: Annual meeting of the American Society for Surgery of the Hand; 1998.
3. Horii E, Gacias-Elias M, An K, et al. A kinematic study of lunatotriquetral dislocations. J Hand Surg Am. 1991;16A:355.
4. Viegas S, Peterson P, et al. Ulnar-sided perilunate instability: An anatomic and biomechanical study. J Hand Surg Am. 1990;15A:268.
5. Trumble T, Bour C, Smith R, et al. Kinematics of the ulnar carpus to the volar intercalated segment instability pattern. J Hand Surg Am. 1990;15A:384.
6. Reagan D, Linscheid R, Dobyns J. Lunatotriquetral sprains. J Hand Surg Am. 1984;9A:502–14.
7. Kleinman W. Physical examination of lunatotriquetral joint. Am Soc Surg Hand Corr Newsletter. 1985;51:74.
8. Kleinman W. Long-term study of chronic scapho-lunate instability treated by scapho-trapezio-trapezoid arthodesis. J Hand Surg Am. 1989;14A:429.
9. Palmer A, Werner F. The triangular fibrocartilage complex of the wrist: anatomy and function. J Hand Surg Am. 1981;6:153.
10. Palmer A. Triangular fibrocartilage complex lesions: a classification. J Hand Surg Am. 1989;14A:594.
11. Palmer A, Glisson R, Werner F. Ulnar variance determination. J Hand Surg Am. 1982;7:376.
12. Gilula L. Posteroanterior wrist radiography: importance of arm positioning. J Hand Surg Am. 1987;12A:504–8.
13. Hulten O. Uber anatomische variationen der hand-Gelenkknochen. Acta Radiol. 1928;9:155.
14. Steyers C, Blair W. Measuring ulnar variance: a comparison of techniques. J Hand Surg Am. 1989;14A:607.
15. Gilula L. Carpal injuries: analytic approach and case exercises. AJR Am J Roentgenol. 1979;133:503–17.
16. Bednar J, Osterman A. Carpal instability: evaluation and treatment. J Am Acad Orthop Surg. 1993;1:10–7.
17. Cooney W, Dobyns J, Linscheid R. Arthroscopy of the wrist: anatomy and classification of carpal instability. Arthroscopy. 1990;6:113–40.
18. Mayfield J. Patterns of injury to carpal ligaments: a spectrum. Clin Orthop. 1984;187:36.
19. Werner F, Palmer A, Fortino M, et al. Force transmission through the distal ulna: effect of ulnar variance, lunate fossa angulation, and radial and palmar tilt of the distal radius. J Hand Surg Am. 1992;17A:423.
20. Melone C Jr, Nathan R. Traumatic disruption of the triangular fibrocartilage complex, pathoanatomy. Clin Orthop. 1992;275:65–73.
21. Green D. Carpal dislocation and instabilities. In: Green D, editor. Operative hand surgery. New York: Churchill Livingston; 1988. p. 878–9.
22. Palmer A, Werner F. Biomechanics of the distal radioulnar joint. Clin Orthop. 1984;187:26.
23. Garcias-Elias M, Domenech-Mateu J. The articular disc of the wrist: limits and relations. Acta Anat. 1987;128:51.
24. Johnson R, Carrera G. Chronic capitolunate instability. J Bone Joint Surg. 1986;68A:1164–76.
25. Viegas S, Wagner K, Patterson R, et al. Medial (hamate) facet of the lunate. J Hand Surg Am. 1990;15A:564–71.
26. Pin P, Young V, Gilula L, et al. Management of chronic lunatotriquetral ligament tears. J Hand Surg Am. 1989;14A:77–83.
27. Osterman A, Sidman G. The role of arthroscopy in the treatment of lunatotriquetral ligament injuries. Hand Clin. 1995;11:41–50.
28. Seradge H, Sterbank P, Seradge E, et al. Segmental motion of the proximal carpal row: their global effect on the wrist motion. J Hand Surg Am. 1990;15A:236–9.

Arthroscopic Management of Dorsal Capsular Lesions

David J. Slutsky

Introduction

Various authors have cast light on the importance of the dorsal radiocarpal ligament (DRCL) in maintaining carpal stability [1–4]. Tears of the DRCL have been linked to the development of both volar and dorsal intercalated segmental instabilities and may be implicated in the development of midcarpal instability [5–7]. In most series, the DRCL is overlooked during the typical arthroscopic examination of the wrist. It is hard to visualize a DRCL tear through the standard dorsal wrist arthroscopy portals since the torn edge of the DRCL tends to float up against the arthroscope while viewing through the 3,4 and 4,5 portals, which makes both identification and repair of the DRCL tear cumbersome. It can be seen obliquely through the 1,2, or 6R portals, but visualization of the DRCL across the radiocarpal joint may be laborious in a tight or small wrist, especially if synovitis is present. Wrist arthroscopy through a volar radial portal (VR) is the ideal way to assess the dorsal radiocarpal ligament due to the straight line of sight [8, 9].

Anatomy/Kinematics

The dorsal radiocarpal ligament is an extracapsular ligament on the dorsum of the wrist. It originates on Lister's tubercle and moves obliquely in a distal and ulnar direction to attach to the tubercle of the triquetrum. Its radial fibers attach to the lunate and lunotriquetral interosseous ligament [10]. The dorsal intercarpal (DIC) ligament originates from the triquetrum and extends radially to attach onto the lunate, the dorsal groove of the scaphoid, and then the trapezium. Viegas et al. observed that the lateral V configurations of the DRCL and the DIC function as a dorsal radioscaphoid ligament. It can vary its length by changing the angle between the two arms while maintaining its stabilizing effect on the scapholunate

joint during wrist flexion and extension [11]. This would require changes in length far greater than any single fixed ligament could accomplish. Elsaidi and Ruch demonstrated the importance of the DRCL on scaphoid kinematics through a series of sectioning studies [12]. They sequentially divided the radioscaphocapitate, long radiolunate, radioscapholunate, and short radiolunate ligaments. They next divided the central and proximal SLIL, then the dorsal SLIL, and finally the dorsal capsule insertion on the scaphoid. There was no appreciable change in the radiographic appearance of this wrist. When the DRCL was then divided, a dorsal intercalated segmental instability (DISI) deformity occurred. In a biomechanical study using 24 cadaver arms, Short et al. determined that the SLIL is the primary stabilizer of the scapholunate articulation and that the DRCL, the dorsal intercarpal (DIC) the scaphotrapezial (ST) ligaments, and the radioscaphocapitate (RSC) ligaments are secondary stabilizers [13]. They found that dividing the DIC or the ST ligaments alone followed by 1000 cycles of wrist flexion–extension and radial–ulnar deviation had no effect on scaphoid and lunate kinematics. Dividing the DRCL alone did cause increased lunate radial deviation when the wrist was in maximum flexion. Dividing the SLIL after any of the ligaments tested produced increased scaphoid flexion and ulnar deviation while the lunate extended. They also hypothesized that cyclic motion appears to cause further deterioration in carpal kinematics due to plastic deformation in the remaining structures that stabilize the scapholunate.

The DRCL tear described in this chapter consists of a detachment of the epiligamentous portion of the ligament. In cases where a dorsal capsulotomy was performed, the dorsal part of the ligament was always intact. I believe that the pain secondary to a DRCL tear represents an impingement phenomenon of the torn DRCL which is caught between the radius and lunate during wrist motion, and that an arthroscopic repair does not necessarily restore normal wrist kinematics—but there are no biomechanical data to support either theory.

D. J. Slutsky (✉)
The Hand and Wrist Institute, Torrance, CA, USA

© Springer Nature Switzerland AG 2022
W. B. Geissler (ed.), *Wrist and Elbow Arthroscopy with Selected Open Procedures*,
https://doi.org/10.1007/978-3-030-78881-0_22

Indications

An arthroscopic repair is indicated for an isolated DRCL tear, which often leads to resolution of the wrist pain. The role of a DRCL repair when associated with other wrist pathology is not well defined.

Contraindications

It is unlikely that performing a DRCL repair when there are two or more intracarpal lesions significantly improves the outcome since the results are inconsistent and appear to be largely determined by the treatment of the associated wrist pathology.

Surgical Technique

The procedure is done under tourniquet control with the arm in 10–15 lb of traction. The operator is seated on the volar aspect of the arm. A volar radial (VR) portal is established by making a 2-cm longitudinal incision in the proximal wrist crease exposing the flexor carpi radialis (FCR) tendon sheath. The sheath is divided, and the FCR tendon is retracted ulnarly. The radiocarpal joint space is identified with a 22G needle. A blunt trochar and cannula are introduced through the floor of the FCR sheath, which overlies the interligamentous sulcus between the radioscaphocapitate ligament and the long radiolunate ligament. A 2.7 mm, 30° arthroscope is inserted through the cannula. The procedure may be done dry, but it is easier to see the torn edges of the DRCL with fluid irrigation. The DRCL is seen just radial to the 3,4 portal, underneath the lunate (Fig. 22.1). The dorsal capsule may often appear redundant and can protrude into the joint, but when a DRCL tear is present the frayed ligamentous fibers can be seen (Fig. 22.2). In long-standing tears, the distal edge of the DRCL becomes rounded (Fig. 22.3). It is helpful to insert a 3 mm hook probe through the 3,4 portal for orientation. The DRCL tear can then be pulled into the joint with the probe which differentiates it from redundant dorsal capsule (Fig. 22.4a, b). The repair is performed by inserting a 22G spinal needle through either the 3,4 or 4,5 portal. A 2–0 absorbable suture is threaded through the spinal needle and retrieved with a grasper or suture snare inserted through the other portal (Fig. 22.5a–c). A curved hemostat is used to pull either end of the suture underneath the extensor tendons, and the knot is tied either at the 3,4 or 4,5 portal. One suture is usually sufficient although an additional suture may be added as necessary to pull the torn edge of the DRCL up against the dorsal capsule. If the plicating suture does not capture the

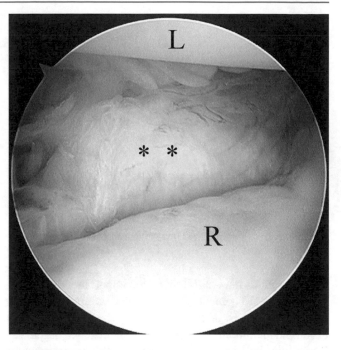

Fig. 22.1 Normal DRCL (*asterisk*) as seen from the VR portal. L lunate, R radius

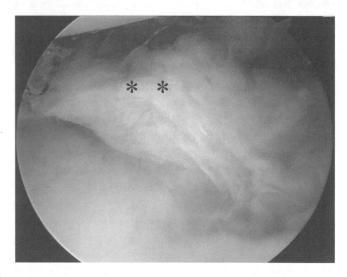

Fig. 22.2 DRCL tear. Note the torn fibers of the distal edge [8]

DRCL tear, the needle can be used to spear the distal edge of the DRCL tear which is then plicated up against the dorsal capsule (Fig. 22.6a–c). The DRCL tear can be seen from the 6R portal (Fig. 22.7), but the obliquity of the view makes this type of repair method arduous.

Following the repair, the patient is placed in a below-elbow splint with the wrist in neutral rotation. Finger motion and edema control are instituted immediately. At the first postoperative visit, the sutures are removed and the patient is placed in a below-elbow cast for a total of 4 weeks, followed by wrist mobilization.

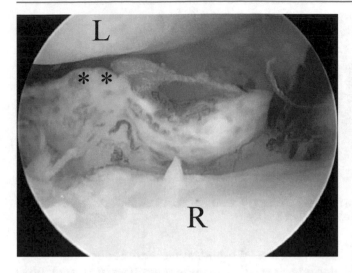

Fig. 22.3 Chronic DRCL tear with rounded edges (*asterisk*). L lunate, R radius

Outcomes

A retrospective chart review of 21 patients who underwent a DRCL repair was published in 2005 [14, 15]. None of the wrists showed a static carpal instability pattern on X-ray. A preoperative MRI was performed by the referring physician in six patients. Preoperative arthrograms were performed as a part of the diagnostic workup for wrist pain in 20 patients. None of the DRCL tears in this series were identified with preoperative arthrography or MRI. A preoperative MRI in one patient with a DRCL tear was misinterpreted as representing a dorsal wrist ganglion. There were 6 men and 16 women. The average patient age was 40 years (range, 25–62 years). All patients failed a trial of conservative treatment with wrist immobilization, cortisone injections, and work restrictions. The average length of conservative treatment was 7 months.

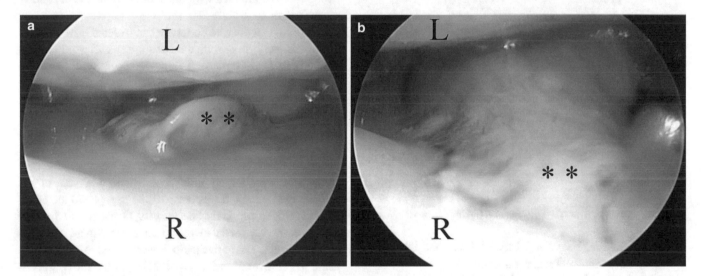

Fig. 22.4 (a) Under dry arthroscopy the DRCL tear appears small and unimpressive (*asterisk*). L lunate, R radius. (b) A hook probe is used to pull the DRCL tear (*asterisk*) into the joint, demonstrating the large amount of tissue that can impinge between the radius and lunate

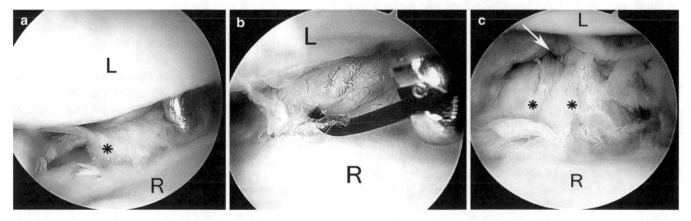

Fig. 22.5 (a) Arthroscopic view of DRCL tear (*asterisk*) from the VR portal. L lunate, R radius. (b) A 2–0 suture has been inserted through a spinal needle in the 4,5 portal and is being retrieved with forceps in the 3,4 portal. (c) Completed repair. Note how the DRCL tear (*asterisk*) has been plicated up against the dorsal capsule (*arrow*)

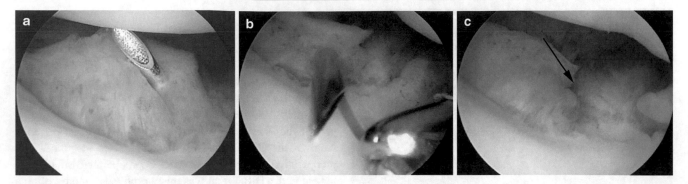

Fig. 22.6 (**a**) A 22G spinal has been inserted through the midsubstance of the DRCL tear. (**b**) A 2–0 suture has been inserted through the spinal needle and is being retrieved with forceps in the 3,4 portal. (**c**) Completed repair (*arrow*)

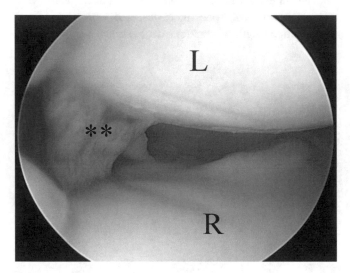

Fig. 22.7 Oblique view of a DRCL tear from the 6R portal

The time interval between injury and surgical intervention averaged 25 months (range, 8–53 months).

At the time of arthroscopy, five patients were found to have an isolated DRCL tear that was solely responsible for their wrist pain. The remaining patients had additional ligamentous pathology. A dorsal capsulodesis was performed in seven patients as the primary treatment for the SLIL instability/tear. Thirteen patients underwent an arthroscopic DRCL ligament repair ± thermal shrinkage (repair = 5, repair + shrinkage = 6, shrinkage = 2). Ten of these patients underwent ancillary procedures for treatment of the coexisting wrist pathology. Lunotriquetral ligament tears were treated with debridement ± pinning. Triangular fibrocartilage tears were debrided or repaired. Scapholunate ligament tears/ instabilities were treated with capsulodesis ± open repair. One patient had generalized arthrofibrosis which precluded a DRCL repair. Concomitant nerve entrapment was a common finding which was treated at the same time.

The average duration of the follow-up period was 16 months (range, 7–41 months), with one patient lost to follow-up at 4 weeks. Pain was graded as none, mild, moder-

ate, and severe. Wrist extension, wrist flexion, radial deviation, ulnar deviation, and grip strength were assessed. Wrist range of motion was compared with presurgical values. Grip strength was compared with the contralateral side at follow-up evaluation.

The five patients who underwent an isolated DRCL repair were satisfied with the outcome of surgery and would repeat the surgery again because it improved their symptoms. All five patients graded their pain as none or mild. None of these patients were taking pain medications. All returned to their previous occupations without restriction. Their wrist motion was unchanged as compared to the preoperative status. Grip strengths were 90–130% of the opposite side.

The patients with coexisting pathology had variable outcomes that were largely influenced by the treatment of the associate pathology. It was not possible to separate the effect of the DRCL repair. At the latest review, 64 patients had undergone arthroscopy for the investigation and treatment of refractory wrist pain. Thirty-five patients were found to have DRCL tears, for an overall incidence of 55%. As such it is prudent that the arthroscopist is diligent in recognizing and treating this condition. Ongoing research into the ideal method of treatment of these combined injuries, however, is still needed.

Arthroscopic Wrist Ganglionectomy

Osterman et al. pioneered the arthroscopic resection of dorsal wrist ganglia and reported on 150 procedures with only one recurrence [16]. Volar wrist ganglia that originate from the radiocarpal joint are amenable to arthroscopic resection, but those that arise from the scaphotrapezial trapezoidal joint are not.

Indications

The indication for arthroscopic removal of a dorsal ganglion is similar to those for an open method. An ideal indication is when patients have concomitant wrist pain and a positive scaphoid shift test where evaluation of any associated SLIL instability is desirable. The occult ganglion that is entirely intracapsular and cannot be visualized during open surgery is another indication. Preoperative X-rays should be performed to rule out intraosseous communication or other carpal pathology. It is important to ensure the lesion is in fact a ganglion either with transillumination, an MRI, or needle aspiration.

Contraindications

Previous scarring in the area due to previous injury or surgery for recurrence may distort the anatomy and make it difficult to establish the portals.

Surgical Technique

Since the ganglion overlies the 3,4 portal, it is the author's preference to view the ganglion through the VR portal, which provides a direct line of sight and allows one to rule out a tear of the DRCL (Fig. 22.8a, b). Alternatively, the 1,2 or 6-R portal can be used. A shaver is then introduced into the ganglion through the 3,4 portal to perforate the ganglion and resect the stalk (Fig. 22.9a, b). The intra-articular ganglion is completely debrided along with a 1-cm area of surrounding dorsal capsule. The extensor tendons may be visible through the defect. Midcarpal arthroscopy should be performed to debride any midcarpal extension of the ganglion and to assess the status of the SL and LT joints (Fig. 22.10).

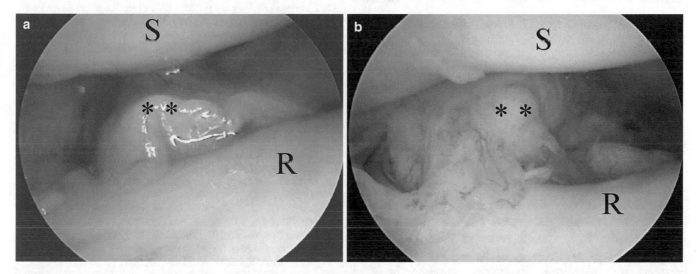

Fig. 22.8 (**a**) View of a dorsal wrist ganglion (*asterisk*) under dry arthroscopy from the VR portal. The appearance can mimic that of a DRCL tear but the ganglion overlies the 3,4 portal and is radial to the DRCL. S scaphoid, R radius. (**b**) Under fluid irrigation the globular structure of the ganglion (*asterisk*) is evident. S scaphoid, R radius

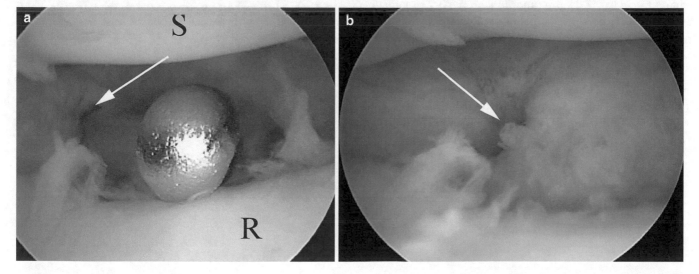

Fig. 22.9 (**a**) View of a shaver from the VR portal which has been introduced through the stalk of the ganglion (*arrow*), which overlies the 3,4 portal. (**b**) Capsular defect (*asterisk*) after resection of the ganglion

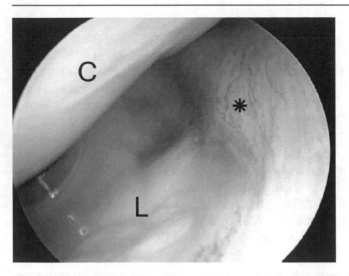

Fig. 22.10 Oblique view from the midcarpal radial portal of a ganglion in the midcarpal joint. C capitate, L lunate

Postoperatively, the wrist is splinted for 1 week for comfort followed by protected range of motion. Loss of wrist flexion following dorsal ganglia excision can be treated with dynamic splinting at 6–8 weeks.

Outcomes

Rizzo and coauthors performed an arthroscopic resection of 41 dorsal ganglia. At 2 years, patients demonstrated improved wrist motion and grip strength, excellent pain relief, and only two recurrences [17]. Good results are not invariable in patients with associated intracarpal pathology, however. Povlsen and Peckett noted an abnormal scapholunate joint in 10/16 patients and an abnormal lunotriquetral joint in 2/16 patients. At a 5-year follow-up, only one patient remained pain free [18]. Edwards and Johansen [19] examined 55 patients with dorsal wrist ganglia following an arthroscopic resection. The ganglion arose from the radiocarpal joint alone in 11 patients and extended into the midcarpal joint in 29 cases. In two patients, it arose exclusively from the midcarpal joint. The preoperative Disabilities of the Arm, Shoulder, and Hand scores improved from 14.2 to 1.7. At a 24-month follow-up, all patients demonstrated motion within 5° of preoperative measurements, and there were no recurrences.

References

1. Short WH, Werner FW, Green JK, Weiner MM, Masaoka S. The effect of sectioning the dorsal radiocarpal ligament and insertion of a pressure sensor into the radiocarpal joint on scaphoid and lunate kinematics. J Hand Surg Am. 2002;27:68–76.
2. Mitsuyasu H, Patterson RM, Shah MA, et al. The role of the dorsal intercarpal ligament in dynamic and static scapholunate instability. J Hand Surg Am. 2004;29:279–88.
3. Viegas SF, Yamaguchi S, Boyd NL, Patterson RM. The dorsal ligaments of the wrist: anatomy, mechanical properties, and function. J Hand Surg Am. 1999;24:456–68.
4. Ruch DS, Smith BP. Arthroscopic and open management of dynamic scaphoid instability. Orthop Clin North Am. 2001;32:233–40. vii
5. Viegas SF, Patterson RM, Peterson PD, et al. Ulnar-sided perilunate instability: an anatomic and biomechanic study. J Hand Surg Am. 1990;15:268–78.
6. Moritomo H, Viegas SF, Elder KW, et al. Scaphoid nonunions: a 3-dimensional analysis of patterns of deformity. J Hand Surg Am. 2000;25A:520–8.
7. Horii E, Garcia-Elias M, An KN, et al. A kinematic study of lunotriquetral dissociations. J Hand Surg Am. 1991;16:355–62.
8. Slutsky DJ. Arthroscopic repair of dorsal radiocarpal ligament tears. Arthroscopy. 2002;18:E49.
9. Slutsky D. Arthroscopic repair of Dorsoradiocarpal ligament tears. J Arthrosc Related Surg. 2005;21:1486e1–8.
10. Slutsky DJ. Management of dorsoradiocarpal ligament repairs. J Am Soc Surg Hand. 2005;5:167–74.
11. Slutsky DJ. Wrist arthroscopy through a volar radial portal. Arthroscopy. 2002;18:624–30.
12. Slutsky DJ. Volar portals in wrist arthroscopy. J Am Soc Surg Hand. 2002;2:225–32.
13. Slutsky DJ. Clinical applications of volar portals in wrist arthroscopy. Tech Hand Up Extrem Surg. 2004;8:229–38.
14. Elsaidi GA, Ruch DS, Kuzma GR, Smith BP. Dorsal wrist ligament insertions stabilize the scapholunate interval: cadaver study. Clin Orthop Relat Res. 2004;425:152–7.
15. Short WH, Werner FW, Green JK, Sutton LG, Brutus JP. Biomechanical evaluation of the ligamentous stabilizers of the scaphoid and lunate: part III. J Hand Surg Am. 2007;32:297–309.
16. Osterman AL, Raphael J. Arthroscopic resection of dorsal ganglion of the wrist. Hand Clin. 1995;11:7–12.
17. Rizzo M, Berger RA, Steinmann SP, Bishop AT. Arthroscopic resection in the management of dorsal wrist ganglions: results with a minimum 2-year follow-up period. J Hand Surg Am. 2004;29:59–62.
18. Povlsen B, Tavakkolizadeh A. Outcome of surgery in patients with painful dorsal wrist ganglia and arthroscopic confirmed ligament injury: a five-year follow-up. Hand Surg. 2004;9:171–3.
19. Edwards SG, Johansen JA. Prospective outcomes and associations of wrist ganglion cysts resected arthroscopically. J Hand Surg Am. 2009;34(3):395–400.

Arthroscopic Management of Dorsal Wrist Syndrome

Rachel E. Hein and Marc J. Richard

Introduction

Dorsal wrist pain is troublesome for both the clinician and the patient. There are several pathologies linked to dorsal wrist pain including ganglion cysts, scapholunate ligament injuries, dorsal radiocarpal ligament injuries, and most recently, dorsal wrist capsular impingement (DWCI). DWCI is defined as pain at the dorsal radiocarpal joint attributed to impingement of dorsal wrist capsular tissue during wrist extension. The entity of dorsal wrist pain without a clear, identifiable source of pathology has been termed dorsal wrist syndrome (DWS) [1].

Historically, unexplained dorsal wrist pain has been attributed to an occult ganglion cyst or a predynamic carpal instability due to ligamentous injury [2, 3]. Many authors described the successful surgical treatment of dorsal wrist pain by open capsulectomy with or without neurectomies and excision of bony ridges [2–6]. This chapter addresses diagnosis of DWCI and arthroscopic treatment which has been clinically successful in the literature and in our practice. This is primarily a clinical diagnosis, although MRI has been shown to be helpful for ruling out other wrist pathologies. Current management includes arthroscopy for definitive diagnosis of redundant dorsal capsular tissue and treatment by limited dorsal capsular debridement. Patients may expect improvement in pain and functional scores [7].

Anatomy, Kinematics, Pathology

The relevant anatomy of the dorsal wrist consists of a system of intrinsic and extrinsic ligaments. The intrinsic ligaments have their origin and insertion on carpal bones. The most important intrinsic ligaments are the scapholunate (SL) and lunotriquetral (LT) ligaments of the proximal carpal row. The extrinsic ligaments link the carpal bones to either the radius or ulna proximally, or the metacarpals distally. There is a volar and dorsal group of extrinsic ligaments. The volar extrinsic ligaments are typically not involved in DWS. The dorsal extrinsic ligaments consist of the radioscaphoid, radiolunate, dorsal radiocarpal (DRC), and dorsal intercarpal (DIC) ligaments (Fig. 23.1).

Many authors have reported on the potential pathology causing DWS. Several studies have identified the intrinsic ligaments, specifically the SL ligament, as the pathologic structure. Watson believed that DWS was the result of underlying predynamic rotatory subluxation of the scaphoid (RSS), secondary to an injury of the SL ligament and often associated with the presence of a ganglion. Because of the RSS, they advocated triscaphe arthrodesis for management of the problem [2]. Yasuda et al. confirmed the association between DWS and SL tears or ganglions. They reported success with open capsulectomy, excision of the ganglion, and posterior interosseous nerve excision [3].

Other authors have identified the dorsal extrinsic ligaments as the cause of DWS. Slutsky reported on the DRC as a cause of DWS [8]. He has advocated arthroscopic repair of this ligament when identified and has reported success with this technique [9, 10]. Swann et al. reported on two cases of DWCI secondary to snapping of the DRC ligament [11]. They successfully treated the patients with open capsular debridement in one case and arthroscopic debridement in the second.

It is our experience that the majority of DWS is DWCI [7]. The pathology typically originates from the dorsal extrinsic wrist ligaments. Microtrauma and chronic injury to

R. E. Hein
Division of Plastic and Reconstructive Surgery, Duke University Medical Center, Durham, NC, USA
e-mail: rhein4989@gmail.com

M. J. Richard (✉)
Department of Orthopaedic Surgery, Duke University Medical Center, Durham, NC, USA
e-mail: marc.richard@duke.edu

© Springer Nature Switzerland AG 2022
W. B. Geissler (ed.), *Wrist and Elbow Arthroscopy with Selected Open Procedures*,
https://doi.org/10.1007/978-3-030-78881-0_23

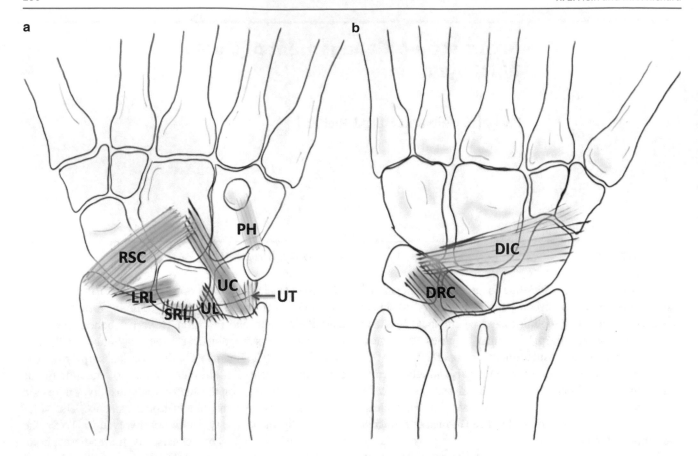

Fig. 23.1 Extrinsic volar (**a**) and dorsal (**b**) wrist ligaments

these dorsal capsular ligaments can cause avulsion, which over time may result in impingement between the extensor carpi radialis brevis and the scaphoid. This causes the patient pain during extremes of wrist extension, especially when loaded [7]. This has been successfully managed with arthroscopic debridement of the dorsal wrist capsule.

Assessment (PE, Imaging)

Assessment of the patient includes a thorough history and physical examination to rule out other causes of dorsal wrist pain. Patients will typically complain of pain with activities that involve axial loading through an extended wrist such as pushups or pushing open a heavy door (Fig. 23.2). Initial radiographs should be obtained to rule out other pathologies such as arthritis, fractures, carpal boss, or findings suggestive of SL ligament pathology.

Physical examination includes a full upper extremity exam with careful attention to the dorsal radiocarpal joint for tenderness. Typically, there is tenderness to palpation at the dorsal radiocarpal joint. Patients will have painful active and passive terminal extension, worsened when loaded. In DWCI, the scaphoid shift test should be nega-

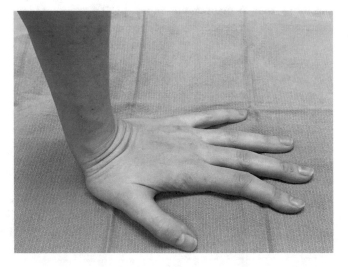

Fig. 23.2 Dorsal wrist syndrome is typically symptomatic at extreme extension and loading

tive. If positive, consideration is given to concomitant or alternative SL pathology as the cause of symptoms. DWCI is not associated with pain on resisted active wrist extension from a neutral position as seen with a diagnosis of tendinitis. Likewise, no masses should be visible or palpable dorsally.

Fig. 23.3 T2-weighted sagittal MRI of the wrist at the level of the scaphoid (**a**) and lunate (**b**). The MRI may reveal dorsal radiocarpal capsular avulsion from its distal attachments or a thickened or redundant capsule at the radiocarpal joint (arrows)

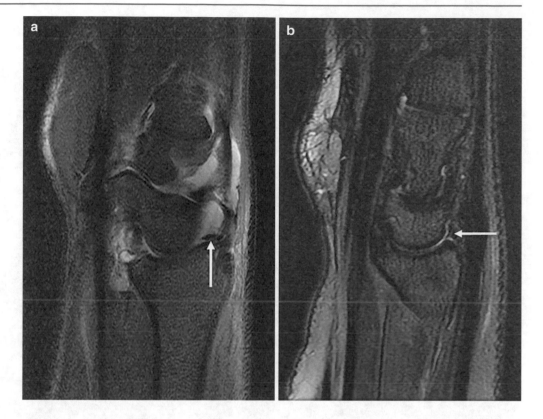

In our practice, this has generally been a clinical diagnosis based upon a careful history and physical examination. Magnetic resonance imaging (MRI) may be obtained in those with unclear history or physical exam, or to look for other concomitant pathology. MRI may or may not reveal DWCI as this is a dynamic process, and thus, a negative MRI does not rule out DWCI. Occasionally, MRI may reveal dorsal radiocarpal capsular avulsion from its distal attachments or a thickened or abundant capsule (Fig. 23.3). Concomitant pathology to carefully rule out includes tendinitis, triangular fibrocartilage complex tears, scapholunate partial or complete tears, dorsal ganglion cysts, wrist arthritis including lunotriquetral arthritis, and os styloideum [7]. Arthroscopy is both diagnostic and therapeutic for the management of DWCI.

Indications

Typically, a trial of conservative therapy is attempted including activity modification, splinting, and anti-inflammatory medications. Patients are counseled to avoid activities that are painful and those that may provoke DWCI including axial loading through an extended wrist. For those unable to avoid all aggravating activities, a removable wrist brace is given. Patients should consider a prescribed trial of non-steroidal anti-inflammatories. If no improvement is seen at 6 weeks, an intra-articular injection of cor-

ticosteroid and local anesthetic into the radiocarpal joint is offered. It is our experience that many patients with DWCI will experience some relief with the injection, even if just short term from the local anesthetic component. For patients who fail nonoperative management, diagnostic arthroscopy with possible debridement of the pathologic dorsal capsule is indicated.

Contraindications

Contraindications for diagnostic arthroscopy and debridement are minimal and include alternative diagnoses that may not be treated arthroscopically, successful conservative treatment with activity modifications and NSAIDs, or general contraindications to anesthesia including significant co-morbidities.

Technique (Authors Preferred: Limited Debridement of Redundant Capsular Tissue)

This procedure is easily performed under a regional interscalene block and monitored anesthesia care. The patient is placed in a supine position with the hand table attached. A non-sterile tourniquet is used in conjunction with a traction tower for wrist arthroscopy. Care is taken to pad all potential points of compression between the upper

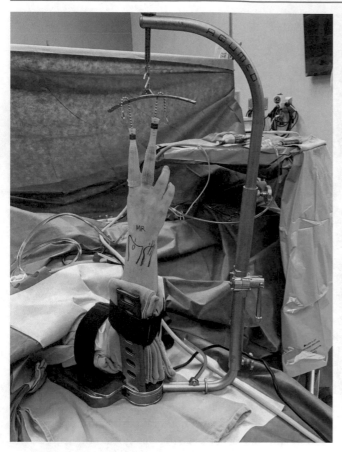

Fig. 23.4 Upper extremity traction tower

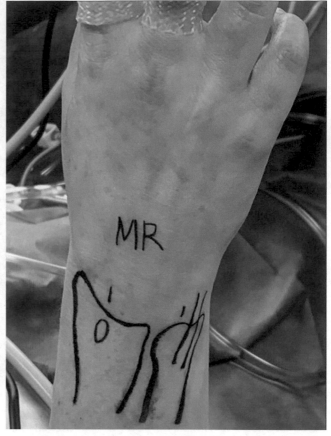

Fig. 23.5 Surface anatomy for wrist arthroscopy

extremity and the traction tower (Fig. 23.4). Twelve pounds of distraction at the radiocarpal joint is sufficient for performing this procedure. The surface anatomy is palpated and drawn to identify the working portals for wrist arthroscopy (Fig. 23.5).

To begin, access is obtained via a dorsal 3,4 portal as previously described. A diagnostic wrist arthroscopy is performed with a 2.7-mm 30-degree arthroscope to assess for other concurrent pathology and to confirm the diagnosis of DWCI. The triangular fibrocartilage complex (TFCC), intercarpal ligaments, and dorsal capsule are carefully evaluated for any potential sources of DWS. Intraoperative diagnosis may be confirmed by the dynamic extension test [7]. This is performed by removing traction intraoperatively while maintaining the arthroscope in the 3,4 portal or 6R portal. The wrist is passively extended; a positive diagnosis occurs when dorsal capsular tissue impinges at the dorsal ridge of the scaphoid during extension.

After the diagnosis is confirmed, a 6R portal is made. Care is taken to avoid the dorsal sensory branch of the ulnar nerve, particularly the transverse branch, which may be 0–6 mm from the portal [12]. While maintaining the arthroscope in the 3,4 portal, a 2.5-mm full radius shaver is employed through the 6R portal for debridement of the dorsal capsule (Fig. 23.6). Debridement continues under direct

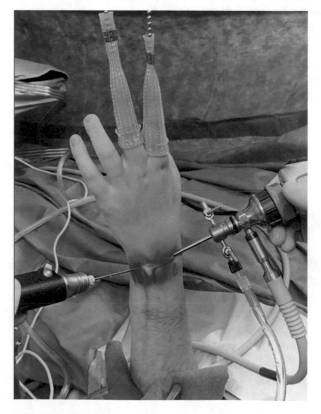

Fig. 23.6 Initial debridement: arthroscope is maintained in 3,4 portal, and 2.5-mm full radius shaver is employed through the 6R portal for debridement of dorsal capsule

visualization working from ulnar to radial until all redundant tissue is removed (Fig. 23.7). The arthroscope is then switched to the 6R portal and the shaver to the 3,4 portal, and debridement of the pathologic dorsal capsule is completed (Fig. 23.8).

Several volar portals for dorsal capsular debridement have been described. Slutsky et al. described the volar ulnar portal for additional visualization of the dorsal capsule, dorsal radial carpal ligament, and the volar scapholunate ligament [13]. These volar portals are useful for completion of debridement when traditional portals are inadequate. In our experience, volar portals are useful for debridement but not for additional visualization and are used in 25% of our cases [7, 13, 14].

Concomitant procedures may be completed prior or after completion of debridement of the redundant dorsal capsular tissue. Slutsky has described an arthroscopic repair of the avulsed DRC ligament when it is present. As previously described, other potential etiologies and concomitant pathologies such as TFCC tear, SL ligament partial or complete tears, and ganglion cysts can be managed in standard fashion per the surgeon's preference.

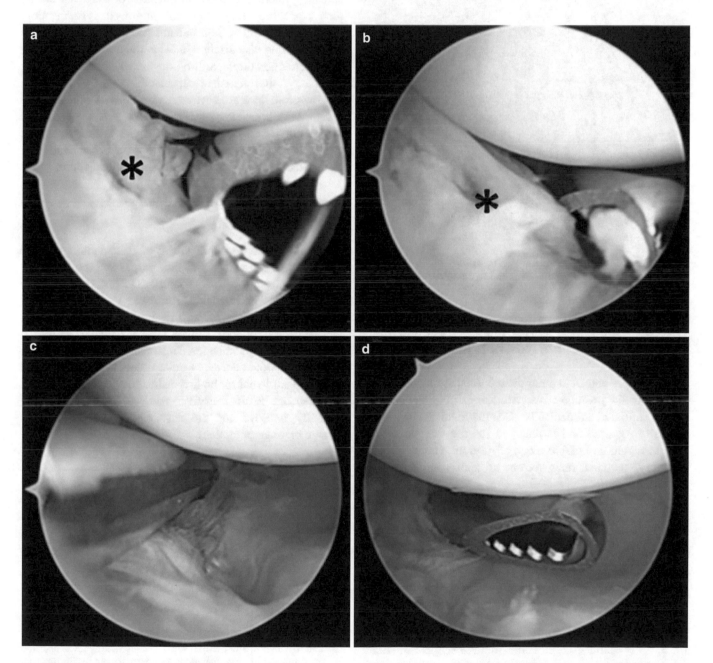

Fig. 23.7 Arthroscopic view of dorsal capsular debridement using a 2.5-mm full radius shaver. The redundant dorsal capsule (*) is first visualized looking ulnar with the arthroscope in the 3,4 portal and the shaver in the 6R portal (**a**). Once the redundant capsule is debrided to a stable edge that does not impinge within the radiocarpal joint (**b**), the arthroscope and shaver are switched to the other portals. Looking radial from the 6R portal, the remaining redundant capsule is visualized (**c**) and debrided (**d**)

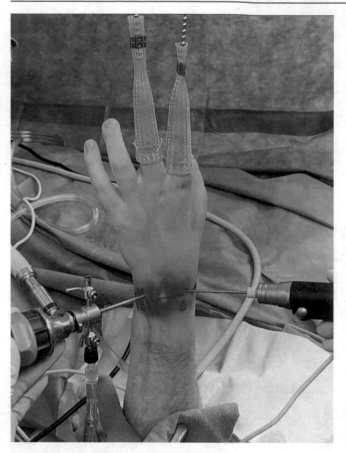

Fig. 23.8 Arthroscopic debridement: The arthroscope is switched to the 6R portal and shaver to the 3,4 portal to complete dorsal capsular debridement

Outcomes: Overall Sustained Improvements in Pain and Function, No Change in ROM

The patient is placed in a removable wrist splint for 2 weeks until their first postoperative visit. Range of motion as tolerated is initiated immediately. Occupational therapy is not typically required and is reserved for the rare patient that fails to regain acceptable range of motion. After 6 weeks of recovery, patients may return to sports or activity as tolerated.

Functional outcomes have been promising in those treated with arthroscopic debridement for DWCI. Many studies have reported improved pain with this procedure [4, 7]. Improvements in range of motion, however, have been inconsistent with some studies reporting significant gains of 17 degrees (61–78 degrees of extension), and others had a range of motion that was similar to preoperative measurements [4, 7]. Disabilities of the Arm, Hand, and Shoulder (DASH) scores have improved in all studies postoperatively [4, 5, 7]. Potential complications include surgical site infection, complex regional pain syndrome, need for repeat debridement for persistent impingement, stiffness, and neu-

ropraxia. Complex regional pain syndrome after arthroscopic debridement has been associated with tethering of the dorsal sensory branch of the ulnar nerve. Overall, these complications are rare, but patients must be counseled about the potential risks of surgical intervention.

Tips and Tricks

Most difficulty from arthroscopic debridement comes from inadequate visualization. In our experience, reassessing and adjusting traction or increasing flexion of the wrist during the procedure may aid in improved visualization. Additionally, if there is an abundance of redundant tissue that is limiting visualization, a 6U portal may be utilized for probe retraction during arthroscopy and debridement. In our experience, the redundant capsular tissue may be chronic and therefore does not always exhibit signs of acute inflammation with injected synovium. Finally, it is imperative to switch portals and assure that the entire dorsal capsule is evaluated for potential pathologic capsule. Consideration of a volar radial portal is advised if visualization is poor.

Conclusion

DWCI is caused by impingement of redundant or avulsed dorsal capsular tissue between the carpus and the dorsal lip of the distal radius, causing pain at the dorsal radiocarpal joint during wrist extension. Arthroscopy is used for both confirmation of diagnosis and treatment. MRI, if obtained, may be negative in the setting of DWCI but can be helpful in evaluating other pathologies. Treatment consists of debridement of redundant dorsal capsular tissue. Dorsal portals are generally sufficient for both visualization and completion of debridement. Postoperatively, pain and functional scores typically improve and are sustained without significant change in range of motion.

References

1. Weinzweig J, Watson HK. Dorsal wrist syndrome: predynamic carpal instability. In: Watson HK, Weinzweig J, editors. The wrist. Philadelphia: Lippincott Williams & Wilkins; 2001. p. 483–90.
2. Watson HK, Rogers WD, Ashmead D. Reevaluation of the cause of the wrist ganglion. J Hand Surg. 1989;14(5):812–7.
3. Yasuda M, Masada K, Takeuchi E. Dorsal wrist syndrome repair. Hand Surg. 2004;09(01):45–8.
4. Srinivasan R, Wysocki R, Jain D, Richard M, Leversedge F, Ruch D. Arthroscopic treatment of dorsal wrist syndrome (DWS) (SS-51). Arthroscopy. 2013;29(6):e25.
5. Jain K, Singh R. Short-term result of arthroscopic synovial excision for dorsal wrist pain in hyperextension associated with synovial hypertrophy. Singap Med J. 2014;55(10):547–9.

6. Henry M. Arthroscopic Management of Dorsal Wrist Impingement. J Hand Surg. 2008;33(7):1201–4.

7. Matson AP, Dekker TJ, Lampley AJ, Richard MJ, Leversedge FJ, Ruch DS. Diagnosis and arthroscopic Management of Dorsal Wrist Capsular Impingement. J Hand Surg. 2017;42(3):e167–74.

8. Slutsky DJ. The incidence of dorsal radiocarpal ligament tears in patients having diagnostic wrist arthroscopy for wrist pain. J Hand Surg. 2008;33(3):332–4. https://doi.org/10.1016/j.jhsa.2007.11.026.

9. Slutsky DJ. Arthroscopic dorsal radiocarpal ligament repair. Arthroscopy. 2005;21(12):1486.

10. Slutsky DJ. Arthroscopic repair of dorsal radiocarpal ligament tears. Arthroscopy. 2002;18(9):1–6. https://doi.org/10.1053/jars.2002.36471.

11. Swann RP, Noureldin M, Kakar S. Dorsal radiotriquetral ligament snapping wrist syndrome – a novel presentation and review of literature: case report. J Hand Surg. 2016;41(3). https://doi.org/10.1016/j.jhsa.2015.12.029.

12. Leversedge FJ, Goldfarb CA, Boyer MI. A pocketbook manual of hand and upper extremity anatomy: primus manus. Philadelphia: Lippincott, Williams and Wilkins; 2012.

13. Slutsky DJ. The use of a volar ulnar portal in wrist arthroscopy. Arthroscopy. 2004;20(2):158–63.

14. Slutsky DJ. Clinical applications of volar portals in wrist arthroscopy. Tech Hand Up Extrem Surg. 2004;8(4):229–38.

Midcarpal Instability

Michael B. Gottschalk and Randy Bindra

Introduction

Midcarpal instability, also known as carpal instability non-dissociative (CIND), is defined as the dissociation between the proximal and distal carpal row under physiologic loads. The incidence is perceived to be low among patients, but this may be secondary to the difficulty in diagnosing the condition as imaging is seldom helpful. Patients with hypermobile joints are more prone to developing midcarpal instability (MCI), but the onset of symptoms often relates to a traumatic event. Pain is usually referred to the ulnar side of the wrist and sometimes specifically to the triquetrohamate joint and is often associated with a clunk on ulnar deviation of the wrist. Several provocative maneuvers are helpful in diagnosing midcarpal instability, and these include the anterior and posterior drawer tests, midcarpal shift test, and forced radial or ulnar deviation tests [1]. Standard wrist radiographs should be performed as part of a routine workup, but the instability between the two carpal rows is only demonstrated on stress views.

The role of wrist arthroscopy in the diagnosis is limited as there is no visible dissociation between the carpal bones. However, arthroscopy is useful to exclude other pathology that may present with ulnar-sided wrist pain.

Treatment of midcarpal instability is also challenging. Therapy to improve the proprioceptive control of the wrist and bracing that corrects the instability should be the first line of management [2, 3]. Arthroscopic thermal capsulorrhaphy may be useful in mild cases. Depending on the type of instability, that is, palmar or dorsal, radiofrequency treatment of the volar or dorsal-involved structures is performed [4, 5]. In more severe cases, especially with multiple joint laxity, or in the presence of degenerative changes, arthroscopic midcarpal fusion can be successful in resolution of symptoms at the expense of some loss of wrist mobility.

Evolution of Midcarpal Instability

The understanding of the mechanisms leading to midcarpal instability has evolved over several years and definition, diagnosis, and treatment of midcarpal instability have not been fully established. What was first described as a "snapping wrist" by Mouchet and Belot in 1934 was likely anterior midcarpal subluxation [6]. While the idea of instability between the carpal rows had yet to be defined, a report by Sutro in 1946 laid the groundwork for the identification of an entity that affected the midcarpal joint and was cured by midcarpal fusion [7]. It was not until almost forty years later that Lichtman and colleagues in 1981 identified volar intercalated segment instability (VISI) as a pattern of ulnar midcarpal instability that occurred secondary to the disruption of the palmar arcuate ligament [8]. A few years later in 1984, its counterpart was described by Louis and colleagues and named the capitate-lunate instability pattern (CLIP), with a demonstrable dorsal subluxation of the capitate relative to the lunate under stress views [9].

Kinematics of Midcarpal Instability

MCI is a collection of several distinct clinical entities differing in the cause and direction of subluxation from abnormal force transmission at the midcarpal joint. Various published small clinical series describe either a palmar, dorsal, or combined palmar and dorsal pattern.

The most common type, palmar MCI results from laxity of the radiocarpal ligament dorsally and the ulnar arcuate

M. B. Gottschalk (✉)
Hand and Upper Extremity, Department of Orthopaedic Surgery, Emory University Hospital, Atlanta, GA, USA
e-mail: mbgotts@emory.edu

R. Bindra
Department of Orthopaedic Surgery, Griffith University School of Medicine, Gold Coast University Hospital, Southport, QLD, Australia

© Springer Nature Switzerland AG 2022
W. B. Geissler (ed.), *Wrist and Elbow Arthroscopy with Selected Open Procedures*,
https://doi.org/10.1007/978-3-030-78881-0_24

ligament of the volar capsule. During normal physiologic loading of the wrist, the proximal row will tend to flex and pronate while being stabilized by the palmar arcuate ligament formed by the radioscaphocapitate and triquetrohamate-capitate ligaments [10]. These ligaments are essential for providing palmar support to the carpus and seamless extension of the proximal carpal row as the wrist moves from radial to ulnar deviation. When the volar arcuate or dorsal radiocarpal ligaments are injured or pathologically lax, the proximal row fails to extend in a synchronous fashion as the wrist moves into ulnar deviation. Complete ulnar deviation causes a sudden reversal of the VISI, as the helicoidal triquetrohamate joint is reengaged and physiologic joint contact forces extend the proximal carpal row, this sudden extension causes the painful clunk – the so-called catch-up clunk. As the wrist moves back to neutral, the ulnar forces are disengaged and the proximal row drops back into a flexed position. The clunk has been reproduced in cadaveric models by sectioning the ulnar arm of the arcuate ligament [11, 12].

In patients with dorsal MCI, attenuation of the palmar radiocapitate ligament allows dorsal subluxation of the capitate on the lunate under load [13].

It should be noted that in both the palmar and dorsal patterns, the proximal row always moves into extension and the distal row translates dorsally with ulnar deviation. When this transition is smooth, it represents normal wrist kinematics. It is the timing and force of this movement that differentiates the two patterns and creates the pathologic clinical patterns of MCI. In palmar MCI, the proximal row sags into a VISI pattern in the neutral wrist and reduces with ulnar deviation. In dorsal MCI, the unloaded wrist is neutral and the dorsal subluxation occurs in ulnar deviation. In either case, the instability is caused primarily by true or relative laxity of selected ligaments supporting the proximal row and their failure to control the complex kinematic relationships between the articular surfaces across the midcarpal joint.

In contrast to the above-described patterns of MCI from intrinsic ligamentous insufficiency, extrinsic causes can also cause MCI when carpal bones adapt to realign the hand in response to abnormal dorsal angulation of the distal radius. As the proximal carpal row tilts dorsally to align with the dorsally angulated distal radius, there is compensatory flexion of the midcarpal joint resulting in an unstable, zigzag pattern of the wrist [14]. The various forms of carpal instability are summarized in Table 24.1.

History and Physical Examination

Diagnosis of midcarpal instability can be perplexing to most physicians. This is in part due to insidious onset of symptoms often without a single traumatic event. Patients present with ulnar-sided pain on loading the wrist, such as getting up from a chair, carrying a tray on the extended wrist or riding a

Table 24.1 Forms of carpal instability

Name	Brief description	Type/example	Alternate nomenclature
Carpal instability dissociative (CID)	Ligamentous disruption *within* the same carpal row	Scapholunate dissociation	
Carpal instability non-dissociative (CIND)	Ligamentous disruption *between* carpal rows	Palmar	(Ulnar MCI) (CIND-VISI)
		Dorsal	(CLIP) (CIND-DISI)
		Combined	
Carpal instability adaptive (CIA)	Sometimes included under CIND	Distal radius with dorsal tilt malunion	
Carpal instability complex (CIC)	Disruption both between and within carpal rows	Perilunate	

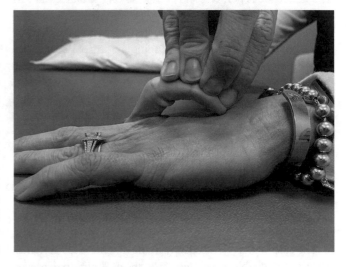

Fig. 24.1 Examination depicting hypermobility of the finger joints associated with Ehlers-Danlos

bicycle. Clunking of the wrist appears later, and in advanced cases, patients can clunk their wrist at will.

The majority of patients with MCI have generalized joint hypermobility secondary to genetic inheritance or acquired it subsequent to years of training or stretching. A history of hypermobile joints with instability in other joints should be sought. General examination should include maneuvers to evaluate hyperlaxity at several common joints (Fig. 24.1). A Beighton score ≥ 4 is suggestive of generalized hypermobility [15]. To further elucidate the type of midcarpal instability, there are several provocative tests that can be performed. These include the anterior and posterior drawer test, and midcarpal shift test [1]. For palmar instability, the anterior drawer test is performed by applying a volar-directed force on the distal carpal row and observing a volar sag on lateral

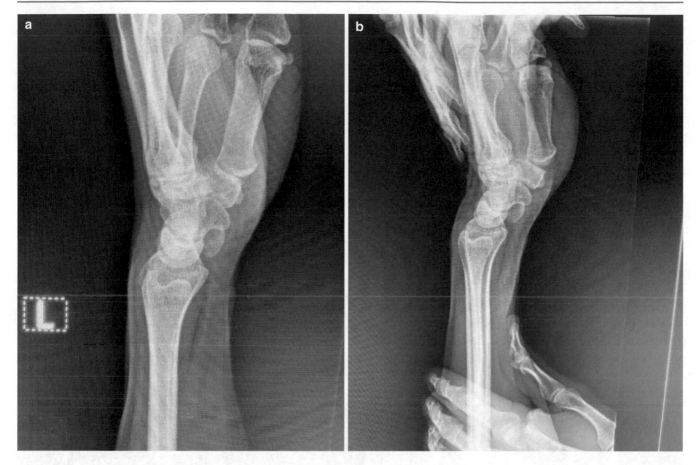

Fig. 24.2 (**a**) Routine lateral radiograph of the wrist without an anterior directed force. (**b**) Lateral radiograph with anterior-directed force and associated volar sag of the midcarpus

radiographs (Fig. 24.2). A midcarpal shift test may also be performed where by a volar-directed force is applied with an addition of an axial load and forced ulnar deviation. In doing so, the proximal carpal row is forced in to extension rapidly, thus creating the "catch-up clunk." For dorsal MCI, the posterior drawer test, also known as dorsal capitate displacement test, is achieved by applying a volar to dorsal-directed force in addition to longitudinal traction. Displacement of the capitate relative to the lunate with dorsal subluxation of the distal carpal row relative to the proximal row is indicative of a positive test. Occasionally, the patients themselves may be able to reproduce their instability. The instability is often demonstrable in the opposite asymptomatic wrist.

Imaging

The diagnosis of MCI is clinical-imaging is helpful when performed under load in dynamic conditions. A standard diagnostic workup should start with a set of radiographs in at

least two planes. A mild VISI pattern with palmar tilt of the lunate may be seen on the lateral projection [1]. Stress views with the wrist in extreme ulnar or radial deviation may demonstrate translation of the capitate either volarly or dorsally depending on the type of instability pattern, with the lunate flexed or extended. PA stress views should also be taken in those patients where there is concern for possible dissociative instability.

Dynamic fluoroscopy, usually performed under anesthesia at the time of wrist arthroscopy will demonstrate the sudden change of position of the lunate from flexion to extension with a clunk in palmar MCI. 4-D CT scanning like cinefluoroscopy allows dynamic imaging of the wrist and can demonstrate subtle cases of wrist instability [16]. The images are particularly helpful in explaining the condition to the patient and solicit their cooperation in rehabilitation.

MR imaging is of limited value as there is no diagnostic sign of MCI. Synovitis at the triquetrohamate joint or marrow edema may be seen in some cases. MR is useful in excluding other causes of ulnar-sided wrist pain.

Conservative Measures

For most patients, including hypermobile patients, the initial treatment for midcarpal instability is most commonly nonoperative, and often takes the form of bracing and therapy focusing on neuromuscular control of the wrist [2, 3]. For patients with palmar MCI, it is recommended that the patient wears a brace that provides a dorsally directed force just proximal to the pisiform. In addition to wearing the brace, neuromuscular modulation in the form of strengthening the wrist flexors and extensors will provide dynamic stabilization to the joints. When this fails to provide adequate relief to the patient, operative intervention should be considered.

Indications

Arthroscopy of the wrist may be utilized for the diagnosis or treatment of MCI. In general, the indications for performing wrist arthroscopy in the setting of midcarpal instability are relatively narrow [17]. There are no arthroscopic findings that are diagnostic of midcarpal instability and arthroscopy is largely performed to rule out other causes of ulnar-sided wrist pain. Laxity of the lunotriquetral interosseous ligament visualized from the 6R portal may be seen. Midcarpal arthroscopy may reveal laxity of the triquetrohamate-capitate ligament, but this is difficult to gauge. There may be an associated tear of the dorsal radiocarpal ligament (DRCL). In advanced cases of MCI, chondral damage may be seen at the triquetrohamate or lunocapitate articulations.

Arthroscopy is helpful in identifying other causes of ulnar-sided wrist pain. Ulnocarpal impaction is easily identified arthroscopically with degeneration or perforation of the central triangular cartilage and corresponding chondromalacia of the ulnar half of the lunate bone. In cases of hamatolunate impaction, arthroscopy of the midcarpal joint demonstrates chondromalacia of the tip of the hamate as it articulates with a distinct facet on the distal lunate (type II lunate) [18].

Therapeutic arthroscopy is directed at treating the lax ligaments with thermal capsulorrhaphy or fusion of the midcarpal joint (Fig. 24.3).

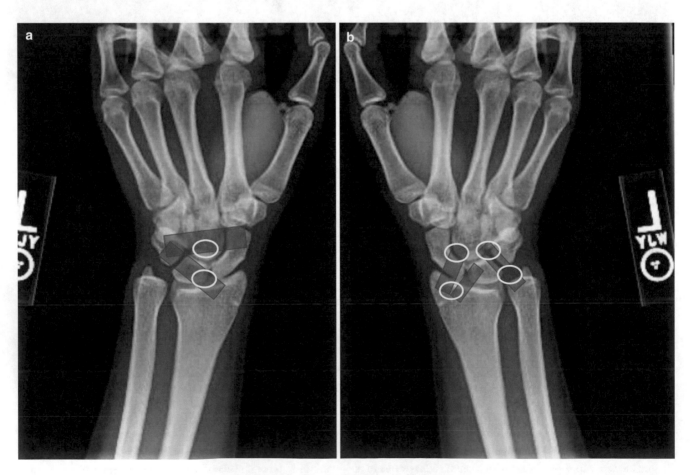

Fig. 24.3 Dorsal (**a**) and volar (**b**) recommended structures (red) of the carpus and subsequent locations of radio frequency ablation (yellow circles)

Contraindications

There are no absolute contraindications to performing a diagnostic arthroscopy with a clinical diagnosis of MCI. When the diagnosis is clear on clinical examination and supported by dynamic imaging, routine arthroscopic examination is of limited value.

Patients that present with a fixed deformities of the carpus are best treated with open procedures to correct their instability. In addition, patients with a combined or mixed volar and dorsal instability often require open surgical intervention with limited carpal fusion. Patients with collagen disorders, such as Ehlers-Danlos or Marfans syndrome and MCI should undergo a bony procedure in lieu of wrist arthroscopy. Lastly, any patient who presents with extrinsic adaptive carpal instability secondary to a malunited distal radius is treated with an osteotomy of the distal radius [17].

Technique

Arthroscopy should start with a standard setup with the patient supine on the table with an associated arm board for stabilization. A traction tower is essential and should provide 10 lb of distraction of the wrist. In addition, the finger traps utilized may be placed more radially or both radially and ulnarly to allow entry in to the various locations of the wrist. Use of a tourniquet allows for better visualization but saline distension is not generally required for diagnostic arthroscopy unless thermal capsulorrhaphy is to be performed. Routine arthroscopy with a 1.9-mm or 2.3-mm arthroscope utilizes standard 3-4 and 6R portals along with the radial and ulnar midcarpal portals. In patients with suspected tears of the dorsal radiocarpal ligament, a volar radial portal may be necessary [19]. The volar radial portal is established by open technique through a 1-cm transverse incision over the flexor carpi radialis tendon at the proximal wrist crease. The tendon is retracted, and the radiocarpal space is identified with a 22-gauge needle and the portal is created by blunt dissection using a hemostat. With the arthroscope in the volar portal, the ligament is visualized just ulnar to the 3-4 portal, dorsal to the lunate. The integrity of the ligament is tested by hooking it with a hook probe inserted from the 3-4 portal.

Therapeutic Arthroscopy

Because the pathology is largely related to ligament laxity rather than a tear, arthroscopic thermal shrinkage is an attractive treatment option. Thermal capsulorrhaphy utilizes a radiofrequency probe to apply heat to affected ligaments. Treated areas of ligament tighten and assume a dull yellow appearance (Fig. 24.4). At a molecular level, the triple helix of collagen "unwinds" and "shrinks" at temperatures around 60 °C. The denatured collagen can potentially shorten to 50% of its resting length. Treatment is carried out by "striping," leaving untreated bands of intact collagen that allows deposition of new collagen fibers over the shortened scaffold of the treated areas of ligament. The tensile strength of heated collagen decreases rapidly and wrist should be protected for up to 12 weeks.

In patients with palmar MCI, the arcuate ligament is amenable to treatment by thermal capsulorrhaphy using a 2.3-mm VAPR end-effect probe (Depuy Mitek, Leeds, UK). The probe is applied to the ulnar arm of the palmar arcuate ligament (ulnocapitate, ulnotriquetral, and triquetrocapitate ligaments) as well as the radial arm (radioscaphocapitate, long and short radiolunate ligaments) and accessible parts of the dorsal capsule in both the radiocarpal and midcarpal joints (Figs. 24.4 and 24.5). The technique for thermal ablation should include a single pass over the ligament in a sweeping manner that causes slight yellowish discoloration of the ligament. This should be repeated as necessary for the area of the ligament in a banding fashion leaving segments of untreated viable ligament in between treated areas. Care is taken to copiously irrigate the joint during the process to avoid thermal damage to cartilage.

In patients with a tear of the dorsal radiocarpal ligament capsular repair of the ligament can be performed arthroscopically. A 2–0 PDS suture is passed through a curved spinal needle that is introduced through the 4/5 portal. The end of

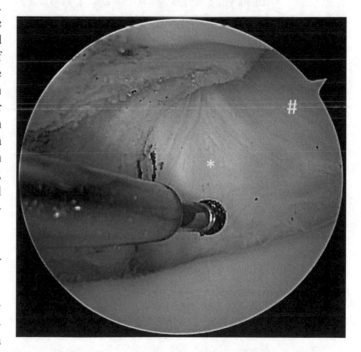

Fig. 24.4 Radiofrequency probe through the 4-5 portal of a left wrist looking radial volar at the volar RL (*) and RSC (#)

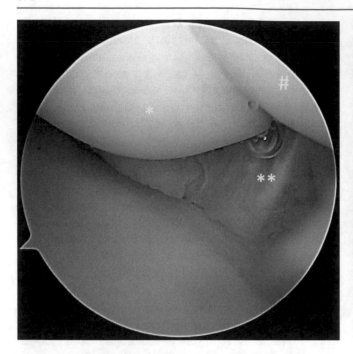

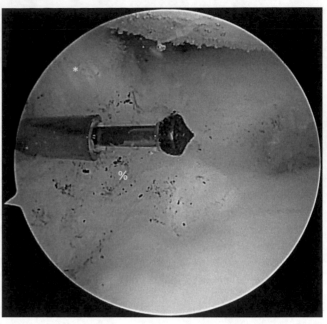

Fig. 24.5 Scope through the radial midcarpal portal of a left wrist looking ulnar volar at the hamate (*), capitate (#), and distal portion of the volar ulnar aspect of the arcuate ligament

Fig. 24.6 Example of normal ligament (*) and caramelized portion (%). Notice the fine tip of the probe that allows for more precise ablation

the suture is retrieved with a grasper in the 3/4 portal. A curved hemostat is used to pull the ulnar end of the suture underneath the extensor tendons and the knot is tied at the 4/5 portal pulling up the torn edge of the ligament against the dorsal capsule One suture is usually sufficient. The repair is augmented with thermal shrinkage if the DRCL is particularly voluminous and protrudes into the joint after the suture is tied.

For dorsal MCI, treatment is directed at the radiocarpal joint. With the arthroscope in the 3-4 portal and the RF probe in the 4-5 or 6R portal, the radioscaphocapitate ligament is treated. This structure is the most radial of the ligaments. Moving from radial to ulnar, the short and long radiolunate ligaments may also be tightened. In addition, the volar ulnar arm of the arcuate ligament, including the ulna-triquetral ligament, may then be cauterized (Fig. 24.6).

Postoperatively, the wrist is immobilized in a below-elbow cast or splint with the wrist in neutral rotation for 4 weeks.

Arthrodesis of the capitolunate joint or the triquetroham-ate joint has been described for the management of MCI. While these are traditionally performed as open surgical procedures, they may be performed arthroscopically or with arthroscopic assistance by surgeons adept at arthroscopic techniques. With the midcarpal joint under distraction for arthroscopy, a 3-mm burr can be introduced into the ulnar midcarpal portal and the joint surfaces denuded

under vision (Fig. 24.7). Dry arthroscopy in particular facilitates the process, with intermittent irrigation for removal of debris. Alternatively, the capitolunate joint is exposed through a small transverse incision and the joint surfaces are excised. Fixation can be achieved with retrograde cannulated screw fixation. Guide wires are passed in a retrograde fashion through the index-middle interosseous space under fluoroscopic guidance. Cancellous graft from the distal radius is inserted into the fusion site via the arthroscope cannula. One or two cannulated screws are then inserted as traction on the hand is released to achieve compression of the arthrodesis [20].

Reported Outcomes of Arthroscopic Management of Midcarpal Instability

Due to the relative low incidence of symptomatic carpal instability and the fact that the arthroscopic management of midcarpal instability is technically demanding, there is a paucity of data on the results of arthroscopic surgical management of the condition [17]. More recently, however, Hargreaves et al. has published on their early and midterm results of arthroscopic capsular shrinkage for PMI [21]. The authors performed a retrospective review of 15 cases in 13 wrists. The mean age of patients was 28 with a predominance of women (77%). The diagnosis was made using the

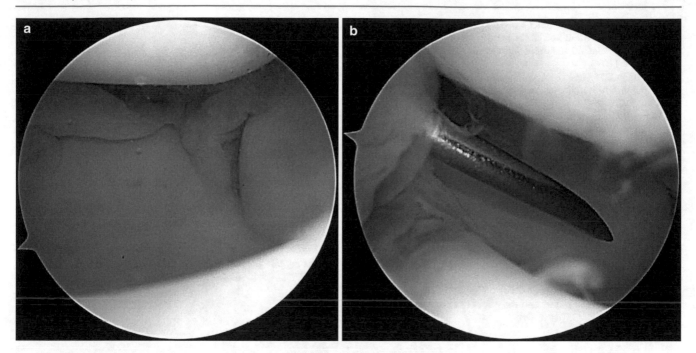

Fig. 24.7 (**a**) Radial midcarpal arthroscopy of a left wrist establishing an ulnar midcarpal portal dorsally under direct visualization (**b**)

ulnar shift and palmar midcarpal drawer. Once diagnosed, those patients who failed conservative measures underwent thermal capsular shrinkage using the technique as described above. Patients were immobilized for 6 weeks and did not receive formal physiotherapy. Only 14 of the wrists were available for follow-up at an average of 42 months. Results demonstrated a statistically significant improvement in Disabilities of the Arm, Shoulder, and Hand (DASH) scores from 34 preoperatively to 12 postoperatively (p = 0.0034). Twelve out of the 14 patients no longer had a positive ulnar shift test on clinical examination. In addition, patients lost on average 16 degrees of flexion and 10 degrees of extension as compared to the contralateral side. The mean reduction of overall arc was 8 degrees comprising 15% of total motion. Lastly, there was no evidence of complication including subsequent arthritis or damage to adjacent tendons or structures.

Tips and Tricks

- Use an arthroscopic tower that allows mobility of the tower relative to the wrist; this grants access to any portal with ease whether it be volar or dorsal.
- Use a designated outflow portal to reduce risk of thermal injury to the cartilage.
- Use a narrow RF wand with a protected tip to more precisely ablate the tissue affected.

Conclusion

Midcarpal instability is a relatively uncommon pathologic entity that requires an astute clinician for diagnosis and treatment. Conservative measures should be employed as the mainstay of treatment and should focus on neuromuscular rehabilitation by a certified hand therapist followed by splinting techniques geared toward the specific type of instability. Should these methods fail, arthroscopic capsular shrinkage remains a viable alternative with relatively good outcomes for those with mild intrinsic instability (e.g., palmar or dorsal). Due to the complexity of the surgery, physicians should be well versed in the various arthroscopic portals necessary to access both volar and dorsal ligaments.

References

1. Wolfe SW, Garcia-Elias M, Kitay A. Carpal instability nondissociative. J Am Acad Orthop Surg. 2012;20(9):575–85.
2. Mulders MAM, Sulkers GSI, Videler AJ, Strackee SD, Smeulders MJC. Long-term functional results of a wrist exercise program for patients with palmar Midcarpal instability. J Wrist Surg. 2018;7(3):211–8.
3. Harwood C, Turner L. Conservative management of midcarpal instability. J Hand Surg Eur Vol. 2016;41(1):102–9.
4. Hargreaves DG. Midcarpal instability. J Hand Surg Eur Vol. 2016;41(1):86–93.
5. Hargreaves DG. Arthroscopic thermal capsular shrinkage for palmar midcarpal instability. J Wrist Surg. 2014;3(3):162–5.

6. Mouchet A, Belot J. Poignet a resault (subluxation mediocarpienne en avant). Bull Mem Soc Natl Chir. 1934;60:1243–4.

7. Sutro CJ. Bilateral recurrent intercarpal subluxation. Am J Surg. 1946;72:110–3.

8. Lichtman DM, Schneider JR, Swafford AR, Mack GR. Ulnar mid-carpal instability-clinical and laboratory analysis. J Hand Surg Am. 1981;6(5):515–23.

9. Louis DS, Hankin FM, Greene TL, Braunstein EM, White SJ. Central carpal instability-capitate lunate instability pattern: diagnosis by dynamic displacement. Orthopedics. 1984;7(11):1693–6.

10. Wolfe SW, editor. Green's operative hand surgery. Philadelphia: Elsevier; 2011.

11. Trumble TE, Bour CJ, Smith RJ, Glisson RR. Kinematics of the ulnar carpus related to the volar intercalated segment instability pattern. J Hand Surg Am. 1990;15(3):384–92.

12. Viegas SF, Patterson RM, Peterson PD, Pogue DJ, Jenkins DK, Sweo TD, et al. Ulnar-sided perilunate instability: an anatomic and biomechanic study. J Hand Surg Am. 1990;15(2):268–78.

13. Johnson RP, Carrera GF. Chronic capitolunate instability. J Bone Joint Surg Am. 1986;68(8):1164–76.

14. De Smet L, Verhaegen F, Degreef I. Carpal malalignment in malunion of the distal radius and the effect of corrective osteotomy. J Wrist Surg. 2014;3(3):166–70.

15. Beighton P. Hypermobility scoring. Br J Rheumatol. 1988;27(2):163.

16. Repse SE, Koulouris G, Troupis JM. Wide field of view computed tomography and mid-carpal instability: the value of the sagittal radius-lunate-capitate axis--preliminary experience. Eur J Radiol. 2015;84(5):908–14.

17. Lindau TR. The role of arthroscopy in carpal instability. J Hand Surg Eur Vol. 2016;41(1):35–47.

18. Thurston AJ, Stanley JK. Hamato-lunate impingement: an uncommon cause of ulnar-sided wrist pain. Arthroscopy. 2000;16(5):540–4.

19. Slutsky DJ. The incidence of dorsal radiocarpal ligament tears in patients having diagnostic wrist arthroscopy for wrist pain. J Hand Surg Am. 2008;33(3):332–4.

20. Slade JF III, Bomback DA. Percutaneous capitolunate arthrodesis using arthroscopic or limited approach. Atlas Hand Clin. 2003;8:149–62.

21. Mason WT, Hargreaves DG. Arthroscopic thermal capsulorrhaphy for palmar midcarpal instability. J Hand Surg Eur Vol. 2007;32(4):411–6.

Internal Brace for Midcarpal Instability

25

Remy V. Rabinovich and Randall W. Culp

Introduction

In the 1980s, the concept of MCI was formally introduced as a pathologic entity [1, 2]. Prior to this, only midcarpal joint laxity and palmar subluxation of the distal carpal row had been described [3]. Since being introduced, the disorder has lacked a consensus agreement on its terminology, etiology, pathomechanics, and subsequently, its approach to treatment. Several distinct clinical entities, each differing in the cause and direction of subluxation, make up the general concept of MCI and together share the common pathology of abnormal force transmission at the midcarpal joint [4]. Midcarpal instability is just one element of a number of different carpal instability patterns [4]. These other patterns of carpal instability include radiocarpal and perilunate dislocation, which can be due to either ligamentous disruption (lesser arc injury), fracture (greater arc injury), or a combination of both as well as proximal carpal instabilities, such as ulnar translocation of the carpus and dorsal/volar Barton shear fractures of the distal radius. Any of these carpal instability patterns can be more broadly categorized as either dissociative (due to ligament disruption between individual carpal bones of the same row) or nondissociative (due to ligamentous laxity and instability between carpal rows). Focusing on MCI, this entity of carpal instability can be further divided into intrinsic or extrinsic forms, depending on whether (1) there is laxity or disruption of the wrist ligaments themselves (intrinsic) or (2) there is a bony abnormality outside the carpus (i.e., distal radius malunion or ulnar-minus variance) contributing to or causing wrist ligament pathology. The intrinsic form can be further subdivided into dorsal, palmar, and combined types.

Pathomechanics

As alluded to previously, the term MCI encompasses several distinct clinical entities, each differing in their etiology, direction of subluxation and ultimately, their pathomechanics. The intrinsic palmar type of MCI (PMCI) is the most common pattern of MCI and is characterized by laxity or disruption of the volar arcuate, the dorsal radiotriquetral, and/or the periscaphoid (STT) ligaments, which leads to the proximal carpal row sagging into volar flexion (VISI) [4]. When the wrist moves along the dart-thrower's trajectory from neutral to ulnar, the normal joint reaction forces are not engaged and the proximal row maintains its flexed (VISI) posture well into ulnar deviation. Meanwhile, the distal row follows the lunate and is settled into a palmarly subluxed position. As maximal ulnar deviation is reached, the helicoidal triquetrohamate (TH) joint is engaged and the physiologic joint reaction forces are reactivated, causing the proximal row to forcefully rotate from flexion into the physiologically extended (DISI) position. Clinically, this is manifested as a loss of the smooth transition of the proximal row from flexion into extension, creating a sudden, painful clunk. This catch-up clunk is shown in Video 25.1. As the wrist moves back to neutral, the ulnar forces are disengaged and the proximal row assumes its VISI posture while the distal row again settles palmarly into its slightly subluxed position. Laboratory investigation by Lichtman and researchers [1, 5] aimed to reproduce MCI in vitro by sectioning various capsular ligaments of the wrist. While sectioning of the dorsal and ulnar TH ligament created subtle midcarpal laxity

Supplementary Information The online version of this chapter (https://doi.org/10.1007/978-3-030-78881-0_25) contains supplementary material, which is available to authorized users.

R. V. Rabinovich
Department of Orthopaedic Surgery, Thomas Jefferson University Hospitals, Philadelphia Hand to Shoulder Center, Philadelphia, PA, USA

R. W. Culp (✉)
Department of Orthopaedic Surgery, Thomas Jefferson University Hospitals, Philadelphia Hand to Shoulder Center, King of Prussia, PA, USA

W. B. Geissler (ed.), *Wrist and Elbow Arthroscopy with Selected Open Procedures*, https://doi.org/10.1007/978-3-030-78881-0_25

and no clunk, division of the more robust ulnar limb of the palmar arcuate ligament produced a clunk similar, but not identical to that observed in their patients with MCI. Additionally, Trumble et al. [6] as well as Viegas et al. [7] were able to produce a VISI deformity and characteristics of PMCI in cadaveric specimens when dividing the ulnar arm of the palmar arcuate ligament or the dorsal radiotriquetral ligament. The less common, intrinsic dorsal type of MCI (DMCI) is more poorly understood and less extensively described. What differentiates the two intrinsic MCI patterns is the timing and force of the sudden change in sagittal plane posture of the proximal carpal row as the wrist is ulnarly deviated. In the PMCI pattern, it is the initial volar translation (subluxation) in neutral that reduces in ulnar deviation whereas in the DMCI pattern, the wrist is reduced in neutral and the dorsal subluxation occurs in ulnar deviation [4]. The dorsal subluxation of the capitate on the lunate with ulnar deviation of the wrist can be attributed to laxity or attenuation of either the dorsal or volar capsular ligaments. Louis and colleagues [2] proposed that the source of instability and symptoms was dynamic laxity of the dorsal capsular ligaments, particularly the radiolunate and dorsal capitolunate, whereas Johnson and Carrera [8] theorized that it was the traumatic attenuation of the palmar radiocapitate ligament that led to this painful instability problem. Wolfe and colleagues [9] eluded to the importance of the dorsal intercarpal ligament (DIC), particularly the thick scaphotriquetral fascicles, as it functions like a pseudolabrum, deepening the ball-and-socket-like scapholunocapitate articulation and preventing dorsal subluxation of the capitate on the lunate. These authors also highlighted that laxity or deficiency of the space of Poirer, formed by the DIC, long radiolunate and radioscaphocapitate ligaments, contributes to dorsal capitate subluxation as well. In either case, the instability is caused primarily by true or relative laxity of selected ligaments supporting the proximal row and their failure to control the complex kinematic relationships between the articular surfaces of the midcarpal joint [4]. Dorsal and palmar instability in patients has also been recognized, particularly among young females with global ligamentous laxity. Apergis [10], in his series on this patient subset, noted VISI alignment in all unstressed wrists that showed dorsal subluxation of the capitolunate and/or radiolunate joints when a dorsal-displacement stress test was performed. When the wrist is placed in radial deviation, lunate flexion and ulnar carpal translation is present. As the wrist is brought into ulnar deviation, the lunate abruptly "clunks" into extension (similar to PMCI) and upon extreme ulnar deviation, dorsal subluxation of the capitate ensues (similarly to DMCI) [9].

Extrinsic MCI is often associated with malunited distal radius fractures or ulna-minus variance plus increased ulnar slope of the lunate fossa. Taleisnik and Watson [11] reported on 13 patients with symptoms of midcarpal pain and insta-bility after sustaining malunited distal radius fractures with an average dorsal tilt of 23°. Upon radiographic evaluation, the authors noted that the lunate (along with the rest of the carpus) had migrated dorsally and was angled palmarly to compensate for the dorsal radial displacement. They attributed the wrist pain and instability to the repetitive overload of the midcarpal joint as a result of reversal of the normal palmar tilt of the distal radius and consequently, intact carpal ligaments that were incapable of preventing excessive dorsal translation of the capitate. Lichtman et al. [4] postulated that reversal of the normal volar tilt of the distal radius effectively slackened the volar extrinsic wrist ligaments, making them less effective in restraining dorsal subluxation of the distal carpal row. The notion that good results were obtained after corrective osteotomy of the distal radius reinforces the theory that reestablishing correct tension of the volar ligaments also corrects the tendency for dorsal subluxation of the lunate and capitate. Wright et al. [12] observed midcarpal instability among patients with ulna-minus variance and an increased ulnar slope of the lunate fossa. The authors speculated that this osseous abnormality led to an increased ulnar translatory force, which stretched the radiolunate and radiocapitate ligaments. When they leveled the distal radioulnar joint in select patients, they felt that the triangular fibrocartilage served as a buttress and provided additional support to the ulnar aspect of the lunate and the triquetrum. This facilitated movement of the proximal carpal row up the radial slope of the distal radius during ulnar deviation of the wrist, providing a smooth, fluid motion of the proximal carpal row rather than the sudden, forceful clunk into DISI.

Patient Evaluation

Presentation and Examination

The typical patient with PMCI is in their third or fourth decade of life and presents with an uncomfortable clunking sensation in the wrist upon performing activities that require twisting, squeezing or ranging the wrist into the extremes of motion [13]. Patients often exhibit global ligamentous laxity and cannot recall a particular injury with the onset of symptoms. It is not uncommon for patients with global, as well as pathologic, ligamentous laxity (Ehlers-Danlos syndrome, Marfan's syndrome, cutis laxa) to have asymptomatic or minimally symptomatic palmar MCI [9]. A volar sag to the wrist is usually noted upon visual inspection. As the patient takes their wrist from radial to ulnar deviation, the classic catch-up clunk can be appreciated as the proximal carpal row rotates from a flexed posture into an extended posture. Lichtman and colleagues [1, 5] described the midcarpal shift test, which helps demonstrate this clunk. It is performed by

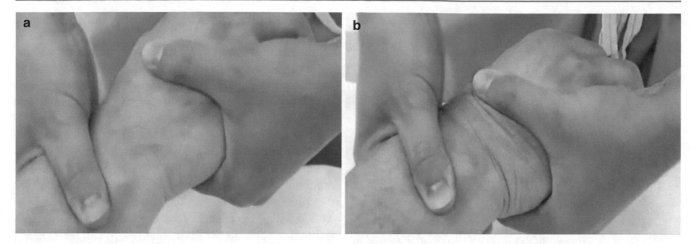

Fig. 25.1 Clinical photos exhibiting a neutrally aligned wrist (**a**) that falls into volar sag (**b**) as an anteriorly directed force to the distal carpus is applied while the forearm held pronated

placing the patient's wrist in neutral with the forearm pronated and then applying a palmar force to the hand at the level of the distal capitate while simultaneously axially loading and ulnarly deviating the wrist (Fig. 25.1a, b). The test result is positive if a painful clunk occurs that reproduces the patient's symptoms. Forearm pronation accentuates the clunk because it increases tension on the ulnar extrinsic ligaments, which resist the extension force on the proximal carpal row as the wrist ulnarly deviates [9]. Patients with DMCI classically report pain and clicking while grasping objects with the forearm supinated, which eventually progresses to weakness with this maneuver [4, 8]. Unlike patients with palmar MCI, history of an extension injury to the wrist may be present. Dorsal MCI can be clinically elicited by the dynamic dorsal displacement test, performed by applying longitudinal traction and a dorsally directed force to the scaphoid tubercle while maintaining the wrist in a flexed and ulnarly deviated position [2]. A positive test recreates the patient's pain as the capitate subluxes dorsally relative to the lunate. Combined palmar and dorsal MCI is often present in ligamentously lax adolescent females that commonly have an extension injury to the wrist. In addition to ligamentous laxity, a volar sag sign of the ulnar carpus may be noted along with positive palmar and dorsal displacement stress tests of the midcarpal joint. The presentation of patients with extrinsic MCI is dependent upon the source of the osseous abnormality contributing to ligamentous imbalance. Patients with malunited distal radius fractures have a history of a wrist injury and fracture. Taleisnik and Watson [11] noted these patients to exhibited tenderness at the lunocapitate and triquetrohamate joints. Roughly half of them demonstrated intermittent midcarpal subluxation and a painful audible snap at the TH joint when the wrist was brought into ulnar deviation while the forearm remained pronated. The authors noted that in all cases, patients reported a period of satisfactory function after the fracture had healed and before the

onset of progressive disability. They reported a gradual onset of symptoms and instability in most patients, which began at least several weeks after the healing of the Colles' fracture and cessation of immobilization. Patients presenting with signs and symptoms of MCI and radiographic evidence of ulna-minus variance with an increased ulnar slope of the lunate fossa have an inconsistent mechanism of injury. These patients tend to be young adults with no predilection to males or females. Many patients exhibit ligamentous laxity with some also reporting a trivial or no history of trauma. Wright and colleagues [12] suggested that ulnar translation of the proximal carpal row increased susceptibility to instability. Thus, physical examination should incorporate a radially directed pressure on the triquetrum, which limits ulnar translation of the proximal row and can prevent the clunk from occurring.

Imaging

Imaging is a vital piece for the work-up of patients with MCI. Initial imaging typically includes bilateral wrist radiographs to compare the osseous architecture and overall alignment. In the evaluation of PMCI, plain radiographs may be normal or they may demonstrate varying degrees of volar tilt of the lunate. Live video fluoroscopy can be more helpful in capturing the dynamic instability of the midcarpal joint as the wrist is moved in radial-ulnar deviation. Lateral video fluoroscopy captures the maintenance of the volar flexed position of the proximal row (Fig. 25.2) until terminal ulnar deviation, when the proximal row abruptly snaps into extension. The anterior drawer stress view can also be performed under live fluoroscopy by applying a volar-directed force to the distal carpal row and observing for either widening of the STT joint or for volar capitolunate subluxation. Diagnostic imaging for DMCI includes performing the dynamic dorsal

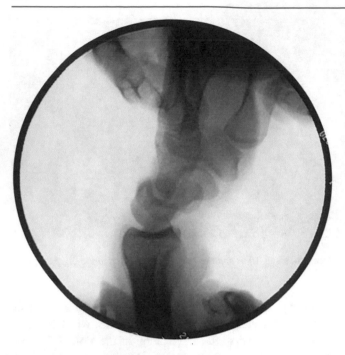

Fig. 25.2 Lateral fluoroscopic image of a wrist in neutral position demonstrating a VISI posture and volar capitolunate subluxation as an anterior stress is applied to the distal carpus

displacement test under video fluoroscopy and directly visualizing dorsal subluxation of the capitate and the reproduction of the patient's pain and clunk. Similar to the assessment of PMCI and DMCI, video fluoroscopy is utilized to evaluate combined MCI by eliciting the VISI deformity in radial deviation or neutral and dorsal capitate subluxation in extreme ulnar deviation.

Indications

Initial management of MCI should be conservative and is primarily nonsurgical. For symptomatic patients, nonsurgical management is usually successful and begins with patient education and avoidance of aggravating activities. Depending on the pattern of MCI, splinting and hand therapy can be helpful for realigning and balancing forces across the wrist. Focusing on the most common pattern of MCI, PMCI, specialized three-point dynamic splints with ulnar volar support can reduce the symptomatic volar ulnar sag. The splint functions by applying a dorsally directed force to the pisiform, taking the proximal carpal row out of VISI and maintaining neutral posture of the lunate [14]. When symptoms occur following an acute injury, the wrist can be casted for 4–6 weeks in neutral flexion and ulnar deviation. With the aid of knowledgeable hand therapists, proprioceptive training can activate the dynamic stabilizers of the wrist to gain stability and relief of symptoms. Isometric strengthening of the flexor carpi ulnaris and extensor carpi ulnaris can help patients pre-

load the wrist to eliminate subluxation and symptomatic clunking [15].

After many months of conservative management without relief of symptoms and instability, surgical treatment is indicated. Options include arthroscopic thermal capsulorrhaphy and/or soft-tissue reconstruction for milder cases and limited radiocarpal or intercarpal fusions for more severe cases. For the palmar intrinsic form of instability, arthroscopic treatment should focus on debridement of any underlying synovitis and shrinkage of the volar extrinsic ligaments [16]. A multitude of soft-tissue reconstruction procedures have been described focusing on stabilizing the triquetrohamate joint by addressing the affected volar arcuate, dorsal radiotriquetral, and/or periscaphoid ligaments [1, 4, 5, 17]. When PMCI is severe and has failed nonsurgical treatment or prior soft-tissue reconstruction, limited radiocarpal or midcarpal fusions should be considered. In this chapter, we focus on mild-to-moderate PMCI amenable to soft-tissue reconstruction using our technique of wrist arthroscopy combined with dorsal radiotriquetral ligament reconstruction with suture tape augmentation.

Contraindications

Relative contraindications to our soft-tissue reconstruction procedure include patients who have not undergone an adequate trial of nonoperative management consisting of activity modification, NSAIDs, splinting, and hand therapy. Careful patient selection is prudent and those unwilling to comply with postoperative management and rehabilitation should not undergo the surgery. Those who display ligamentous laxity and the presence of a clunk but do not have pain are contraindicated to undergo surgery as well. Furthermore, the procedure is relatively contraindicated in patients who have failed a prior attempt at soft-tissue reconstruction and those with mild degenerative changes at the midcarpal joint(s). Finally, absolute contraindications are active infection and patients with end-stage chronic instability who have failed multiple soft-tissue reconstruction attempts and those with severe degenerative changes requiring arthrodesis.

Surgical Technique

Our technique of dorsal radiotriquetral ligament reconstruction with suture tape augmentation is a novel concept that abides to the principal of internally bracing the repair or reconstruction construct. This method of ligament repair or reconstruction overcomes delayed rehabilitation and accelerates return to work and activity. Although its reported use in hand and wrist surgery has been limited, recent literature encompassing its use in foot and ankle, shoulder and elbow surgery has been promising [18–21]. Biomechanical studies in hand surgery as well as in other realms of orthopedic surgery have shown superior results with this technique of ligament repair. Shin et al. [22] recently demonstrated the biomechanical superiority of thumb ulnar collateral ligament (UCL) repair with suture tape augmentation when compared with non-augmented repair at time 0. Dugas et al. [21] compared elbow UCL repair with suture tape augmentation to the modified Jobe reconstruction and demonstrated less gap formation in the repair group upon testing with no difference between the groups for the maximum torque at failure, torsional stiffness, or gap formation during the failure test. Biomechanical superiority of ligament or tendon repair with suture tape augmentation has been reported in the shoulder [20] and ankle [23] as well. De Giacomo and Shin [24] have reported their technique of thumb UCL repair with suture tape augmentation. They noted that the use of suture tape provides immediately enhanced strength and support allowing for an expedited recovery and rehabilitation process with earlier return to activities, work or play. Another advantage with this technique is obviating the need for supplemental fixation with Kirschner (K) wires. This can theoretically avoid pin-site-related complications (wire breakage, superficial, and deep infections).

General or regional anesthesia can be used for the procedure. Prior to induction of anesthesia, we evaluate the patient's affected wrist for the presence of a palmaris longus (PL) tendon, as this is the preferred graft for dorsal radiotriquetral ligament reconstruction. If not present, we use a slip of the abductor pollicis longus (APL) tendon. We position the patient supine on an operating room table with an arm table on the operative side. The patient's arm should be centered on the arm table and a well-padded, nonsterile pneumatic tourniquet is placed on the upper arm. We typically begin our procedure with a diagnostic wrist arthroscopy and perform thermal shrinkage of the affected ligamentous structures. After sterilizing the entire upper extremity, the traction tower is assembled and the arm is positioned, well-padded over folded towels, so that the ulna is parallel to the longitudinal axis of the traction tower. Sterile finger traps are placed on the index, long, ring, and small fingers. After the arm is adequately positioned, 10 lbs of traction is applied to the wrist joint. The 3–4 portal is established first by placing an 18G needle to ensure appropriate location and insufflating with 5–10 milliliters of normal saline; this portal is created as a visualization portal. A stab incision is made through the skin; this is followed by blunt dissection with a small, curved hemostat. A capsulotomy is performed with the hemostat by gently pushing through the capsule and spreading on the way out. A 2.3-mm arthroscope is then inserted and a diagnostic examination is performed. In a similar fashion, a 6R portal is established as a working portal through which the arthroscopic thermal probe is introduced. Typically, laxity

and synovitis is evident upon probe evaluation of the volar ulnolunate and ulnotriquetral ligaments. Electrothermal shrinkage of the affected ligaments is performed using the stripe technique. After assessment of the radiocarpal joint, radial and ulnar midcarpal portals are established using the same technique for assessment of the midcarpal joint. Careful inspection of the TH joint is performed along with evaluation of the arcuate ligament. In most patients with PMCI, laxity of the ligament is noted and synovitis is present around the TH joint. In similar fashion, electrothermal shrinkage and debridement of the affected structures is performed.

After arthroscopic examination and treatment, the arm is taken off the traction tower, the limb is exsanguinated using an Esmarch bandage and the tourniquet is inflated to 250 mm Hg. A 2-cm longitudinal incision is made over the origin of the dorsal radiotriquetral ligament, just proximal and ulnar to Lister's tubercle. Dissection is carried down to the level of the periosteum taking care not to injure branches of the superficial radial sensory nerve and the extensor tendons. A similar size incision is made directly over the dorsal aspect of the triquetrum and dissection is carried down to the level of the insertion of the radiotriquetral ligament on the dorsal aspect of the triquetrum. Dissection is performed with caution so as to not injure branches of the dorsal ulnar sensory nerve and the extensor tendons. Next, if the PL tendon is present, we harvest it using three separate 1- to 2-cm transverse incisions along the volar wrist and forearm, with the most distal incision being just proximal to the wrist crease. A maximal length graft is harvested, with care not to injure the median nerve and adjacent flexor tendons. When the PL tendon is absent, we prefer taking a slip of APL. A separate 2-cm longitudinal incision is made over the first extensor compartment, centered just distal to the radial styloid. Dissection is carried down through the subcutaneous tissue with caution to not injure the dorsal radial sensory nerve. The first extensor compartment tendon sheath is then completely released, exposing the EPB tendon and the multiple slips of APL. A 2-mm slip of APL is harvested off its insertion on the thumb metacarpal base, maintaining as much length as possible. Whether using PL or APL, the tendon is contoured into a 2-mm diameter graft, as shown in Fig. 25.3. Each end is then whipstitched using a 2-0 FiberLoop® (Arthrex Inc., Naples, FL, USA) or equivalent nonabsorbable suture. The graft is then wrapped with a damply moistened sponge to prevent desiccation. A 1.35 mm guidewire is then placed into the triquetrum at the ligament insertion; the position is confirmed using mini C-arm fluoroscope. The guidewire is then overdrilled using a cannulated 3.0-mm drill bit, 1 cm into the bone, as limited by the depth stop. The graft along with 1.3-mm SutureTape™ (Arthrex Inc.) is then loaded onto a forked-tip, fully threaded, twist-in, knotless 3.5 mm × 8.5 mm suture anchor (Arthrex Inc.) and subsequently inserted into the drill hole. Using a small curved

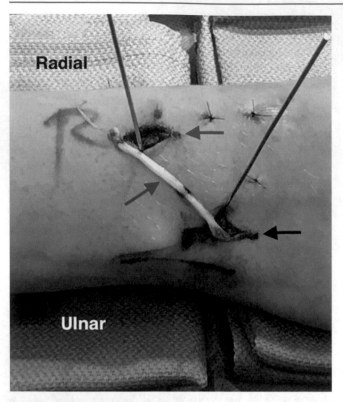

Fig. 25.3 Intraoperative photo demonstrating the two incisions used to gain access to the origin (blue arrow) and insertion (black arrow) of the dorsal radiotriquetral ligament. K-wires, as shown, are placed to fluoroscopically confirm satisfactory placement of the planned bony sockets in the distal radius and triquetrum for anatomic ligament reconstruction. The harvested and contoured tendon graft (red arrow) is shown, in its planned position, prior to bony fixation and passage along the dorsal wrist capsule

hemostat, a path is created from the more distal wound to the more proximal wound staying deep to the extensor tendons and onto the origin of the dorsal radiotriquetral ligament. The wrist is held in 20° ulnar deviation when creating the soft tissue tunnel for later achieving appropriate tension of the reconstructed ligament construct. The proximal end of the graft and SutureTape™ are then shuttled into the proximal wound through the newly created soft tissue tunnel, making sure to stay deep to the extensor tendons. A 1.35-mm guidewire is then placed into the distal radius at the dorsal radiotriquetral ligament origin. Appropriate position is confirmed using the mini C-arm fluoroscope. In similar fashion, as the creation of the triquetral bony socket, a second bony socket is made over the guidewire entering the distal radius. The proximal end of the graft and SutureTape™ is then loaded onto a second forked-tip anchor and under appropriate tension, with the wrist held in 20° ulnar deviation, the anchor is inserted and fixed into the bony socket. A midcarpal shift test, as described earlier, is performed to confirm the absence of a clunk, as shown in Video 25.2. The tourniquet is

then deflated and adequate hemostasis is achieved. After copious irrigation, the wounds are closed in layers and a well-padded, volar slab postoperative splint is applied.

Postoperative Management

Initial postoperative management consists of the application of a well-padded, volar plaster slab wrist splint, with the wrist positioned in roughly 30° extension. The patient returns to the outpatient office for a wound check and suture removal 10–14 days following surgery. At this time, the postoperative splint is converted to a wrist-based, removable splint that is worn for 4 weeks. Active ROM is begun 6 weeks after surgery and strengthening commences 10–12 weeks postoperatively. Full, unrestricted activity is allowed 16 weeks after surgery. Video 25.3 shows a stable midcarpal joint in a patient 2 years following our stabilization procedure.

Tips and Tricks

Upon utilizing this surgical technique to restore midcarpal stability, several points should be considered to facilitate the surgical steps and achieve a sound reconstruction. Firstly, using SutureTape™ to augment and internally brace the reconstruction requires attention to certain technique principles. Whether using a PL or APL autograft, a 2-mm slip must be obtained to reconstruct the dorsal radiotriquetral ligament. Tendency is to use a larger diameter graft, however, this does not allow proper fit into the forked-tip suture anchor. As a result, anchor placement into bone will not be possible or may result in suboptimal fixation (due to a protruding graft). Secure fixation of the anchor into the bone must be obtained by following several steps. These include (1) proper use of the depth stop soft tissue sleeve for the 3.5-mm drill bit and (2) ensuring complete placement of the anchor into the bone. Overdrilling too long of a bony socket and incomplete placement of the anchor will likely result in poor fixation and risks anchor pullout. Proper tensioning is critical to restore the dynamic forces brought forth by the reconstructed dorsal radiotriquetral ligament. Therefore, when creating the bony socket at the origin of the ligament in the distal radius, a position of 20° of ulnar deviation must be maintained. This position is again replicated when securing the proximal anchor. Caution must also be pertained to when creating the soft tissue tunnel prior to shuttling the graft from distal to proximal. The tunnel must be deep to the extensor tendons and along the dorsal wrist capsule to recreate the anatomic position of the dorsal radiotriquetral ligament.

Conclusion

The diagnosis and management of MCI has made tremendous advancements. In the last 15–20 years, a multitude of treatment principles spanning from splints and hand therapy exercises to various surgical techniques have been elucidated. This, along with larger collections of treated patients has allowed us to better grasp what it takes to obtain successful outcomes among this group of challenging cases. All that considered, the current understanding of MCI is still limited by an incomplete awareness of the complex joint reaction forces and soft tissue constraints that come into play during wrist motion [13]. Advancements in ligament repair and reconstruction techniques are constantly evolving and the novel application of SutureTape™ with anchors to internally brace the construct has changed the current landscape in many specialties, including shoulder, foot and ankle, and elbow and hand surgery. The utilization of an internal brace to reconstruct the affected dorsal radiotriquetral ligament is the focus of this chapter in that we believe this entity is a result of laxity or injury to both radiocarpal and midcarpal ligaments. We review the indications and contraindications for soft-tissue reconstruction in MCI, describe our surgical steps and provide key points of the technique that should be carefully pertained to in order to achieve a sound reconstruction. The advantage of this technique is its relative technical ease compared to other surgical options and the ability to expedite postoperative rehabilitation for faster return to work or sport.

Conflict of Interest No benefits in any form have been received or will be received from a commercial party related directly or indirectly to the subject of this chapter. No funds were received in support of this study.

References

1. Lichtman DM, Schneider JR, Swafford AR, Mack GR. Ulnar midcarpal instability-clinical and laboratory analysis. J Hand Surg Am. 1981;6(5):515–23.
2. Louis DS, Hankin FM, Greene TL, Braunstein EM, White SJ. Central carpal instability-capitate lunate instability pattern: diagnosis by dynamic displacement. Orthopedics. 1984;7(11):1693–6.
3. Sutro CJ. Bilateral recurrent intercarpal subluxation. Am J Surg. 1946;72:110–3.
4. Lichtman DM, Wroten ES. Understanding midcarpal instability. J Hand Surg Am. 2006;31(3):491–8.
5. Lichtman DM. Management of chronic rotary subluxation of the scaphoid by scapho-trapezio-trapezoid arthrodesis. J Hand Surg Am. 1983;8(2):223.
6. Trumble TE, Bour CJ, Smith RJ, Glisson RR. Kinematics of the ulnar carpus related to the volar intercalated segment instability pattern. J Hand Surg Am. 1990;15(3):384–92.
7. Viegas SF, Patterson RM, Peterson PD, Pogue DJ, Jenkins DK, Sweo TD, et al. Ulnar-sided perilunate instability: an anatomic and biomechanic study. J Hand Surg Am. 1990;15(2):268–78.
8. Johnson RP, Carrera GF. Chronic capitolunate instability. J Bone Joint Surg Am. 1986;68(8):1164–76.
9. Wolfe SW, Garcia-Elias M, Kitay A. Carpal instability nondissociative. J Am Acad Orthop Surg. 2012;20(9):575–85.
10. Apergis EP. The unstable capitolunate and radiolunate joints as a source of wrist pain in young women. J Hand Surg Br. 1996;21(4):501–6.
11. Taleisnik J, Watson HK. Midcarpal instability caused by malunited fractures of the distal radius. J Hand Surg Am. 1984;9(3):350–7.
12. Wright TW, Dobyns JH, Linscheid RL, Macksoud W, Siegert J. Carpal instability non-dissociative. J Hand Surg Br. 1994;19(6):763–73.
13. Niacaris T, Ming BW, Lichtman DM. Midcarpal instability: a comprehensive review and update. Hand Clin. 2015;31(3):487–93.
14. Chinchalkar S, Yong SA. An ulnar boost splint for midcarpal instability. J Hand Ther. 2004;17(3):377–9.
15. Salva-Coll G, Garcia-Elias M, Hagert E. Scapholunate instability: proprioception and neuromuscular control. J Wrist Surg. 2013;2(2):136–40.
16. Mason WT, Hargreaves DG. Arthroscopic thermal capsulorrhaphy for palmar midcarpal instability. J Hand Surg Eur Vol. 2007;32(4):411–6.
17. Garcia-Elias M. The non-dissociative clunking wrist: a personal view. J Hand Surg Eur Vol. 2008;33(6):698–711.
18. Cho BK, Park KJ, Park JK, SooHoo NF. Outcomes of the modified Broström procedure augmented with suture-tape for ankle instability in patients with generalized ligamentous laxity. Foot Ankle Int. 2017;38(4):405–11.
19. Cho BK, Park KJ, Kim SW, Lee HJ, Choi SM. Minimal invasive suture-tape augmentation for chronic ankle instability. Foot Ankle Int. 2015;36(11):1330–8.
20. Edgar CM, Singh H, Obopilwe E, Voss A, Divenere J, Tassavor M, et al. Pectoralis major repair: a biomechanical analysis of modern repair configurations versus traditional repair configuration. Am J Sports Med. 2017;45(12):2858–63.
21. Dugas JR, Walters BL, Beason DP, Fleisig GS, Chronister JE. Biomechanical comparison of ulnar collateral ligament repair with internal bracing versus modified Jobe reconstruction. Am J Sports Med. 2016;44(3):735–41.
22. Shin SS, van Eck CF, Uquillas C. Suture tape augmentation of the thumb ulnar collateral ligament repair: a biomechanical study. J Hand Surg Am. 2018;43(9):868.e1–6.
23. Viens NA, Wijdicks CA, Campbell KJ, Laprade RF, Clanton TO. Anterior talofibular ligament ruptures, part 1: biomechanical comparison of augmented Broström repair techniques with the intact anterior talofibular ligament. Am J Sports Med. 2014;42(2):405–11.
24. De Giacomo AF, Shin SS. Repair of the thumb ulnar collateral ligament with suture tape augmentation. Tech Hand Up Extrem Surg. 2017;21(4):164–6.

Arthroscopic-Assisted and Limited Open Approach to Perilunate Dislocations

Bo Liu and Feiran Wu

Abbreviations

LT   Lunotriquetral
PLD   Perilunate dislocation
PLFDs   Perilunate fracture-dislocations
RL   Radiolunate
SL   Scapholunate
TFCC   Triangular fibrocartilage complex

Introduction

Perilunate injuries are severe wrist injuries, commonly as a consequence of high-energy trauma. Such injuries represent a spectrum of conditions that includes purely ligamentous injuries through the lesser arc in the so-called perilunate dislocations (PLDs), through to greater arc injuries caused by trans-scaphoid perilunate fracture-dislocations (PLFDs) [1–3].

Accurate and early identification of these injuries is essential because delayed or neglected treatment usually leads to poor post-injury outcomes. The key to success is to achieve early anatomical reduction and maintain the carpal alignment in both fractures and dislocations [4]. Closed reduction and cast treatment of perilunate injuries have been shown to have unacceptable outcomes; therefore, surgical management with open reduction, ligament repair or reconstruction and internal fixation of fractures is the current gold standard [3–12].

Open procedures, however, could impair the limited blood supply to the scaphoid [13], and could jeopardize important capsuloligamentous structures, which may then result in fur-ther carpal malalignment, capsular scarring and joint stiffness [14]. To minimize morbidity, arthroscopic-assisted minimally invasive surgery of PLDs and PLFDs has been efficaciously demonstrated by multiple investigators [3, 4, 14–20]. An arthroscopic technique facilitates precise anatomic reduction and accurate percutaneous internal fixation of the carpus with minimal tissue disruption. This may encourage healing with reduced stiffness, and recent studies have shown promising results [14, 19, 20].

In this chapter, we discuss the surgical techniques of the arthroscopic management of PLDs and PLFDs in detail. We aim to describe refinements of the existing published methods in order to present the most up-to-date technique for the treatment of this condition.

Indications

The majority of patients who present with acute or early sub-acute perilunate dislocations (within 4 weeks of injury) are suitable for arthroscopic-assisted intervention.

Contraindications

For patients presenting >4 weeks after injury, the existing scarring would impede the likelihood of arthroscopic-assisted fracture reduction for the capitolunate joint, limiting the success of this technique and contraindicating its use. For lunate dislocations, if the lunate has migrated a significant distance away from the lunate fossa, such as into the forearm, arthroscopic-assisted surgery is not viable, necessitating an open approach. Open injuries with severe soft tissue damage are also unsuitable for this method.

B. Liu (✉)
Department of Hand Surgery, Beijing Ji Shui Tan Hospital, The Fourth Clinical College of Peking University, Beijing, China

F. Wu
Department of Orthopaedics, Queen Elizabeth Hospital, University Hospitals Birmingham, Birmingham, UK

© Springer Nature Switzerland AG 2022
W. B. Geissler (ed.), *Wrist and Elbow Arthroscopy with Selected Open Procedures*,
https://doi.org/10.1007/978-3-030-78881-0_26

Surgical Technique

Arthroscopic Inspection of Capitolunate Joint Dislocations

At initial presentation, we recommend a single attempt of closed manual reduction in capitolunate joint dislocations. For acute perilunate dislocations, usually more than 50% of cases are successfully reduced with one attempt. If reduction fails, further repeated attempts are generally unsuccessful and should be avoided. Repeated blind and forceful attempts can lead to further damage of the proximal capitate cartilage, an area that is already vulnerable from the index injury (Fig. 26.1). In this scenario, arthroscopic surgery should be arranged without delay, ideally within 48 hours. In our experience, the rate of successful closed manual reductions in capitolunate dislocations significantly reduces when there is a delay of 3 days or longer following initial injury. For presentations after 3 days, we recommend using arthroscopic-assisted reduction (AAR) as the primary attempt.

In the operating room under a regional brachial plexus anaesthetic block, the arm is positioned in a wrist arthroscopy traction tower with traction applied by sterile finger traps. We use a dorsal 3–4 radiocarpal portal for initial inspection of the joint. There is usually sufficient space for scope placement because the lunate is commonly tilted volarly and impinged against the proximal volar aspect of the capitate. It can also be trapped by interposed torn palmar capsular ligaments, which is another cause for the failure of closed reduction. The initial arthroscopic view is usually obscured by the traumatic synovitis, intra-articular haematoma, bony/chondral debris and torn capsuloligamentous tissue. Therefore, a wet arthroscopy technique is required for initial joint debridement to facilitate establishment of a working view. Joint insufflation also helps to compress small capillaries within the capsule and synovium, further aiding the control of intra-articular bleeding and achieving clearer vision.

Reduction and Fixation of PLDs

The dorsal 3–4 and 4–5 portals are utilized to examine the radiocarpal joint. The triangular fibrocartilage complex (TFCC), volar and intercarpal ligaments are assessed by direct inspection and manual probing. TFCC tears are addressed concurrently according to their injury type. The volar ligament injuries are treated with debridement after the dislocations and/or fractures have been reduced and fixed. The radial and ulnar midcarpal portals are used to examine the midcarpal joint. The scapholunate (SL) and lunotriquetral (LT) ligaments are assessed by manual probing and concomitant chondral injuries are identified and debrided. Any soft tissue or bony fragments interposed between the SL and LT intervals are debrided or excised to facilitate reduction in the intercarpal joint.

Once the radiocarpal and midcarpal joints have been fully assessed, an arthroscopic probe is introduced into the radiocarpal joint through the dorsal 4–5 portal. We found this portal to be the most convenient for this manoeuvre because it allows

Fig. 26.1 Further damage of the capitolunate articular cartilage from blind repeated forceful reduction attempts

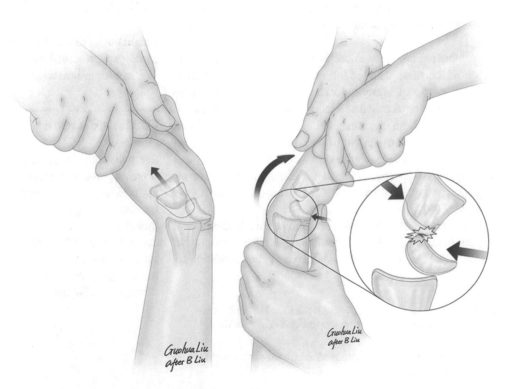

the probe to directly face the subluxated lunate. The force of wrist traction is gently increased at the point, up to a maximum of 15 lb, such that the tip of the probe can be hooked onto the dorsal rim of the lunate (Fig. 26.2). Two K-wires are advanced towards the lunate from the scaphoid and triquetrum, initially without crossing the SL and LT intercarpal intervals (Fig. 26.3). Next, the surgeon gently pulls and reduces the dislocated lunate back under the capitate using a 'shoehorn manoeuvre'. This can be conducted entirely under direct arthroscopic visualization without requiring any forceful movements, which protects against further compromise of the articular cartilage. When the capitolunate joints are reduced, the position of the lunate is assessed. If it is not neutral (i.e. in volar or dorsal tilt), reducing traction force on the traction tower and passively flexing or extending the wrist will restore the neutral radiolunate (RL) angle. The RL joint can then be temporarily transfixed with a percutaneous K-wire, advanced through the dorsal distal radius. Further correction of the rotation deformity of the SL and LT intervals can be obtained by using a probe or depressor through the midcarpal portals. Once the RL and SL intervals are reduced, the K-wires in the scaphoid and triquetrum are advanced under direct vision into the lunate and the alignment verified by fluoroscopy.

Augmentation of the SL Ligament for Grossly Unstable PLDs

In our experience, more than half of the PLDs will have grossly unstable SL joints that are easily redislocated, signifying incompetence of both the primary and secondary stabilizers of the SL interval. In this situation, we advocate augmentation of the SL ligament through a dorsal mini-open approach, by reinforcing the dorsal scapholunate complex. The dorsal scapholunate complex, including dorsal capsuloscapholunate septum (DCSS) and the dorsal extrinsic ligament, is regarded as one of the most important structures for SL stability [21, 22].

The 3–4 portal is extended transversely along the skin crease, creating a 2-cm opening. The extensor tendons are retracted to expose the capsule. A suture anchor is placed into the scaphoid and lunate at a distance of 1 cm from the SL interval under fluoroscopic guidance. Following joint fixation using two K-wires as described, both sutures are delivered through the dorsal capsule and tied together on top of the dorsal capsule (extra-articularly), creating a reinforcement of the scapholunate complex (Fig. 26.4).

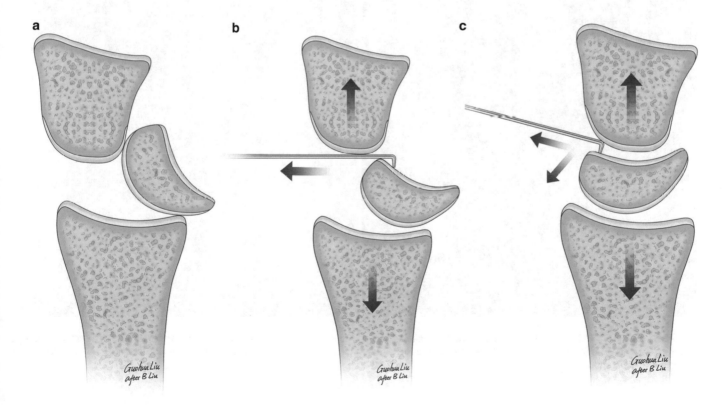

Fig. 26.2 The 'shoehorn manoeuvre' in reducing perilunate dislocations. (**a**) Diagram of a wrist in sagittal profile demonstrating a dislocated lunate. (**b**) The wrist traction force is increased and an arthroscopic probe is introduced to hook onto the dorsal rim of the lunate. (**c**) The lunate is gently reduced under the capitate using the shoehorn manoeuvre

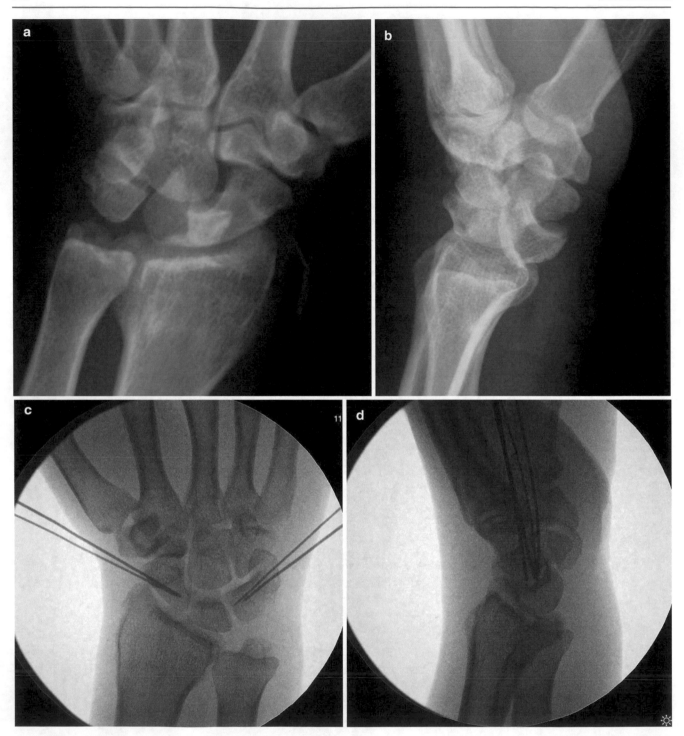

Fig. 26.3 (**a**, **b**) PA and lateral radiographs demonstrating a lunate dislocation. (**c**, **d**) PA and lateral radiographs showing the position of the K-wires before fixation of the SL and LT intervals. Note the dorsal tilting of the lunate. (**e**) Transfixion of the lunate in a neutral angle through the distal radius. (**f**, **g**) Using a depressor to aid intercarpal reduction in the LT interval. C capitate, T triquetrum, L lunate. (**h**) Final fixation position of the PLD

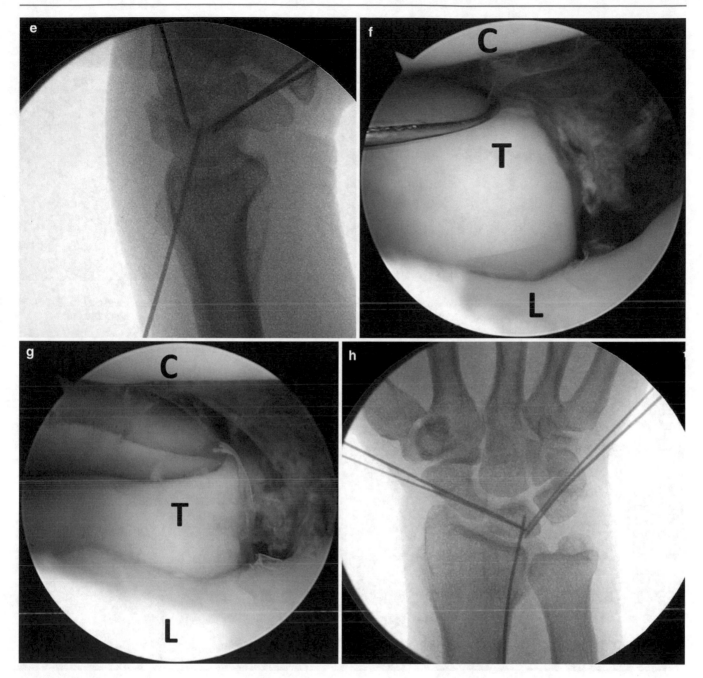

Fig. 26.3 (continued)

Management of Associated Injuries in PLDs

Traditionally, PLDs are thought of as 'purely ligamentous' injuries. However, in our experience, it is not uncommon to find concomitant carpal fractures in patients with PLDs, particularly following high-energy trauma. Associated displaced fractures of the triquetrum or capitate require arthroscopic-assisted reduction and percutaneous fixation (Figs. 26.4 and 26.5). Other associated injuries that are typically seen include tears of the TFCC. These can be debrided or repaired as appropriate.

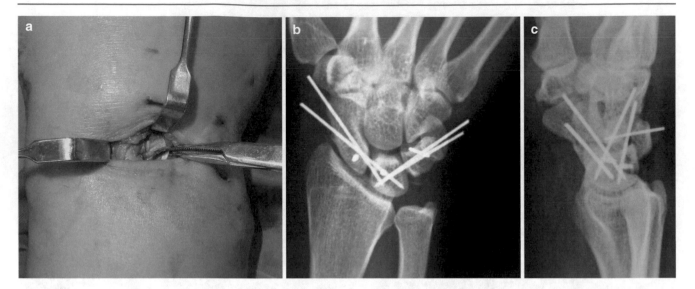

Fig. 26.4 (**a**) Using a mini-invasive dorsal approach to reinforce the dorsal scapholunate complex. (**b, c**) Post-operative AP and lateral radiographs of the same patient demonstrating arthroscopy-assisted percutaneous fixation of a PLD, with K-wire fixation of the triquetrum fracture

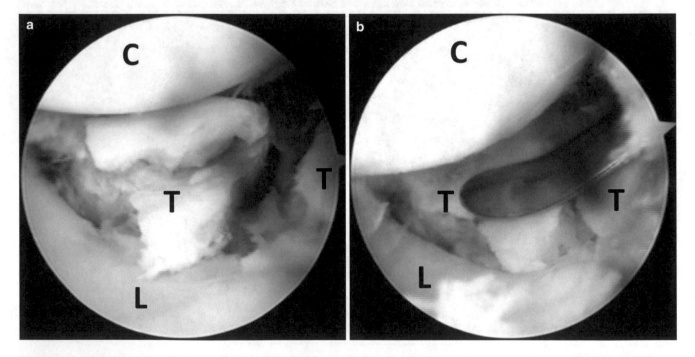

Fig. 26.5 (**a, b**) Reduction in a displaced triquetrum fracture arthroscopically using an arthroscopic depressor. C capitate, T triquetrum, L lunate

Reduction and Fixation for Trans-Scaphoid PLFDs

Similar to the treatment of PLDs, a thorough arthroscopic examination and debridement of the radiocarpal and midcarpal joints are initially performed in trans-scaphoid PLFDs. AAR of the dislocated capitolunate joint is performed for patients who failed closed reduction or presented 3 days or later after the initial injury. An arthroscopic probe is introduced into the radiocarpal joint through the 3–4 portal, while the scope is placed in the 4–5 portal. The hook of the probe

is positioned onto the dorsal edge of the scapholunate ligament (Fig. 26.6). The wrist traction force is then gently increased, up to a maximum of 15 lb, while the surgeon gently pulls and reduces the volarly dislocated proximal scaphoid fragment-lunate complex back under the capitate using the 'shoehorn manoeuvre' (Fig. 26.7). In these injuries, the scaphoid fracture is the initial surgical target after reduction. This fracture frequently remains significantly displaced with varying degrees of comminution even after the capitolunate dislocation is reduced (Fig. 26.8). Arthroscopic-assisted scaphoid fracture reduction and percutaneous fixation are

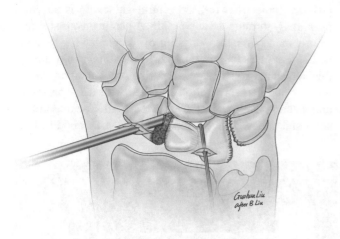

Fig. 26.6 The probe hooking on the scapholunate ligament for reducing perilunate fracture dislocations

typically the most technically demanding steps and critical in the success of the overall surgical outcome. Manual closed reduction is often unsatisfactory. In such circumstances, a guidewire is advanced along the central axis of the distal fragment from the scaphoid tubercle in a retrograde direction, not crossing the fracture line. Further K-wires can be inserted into the distal and proximal fragments in grossly unstable fractures. Using the ulnar midcarpal portal for visualization, the scaphoid fracture is reduced by manipulating these K-wire 'joysticks'. Care should be paid to both the sagittal and coronal planes when checking the adequacy of reduction to ensure both the rotational and translational displacements are corrected. Once the scaphoid is reduced anatomically, the surgical assistant drives the central axis guidewire and a further anti-rotation K-wire across the fracture site into the proximal scaphoid fragment.

a   b

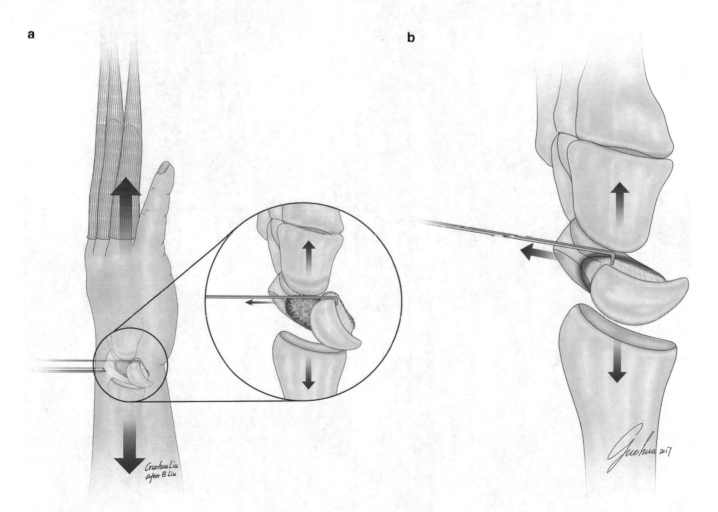

Fig. 26.7 (**a**) The probe hooking on the scapholunate ligament for reducing perilunate fracture dislocations. (**b**) With the force of wrist traction gently increased, the volarly dislocated proximal scaphoid fragment-lunate complex is pulled dorsally under the capitate using the 'shoehorn manoeuvre'

If a residual gap persists between the proximal and distal fragments after K-wire reduction, a cannulated headless compression screw may be implanted after reduction and fixation of the intercarpal dislocation for further compression. In such cases, the traction is released and the wrist placed on the operating table to allow ease of fluoroscopic guidance. The scaphoid is reamed over the central guidewire and the screw advanced retrograde. For proximal third or proximal pole fractures, the central guidewire is advanced proximally through the dorsal skin. A percutaneous stab incision is made over the exit point of the guidewire. Reaming and screw insertion are then performed antegrade through this dorsal incision. In cases requiring screw fixation, we frequently supplement fixation stability with a further single anti-rotation K-wire in the scaphoid. All K-wires are cut short and buried under the skin for both PLDs and PLFDs.

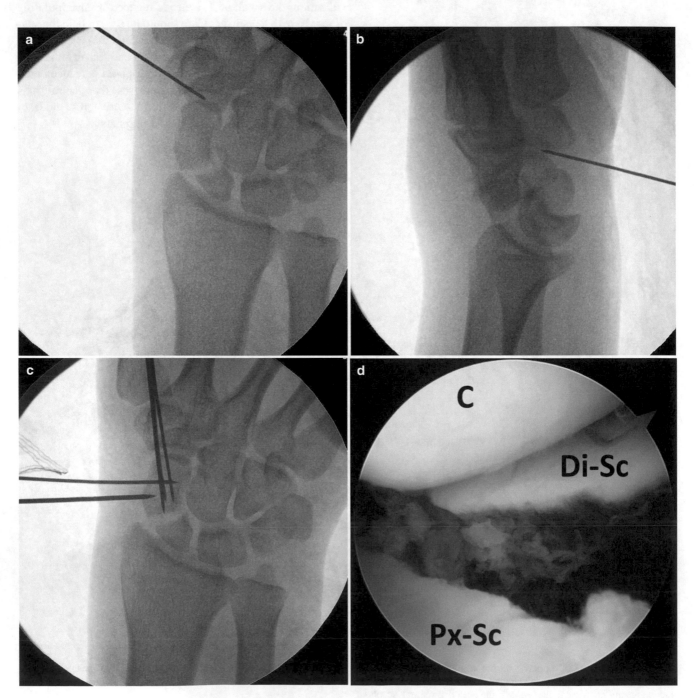

Fig. 26.8 (**a**, **b**) Postero-anterior and lateral radiographs of a transscaphoid PLFD. (**c**) Position of K-wire 'joystick' in the reduction in the scaphoid fracture. (**d**) Arthroscopic view of the displaced scaphoid fracture from the midcarpal portal. (**e**, **f**) Post-reduction view of the scaphoid fracture. C capitate, Di-Sc distal scaphoid, Px-Sc proximal scaphoid

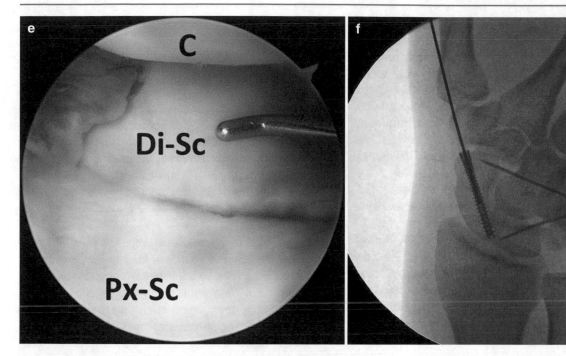

Fig. 26.8 (continued)

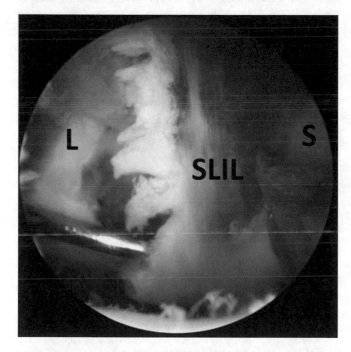

Fig. 26.9 Scapholunate ligament avulsion from the lunate in a patient with trans-scaphoid PLFD. L lunate, S scaphoid

Associated Injury Management in PLFDs

Contrary to the commonly held belief that the SL ligaments remain intact in PLFD injuries, haemorrhage and attenuation of this ligament can be observed arthroscopically in almost all patients. However, most of these are Geissler grade I or II injuries, which can be managed with immobilization only. A few patients will have more severe SL ligament avulsions from the lunate or gross ruptures of the SL ligament (Fig. 26.9). In these cases, a Geissler grade III or IV disruption will be revealed during arthroscopic midcarpal inspection, and scapholunate pinning is required following an accurate reduction in the SL interval.

Post-operative Care

Post-operatively, the wrists are immobilized in a short-arm thermoplastic splint. We include the proximal phalanx of the thumb in the splint for PLFDs, but left free in PLDs. In those with TFCC injuries, long-arm thermoplastic splints are used with the forearm at semi-supination rotation for 6 weeks, followed by short-arm splints for a further 2 weeks.

K-wires are removed at 8 weeks post-operatively. Active wrist motion is initiated at this point under the guidance of hand therapy. In PLFDs, weight loading and sporting activities can be initiated following confirmation of scaphoid union.

Clinical Results

Thirty-one patients presenting with perilunate injuries were treated using the described arthroscopic-assisted method. There were 26 trans-scaphoid PLFDs and 5 dorsal PLDs. The mean duration from injury to surgery was 8 days (range 2–20). The mean surgical time was 155 minutes (range

90–300). In all 31 patients, arthroscopic-assisted reduction and percutaneous fixation were successful. Nine patients had median nerve symptoms post-operatively, which resolved spontaneously after 2 weeks. None required carpal tunnel decompression.

At a mean final follow-up of 14.8 months (range 12–32), normal carpal alignment was restored and maintained for all patients. The mean flexion-extension arc of the wrist was 115 degrees (range 80–150), which was 86% of the contralateral wrist. The mean grip strength was 33 kg using a calibrated Jamar dynamometer (range 8–48 kg), which was 83% of the contralateral wrist. Patient-reported outcome measures were also assessed. The mean Mayo wrist score was 87 (range 40–100) – excellent in 17 patients, good in 9, fair in 4 and poor in 1. The mean Disabilities of the Arm, Shoulder and Hand (DASH) score was 7 (range 0–65). The mean Patient-Rated Wrist Evaluation (PRWE) score was 10 (range 0–63). All patients returned to their pre-injury occupations at a mean of 4 months after surgery (range 1–12 months). There were 15 manual labourers, of whom only 3 required reduced workloads.

Tips and Tricks

The arthroscopic management of perilunate injuries can be highly technically challenging. This technique has a steep learning curve, even for experienced hand surgeons and arthroscopists.

Our experience shows that the success rate decreased significantly if traditional closed manual reduction in capitolunate dislocations is executed more than 3 days after the initial injury. For this reason, we recommend AAR of the capitolunate joint as the primary treatment method to reduce morbidity and preserve articular cartilage for delays in presentation of 72 hours or longer.

Surgeons attempting this method should be proficient in the open management of such injuries and be ready to convert from arthroscopic to open surgery if difficulties are encountered intra-operatively. In particular, a poorly reduced scaphoid fracture in trans-scaphoid PLFDs is unacceptable and an open reduction and internal fixation should be performed if the scaphoid cannot be reduced arthroscopically.

The reduction in the scaphoid is often the most time-consuming step, and proficient conversion of wet to dry arthroscopy techniques may be helpful in facilitating fracture reduction and fixation. Wrist traction should be used selectively, and the surgeon should clearly recognize the specific situations where wrist traction would be helpful, for example, increasing wrist traction for AAR of the capitolunate joint, and releasing traction when reducing and fixing the scaphoid fracture in trans-scaphoid PLFDs.

Conclusion

The optimal management of perilunate injuries is challenging and remains controversial. It is our philosophy to employ the method that is associated with the least surgical morbidity in order to achieve a successful outcome. Open surgery involves extensive soft tissue dissection, which could lead to capsular scarring, joint stiffness and further impair the already tenuous vascular supply to the scaphoid and intrinsic ligaments. Arthroscopic treatment of such injuries, when combined with intra-operative fluoroscopy, offers a more precise alternative to assist with anatomic reduction and percutaneous fixation.

It is important to appreciate that repeated forceful reduction in the capitolunate joint can lead to further articular damage of the capitate, an area already weakened or injured during the initial dislocation. Arthroscopic-assisted reduction occurs under direct vision at all times and requires no manoeuvres that may further compromise the cartilage.

The early outcomes of arthroscopic management of perilunate injuries are encouraging. Despite the technical challenges, this minimally invasive approach is clinically reliable and offers a favourable alternative to the traditional open treatment of this condition.

Conflict of Interest The authors declare no potential conflicts of interest with respect to the research, authorship and/or publication of this manuscript.

Ethical Approval The local ethical committee approved the research protocol in advance.

References

1. Mayfield JK, Johnson RP, Kilcoyne RK. Carpal dislocations: pathomechanics and progressive perilunar instability. J Hand Surg. 1980;5(3):226–41.
2. Johnson RP. The acutely injured wrist and its residuals. Clin Orthop. 1980;NA(149):33–44.
3. Herzberg G. Perilunate and axial carpal dislocations and fracture–dislocations. J Hand Surg. 2008;33(9):1659–68.
4. Weil WM, Slade JF, Trumble TE. Open and arthroscopic treatment of perilunate injuries. Clin Orthop. 2006;445:120–32.
5. Cooney WP, Bussey R, Dobyns JH, Linscheid RL. Difficult wrist fractures. Perilunate fracture-dislocations of the wrist. Clin Orthop. 1987;214:136–47.
6. Herzberg G, Forissier D. Acute dorsal trans-scaphoid perilunate fracture-dislocations: medium-term results. J Hand Surg. 2002;27(6):498–502.
7. Budoff JE. Treatment of acute lunate and perilunate dislocations. J Hand Surg. 2008;33(8):1424–32.
8. Trumble T, Verheyden J. Treatment of isolated perilunate and lunate dislocations with combined dorsal and volar approach and intraosseous cerclage wire. J Hand Surg. 2004;29(3):412–7.
9. Knoll VD, Allan C, Trumble TE. Trans-scaphoid perilunate fracture dislocations: results of screw fixation of the scaphoid and lunotriqu-

etral repair with a dorsal approach. J Hand Surg. 2005;30(6):1145. e1–e11.

10. Forli A, Courvoisier A, Wimsey S, Corcella D, Moutet F. Perilunate dislocations and transscaphoid perilunate fracture–dislocations: a retrospective study with minimum ten-year follow-up. J Hand Surg. 2010;35(1):62–8.

11. Kremer T, Wendt M, Riedel K, Sauerbier M, Germann G, Bickert B. Open reduction for perilunate injuries—clinical outcome and patient satisfaction. J Hand Surg. 2010;35(10):1599–606.

12. Souer JS, Rutgers M, Andermahr J, Jupiter JB, Ring D. Perilunate fracture–dislocations of the wrist: comparison of temporary screw versus K-wire fixation. J Hand Surg. 2007;32(3):318–25.

13. Botte MJ, Mortensen WW, Gelberman RH, Rhoades CE, Gellman H. Internal vascularity of the scaphoid in cadavers after insertion of the Herbert screw. J Hand Surg. 1988;13(2):216–20.

14. Liu B, Chen S, Zhu J, Tian G. Arthroscopic management of perilunate injuries. Hand Clin. 2017;33(4):709–15.

15. Wong T-C, Ip F-K. Minimally invasive management of trans-scaphoid perilunate fracture-dislocations. Hand Surg. 2008;13(03):159–65.

16. Kim JP, Lee JS, Park MJ. Arthroscopic reduction and percutaneous fixation of perilunate dislocations and fracture-dislocations. Arthrosc J Arthrosc Relat Surg. 2012;28(2):196–203.e2.

17. Jeon I-H, Kim H-J, Min W-K, Cho H-S, Kim P-T. Arthroscopically assisted percutaneous fixation for trans-scaphoid perilunate fracture dislocation. J Hand Surg Eur Vol. 2010;35(8):664–8.

18. Liu B, Chen S-L, Zhu J, Wang Z-X, Shen J. Arthroscopically assisted mini-invasive management of perilunate dislocations. J Wrist Surg. 2015;04(02):093–100.

19. Herzberg G, Burnier M, Marc A, Merlini L, Izem Y. The role of arthroscopy for treatment of perilunate injuries. J Wrist Surg. 2015;04(02):101–9.

20. Kim J, Lee J, Park M. Arthroscopic treatment of perilunate dislocations and fracture dislocations. J Wrist Surg. 2015;04(02):081–7.

21. Wahegaonkar A, Mathoulin C. Arthroscopic dorsal capsuloligamentous repair in the treatment of chronic scapho-lunate ligament tears. J Wrist Surg. 2013;02(02):141–8.

22. Mathoulin C. Treatment of dynamic scapholunate instability dissociation: contribution of arthroscopy. Hand Surg Rehabil. 2016;35(6):377–92.

Arthroscopic Arthrolysis

27

Duncan Thomas McGuire, Riccardo Luchetti, Andrea Atzei, and Gregory Ian Bain

Introduction

Wrist stiffness is a multifactorial condition that is debilitating for those whom it affects. The etiology may be classified as either intra-articular or extra-articular. Intra-articular and capsular injuries as well as prolonged immobilization may stimulate arthrofibrosis. This may be seen after conservative and surgical management of injuries (Table 27.1) [1, 2].

Conservative treatment with physiotherapy and splinting is the treatment of choice. Surgery is reserved for those cases refractory to conservative treatment. Arthroscopic treatment of arthrofibrosis of the knee, shoulder, and elbow is well established and commonly used.

Frequently, incorrect or incomplete reduction in a distal radius fracture is the cause of a stiff and painful wrist. Intra-articular and extra-articular malunions need to be corrected with osteotomies to restore normal anatomy and alignment of the articular surface of the distal radius [3]. Following distal radius fractures, two main conditions can contribute to painful limitation of ROM: (1) capsular contracture with intra-articular adhesions (most commonly), and (2) radiocarpal impingement caused by either malunion of fractures involving the dorsal rim of the distal radius (Figs. 27.1 and 27.2) or an increase in volar tilt of the distal radius articular surface. The two conditions can sometimes coexist and must

Table 27.1 Possible causes of secondary wrist stiffness (extra- and/or intra-articular)

Posttrauma	Postsurgery
1. Fracture	1. Dorsal wrist ganglia
2. Fracture-dislocation	2. Treatment of scaphoid fractures or nonunion
3. Dislocation	3. Intercarpal arthrodeses
4. Ligament injuries	4. Ligament reconstruction
	5. Proximal row carpectomy
Prolonged immobilization	

be treated at the same time. It is important to note the rehabilitation protocol for the various surgical procedures that may need to be performed. Any procedure that would involve postoperative immobilization such as ligament reconstructions must be avoided. Immediate mobilization following surgery is mandatory.

Other potential causes of wrist pain and stiffness include neuroma of the posterior interosseous nerve (PIN), extensor and/or flexor tendons adhesions, and chronic regional pain syndrome (CRPS).

Traditionally, wrist manipulation under anesthesia (MUA) is commonly used when the rehabilitation regime has failed to improve wrist ROM. However, this procedure can be detrimental by causing traumatic ligamentous injuries, chondral or osteochondral damage (especially in cases with dorsal radiocarpal [RC] impingement), or even fractures. Surgical arthrolysis is a gentler and more controlled option that can be performed via open or arthroscopy surgery [4, 5]. This is already a successful treatment option in other joints [6–8].

Arthroscopic arthrolysis of the wrist allows the surgeon to treat the RC and intercarpal joints, while minimizing the risk of secondary damage to other articulations, and at the same time permitting immediate postoperative mobilization [9–15].

D. T. McGuire (✉)
Department of Orthopaedic Surgery, Groote Schuur Hospital, Cape Town, South Africa

R. Luchetti
Rimini Hand & Rehabilitation Center, Rimini, Italy

A. Atzei
Fenice HSRT Hand Surgery and Rehabilitation Team, Centro di Medicina, Treviso, Italy

Policlinico San Giorgio, Pordenone, Italy

G. I. Bain
Department of Orthopaedic Surgery, Flinders University of South Australia, Adelaide, SA, Australia
e-mail: greg@gregbain.com.au

© Springer Nature Switzerland AG 2022
W. B. Geissler (ed.), *Wrist and Elbow Arthroscopy with Selected Open Procedures*,
https://doi.org/10.1007/978-3-030-78881-0_27

Fig. 27.1 Drawing showing malunion of the dorsal rim of the distal radius following fracture (**a**). Note the impingement between the dorsal rim and the carpus (**b**)

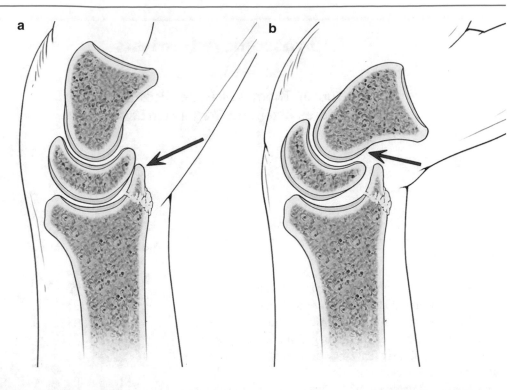

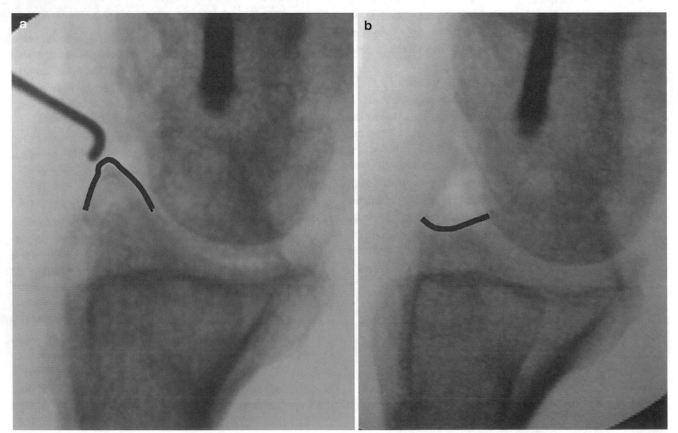

Fig. 27.2 Lateral radiograph of a wrist showing dorsal impingement (*arrow*) of the distal radius following malunion of a fracture. (**a**) Before and (**b**) after arthroscopic debridement of dorsal rim. Courtesy of Francisco del Piñal

Table 27.2 Instruments for arthroscopic arthrolysis

Motor powered
  Full radius blade
  Cutter blade/incisor
  Razor cut blade
  Barrel abrader
Suction punch
Miniscalpel (banana blade)
Laser
Radiofrequency
Dissector and scalpel

Technique

Traditional RC portals are used for arthroscopic arthrolysis of the wrist. Two volar portals (radial and ulnar) may also be used for the RC and ulnocarpal (UC) joint [6]. The distal radioulnar joint (DRUJ) may also be involved in the pathological process, and may also be debrided arthroscopically. The midcarpal (MC) joint is rarely involved; however, if it is affected, traditional MC portals are used.

Arthrolysis may be performed using a variety of instruments (Table 27.2). Dry arthroscopy is utilized more frequently for this condition as it has the benefit of avoiding fluid extravasation into the soft tissues [16, 17].

Articular distraction is obtained using the traditional vertical position with countertraction at the elbow of about 3 kg. Occasionally the articular distraction is not sufficient enough to permit the use of a 2.7-mm scope even when more traction weight is applied. In these cases, a 1.9-mm scope is recommended.

Although arthroscopy starts at the level of the RC joint, the MC joint should always be assessed. When there is a loss of pronation and supination, arthrolysis of the DRUJ should also be performed.

In the most difficult cases, it is impossible to recognize the normal arthroscopic anatomy of the wrist due to the presence of fibrosis that completely encloses the joint space. Difficulties could be encountered in performing triangulation with the instruments. Synovitis, fibrosis, and adhesions that obstruct the visual field, must be resected with caution, ensuring that no damage occurs to the surrounding structures. Obviously, the surgeon's surgical ability is of utmost importance here.

Radiocarpal Joint

All the portals (1–2, 3–4, 4–5, 6R, and 6U) may be used, including the volar ones, if needed. Inflow is permitted through the scope. Outflow by 6U portal or none. When dry arthroscopy is used, the trocar inflow portal is left open per-

mitting the entrance of air as the shaver is used with constant aspiration. This allows removal of synovial fluid, blood, and debris. Furthermore, a 5-cc syringe can be used to inject fluid in order to wash the joint debris and blood, which is then removed by the suction of the shaver. Only when the radiofrequency instrument is used, does fluid become necessary. Once the radiofrequency is no longer required, it is possible to return to dry arthroscopy by using the shaver to aspirate fluid and debris in the joint.

The procedure is divided into two steps to permit a better understanding of the technique.

Step One: Fibrosis and Fibrotic Band Resection

Arthroscopic arthrolysis always starts from the radial side of the RC joint (Fig. 27.3). The starting portal is usually the 3–4 and the 1–2 is used as a working portal; however, portals are switched frequently.

Adhesions are initially removed from the radial side of the joint using the shaver (full radius: 2.9 mm, and aggressive or incisor: 3.2 mm) and radiofrequency instruments. However, not infrequently, difficulties are encountered in triangulation due to intense intra-articular fibrosis. In these circumstances, it is better to switch the scope from the 3–4 portal to the 1–2 portal and use the 3–4 portal as the working

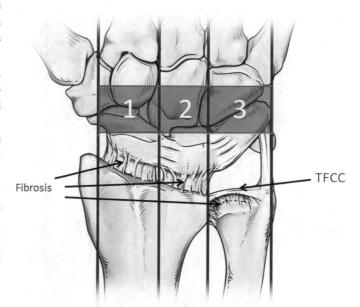

Fig. 27.3 Drawing showing the division of the radiocarpal joint into three parts. The proper radiocarpal joint is divided into two parts by a *longitudinal line* passing through the scapholunate joint. The ulnocarpal joint is separated from the radiocarpal joint by a *longitudinal line* through the medial border of the radius at the sigmoid notch. The ulnocarpal joint is rarely involved. In this drawing, fibrosis is located in the radiocarpal joint, the DRUJ, and under the TFCC ligament

portal. The 1–2 portal is established with an outside-in technique using a needle. A longitudinal skin incision is made and blunt dissection with a mosquito forceps is performed to gain access to the joint. Shaving should only be started after ensuring that the full radius is turned toward the scope and not to the articular surface. As the intra-articular vision improves, the resection of fibrosis becomes easier.

Once fibrosis is completely removed from the radial side of the RC joint, the arthroscopic procedure is shifted to the ulnar side (Fig. 27.4). The scope is introduced through the 3–4 portal and the shaver through the 6R. Visualization of the shaver is frequently limited by the presence of the fibrotic band. Traditionally the fibrotic band [14] is localized between the scapholunate (SL) ligament and the ridge between the scaphoid and lunate facet of the distal radius (Figs. 27.5 and 27.6). It may be partial or complete. When it is complete, it divides the radiocarpal joint into two separate spaces. The fibrotic band may be incised using a small dissector introduced via the 6R portal in the direction of the scope. The band is carefully detached from the articular surface using the dissector. The fibrotic band may then be resected using a basket forceps or a shaver from the 6R portal (Fig. 27.7). To obtain a complete resection of the band, instruments must be switched from the 6R to 3–4 portal and scope from 3–4 to 6R. Radiofrequency instruments may also be used to resect the fibrotic bands. Multiple fibrotic bands may be encountered in a joint with osteochondral damage to the articular

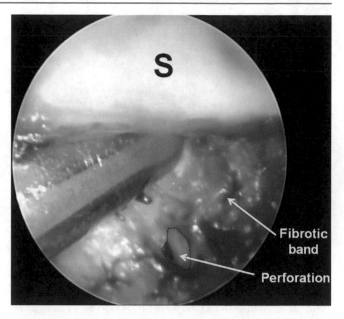

Fig. 27.5 Arthroscopic view of the fibrotic band that has resulted in a virtually complete separation of the radiocarpal joint in two compartments. A shaver is being used to excise the fibrotic band (S scaphoid)

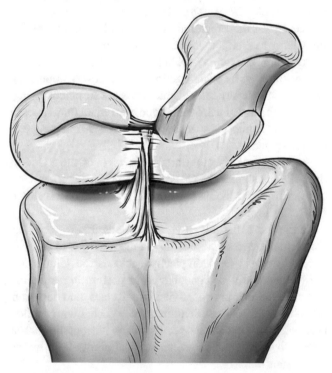

Fig. 27.6 Drawing showing the location of the fibrotic band

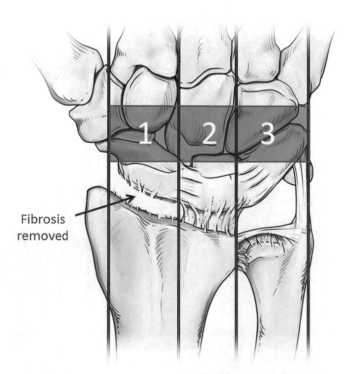

Fig. 27.4 Drawing showing division of the radiocarpal joint into three parts, where fibrosis in the radial side has been removed (step one)

surface of the distal radius (Fig. 27.8), with all of them originating from the defect.

Resection of this intra-articular fibrosis is often sufficient to improve passive wrist ROM. However, on occasion, this fibrosis may be much more complex making arthrolysis

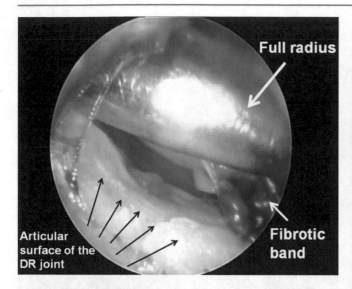

Fig. 27.7 Arthroscopic view of the wrist joint after fibrotic band resection. Note the irregularity of the articular surface of the distal radius due to a previous fracture

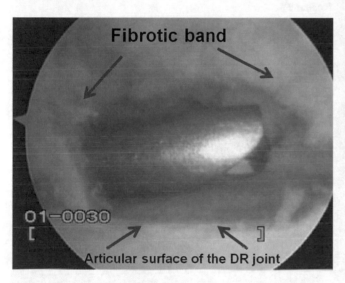

Fig. 27.8 Cartilage damage to the articular surface of the distal radius becomes evident after resection of the fibrosis

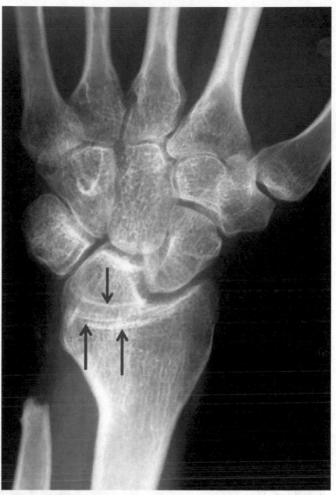

Fig. 27.9 X-ray of a wrist showing an ankylosis of the radiolunate joint due to progression of an osteofibrotic band

much more difficult. Rarely these bands may ossify and form an osteofibrotic band, and with progression may result in an ankylosis of the RC joint (Fig. 27.9). In this situation it is very difficult to remove the band and may sometimes be impossible. Resection of these osteofibrotic bands may not be indicated if it will cause an osteochondral defect that would then result in persistence of pain and recurrent formation of the bands.

When fibrosis in the ulnar side of the RC joint has been completely excised, the procedure continues into the ulnocarpal joint (Fig. 27.10). This part of the wrist joint is rarely affected by fibrosis, and arthroscopy is often diagnostic only. Occasionally, peripheral TFCC tears may be found; however, the treatment of these should be limited to a debride-

ment in order to avoid the need for postoperative immobilization.

Before moving to the second step of the procedure, it is mandatory to evaluate the wrist ROM (Fig. 27.11). This should be performed out of traction.

Step Two: Volar and Dorsal Capsule Resection

Depending on the ROM obtained after step one, the volar and/or dorsal capsule and RC ligaments may need to be released. A miniscalpel, such as a banana blade for peripheral nerve surgery or microscalpel for ocular surgery, is used. Radiofrequency instruments may also be used. Volar capsulotomy is easier than dorsal because the structures are immediately in the field of vision when viewing from the dorsal arthroscopy portals. Initially, the shaver is used to debride the intra-articular portion of the volar ligaments in order to see the entrance point of the miniscalpel. Once inside the joint, the surgeon addresses each affected ligament (Fig. 27.12). Often this is made difficult by articular incon-

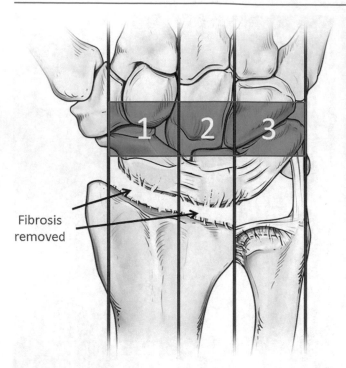

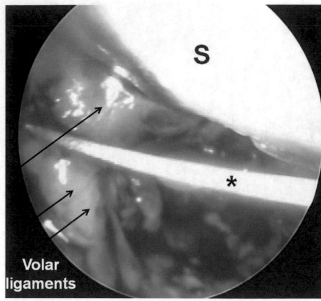

Fig. 27.12 Sectioning of the volar capsule using a miniscalpel (S scaphoid)

Fig. 27.10 Drawing showing complete resection of fibrosis in the radiocarpal joint

Fig. 27.11 Wrist ROM evaluation after step one of the arthroscopic arthrolysis procedure (a) Wrist extension (b) Wrist flexion

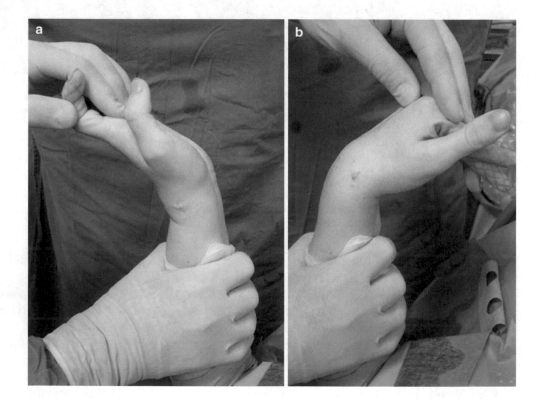

a
b

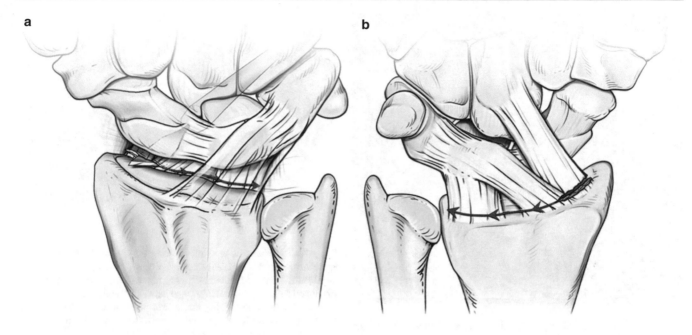

Fig. 27.13 Drawing illustrating the site of sectioning of the volar capsule and ligaments of the wrist (*red arrows*) (**a**) Wrist extension (**b**) Wrist flexion

gruity, making it impossible to reach all areas of the capsule. This may be made easier by smoothing off the articular steps using a shaver (burr) that helps in reaching the volar capsule. It is much easier to cut the radial side of the capsule from the 1–2 portal with the scope in the 3–4 portal.

Radioscaphocapitate and radiolunate ligaments are resected at their base and the procedure continues through to the ulnar side (Fig. 27.13). The ulnar side of the volar capsule is released through the 6R portal (scope in 3–4). Identification of the volar ulnar limit of the distal radius permits the surgeon to stop the ligament dissection at this point to prevent resection of the volar UC ligament. At this point, traction is removed, and a gentle manipulation is performed.

Traction is now reapplied and the procedure continues with resection of the dorsal wrist capsule (Fig. 27.14). This is performed with the scope through the 1–2 portal and the instruments through the 6R portal. The dorsal central part of the capsule is sectioned first. By switching the scope to the 6R portal, the capsule can be further resected by introducing the instruments through the 1–2 portal. The intra-articular position of the 3–4 portal is located and, from this point, the resection of the capsule starts by using a miniscalpel, shaver, or radiofrequency with a hook tip (Fig. 27.15). The radial part of the capsule is easily resected through the 1–2 portal with the scope in the 6R portal. The ulnar part of the dorsal capsule contains the strong dorsal radiocarpal ligament. Here, the procedure becomes more difficult due to the firm consistency of this ligament. In this case, a volar radial portal may be used [18–20]. Bain et al. have described a safe method to resect the dorsal capsule with minimal risk to the

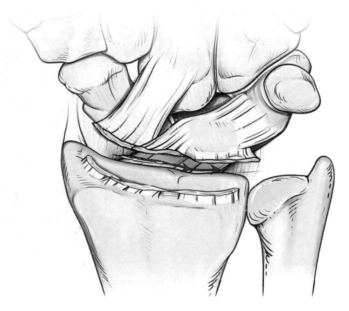

Fig. 27.14 Drawing illustrating the site of section of the dorsal capsule and ligaments (*red arrows*)

extensor tendons [21, 22]. This technique involved the use of an intracapsular nylon tape that is used as a retractor to pull the extensor tendons out of harm's way (Fig. 27.16).

It is very important to remember that the volar UC ligaments and dorsal capsule of the UC joint must not be resected (Fig. 27.17). The dorsal capsule of the UC joint is without a proper ligament but is reinforced by the floor of the ECU tendon sheath. The two volar UC ligaments are the ulnolu-

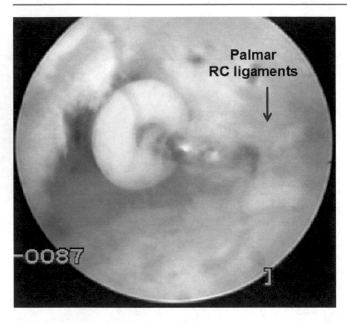

Fig. 27.15 Use of a hook tip of a radiofrequency device to section the dorsal capsule. Care should be taken to avoid injury to the structures dorsal to the capsule

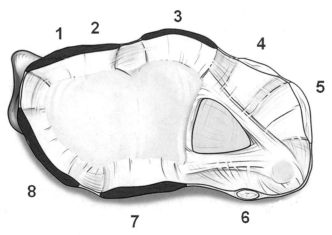

Fig. 27.17 Schematic drawing showing the extrinsic ligaments of the radiocarpal joint. (*1*) Radioscaphocapitate, (*2*) long radiolunate, (*3*) short radiolunate, (*4*) ulnolunate, (*5*) ulnotriquetral, (*6*) ECU tendon, (*7*) dorsal radiocarpal, and (*8*) dorsal capsule. The ligaments (*1–2–3–7*) that can be sectioned during the arthroscopic volar and dorsal capsulotomy are shown in *red* (according to Verhellen and Bain [15]). The ulnocarpal ligaments (*4* and *5*) must be preserved

Fig. 27.16 Drawings illustrating the use of nylon tape to retract the extensor tendons during dorsal wrist capsule resection

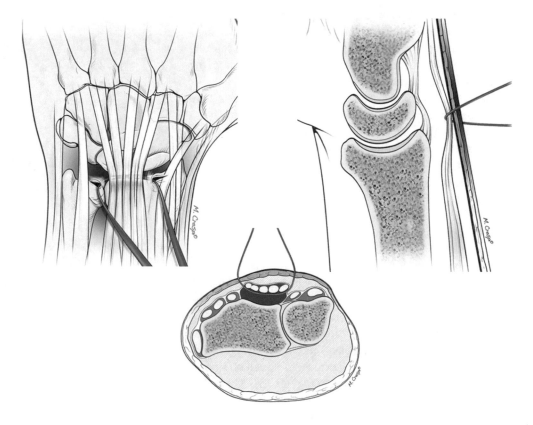

nate and the ulnotriquetral ligament. Moritomo et al. showed that the volar UC ligaments insert into the volar aspect of the TFCC ligament and both run proximally attaching to the ulnar head [23]. He demonstrated that a TFCC detachment produces both DRUJ and UC instability. Viegas reported that section of the radioscaphocapitate and radiolunate ligaments does not lead to significant ulnar translation of the carpus, and that either the volar ulnar ligament or the dorsal ulnar ligament complex alone can prevent ulnar translation [24]. The arthroscopic capsulotomy leaves the volar ulnar ligament and dorsal ulnar ligament complex intact.

Resection of a portion of the dorsal rim of the distal radius is mandatory when wrist extension is limited due to dorsal radiocarpal impingement secondary to malunion of a distal radius fracture (see Fig. 27.1). This may be performed arthroscopically and improves wrist extension. After dorsal capsule resection, the dorsal rim of the distal radius is resected by using a burr of 2.9–3.2 mm introduced through the 6R or 1–2 portal. Sometimes a volar radial portal is used but the ulnar-most side of the dorsal rim cannot be completely reached due to the carpal bones even if wrist distraction is increased. Therefore, the ulnar-most side of the dorsal rim of the distal radius is resected mostly through the 6R portal.

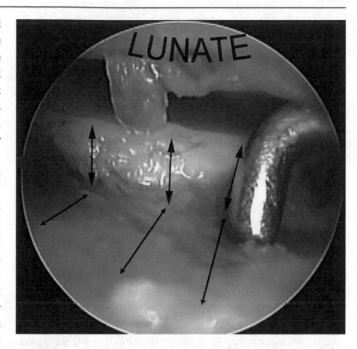

Fig. 27.18 Arthroscopic view showing an articular step of the distal radius that became evident during arthrolysis. Courtesy of Francisco del Piñal

Ancillary Procedures

During arthroscopy one may identify other occult articular, DRUJ, and carpal bone problems. Some of these may be treated during the same procedure but others may need to be treated later due to different rehabilitation programs, in order to avoid postoperative immobilization.

Small articular steps (<1 mm) of the distal radius may be addressed (Fig. 27.18). A burr of 2.9–3.2 mm is used at 500 revolutions per second introduced through the 6R portal with the scope in the 3–4 or 1–2 portal. Larger steps can also be treated but this often results in fibrotic band recurrences and ongoing wrist pain.

TFCC central tears are debrided: the flap is removed and the edges are resected. TFCC peripheral lesions or foveal detachments must be treated later because of the necessity for postoperative immobilization. Positive ulnar variance may be treated with arthroscopic wafer resection. Loose bodies, an extremely rare occurrence, should be removed if they are found.

This concludes the RC arthroscopy and, at this point, the ROM should be assessed before proceeding to the MC joint. Traction is temporarily removed and passive wrist ROM is evaluated.

Midcarpal Joint

If there is no appreciable change in passive wrist ROM after the RC arthrolysis, a MC arthroscopy should be carried out. The approach for this articulation is via the two portals (RMC and UMC) but if needed, more portals can be used (scapho-trapezio-trapezoid [STT] and triquetrohamate [TH]). Arthroscopy of this joint is much easier to perform and synovitis is the most frequently found pathology. It is usually localized at the level of the STT and TH joints. Commonly, one tends to see cartilage degeneration between the capitate and hamate. This may well be responsible for wrist pain. Debridement of the MC joint is performed and may improve pain and ROM. MC joint arthroscopy does not require any ligament resection.

Dorsal radiomidcarpal impingement is suspected when wrist extension is limited and painful, with the pain localized to the capitate, with radiographs demonstrating deformity of the dorsal rim of the radius. The degree of chondral damage to the capitate due to impingement may be assessed. After a synovectomy and debridement, a burr is used to remove excess bone from the dorsum of the neck of the capitate to facilitate acceptance of the remodeled dorsal rim of the distal radius during wrist extension. The procedure is similar to that performed in the elbow for humeral-olecranon impingement in which osteophytes on the tip of the olecranon and the olecranon fossa are arthroscopically removed.

Distal Radioulnar Joint

A prerequisite to ensure a good outcome for the DRUJ is the preservation of a normal articular surface (sigmoid notch and ulnar head). Malunion of the sigmoid notch due to fracture of the ulna aspect of the distal radius should be treated by osteotomy if there are no signs of arthritis [3]. Salvage procedures are recommended for DRUJ incongruity with secondary arthritis of the joint.

Arthroscopy of the DRUJ is difficult. It is very unusual to have good visibility in the DRUJ even in normal conditions. Stiffness of this joint is due to capsular contraction, intra-articular fibrosis, and synovitis, which makes arthroscopy more difficult.

DRUJ arthroscopy is performed through distal and proximal portals. The scope is introduced in the proximal portal and the instruments in the distal portal. Normally, fibrosis does not permit any visualization. Fluid is constantly used to try to expand the joint and improve visualization. Once visualization is achieved and the tips of the instruments are seen, fibrosis is progressively removed using a full radius or aggressive resector.

From an arthroscopic point of view, the DRUJ comprises two spaces (Fig. 27.19): one between the TFCC ligament and the ulna head, and the other between the ulna head and the radius (sigmoid notch). In posttraumatic conditions, both spaces are involved. Fibrosis under the TFCC precludes any visualization by arthroscopy, and in the absence of a central

perforation of the TFCC, good visualization is difficult. In these cases, we suggest introducing a blunt dissector between the TFCC and the ulnar head, and gently dissecting the adhesions. It can also be done using an arthroscopic shaver through the traditional DRUJ portals or just below the 6U portal (direct foveal portal) or lateral to the 6U portal. Fibrosis can be completely removed through these portals (Fig. 27.20) and it is also possible to perform a wafer resection.

The second space, lying between the ulnar head and radius in the sigmoid notch, is affected by contraction of the volar and dorsal capsule causing a restriction in pronation and supination. Arthroscopic arthrolysis of this space starts with the scope in the distal portal and instruments in the proximal portal. It is difficult to visualize the tip of the instrument introduced in the DRUJ proximal portal. The dorsal and the volar capsule must be detached and/or resected (Fig. 27.21). Volar capsulectomy would improve the supina-

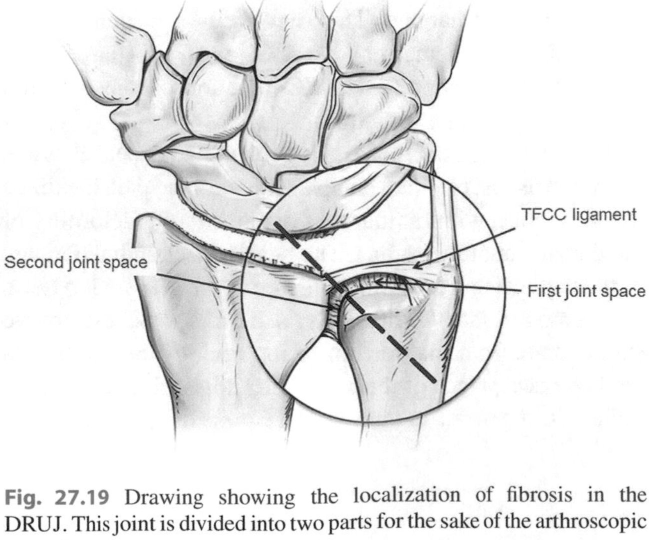

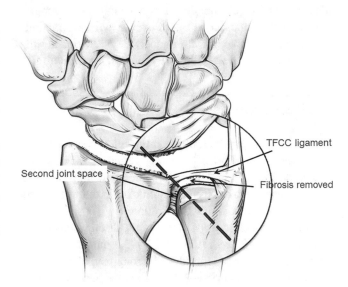

Fig. 27.20 Drawing showing removal of the fibrosis under the TFCC

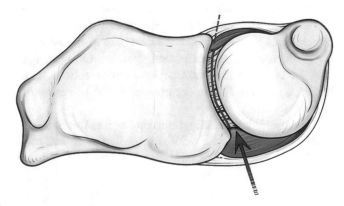

Fig. 27.19 Drawing showing the localization of fibrosis in the DRUJ. This joint is divided into two parts for the sake of the arthroscopic procedure

Fig. 27.21 Drawing showing an axial view of the DRUJ. Dorsal and volar capsules are sectioned (*red arrows* and *red line*)

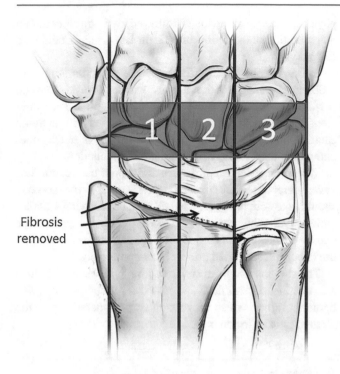

Fibrosis
removed

Fig. 27.22 Drawing showing complete removal of fibrosis in the DRUJ and radiocarpal joint

tion, and dorsal capsulectomy the pronation. To improve the visualization and speed of this last part of the procedure, a curved dissector is introduced into the joint from the proximal portal. By passing from dorsal to volar, it is possible to detach the ligament from the sigmoid notch (Fig. 27.22). The volar and the dorsal parts of the TFCC ligament must not be detached from the bony origin (radius and ulnar fovea). If this happens, DRUJ instability will follow. The articular surface of the ulna head or sigmoid notch must not be damaged. Dry arthroscopy is rarely used for the DRUJ. Finally, out of the traction, gentle pronation, and supination maneuvers are performed to evaluate the improvement in ROM.

Postoperative Rehabilitation

Rehabilitation is started immediately after surgery [25]. Routine analgesics are used for postoperative pain control. Active and passive pronation-supination and flexion-extension exercises are performed, gradually increasing the passive mobilizing force, under the guidance of a therapist.

Return to work is delayed up to 3 months as per the work requirements of the patient. A volar wrist splint is used for protection while performing heavy activities. Endurance and strengthening exercises using isokinetic and isotonic rehabilitation equipment can be initiated 1 month after surgery under the strict supervision of a physical therapist. The

patient protocol is individualized depending on strength requirements for each individual patient and their job requirements [25].

Discussion

Arthroscopic wrist arthrolysis is a difficult and time-consuming procedure. Occasionally, the technique requires mini-open surgery or conversion into an open procedure to obtain the best result. This is particularly true for the DRUJ, where resection of the volar and dorsal capsule is difficult to perform arthroscopically. However, arthroscopic arthrolysis is a suitable and effective surgical option for the treatment of wrist stiffness after trauma or surgery. It is a safe and minimally invasive procedure and allows the surgeon to identify the intra-articular pathology.

Comparison between published series regarding the improvement of wrist ROM after arthroscopic wrist arthrolysis is reported in Table 27.3. All series showed a significant improvement in wrist ROM.

Arthroscopy may identify associated lesions that contribute to the patient's pain. Loose bodies, arthrofibrosis, radiocarpal septae, arthritis, partial, or complete tears of the intercarpal ligaments and TFCC, and articular incongruity that may not had been evident on radiographs or MRI may also be identified arthroscopically. This is one of the advantages of performing this procedure arthroscopically [26, 27]. Moreover, it is often possible to treat all the pathologies at the same time, thereby improving outcomes.

Conversion into open surgery is only indicated when it is necessary to surgically treat the DRUJ and when difficulty is encountered during arthroscopy. Other surgical procedures may be performed at the same time to treat associated pathologies, such as carpal tunnel syndrome and partial or total wrist denervation.

Table 27.3 Comparison between studies in literature

Publications	Cases No.	F-up Months	Preop Flex/ext (mean degrees)	Postop Flex/ext (mean degrees)
Pederzini et al. [5]	5	10	44/40	54/60
Verhellen and Bain [15]	5	6	17/10	47/50
Osterman and Culp [14]	20	32	9/15	42/58
Luchetti et al. [2, 12]	19	32	46/38	54/53
Hattori et al. [28]	11	Unsure	29/47	42/56

Based on our experience, we suggest that TFCC tears type 1B or a complete tear of the SL ligament must not be treated simultaneously with arthrolysis since they require prolonged postoperative immobilization, and the rehabilitation protocol is contrary to that of arthrolysis. Therefore, before arthroscopy, it is important to discuss with the patient, the surgical procedure indicated based on a thorough clinical evaluation and to plan the optimal timing of the surgery, since it is mandatory that the wrist is mobilized and that the patient initiates rehabilitation immediately after an arthroscopic arthrolysis procedure.

One must remember that if there is an underlying SL ligament tear, in addition to the presence of wrist stiffness, the surgeon may not be able to obtain a good result by performing an arthroscopic arthrolysis. The injury to this ligament is often concealed by the wrist stiffness and, only after wrist arthrolysis has been performed, instability due to ligament injury will be manifested. The improvement in pain and ROM that is obtained following wrist arthrolysis may be inconsistent.

It may be seen that an intra-operative increase in wrist flexion-extension ROM is followed by a temporary decrease soon after surgery, but is regained over time. On the contrary, pronation-supination improvement that has been obtained during surgery is almost always maintained postoperatively [5].

DRUJ (pronation-supination) stiffness is more frequently encountered than RC stiffness, and may be isolated or in conjunction with RC joint stiffness. When DRUJ stiffness is isolated, ROM recovery after surgery is easier to obtain than when it is associated with RC stiffness, and this improvement is maintained.

Failures and Complications

Unfortunately, it may happen that the surgeon is unable to perform a wrist arthroscopic arthrolysis due to the presence of an osteofibrotic band (RC septum) that is too thick and dense and obstructs the field of view. This may result in a radiolunate ankylosis (Fig. 27.9). These are the types of cases that should not be treated arthroscopically since they tend to end up with residual wrist stiffness.

Radiographs may not demonstrate all of the pathology, and when the surgeon sees a preserved joint space, they tend to be eager to perform an arthroscopic arthrolysis. Unfortunately, the underlying difficulties become quite evident during the surgery, and if one is able to perform the wrist arthrolysis, they have to first detach the adherent bands and the osteofibrotic band in order to improve the visual field and, ultimately, ROM. At the same time osteochondral lesions may become evident. In these cases, even if a proper physical therapy protocol is followed, it is quite common that fibrotic bands reform and result in partial or complete RC ankylosis.

Extra-articular wrist stiffness due to CRPS is a difficult problem to manage. In these cases, wrist arthrolysis must be performed with release of extra-articular soft tissue adhesions. Surgery in these cases must be planned with extreme caution since the root of the wrist stiffness is much more complex than just a localized articular dysfunction.

When the patient reports that wrist pain has recurred or never completely disappeared after surgery, the surgeon should take note that there can still be an underlying articular pathology that has not been diagnosed. Often the pain can be due to intrinsic ligament tears (scapholunate or lunotriquetral) not been identified pre- or intra-operatively.

The surgeon should exercise caution with the use of intra-articular instruments that can cause osteochondral damage or ligament injury, which may manifest postoperatively in the form of pain or instability.

References

1. Altissimi M, Rinonapoli E. Le rigidità del polso e della mano. Inquadramento clinico, valutazione diagnostica e indicazioni terapeutiche. Giornale Italiano di Ortopedia e Traumatologia. 1995;21(3):187–92. suppl, LXXX Congresso SIOT
2. Luchetti R, Atzei A, Fairplay T. Arthroscopic wrist arthrolysis after wrist fracture. Arthroscopy. 2007;23:255–60.
3. del Piñal F, Garcia-Bernal FJ, Delgado J, Sanmartin M, Regalado J, Cerezal L. Correction of malunited intra-articular distal radius fractures with an inside-out osteotomy technique. J Hand Surg. 2006;31A:1029–34.
4. af-Ekenstam FW. Capsulotomy of the distal radio-ulnar joint. Scand J Plast Surg. 1988;22:169–71.
5. Pederzini L, Luchetti R, Montagna G, Alfarano M, Soragni O. Trattamento artroscopico delle rigidità di polso. Il Ginocchio. 1991;XI–XII:1–13.
6. Jones GS, Savoie FH. Arthroscopic capsular release of flexion contractures of the elbow. Arthroscopy. 1993;9:277–83.
7. Warner JJ, Answorth A, Marsh PH, Wong P. Arthroscopic release for chronic, refractory adhesive capsulitis of the shoulder. J Bone Joint Surg. 1995;78A:1808–16.
8. Warner JJ, Allen AA, Marks PH, Wong P. Arthroscopic release of post-operative capsular contracture of the shoulder. J Bone Joint Surg. 1996;79A:1151–8.
9. Bain GI, Verhellen R, Pederzini L. Procedure artroscopiche capsulari del polso. In: Pederzini L, editor. Artroscopia di Polso. Milano: Springer; 1999. p. 123–8.
10. Luchetti R, Atzei A. Artrolisi artroscopica nelle rigidità post-traumatiche. In: Luchetti R, Atzei A, editors. Artroscopia di Polso, vol. 2001. Fidenza: Mattioli; 1885. p. 67–71.
11. Luchetti R, Atzei A, Fairplay T. Wrist arthrolysis. In: Geissler WB, editor. Wrist arthroscopy. New York, NY: Springer; 2004. p. 145–54.
12. Luchetti R, Atzei A, Mustapha B. Arthroscopic wrist arthrolysis. Atlas Hand Clin. 2001;6:371–87.
13. Luchetti R, Atzei A, Papini-Zorli I. Arthroscopic wrist arthrolysis. Chir Main. 2006;25:S244–53.

14. Osterman AL, Culp RW, Bednar JM. The arthroscopic release of wrist contractures. Scientific Paper Session A1. Presented at the American Society of Hand Surgery Annual Meeting, Boston, MA, 2000.

15. Verhellen R, Bain GI. Arthroscopic capsular release for contracture of the wrist. Arthroscopy. 2000;16:106–10.

16. Atzei A, Luchetti R, Sgarbossa A, Carità E, Llusa M. Set-up, portals and normal exploration in wrist arthroscopy. Chir Main. 2006;25:S131–44.

17. del Piñal F, Garcìa-Bernal FJ, Pisani D, Regalado J, Ayala H, Studer A. Dry arthroscopy of the wrist. Surgical technique. J Hand Surg. 2007;32A:119–23.

18. Doi K, Hattori Y, Otsuka K, Abe Y, Yamamoto H. Intra-articular fractures of the distal aspect of the radius: arthroscopically assisted reduction compared with open reduction and internal fixation. J Bone Joint Surg. 1999;81A:1093–110.

19. Slutsky DJ. Wrist arthroscopy through a volar radial portal. Arthroscopy. 2002;18:624–30.

20. Tham S, Coleman S, Gilpin D. An anterior portal for wrist arthroscopy. Anatomical study and case reports. J Hand Surg. 1999;24B:445–7.

21. Bain GI, Munt J, Bergman J. Arthroscopic dorsal capsular release in the wrist: a new technique. Tech Hand Up Extrem Surg. 2008;12:191–4.

22. Bain GI, Munt J, Turner PC. New advances in wrist arthroscopy. Arthroscopy. 2008;24:355–67.

23. Moritomo H, Murase T, Arimitsu S, Oka K, Yoshikawa H, Sugamoto K. Change in the length of the ulnocarpal ligaments during radiocarpal motion: possible impact on triangular fibrocartilage complex foveal tears. J Hand Surg. 2008;33A:1278–86.

24. Viegas SF, Patterson RM, Eng M, Ward K. Extrinsic wrist ligaments in the pathomechanics of ulnar translation instability. J Hand Surg Am. 1995;20:312–8.

25. Travaglia-Fairplay T. Valutazione ergonomica dell'ambiente industriale e sua applicazione per screening di pre-assunzione e riabilitazione work-hardening. In: Bazzini G, editor. Nuovi approcci alla riabilitazione industriale. Pavia: Fondazione Clinica del Lavoro Edizioni; 1993. p. 33–48.

26. Cerofolini E, Luchetti R, Pederzini L, Soragni O, Colombini R, D'Alimonte P, Romagnoli R. MRI evaluation of triangular fibrocartilage complex tears in the wrist: comparison with arthrography and arthroscopy. J Comput Assist Tomogr. 1990;14:963–7.

27. Zlatkin MB, Chao PC, Osterman AL, Schnall MD, Dalinka MK, Kressel HY. Chronic wrist pain: evaluation with high-resolution MR imaging. Radiology. 1989;173(3):723–9.

28. Hattori T, Tsunoda K, Watanabe K, Nakao E, Nakamura R. Arthroscopic mobilization for post-traumatic contracture of the wrist. J Jpn Soc Surg Hand. 2004;21:583–6.

Wrist Arthritis: Arthroscopic Techniques of Synovectomy, Abrasion Chondroplasty, Radial Styloidectomy, and Proximal Row Carpectomy of the Wrist

28

Kevin D. Plancher, Michael L. Mangonon, and Stephanie C. Petterson

Introduction

In the eyes of most people, the wrist is a single joint connecting the forearm and the hand. To the surgeon, we know that the wrist is a more intricate entity than our eyes can see. Thus, treatment of such a complex structure is not easily undertaken and the limitations caused by a loss of wrist function due to arthritis can greatly change the daily lives of patients.

With the introduction of arthroscopy, orthopedic and hand surgeons have reinvented old techniques to provide the same gold standard of care using minimally invasive means. Some procedures are enhanced and more successful with the use of arthroscopy than traditional open techniques. Innovations such as new portals and smaller arthroscopes have led to the expansion of arthroscopic procedures [1–3].

Wrist arthroscopy has become an important tool for the examination and treatment of intra-articular abnormalities. Arthroscopy of the wrist is most useful as a diagnostic tool to examine the joint articular surfaces, diagnose degenerative triangular fibrocartilage lesions, and perform synovial biopsy. It can also be used as a therapeutic modality to remove loose bodies and debride the wrist in early-stage arthritis.

Early results for arthroscopic synovectomy demonstrated a reduction in pain and swelling and improved joint function [4–6]. The effectiveness of arthroscopic synovectomy is dependent on the preoperative level of activity as well as the underlying cause of the disease. Arthroscopic synovectomy may be effective in delaying more complex procedures such as arthrodesis or total wrist arthroplasty in select cases [7]. With abrasion chondroplasty of the wrist, it is known that "repair" (type I) fibrocartilage, which replaces articular cartilage, allows for defects to be recontoured, as demonstrated in several animal models [8, 9]. Abrasion chondroplasty has been found to be effective in patients with proximal pole hamate arthrosis and radiocarpal arthrosis, with positive results obtained [10–12]. Radial styloidectomy has been shown to be a suitable alternative for treatment of arthritis of the wrist when a patient does not want to undergo more complex procedures such as a proximal row carpectomy (PRC) or a partial or complete fusion. It is a target-specific procedure with excellent outcomes. Finally, when needed due to severity of the arthritis, PRC is a good salvage procedure, and when performed arthroscopically, the soft tissue envelope and capsular ligaments of the wrist are preserved, making this a more desirable option [13]. This review will discuss the indications and techniques for arthroscopic synovectomy, abrasion chondroplasty, radial styloidectomy, and proximal row carpectomy.

K. D. Plancher (✉)
Montefiore Medical Center/Albert Einstein College of Medicine, New York, NY, USA

Weill Cornell Medical College, New York, NY, USA

Plancher Orthopaedics & Sports Medicine, New York, NY, USA

Orthopaedic Foundation, Stamford, CT, USA
e-mail: kplancher@plancherortho.com

M. L. Mangonon
Plancher Orthopaedics & Sports Medicine, New York, NY, USA

S. C. Petterson
Orthopaedic Foundation, Stamford, CT, USA

Anatomy

Fifteen bones form connections from the end of the forearm to the hand including the radius, ulna, eight carpal bones, and five metacarpals. The carpal bones are grouped in two rows across the wrist. Beginning with the thumb side of the wrist, the proximal row of carpal bones is made up of the scaphoid, lunate, and triquetrum. The distal row is made up of the trapezium, trapezoid, capitate, hamate, and pisiform.

The radiocarpal joint is the primary joint of the wrist formed by the articulations between the radius and the proxi-

© Springer Nature Switzerland AG 2022
W. B. Geissler (ed.), *Wrist and Elbow Arthroscopy with Selected Open Procedures*,
https://doi.org/10.1007/978-3-030-78881-0_28

mal row of carpal bones. The primary motion that occurs at the radiocarpal joint is wrist flexion and extension. The distal radioulnar joint, the articulation between the ulnar head and the ulnar notch of the radius, allows for rotary movements of supination and pronation. The intercarpal joints are small synovial joints that create the transverse arch of the wrist, which is concave on the palmar side. The intercarpal joints, namely the scaphoid-capitate joint and the lunate-capitate joint, contribute to the total range of motion of the wrist [14]. When the wrist flexes, the transverse arch deepens, and when the wrist is extended, the transverse arch flattens. Radial and ulnar deviations occur primarily through the midcarpal joints with a smaller contribution from the radiocarpal joint [15].

The intricate set of ligaments surrounding the bones of the wrist provides stability to the osseous structures and aid in maintaining alignment during wrist movements. The ligaments on the palmar side are stronger than the stabilizing ligaments on the dorsal side. The triangular fibrocartilage complex (TFCC) is the major stabilizer of the distal radioulnar joint (DRUJ). It also improves the gliding motion of the wrist. Housed within the TFCC is an articular disc, which serves to distribute forces to the ulna from the carpus. Medial and lateral wrist stability are provided by the ulnar and radial collateral ligaments which connect the ulna and radius, respectively, to the carpal bones. The palmar radiocarpal ligament stabilizes the radius and carpals on the palmar side and limits excessive wrist extension, whereas the dorsal radiocarpal ligament stabilizes the radius and carpals on the dorsal side and limits excessive wrist flexion. The intrinsic dorsal and palmar midcarpal ligaments stabilize the proximal and distal rows of carpal bones and the intrinsic interosseous ligaments stabilize the individual intercarpal joints. Lastly, the accessory, transverse carpal ligament supports the transverse carpal arch.

The articular surfaces of the wrist bones are covered with a white, shiny material known as articular cartilage. Articular cartilage aids in facilitation of joint motion between two joint surfaces. Articular cartilage can be up to ¼-inch thick in the large, weight-bearing joints, and is thinner in joints such as the wrist that do not support as much weight. Its rubbery consistency contributes to its function as a shock absorber. In the wrist, articular cartilage covers a much larger surface area due to the many joint surfaces involved.

Physiology

Osteoarthritis (OA) is a complex cascade of events leading to degeneration of articular cartilage, which may be accelerated with injury or trauma. Chronic injuries of the scapholunate ligament and in scaphoid nonunions are often initiated with OA of the radial styloid, which then progresses to the radiocarpal and capitolunate joints, and finally, results in collapse of the capitate into the scapholunate interval [16].

Matrix metalloproteinases and proinflammatory cytokines (e.g., interleukin-1) have been found to be important mediators of cartilage destruction in patients with primary OA. Interleukin-1 increases the synthesis of matrix metalloproteinases and, thereby, plays an important role in OA. During the initial stages of OA, the superficial layers of the articular cartilage fibrillate and crack. As degeneration progresses, deep layers become involved, resulting in erosions that produce bare subchondral bone. Denatured type II collagen is found in abundance in OA articular cartilage, with decreased water content and decreased ratio of chondroitin sulfate-to-keratin sulfate constituents.

Rheumatoid arthritis (RA) is a progressive inflammatory disease characterized by synovitis and joint destruction. Synovial cell proliferation results in pannus formation and fibrosis, which in turn results in erosion of cartilage and bone. Cytokines, prostanoids, and proteolytic enzymes mediate this process. A cell-mediated immune response to an unidentified antigen appears essential in the pathogenesis of RA. Proinflammatory cytokines, such as interleukin-1 and tumor necrosis factor alpha, and T-cell initiation are the central mediators in RA.

In gouty arthritis, allantoin, the enzyme uricase that breaks down uric acid into a more soluble product, is deficient and leads to tissue deposition of crystalline forms of uric acid. Hyperuricemia is a risk factor for the development of gout; however, hyperuricemia does not implicate the development of gout and acute gouty arthritis can occur in the presence of normal serum uric acid concentrations. Gout appears as crystal deposition on the scapholunate and lunotriquetral ligaments when viewed arthroscopically [17].

Secondary OA may emerge as a result of injury to the ligamentous stabilizers. Loss of joint stability contributes to loss of coupled motion in the wrist, abnormal wrist mechanics, and altered joint reaction and loading forces. This process produces degeneration of the articular cartilage, resulting in radiocarpal arthritis, selective intercarpal arthritis, or pancarpal arthritis, depending on the nature and extent of the initial injury and subsequent healing.

Scaphoid fractures, in particular, can result in OA by three different mechanisms:

1. *Nonunion*. A nonunion fracture leads to abnormal movement between the bone fragments. Consequently, the normal distribution of forces across the wrist is altered and can result in early degeneration of the radioscaphoid joint if not treated properly.
2. *Malunion*. Malunion fractures may reduce the height of the scaphoid and restrict the range of motion in one or more planes. Altered range of motion can cause increased strain and lead to OA changes over time.
3. *Avascular Necrosis*. Scaphoid fractures resulting in avascular necrosis of the proximal pole can lead to collapse and degeneration of the radioscaphoid joint. Progression to the lunate and, then, the entire wrist is also possible.

Regardless of the type of arthritis in question, the main reason for symptoms is the underlying inflammatory processes. Knowledge of the underlying disease process will allow for directed treatment to resolve symptoms and minimize the chance of further disease progression.

Patient Evaluation

History

With proper history, one can elicit certain "historical" facts that can aid in the diagnosis of wrist arthritis. Symptoms typically emerge gradually over time and often do not involve an acute injury. The most commonly reported complaint is pain throughout the arc of motion, which is aggravated at extremes of motion. Pain is often improved with rest and gradually worsens with length of activity. As the disease worsens, the functional range of motion of the wrist decreases and in severe cases patients may experience a complete loss of movement.

Physical Examination

Physical deformity is a key feature of wrist arthritis, particularly in RA. Patients with RA may exhibit enlargement of the wrist and metacarpophalangeal joints as well as subluxation of the radiocarpal and inferior radioulnar joints. Enlargement of the proximal interphalangeal joints (Bouchard's nodes) may be present; however, Bouchard's nodes are more commonly found in patients with OA. Enlargement of the distal interphalangeal joints of the hand, or Heberden's nodes, are also characteristic of OA.

Classically in RA, wrist deformity begins with wrist radial deviation and resultant ulnar head prominence and progresses to supination and ulnar translation of the carpus and volar subluxation of the radiocarpal joint. Swelling of the wrist is also a common manifestation of RA due to synovial thickening. If left untreated, the synovitis can lead to tendon weakening rupture and collapse resulting in the aforementioned characteristic deformities.

Palpation of the wrist would reveal crepitus with motion, capsular edema dorsally without any fluctuance, and localized tenderness. The wrist acts as a stabilizer of the hand for function. Therefore, resultant arthritis-related pain and deformity can lead to decreased grip strength. Wrist deformity and instability reduce support for the hand to grasp; thus, impairing fine motor movements. Loss of wrist extension due to stiffness will also hinder the ability to properly evaluate for the tenodesis effect (passive flexion of the digits with passive wrist extension and passive extension of the digits with passive wrist flexion) during examination.

Diagnostic Imaging

Plain radiographs are the mainstay and most accurate modality for imaging and diagnosing arthritis. Radiographs should not be a substitute for the physician's clinical examination. Radiographs may only show the picture in the late stages of disease when bone tissue is already affected [18] and findings are not always indicative of symptoms [19]. Appropriate radiographic workup can provide insight into areas of localized pain in the wrist.

Common wrist radiographic views, include zero postero-anterior, zero lateral, oblique, ulnar and radial deviation, and grip views for a complete evaluation of the wrist (Fig. 28.1). Characteristic findings that lead to a diagnosis of arthritis include reduction in articular height, sclerosis, osteophyte formation, bone erosions, intra-articular calcifications, and joint deformity.

Magnetic resonance imaging (MRI) correlations with an appropriate clinical history and confirmatory arthroscopic findings is a useful diagnostic tool for articular cartilage. However, others refute the role of MRI as a diagnostic tool. Haims and colleagues concluded that wrist MRI (41 indirect MR arthrograms and 45 unenhanced [nonarthrographic] MR images) is not adequately sensitive or accurate for diagnosing cartilage defects in the distal radius, scaphoid, lunate, or triquetrum, as demonstrated compared to arthroscopic findings [20]. This was also supported by Multimer et al., who demonstrated that MRI and arthroscopy are not correlated and, therefore, arthroscopy continues to have a role in the diagnosis of an arthritic wrist [21]. While true for the radiologist who sees a rare MRI of the wrist, a trained musculoskeletal radiologist well versed in wrist anatomy can be enormously helpful in treatment planning with an accurate reading of the cartilage status of the wrist.

In cases of synovitis and ulnar-sided pathology, MRI remains a strong indicator for which areas need to be addressed with the arthroscope to treat successfully. Signs of synovitis, enhancement with bone erosion-like changes, and of bone marrow edema are strong indicators of an evolving arthritic disease process [22, 23].

MRI is also a sensitive method for excluding the diagnosis of early avascular necrosis and for evaluating the extent to which fibrocartilaginous repair tissue has formed postoperatively. The utilization of MRI after microfracture or cartilage repair procedures is common in knee pathologies after surgery, and we have established the same protocols for wrist defects [20, 24].

Fig. 28.1 Wrist radiographs demonstrating wrist arthritis. (*Left*) Scapholunate advanced collapse (SLAC) wrist stage III/IV with styloscaphoid arthritis, radiocarpal arthritis, and joint space narrowing of the capitolunate junction. (*Right*) Scaphotrapeziotrapezoidal (STT) arthritis with joint space narrowing and sclerotic changes

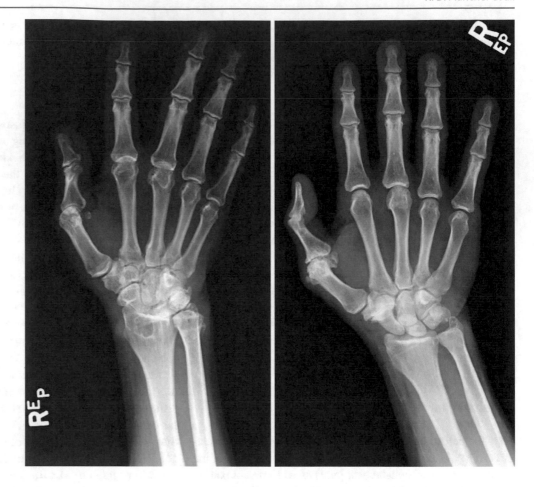

Treatment Options

Conservative Management

Nonoperative measures for wrist arthritis are typically the first line of defense and are primarily aimed at relieving pain in the wrist. Rest in the form of splinting with removable thermoplastic splints constructed by a certified hand therapist may be useful during periods of exacerbation. The wrist is usually maintained in a functional position of neutral or slight dorsiflexion. While providing pain relief, the disadvantages of splinting include stiffness and wrist weakness as a result of overuse or prolonged immobilization, which should always be avoided. Therefore, splinting should be used in conjunction with alternative therapies such as exercise and occupational hand therapy.

Pharmacologic management should also be used during inflammatory periods to control pain and swelling. For patients with inflammatory arthritis, nonsteroidal anti-inflammatory drugs (NSAIDs) are indicated to assist in controlling inflammation and reducing synovitis. Topical NSAIDs can also control acute and chronic symptoms and eliminates the adverse, systemic complications associated with prolonged, oral NSAID use. Topical formulations can be compounded with ingredients such as muscle relaxants, calcium-channel blockers, anesthetics, and GABA-receptor blockers to provide a broader coverage of symptoms. Antirheumatic medications, including systemic steroids, methotrexate, and antitumor necrosis factor, are indicated for patients with RA and allopurinol, a xanthine oxidase inhibitor, which may be useful in patients with gouty arthritis of the wrist.

Steroid injections, with or without local anesthetic into the joint, may also be performed. Methylprednisolone acetate injection into the wrist can play a role in treating degenerated triangular fibrocartilage. Local steroid injections using a 1½″, 25- or 27-gauge needle when combined with local anesthetic may provide both a diagnostic and therapeutic effect. The effects of steroid injections are transient and, therefore, repeat injections may be needed. However, repeat injections should be used sparingly (our recommended maximum is two) due to the associated risk of soft tissue weakening and thinning of the cartilage in an already compromised joint.

Surgical Management

When conservative options have failed, arthroscopic intervention may be a viable option for some patients. Indications for surgical management are dependent on the severity and the extent of wrist arthritis. MRI in conjunction with clinical assessment of the patient aids surgical decision-making. Arthroscopic procedures are more favorable compared to their parent open procedures due to less joint capsule and ligament damage. In general, arthroscopic procedures are safe procedures with no major complications being reported [25–27].

In the earliest stages, when the problems are mainly caused by carpal instability (i.e., prearthritic stage), the aim of surgery is to restore the anatomic position and correct carpal instability to prevent degeneration. In the intermediate stages, when the patient has well-established arthritis but a well-preserved range of motion, no proven standard treatment has been established. The available options are geared toward less invasive, arthroscopic procedures with fewer complexities such as synovectomy, abrasion chondroplasty, radial styloidectomy, and proximal row carpectomy. In the late stages of arthritis, a partial or total wrist arthrodesis, a PRC, or a total wrist arthroplasty may be contemplated. Patients with severe dorsal tenosynovitis have weakened tendons and are not usually candidates for arthroscopy due to the risk of tendon injury when establishing portals.

Arthroscopic synovectomy has become a well-described procedure. Aggressive arthroscopic debridement, including radial styloidectomy and partial resection of the scaphoid, has been reported. Resection of the lunate in patients with Kienböck's disease may also be performed arthroscopically. In the DRUJ, arthroscopy can be used for debridement of the TFCC and for a modified Darrach procedure that involves distal ulna resection. Arthroscopic reconstructive procedures have been described for repair of the lunate-triquetrum ligament and ulnocarpal ligament complex, as well as for capsular placation. More recently, arthroscopy has seen increased use for the removal of single or multiple bones in the proximal carpal row and for partial wrist fusions, procedures that are traditionally performed using open techniques.

Arthroscopic Synovectomy

Arthroscopic synovectomy provides effective treatment of patients with RA, juvenile RA, systemic lupus erythematosus (SLE), and postinfectious arthritis when conservative measures have failed [4–6, 27]. Patients with posttraumatic joint contractures and septic arthritis of the wrist after failed systemic antibiotics and lavage also benefit from arthroscopic synovectomy. Patients requiring more extensive, open wrist procedures would not be an ideal candidate for arthroscopic synovectomy. The goal of the procedure is to decrease pain and improve joint function by excising the inflamed synovium and, thereby, removing or eliminating the effusion and inflammatory substrate.

The protocol for arthroscopic synovectomy in patients with RA was established by Adolfsson [4]. Indications include persistent joint symptoms following a 6-month course of pharmacologic treatment and the presence of radiographic changes in grade 0, I, or II according to the staging system by Larsen and colleagues [28]. Synovectomy for RA is indicated in the early stages of development when complete synovectomy is more feasible and has been shown to slow and even halt the progression of the disease [6, 29]. It allows for significant improvement in pain, joint motion, inflammatory markers, and disability score [5].

In noninflammatory disease, the Outerbridge classification system, originally developed for patients with chondromalacia patellae, can be used (Fig. 28.2) [30]. Patients with early presentation of SLE or reactive arthritis (bacterial or viral) and those with OA with nominal radiographic changes and florid synovitis are also considered good candidates for wrist synovectomy. Patients after intra-articular fractures or multiple previous wrist interventions also benefit from capsular release, removal of adhesions, and synovectomy.

Arthroscopic Abrasion Chondroplasty

Chondral defects are a common source of occult pain. Fibrocartilage forms in locations of disrupted subchondral bone (Outerbridge grade IV). Abrasion and drill chondroplasty take advantage of this phenomenon and are used to fill articular defects with the goals of reducing mechanical symptoms and minimizing intra-articular debris by smoothing out the chondral lesions [9, 24, 30].

Abrasion chondroplasty is effective in patients with proximal pole hamate arthrosis, a cause of ulnar-sided wrist pain when loaded during ulnar deviation. Lunate morphology plays a key role in this condition. Patients with a type II lunate defect have a particularly positive outcome. The type II lunate and its medial facet during contact loading of the proximal pole of the hamate can lead to arthritis. 44% of patients with type II lunates develop arthritis compared to only 2% of patients with type I lunates [11, 31–37]. In cases of advanced arthrosis and an Outerbridge grade IV lesion, Yao and coworkers recommend excision of the proximal pole [31]. Abrasion arthroplasty is contraindicated for patients with active rheumatoid disease, those who are medically unfit, and patients with active infections not located in the wrist.

Also, with ulnar-sided wrist pain, it is common for patients to have concomitant injuries that also require treat-

Fig. 28.2 The Outerbridge classification of articular cartilage lesions: grade 0: normal cartilage; (**a**) grade I: superficial softening; (**b**) grade II: fibrillation; (**c**) grade III: fissuring; and (**d**) grade IV: loss of all cartilage layers and exposure of subchondral bone

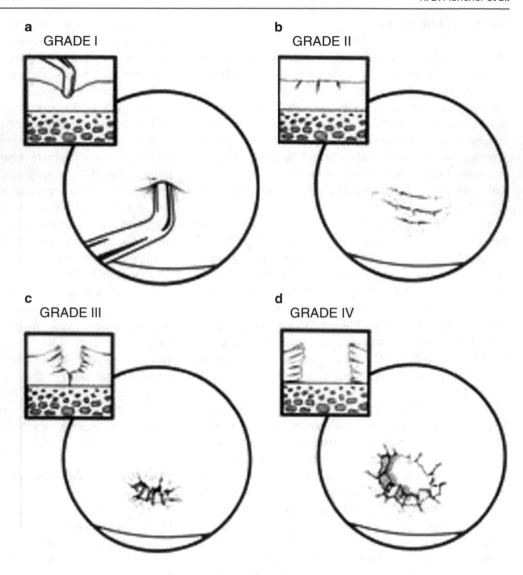

ment including TFCC tears, lunotriquetral interosseous ligament tears, ulnar impaction, and radial-sided pathology. When synovitis is noted on the ulnar side of the wrist, a TFCC injury is almost always noted in the absence of any other structural problem.

Arthroscopic Radial Styloidectomy

Radial styloid arthritis as a result of scapholunate advanced collapse (SLAC), scaphoid nonunion advanced collapse (SNAC), Kienböck's disease, or impingement after scaphotrapeziotrapezoidal (STT) fusion, PRC, or four-corner fusion is the primary indication for radial styloidectomy. Arthroscopic intervention is indicated and highly effective when a PRC or fusion is not yet indicated or when patients are not ready to undergo a more extensive procedure. Arthroscopic radial styloidectomy ensures preservation of

the volar ligaments, which provide radial stability of the wrist and enhance precision when determining the appropriate amount of styloid to be removed [31].

Arthroscopic Proximal Row Carpectomy

PRC has long been considered a salvage procedure for advanced wrist arthritis because of its association with decreased range of motion, decreased strength, and progression of arthritis. Recent studies have shown its reliability to be equal to that of the four-corner fusion, which has been a well-established standard of treatment [38]. Arthroscopic PRC, thus, can be viewed as beneficial over the open technique because it does not require capsulotomy, does not disrupt the stabilizing ligaments, and allows for early mobilization [13]. PRC is contraindicated in the presence of arthritis at the head of the capitate or in the lunate fossa of the radius.

General Technique and Instrumentation for Arthroscopy of the Wrist

The preferred method of anesthesia in patients with arthritic changes is general or regional anesthesia. The patient is positioned supine on the operating table with the shoulder along the edge of the table. A tourniquet is placed above the elbow and inflated to 250 mmHg. The shoulder is abducted 70–90°, and finger traps from an articulating arm attached to the operating table suspend the forearm vertically. We routinely use the long and index fingers; however, all the digits may be placed in the finger traps to distribute the traction load particularly for patients with rheumatoid arthritis whose skin is delicate. A traction force of approximately 10–15 lb is applied to help open the joint and improve access during the surgical procedure (Fig. 28.3). In addition, a sling with 7–10 lb of weight is placed over the tourniquet to provide downward countertraction and distraction of the wrist joint.

Following patient setup, the wrist is thoroughly examined, and relevant anatomical landmarks are palpated. The arthroscopic wrist portals are described in Table 28.1. The 3–4 portal is established in the soft spot, 1 cm distal to Lister's tubercle (Fig. 28.4). To minimize the risk of articular cartilage damage, a 22-gauge needle is first inserted and angled 10° volar to be parallel to the radiocarpal joint surface. The wrist is then distended with 5–7 mL of saline solution. If insufflation of the joint does not occur, this is indicative of a torn TFCC. A vertical stab incision is made with a No. 15 scalpel blade through the dermis only and then a blunt trocar is intro-

Table 28.1 Arthroscopic wrist portals: technique and comments

Portal Dorsal	Technique	Comment
1–2	Inserted in the extreme dorsum of the snuffbox just radial to the EPL tendon to avoid the radial artery	Provides access to the radial styloid, scaphoid, lunate, and articular surface of the distal radius
3–4	The portal is 1-cm distal to Lister's tubercle between the tendons of the third and fourth compartments	Primary working portal. Gives a wide range of movement and view
4–5	Between the common extensor fourth compartment and EDQ in the fifth compartment	Alternative to the 6R portal
6R	Located distal to the ulna head and radial to the ECU tendon. Established under direct vision of the arthroscope by use of a needle. Avoids damage to the TFCC	Primary working portal
6U	Established under direct visualization similar to the 6R portal. Blunt dissection is always used to avoid the dorsal branches of the ulnar nerve	6U and 6R portals allow visualization back toward the radial side and access to the ulnar-sided structures
MCR	The portal is created 1-cm distal to the 3–4 portal	Allows instrument access to the ulnar midcarpal joint
MCU	The portal is created 1-cm distal to the 4–5 portal	Allows instrument access to the radial midcarpal joint

EPL extensor pollicis longus, *EDQ* extensor digiti quinti proprius, *6R* 6-radial, *ECU* extensor carpi ulnaris, *TFCC* triangular fibrocartilage complex, *6U* 6-ulnar, *MCR* midcarpal radial, *MCU* midcarpal ulnar

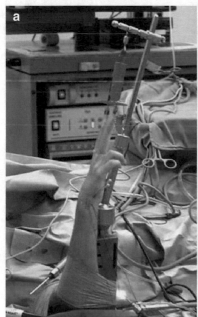
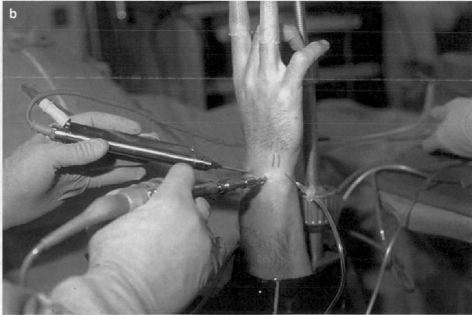

Fig. 28.3 (**a**) Wrist arthroscopy setup. Note the index and long fingers are placed in finger traps. 10–15 lb of traction is applied to allow for better access and mobility inside the wrist joint. (**b**) Wrist arthroscopy setup with instrumentation. Note the arthroscope and instruments can be interchanged between portals to obtain the proper vantage point

Fig. 28.4 Dorsal portal anatomy. (**a**) Cadaver dissection of the dorsal aspect of a left wrist, demonstrating the relative positions of the dorsoradial portals. (**b**) Relative positions of the dorsoulnar portals. EPL extensor pollicis longus, * Lister's tubercle, EDC extensor digitorum communis, EDM extensor digiti minimi, DCBUN dorsal cutaneous branch of the ulnar nerve, MCU midcarpal ulnar portal, SRN superficial radial nerve, MCR midcarpal radial portal

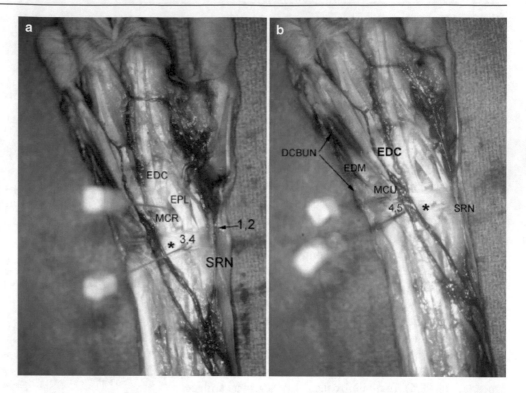

duced into the joint. To maintain orientation, the thumb is kept on Lister's tubercle until the arthroscope is introduced. Inflow of lactated Ringer's solution is gravity fed (i.e., no pump required).

Subsequent portals are made using an outside-in technique. A needle is first introduced into the joint to establish these portals. Introduction of the needle should be distal to the TFCC and either radial to the extensor carpi ulnaris tendon or ulnar to the common extensor tendons. Both the 4–5 and 6R portals can be used for a radiocarpal portal. The 4–5 or 6R portals are identified by use of transillumination. A 2.5-mm arthroscope is used with a 30° viewing angle. A short-bridge arthroscope (lever arm of 100 mm) allows better control. The 6U portal can be used when necessary but caution to the dorsal sensory branch of the ulnar nerve is taken.

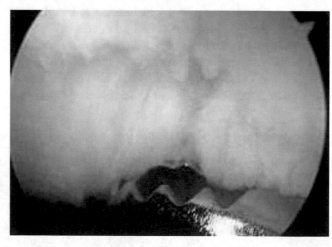

Fig. 28.5 The rotator shaver is used to perform the synovectomy and removes all the fibrillated cartilage

Arthroscopic Synovectomy

To perform an arthroscopic synovectomy, a 2.5-mm-diameter, 30° arthroscope is inserted through the 3–4, 4–5, or 6R working portals for the radiocarpal joint. The 6U portal is used for outflow. The radial and ulnar midcarpal portals are used to access the midcarpal joint. Efficiency and speed are important to decrease wrist swelling. In cases of severe STT arthritis, a separate STT portal can be established to provide better access and visualization of the joint.

A motorized shaver system with a 3.5-mm-diameter synovial resector blade and 3.5-mm flexible shaver is used to

remove the inflamed tissue (Fig. 28.5). We routinely use thermoregulation, which aids in decreasing bleeding. Great care must be taken to avoid touching the articular surfaces. Flow must be maintained within the wrist joint when using thermoregulation to avoid heat buildup.

It is important to inspect the radial styloid, the radioscapholunate and radioscaphocapitate ligaments, ulnar prestyloid recess, and the dorsoulnar region underneath the extensor carpi ulnaris subsheath. Midcarpal space synovitis is often found along the dorsoulnar region, volarly underneath the capitohamate joint, and in the STT joint. Inspection of the DRUJ can be performed through a central defect in the horizontal portion of the TFCC, and synovectomy can be carried out through the 6R portal. In circumstances where there is no central defect in the TFCC, a separate DRUJ portal immediately proximal to the TFCC can be used for shaving while viewing through the radiocarpal joint.

Incisions are closed with dermabond and augmented with steri-strips or with subcuticular monocryl. A light dressing is placed with a volar short-arm splint and is used for approximately 7–10 days. Patients return for a wound check and suture removal at 2 weeks postoperatively. Immediate wrist motion with a certified hand therapist and home exercise program is encouraged. Patients are instructed to avoid vigorous activity for 6 weeks.

Complications of arthroscopic synovectomy are similar to those of any arthroscopic procedure. When making a skin incision for the 6U portal, the surgeon must use caution to avoid laceration or a painful neuroma of the dorsal sensory branch of the ulnar nerve. Meticulous care must be used at all times to avoid chondral damage to the articular surfaces. Blunt dissection, direct visualization, and transillumination are used to minimize the risk of injury to tendons and vessels.

Results of arthroscopic synovectomy for wrist arthritis are favorable. Chung et al. evaluated 21 patients with rheumatoid arthritis in the wrist. Arthroscopic synovectomy following failed conservative management resulted in improved pain, joint motion, inflammatory markers, and decreased disability at an average of 30 months [5]. None of the study patients were taking long-term pain medications at the latest follow-up. Similarly, Adolfsson and colleagues reported improved wrist arc of motion from 69.5° to 90° and an 87% increase in grip strength in 18 wrists 6 months following arthroscopic synovectomy [25]. A second study by the same group reported similar increase in wrist arc of motion and improved pain in 24 wrists at an average of 3.8 years following surgery [26]. Therefore, arthroscopic synovectomy should be considered as an option for patients with mild-to-moderate stages of arthritis as an effective treatment to decrease pain and improve functional status in patients with arthritis [39, 40].

Arthroscopic Abrasion Chondroplasty

Radiocarpal arthritis treated with abrasion chondroplasty follows the same principles that have been described by Steadman and coworkers for the knee [12]. Working portals in the wrist and instrumentation setup are established as previously described for arthroscopic synovectomy. During the diagnostic arthroscopy, loose bodies are removed and areas of focal chondral damage are identified. Specially designed awls (2.5 and 3.5 mm) are used to make multiple perforations, or microfractures, into the subchondral bone

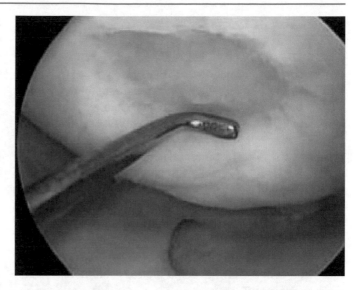

Fig. 28.6 Chondral lesion is debrided and ready for chondroplasty

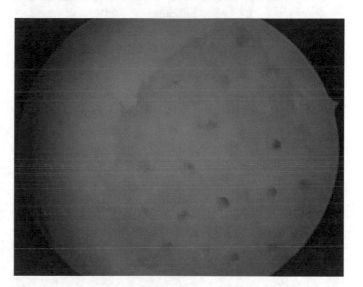

Fig. 28.7 Microfractures created in the subchondral bone 1–2 mm apart using specially designed awls

plate (Fig. 28.6). Perforations are made as close together as possible, approximately 1–2 mm apart, but not so close that one breaks into another (Fig. 28.7). The integrity of the subchondral bone plate should be maintained. The released marrow elements (i.e., mesenchymal stem cells, growth factors, and other healing proteins) form a surgically induced superclot that provides an enriched environment for new tissue formation [12].

Dressings and closure are carried out as previously described for arthroscopic synovectomy. Early range of motion is recommended with a continuous passive motion device to avoid postoperative complications such as stiffness. Rehabilitation is crucial to optimize the results of the surgery.

Arthroscopic Radial Styloidectomy

Arthroscopic radial styloidectomy enhances visualization to ensure complete resection of the arthritic portion of the styloid without sacrificing the ligamentous support of the wrist. This is best done with a short oblique osteotomy [31].

A small 3.5-mm burr is used by entering the 1–2 portal. The diameter of the burr is a good benchmark to gauge the amount of styloid to be removed; ideally this is less than 4 mm. An 18-gauge needle can be introduced into the bone to mark the end point of the styloid resection. Fluoroscopy is used for verification. Following excision of the styloid, a shaver is used to remove debris and loose bodies from the wrist joint (Figs. 28.8 and 28.9). Wounds are closed as previously described. Postoperative management includes the use of a short-arm splint. Protected motion is initiated immediately to avoid stiffness.

Complications of radial styloidectomy include incomplete resection, loss of radial support, and excessive resection. Excessive resection can lead to the loss of the radioscaphocapitate and long radiolunate ligaments yielding subsequent instability and eventual ulnar translocation of the carpus.

A report of three patients with scaphoid nonunion fracture and associated avascular necrosis that underwent arthroscopic resection of the distal pole of the scaphoid and radial styloidectomy showed complete relief of pain and improved wrist

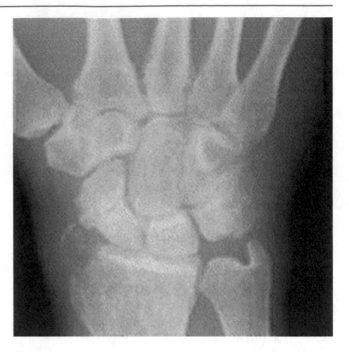

Fig. 28.9 Radial styloidectomy performed. Note that approximately 4 mm was removed off the radial styloid decompressing the articular surface of the scaphoid and the radius

range of motion [41]. Patient-reported satisfaction was also high and a 28-point improvement of the Modified Mayo Wrist Score was also reported. Postoperative X-rays did not reveal progression of degeneration; however, the capitolunate angle increased 10°. Long-term outcome studies are needed to determine any possible chronic sequelae of this procedure.

Arthroscopic Proximal Row Carpectomy

For arthroscopic proximal row carpectomy, a fluoroscopy unit is used and placed in a horizontal position. Diagnostic radiocarpal and midcarpal arthroscopy is initially performed.

The midcarpal portals are used for the arthroscopic PRC. A small joint arthroscopic burr or shaver is inserted into a midcarpal radial (MCR) portal and the scope into the midcarpal ulnar (MCU) portal. A burr is first used to decorticate the medial corner of the scaphoid at the midcarpal scapholunate joint. Once an adequate portion of the corner of the scaphoid is removed, the MCR portal is slightly enlarged and a 4.0-mm hooded burr is used to remove the remaining scaphoid moving ulnar to radial and distal to proximal. The portals are then switched and the hooded burr is inserted into the MCU portal. Excision of the lunate and triquetrum is performed sequentially moving radial to ulnar and distal to proximal. Facilitation of removal may be performed through the MCR portal while viewing through the STT portal. Once

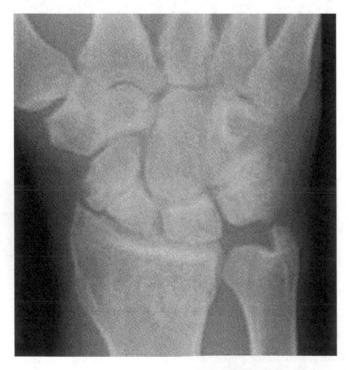

Fig. 28.8 Radiocarpal arthritis secondary to a scaphoid nonunion fracture (SNAC wrist). Note the penciling of the radial styloid, which is pathoneumonic of this condition

the proximal pole is completely excised, a fine synovial rongeur may be used under direct visualization to remove any remaining bone or cartilage adherent to the capsule. If significant impingement of the radial styloid with the trapezium is encountered, arthroscopic styloidectomy is also performed. Portals are then closed with Monocryl. Early motion is initiated postoperatively [13].

Complications of arthroscopic PRC include damage to the articular surfaces of the capitate or lunate fossa on the radius during instrumentation, disruption of the volar extrinsic ligaments, and nerve damage to the dorsal and ulnar sensory branches [38, 42].

Weiss et al. reported 2-year outcomes of 16 patients following arthroscopic PRC. The investigators reported favorable results including improved wrist range of motion and improved grip strength. Patients achieved 80% of the grip strength and 80% of wrist range of motion compared to their contralateral side at final follow-up. Eighty-one percent of patients returned to the previous employment. While long-term data at 15 years post-PRC in one study suggest poor patient satisfaction with progression of degenerative changes, and persistent pain follow PRC [43], we have not had the same experience. The senior surgeon, KDP, has found great success to return athletes to the field for golf and tennis at 25 years. We agree caution should be used for this procedure especially in high demand, manual labor populations (e.g., firefighters), and in persons younger than 35 years of age [44].

Pearls and Pitfalls

Pearls

- When using the traction device, ensure at least 15 lbs of traction to aid in visualization in an already compromised joint space.
- Remove all loose bodies in the radial carpal and midcarpal joints.
- When performing microfracture or chondroplasty, use commercially available picks, and separate holes to avoid defects. Remove the calcified layer with a curette.
- Versatile use of the many portal options can facilitate visualization of the complete wrist.

Pitfalls

- Place the arthroscope with a blunt trocar to avoid penetration of the articular cartilage.
- Avoid ligament injury by understanding the wrist anatomy.

- Avoid debridement and resection of the radial styloid below the level of the radial scaphocapitate ligament; failure to do so can lead to instability of the wrist.
- Avoid damage to the chondral surfaces on the head of the capitate or in the lunate fossa on the radius during arthroscopic PRC.

References

1. Ekman EF, Pochling GG. Principles of arthroscopy and wrist arthroscopy equipment. Hand Clin. 1994;10:557–66.
2. Gupta R, Bozentka DJ, Osterman AL. Wrist arthroscopy: principles and clinical applications. J Am Acad Orthop Surg. 2001;9:200–9.
3. Wolf JM, Dukas A, Pensak M. Advances in wrist arthroscopy. J Am Acad Orthop Surg. 2012;20:725–34.
4. Adolfsson L. Arthroscopic synovectomy in wrist arthritis. Hand Clin. 2005;21:527–30.
5. Chung CY, Yen CH, Yip ML, Koo SC, Lao WN. Arthroscopic synovectomy for rheumatoid wrists and elbows. J Orthop Surg (Hong Kong). 2012;20:219–23.
6. Adolfsson L. Arthroscopic synovectomy of the wrist. Hand Clin. 2011;27:395–9.
7. Feldkamp G. Possibilities of wrist arthroscopy. Even for patients with arthritis? Z Rheumatol. 2008;67:478–84.
8. Altman RD, Kates J, Chun LE, et al. Preliminary observations of chondral abrasion in a canine model. Ann Rheum Dis. 1992;51:1056–62.
9. Kuo AC, Rodrigo JJ, Reddi AH, Curtiss S, Grotkopp E, Chiu M. Microfracture and bone morphogenetic protein 7 (BMP-7) synergistically stimulate articular cartilage repair. Osteoarthr Cartil. 2006;14:1126–35.
10. Steadman JR, Biggs KK, Rodrigo JJ, et al. Outcomes of microfractures for traumatic chondral defects of the knee: average 11-year follow-up. Arthroscopy. 2003;19:477–84.
11. Harley BJ, Werner FW, Boles SD, Palmer AK. Arthroscopic resection of arthrosis of the proximal hamate: a clinical and biomechanical study. J Hand Surg Am. 2004;29:661–7.
12. Steadman JR, Rodkey WG, Rodrigo JJ. Microfracture: surgical technique and rehabilitation to treat chondral defects. Clin Orthop Relat Res. 2001;391(Suppl):S362–9.
13. Weiss ND, Molina RA, Gwin S. Arthroscopic proximal row carpectomy. J Hand Surg Am. 2011;36:577–82.
14. Seradge H, Owens W, Seradge E. The effect of intercarpal joint motion on wrist motion: are there key joints? An in vitro study. Orthopedics. 1995;18(8):727–32.
15. Kaufmann R, Pfaeffle J, Blankenhorn B, Stabile K, Robertson D, Goitz R. Kinematics of the midcarpal and radiocarpal joints in radioulnar deviation: an in vitro study. J Hand Surg Am. 2005;30(5):937–42.
16. Watson HK, Ballet FL. The SLAC wrist: scapholunate advanced collapse pattern of degenerative arthritis. J Hand Surg Am. 1984;9(3):358–65.
17. Wilczynski MC, Gelberman RH, Adams A, Goldfarb CA. Arthroscopic findings in gout of the wrist. J Hand Surg Am. 2009;34:244–50.
18. Sankowski AJ, Lebkowska UM, Cwikla J, Walecka I, Walecki J. The comparison of efficacy of different imaging techniques (conventional radiology, ultrasonography, magnetic resonance) in assessment of wrist joints and metacarpophalangeal joints in patients with psoriatic arthritis. Pol J Radiol. 2013;78:18–29.

19. Feydy A, Pluot E, Guerini H, Drape JL. Role of imaging in spine, hand, and wrist osteoarthritis. Rheum Dis Clin N Am. 2009;35:605–49.

20. Haims AH, Moore AE, Schweizer ME, et al. MRI in the diagnosis of cartilage injury in the wrist. AJR Am J Roentgenol. 2001;182:1267–70.

21. Mutimer J, Geen J, Field J. Comparison of MRI and wrist arthroscopy for assessment of wrist cartilage. J Hand Surg Eur Vol. 2008;33:380–2.

22. Ejbjerg B, Narvestad E, Rostrup E, Szkudlarek M, Jacobsen S, Thomsen HS, Ostergaard M. Magnetic resonance imaging of wrist and finger joints in healthy subjects occasionally shows changes resembling erosions and synovitis as seen in rheumatoid arthritis. Arthritis Rheum. 2004;50:1097–106.

23. Kosta PE, Voulgari PV, Zikou AK, Drosos AA. Argyropoulou MI. Arthritis Res Ther. 2011;9:R84.

24. Amrami KK, Askan KS, Pagnano MW, Sundaram M. Radiologic case study. Abrasion chondroplasty mimicking avascular necrosis. Orthopedics. 2002;25(1018):1107–8.

25. Adolfsson L, Nylander G. Arthroscopic synovectomy of the rheumatoid wrist. J Hand Surg Br. 1993;18:92–6.

26. Adolfsson L, Frisen M. Arthroscopic synovectomy of the rheumatoid wrist. A 3.8 year follow-up. J Hand Surg Br. 1997;22:711–3.

27. Park MJ, Ahn JH, Kang JS. Arthroscopic synovectomy of the wrist in rheumatoid arthritis. J Bone Joint Surg Br. 2003;85:1011–5.

28. Larsen A, Dale K, Eek M. Radiographic evaluation of rheumatoid arthritis and related conditions by standard reference films. Acta Radiol Diagn (Stockholm). 1977;18:481–91.

29. Carl HD, Swoboda B. Effectiveness of arthroscopic synovectomy in rheumatoid arthritis. Z Rheumatol. 2008;67:485–90.

30. Outerbridge R. The etiology of chondromalacia patellae. J Bone Joint Surg Br. 1961;43:752–7.

31. Yao J, Osterman AL. Arthroscopic techniques for wrist arthritis (radial styloidectomy and proximal pole hamate excisions). Hand Clin. 2005;21:519–26.

32. Nakamura K, Patterson RM, Moritomo H, Viegas SF. Type I versus type II lunates: ligament anatomy and presence of arthrosis. J Hand Surg Am. 2001;26:428–36.

33. Nakamura K, Beppu M, Patterson RM, et al. Motion analysis in two dimensions of radial-ulnar deviation of type I versus type II lunates. J Hand Surg Am. 2000;25:877–88.

34. Malik AM, Schweitzer ME, Culp RW, et al. MR imaging of the type II lunate bone: frequency, extent, and associated findings. AJR Am J Roentgenol. 1999;173:335–8.

35. Dautel G, Merle M. Chondral lesions of the midcarpal joint. Arthroscopy. 1997;13:97–102.

36. Viegas SF, Wagner K, Partterson R, Peterson P. Medial (hamate) facet of the lunate. J Hand Surg Am. 1990;15:564–71.

37. Viegas SF. The lunatohamate articulation of the midcarpal joint. Arthroscopy. 1990;6:5–10.

38. Atik TL, Baratz ME. The role of arthroscopy in wrist arthritis. Hand Clin. 1999;15:489–94.

39. Kim SJ, Jung KA, Kim JM, Kwun JD, Kang HJ. Arthroscopic synovectomy in wrists with advanced rheumatoid arthritis. Clin Orthop Relat Res. 2006;449:262–6.

40. Kim SM, Park MJ, Kang HJ, Choi YL, Lee JJ. The role of arthroscopic synovectomy in patients with undifferentiated chronic monoarthritis of the wrist. J Bone Joint Surg Br. 2012;94(3):353–8.

41. Ruch DS, Chang DS, Poehling GG. The arthroscopic treatment of avascular necrosis of the proximal pole following scaphoid nonunion. Arthroscopy. 1998;14(7):747–52.

42. Wall LB, Stern PJ. Proximal row carpectomy. Hand Clin. 2013;29:69–78.

43. Ali MH, Rizzo M, Shin AY, Moran SL. Long-term outcomes of proximal row carpectomy: a minimum of 15-year follow-up. Hand (N Y). 2012;7(1):72–8.

44. Diao E, Andrews A, Beall M. Proximal row carpectomy. Hand Clin. 2005;21(4):553–9.

Arthroscopic Proximal Row Carpectomy

29

Noah D. Weiss and Aaron H. Stern

Abbreviations

APRC	Arthroscopic proximal row carpectomy
CRPS	Chronic regional pain syndrome
MCR	Midcarpal radial portal
MCU	Midcarpal ulnar portal
PRC	Proximal row carpectomy
SLAC	Scapholunate advanced collapse
SNAC	Scaphoid nonunion
STT	Scaphotrapezial trapezoid portal

Historical Perspective

Proximal row carpectomy is a well-recognized treatment option to treat a variety of degenerative and posttraumatic conditions of the wrist, including progressive carpal collapse, scaphoid nonunion, Kienbock's avascular necrosis of the lunate, and posttraumatic radioscaphoid arthritis [1].

Proximal row carpectomy (PRC) involves the excision of the entire proximal row of the carpus (the scaphoid, lunate, and triquetrum), so that the majority of radiocarpal motions take place between the head of the capitate and the lunate fossa of the distal radius [2]. The removal of the proximal carpal row clearly alters the normal kinematics of the wrist, simplifying the radiocarpal articulation into a "sloppy hinge" joint [3, 4]. This change in wrist kinematics necessitates a loss of range of motion, shortening of the height of the carpus, and an incongruent radiocapitate joint. This procedure, along with the four-corner fusion, has long been considered a "salvage" procedure because of the concern for permanent loss of motion, consistent loss of grip strength, possible progression of degenerative arthritis, and unreliable outcomes [5].

N. D. Weiss (✉) · A. H. Stern
Weiss Orthopaedics, Sonoma, CA, USA
e-mail: nweiss@weissortho.com

Recent outcome studies [6–8], however, have consistently shown that the PRC is a reliable procedure with high patient satisfaction, good pain relief, reasonable long-term outcomes, and a relatively low rate of complications. Multiple studies have consistently produced results demonstrating retention of approximately 75% of grip strength and range of motion [7, 8]. The incidence of late arthritis appears to be low [8]. PRC permits some degree of both radial-ulnar deviation and dorsal-ulnar translation, which may help dissipate the load across the radiocapitate joint, decreasing the expected wear of this new incongruous joint, and improving the long-term durability of the procedure.

While long-term results between the PRC and four-corner fusion are very similar [9], the PRC typically does not require long-term immobilization, and there are fewer complications than the four-corner fusion, with no need for subsequent hardware removal, and zero risk of nonunion.

Until recently, the PRC has been described only as an open procedure performed through a dorsal wrist arthrotomy, dividing (and repairing) the wrist capsule and dorsal ligaments [10]. Patients are typically immobilized for several weeks postoperatively to allow for soft tissue healing. Recently, an all-arthroscopic proximal row carpectomy (APRC) has been described [11] with results equal to, or exceeding, those results from previously published studies on the open technique. With an arthroscopic PRC, an open capsulotomy is avoided and dorsal capsular ligaments are spared, potentially allowing for increased postoperative stability of the wrist. Less soft tissue disruption also allows for earlier postoperative motion, less postoperative pain and scarring, and potentially increased motion.

Indications and Contraindications

The indications for the arthroscopic proximal row carpectomy are the same as those for the open technique. These include patients with disabling wrist pain, not relieved by other conservative measures. Common diagnoses treated with the PRC include carpal instability, scapholunate advanced collapse (SLAC), scaphoid nonunion (SNAC), Kienbock's disease, and radioscaphoid arthritis. Good-quality cartilage on both the head of the capitate and on the lunate fossa of the distal radius is essential, as this will be the new radiocarpal articulation.

Contraindications include arthrosis on either the head of the capitate or lunate fossa, preexisting ulnar translocation of the carpus, and possibly rheumatoid arthritis [12, 13]. We have successfully performed this operation on patients with Ehlers-Danlos syndrome, and hypermobility or ligamentous laxity does not appear to be a contraindication.

Surgical Technique

The patient is placed in a supine position. The involved wrist is secured to a standard wrist arthroscopy tower, with 5 kg of longitudinal traction applied throughout the procedure. Good access to the dorsum of the wrist is essential, and adequate radiographic visualization of the wrist with the fluoroscopy arm in the horizontal position should be confirmed prior to draping of the patient. A well-padded tourniquet is always applied preoperatively as a precaution, although the tourniquet is inflated at the discretion of the surgeon. Standard small-joint arthroscopy instruments (arthroscope, shaver, and probe) are used. In addition, the large-joint shaver with a 4.0 m bur and fine synovial rongeurs should be available.

Routine radiocarpal portals (3/4, 4/5, 6R, and 6U) and midcarpal portals (MCR, MCU, and STT) are established. Standard radiocarpal and midcarpal arthroscopy is per-

formed, and additional procedures (debridement, synovectomy, etc.) are performed as necessary. Adequate articular cartilage of the lunate fossa of the distal radius and of the head of the capitate should be confirmed, as significant arthritic changes would be a contraindication to continuing with APRC.

After diagnostic and operative radiocarpal arthroscopy, the APRC is then performed exclusively through the midcarpal portals, including the scaphotrapezial trapezoid (STT) portal. With the arthroscope placed ulnarly in the midcarpal ulnar(MCU) portal, the small-joint arthroscopic shaver or bur is introduced into the midcarpal joint through the midcarpal radial(MCR) portal. At all times, great care should be taken to avoid any articular injury to the head of the capitate, which is at risk throughout the procedure. The hood of the bur and shaver should always be directed at the head of the capitate to avoid articular cartilage injury. The small shaver or bur is then used to remove the ulnar distal corner of the scaphoid at the scapholunate joint (Fig. 29.1). Once an adequate portion of the distal ulnar scaphoid is removed, the MCR portal is slightly enlarged, and the large shaver with a 4.0 hooded bur is introduced into the MCR portal. The use of the larger bur facilitates more rapid removal of bone.

With the arthroscope in the ulnar viewing (MCU) portal, the scaphoid is excised with the bur, moving from ulnar to radial, and distal to proximal. The bur is then typically placed more radially in the STT portal to remove the distal pole of the scaphoid. Under direct arthroscopic visualization, a fine synovial rongeur is useful to remove small fragments of bone or cartilage that remain adherent to capsule (Fig. 29.2). Complete excision of the distal pole of the scaphoid is left to the discretion of the surgeon (Fig. 29.3).

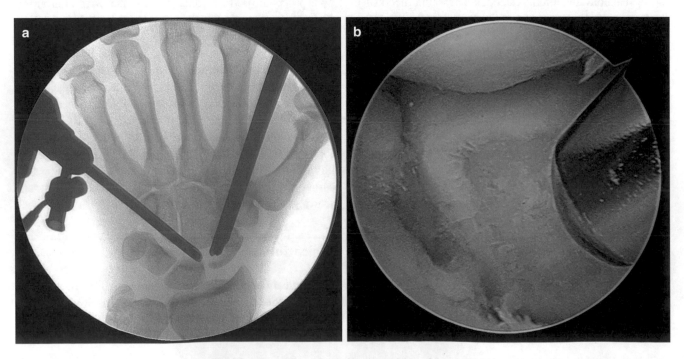

Fig. 29.1 Fluoroscopic (**a**) and arthroscopic (**b**) imaging of the wrist during the excision of the scaphoid

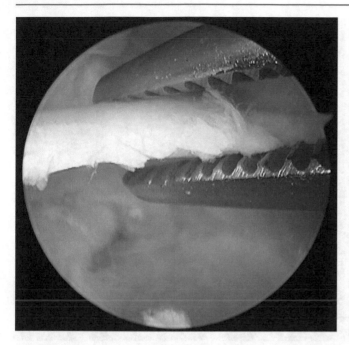

Fig. 29.2 Arthroscopic imaging of bone fragment excision using a fine synovial rongeur

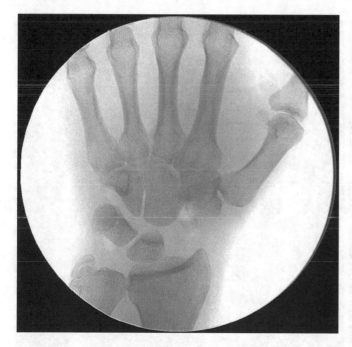

Fig. 29.3 A fluoroscopic image of the wrist following the scaphoid excision

Following scaphoid excision, the arthroscope is then placed in the STT portal. With the arthroscope placed radially, and viewing ulnarly, the bur is placed in an enlarged MCR portal. The lunate is then excised with the bur, now working radial to ulnar, and distal to proximal (Fig. 29.4). Great care should be taken when removing the proximal

layer of articular cartilage of the lunate, but traction usually creates a safe space above the distal radius. Again, the use of fine synovial rongeurs facilitates removal of small fragments of bone and cartilage that remain adherent to the capsule. Following removal of the lunate, the arthroscope is moved to the MCR portal, the bur is placed in the MCU portal, and the triquetrum is excised. Confirmation of a complete APRC is made with fluoroscopy (Fig. 29.5).

The limb is then taken out of traction, and the radiocapitate joint is reduced. Seating of the head of the capitate in the lunate fossa of the radius is confirmed both arthroscopically and with fluoroscopy (Fig. 29.6). Range of motion of the wrist under fluoroscopy will confirm stability, and also reveal occasional radial styloid impingement, which can be treated with arthroscopic radial styloidectomy (performed with the bur in the 1/2 portal).

Postoperatively, the wrist is injected with bupivacaine, and a bulky dressing and volar splint are applied, allowing for immediate finger range of motion. The patient is seen in the office 2 days postoperatively, when the bandage is removed, and a removable volar splint is applied for comfort. Early active and passive range of motion of the wrist is encouraged, and return to activity is within the limits of patient comfort. Formal hand therapy is prescribed on an individual basis as needed.

Complications

There are several potential complications that exist when performing the arthroscopic proximal row carpectomy. As with any wrist arthroscopy, sensory nerve injury during portal placement is a concern, and the portals must be developed by careful skin incision, blunt dissection down to the capsule, and careful introduction of a blunt trochar into the joint. When expanding the midcarpal portals to allow the introduction of the large joint bur, the portals must similarly be enlarged using careful technique. With the APRC, it is essential to avoid injury to either the head of the capitate or the lunate fossa of the distal radius, and the hood of the bur should be directed toward those surfaces at all times. Careful fluoroscopic evaluation of the wrist is important at the end of the procedure to confirm a complete proximal row carpectomy. While it may be desirable to leave the distal pole of the scaphoid, occasionally fragments of bone remain adherent to the dorsal capsule, and may not be seen arthroscopically.

Results

Review of our first 35 patients, with an average of 33-month (minimum of 1 year) follow-up, was recently performed. There were no surgical complications, and no patient

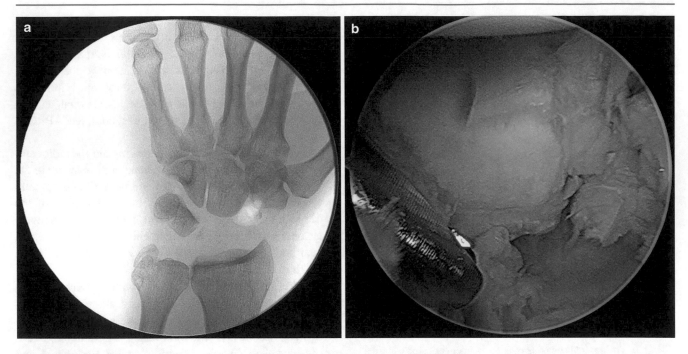

Fig. 29.4 Fluoroscopic (**a**) and arthroscopic (**b**) imaging of the wrist following removal of the lunate

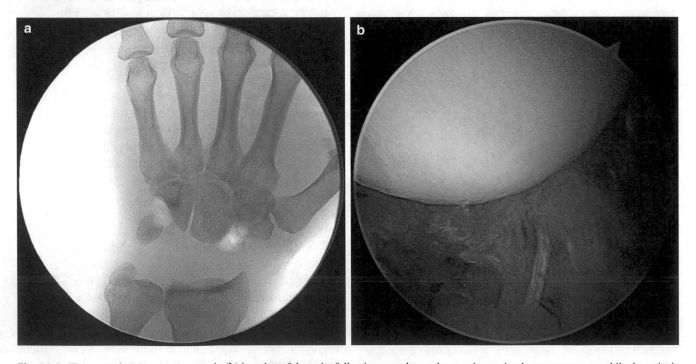

Fig. 29.5 Fluoroscopic (**a**) and arthroscopic (**b**) imaging of the wrist following complete arthroscopic proximal row carpectomy while the wrist is in traction

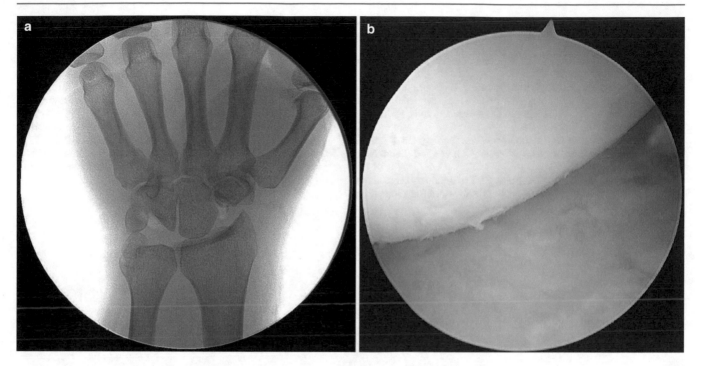

Fig. 29.6 Fluoroscopic (**a**) and arthroscopic (**b**) imaging of the newly formed wrist joint after the wrist is released from traction

required conversion to an open procedure. There were no instances of radiocarpal subluxation, despite immediate mobilization. One patient did subsequently progress to radiocarpal arthritis, and one patient developed chronic regional pain syndrome (CRPS) type 2. The average length of surgery was 61 min. Patients retained an average of 78% of the flexion/extension arc of the wrist, and 70% of radial and ulnar deviation. Grip strength averaged 83% of the contralateral wrist, and patient satisfaction was high (94% satisfied or very satisfied).

Advantages

The APRC has been shown to have several potential advantages over the open procedure with few disadvantages, and provides results that are similar to the open procedure, with maintenance of reasonable range of motion and strength and high patient satisfaction. By preserving the dorsal capsular ligaments, there is potentially improved postoperative motion. As in other joints, the advantages of arthroscopic surgery over an open arthrotomy include less postoperative pain, decreased scarring, less soft tissue damage, no unsightly scars, and often earlier range of motion leading to a quicker recovery. Additionally, this arthroscopic procedure allows for optimum evaluation of the wrist joint, and the identification and treatment of other pathologies.

Conclusion

Arthroscopic proximal row carpectomy is a reproducible and effective new arthroscopic procedure that compares favorably to the established open technique. The APRC can be accomplished in a reasonable amount of surgical time, with routine small-joint and large-joint arthroscopic instrumentation. Arthroscopic proximal row carpectomy patients have similar long-term objective strength and possibly improved range of motion as well as high subjective satisfaction when compared to open proximal row carpectomy patients. It is a technically complex procedure, but one that can be performed relatively quickly and successfully using standard arthroscopic techniques and equipment. Patients may be mobilized immediately, and the APRC provides many of the benefits typically associated with arthroscopic surgery such as less scarring and less trauma to the area without any identifiable drawbacks.

References

1. Richou J, Chuinard C, Moineau G, Hanouz N, Hu W, Le Nen D. Proximal row carpectomy: long-term results. Chir Main. 2010;29:10–5.
2. Stamm TT. Excision of the proximal row of the carpus. Proc R Soc Med. 1944;38:74–5.
3. Sobczak S, Rotsaert R, Vancabeke M, Jan SV, Salvia P, Feipel V. Effects of proximal row carpectomy on wrist biomechanics: a cadaveric study. Clin Biomech (Bristol, Avon). 2011;26:718–24.

4. Blankenhorn BD, Pfaeffle HJ, Tang P, Robertson D, Imbriglia J, Goitz RJ. Carpal kinematics after proximal row carpectomy. J Hand Surg. 2007;32A:37–46.

5. Neviaser RJ. On resection of the proximal carpal row. Clin Orthop Relat Res. 1986;202:12–5.

6. Vanhove W, De Vil J, Van Seymortier P, Boone B, Verdonk R. Proximal row carpectomy versus four-corner arthrodesis as a treatment for SLAC (scapholunate advanced collapse) wrist. J Hand Surg. 2008;33B:118–25.

7. Croog AS, Stern PJ. Proximal row carpectomy for advanced Kienbock's disease: average 10-year follow-up. J Hand Surg. 2008;33A:1122–30.

8. DiDonna ML, Kiefhaber TR, Stern PJ. Proximal row carpectomy: study with a minimum of ten years of follow-up. J Bone Joint Surg. 2004;86A:2359–65.

9. Bisneto ENF, Freitas MC, de Paula EJL, Mattar R, Zumiotti AV. Comparison between proximal row carpectomy and four-corner fusion for treating osteoarthrosis following carpal trauma: a prospective randomized study. Clinics. 2011;66:51–5.

10. Wall LB, Stern PJ. Proximal row carpectomy. Hand Clin. 2013;29:69–78.

11. Weiss ND, Molina RA, Gwin S. Arthroscopic proximal row carpectomy. J Hand Surg. 2011;36A:577–82.

12. Culp RW, McGuigan FX, Turner MA, et al. Proximal row carpectomy: a multicenter study. J Hand Surg. 1993;18A:19–25.

13. Ferlic DC, Clayton ML, Mills MF. Proximal row carpectomy: review of rheumatoid and non-rheumatoid wrists. J Hand Surg Am. 1991;16A:420–4.

Arthroscopic Partial Wrist Fusion

30

Pak-cheong Ho

Introduction

Partial wrist fusion or limited carpal fusion is considered as a motion-preserving salvage procedure for multiple painful wrist conditions. It is a good alternative, particularly for those patients who would prefer a mobile functional wrist rather than a solid total wrist fusion [1]. The wrist consists of multiple bony linkages from the forearm to the metacarpus via the carpal bones, and this anatomical peculiarity offers an opportunity to allow fusion of the painful segments of the wrist while preserving motion in the other unaffected segments. It also helps to halt any predictable mechanical collapse of the carpal column and maintain carpal height in the carpal instability conditions due to failure of the ligament constraint or loss of the bony integrity such as in scaphoid nonunion and Kienbock's disease.

A wide variety of partial wrist fusion has been designed in the past to address problems arising from various parts of the wrist [2–5]. Essentially all carpal bones and intervals can be fused selectively, and the resulting motion loss and the biomechanical effect have been studied extensively in laboratory and in the clinical settings [6–11]. The fusion can take place between the radius and the proximal carpal row such as radiolunate fusion and radioscapholunate fusion; between the two carpal rows such as the scaphotrapeziotrapezoid fusion, scaphocapitate fusion, capitolunate fusion, triquetrohamate fusion, and the four corner fusion involving the medial carpal bones; and within the proximal carpal row such as scapholunate fusion and lunotriquetral fusion. The operations being described in the literature and commonly in use are open surgery requiring much soft tissue dissection including capsular and ligament incisions around the wrist to expose the carpal intervals. This may lead to iatrogenic stiffness of the joint on top of the mechanical constraint rendered by the selected carpal fusion. The expected loss of motion can be predicted theoretically from the biomechanical models, though in practice, the final range of motion retained clinically will also rely on the degree of soft tissue contracture and the amount of compensatory hypermobility of the adjacent mobile segments. Thus, it is desirable to minimize surgical insult to soft tissue so as to maximize the motion preservation which is always the interest of both the patients and the surgeons.

Arthroscopic intervention in partial wrist fusion has potential advantages of a minimal surgical damage to the supporting ligaments and the capsular structures of the wrist while allowing an unimpeded view to most articular surfaces of the joints and the important soft tissue elements. This ensures a more accurate staging of the arthritis and facilitates clinical decision making on the most appropriate choice of fusion. The remaining carpal motion can be maximized and postoperative pain reduced, which favors rehabilitation. There is also cosmetic benefit with the minimal surgical scar.

This chapter describes our pioneer experience in the past 15 years in developing this surgical concept and technique for various clinical conditions.

Indications and Contraindications

The main indication for a partial wrist fusion is the painful arthritic conditions of the wrist which affect part of the articulating system and the patient would like to have adequate pain control as well as preservation of a useful functional arc of motion. This is best indicated in posttraumatic arthritis and osteoarthritis. Common indications include scapholunate advanced collapse (SLAC), scaphoid nonunion advanced collapse (SNAC), Kienbock's disease, post-distal radius fracture radiocarpal joint arthrosis, and scaphotrapeziotrapezoid (STT) arthritis. Chronic painful carpal instabilities with or without secondary arthritic change are also good indications. These include chronic

P.-c. Ho (✉)
Department of Orthopaedics and Traumatology, Prince of Wales Hospital, Hong Kong, China
e-mail: pcho@cuhk.edu.hk

© Springer Nature Switzerland AG 2022
W. B. Geissler (ed.), *Wrist and Elbow Arthroscopy with Selected Open Procedures*,
https://doi.org/10.1007/978-3-030-78881-0_30

lunotriquetral instability, capitolunate instability, palmar midcarpal instability, and radiocarpal translocation. In inflammatory arthritis such as rheumatoid arthritis and crystal deposition disease, the disease progression should be optimally controlled by the pharmacological mean and should not be at an active proliferative phase. This can avoid a rapid deterioration of the clinical improvement due to a progressive involvement of the unfused segments of the wrist. Patients with multiple joint involvement of the same upper limb may have stronger desire to preserve motion over the wrist to compensate for the stiffness over the other joints. Arthroscopic version of partial wrist fusion is a particular good option for patient conscious of a surgical scar and would like to have less postoperative pain and a potential faster rehabilitation.

Partial wrist fusion is contraindicated when there is an active ongoing sepsis over the wrist joint, panarthritis involving all or most compartments of the wrist, and rapidly progressive inflammatory arthritis at a proliferative stage. Partial wrist fusion is also not a guarantee for pain relief. The potential advantage of partial wrist fusion in preserving a useful arc of motion may be offset by the risks of nonunion or by a continuing pain despite a successful fusion [12]. Nagy and Büchler reviewed a cohort of 15 cases of radioscapholunate fusion and reported a nonunion rate of 27% [13]. Nearly half of them showed secondary degenerative changes of the midcarpal joint, two of which were progressive. Four patients had continuing symptoms despite a sound radiological union of the partial wrist fusion. Revision of total wrist fusion was required in 33% of cases ultimately. Thus, those patients who prefer a more guaranteed outcome on the pain control, do not want multiple surgical procedures, and do not bother a loss of wrist motion may be better candidates for a total wrist fusion. Chronic smoker has higher incidence of nonunion after partial wrist fusion and required more revision surgery to achieve a union. Alternative for pain control treatment such as a wrist denervation can be considered. Total wrist arthroplasty can be considered in the older patients with limited functional demand. Accompanying distal radioulnar joint pathology would not be altered by the partial wrist fusion and needs to be tackled separately or concomitantly. Arthroscopic partial wrist fusions are technically demanding procedures and should not be lightly taken by surgeons without much experience in therapeutic arthroscopy of the wrist. Patients with preexisting extensor tendon pathology over the wrist region may have higher incidence of tendon complications associated with complex arthroscopic wrist reconstruction procedures. Severe arthrofibrosis, joint contracture, and long-standing carpal collapse or wrist deformity may also pose additional difficulty and risk for the surgeons in using the arthroscopic approach.

Technique

The general principles in all forms of arthroscopic partial wrist fusion should include the following steps:

1. Set up and instrumentation
2. Arthroscopic surveillance for final staging of the disease
3. Cartilage denudation
4. Correction of carpal malalignment
5. Provisional fixation of the fusion intervals
6. Augmentation of the fusion segment(s) with bone graft or bone substitute in selected indications
7. Definitive fixation

General Approach

Set Up and Instrumentation

The operation is typically performed under general anesthesia for convenience and patient comfort in harvesting the bone graft if it deems necessary. It can be done under regional anesthesia if bone substitute is employed, or when no bone graft or substitute augmentation is needed. Either injectable or small granule form of the bone substitute is suitable for the purpose. There is a tendency of not using any bone graft or bone substitute augmentation if a rigid fixation device such as cannulated compression screws can be applied to the fusion site, and the fusion surfaces are congruent enough without excessive dead space. C-arm fluoroscopy should be available in all cases for intraoperative assessment. The list of essential instruments includes a motorized full-radius shaver and burr system of diameters ranging from 2.0 to 3.5 mm, small angled curette and ring curette, 2.5 mm suction punch, radiofrequency thermal ablation system, K-wires, and small cannulated screw system.

The patient is put in supine position while the operated arm is supported on a hand table. Either side of the iliac crest region is draped for bone graft harvesting depending on the patient's preference. An arm tourniquet is applied, but need not be inflated routinely. A tight application of the tourniquet without inflation leads to venous engorgement and can induce more troublesome bleeding. Most of the procedures can be done without the use of a tourniquet. Piñal advocates the use of dry arthroscopy to avoid the problem of swelling and the extravasation of fluid, but the use of tourniquet becomes mandatory throughout the procedure which may take extended time [14]. A vertical traction of 4–6 kgf is applied through plastic finger trap devices to the middle three fingers for joint distraction via a wrist traction tower. We employ continuous saline irrigation and distension of the joint by using a 3-liter bag of normal saline solution suspended at 1–1.5 m above the operating table and instill with the aid of gravity to maintain a clear arthroscopic view. Infusion pump is not necessarily and is potentially harmful in causing an extravasation of fluid. In wrist arthroscopy, it is mainly the distraction device that keeps the joint opened, not the fluid irrigation like in the shoulder joint.

Arthroscopic Surveillance

We perform routine inspection of both radiocarpal joint through 3/4 portal and midcarpal joint through MCR portal using a 2.7- or 1.9-mm video arthroscope. The aim of the examination is to establish a precise arthroscopic staging of the pathology. Adrenaline solution of 1 in 200,000 dilution is injected to the portal site skin and capsule to reduce bleeding associated with incision [15] (Fig. 30.1). Intra-articular injection is optional and may reduce bleeding associated with the arthroscopic procedures. The outflow is established at 6U portal just volar to the ECU tendon using an 18G needle. In general, all portals should be marked after careful palpation with surgeon's thumb tip and the wrist being distracted on the traction device before saline was injected intra-articularly.

Once the arthroscope is being inserted, particular attention is paid to assess the status of the interosseous ligaments, the degree of synovitis, and the articular cartilage condition of the joints intended to be fused and the other uninvolved joint compartments of the wrist. The latter is essential to determine whether the proposed fusion is appropriate or not. The dorsal rim of the radial styloid is a common site of occurrence of the early SLAC or SNAC wrist arthritic changes and should be assessed in all cases by rotating the 30° forward slanting lens downward to reach the area. The frequently associated localized posttraumatic synovitis in

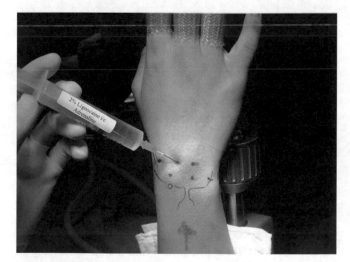

Fig. 30.1 Lignocaine 2% with adrenaline solution in 1:200,000 dilution is injected to portal sites for hemostasis effect

this area may obscure the observation of cartilage condition. The synovial growth needs to be eliminated by using a 2.0-mm shaver or a radiofrequency probe inserted from 4/5 portal. It may be necessary to swap the portal of the arthroscope and instrument in order to obtain a better attacking angle of the instrument for a more efficient synovectomy. The ulnocarpal joint should also be routinely inspected and the status of TFCC ascertained. Any central perforation of the TFCC without peripheral involvement should be debrided of any unstable flap tear at the same operation to avoid possible new source of pain after the definitive index procedure.

The midcarpal joint is approached through the MCR portal. Routinely the STT joint, scaphocapitate joint, capitolunate joint, and triquetrohamate joint are inspected for cartilage lesion and synovitis. The scapholunate and lunotriquetral joints are assessed for stability with a 2-mm probe introduced from the MCU portal. Any instability is graded according to the Geissler classification. Synovial overgrowth should be debrided by using a shaver or radiofrequency probe to adequately expose the underlying cartilage area for assessment of the true extent of chondral damage and subchondral bone exposure. In posttraumatic arthritis, difficulty may be encountered when developing the radial portal at the midcarpal joint due to the intra-articular adhesion and periarticular soft tissue contracture. Under this circumstance, one should not hesitate to shift to the midcarpal ulnar portal where joint space is usually more generous. Once the joint is entered, the other portal can be developed more easily by applying an 18G needle through the skin under direct vision. This greatly helps the localization of any difficult portal. A prerequisite for a successful radiocarpal fusion is a relatively intact articular surface at the midcarpal and STT joints. If significant arthritic change is present, one may need to abandon the planned procedure and consider other salvage option such as total wrist fusion. Two accessory portals may also be recruited during any midcarpal procedure. The triquetrohamate (TH) portal can be located by palpating the tendon of ECU and moving distally until the palpating finger reaches the hamate bone. The portal is then located at the axilla between the ECU tendon and the hamate. It is most useful as an outflow portal. The scaphotrapeziotrapezoid (STT) portal is situated about 1 cm radial and slightly distal to the MCR portal just ulnar to the EPL tendon slightly distal to the MCR portal. The portal is located at the junction between the scaphoid, trapezoid, and trapezium. Care should be taken in avoiding injury to the radial artery which is radial to the EPL tendon.

Cartilage Denudation

The articular surfaces of the joint compartments to be fused are then prepared. The extent and depth of cartilage denudation should be precisely controlled using a 2.9-mm arthroscopic burr. In debriding the carpal interval of the same carpal row, such as lunotriquetral or capitohamate interval, a smaller burr such as 2 mm sized should be used to cater for the narrower joint space to avoid excessive cartilage and subchondral bone removal. Either forward or reverse blade rotation mode should be adopted at a speed of 2000–3000 rpm. Oscillating mode is not as effective as compared to the unidirectional mode. One should be cautious about the jumping phenomenon when using a burr to attack a particularly sclerotic bone surface. The burr may get caught in the area of hard subchondral bone during the high-speed revolution. The resultant force will bounce the burr off the bone and may lead to accidental damage of the articular surface of the surrounding or opposing carpal bones. To have better control of the instrument, the surgeon is recommended to hold the arthroscopic burr near the far end with the surgeon's thumb and index finger, while using the middle finger to firmly anchor the burr over the skin around the portal site (Fig. 30.2). There should be maximal preservation of the subchondral bone so as to maintain carpal height. Burring is completed when the subchondral cancellous bone with healthy punctate

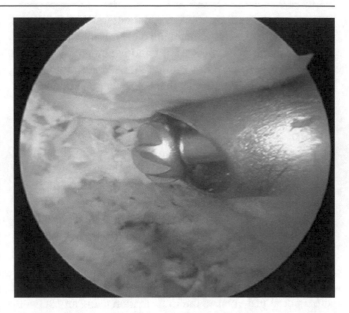

Fig. 30.3 Punctate bleeding can be readily seen from the subchondral bone during burring without the use of tourniquet

bleeding is reached. This phenomenon can be easily observed if a tourniquet is not used during this process (Fig. 30.3). Usually, bleeding is limited and can be well controlled with the hydrostatic pressure applied through the irrigation system. If bleeding is profuse, one may further elevate the suspension of the instilling saline bag to increase the hydrostatic pressure, or use the coagulation mode of the radiofrequency apparatus. During the burring process, suction is switched on and off intermittently to remove any accumulated bone debris which may block the visual field. If suction is applied continuously during the burring process, excessive air bubbles drawn in will severely compromise the visibility of the operating site.

Correct Carpal Deformity

DISI deformity is commonly present in many posttraumatic wrist arthritis conditions. It is prudent to correct the deformity as far as possible during the process of partial wrist fusion involving the capitate-lunate joint in order to maximize the motion and to reduce abnormal loading through the lunate fossa. A close reduction can be accomplished by correcting the radiolunate angle to zero degree using a K-wire to transfix the radiolunate joint with the wrist in moderate flexion and slight ulnar deviation (Fig. 30.4). A 1.1-mm K-wire is introduced percutaneously through a small stab wound over the distal radius slightly proximal to the sigmoid notch level, aiming at the level between the 3/4 and 4/5 portals. A fine tip hemostat or stitch scissor should be used to dissect bluntly the extensor tendons to avoid iatrogenic injury or tethering of the extensor tendons during the introduction of K-wire through the skin. The precise location of the insertion point and insertion angle should be guided by an image

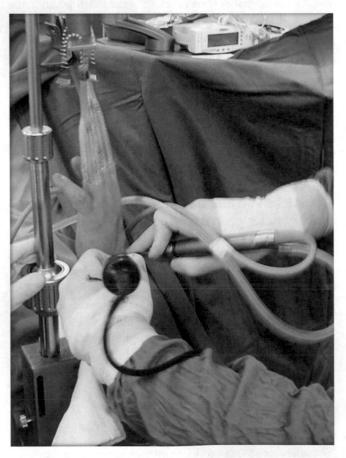

Fig. 30.2 To have better control of the instrument, the arthroscopic burr is being held near the far end with the surgeon's thumb and index finger, while the middle finger firmly anchors the burr over the skin around the portal site

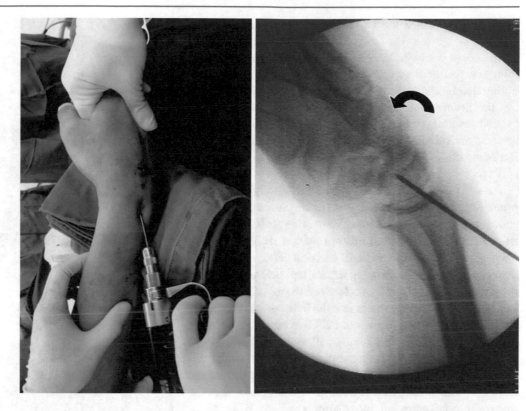

Fig. 30.4 DISI deformity of the lunate can be closely reduced by flexing the wrist and transfixing radiolunate interval at an anatomical alignment before reduction of other carpal bones in relation to lunate

intensifier both in the anteroposterior and lateral projection. The K-wire should not perforate through the distal cortex of lunate so as to leave a space at the capitate-lunate joint. Before the final fusion progress, the other carpal bones are realigned manually in relation to proper lunate position.

Provisional Fixation of the Carpal Fusion

The wrist is dislodged from the wrist traction tower and is placed horizontally over a hand table for the provisional fixation. The carpal interval(s) to be fused is temporarily fixed with 1.0 or 1.1 mm K-wire percutaneously using a powered driver in an anatomical position as far as possible. Alignment is confirmed with an intraoperative image intensifier. The K-wires can be used as definitive fixation device or they can be used as the guide pins for the subsequent conversion into percutaneous cannulated screw fixation. The pins are then withdrawn to free from the joint to be fused while they are maintained in position in the carpal bone or distal radius. Externally the pins should be protected with pin caps to avoid accidental injury to the surgeon's hand in the remaining process. The joint is then ready for grafting with autogenous cancellous bone or bone substitute.

Augmentation of the Fusion Segment(s) with Bone Graft or Bone Substitute

Autogenous bone graft or bone substitute is frequently required to fill up the voids between the articular surfaces to be fused. As the vascularity and the bone quality of the fusing bones are usually adequate, cancellous chip graft from

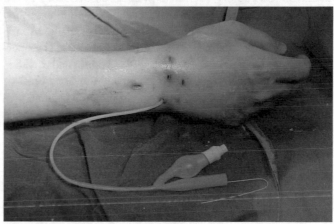

Fig. 30.5 Foley catheter blocking technique to avoid spillage of bone graft/substitutes to the uninvolved space

iliac crest may not be essential and there is an increasing role of using bone substitute to reduce the potential donor site morbidity with similar outcome. Both injectable form and small granule form are suitable for the purpose. In order to prevent spillage of the graft inside the joint to the undesirable compartments, special Foley catheter balloon blocking technique has been developed (Fig. 30.5). A French size 6 Foley catheter with a stylet on is introduced through the arthroscopic portal. The tip of the catheter is usually cut short to allow better placement of the balloon. Advancement of the catheter into the joint can be facilitated by grasping the tip of the catheter using a small arthroscopic grasper introduced from a third portal. Once the balloon portion of the catheter is completely inside the joint as monitored through the arthroscope, it can be inflated with saline solution until the joint compartment away from the fusion interval is largely obliterated by the balloon. The balloon remains inflated during the arthroscopic bone graft process so that redundant cancellous graft or bone substitute will not fall into and be trapped in other compartments not going to be fused. Reducing fluid inflow is also a useful trick to avoid graft spillage.

An arthroscopic cannula is introduced through the appropriate portal directly opposing the fusing surfaces. If autogenous graft is to be used, cancellous bone graft is harvested from the iliac crest using either trephine technique or an open approach through a small incision. The bone graft is then cut into small chips using scissor and delivered through the cannula with a slightly undersized trocar with a flat end such as the bone biopsy trocar into the joint cavity (Fig. 30.6). Trocar with roundish end is not effective enough. Too exact fitting of the trocar in the cannula will cause an easy trapping of bone graft substance between the trocar and cannula wall and may lead to delivery problem. So a slightly undersized trocar is more desirable. The bone graft is impacted with the trocar till satisfactory volume of graft is achieved (Fig. 30.7). This process requires two assistants to execute smoothly. One assistant helps to maintain the position of the arthroscope to provide optimal vision of the fusion site. The operating surgeon controls the arthroscopic cannula and trocar. A second assistant is responsible to deliver the bone graft or bone substitutes into the opening of the cannula in small volume every time. The operating surgeon then drives the bone

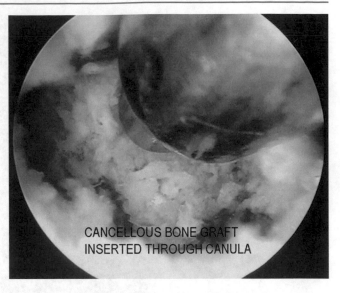

Fig. 30.7 Impaction of graft with blunt trocar at fusion site

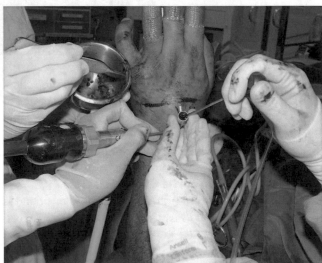

Fig. 30.8 With the help of two assistants, the operating surgeon controls the arthroscopic cannula and trocar and drives the bone graft or substitute into the fusion site under direct arthroscopic monitor

graft or substitute into the fusion site under direct arthroscopic monitor (Fig. 30.8). The speed of the process can be enhanced by using a cannula of wider bore such as 4.5 or 5 mm so that each time more graft can be accommodated. If injectable bone substitute is to be used, joint irrigation should be ceased and all joint fluid evacuated with suction. A wide bore needle connecting the syringe containing the bone substitute is inserted through appropriate portal to reach the fusion site. Injection of the bone substitute can then be performed under direct vision till the cavity is filled up completely. If necessary, intraoperative fluoroscopy can help to confirm the completeness of the filling process.

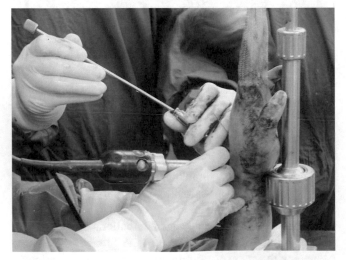

Fig. 30.6 Bone graft is delivered through a cannula with a slightly undersized trocar of flat end such as the bone biopsy trocar into the joint cavity

Definitive Fixation

The wrist is taken off from the traction tower again and placed in the hand table. Definitive fixation is performed by driving the K-wires across the bony interval to be fused and in a correct carpal alignment. If cannulated screw is preferred, the K-wires will then serve as the guide pins. After measuring the length of the screw required, the pin tract is drilled using a cannulated drill bit. Stable internal fixation can then be achieved with compression screw using appropriate percutaneous cannulated screw system, preferably a headless screw system to avoid screw head impingement. The final carpal alignment, screw position, and length should be assessed by using an image intensifier. In older patient with osteoporotic bone, multiple K-wires fixation is preferred over screw fixation to avoid hardware problem, such as the protrusion of screw tip into the joint (Fig. 30.9). Percutaneous K-wires should be cut short and buried underneath the skin. They are removed under local anesthesia when the bone healing is complete. Exposing pins outside skin may predispose to pin tract infection. The wrist is then immobilized with a plaster slab.

Specific Fusion Technique and Rehabilitation

STT Fusion

STT fusion is commonly indicated in stage I or II SLAC wrist, Kienbock's disease stage IIIa or IIIb, and STT joint arthritis [16–18]. It is frequently performed together with a radial styloidectomy, which can also be accomplished under an arthroscopic mean. The best indication for arthroscopic STT fusion is STT joint arthritis, with or without association with SLAC wrist. Under such circumstance, there is usually no scaphoid malalignment and hence no DISI deformity needed to be correct.

Radiocarpal joint arthroscopy should be routinely performed to look for arthritic changes over the radioscaphoid and radiolunate joints. Arthritic change in the former compartment may make the radial styloidectomy a necessary accompanying procedure, while change in the latter compartment may constitute a contraindication of the procedure.

Arthroscopic STT fusion is then performed at the midcarpal joint. The STT portal is often required to provide a direct access to the STT joint. The arthroscope is inserted in the MCR portal and directed toward the STT joint by climbing up the slanting articular surface of the scaphoid over the waist portion opposing the capitate till the scaphotrapezoid-capitate junction is reached. The latter is signified by an inverted Y-shaped joint interval, which I call it as "Mercedes Benz" sign (Fig. 30.10). In STT arthritis condition, the joint is frequently obliterated by synovial overgrowth and joint debris (Fig. 30.11). They need to be cleared up with a shaver and/or radiofrequency probe before the articular cartilage condition can be verified. The joint space may also be contracted with the periarticular soft tissue fibrosis. Joint entry

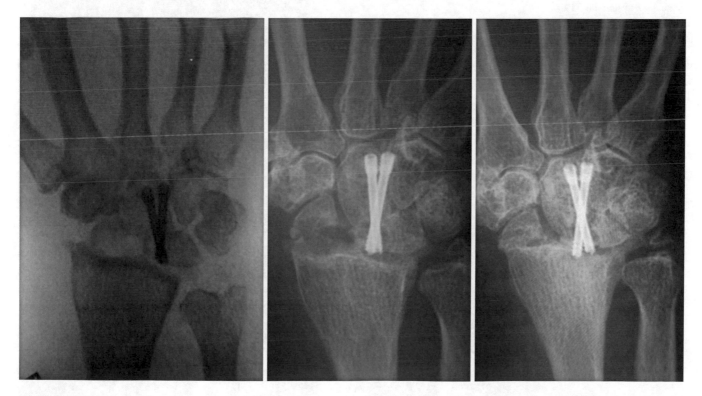

Fig. 30.9 Self-tapping headless screw may protrude into the joint gradually during healing process of the fusion site in old patient with osteopenic bone

can be facilitated by using a smaller arthroscope such as 1.9 mm. Sometimes the joint space in the whole radial compartment of the midcarpal joint may be compromised and one should not hesitate to start the joint exploration through

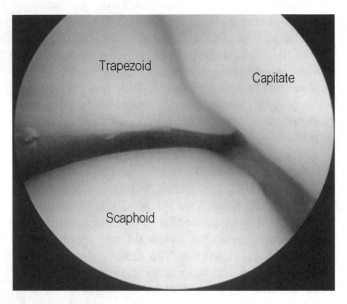

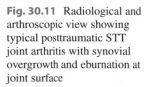

Fig. 30.10 Mercedes Benz sign at junction between capitate, trapezoid, and scaphoid

the ulnar midcarpal portal, which is always less affected under such circumstances. Nevertheless, joint space usually gets enlarged after a period of joint debridement procedure and manipulation to allow sufficient access for the subsequent grafting procedure with bigger instruments. The arthritic joint surface is then debrided of the remaining articular cartilage till subchondral bone is exposed. Initially the trapezium may be difficult to reach as it is situated in deeper space at the STT joint. As long as the cartilage surface of the distal scaphoid and trapezoid is removed with arthroscopic burr, there is progressively more space for the burr to reach the surface of the trapezium. Due to the relatively tight space, bleeding from bone ends may obscure the operative field and tourniquet may be required to control bleeding at this junction temporarily. The proximal part of the articular surface between the trapezium and trapezoid should also be denuded of cartilage with an arthroscopic burr. However, complete take down of the articular surface is probably not necessary as normally the TT joint is very tight and stable.

Once the articular surface for fusion is well prepared, a percutaneous fixation of the STT joint can be performed. Fixation can be in the form of K-wires transfixing scaphotrapezial, scaphotrapezoid, and trapeziotrapezoid joints. I prefer to employ rigid fixation using a cannulated screw with compression inserted from trapezium to scaphoid percutane-

Fig. 30.11 Radiological and arthroscopic view showing typical posttraumatic STT joint arthritis with synovial overgrowth and eburnation at joint surface

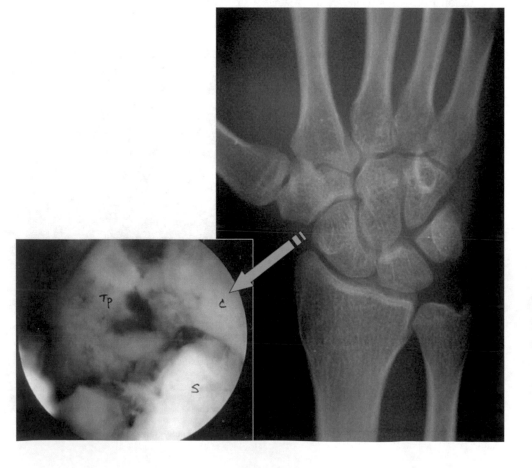

Fig. 30.12 Intraoperative X-ray view showing placement of starting awl over the distal tubercle of trapezium and the guide pin insertion across scaphotrapezial joint

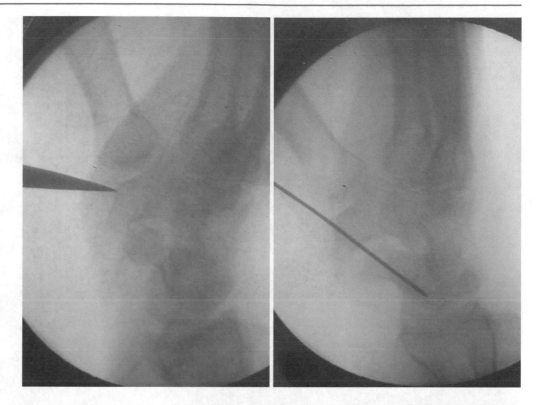

ously. Fixation of the scaphotrapezoid and trapeziotrapezoid joints then becomes nonessential. With the hand placed horizontally in hand table, a guide pin is inserted through a small stab wound at junction between base of first metacarpal and the trapezium under an image guidance with the aim toward the proximal pole of the scaphoid (Fig. 30.12). Alignment should be confirmed by at least four radiological views of AP, lateral, semisupinated AP, and semipronated PA view. If scaphoid is abnormally flexed and pronated due to scapholunate instability, a 1.6-mm K-wire can be inserted percutaneously to be used as joystick to correct the alignment of scaphoid. With the arthroscope in MCR portal, a small probe can also be inserted through STT portal to assist the reduction of scaphoid alignment by hooking onto the distal part of the scaphoid to extend and derotate the scaphoid. The K-wire inserted through trapezium can then be driven through to reach the proximal scaphoid.

The arthroscope is then inserted again into the joint through MCR portal to verify the position of K-wire (Fig. 30.13). If the joint space at STT joint becomes too tight to allow bone grafting through an arthroscopic cannula, the K-wire can be withdrawn from the scaphoid but remains attached to the trapezium. Autogenous bone graft or bone substitute can be inserted through a small cannula as described earlier to fill up the void (Fig. 30.14). The K-wire is then driven back into the scaphoid till the subchondral surface of proximal scaphoid is reached. Length of the inserted portion of the K-wire is measured. The screw length should be 2 mm short of the measured length to reduce the possibil-

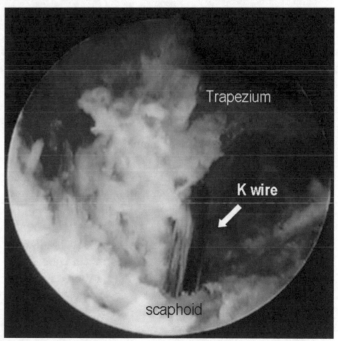

Fig. 30.13 Verification of the guide pin position at the STT joint as viewed through the arthroscope

ity of perforation of the proximal articular surface of scaphoid. The K-wire is then driven further proximally, perforating the proximal pole of scaphoid and exiting outside skin near the 3/4 portal of radiocarpal joint. The tip of the K-wire is grabbed with a hemostat. This trick helps to prevent accident

Fig. 30.14 Delivery of autogenous bone graft through cannula to the fusion site, impaction, and final appearance

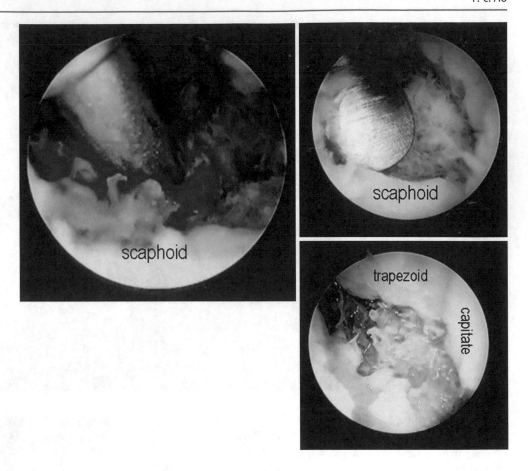

pull off of the K-wire during subsequent drilling process with the small cannulated drill. The bone is then drilled with a cannulated drill bit and finally the trapezioscaphoid joint is transfixed with an appropriate cannulated screw with compression for added stability (Fig. 30.15). The guide wire can be removed afterward. Final alignment of the screw should be confirmed using an image intensifier. The midcarpal joint is then surveyed with an arthroscope to check for any spilled-out graft material, which should be removed by using a mosquito grasper or flushed out from the cannula with saline.

Wounds are closed with steri-strips and a comfortable bulky dressing is applied supported with a short arm plaster slab. The slab is changed to a removable scaphoid splint after the first week. Active mobilization of the wrist is allowed out of splint under supervision of a hand therapist. Passive wrist mobilization and strengthening exercise can be offered when radiological and clinical union is evidenced, usually around 10–12 weeks postoperative (Fig. 30.16).

Four Corners Fusion

Four corners fusion is indicated when there is significant periscaphoid arthritis in the presence of a relatively intact radiolunate joint (Fig. 30.17). Under these circumstances, the scaphoid is usually removed surgically as a concomitant procedure with the four corners fusion. Presence of severe arthritic change at the midcarpal joint will exclude the alternative option of proximal row carpectomy and makes the operation a procedure of choice [19, 20]. For pathology that does not involve radioscaphoid arthritis, the indications include midcarpal instability, isolated midcarpal arthritis, or lunotriquetral dissociation with fixed volar intercalated segmental instability alignment of the lunate. When performing four corners fusion in cases without radioscaphoid arthritis, Taleisnik favored scaphoid inclusion [21] and Weiss et al. preferred scaphoid retention [22]. In a cadaveric study carried out by Kobza et al. [10], it was shown that simple four

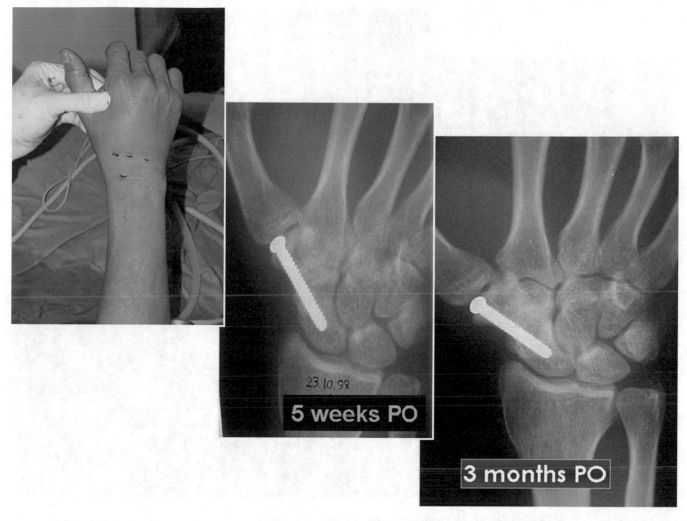

Fig. 30.15 Final wound appearance and progress of radiological changes showing early union at 5 weeks and consolidation over 3 months postoperative

corners fusion with scaphoid retention led to a significant decrease in extension, radial deviation, and ulnar deviation. Four corners fusion with scaphoid excision not only allowed significantly greater radial deviation but also led to significant increase in radiolunate contact area and the mean contact pressure. However, the clinical impact was not known.

We reported four cases of arthroscopic four corners fusion with scaphoidectomy in 2008 [23]. The operation should begin with a surveillance of the radiocarpal joint to confirm an intact radiolunate articulation and preferably an intact proximal articular surface of triquetrum. Arthroscopic scaphoidectomy is then performed from the midcarpal joint. The operation can be performed without a tourniquet provided that the portal sites and joint space are infiltrated with adrenaline solution in lignocaine. With the arthroscope introduced from the MCU portal, an arthroscopic burr of 2.9 mm is inserted into MCR portal and directed toward the proximal and midscaphoid region. The scaphoid is burred at high speed from the articular surface down to the core cancellous bone. Bone debris is removed by intermittently applied suction. To avoid accidental damage of the adjacent articular surfaces to be preserved, a shell of cartilage can be left intact until majority of the cancellous bone is removed. This shell of cartilage can help to separate the burr from the adjacent carpal bone during the burring process (Fig. 30.18). This can be removed piecemeal at the end of the scaphoidectomy procedure by using a small pituitary rongeur or an arthroscopic punch (Fig. 30.19). When taking out the larger piece of bone fragment, it is advisable not to use excessive violence in order to avoid damage to the attaching ligament and soft tissue structure. One trick is to firmly grip on the bone fragment with the small rongeur using both hands while to twist

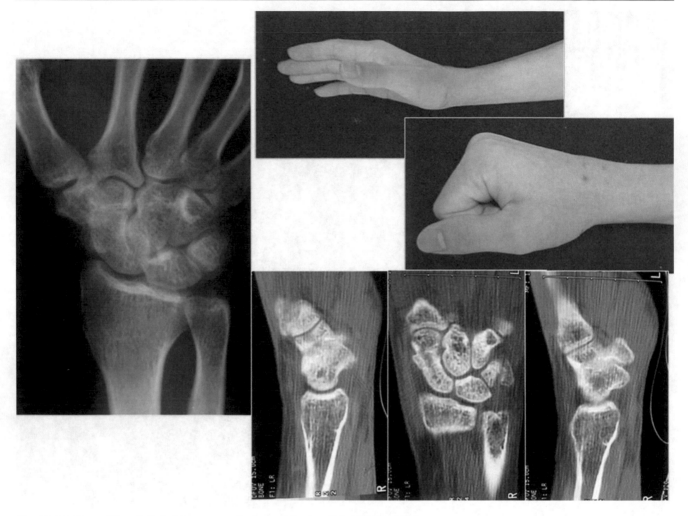

Fig. 30.16 X-ray, CT, and clinical features confirming solid union of the STT joint fusion

around its own axis and maintain a gentle pulling force. The fragment will gradually lose its connection to the soft tissue and can be delivered smoothly out of the joint. During the delivery process, the surgeon has to maintain a sustained and firm grip on the bony fragment or otherwise it may get lost in the juxta-articular or subcutaneous tissue plane. Under such situation, the surgeon may be forced to enlarge the surgical wound in order to remove the retained bony fragment, which is not desirable (Fig. 30.20). In order to speed up the process, an arthroscopic burr of progressive increase in size such as 3.5 mm and even 4.5 mm can be used when there is more space opened up after part of the scaphoid is removed (Fig. 30.21). The speed of scaphoid excision can often be doubled or even tripled. Alternatively a small osteotome can also be used to break the bone into piecemeal for easier removal. Extreme care has to be exercised during insertion of the larger burr or osteotome to avoid iatrogenic injury to the extensor tendon and cutaneous nerve. The distal few milli-

meters of the scaphoid can be left in situ so as to preserve the scaphotrapezial ligament. The distal scaphoid tubercle does not normally articulate with the radial styloid and hence its preservation will not cause impingement pain postoperatively.

Once scaphoid is cleared, attention can be paid to the fusion of the midcarpal joint at the four corners region. The arthroscope is now inserted through MCR portal, while the MCU portal is reserved for the arthroscopic instruments. The articular surface between the capitate, lunate, triquetrum, and hamate is denuded of cartilage with 2.9 mm burr. The joint surface of the lunotriquetral joint is also burred. I do not routinely burr the articulation between hamate and capitate as the joint is very rigid normally.

After an adequate cartilage destruction, provisional fixation is performed under an image intensifier's guide. If there is significant ulnar translocation and DISI deformity of the lunate and radial subluxation of the capitate off the lunate

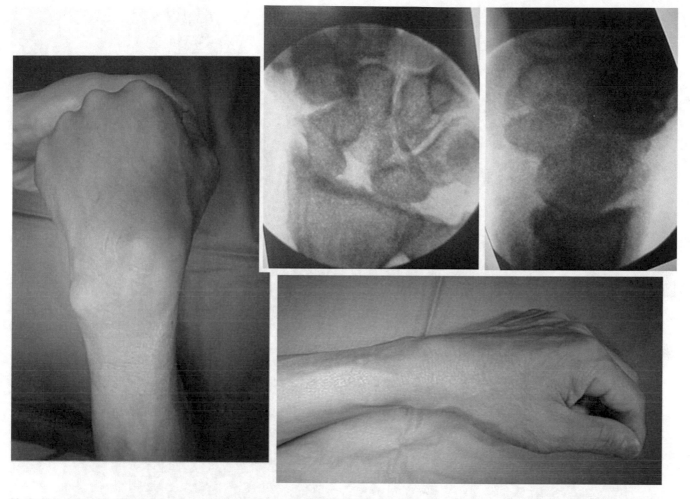

Fig. 30.17 A 47-year-old manual worker with SLAC wrist stage III undergoing arthroscopic scaphoidectomy and four corners fusion at September 2000

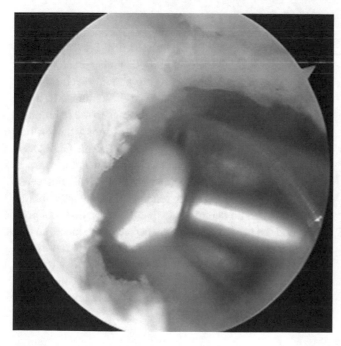

Fig. 30.18 Shell of cartilage left intact during burring of scaphoid to protect other uninvolved articular surfaces

margin, the lunate is reduced by gentle flexion and radial translation of the wrist so as to restore the normal radiolunate relationship. The aim is to have at least half of the lunate sitting over the distal radius. The lunate is then fixed to the radius with a percutaneous K-wire of 1.1 or 1.6 mm inserted from the distal radius.

The capitate is then reduced by ulnar translation of the wrist so that it sits as much as possible on the distal lunate articular surface (Fig. 30.22). A percutaneous K-wire is inserted from the dorsal surface of the capitate at the distal junction with the base of the third metacarpal under an image guide (Fig. 30.23). The ministab wound should be bluntly dissected to avoid iatrogenic injury to the extensor tendon. With the help of a lateral projection on the image guide, the K-wire is driven across the capitolunate joint to anchor into the lunate. The angle of attack has to be acute enough in order to catch the central part of the lunate to have a better purchase of the bone. It is most crucial to obtain a good surface contact of the capitolunate joint as the key point of the operation is to achieve solid fusion of the CL joint to avoid late collapse of the midcarpal joint and hence loss of the carpal height.

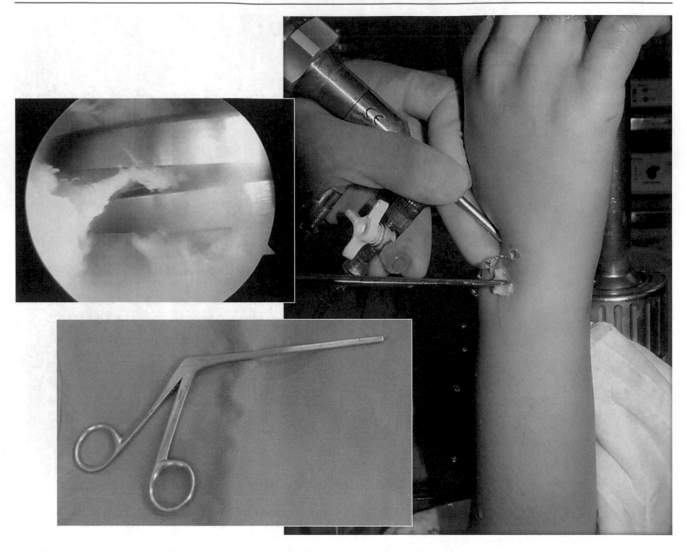

Fig. 30.19 Cartilage shell removed in piecemeal using small pituitary rongeur inserted through portals

If satisfactory alignment can be achieved, the K-wire is withdrawn from lunate while still attaching to the capitate. This is then followed by the bone grafting procedure at the midcarpal joint as described in session before. With the arthroscope held at MCR portal, the cannula can be inserted through the MCU portal for bone graft or substitute delivery. If scaphoidectomy is included, a French size 6 Foley catheter is inserted via the 3/4 portal to completely obliterate the empty space left after the scaphoidectomy procedure. The balloon is inflated while bone graft or substitute is being delivered to the ulnar midcarpal space (Fig. 30.24). The catheter can be removed after the bone grafting procedure, or can be left in situ for a day or two to serve as a surgical drain.

After completion of the bone grafting, the K-wire over the capitate is driven back to lunate at the reduced position. Length of the K-wire inserted is measured. This is followed

by drilling of bone with a cannulated drill bit and the final insertion of a headless self-tapping cannulated screw to fix the capitolunate joint. The screw tip should reach no more than 2 mm from the proximal surface of the lunate to avoid screw tip protrusion and iatrogenic damage to the radiolunate articulation. To avoid loss of reduction during the drilling action, an additional K-wire can be inserted to the CL interval for temporary fixation. One has to be sure that the screw is completely buried in the capitate so that it will not cause impingement to the extensor tendons. Lateral and oblique X-ray views should demonstrate that the screw does not project beyond the proximal articular surface of the lunate so that no scratching of the articular surface of the distal radius will occur. This can also be checked with a gentle passive movement of the wrist after the fixation procedure, or more definitely with an arthroscopic evaluation at the radiocarpal joint.

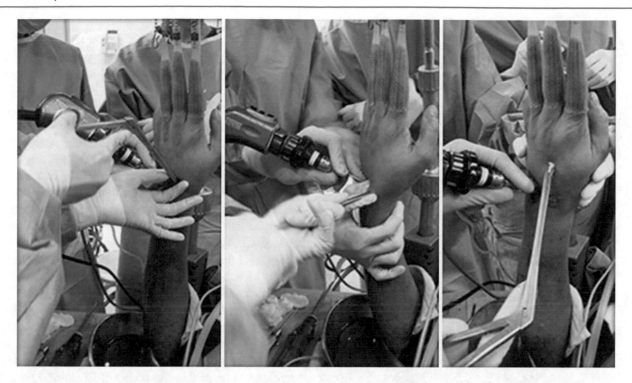

Fig. 30.20 The surgeon firmly grips on the bone fragment with the small rongeur using both hands while to twist around its own axis and maintain a gentle pulling force. The fragment will gradually lose its connection to the soft tissue and can be delivered smoothly out of the joint

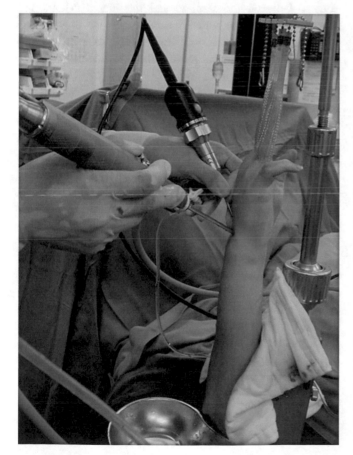

Fig. 30.21 Use of large 4.5-mm arthroscopic burr helps to speed up the burring process

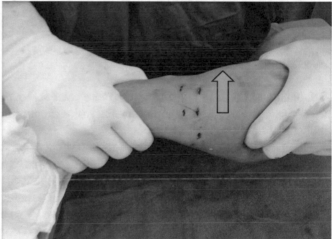

Fig. 30.22 The capitate is reduced by ulnar translation of the wrist so that it sits as much as possible on the distal lunate articular surface

The lunotriquetral joint and the capitohamate joint are then fixed with percutaneous K-wires through small stab incisions (Fig. 30.25). If the positions of the K-wires are satisfactory, headless screws are inserted from ulnar aspect of the hand to fix the carpal intervals (Fig. 30.26). Structures at risk include the dorsal branches of ulnar nerve, EDM, and ECU tendons. Blunt dissection of the stab wounds should be a routine before the insertion of guide wire to avoid iatrogenic injury to these important structures. In order to reduce the chance of hitting onto the screw fixing capitolunate joint, the guide wire for

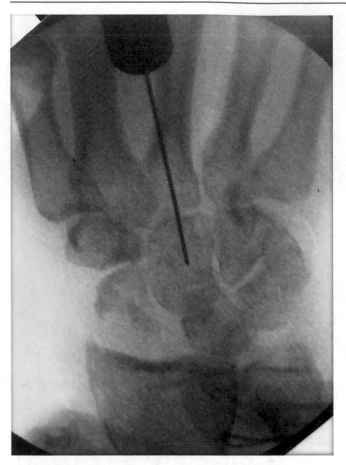

Fig. 30.23 Guide pin inserted through distal capitate to transfix capitolunate joint

capitohamate fusion should aim at the more volar aspect of the capitate, while that of the lunotriquetral fusion should aim at the more dorsal aspect of lunate.

After solid fixation of the four corners bones, any K-wire over the radiolunate joint can be left in situ for 2 weeks. The wire end is cut short and bent outside the skin. Wounds are approximated with steri-strips and a comfortable bulky dressing is applied supported with a short arm plaster slab (Fig. 30.27). The plaster slab is changed to a removable wrist splint after the first week. After removal of the K-wire over the radiolunate joint, active mobilization of the wrist can be initiated out of splint under the supervision of a hand therapist. Passive wrist mobilization and strengthening exercise can be offered when radiological and clinical union is evidenced, usually around 10–12 weeks postoperative (Figs. 30.28, 30.29 and 30.30).

Capitolunate Fusion

Capitolunate (CL) fusion and scaphoidectomy are now the preferred solution for me in managing stage II or III SLAC or SNAC wrist condition, unless there is concomitant arthritis at the ulnar midcarpal joint. This allows a shorter operating time and preservation of the relatively normal ulnar component of the midcarpal joint, while adequately preventing carpal collapse after the removal of the scaphoid in arthritic condition. CL fusion has historically bad reputation for high nonunion rate due to the limited bony fusion surface and masses. Nevertheless, Slade and Bomback demonstrated a high union and satisfaction rate with an arthroscopic assisted CL fusion, accountable by the minimal invasive method and the rigid percutaneous fixation [24]. The more conservative bone resection also eliminates the potential drawback of triquetral hamate impingement.

The operation begins with a surveillance of the radiocarpal joint to confirm an intact radiolunate articulation. Arthroscopic scaphoidectomy can then be performed at the midcarpal joint as described earlier. Once scaphoid is cleared, attention can be paid to the fusion of CL joint. The arthroscope is now inserted through MCR portal, while the MCU portal is reserved for arthroscopic instruments. The articular surface between the capitate and the lunate is carefully denuded of cartilage with 2.9 mm burr, while those of the triquetrum and hamate should be carefully protected and preserved. For type I lunate, the whole distal articulating surface of the lunate should be debrided. For type II lunate, the typical small ulnar facet need not be debrided as it will not be involved in the fusion process. If the ulnar facet is of considerable size and proportion, one may consider more aggressive flattening of the articular surface by removing the central wedge in between the two facets before attempting the fusion. However, the chance of subsequent triquetrohamate impingement may become higher such that one may consider switching to a formal four corners fusion.

If there is significant ulnar translocation and DISI deformity of the lunate and radial subluxation of the capitate off the lunate margin, the lunate should be reduced and fixed to the radius temporarily as described earlier.

The wrist is taken off from the wrist tower. A small stab wound is being made over the distal dorsal surface of the capitate at the junction with the radial aspect of the base of third metacarpal (see Fig. 30.13). The ministab wound should be bluntly dissected to avoid iatrogenic injury to the

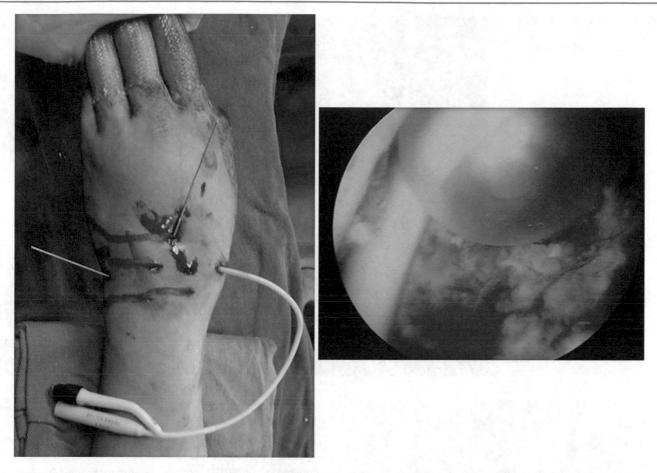

Fig. 30.24 A French size 6 Foley catheter is inserted via the 3/4 portal to completely obliterate the empty space left after the scaphoidectomy procedure

Fig. 30.25 The lunotriquetral joint and the capitohamate joint are fixed with percutaneous K-wires

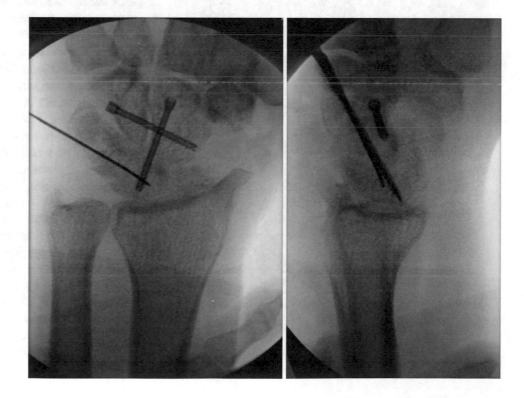

Fig. 30.26 Fusion of the four corners bones with percutaneous headless screws

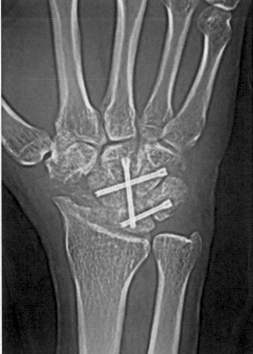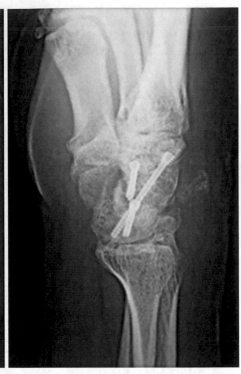

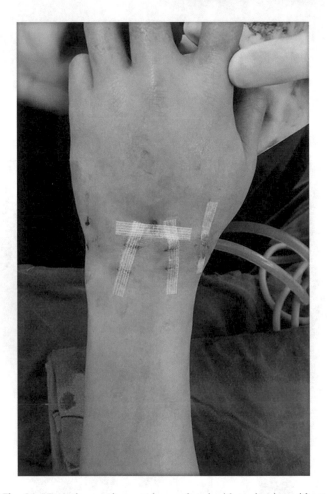

Fig. 30.27 Arthroscopic wounds are closed with steri-strips without stitch

extensor tendon until the bony cortex is reached. With the help of an anteroposterior and lateral projection under an image intensifier, a guide wire of a small cannulated screw system is inserted and driven across the capitate toward lunate and parallel to the radial border of capitate. A small metal awl is helpful to establish the entry point over the capitate prior to the insertion of the guide pin (Fig. 30.31). The angle of attack has to be acute enough with an aim to catch the central part of the lunate to have better purchase of the bone. Before the first guide wire is being fired across the CL joint, the second one should be placed to the ulnar side of the capitate-metacarpal joint. With a second small stab wound over the distal dorsal surface of the capitate at the junction with the ulnar aspect of the base of third metacarpal, the guide wire is driven across the capitate, with an aim to catch the dorsal third of the lunate at the CL junction. The slightly different angle of attack of the two guide pins can avoid crowding of the screws upon final definitive fixation.

With the two pins on the capitate, the capitate is manually reduced to the lunate by ulnar translation of the wrist so that it sits as much as possible on the distal lunate articular surface (Fig. 30.32). The pins are then driven through the lunate until they reach the subchondral surfaces (Fig. 30.33). It is most crucial to obtain good surface contact of the capitolunate joint as the key point of the operation is to achieve a solid fusion of the CL joint to avoid late collapse of the midcarpal joint and hence loss of the carpal height.

In CL fusion, the articular congruency achieved between the capitate and lunate is typically very good. There is no

Fig. 30.28 The 47-year-old manual worker with SLAC wrist stage III as shown in Fig. 30.17 undergone arthroscopic scaphoidectomy and four corners fusion showed solid fusion 3 months postoperative

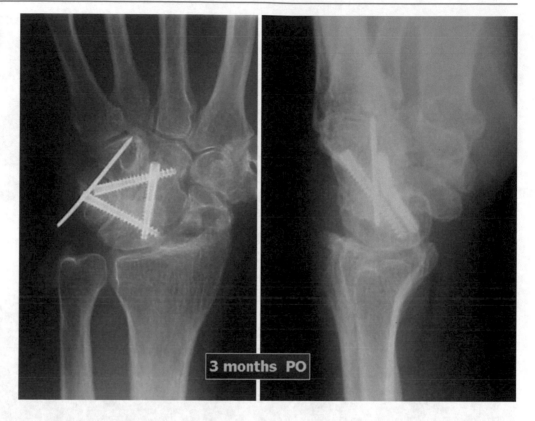

need for added bone graft or substitute. Conversion of the K-wires fixation with cannulated screws is then followed as described previously (Fig. 30.34). Lateral and oblique X-ray views are taken to confirm that no screw should project beyond the proximal articular surface of the lunate (Fig. 30.35). The stability and range of motion of the wrist can be checked under fluoroscopic guidance. Passive finger movement should be checked to confirm no impingement by the screws.

Wounds are then closed with steri-strip and a comfortable bulky dressing is applied supported with a short arm plaster slab. The slab is changed to a removable wrist splint after the first week, when gentle active mobilization of the wrist can be initiated out of splint under supervision of hand therapist. Passive wrist mobilization and strengthening exercise can be offered when radiological and clinical union is evidenced, usually around 8–10 weeks postoperative (Figs. 30.36 and 30.37).

Radioscapholunate Fusion

Radioscapholunate fusion is indicated for severe painful posttraumatic arthritis involving the whole radiocarpal joint, while the midcarpal joint is relatively preserved [25] (Fig. 30.38). For inflammatory arthritis, the disease should not be at the height of progression and better be adequately controlled with medication [26]. It has been shown that an accompanying distal scaphoidectomy procedure can help to improve midcarpal motion especially on ulnar radial deviation [27]. This can also be accomplished by arthroscopic mean.

A general surveillance of the midcarpal joint to confirm its relative integrity is a prerequisite for a successful radioscapholunate fusion. Arthroscopic distal scaphoidectomy can also be performed at the same time. With the arthroscope placed at the MCU portal, a 2.9-mm burr is inserted into the MCR portal and directed toward the distal scaphoid portion articulating with the trapezoid. Burring of the scaphoid is started at this point toward the distal pole from dorsoulnar to volar-radial direction. Caution has to be taken to avoid iatrogenic damage to the articular cartilage of trapezoid, trapezium, and capitate. The junction between capitate, scaphoid, and trapezoid forms the landmark of the proximal extent of resection. A shell of cartilage can be left intact until majority of the cancellous bone of the distal scaphoid pole is removed. This shell of cartilage can help to separate the burr from the adjacent carpal bones during the burring process. This can be removed piecemeal at the end of the distal scaphoidectomy procedure by using a small pituitary rongeur or an arthroscopic punch. The STT portal can also be employed to facilitate burring of the most distal part

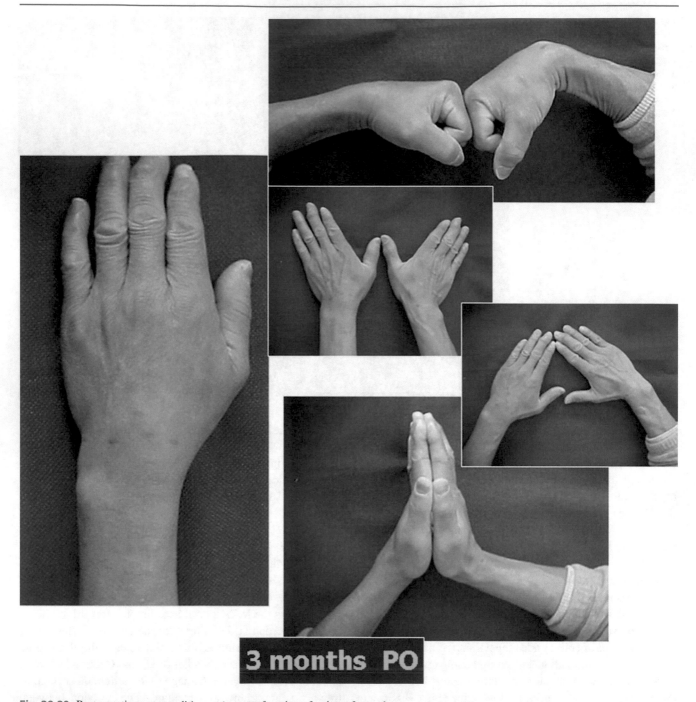

Fig. 30.29 Postoperative scar condition and range of motion of wrist at 3 months

of the scaphoid. At the end of the procedure, there should be a void opposing the trapezium and trapezoid bone, while the waist of scaphoid is preserved and is articulating with capitate. The precise extent of distal scaphoid resection can be checked with intraoperative fluoroscopy (Fig. 30.39).

After the distal scaphoidectomy is complete, the arthroscope can be directed to the radiocarpal joint. The remaining articular cartilage of the radiocarpal joint is denuded. With the arthroscope in 3/4 portal, a 2.9-mm burr is inserted into 4/5 portal and both the lunate fossa and the proximal surface of the lunate are debrided of articular cartilage. The degree of cartilage denudation should be well controlled so that no excessive subchondral cancellous bone is being removed. Burring is completed when the subchondral bone with healthy punctate bleeding is reached. This phenomenon can be easily observed if tourniquet is not used during this pro-

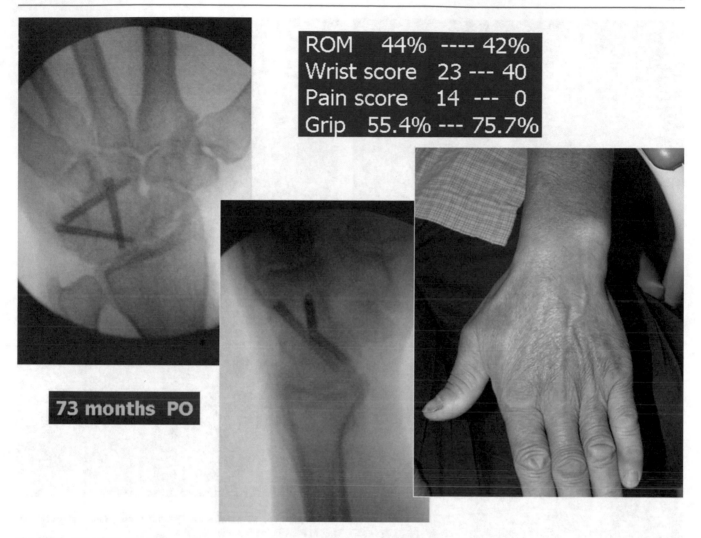

ROM   44% ---- 42%
Wrist score   23 --- 40
Pain score   14 --- 0
Grip   55.4% --- 75.7%

73 months PO

Fig. 30.30 Final follow-up at 73 months postoperative: Wrist ROM similar to preoperative (42% vs. 44% of opposite wrist), full wrist function score, no pain, grip power increased from 55.4% to 75.7% of opposite side. Scar was invisible

cess. Usually, bleeding is limited and can easily be controlled with hydrostatic pressure applied through the irrigation system. If bleeding is profuse, one may use the coagulatory role of radiofrequency apparatus. Use of a tourniquet is optional depending on the degree of bleeding. During the burring process, suction can be switched on and off intermittently to remove any accumulated bone debris which may block the visual field. If suction is applied continuously during the burring process, excessive air bubbles drawn in will severely compromise the visibility of the operating site. The portals are then switched so that the burr is introduced from the 3/4 portal to have a better clearance of the articular cartilage of the proximal scaphoid and the scaphoid fossa including the radial styloid area.

After completion of the burring process, the hand is taken off the wrist traction tower and placed horizontally on the operating hand table. An image intensifier is moved in.

Percutaneous K-wires are inserted from distal radius to transfix the radiolunate and radioscaphoid joint (Fig. 30.40). A small longitudinal incision is made at the distal radius about 2 cm proximal to the midpoint between the 3/4 and 4/5 portals. This is corresponding to the direct articulation between radius and lunate. The extensor tendons are bluntly dissected off from the potential wire insertion point using a fine-pointed stitch scissor. With the wrist placed in neutral position both in flexion-extension plane and radioulnar deviation plane, two 1.1 mm K-wires are inserted using a protective sheath one after the other from distal radius to fix the lunate. If small cannulated screw is being used, the guide pin is inserted in the same manner. One or two guide pins are used according to the size of the carpal bone. The two wires should aim at the radial and ulnar border of the lunate so as to have even purchase of the bone. The radiolunate angle should be maintained at zero degree. This requires

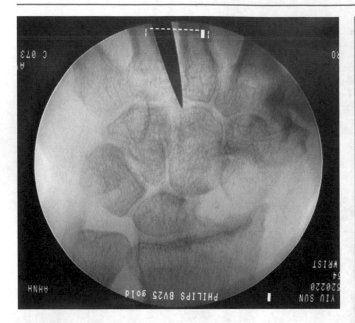

Fig. 30.31 A small metal awl inserted through a stab wound at the ulnar border of the base of the third metacarpal and the capitate to establish an entry point for the guide pin

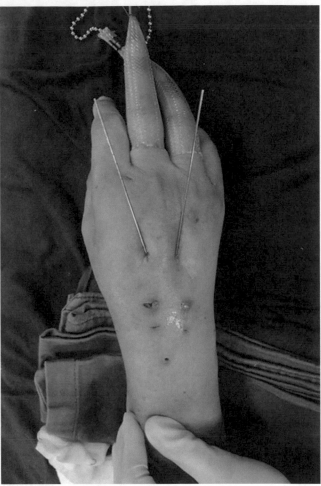

Fig. 30.33 Two pins are inserted percutaneously under image intensifier to transfix the capitolunate joint

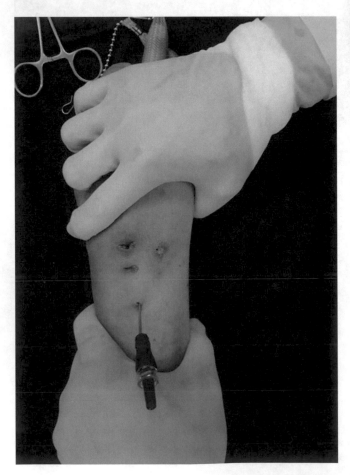

Fig. 30.32 The wrist is manually ulnar translated to reduce the capitate as much as possible to the distal articular surface of the lunate

confirmation using both AP and lateral view of X-ray. On the lateral projection, the wire should target on the anterior horn of the lunate bone. To optimize the bone purchase, the angle of insertion of the K-wire should be quite acute at 20–30° with reference to the long axis of the forearm. Another incision is made over the radial styloid at the bare area between the first and second extensor compartments. After careful blunt dissection of the superficial branches of radial nerve, the two K-wires or guide wires are inserted in sequence to transfix the distal radius to the scaphoid. After verification of the wire position, they can be back out from the carpal bones while attaching to the distal radius. The protruded ends of the K-wire are capped to avoid injury to the surgeon. The wrist is then put back to the wrist traction tower for the arthroscopic grafting procedure.

With arthroscope introduced at 4/5 portal, an arthroscopic cannula is inserted through 3/4 portal to reach the radial side of the scaphoid fossa. Autogenous bone graft or bone substitute can be inserted to fill up the radial side of the radioscaphoid joint. As the fusion surfaces are usually well vascularized,

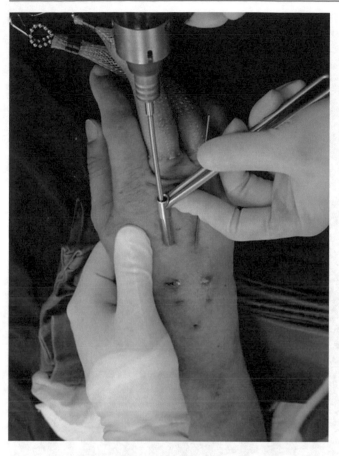

Fig. 30.34 Cannulated drill is inserted through the percutaneous pin to prepare track for the cannulated screw

I prefer the use of bone substitute to reduce donor site morbidity on the patient (Fig. 30.41). To achieve better vision on the operative field, the tourniquet is inflated at this junction to reduce bleeding inside the joint (Fig. 30.42). When the radioscaphoid joint is half filled with bone substitute, the arthroscope is switched to 3/4 portal and the cannula is inserted at the 4/5 portal. Grafting process is continued at the radiolunate joint. To prevent spilling of the graft to the ulnocarpal compartment, a size 6 Foley catheter is inserted through the 6R portal and is inflated with saline so as to obliterate the space there.

When the grafting procedure is complete, the hand is again taken off the tower and tourniquet deflated. Under image guide, the K-wires are driven back into the carpal bones just short of the articulating surface at the midcarpal joint. For posttraumatic arthritis in the younger patients, I prefer using percutaneous compression screws to enhance fusion rate. After measuring the length of the inserted portion of the K-wires, the wire tracks are drilled with cannulated drill bit. Definitive fixation is performed with 3.0 mm cannulated screws with the head firmly anchored over the dorsal cortex of the distal radius. Alternatively, a headless cannulated screw system can also be used (Figs. 30.43 and 30.44). X-ray is required to confirm that the thread of the screws should not perforate the midcarpal joint surface to impinge on the distal carpal row. This can also be verified arthroscopically. In osteopenic bone where screw purchase can be suboptimal, the four K-wires can serve as the defini-

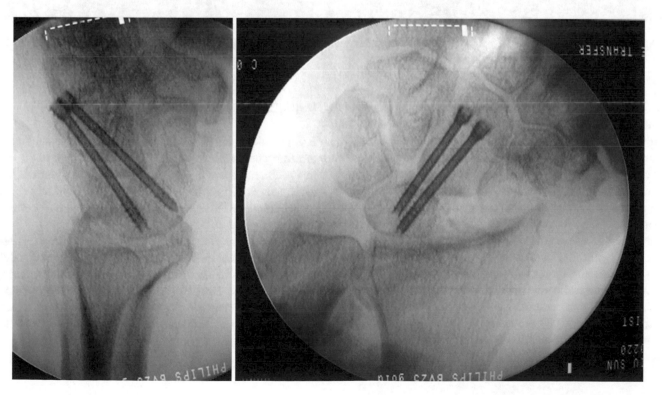

Fig. 30.35 The position of the two headless cannulated screws is being checked radiologically to ensure no violation of the articular surface at the radiolunate joint

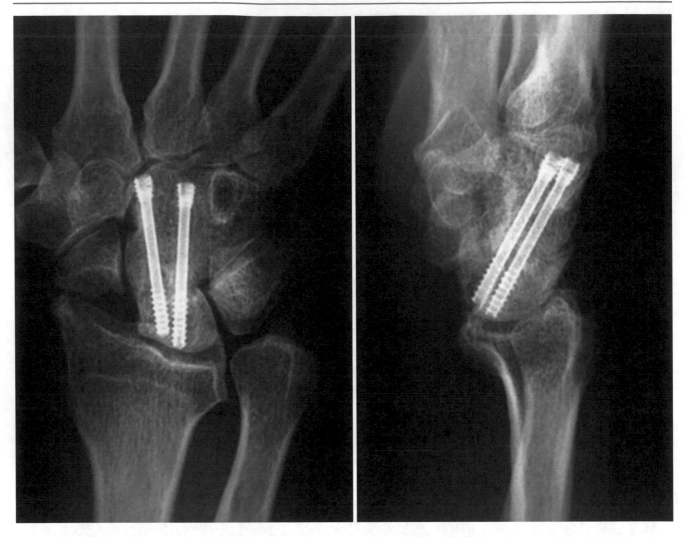

Fig. 30.36 A 55-year-old man with SLAC wrist stage III underwent arthroscopic scaphoidectomy and capitolunate fusion. X-ray at 12 months postoperative showed solid fusion and good carpal alignment

tive mean of fixation (Figs. 30.45, 30.46 and 30.47). They are cut short and buried underneath skin. The wrist should be moved gently to confirm the smooth articulation at the midcarpal joint and a stable fixation at the radiocarpal joint. The incision wounds are then opposed with steri-strips or simple stitches. Comfortable compression dressing with a short arm plaster slab is applied. It is changed to a removable wrist splint at 1–2 weeks of time. For K-wire fixation cases, active mobilization of the wrist is initiated after the fusion is united radiologically and clinically. The K-wires can be removed under local anesthesia through the original skin incisions. For compression screw fixation cases, gentle active wrist mobilization can be started at 2 weeks postoperative under supervision. More vigorous mobilization can be performed when radiological and clinical union is achieved.

Radiolunate Fusion

Radiolunate fusion is most commonly utilized in rheumatoid arthritis where there is painful ulnar translocation of the carpus at the radiocarpal joint. In posttraumatic situation, it is indicated when the articular cartilage destruction is confined to the radiolunate joint, such as in postdistal radius die-punch fracture (Fig. 30.48).

The operation is essentially similar to radioscapholunate fusion, except that the radioscaphoid joint is spared. In addition, distal scaphoidectomy is not necessary. Thus, during the burring procedure, the articular surface of the proximal scaphoid and scaphoid fossa should be well protected. During the graft insertion procedure, a second Foley catheter can be inserted at the 1/2 portal to obliterate the space at the

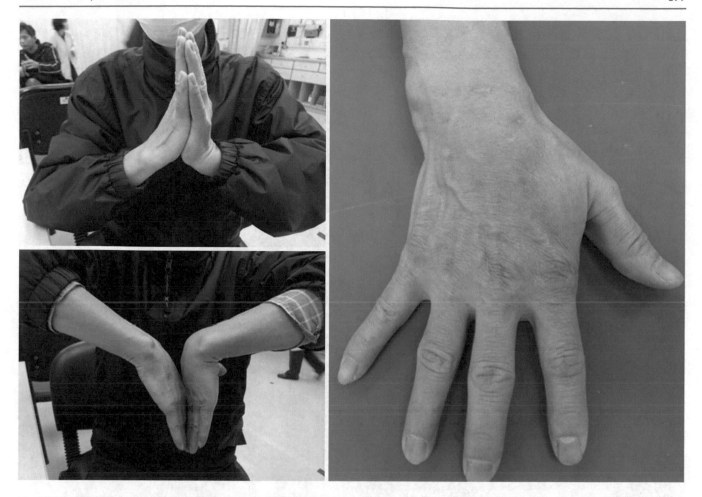

Fig. 30.37 Clinically the patient got 35° extension and 40° flexion at the wrist. Operative scars were inconspicuous

radioscaphoid articulation so as to isolate the space at the RL joint (Fig. 30.49). The arthroscope is placed at the 3/4 portal, while the bone substitute is delivered to the radiolunate joint through a cannula at the 4/5 portal (Fig. 30.50). The fixation can be accomplished by two K-wires or two compression cannulated screws inserted percutaneous from distal radius as described earlier (Figs. 30.51 and 30.52). In patient with significant ulnar-positive variance, an accompanying ulnar shortening osteotomy is performed to unload the ulnocarpal joint as well as to avoid potential ulnocarpal impaction after the radiolunate fusion which may shorten the proximal carpal row. The postoperative care and rehabilitation is same as radioscapholunate fusion as described earlier. However, the period of immobilization may need to be extended due to the limited contact area between lunate fossa and proximal lunate. Postoperatively close radiological monitoring is essential to determine the pacing of rehabilitation (Figs. 30.53, 30.54, 30.55, 30.56, 30.57, 30.58, 30.59 and 30.60). The author favors the granule form of bone substitute rather than injectable form, though the latter is very convenient for administration through the arthroscopic cannula.

Lunotriquetral Fusion

Lunotriquetral (LT) fusion is indicated for symptomatic chronic LT instability with or without ulnocarpal impaction syndrome [28, 29]. In the latter condition, ulnar shortening osteotomy is often an accompanying procedure to decompress the ulnocarpal joint. In the absence of secondary chondral damage, an alternative option of LT ligament reconstruction can be considered, since failure to unite is common in surgical fusion of the LT joint, according to the literature. In a meta-analysis of the outcome of intercarpal arthrodesis conducted by Siegel and Ruby, the overall reported nonunion rate in 81 patients of a total of 143 cases of LT fusion by open surgery in seven clinical series was 26% [6]. Where reported, 46% of patients has persistent postoperative symptom. Sennwald et al. also found disappointing high rate of pseudarthrosis of 5% in 23 patients receiving LT fusion [30]. In their open procedures from a dorsoulnar approach, they recommended the routine use of corticocancellous bone graft to enhance union. They cautioned about prolonged rehabilitation with 6 months out of

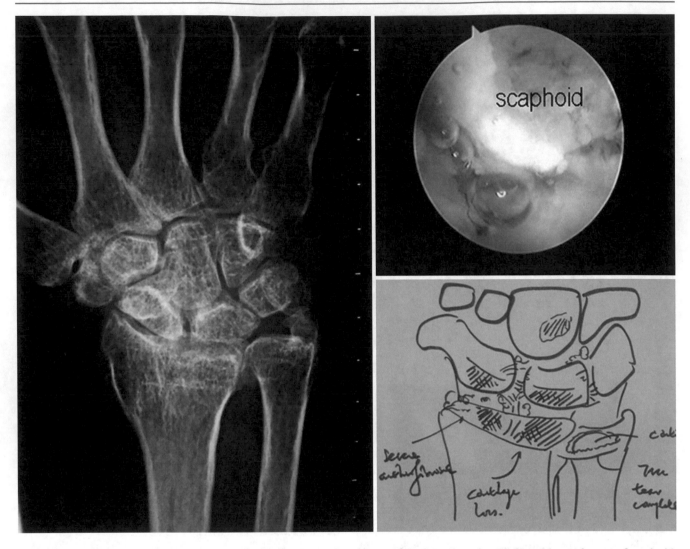

Fig. 30.38 Postdistal radius fracture arthrosis of the radiocarpal joint with complete eburnation of scaphoid and lunate fossa confirmed with arthroscopy. The midcarpal joint was preserved

work at best and the significant loss of grip power particularly in male subjects, which might force them to change their job nature.

Arthroscopic fusion of the LT joint can be performed with midcarpal arthroscopic approach (Fig. 30.61). Routine radiocarpal joint arthroscopy is performed to evaluate the status of the TFCC, associated chondral lesions of the ulnar head, proximal lunate and triquetrum, and the LT ligament. If significant chondral lesion is present at the carpal bone surface, ulnar shortening or arthroscopic Wafer procedure should be done in association with the LT fusion procedure.

The arthroscope is then directed to the midcarpal joint. With the arthroscope placed at the MCR portal, a small probe is inserted at the MCU portal to reach the LT joint to confirm instability. This is then replaced by a 2.0- or 2.9-mm arthroscopic burr and debridement of the articular cartilage is performed from distal to proximal direction (Fig. 30.62). Attention should be paid at the dorsal aspect of the joint by

rotating the 30° forward slanting lens to a downward position. Difficulty may be encountered in burring this portion as the angle of attack of the burr is frequently restricted by the dorsal soft tissue of the wrist. A small angled curette or ring curette may be useful in removing the cartilage at this area.

When burring is complete, provisional fixation of the LT interval is performed. A small wound is made opposing the ulnar surface of triquetrum and blunt dissection is performed to free the overlying terminal branch of the dorsal sensory branch of ulnar nerve. Under an image guide, a guide wire is inserted from the triquetrum across the LT joint to reach the lunate bone. The length of the guide wire is measured. Whenever feasible, two parallel guide pins are inserted to aim for two cannulated screws. If alignment is satisfactory, the guide pins are withdrawn from the lunate to free the joint space. The joint gap is then filled with bone graft or bone substitute through a cannula inserted at the MCU portal. The former is preferred as nonunion of the

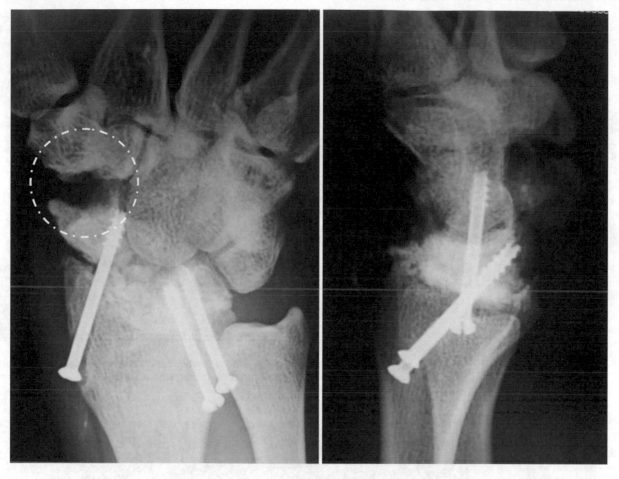

Fig. 30.39 X-ray showing the extent of distal scaphoidectomy in patient receiving arthroscopic radioscapholunate fusion (*circle of dotted line*)

Fig. 30.40 Arthroscope being inserted into the radiocarpal joint after the two percutaneous K-wires were back out from the joint

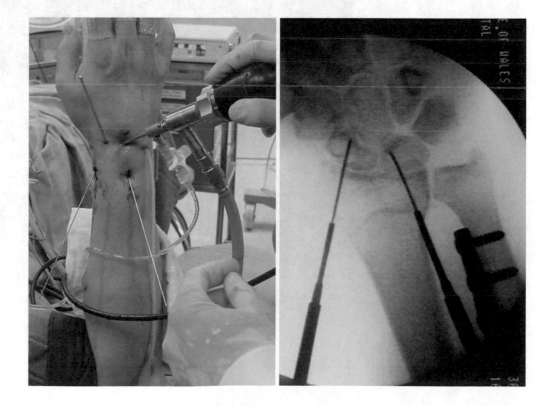

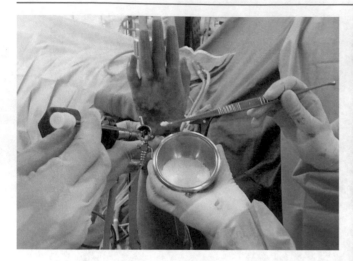

Fig. 30.41 Fine granules of artificial bone substitutes are being inserted into the radiocarpal joint space through a cannula before the definitive bony fixation

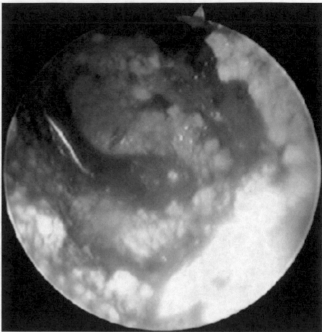

Fig. 30.42 Bone substitute granules are being impacted with a small impacter monitored through the arthroscope

Fig. 30.43 Intraoperative X-ray shows the final fixation of radioscapholunate intervals with two percutaneous AO screws. Noted that the ulnar shortening was performed before the indexed procedure

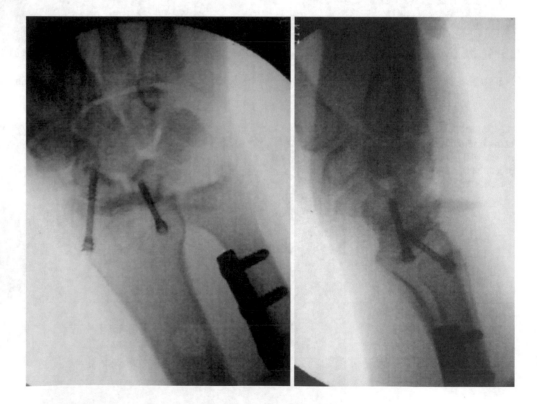

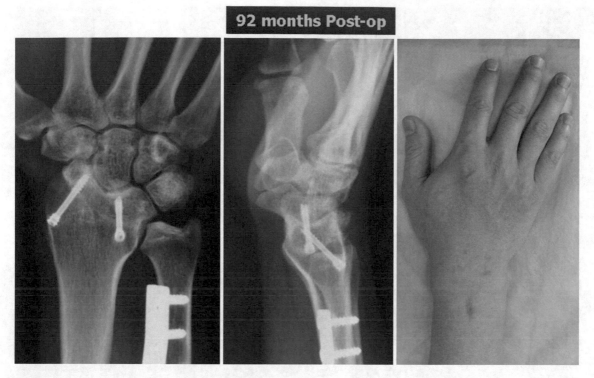

Fig. 30.44 Solid union of radioscapholunate fusion site at 92 months postoperative. Surgical scar was minimal

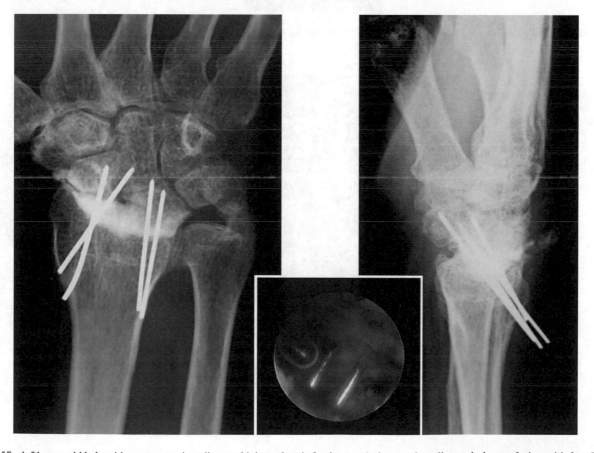

Fig. 30.45 A 51-year-old lady with posttraumatic radiocarpal joint arthrosis for 4 years. Arthroscopic radioscapholunate fusion with four K-wires and bone substitutes was done. Position of K-wires could be verified through arthroscopy at radiocarpal joint

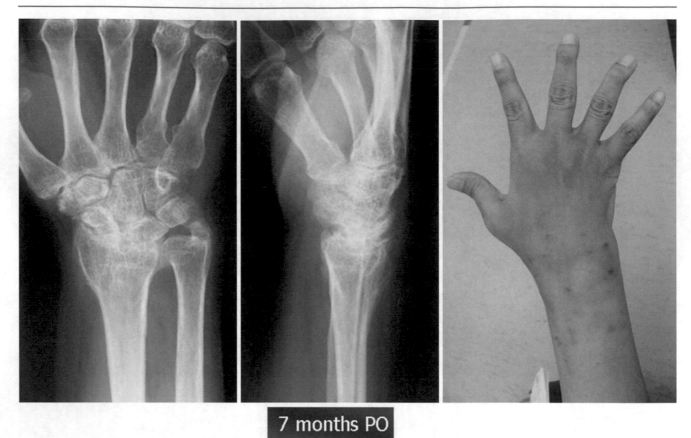

Fig. 30.46 X-ray at 7 months postoperative shows good fusion; scars on patients are minimal

Fig. 30.47 Solid
radioscapholunate fusion at
88 months postoperative.
There was also spontaneous
lunotriquetral fusion.
Midcarpal joint was
preserved. Patient had no pain

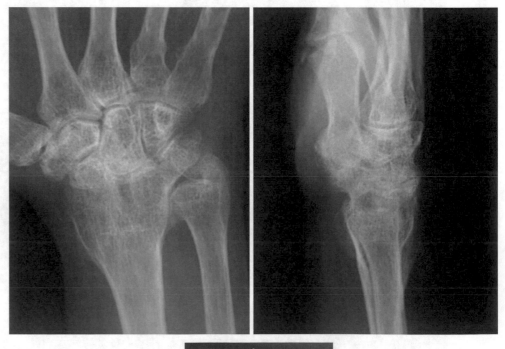

Fig. 30.48 A 34-year-old man with severe painful postdistal radius fracture arthrosis at radiolunate joint

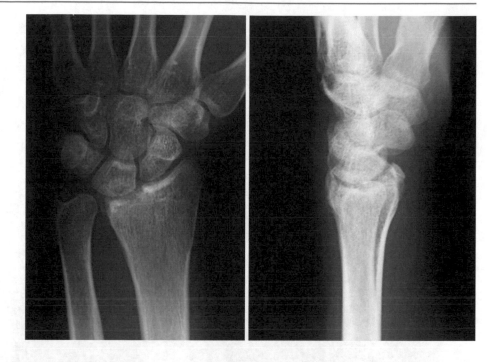

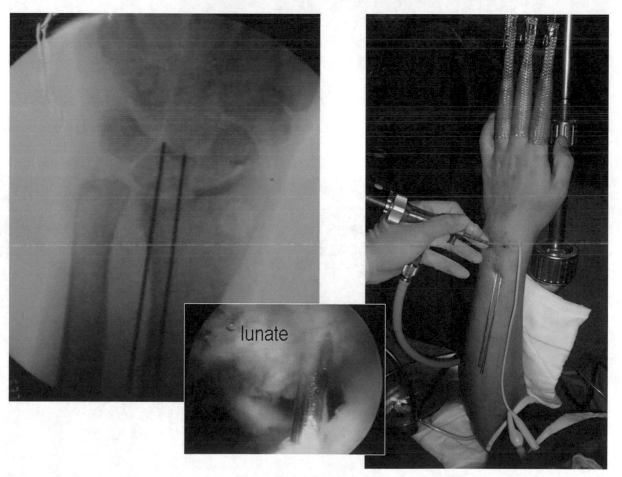

Fig. 30.49 Percutaneous pinning of the radiolunate joint under X-ray and arthroscopic guidance. A Foley catheter had been placed to obliterate the space at the radioscaphoid joint

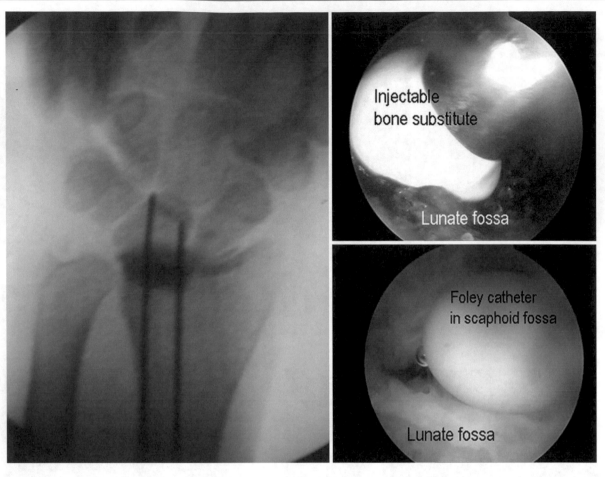

Fig. 30.50 Filling of radiolunate joint space with injectable bone substitute. Spilling of bone substitutes to adjacent space was blocked with inflated Foley catheter

Fig. 30.51 Definitive fixation with two percutaneous AO screws at radiolunate joint

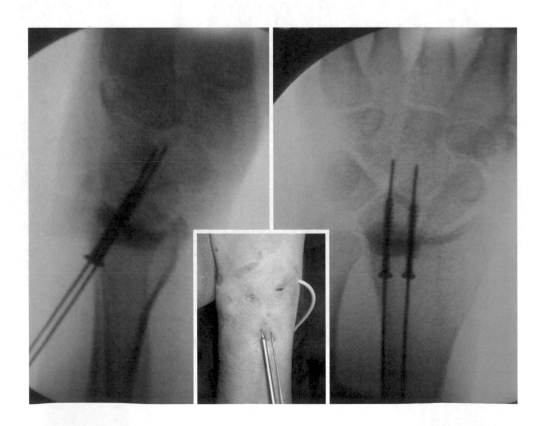

Fig. 30.52 Postoperative
X-ray appearance of the
radiolunate fusion with good
capitolunate alignment. Noted
that the bone substitutes were
well contained at the
radiolunate joint

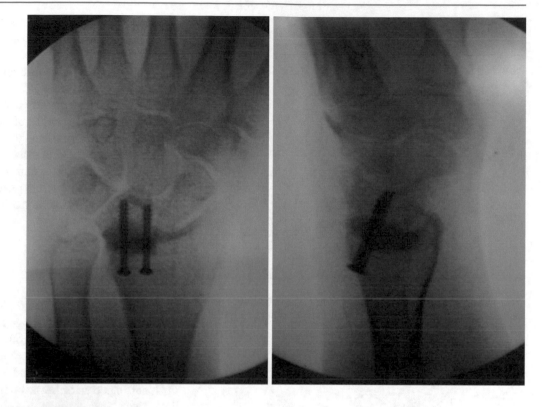

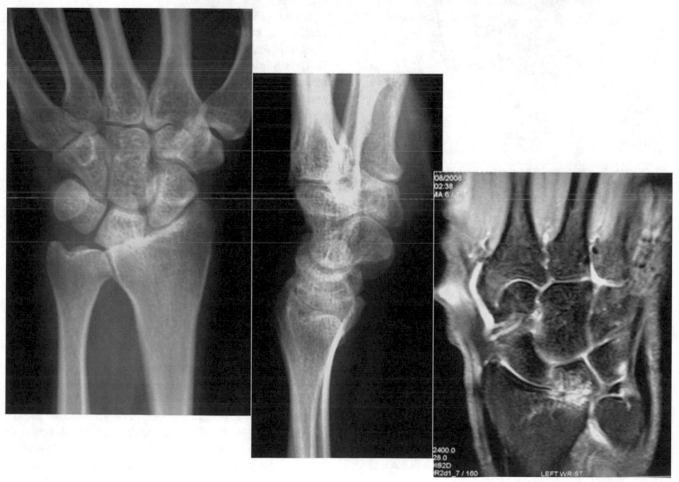

Fig. 30.53 A 53-year-old lady developed severe radiolunate arthrosis without history of trauma

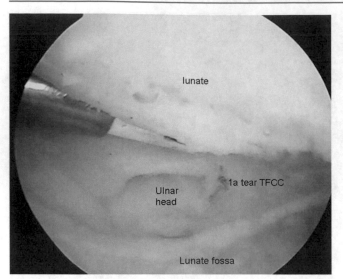

Fig. 30.54 Wrist arthroscopy shows complete eburnation of lunate fossa and proximal lunate, old 1a tear of TFCC with preserved ulnar head cartilage

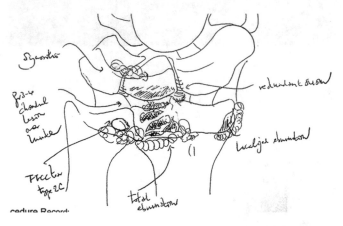

Fig. 30.55 Operative diagram depicts extent of joint pathology. There is associated small osteochondral lesion over scaphoid fossa. The midcarpal joint is normal

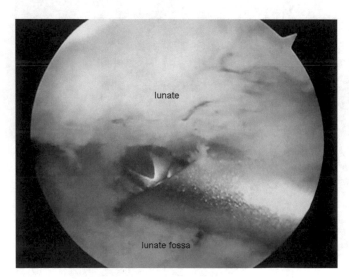

Fig. 30.56 Without tourniquet on, burring of proximal lunate revealed good subchondral punctate bleeding

fusion site is notoriously common. This is then followed by percutaneous fixation with compression cannulated screws inserted from the ulnar aspect of the hand. A cannulated drill bit is applied and a compression headless and self-tapping cannulated screw is inserted to compress the fusion site (Fig. 30.63). Preferably two screws should be inserted to obtain maximal stability of the fusion site (Fig. 30.64). Alternatively, a K-wire can be used to augment the strength of a single screw fixation if the bone is too small to accommodate two screws. All wounds are closed with steri-strips and a short arm plaster is applied to protect the fusion site until radiological union or stable fibrous union is achieved (Fig. 30.65).

Scaphocapitate Fusion

Scaphocapitate (SC) fusion is indicated in advanced Kienbock's disease as a salvage solution [31]. It is best indicated when the lunate has collapsed and the articular surfaces become fragmented, such as in Lichtman stage IIIa or IIIb situation (Figs. 30.66 and 30.67). I routinely removed the lunate since an ischemic bone can be a source of pain in the patient.

Routine surveillance of the radiocarpal joint is required to confirm an intact radioscaphoid articulation and the damaged articular cartilage of the lunate. When there is a fixed DISI deformity, the radial volar ligament and capsule can be released with the aid of shaver or radiofrequency apparatus to improve the scaphoid extension. Arthroscopic lunate excision is then performed from the midcarpal joint. With the arthroscope introduced from MCR portal, an arthroscopic burr of 2.9 mm is inserted into MCU portal and directed toward the distal surface of the lunate. The lunate is burred at high speed from articular surface down to the core cancellous bone. Bone debris is removed by intermittently applied suction. To avoid accidental damage of the adjacent articular surfaces to be preserved, a shell of cartilage can be left intact until majority of the cancellous bone is removed. This shell of cartilage can help to separate the burr from the adjacent carpal bone during the burring process. This can be removed piecemeal at the end of the lunate excision procedure by using a small pituitary rongeur or an arthroscopic punch. In order to speed up the process, arthroscopic burr of progressive increase in size such as 3.5 mm and even 4.5 mm can be used when there is more space open up after part of the lunate is removed.

Once the lunate is cleared, attention can be paid to the fusion of the scaphocapitate joint. The arthroscope is now inserted through MCU portal while the MCR portal is reserved for arthroscopic instruments. The articular surface between the scaphoid and capitate is denuded of cartilage with 2.9 mm burr with the principle as described earlier. The articular cartilage at the STT joint area should remain intact.

Fig. 30.57 Intraoperative fluoroscopy shows good position of the guide pins across the radiolunate joint

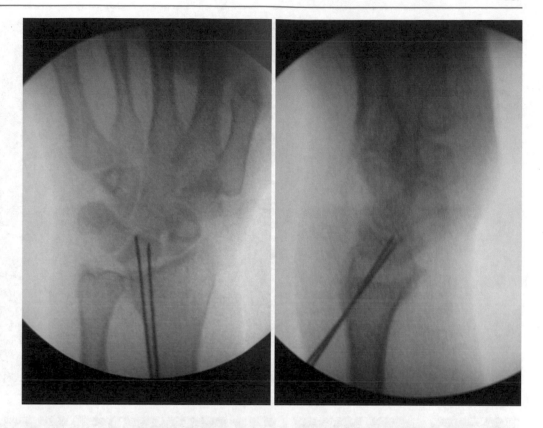

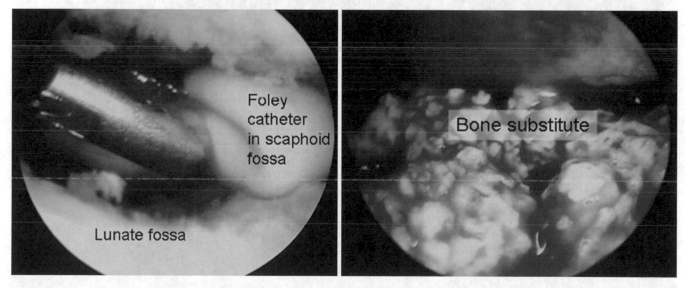

Fig. 30.58 Arthroscopic view showing position of Foley catheter at the scaphoid fossa and granule form of bone substitute at radiolunate joint space

The wrist is taken off from the wrist tower. A small stab wound is being made at the anatomical snuff box area. The ministab wound should be bluntly dissected to avoid iatrogenic injury to the radial artery and terminal branches of the radial nerve until the bony cortex of scaphoid is reached. With the help of an anteroposterior and lateral projection under an image intensifier, two guide wires of a small cannulated screw system with adequate space in between are being inserted and driven across the scaphoid toward capitate. To avoid injury to the vessel, the guide pins can be inserted through a metal sheath of a 14G angiocatheter serving as a guide.

In SC fusion, the articular congruency achieved between the scaphoid and the capitate is typically good. The use of bone graft or substitute is optional. Conversion of the K-wire fixation with cannulated screws is then followed as described

Fig. 30.59 Final definitive fixation of radiolunate joint with two percutaneous bold screws. Noted that both radioscaphoid and ulnocarpal joint were free of bone substitute due to blockage by Foley catheter

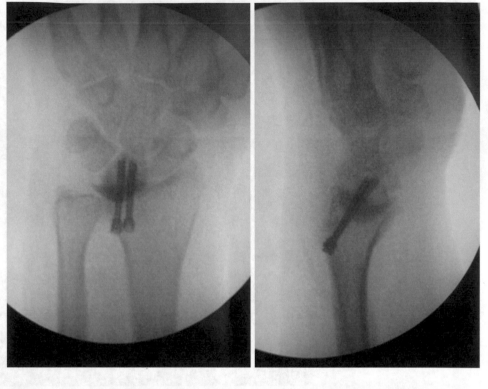

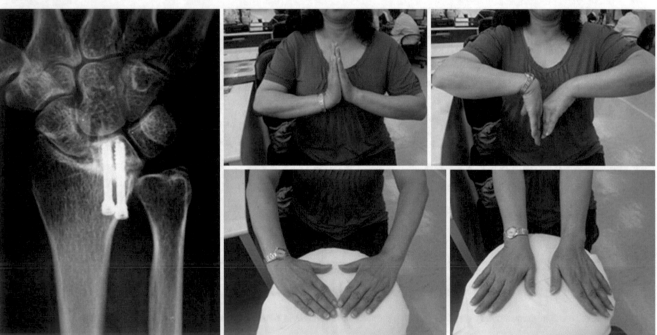

Fig. 30.60 Solid bone union at 6 months postoperative and clinical range of motion of the left wrist. Patient was pain free and returned to normal duty as office assistant

Fig. 30.61 Patient with chronic ulnar wrist pain for 2 years. X-ray reviewed an increased lunotriquetral interval. Arthroscopy confirmed Geissler grade 3 lunotriquetral instability

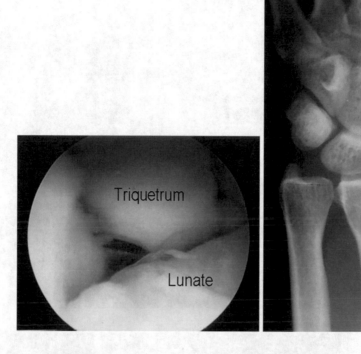

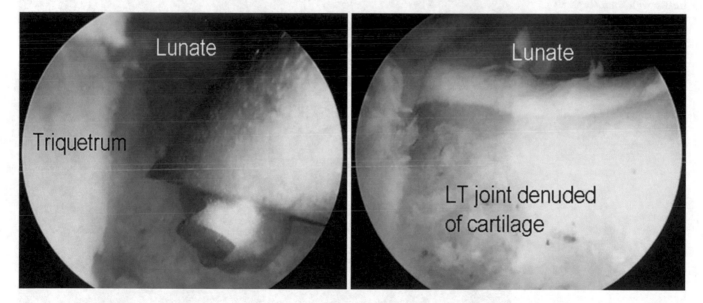

Fig. 30.62 Burring of the lunotriquetral joint before fusion

Fig. 30.63 Arthroscopic view of the screw in the lunotriquetral joint, which is eventually covered with arthroscopic bone graft. X-ray shows good fusion position

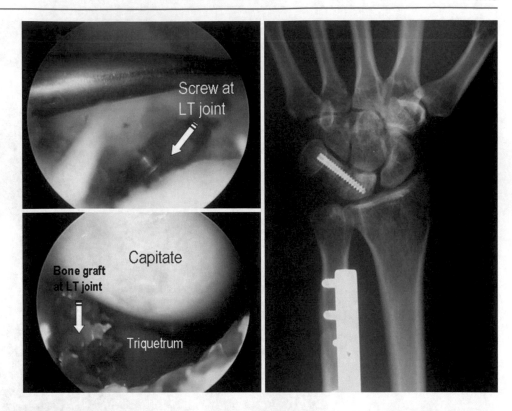

Fig. 30.64 Another patient with complete LT dissociation treated with arthroscopic LT fusion using two compression screws

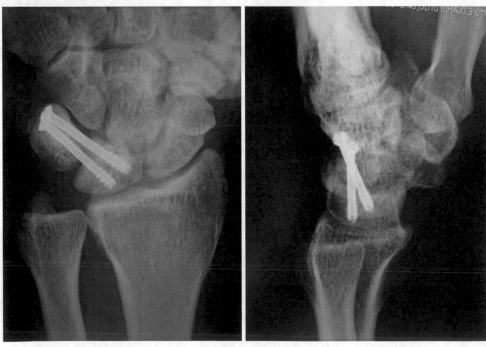

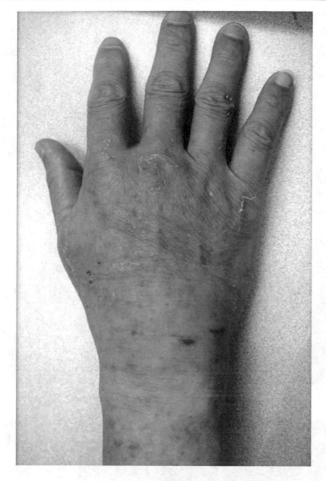

Fig. 30.65 Minimal scarring over surgical wounds

Fig. 30.66 A 22-year-old male semiprofessional tennis player with right dominant wrist Kienbock's disease stage IIIb for 5 years

previously (Fig. 30.68). Stability and range of motion of the wrist can be checked under fluoroscopic guidance.

Wounds are then closed with steri-strips and a comfortable bulky dressing is applied supported with a short arm plaster slab. The slab is changed to a removable wrist splint after the first week, when gentle active mobilization of the wrist can be initiated out of splint under the supervision of a hand therapist (Fig. 30.69). Passive wrist mobilization and strengthening exercise can be offered when radiological and clinical union is evidenced, usually around 8–10 weeks postoperative (Figs. 30.70 and 30.71).

Outcome and Complications

From November 1997 to October 2011, we had performed arthroscopic partial wrist fusion in 23 patients, including 19 males and 4 females. The indications were SLAC wrist in six, SNAC wrist in five, chronic LT instability in two, Kienbock's disease in three, posttraumatic arthrosis in five, and inflammatory arthritis in two. The average duration of symptom was 34.2 months (range 9–82 months). These procedures included STT fusion in three, scaphoidectomy plus four corners fusion in five, scaphoidectomy plus capitolunate fusion in four, lunatectomy plus scaphocapitate fusion in three, radioscapholunate fusion in four, radiolunate fusion in two, and lunotriquetral fusion in two. The average age of the patients at time of surgery was 42 (range 18–68 years old). Concomitant arthroscopic procedures were performed in

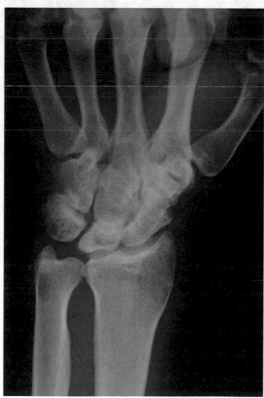

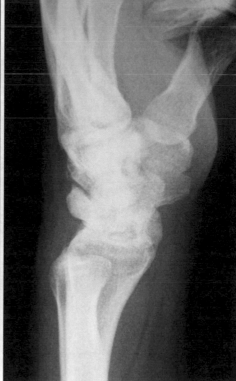

Fig. 30.67 MRI images of
the right wrist show severe
avascular necrosis and
complete fragmentation
collapse of the lunate

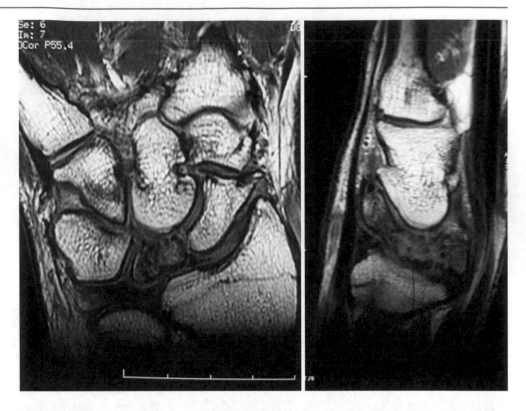

Fig. 30.68 The patient
underwent arthroscopic lunate
excision and scaphocapitate
fusion with two headless
cannulated screws augmented
with injectable demineralized
bone matrix at the fusion
interface

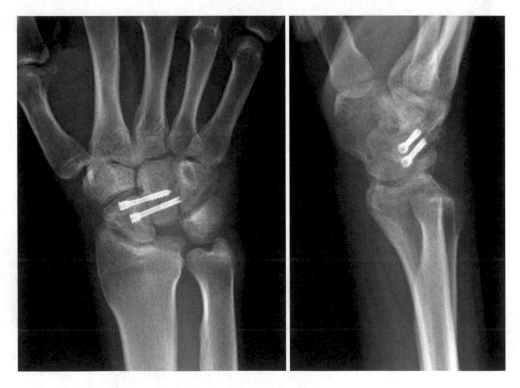

four patients and they included radial styloidectomy, TFCC reconstruction with palmaris longus graft, Wafer procedure, and endoscopic carpal tunnel release. Autogenous bone graft was used in nine patients, while bone substitute was employed in another nine patients. Radiological union of the fusion site was obtained in 19 cases, stable asymptomatic fibrous union in three cases, and definite nonunion requiring

revision in one case. Break down of union rate according to the surgical types is shown in Table 30.1.

The median time of radiological union in the united cases was 10 weeks (range 5–50 weeks). The average follow-up time was 59.9 months (range 11–112 months). The three cases of fibrous union remained asymptomatic and no further surgery or treatment was required. It was notable that both cases of LT fusion ended up in fibrous union. Among the bony union cases, three patients had continuing pain and required further treatment including wrist fusion in two and Amandy interposition arthroplasty in one patient. Two patients required a combined anterior and posterior interosseous nerve neurectomy as secondary procedure for complete pain relief. At final follow-up, all except one patient had no pain or minimal residual pain (Figs. 30.72 and 30.73). The case of RL fusion using percutaneous screw fixation and injectable bone substitute failed to heal in 9 months despite optimal internal fixation and was revised successfully with open RL fusion using iliac crest block bone graft and plating. Intraoperatively marked osteolysis was noted at the fusion site though no evidence of infection was obtained. The final outcome was excellent (Figs. 30.74, 30.75, 30.76, 30.77 and 30.78). All arthroscopic surgical scars were almost invisible

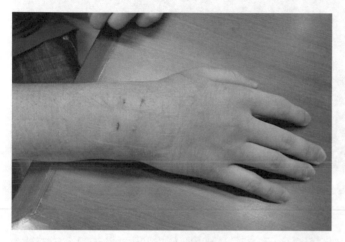

Fig. 30.69 Right wrist condition at 2 weeks postoperative showing minimal swelling and scars

Fig. 30.70 Solid fusion and excellent aesthetic result at 11 months postoperative

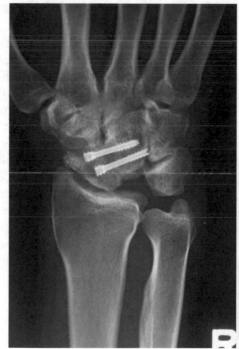

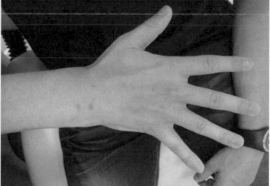

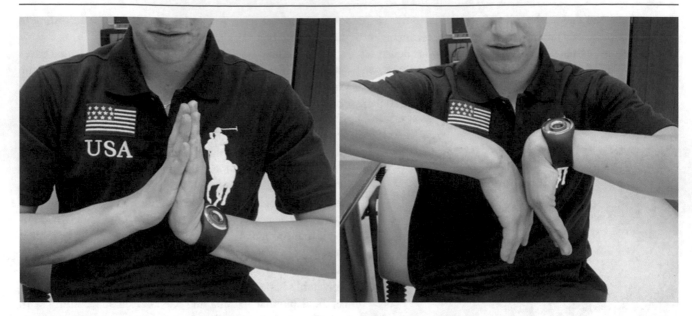

Fig. 30.71 Patient retained 45° extension and 55° flexion at the wrist. He resumed competitive tennis sport activities at 6 months postoperative

Table 30.1 Break down of union rate according to the surgical types

	Bony union	Fibrous union	Nonunion
STT fusion	2	1	
LT fusion		2	
Scaphoidectomy + four corners fusion	5		
Scaphoidectomy + CL fusion	4		
Lunatectomy + SC fusion	3		
RSL fusion	4		
RL fusion	1		1
Total	19	3	1

at the final follow-up and all patients were satisfied with the clinical result.

Complications in our small series of 23 patients were limited. Early complication included two cases of pin tract infection which responded to dressing, antibiotic, and early pin removal. There was one case of superficial second-degree skin burn due to the use of a high-speed burr without a good protective sheath, and one case of delayed union of the radioscapholunate fusion which required 50 weeks to complete the radiological union. One old and osteoporotic patient required removal of the screws at 8 months postoperation due to protrusion of screw threads at the proximal lunate articular surface.

Technically there are potential drawbacks of arthroscopic approach compared to the conventional open techniques. Use of additional bone graft or bone substitute to augment fusion may become mandatory in some cases due to inability to recycle the excised carpal bone as bone graft in situations such as concomitant scaphoidectomy. The small surgical access also limits the choice of use of implant for fixation. K-wire or cannulated screw becomes the usual armamentarium. It can be technically demanding and time-consuming for those less experienced with small joint arthroscopy. Our average operating time was 185 min. Efficiency of current commercially available instruments can also be one of the limiting factors on the speed of the operation.

In conclusion, arthroscopic partial wrist fusion is a viable option for patients suffering from posttraumatic or nonprogressive wrist arthritis who would like to preserve useful wrist motion with good aesthetic outcome. Union rate is high and complication uncommon. However, it is a technically demanding procedure with steep learning curve. Proper training in small joint arthroscopy and further improvement in design and efficacy of the arthroscopic instruments will be helpful in popularizing the technique.

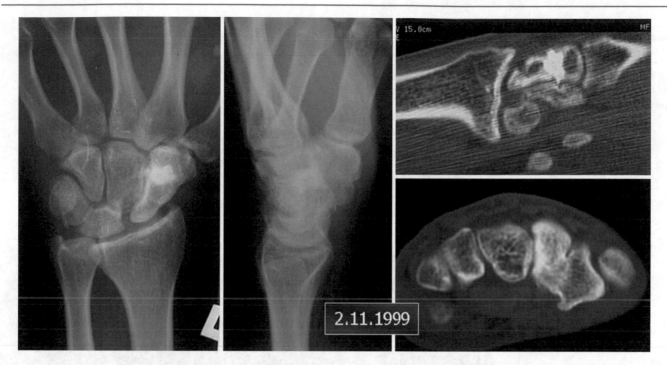

Fig. 30.72 A 22-year-old man with 34 months history of chronic SL dissociation. Arthroscopic STT joint fusion was performed on November 24, 1997. Solid radiological union on X-ray and CT scan was seen 24 months postoperative

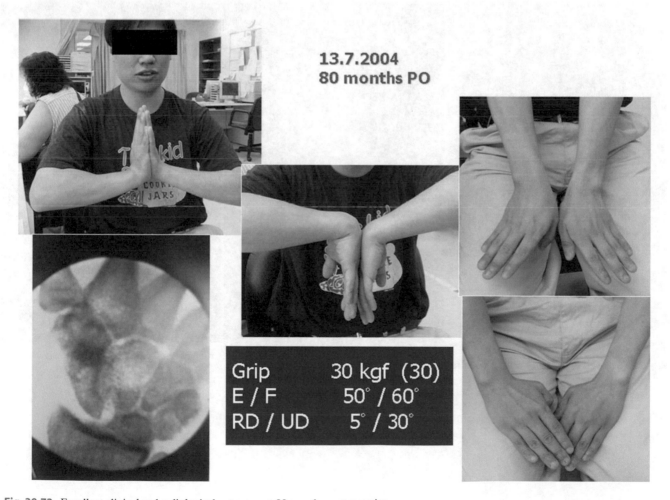

Fig. 30.73 Excellent clinical and radiological outcomes at 80 months postoperative

Fig. 30.74 A 31-year-old man with postdistal radius fracture radiolunate arthrosis. Good alignment and fixation of the arthroscopic radiolunate fusion at 6 weeks postoperative was shown

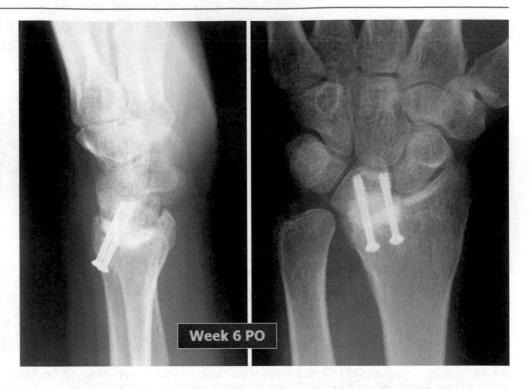

Week 6 PO

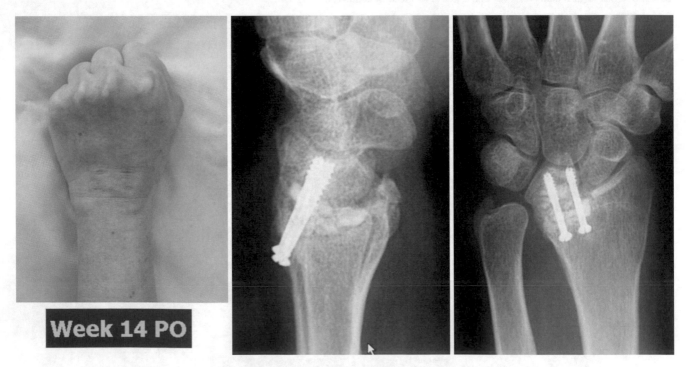

Week 14 PO

Fig. 30.75 Evidence of early osteolysis of fusion site at 14 weeks postoperative

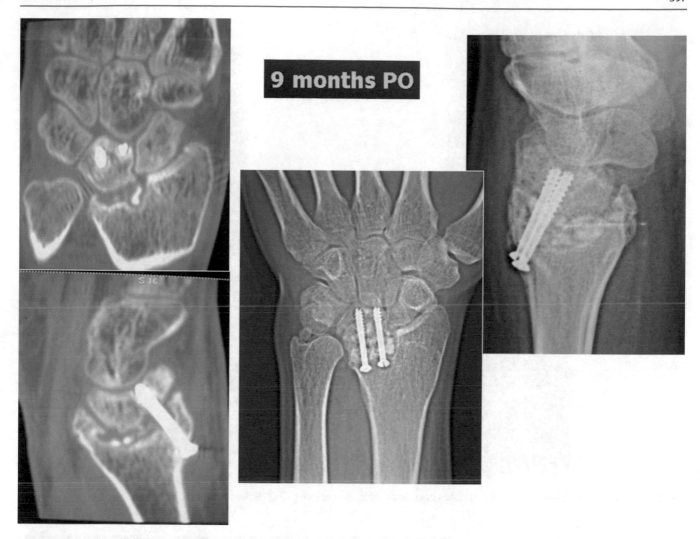

Fig. 30.76 Definite nonunion at 9 months postoperative as shown by X-ray and CT scan

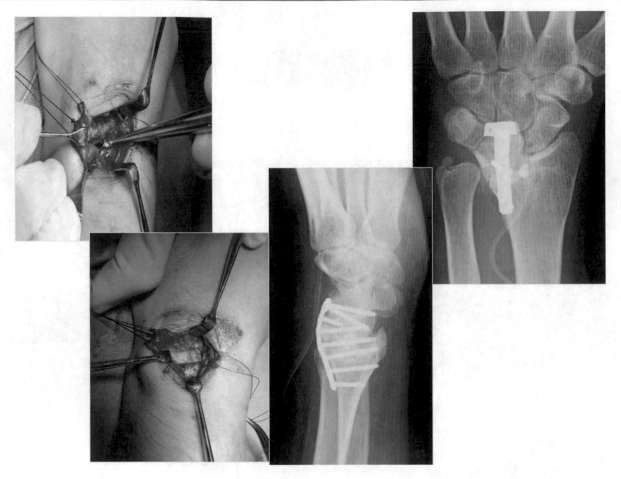

Fig. 30.77 Aseptic nonunion confirmed at revision operation with fusion converted to open iliac crest block bone grafting and plating

Fig. 30.78 Final X-ray at
8.5 years postoperative
showing no ongoing arthrosis
of the wrist

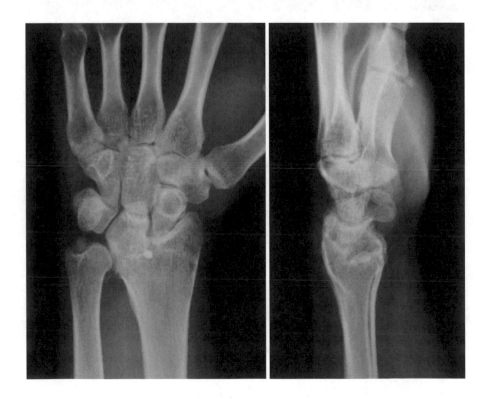

References

1. Krimmer H, Wiemer P, Kalb K. Comparative outcome assessment of the wrist joint-mediocarpal partial arthrodesis and total arthrodesis. Handchir Mikrochir Plast Chir. 2000;32:369–74.
2. Peterson HA, Lipscomb PR. Intercarpal arthrodesis. Arch Surg. 1967;95:127–34.
3. Hasting DE, Silver RL. Intercarpal arthrodesis in the management of chronic carpal instability after trauma. J Hand Surg Am. 1984;9:834–40.
4. Minami A, Kato H, Iwasaki N. Limited wrist fusions: comparison of results 22 and 89 months after surgery. J Hand Surg Am. 1999;24:133–7.
5. Tomaino M. Intercarpal fusion for the treatment of scaphoid nonunion. Hand Clin. 2001;17(4):671–86.
6. Siegel LM, Ruby LK. A critical look at intercarpal arthrodesis: review of literature. J Hand Surg Am. 1996;21:717–23.
7. Douglas DP, Peimer CA, Koniuch MP. Motion of the wrist after simulated limited intercarpal arthrodesis: an experimental study. J Bone Joint Surg Am. 1987;69:1413–8.
8. Garcia-Elias M, Cooney WP, An KN. Wrist kinematics after limited intercarpal arthrodesis. J Hand Surg Am. 1989;14A:791–9.
9. Iwasaki N, Genda E, Barrance PJ, et al. Biomechanical analysis of limited intercarpal fusion for the treatment of Kienbock's disease: a three-dimensional theoretical study. J Orthop Res. 1998;16(2):256–63.
10. Kobza PE, Budoff JE, Yeh ML. Management of the scaphoid during four-corner fusion—a cadaveric study. J Hand Surg Am. 2003;28(6):904–9.
11. Middleton A, MacGregor D, Compson JP. An anatomical database of carpal bone measurements for intercarpal arthrodesis. J Hand Surg Br. 2003;28(4):315–8.
12. Hastings H. Arthrodesis (partial and complete). In: Pederson WC, Wolfe SW, editors. Green's operative hand surgery, vol. 1. 5th ed. Philadelphia: Elsevier; 2005.
13. Nagy L, Büchler U. Long-term results of radioscapholunate fusion following fracture of the distal radius. J Hand Surg Am. 1997;22B:705–10.
14. del Piñal F. Dry arthroscopy and its applications. Hand Clin. 2011;27:335–45.
15. Ho PC, Lo WN. Arthroscopic resection of volar ganglion of the wrist: a new technique. Arthroscopy. 2003;19(2):218–21.
16. Sauerbier M, Trankle M, Erdmann D. Functional outcome with scaphotrapeziotrapezoid arthrodesis in the treatment of Kienbock's disease stage III. Ann Plast Surg. 2000;44(6):618–25.
17. Minami A, Kato H, Suenaga N. Scaphotrapeziotrapezoid fusion: long-term follow-up study. J Orthop Sci. 2003;8(3):319–22.
18. Wollstein R, Watson HK. Scaphotrapeziotrapezoid arthrodesis for arthritis. Hand Clin. 2005;21(4):539–43.
19. Sauerbier M, Trankle M. Midcarpal arthrodesis with complete scaphoid excision and interposition bone graft in the treatment of advanced carpal collapse (SNAC/SLAC wrist): operative technique and outcome assessment. J Hand Surg Br. 2000;25(4):341–5.
20. Enna M, Hoepfner P, Weiss AP. Scaphoid excision with four-corner fusion. Hand Clin. 2005;21(4):531–8.
21. Taleisnik J. Subtotal arthrodesis of the wrist joint. Clin Orthop. 1984;187:81–8.
22. Weiss LE, Taras JS, Sweet S, Osterman AL. Lunotriquetral injuries in athletes. Hand Clin. 2000;16:433–8.
23. Ho PC. Arthroscopic partial wrist fusion. Tech Hand Up Extrem Surg. 2008;12:242 65.
24. Slade JF III, Bomback DA. Percutaneous capitolunate arthrodesis using arthroscopic or limited approach. In: Osterman A, Slade III JF, editors. Scaphoid injuries, Atlas of the hand clinics: scaphoid injuries, vol. 8:1; 2003. p. 149–62.
25. Yajima H, Kobata Y, Shigematsu K. Radiocarpal arthrodesis for osteoarthritis following fractures of the distal radius. Hand Surg. 2004;9(2):203–9.
26. Ishikawa H, Murasawa A, Nakazono K. Long-term follow-up study of radiocarpal arthrodesis for the rheumatoid wrist. J Hand Surg Am. 2005;30(4):658–66.
27. Garcia-Elias M, Lluch AL. Resection of the distal scaphoid for scaphotrapeziotrapezoid arthritis. J Hand Surg Br. 1999;24(4):448–52.
28. Guidera PM, Watson HK, Dwyer TA. Lunotriquetral arthrodesis using cancellous bone graft. J Hand Surg Am. 2001;26(3):422–7.
29. Vandesande W, De Smet L, Van Ransbeeck H. Lunotriquetral arthrodesis, a procedure with a high failure rate. Acta Orthop Belg. 2001;67(4):361–7.
30. Sennwald GR, Fischer M, Mondi P. Lunotriquetral arthrodesis: a controversial procedure. J Hand Surg Br. 1995;20(6):755–60.
31. Pisano SM, Peimer CA, Wheeler DR. Scaphocapitate intercarpal arthrodesis. J Hand Surg Am. 1991;9:501–4.

Partial Wrist Fusion

William B. Geissler and Wood W. Dale

Introduction

Wrist pain resulting from degenerative, post-traumatic, or metabolic disease can be debilitating to the patient's ability to perform activities of daily living (ADL) by reducing range of motion (ROM) and grip strength. Degenerative disease from primary osteoarthritis is common, but wrist arthrosis usually is the result of trauma to the wrist or inflammatory conditions such as rheumatoid arthritis (RA). However, other metabolic derangements can also lead to degenerative changes, including avascular necrosis (such as Keinbock's), hemophilia, giant cell tumors of distal radius, and idiopathic chondrolysis [1]. Ligamentous and bony trauma to the wrist can result in carpal instability and, ultimately, degenerative changes. An example of ligamentous injury, such as an injury to the dorsal scapholunate (SL) interosseous ligament (SLIL), can lead to dorsal intercalated segmental instability (DISI) of the carpus, which can ultimately lead to scapholunate advanced collapse (SLAC). An example of bony injury is an injury to the proximal scaphoid, which can disrupt the dorsal carpal arterial branch feeding the proximal pole, ultimately leading to scaphoid nonunion advanced collapse (SNAC). These degenerative conditions can be quite painful to the patient, which can lead to a loss in grip strength and, ultimately, a decrease in function of the affected limb.

Treatments of wrist pain may consist of nonsurgical means such as therapy, splinting, and injections, while minimally invasive surgical techniques include sensory nerve neurectomy (posterior interosseous nerve (PIN) neurolysis) and metaphyseal decompressions. However, the mainstay of surgical treatments includes partial carpal fusions or arthrodesis of affected joints. The intended outcomes of partial wrist fusions are an alleviation of pain and partial preservation of wrist ROM while maintaining as much grip strength as possible. Another alternative surgical treatment is the proximal row carpectomy (PRC), in which the proximal row is excised. The PRC relies on intact proximal capitate and lunate fossa articular surfaces without degenerative changes, as once the proximal row is excised, a new radiocapitate joint will be constructed. The PRC also depends upon an intact radioscaphocapitate ligament to prevent capitate shift. The PRC does provide ROM, grip strength, and pain relief similar to the partial wrist arthrodesis but is routinely not recommended for younger patients; however, Rhagozar and colleagues have recently debated this paradigm [2].

The preservation of wrist strength and ROM seen in partial fusions is meant to allow the patient the highest functional outcome while alleviating pain. Several studies have been done that attempt to define wrist ROM in which activities of daily living (ADL) are still able to be performed. Palmer et al. and Ryu et al. found that 30–60° of wrist extension, 5–54° of wrist flexion, 15–40° of ulnar deviation, and 10–16° of radial deviation are necessary to perform high-function ADLs [3, 4]. However, Nelson showed that ADLs could still be achieved to some degree with only 6° of extension, 5° of flexion, 7° of radial deviation, and 6° of ulnar deviation with the patient compensating through the elbow and shoulder [5]. However, this is very patient-dependent, and post-surgical expectations should be discussed with the patient in depth regarding an intended outcome.

Fusion Subtypes and Techniques

Radiolunate Arthrodesis

Indications for radiolunate (RL) arthrodesis include injuries to the chondral surface of the radiolunate joint that can derive

W. B. Geissler (✉)
Division of Hand and Upper Extremity Surgery, Section of Arthroscopic Surgery and Sports Medicine, Department of Orthopedic Surgery and Rehabilitation, University of Mississippi Medical Center, Jackson, MS, USA

W. W. Dale
Department of Orthopaedic Surgery and Rehabilitation, University of Mississippi Medical Center, Jackson, MS, USA

© Springer Nature Switzerland AG 2022
W. B. Geissler (ed.), *Wrist and Elbow Arthroscopy with Selected Open Procedures*,
https://doi.org/10.1007/978-3-030-78881-0_31

from the "die punch" deformity seen in some types of distal radius fractures but can also be seen, less commonly, in inflammatory conditions such as rheumatoid arthritis (RA). It can be corrected by partial fusion at the radiolunate surface. This can be done with screws, plates, or staples. It is important to restore anatomic height to the lunate, and grafting may be necessary [1]. Contraindications to RL arthrodesis include midcarpal and radioscaphoid degenerative changes. Patients should be counseled to expect ~50% ROM loss to the surgical side, a 9–12-month recovery, and a risk of progression to midcarpal degeneration.

Scaphocapitate Arthrodesis

Indications for scaphocapitate arthrodesis include injuries to the scaphoid and scapholunate ligaments. It can cause dynamic and rotatory subluxation of the scaphoid in relation to the other carpal bones, scaphoid fracture nonunions, and lunate avascular necrosis (Keinbock's). Contraindications to Scaphocapitate (ScC) arthrodesis include any radioscaphoid and scaphotrapeziotrapezoid (STT) degeneration. Arthrodesis can be achieved by using cannulated compression screw fixation or staples. Patients should be counseled to expect ~50% ROM loss and ~20% loss of grip strength as well as ~4-month recovery time.

Radioscapholunate Arthrodesis

Indications for radioscapholunate arthrodesis include injuries to the chondral surfaces from post-traumatic proximal row destruction, chondrolysis, infection, and inflammatory arthritis such as RA. Contraindications include midcarpal degenerative changes. Patients should be counseled to expect ~50% ROM loss.

Scapholunate Arthrodesis

Indications for scapholunate arthrodesis mainly consist of SLIL injuries leading to SL disassociation. It is important to anatomically reduce both the scaphoid and lunate before arthrodesis. Motion at the scaphoid can be unpredictable and, as such, arthrodesis of the SL joint has varying results [6]. SL arthrodesis has fallen out of favor for its unpredictable outcomes and 50–85% nonunion rates [6, 7].

Lunotriquetral Arthrodesis

Indications for lunotriquetral arthrodesis include lunotriquetral disassociation leading to instability and a painful joint [8]. Contraindications are midcarpal arthritis or instability and ulnocarpal impingement in the presence of lunotriquetral dissociation. Nonunion rates can be as high as 30% [7], and patients should be counseled to expect a 30–40% loss of ROM with a recovery of ~9–12 months.

Scaphotrapeziotrapezoid Arthodesis

Indications for scaphotrapeziotrapezoid (STT) arthrodesis not only include a myriad of pathologies, such as obvious STT arthritis, but also include scaphoid instability and subluxation, SL disassociation, midcarpal instability, Keinbock's, and congenital synchondrosis of the STT joint. Contraindications include radioscaphoid degenerative changes and carpometacarpal (CMC) arthritis. Fixation techniques involve removable Kirschner wires (K-wires), staples, circular plates, and headless compression screws. Watson has reported results of only 20–20% loss of ROM, only 10–30% loss of grip strength, as well as a 20% nonunion rate [9]. Radial styloid impingent on the scaphoid is a concern with this surgery and a radial styloidectomy is recommended [10].

Capitate-Hamate-Lunate-Triquetrum Arthrodesis (4-Corner Fusion or 4CF) with Scaphoid Excision

Indications for the 4-corner fusion include the SLAC and SNAC midcarpal arthritic patterns. Contraindications include any degenerative changes to the radiolunate joint. After excision of the scaphoid, the lunate, capitate, hamate, and triquetrum form 4-bone, cross-shaped mass that is then fused. The radiolunate surface must not show any degenerative changes. The 4-corner fusion is thought to be superior to the capitolunate arthrodesis (2-corner fusion) by some [1] and is preferred over PRC in younger patients. The arthrodesis is generally achieved with a circular plate and screw fixation after the scaphoid is excised. This circular plate can be radiolucent or radiopaque. The excised scaphoid can be used as bone grafting between the four carpi to achieve a greater fusion rate. Removable Kirschner wire fixation is also an option in which the pins can be buried in the subcutaneous tissues or left exposed and are generally removed around 8 weeks. Staple fixation is another option with staples placed between hamate-capitate, hamate-triquetrum, and lunate capitate, respectively. Headless compression screws are another option of treatment. Patients should be told to expect a 30% loss of ROM of the affected wrist, 10% loss in grip strength, as well as an 11% nonunion rate and a 9–12-month recovery depending on treatment modality [11]. As mentioned in the introduction, Rhagozar and colleagues showed that conversion rates to total wrist arthroplasty are significantly higher with a partial wrist arthroplasty (19.2%) than with a PRC (4.9%) and have a greater associated direct cost. Moreover, this included younger patients, who were considered better surgical candidates for partial wrist arthroplasty (PWA) over PRC [2].

Capitolunate Arthodesis (2-Corner Fusion, 2CF, or CLF) with Scaphoid and Possible Triquetral Excision

Indications for the 2-corner fusion are essentially the same as for the 4-corner fusion. It is used for SLAC and SNAC reconstruction. The scaphoid is excised and the lunate and capitate are brought together and fused. The 2-corner fusion is considered less invasive than the 4-corner fusion, but it is thought that the 2-corner fusion has less fusion area and should have a higher rate of nonunion. Gaston et al. showed a 50% loss or ROM compared to the contralateral side and a 30% loss in grip strength. Dunn and colleagues recently showed a nonunion rate of only 4% in an analysis of 80 patients. They also showed only an 8% loss in grip strength and a well-preserved arc or ROM (71° flexion-extension). The triquetrum can be excised for ease of lunate reduction, elimination of the risk for pisotriquetral arthritis, and decreased articulations that require preparation and grafting. Moreover, Gaston et al. found that in three of four CLA patients in whom the triquetrum was not excised, the headless compression screw fixation became loose and required removal. One limitation of triquetral excision is the decreased area available for arthrodesis.

Partial Wrist Fusions

Surgical Technique: Plate 4-Corner Arthrodesis

Plate fixation for partial wrist fusion has an inherit high complication rate, but by following attention to detail, this can help decrease the complication rate (Fig. 31.1). A standard dorsal approach is made to the wrist. The extensor pollicis longus is initially identified and retracted and released through the third compartment. The second and fourth dorsal compartments are then elevated, exposing the dorsal capsule. A radial-based flap is made to expose the carpus. It is important to identify and release the extensor digiti minimi so it will not be injured when one opens the capsule to avoid injury. A wide exposure has to be made for the 4-corner fusion. The first step is to incise and remove the scaphoid. The scapholunate interosseous ligament is completely incised and the wrist is hyper-flexed. Again, a wide capsule release allows the wrist to be easier flexed to remove the scaphoid. Small retractors are placed around the scaphoid to

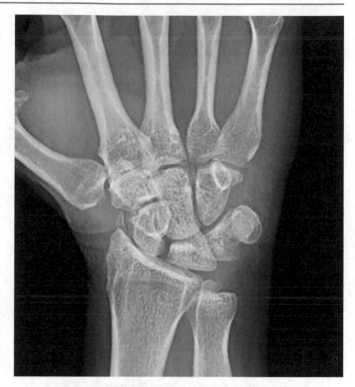

Fig. 31.1 Anterior–posterior radiograph demonstrating chronic scapholunate instability with radioscaphoid arthritis

help lever out the bone. The key is not to cut the radioscapholunate ligament. If this is cut, it will result in ulnar translation.

A large 0.062 Kirschner wire is inserted into the lunate. This gives good control and rotation of the lunate so the midcarpal space can be opened and the articular cartilage of the distal aspect of the lunate, triquetrum, and the proximal aspect of the capitate and hamate is totally removed. It's very important to remove all of the articular cartilage for a successful fusion.

The key in a partial fusion is to fuse the lunate in neutral or slightly over corrected. A K-wire jail is made (Figs. 31.2 and 31.3). The key step is to pin the lunate to the radius in this neutral or overcorrected position; this should be maintained during the reaming of the plate. The Kirschner wires should be placed in the volar aspect of the carpus so that the reams for the plate will not engage in the Kirschner wires and disrupt the provisional fixation. The Kirschner wires are placed in oscillation mode to avoid damage or injury to the sensory branches of the nerve throughout the wrist. The lunate should not be overcorrected radially on the capitate but should be pinned in its normal anatomic relationship to the capitate. This potentially allows improved ROM to the wrist. When reaming the carpus, it's important that the plate sits below the dorsal aspect of the carpus (Figs. 31.4 and 31.5). If the plate is not recessed below the carpus, it can block wrist extension. Additionally, it is important not to

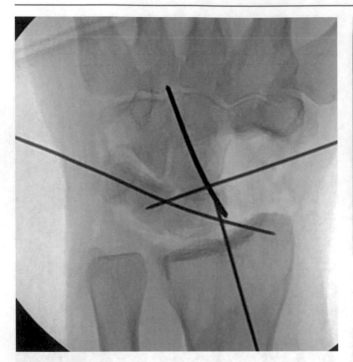

Fig. 31.2 Fluoroscopic view showing pinning of the lunate in a neutral position in the anterior–posterior plane under fluoroscopy

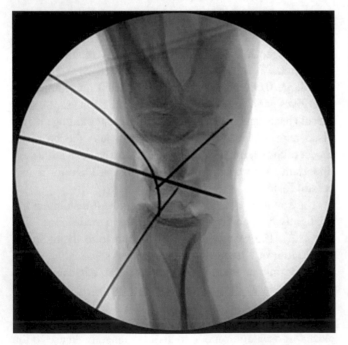

Fig. 31.3 Lateral radiograph showing the lunate pinned in a neutral position under fluoroscopy

over-ream for the plate so that if there is not enough bone along the volar aspect for the screws to get purchase. It is important when the plate is placed and the screws are inserted that they are not too long to avoid injury to the ulnar neuro-vascular structures (Fig. 31.6). Particularly on inserting the screws to the hamate, beware of injury to the ulnar nerve. Usually, screws of 10–12 mm are being used.

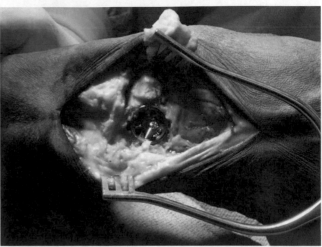

Fig. 31.4 Intra-operative photograph showing placement of the 4-corner partial fusion plate

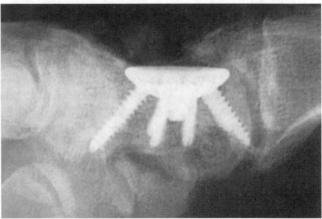

Fig. 31.5 Lateral radiograph demonstrating placement of the 4-corner fusion plate resected below the dorsal aspect of the carpus to prevent impingement with wrist extension

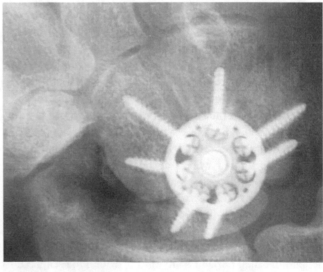

Fig. 31.6 Anterior–posterior radiograph demonstrating the successful union of a 4-corner fusion with plate fixation

To improve ROM, only close the ulnar edge of the capsule. Leaving the proximal and distal edges open will potentially allow for more flexion. The second and fourth dorsal compartments, are closed and the extensor pollicis longus is left free.

Surgical Technique: Headless Screw Stabilization for 4-Corner Fusion

A standard dorsal approach to the wrist is made as described above. A wide radial-based capsule flap is performed to expose the carpus (Fig. 31.7). Again, the scaphoid is removed (Fig. 31.8). The articular cartilage is removed from the midcarpal space with a large Kirschner wire in the lunate to control rotation and open up the midcarpal space (Fig. 31.9). Demineralized bone matrix is placed at the fusion site (Fig. 31.10). The joystick is then used to pull the lunate dorsally and reduce the rotation to neutral or slightly overcorrected and a guidewire is placed down the center of the axis of the lunate into the capitate (Fig. 31.11). Two guidewires are placed to help hold rotation as the carpus is drilled so the reduction is not lost as the first guidewire is drilled

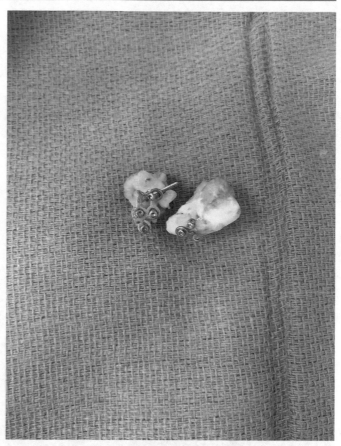

Fig. 31.8 Intra-operative radiograph showing nonunion of the scaphoid despite vascularized bone fixation

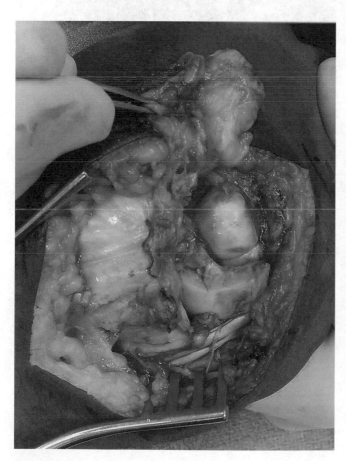

Fig. 31.7 Intra-operative radiograph demonstrating a radial-based flap exposing the carpus in a scaphoid nonunion

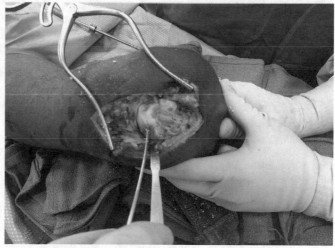

Fig. 31.9 Intra-operative photograph using control of the guidewire into the lunate to expose the midcarpal joint. The articular cartilage off the proximal aspect of the lunate, triquetrum, and the distal aspect of the capitate and hamate has been removed

(Fig. 31.12). The guidewire is measured, and a headless screw at least 4-mm shorter is inserted from the lunate into the capitate (Fig. 31.13). It is important to insert these screws

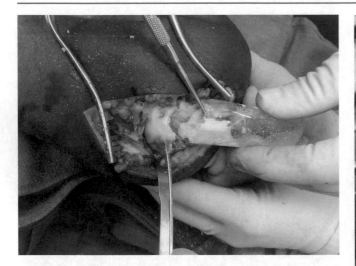

Fig. 31.10 Vivigen allograft bone grafting (Virginia Beach, VA) is added at the fusion sight

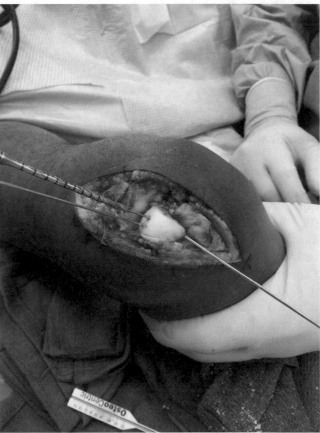

Fig. 31.12 Cannulated drilling of the lunate capitate fusion with the osteocentric drill (Austin, TX)

This capsule is closed on the ulnar aspect, leaving the proximal and distal edges open for improved ROM, particularly in flexion.

Digital ROM exercises are immediately started and the patient is placed in a removable splint 2 weeks post-operatively. Range- and motion-strengthening exercises are initiated at 4 weeks post-operatively (see Fig. 31.14).

Surgical Technique: Radioscapholunate Fusion

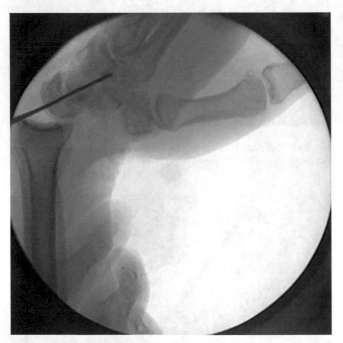

Fig. 31.11 Fluoroscopic view showing provisional pinning of the lunate neutral to the capitate

far up into the carpus, as they can potentially back out. In general, one screw is placed in the lunocapitate interval, one is placed in the lunate-hamate interval, and a third screw is placed from the triquetrum into the hamate (Figs. 31.14 and 31.15). All screws are fully inserted into the carpus to avoid them backing out (Figs. 31.16 and 31.17). The concern for traditional headless screws is that they can back out, causing injury to the articular cartilage of the distal radius (Fig. 31.18).

The standard dorsal approach is made to the wrist as described previously (Fig. 31.19). A wide radial-based flap is made to expose the dorsal carpus. A joystick is placed into the scaphoid to help dorsiflex the bone. This allows for easier excision of this distal pole. The triquetrum is excised as well. The articular cartilage of the distal radius and proximal scapholunate is then removed to subchondral bone. Joysticks are then used to provisionally pin the scaphoid and lunate to the distal radius (Fig. 31.20). It's important not to overcor-

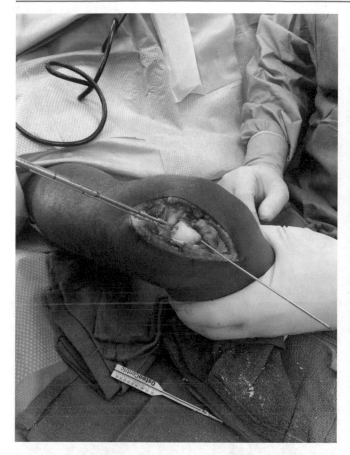

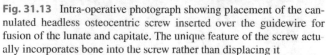

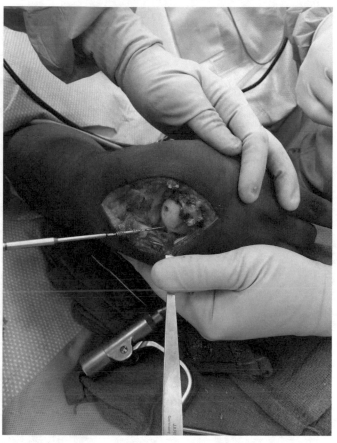

Fig. 31.13 Intra-operative photograph showing placement of the cannulated headless osteocentric screw inserted over the guidewire for fusion of the lunate and capitate. The unique feature of the screw actually incorporates bone into the screw rather than displacing it

Fig. 31.14 A second osteocentric screw (Austin, TX) is placed from the triquetrum into the hamate for the 4-corner fusion

rect the interval between the scaphoid and lunate in order to allow the normal relationship of the capitate to sit in the fossa. The lunate should be pinned at neutral position or a slightly volar tilt. A headless cannulated screw is then placed over the guidewire from the scaphoid into the radius, and a second headless screw from the lunate is placed into the distal radius (Figs. 31.21 and 31.22). Excision of the distal portion of the scaphoid and triquetrum allows easy access for placement of the cannulated screws. Demineralized bone matrix is placed at the fusion site prior to the fusion. The dorsal capsule is then closed in its most ulnar aspect, leaving the dorsal and proximal edges free to help improve wrist flexion. The second and fourth dorsal compartments are closed, and the extension pollicis longus is let free (Figs. 31.23 and 31.24).

Tips and Tricks

Partial Wrist Fusion: Plate Fixation

- It is important to reduce the lunate in neutral or slightly overcorrected with a volar tilt. An easy way to do this is to pin the lunate from itself to the radius utilizing a joystick. Increased volar tilt allows for more wrist extension.
- It is important to place the provisional fixation in the volar aspect of the carpus so as one reams for the plate, it does not disrupt the provisional fixation.
- It is important to place the plate volar to the dorsal carpus so the plate does not block dorsal extension.
- It is important not to over-ream the carpus so there is adequate bone left for screw purchase.

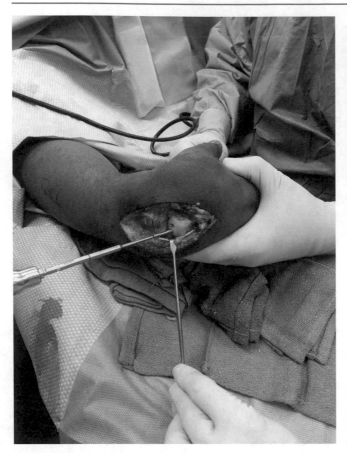

Fig. 31.15 A third osteocentric screw (Austin, TX) is placed from the lunate into the hamate to complete the 4-corner fusion

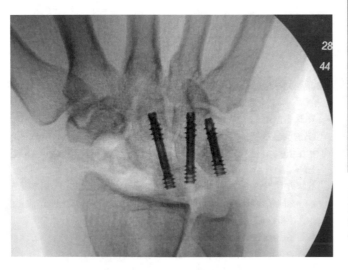

Fig. 31.16 Fluoroscopic view in the anterior–posterior plane showing the 4-corner fusion with screws placed from the lunate into the capitate lunate, into the hamate, and triquetrum into hamate

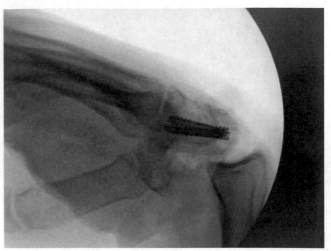

Fig. 31.17 Lateral radiograph showing placement of the osteocentric screws in the 4-corner fusion

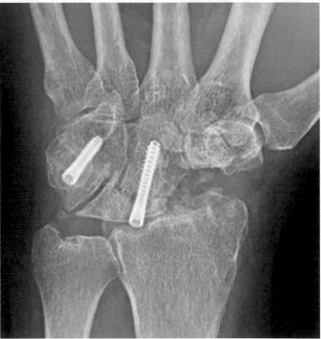

Fig. 31.18 Anterior–posterior radiograph showing headless cannulated screws backing out from the previous 4-corner fusion with potential injury to the articular cartilage of the distal radius. This is the concern of headless screws in 4-corner fusion

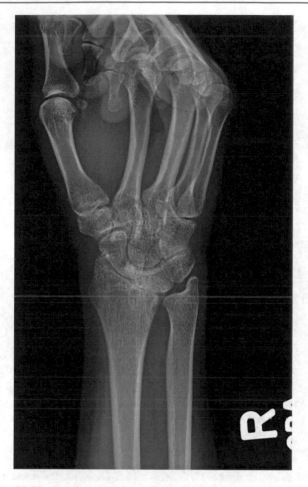

Fig. 31.19 Anterior–posterior radiograph of a young patient with rheumatoid arthritis involving the radiocarpal joint

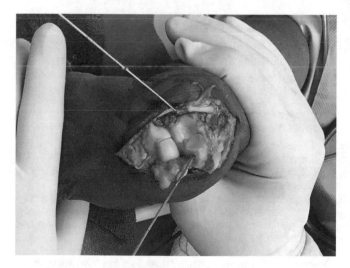

Fig. 31.20 The carpus is provisionally pinned after excision of the distal pole of the scaphoid and excision of the triquetrum. This allows for increased ROM to the wrist joint following unlocking the midcarpal joint

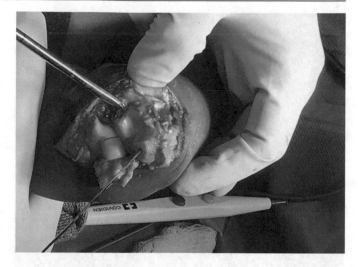

Fig. 31.21 A cannulated drill is used to drill the hole for the headless cannulated screws

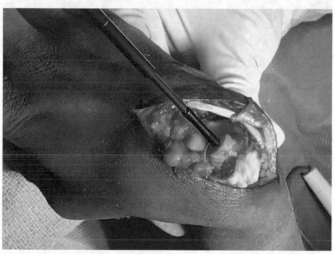

Fig. 31.22 The Acutrak (Beaverton, OR) headless cannulated screw is then inserted over the headless cannulated guidewire

Headless Screw Fixation

- It is important to use a guidewire to reduce the lunate onto the capitate. The goal is not to over-reduce the lunate to the radial in relation to the capitate, but to its normal anatomic position. The goal is to reduce the lunate to neutral, or slightly over-corrected in a volar tilt position.
- It is very important to always use a screw at least 4-mm shorter than it was measured so the headless screw can be inserted fully up into the carpus and not back out to violate the articular cartilage of the distal radius. Usually three screws are utilized: one from the lunate to the capitate, one from lunate into the hamate, and one from the triquetrum into the hamate.

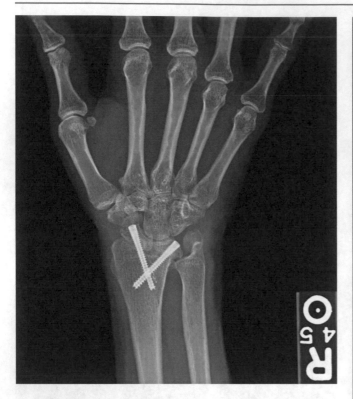

Fig. 31.23 Anterior–posterior radiograph at final follow-up showing successful fusion of the radiocarpal space

Radioscapholunate Fusion

- It is helpful to excise the distal pole of the scaphoid and the triquetrum in a radial scapholunate fusion. This will allow more motion through the midcarpal space. It also allows easier access for headless cannulated screws to be placed from the scaphoid and lunate into the distal radius.
- It is important not to over-compress the scapholunate interval to allow for the normal articulation for the capitate. The headless screws are placed and recessed below the distal aspect for the scaphoid and the remaining lunate.

Conclusion

Partial wrist fusions can be achieved using a variety of methods depending on the pathology. The goals of the partial fusions are to essentially preserve as much natural ROM and strength as possible while alleviating pain when compared to the total wrist arthrodesis or arthoplasty. Complication rates and nonunion rates vary with the type of fusion and pathol-

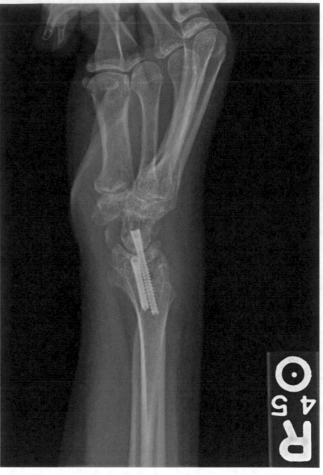

Fig. 31.24 Lateral radiograph showing successful fusion of the radiocarpal space

ogy. Recent data have shown that the PRC may have a lower conversion rate to the PWA and may be considered for younger patients. The 2-corner fusion has recently shown similar outcomes as the 4-corner fusion.

References

1. Rizzo M, Wolfe SW, Pederson WC, Hotchkiss RN, Kozin SH, Cohen MS. Green's operative hand surgery. 7th ed. Philadelphia: Elsevier Health Sciences; 2016.
2. Rahgozar P, Zhong L, Chung KC. A comparative analysis of resource utilization between proximal row carpectomy and partial wrist fusion: a population study. J Hand Surg Am. 2017;42(10):773–80.
3. Palmer AK, Werner FW, Murphy D, Glisson R. Functional wrist motion: a biomechanical study. J Hand Surg Am. 1985;10(1):39–46.

4. Ryu JY, Cooney WP 3rd, Askew LJ, An KN, Chao EY. Functional ranges of motion of the wrist joint. J Hand Surg Am. 1991;16(3):409–19.

5. Nelson DL. Functional wrist motion. Hand Clin. 1997;13(1):83–92.

6. Hom S, Ruby LK. Attempted scapholunate arthrodesis for chronic scapholunate dissociation. J Hand Surg Am. 1991;16(2):334–9.

7. Larsen CF, Jacoby RA, McCabe SJ. Nonunion rates of limited carpal arthrodesis: a meta-analysis of the literature. J Hand Surg Am. 1997;22(1):66–73.

8. Kirschenbaum D, Coyle MP, Leddy JP. Chronic lunotriquetral instability: diagnosis and treatment. J Hand Surg Am. 1993;18(6):1107–12.

9. Watson HK, Wollstein R, Joseph E, Manzo R, Weinzweig J, Ashmead D 4th. Scaphotrapeziotrapezoid arthrodesis: a follow-up study. J Hand Surg Am. 2003;28(3):397–404.

10. Rogers WD, Watson HK. Radial styloid impingement after triscaphe arthrodesis. J Hand Surg Am. 1989;14(2 Pt 1):297–301.

11. Neubrech F, Mühldorfer-Fodor M, Pillukat T, van Schoonhoven J, Prommersberger KJ. Long-term results after midcarpal arthrodesis. J Wrist Surg. 2012;2:123–8.

Total Wrist Fusion

William B. Geissler and Wood W. Dale

Introduction

In advanced disease, the wrist pain resulting from degenerative, post-traumatic, or metabolic disease can be debilitating due to the patient's ability to perform activities of daily living. Primary osteoarthritis, post-traumatic arthritis, inflammatory conditions such as rheumatoid arthritis, and other metabolic derangements can also lead to degenerative changes. This degeneration is often the cause of pain and loss of grip strength, which can be debilitating to the patient.

Treatments of wrist pain may consist of nonsurgical means such as therapy, splinting, and injections, while minimally invasive surgical techniques include posterior interosseous nerve (PIN) sensory nerve neurectomy and metaphyseal decompressions. Partial wrist fusions and proximal row carpectomies may be considered in localized changes but in many cases the conversion to total wrist arthrodesis or arthroplasty is significant, nearly 20% in some cases of partial wrist fusion [1]. Total wrist arthroplasty may be indicated if the bone stock is retained and the patient is low demand. The total wrist arthroplasty carries the risk of loosening and dislocation with overuse and the patient must be educated in protected use of that wrist. Total wrist arthroplasty also carries a high complication and reoperation rate in which total wrist fusion may be the only salvage before amputation. Pong and colleagues found that the total wrist arthroplasty had a reoperation rate of 29% at 5 years and the largest predictor of a poor outcome for arthroplasty was prior wrist surgeries [2], although this number is significantly lower in other studies such as the ~1% complication rate

seen by Boeckstyns and colleagues, where only 5 of 65 wrists needed revision after total wrist arthroplasty. However, they did find a higher complication rate in patients with rheumatoid arthritis [3]. This high complication rate with rheumatoid arthritis agrees with other studies, such as that of Ward and colleagues, which show up to a 50% complication rate, predominantly consisting of carpal loosening [4].

When the disease has progressed to the point of loss of bone stock, then arthrodesis of the wrist may provide the patient with the best functional outcome with the reduction of pain (Figs. 32.1, 32.2, and 32.3). Pancarpal arthrosis or the failure of prior partial wrist arthrodesis can be an indication for total wrist fusion. Another indication can be paralysis of the wrist joint (such as wrist drop) where a fusion may lead to a better functional outcome.

Function after a total wrist arthrodesis can be obtained but may be patient-specific, as there will be a total loss of wrist range of motion (ROM). Some surgeons recommend having the patients wear a brace prior to surgery to replicate the motion loss they will experience. This loss of ROM can be compensated for by utilization of the elbow and shoulder. Murphy and colleagues found that persons who received arthroplasty over arthrodesis reported a trend toward greater ease with personal hygiene and fastening buttons and that persons who had an arthroplasty on one side and a fusion on the other preferred the arthroplasty over the fusion [5].

Considerations for total wrist fusion may include a carpal tunnel release. Carpal tunnel syndrome can be a complication if the carpal reduction impinges on the carpal tunnel or the carpal tunnel is not adequately reconstructed. Carpal tunnel syndrome has shown to have a rate of almost 10%, with almost 67% requiring a carpal tunnel release [6]. However, using the third metacarpal-to-radius fusion can both radial translate and distract, a complication of pain from ulnocarpal abutment and impingement. The carpal bone usually involved is the triquetrum. If there does not seem to be adequate spacing between the ulna and the triquetrum, the triquetrum should be excised [7]. A proximal row carpectomy has been

W. B. Geissler (✉)
Division of Hand and Upper Extremity Surgery, Section of Arthroscopic Surgery and Sports Medicine, Department of Orthopedic Surgery and Rehabilitation, University of Mississippi Medical Center, Jackson, MS, USA

W. W. Dale
Department of Orthopaedic Surgery and Rehabilitation, University of Mississippi Medical Center, Jackson, MS, USA

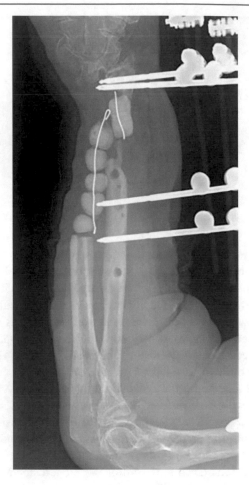

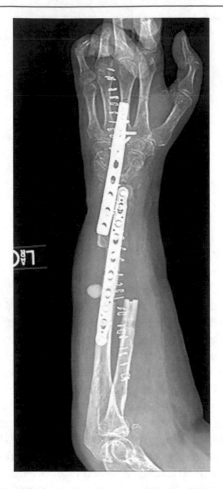

Fig. 32.1 Anterior–posterior radiograph of a patient who had approximately 20 previous operations to the forearm. The patient currently has an external fixator and antibiotic beads. Note the severe bone loss of the distal ulna and ulna translation of the carpus on the radius

Fig. 32.2 Anterior–posterior radiograph demonstrating reconstruction to the forearm. A one bone forearm was created utilizing iliac crest bone graft, and a wrist fusion was performed

successfully described prior to performing the total wrist fusion to prevent ulnocarpal abutment [8].

Fusion Subtypes and Techniques

Several methods provide adequate fusion of the wrist. A successful wrist fusion involves preparation and arthrodesis of the radiolunate, radioscaphoid, lunocapitate, scaphocapitate, and the third or long finger carpometacarpal (CMC) joints.

Plate Fixation

Total wrist fusion utilizing plates involves the preparation of the above joints and a wrist-spanning plate. Modern plates are low-profile, precontoured, and may utilize 3.5-mm screws proximally and 2.7-mm screws distally on the third metacarpal (Fig. 32.4). Locking screws can empower the fixation in patients with poor bone stock. Union rates can be

100% in some studies [6]. Geissler recently designed a wrist fusion plate that curves radial to the index metacarpal. In this manner, it decreases irritation to the extensor tendons. Some surgeons prefer to do a proximal row carpectomy with a wrist fusion. In this technique, only one row at the carpus needs to heal to the distal radius. This may decrease the nonunion note in the wrist fusion as compared to having both carpal rows having to fuse. Geissler designed a wrist fusion plate for surgeons who do a proximal row carpectomy with wrist fusion so the plate size on the long metacarpal. The dorsal distal aspect of the plate is smooth and the screws are placed in an offset direction rather than straight posterior to anterior. In this manner, there is decreased extensor tendon irritation and stronger biomechanically to anterior–posterior wrist arthrodesis.

Intramedullary Pin Fixation

Intramedullary pin fixation can also be utilized, especially in patients with rheumatoid arthritis and poor bone stock.

carpal and is advanced through the carpi and into the distal radius. An additional pin, staple, or plate may be necessary for rotational control.

Surgical Technique

Curved Plate Index Wrist Fusion

The standard dorsal approach is made to the wrist. The extensor pollicis longus is released in the third compartment, and the second and fourth dorsal compartments are elevated (Fig. 32.5). The extensor digiti minimi is identified separately to the fifth compartment and protected. A wide radial base flap is made exposing the carpus. Joysticks are replaced in the proximal row to control rotation and gain access between the midcarpal and radiocarpal spaces (Fig. 32.6). Utilizing a burr, the articular cartilage is removed from both the proximal and distal rows as well the distal aspect of the distal radius. Demineralized bone matrix is placed at the fusion sites. The Acumed curved index plate (Beaverton, OR) is placed on the index metacarpal (Fig. 32.7). There are two different sizes to

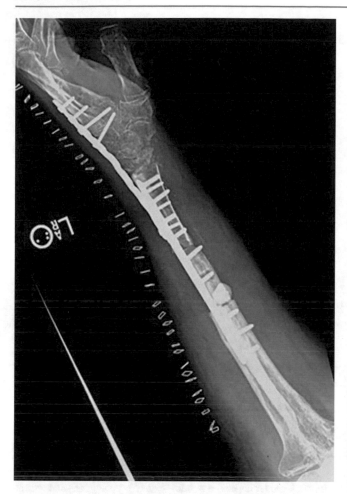

Fig. 32.3 Lateral radiograph following reconstruction of the forearm

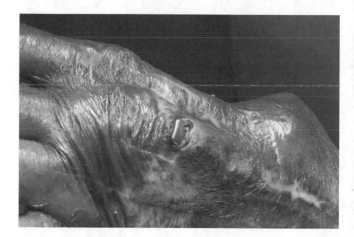

Fig. 32.4 Photograph demonstrating prominence of a wrist fusion plate on the long metacarpal. This caused extensive extensor tendon irritation and problems with the plate protruding through the skin

Clayton first described this method, and Millander and Nailbuff brought it to popularity using a Steinmann pin [9, 10]. The pin is inserted through the head of the third meta-

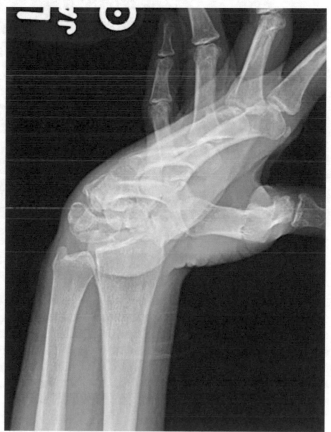

Fig. 32.5 Anterior–posterior radiograph of a patient with multiple distal nerve palsies

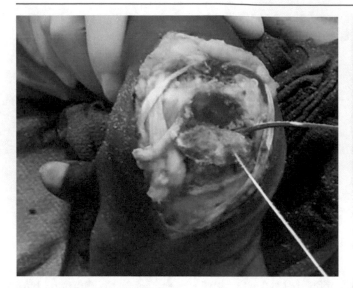

Fig. 32.6 Intra-operative photograph demonstrating removal of the articular cartilage from the proximal and distal rows of the carpus and the distal aspects of the distal radius

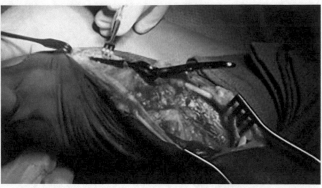

Fig. 32.8 Lateral intra-operative photograph demonstrating placement of the Acumed (Beaverton, OR) curved wrist fusion plate placed on the dorsal aspect of the index metacarpal

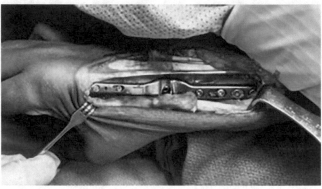

Fig. 32.9 Anterior–posterior intra-operative photograph demonstrating placement of the Acumed (Beaverton, OR) curved fusion plate on the dorsal aspect of the index metacarpal and the distal radius

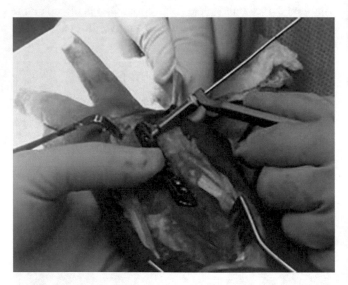

Fig. 32.7 Intra-operative photograph demonstrating placement of the Acumed (Beaverton, OR) curved wrist fusion plate placed on the distal aspect of the index metacarpal

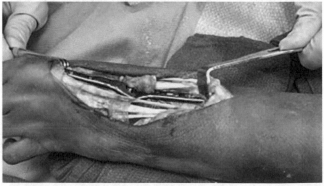

Fig. 32.10 Intra-operative photograph from a lateral view showing placement of the curved wrist fusion plate

correlate with smaller and larger patients. The plate is placed in the dorsal aspect of the index metacarpal and fits along the distal edge of the carpus. The first screw placed is in the oblong hole, which is non-locking to compress the plate down to the index metacarpal. The remaining four locking screws are placed (Fig. 32.8). The wrist is then reduced to the radius, and the first screw placed is in the slot with a 3.5-mm non-locked screw (Figs. 32.9 and 32.10). The second screw is placed in the offset screw to further compress the wrist arthrodesis site. The two remaining 3.5-mm locking screws are placed into the distal radius. The last screw placed with the 3.5-mm locking screw runs across the capitate into a por-

tion of the hamate. It is important not to over-drill this or place a screw too long, which could injure the ulnar neurovascular structures (Figs. 32.11 and 32.12). The dorsal capsule is then closed over the plate to help protect the wrist extensor tendons. The second and fourth dorsal retinaculum is then closed and the extensor pollicis longus is left free.

Neutral Plate Fusion

The standard dorsal approach is made as described and a wide radial base flap is made. With the wrist neutral fusion plate, a proximal row carpectomy is performed. This is particularly useful in patients who have spastic wrist and finger contractures to help gain some length to the contracture (Figs. 32.13 and 32.14). The articular cartilage is removed off the proximal aspect of the capitate, hamate, and the distal aspect for the distal radius. The Acumed neutral wrist fusion plate (Beaverton, OR) is then placed on the dorsal of the long metacarpal (Fig. 32.15). The first screw placed will be on the oblong hole, which is non-locking and compresses the plate to the bone. The remaining four locking screws are then inserted. Notice how the screws are placed at an oblique

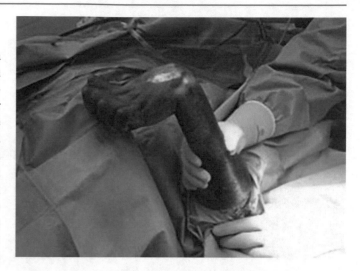

Fig. 32.13 Intra-operative photograph showing severe wrist and finger spastic flexion deformities

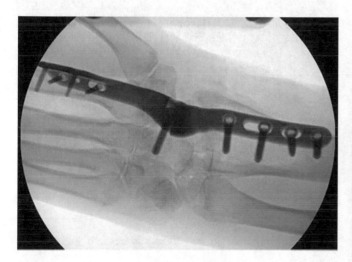

Fig. 32.11 Anterior–posterior fluoroscopic view of the curved wrist fusion plate centered on the index metacarpal. Note good compression of the carpal fusion

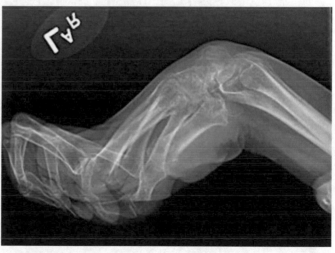

Fig. 32.14 Lateral radiograph demonstrating the severe wrist and finger flexion deformities

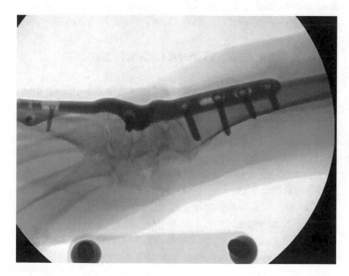

Fig. 32.12 Lateral fluoroscopic view with the curved index fusion plate showing good compression of the radiocarpal space

angle, rather than straight dorsally to decrease extensor tendon irritation. Once the distal portion of the plate has been placed, the wrist is reduced onto the distal radius. Demineralized bone matrix had been placed in prior to this, to help facilitate fusion (Fig. 32.16). The first screw placed will be the 3.5-mm non-locking screw in the slot, and then the offset hole the second 3.5-mm non-locking screw to further compress the fusion site on the distal radius. The remaining two 3.5-mm non-locking screws are inserted onto the plate through the distal radius (Fig. 32.17). The last screw inserted is from the plate into the capitate that decreases micromotion between the remaining carpus and the metacarpals.

The dorsal capsule is then closed over the plate to protect the extensor tendons from irritation, and the second and fourth dorsal compartments are closed (Figs. 32.18 and

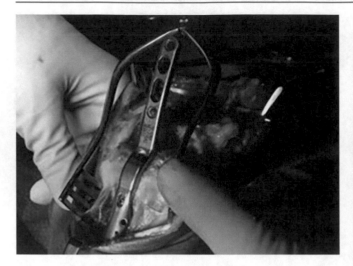

Fig. 32.15 A proximal row carpectomy has been performed to help decrease the length of the wrist to help decrease the spacity of the finger flexors. The neutral wrist fusion plate is initially placed on the long metacarpal. The wrist is reduced and the remaining 3.5-mm locking and non-locking screws are placed through the plate of the distal radius

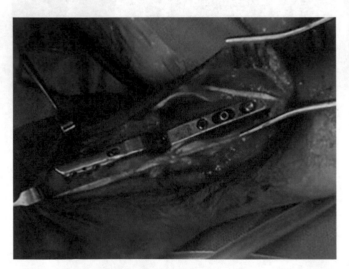

Fig. 32.16 Intra-operative photograph demonstrating the smooth dorsal surface of the neutral fusion plate on the long metacarpal and distal radius

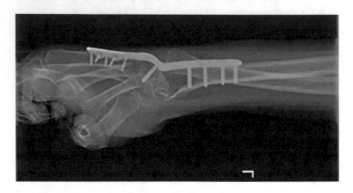

Fig. 32.17 Lateral photograph with the neutral wrist fusion plate. Note good bony contact of the remaining carpus to the distal radius

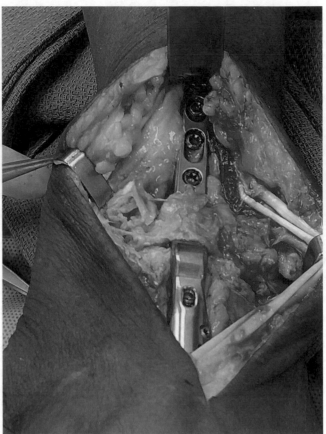

Fig. 32.18 The dorsal capsule is closed over the plate to decrease extensor tendon irritation

32.19). The extensor pollicis longus is left free, and the skin is closed.

Digital range and motion are started immediately, and grip strengthening exercises at 4 weeks.

Tips and Tricks

Total Wrist Fusion: Curved Index Plate

- It is important to place the first screw in the oblong hole, which is a non-locking slot. This compresses the plate to the bone.
- The remaining distal locking screws are placed.
- The carpus is introduced, the distal radius with the first screw placed in a 3.5-mm oblong hole to compress the plate to the bone.
- The offset 3.5-mm screw is then placed to further compress the carpus.
- It is important to place the carpal screw from the capitate in the hamate to decrease micromotion between the carpus and meta-carpus.
- It is important not to over-drill the carpal screw to avoid injury to the ulnar nerve vascular bundle.

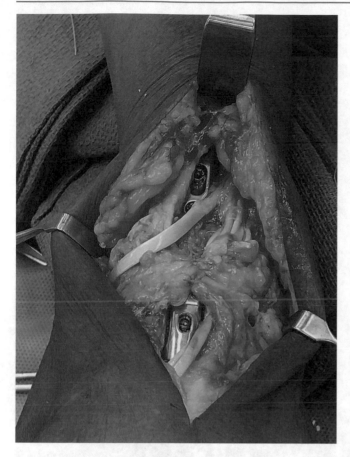

Fig. 32.19 The second and fourth dorsal compartments are closed and the EPL is left free

Neutral Plate

- It is important to remove all of the bones of the proximal carpal row.
- As before, the demineralized bone matrix is placed between the distal carpal row and the radius to potentially improve the fusion rate.
- The neutral wrist fusion plate is placed on the long metacarpal. The first screw inserted will be in the slot to compress the plate against the bone.
- The remaining distal locked screws are placed.
- The carpus is then reduced to the distal radius, and the first screw placed is the 3.5-mm non-locking screw in its slot.
- Further compression is provided by the offset screw in the neutral fusion plate.
- It is important to close the dorsal capsule on top of the plate to decrease extensor tendon irritation.
- The extensor retinaculum is then closed over the extensor tendons of the second and fourth dorsal compartments to prevent bowstringing.

Conclusion

The total wrist fusion is usually considered a last option after pan-carpal degeneration that cannot be corrected with a partial wrist fusion in the patient who is not a candidate for a total wrist arthroplasty or as a salvage procedure after the failure of a partial wrist fusion or total wrist arthroplasty (Figs. 32.20, 32.21, and 32.22). It should be considered in the rheumatoid patient because the chances of complications with a total wrist arthroplasty are significant. More recent designed plates are angled over the index metacarpal in order to decrease extensor tendon irritation as compared to straight dorsal plates (Figs. 32.23, 32.24, 32.25, and 32.26). For surgeons who prefer a proximal row carpectomy with wrist fusion, a new plate has been designed with a smooth dorsal surface to decrease extensor tendon irritation. Although the loss of ROM from the arthrodesis can be irritating to the patient, the total wrist fusion can be an excellent method to alleviate pain in pan-carpal arthrosis. It has a high union rate as well with early use. The decreased function can be overcome in many patients, but the patients should receive adequate presurgical counseling on the loss of fine wrist control. However, when done correctly, it can lead to pain relief and stabilization of the degeneration of the traumatized wrist.

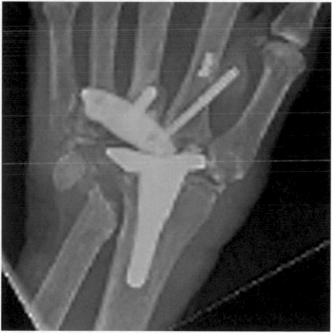

Fig. 32.20 Anterior–posterior radiograph demonstrating a fracture dislocation to a total wrist arthroplasty

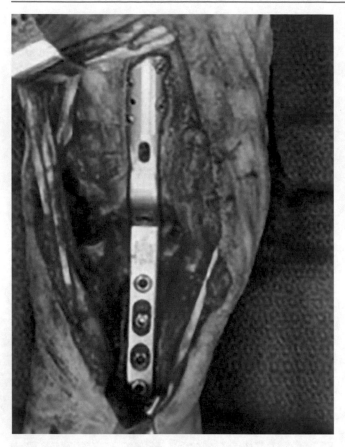

Fig. 32.21 Intra-operative photograph showing removal of the prosthesis and fusion of the remaining wrist with the neutral wrist fusion plate

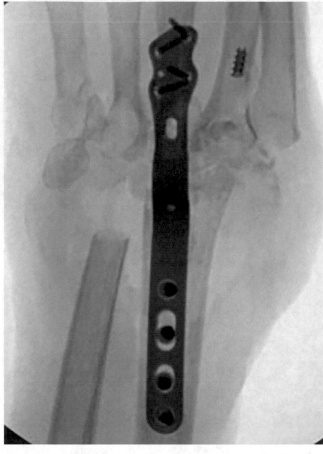

Fig. 32.22 Intra-operative fluoroscopy in the anterior posterior plane showing removal of the wrist prosthesis and fusion with the neutral wrist fusion plate

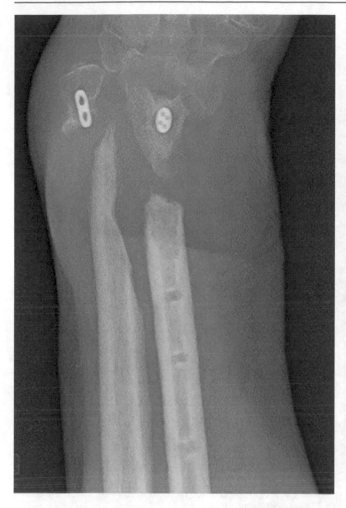

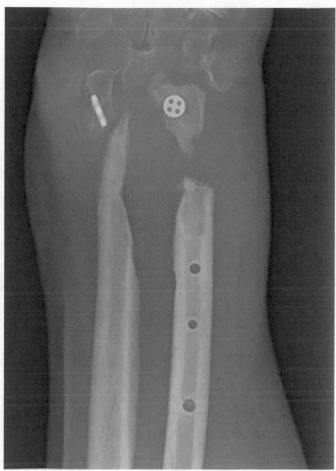

Fig. 32.24 Lateral radiograph of the same patient demonstrating marked bone loss with a tightrope device between the radius and ulna

Fig. 32.23 Anterior–posterior radiograph of a patient who has had approximately 25 surgeries to the wrist, resulting in marked bone loss and nonunion

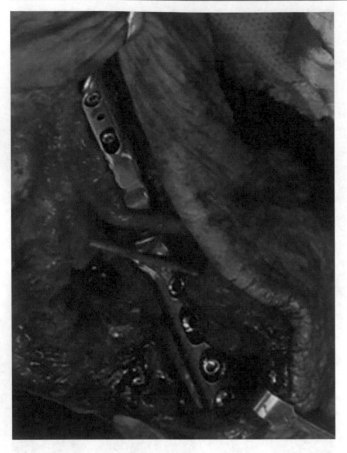

Fig. 32.25 Intra-operative photograph demonstrating wrist fusion with a curved fusion plate placed underneath the extensor tendons

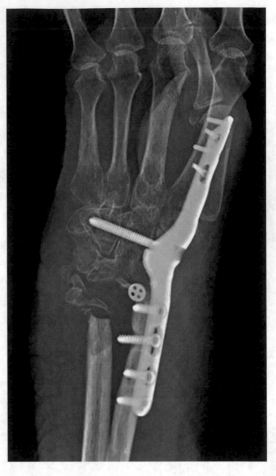

Fig. 32.26 Anterior–posterior radiograph showing successful fusion in this complex case

References

1. Rahgozar P, Zhong L, Chung KC. A comparative analysis of resource utilization between proximal row Carpectomy and partial wrist fusion: a population study. J Hand Surg. 2017;42(10):773–80.
2. Pong TM, van Leeuwen WF, Oflazoglu K, Blazar PE, Chen N. Unplanned reoperation and implant revision after total wrist arthroplasty. Hand. 2020:1558944719898817.
3. Boeckstyns MEH, Herzberg G, Merser S. Favorable results after total wrist arthroplasty: 65 wrists in 60 patients followed for 5–9 years. Acta Orthop. 2013;84(4):415–9.
4. Ward CM, Kuhl T, Adams BD. Five to ten-year outcomes of the universal total wrist arthroplasty in patients with rheumatoid arthritis. J Bone Joint Surg Am. 2011;93(10):914–9.
5. Hinds RM, Capo JT, Rizzo M, Roberson JR, Gottschalk MB. Total wrist arthroplasty versus wrist fusion: utilization and complication rates as reported by ABOS part II candidates. Hand. 2017;12(4):376–81.
6. Hastings H 2nd, Weiss AP, Quenzer D, Wiedeman GP, Hanington KR, Strickland JW. Arthrodesis of the wrist for post-traumatic disorders. J Bone Joint Surg Am. 1996;78(6):897–902.
7. Trumble TE, Easterling KJ, Smith RJ. Ulnocarpal abutment after wrist arthrodesis. J Hand Surg. 1988;13(1):11–5.
8. Louis DS, Hankin FM, Bowers WH. Capitate-radius arthrodesis: an alternative method of radiocarpal arthrodesis. J Hand Surg. 1984;9(3):365–9.
9. Clayton ML. Surgical treatment at the wrist in rheumatoid arthritis: a review of thirty-seven patients. J Bone Joint Surg Am. 1965;47:741–50.
10. Millender LH, Nalebuff EA. Arthrodesis of the rheumatoid wrist. J Bone Joint Surg Am. 1973;55:1026–34.

Capitate Resurfacing

33

Jessica M. Intravia and Randall W. Culp

Introduction

Arthritis of the wrist can be functionally limiting. After non-operative treatment options such as injections and bracing have been exhausted, a variety of surgical options are available. Early surgical treatment of radiocarpal arthritis allows for motion-sparing procedures such as proximal row carpectomy (PRC) and intercarpal arthrodesis to be performed. Proximal row carpectomy is effective in the treatment of post-traumatic degenerative osteoarthritis such as scaphoid nonunion advanced collapse (SNAC), scapholunate advance collapse (SLAC), scaphoid chondrocalcinosis advanced collapse (SCAC), and advanced Keinbock's disease. It has several advantages including its technical ease, maintenance of functional range of motion and grip strength, pain relief, ease of recovery and rehabilitation, and high patient satisfaction.

However, a successful proximal row carpectomy requires that both the proximal surface of the capitate and distal radius have normal cartilage. If there is lunocapitate osteoarthritis, a PRC is not recommended. Traditional teaching has included an intercarpal arthrodesis such as a four-corner fusion in this situation. Other alternatives include partial or total wrist fusion, resection-interposition arthroplasty, or total wrist prosthesis. Recent developments have led to the development of a capitate resurfacing arthroplasty to address this situation. Commercially available products include the Resurfacing Capitate Pyrocarbon Implant (RCPI, Tournier, Grenoble, France) and the Hemicapitate Wrist Hemiarthroplasty System (Arthrosurface, Franklin MA).

One advantage of a capitate resurfacing arthroplasty is that the implant may restore some carpal height leading to improved wrist biomechanics. Furthermore, a capitate resurfacing does not preclude any further salvage procedures. Patients younger than age of 40 tend to have increased wear after a PRC and may require future revision. Capitate resurfacing can be a useful option for these patients.

The remainder of the chapter will detail the PRC+ procedure or the technique of capitate resurfacing with the Hemicapitate Wrist Hemiarthroplasty System (Arthrosurface, Franklin MA). This may also be augmented with a capsular interpositional arthroplasty or dermal allograft.

Indications

Main indications for traditional PRC:

- SLAC wrist (Stage 2, not Stage 3)
- SNAC wrist
- Kienbock's disease

Additional indications for capitate resurfacing:

- SLAC wrist (Stage 3)
- Failed PRC with capitate wear
- Failed fusions (at surgeon's discretion)

Contraindications

- Active infection
- Advanced inflammatory arthritis
- Extensive bone loss of distal radius or carpus
- Inadequate soft tissue coverage
- Loss of extensor tendons
- Allergy or sensitivity to cobalt chrome and titanium alloys

J. M. Intravia
Donald and Barbara Zucker School of Medicine at Hofstra, Long Island Jewish Medical Center and North Shore University Hospital, Northwell Health Orthopaedic Institute, New Hyde Park, NY, USA

R. W. Culp (✉)
Department of Orthopaedic Surgery, Thomas Jefferson University Hospitals, Philadelphia Hand to Shoulder Center, King of Prussia, PA, USA

© Springer Nature Switzerland AG 2022
W. B. Geissler (ed.), *Wrist and Elbow Arthroscopy with Selected Open Procedures*, https://doi.org/10.1007/978-3-030-78881-0_33

Technique in Detail

1. The patient is placed supine with the hand on extended on a hand table. A midline incision is marked over the wrist (Fig. 33.1).

2. Tourniquet is inflated to 250 mmHg mercury and sharp dissection is made through skin. The extensor pollicis longus (EPL) is identified crossing over the second extensor compartment. The third compartment is then released and transposed radially. The radial wrist extensors along with the EPL are retracted radially while the extensor digitorum communis (EDC) tendons are retracted ulnarly (Fig. 33.2). The wrist is approached between the second and fourth extensor compartments. The posterior interosseous nerve (PIN) resides on the floor of the fourth extensor compartment and can be resected to perform a PIN neurectomy.

3. The capsule is approached through either a dorsal ligament sparing or sacrificing incision. It is the author's preference to use an inverted T incision to enter the capsule (Fig. 33.3). A longitudinal incision is made in the capsule in line with the third metacarpal and a transverse arm is made at the level of the radiocarpal joint. Care is taken not to plunge into the underlying hyaline cartilage of the carpal bones. Full thickness radial and

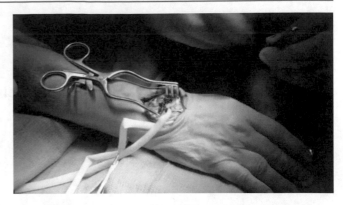

Fig. 33.3 A inverse T-type incision is made over the capsule

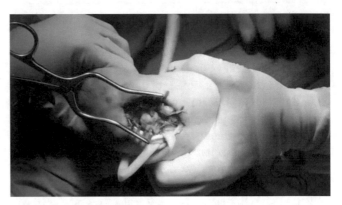

Fig. 33.4 View of the proximal capitate arthrosis after a proximal row carpectomy has been performed

ulnar capsular flaps are then developed from proximal to distal.

4. The lunate fossa and head of the capitate are inspected for degenerative changes. If no degenerative changes are seen, proceed to proximal row carpectomy. If any changes of the capitate are seen, consider a capitate resurfacing procedure and/or capsular interposition in addition to PRC (PRC+ procedure).

5. Perform a proximal row carpectomy removing the scaphoid, lunate, and the triquetrum (Fig. 33.4). Typically, the scaphoid is removed first after dividing the scapholunate ligament. A K-wire may be drilled into the scaphoid as a joystick in order to facilitate its removal. McGlamery elevators may also aid in the excision of the carpal bones. Take care to avoid injury to volar radiocarpal ligaments including the radioscaphocapitate ligament; triangular fibrocartilage complex (TFCC); capitate; and pisiform.

6. Determine the appropriate curvatures of the articular surfaces of the distal radius and capitate. Use the manufacturer's guidelines to select the appropriate implant size. A series of mapping templates is available to measure the radius of curvature of the lunate fossa in both the sagittal and coronal plane (Figs. 33.5 and 33.6).

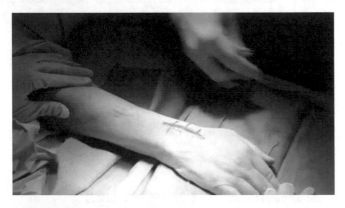

Fig. 33.1 Mid-line wrist incision

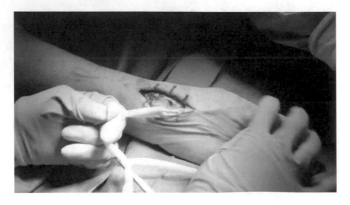

Fig. 33.2 A Penrose drain is used to retract the EDC tendons ulnarly

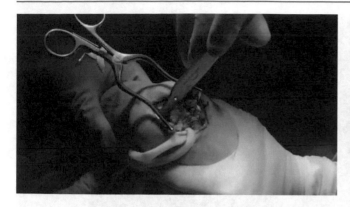

Fig. 33.5 Determine the coronal size of the lunate fossa using the guide

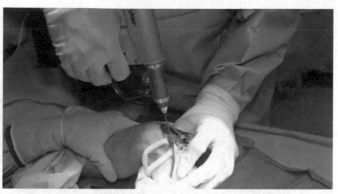

Fig. 33.8 The K-wire may need to be adjusted freehand in order to get a center-center position

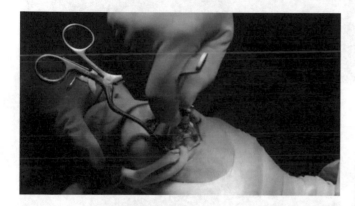

Fig. 33.6 Determine the sagittal size of the lunate fossa using the guide

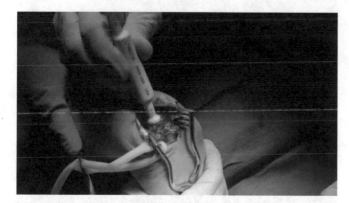

Fig. 33.7 Size the capitate using the appropriate-sized guide and insert a K-wire through the center of the capitate

7. Place the appropriate capitate sizer on the proximal aspect of the capitate (Fig. 33.7). Advance a 1.5-mm guide pin in the center of the capitate. Confirm the appropriate position using fluoroscopy in the anterior–posterior (AP) and lateral plane. Use the long finger metacarpal as a surface marker. The drill guide should be seated so that all four points of contact are flush with

the articular surface. The K-wire may be adjusted using a free-hand technique in order to confirm a center-center position (Figs. 33.8 and 33.9).

8. Place the cannulated drill over the guidewire (Fig. 33.10). Advance the drill so that all of the threads are buried. Remove any loose bone fragments.

9. Advance the tap until the black laser line (Figs. 33.11 and 33.12).

10. Advance the taper post screw until the black laser line is flush with the capitate surface (Fig. 33.13).

11. Choose the appropriate-sized capitate reamer based on your initial measurements. Start the capitate reamer off of the bone and ream the capitate over the guide pin until it contacts the taper post (Figs. 33.14 and 33.15). Remove the guide pin.

12. Place the dorsal reamer guide into the taper of the taper post. It should be oriented so that the dorsal ream is at the 12 o'clock position. Advance the dorsal reamer until its predetermined stop depth (Fig. 33.16).

13. Clean the wrist of any bone debris and place the appropriate-sized trial on the taper post. Confirm the fit of the sizing trial so that it is congruent with the edge of the surrounding articular surface or slightly recessed (Figs. 33.17 and 33.18). Use fluoroscopy to confirm size.

14. Remove the trial and irrigate the wrist (Fig. 33.19).

15. Place the implant on the taper post. Use the impactor to set the implant and engage the morse taper (Figs. 33.20 and 33.21).

16. Confirm implant position with fluoroscopy. Take the wrist through a range of motion to confirm implant position under live fluoroscopy (Fig. 33.22).

17. Consider capsular interposition or dermal allograft on distal radius (Arthrex, Naples FL).

18. Close the capsule with vicryl sutures and the skin with nylon. Leave the EPL transposed radially (Fig. 33.23). Apply a volar splint with the wrist in 10–15 degrees of extension.

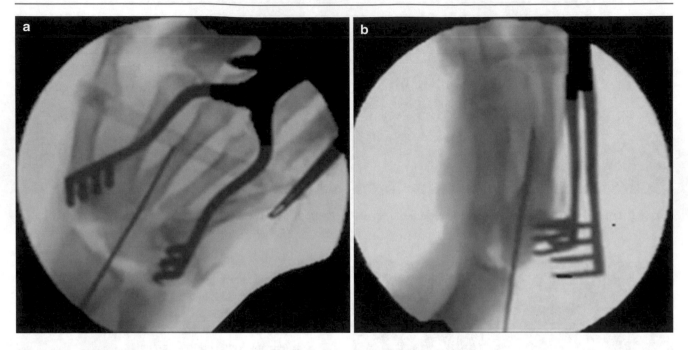

Fig. 33.9 (**a, b**) AP and lateral images showing correct K-wire position

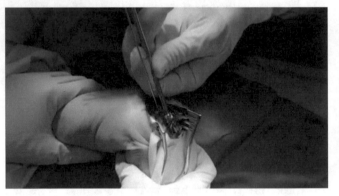

Fig. 33.10 Demonstration of the appropriate depth of the cannulated drill

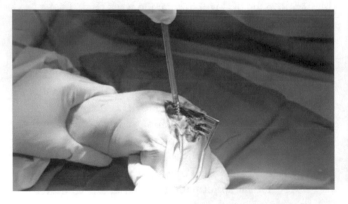

Fig. 33.11 Tap placement over the guidewire

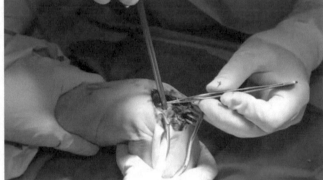

Fig. 33.12 Advance the tap until the black laser line

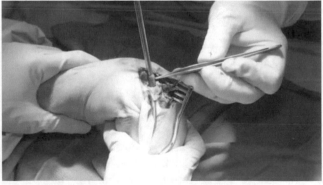

Fig. 33.13 Advance the taper post screw until the black laser line

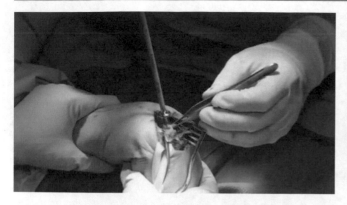

Fig. 33.14 Place the reamer over the guidewire

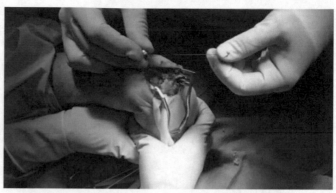

Fig. 33.17 Tie a string around the trial implant for ease of removal

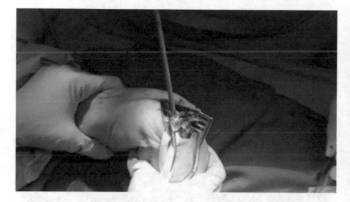

Fig. 33.15 Advance the reamer until it contacts the taper post

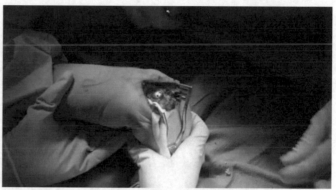

Fig. 33.18 Place the trial implant and check implant fit

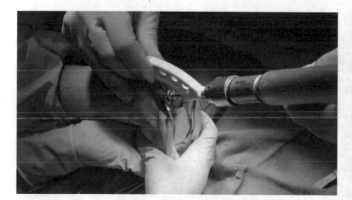

Fig. 33.16 Advance the dorsal reamer

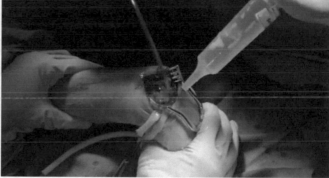

Fig. 33.19 Irrigate wrist

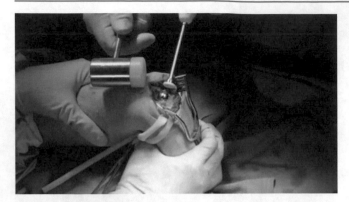

Fig. 33.20 Final implant will need to engage the morse taper. Ensure small mallet and impactor are available

Tips and Tricks

- Protect the extensor tendons throughout your approach, consider tying a Penrose drain around the EDC tendons to aid in your retraction
- Make sure that your initial guidewire is in the center of the capitate, lined up with the third metacarpal
- Always start the reaming off the bone
- Tie a suture around the base of the trial for easy removal of the trial implant

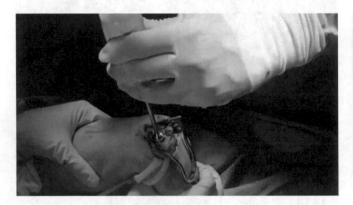

Fig. 33.21 Impact the final implant to engage the morse taper

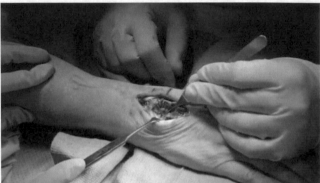

Fig. 33.23 Capsular closure

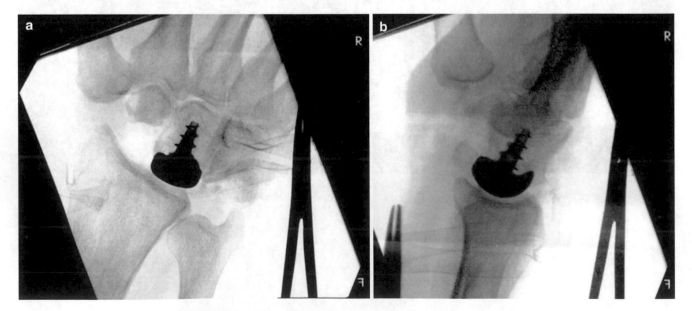

Fig. 33.22 (**a, b**) Final fluoroscopic images

Conclusion

Proximal row carpectomy with capitate resurfacing provides a useful alternative for patients with lunocapitate arthritis. The Hemicapitate Wrist Hemiarthroplasty System (Arthrosurface, Franklin MA) was launched in September of 2015. Given its relatively recent introduction, no long-term results have been published yet. However, short-term results seem promising. Preliminary, single surgeon, results of 17 patients who underwent a hemicapitate wrist hemiarthroplasty from September 2015 to April 2017 with an average of 70 week follow-up (1–78 wk) shows an average improvement in grip strength from 56 to 72 pounds. Average improvement in wrist range of motion increased from a 43- to 62-degree arc. Average QuickDASH score improved from 41 to 21. One patient in this cohort had a complication and no revisions were performed. The Resurfacing Capitate Pyrocarbon Implant (Tournier, Grenoble, France) has published mid-size studies showing comparative results to proximal row carpectomy for those patients with lunocapitate arthritis at minimum of 2-year follow-up.

Post-Operative Protocol

- Short arm splint with wrist in 10 to 15 degrees of extension 7 to 10 days
- Short arm cast or splint for 3 weeks
- Removable wrist splint and range of motion at 4 weeks
- Weight bearing at 3 months
- Impact activities at 6 months

Suggested Reading

Giacalone F, Summa P, Fenoglio A, Sard A, Dutto E, Ferrero M, et al. Resurfacing capitate pyrocarbon implant versus proximal row carpectomy alone: a comparative study to evaluate the role of capitate prosthetic resurfacing in advanced carpal collapse. Plast Reconstr Surg. 2017;140:962–9.

Goubier J, Vogels J, Teboul F. Capitate pyrocarbon prosthesis in radiocarpal arthritis. Tech Hand Surg. 2011;15:28–31.

Kirker-Head CA, Van Sickle DC, Ek SW, McCool JC. Safety of, and biological and functional response to, a novel metallic implant for the management of focal full thickness cartilage defects: preliminary assessment in an animal model out to 1 year. J Orthop Res. 2006;24(5):1095–108.

Marcuzzi A, Ozben H, Russomando A. The use of a pyrocarbon capitate resurfacing implant in chronic wrist disorders. J Hand Surg Eur. 2014;39E(6):611–8.

Rabinovich R, Lee S. Proximal row carpectomy using decellularized Dermal Allograft. J Hand Surg Am. 2018;43(4):392. e1–e9.

Yi IS, Culp R. PRC+ an augmented alternative to four corner fusion. Expert Opinions in Joint Preservation. 2015;

Total Wrist Arthroplasty

34

Greg Packer

Introduction

Evolution of the human wrist has taken a long period spanning approximately 60 million years from the simple flipper that our most distant ancestors, marine reptiles such as the Kronosaurus, required for alignment of the forelimb to facilitate passage through water in pursuit of prey. Essentially, the forelimb acted as a flipper, strong but flexible. As our ancestors adapted to life on land, the requirements for the forelimb became greater; the hind limb was used for propulsion and the forelimb, while often also used for propulsion, required more complexity and in particular movement, to cope with the extra burdens placed upon it, such as to find and manipulate food, as our ancestors, such as the giant ground sloth (approximately 6 million years ago), demonstrate [1].

Humans require a great deal from their wrists, including significant weight bearing in both compression and distraction (unlike in the lower limb), but also a great range of movement, some of it fine and very specific for work, sporting and normal social activities, as well as personal care and hygiene.

The evolution of dart thrower's motion along with other adaptations to the upper limb, including our long clavicle and opposable thumbs, was key in providing the evolutionary advantages that have resulted in our species being so successful [2].

Following injury and arthritis of the wrist, arthrodesis has remained the gold standard for the treatment of patients with end-stage arthritis of the wrist, but although it is often successful in relieving pain, it is clearly a compromise and effectively reverts the human wrist back to the design of its distant ancestor.

For this reason, the history of wrist arthroplasty is surprisingly long, with designs dating as far back as the 1800s that used the available materials of the time such as ivory and were, not surprisingly, unsuccessful.

This was, of course, very similar to the experience in other joints, and it was not until the benefits of joint arthroplasty as a treatment for arthritis by abolishing pain while retaining movement were demonstrated by the invention of the low friction arthroplasty for the hip by Sir John Charnley in the 1960s [3] that, as in many other joints, there was a new stimulus to design a suitable form of arthroplasty for the wrist.

In the wrist, the initial generation of implants was the silastic replacements pioneered by Swanson in the 1960s, which although they demonstrated initial good results, suffered from the problems of breakage and silicone synovitis, which resulted in poor medium-term outcomes [4].

In the 1970s, ball and socket designs, such as those designed by Meuli, were introduced, but these fared little better, as they were prone to the problems associated with more constrained forms of implants such as peri-prosthetic fractures and loosening [5].

By the third generation of implants, there was a move toward less bony resection and better soft tissue balance by the use of offset articulating surfaces [6].

The fourth generation of wrist implants marked the move toward screw fixation of the carpus and the use of porous surfaces to provide osseo-integration. This is associated, of course, with a move away from the cemented implants of the previous generation, and these are the implants that remain in use today.

These implants include the Maestro (recently discontinued), the Re-motion, and the Universal 2, more recently re-designed as the Freedom and the Motec.

As impacts have moved toward less bone resection and uncemented design, there has been a move toward using these implants, not in the traditional inflammatory low-demand patient but in higher-demand patients such as those in middle age affected by the long-term effects of wrist fractures, ligamentous injury (SLAC), scaphoid non-union

G. Packer (✉)
Department of Orthopaedic Surgery, Southend University Hospital, Westcliff-on-Sea, Essex, UK

© Springer Nature Switzerland AG 2022
W. B. Geissler (ed.), *Wrist and Elbow Arthroscopy with Selected Open Procedures*,
https://doi.org/10.1007/978-3-030-78881-0_34

(SNAC), and Keinbock's disease as well as those with osteo-arthritis.

There has also been a move toward modularity of these implants, which is of benefit in a population that may require revision of the articulation utilizing the remaining stable fixation in the carpus and radius.

One alternative method to deal with the younger and more active population, particularly in disease processes that spare the mid-carpal joint, is to perform a partial wrist fusion or a wrist hemi-arthroplasty in order to retain movement within the joint while not requiring a full fusion or total wrist arthroplasty. These hemi-arthroplasties include the Universal 2 [4] and the Freedom, as well as the KinematX [7]. These forms of fusion and implants are relatively easy to convert to total wrist replacement, especially whereas in the Freedom and the KinematX, they are part of a system facilitating replacement of the carpal side while retaining the radial fixation. The later operation is the other half of the hemi-arthroplasty.

Although these forms of fusion and implants have proved useful in these patients, they are limited by the need for the mid-carpal joint to be spared from the arthritic process, which is not always the case, especially in some subgroups such as those with SNAC, some SLACs, and Keinbock's disease wrists.

These fourth-generation implants now have published results that support their use in both an inflammatory and a non-inflammatory population and with results that are reaching levels of the effectiveness and survivorship of other joint replacements.

Boeckstyns has published results of the Re-motion, demonstrating the results of 65 wrists in 60 patients with a follow-up of 5–9 years. While these patients were mainly those with rheumatoid arthritis, 20% of patients had post-traumatic or osteoarthritis and one Keinbock's disease. They reported implant survival of 90% at 9 years with no difference between those with rheumatoid or other conditions. Scores for pain and quick DASH and grip strength all improved, and the range of movement remained similar to that recorded preoperatively, with the exception of supination (which they noted was probably a function of the other operations performed on the DRUJ) [8].

The Motec has published results with a similar duration to the Re-motion, with 5- to 10-year results from the designing surgeon [9] and 4-year results from an independent center [10]. These results demonstrate that the results for pain, Quick DASH, and grip strength were all significantly improved. As opposed to the Re-motion study, the arc of range of movement within the Motec patients also significantly improved from an average of 97 degrees to 126 degrees. This should be seen against the context of an arc of 120 degrees being regarded as normal with regard to wrist function. This result is supported by the independent center

results, which also demonstrated a significant increase in the flexion extension arc.

One other important result of the Motec study is that all of the patients were high demand and relatively young (average age 47 years); no inflammatory arthritis patients were included in this study. The survival curve for the implant in these patients is 86% at 10 years.

One other benefit of the Motec is that it has an integrated fusion system that allows for conversion to fusion either inter-operatively or later, if required; the system is compatible with the radial and metacarpal screws.

The following sections describe the indications, contraindications, operative technique, and tips and tricks for the Motec total wrist replacement system.

Indications

The Motec total wrist replacement is indicated in patients who have pan carpal wrist arthritis, which may arise from osteoarthritis, inflammatory arthritis, post-traumatic arthritis, SLAC, and SNAC stage IV (including SLAC/SNAC stage III where the arthritis affects the articular part of the capitate). The implant can also be used for patients who have had a pre-existing treatment to the wrist including RSL, four-corner, and PRC. The implant may also be used as a revision prosthesis from other hemi-arthroplasties and total wrist implants and for conversion of total wrist fusion to total wrist replacement.

The implant may also be used for the immediate treatment of fractures of the distal radius in the presence of pre-existing wrist arthritis.

Contraindications

The contraindications to wrist arthroplasty are those standard to any form of arthroplasty, especially the presence of any form of active infection.

Another important contraindication is neurological imbalance in the affected limb such as may occur post-CVA and for neurological disorders such as may occur post-head injury and with other neurological conditions. A wrist fusion is more appropriate for these patients.

The Motec wrist, in particular, has a very wide potential for movement due to the nature of the ball and socket joint used; therefore, a relative contraindication is where the soft tissues of the wrist are poor, especially the extensor tendons. This is particularly important in patients with inflammatory arthritis in which another implant such as the Re-motion may be more appropriate, or the soft tissues may be reconstructed prior to the total wrist arthroplasty being undertaken. In such circumstances, if a Motec total wrist is considered an appropriate implant, the Motec arthrodesis system may be utilized as a temporary stabilizing device until the soft tissues are suitable.

Technique

Pre-operatively the patient needs to be suitably assessed and counseled for the contraindications above and suitable pre-operative imaging undertaken. Generally radiographs alone are sufficient, but other imaging such as MRI and CT scan may be required if the diagnosis is uncertain or there has been previous injury or surgery.

Wrist arthroscopy may be required in case of uncertainty because it remains the gold standard for the assessment of the wrist joint, in particular to assess the state of the mid-carpal joint.

The operation is undertaken in a suitable laminar flower theater, and general or, more commonly, regional anesthesia is employed. With the use of suitable regional anesthetic techniques, many patients can have this operation on an ambulatory or day-stay basis.

The patient is supine on a standard operation table and a tourniquet with exsanguination is used. A radio-lucent hand table and image intensification (preferably a mini C-arm) are required. Appropriate antibiotic prophylaxis and prophylactic anti-coagulation measures, mechanical and/or chemical, are used.

A longitudinal incision approximately 10 cm in length centered over the wrist joint in both transverse and longitudinal planes is made (Fig. 34.1) and thick flaps developed to expose the extensor retinaculum. The fourth extensor compartment is divided in the mid-line protecting the extensor

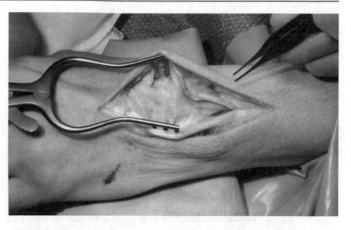

Fig. 34.2 Approach through forth extensor compartment

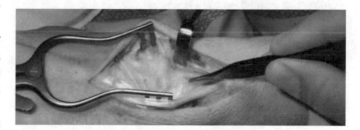

Fig. 34.3 Identification and resection posterior interosseous nerve

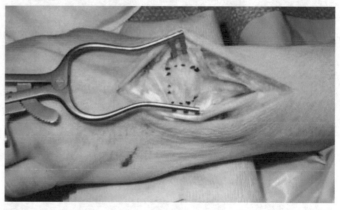

Fig. 34.4 Margins of proximally based flap

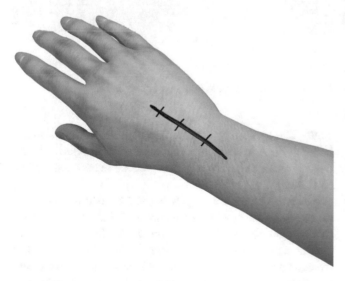

Fig. 34.1 Incision for wrist arthroplasty

tendons beneath and the contents of the compartment retracted ulnarly. The bed of the second compartment (ECRL) is incised and a self-retaining retractor inserted beneath both sets of tendons (Fig. 34.2). The posterior interosseous nerve is identified and resected with hemostasis (Fig. 34.3).

A proximally based wrist flap is created with the following boundaries: radially, the bed of ECRL; distally, the mid-section of the capitate, just distal to the articular surface; and ulnarly, as close to the fifth compartment as possible (Fig. 34.4). The flap is developed from the distal radial corner first (Fig. 34.5) and then developed proximally to the radius both radially and ulnarly. In the ulnar corner as the flap thins, it is useful to take a sliver of triquetrum with an osteotome (Fig. 34.6). The edges of the flap are then developed radial, ulnarly and proximally to the radius and the flap secured with a stay suture (Fig. 34.7).

In order to assess the third carpo-metocarpal joint (3rd CMC), the distal part of the flap is divided longitudinally in the mid-line and the soft tissue dissected to the edges of the joint.

A full proximal row carpectomy is undertaken in the usual fashion.

The wrist is placed over a padded kidney dish or bowl to facilitate flexion of the distal part, and a double retractor from the set is used to lift the capitate; using a saw approximately 1–2 mm of capitate is resected.

The 3rd CMC joint is identified by means of a needle supplemented by image intensification, if necessary. It is worth remembering that the joint is oblique and more distal in the radial direction.

A closing wedge osteotomy is undertaken by resecting 1 mm from each side of the 3rd CMC joint at a 45-degree

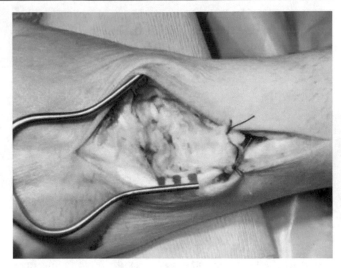

Fig. 34.7 Stay suture to flap

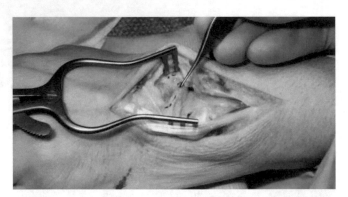

Fig. 34.5 Starting resection at distal radial margin of flap

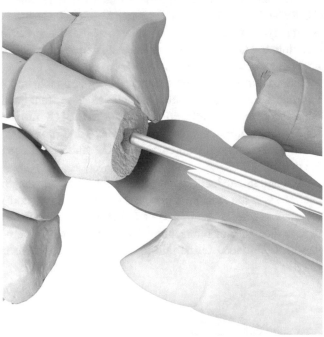

Fig. 34.8 Claw retractor to lift and position capitate

angle. The osteotomy is completed with osteotomes and/or bone nibblers to allow the capitate to lift up relative to the metacarpal and remove the 15-degree angle between the two (Fig. 34.8).

Once the capitate and metacarpal are lined up, the sharp guide wire is inserted into the center of the capitate, aiming for the center of the third metacarpal (Fig. 34.9).

The sharp guide wire is driven through the distal part of the capitate and the base of the third metacarpal into the center of the shaft. Image intensifier control is used to ensure correct placement of the wire (Fig. 34.10). Once the wire has been positioned, the blunt guide wire is used and driven into

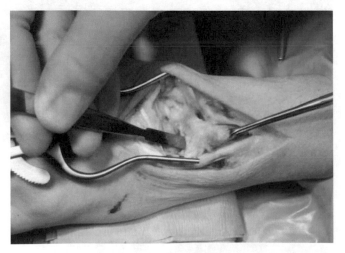

Fig. 34.6 Removing bone sliver from triquetrum

the third metacarpals ensuring that it passes beyond the isthmus and the position checked on image intensifier (Fig. 34.11).

Once the wire is positioned correctly, the cannulated metacarpal reamer is selected (two are available, always start with the smaller of the two). It should be noted that the small metacarpal reamer is sufficient in approximately 95% of cases; the large metacarpal reamer is only ever used after the small and is necessary in only 5% of cases. The reamer is marked in 5-mm increments from 45 mm to 60 mm, and there are two more marks corresponding with 65 and 70 mm (Fig. 34.12). The metacarpal is reamed over the guide wire and under image intensifier control until the retired depth. Take care with the reaming not to overheat the bone, and stop frequently to clean the reamer of debris and use copious amounts of normal saline to cool. The reaming should ensure

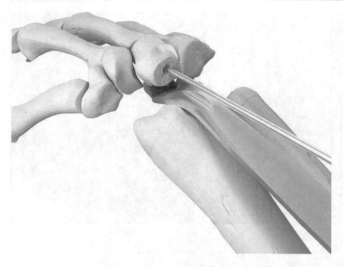

Fig. 34.9 Insertion of guide wire

Fig. 34.10 Insertion of sharp guide wire

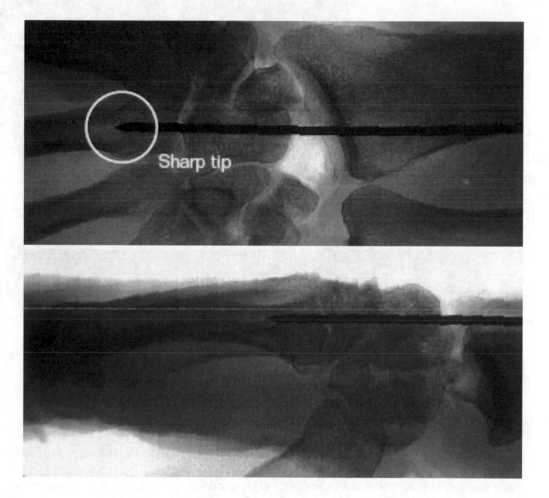

Fig. 34.11 Blunt wire in center of medullary canal of metacarpal

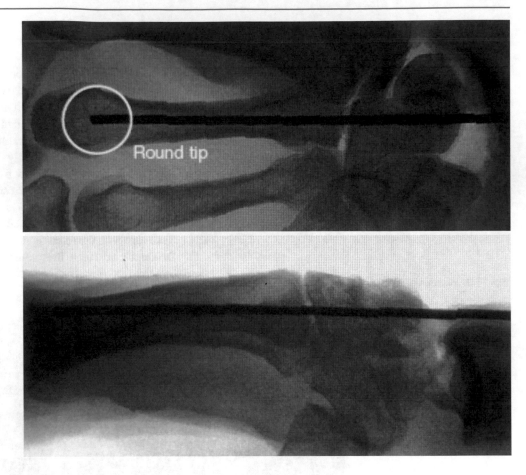

Round tip

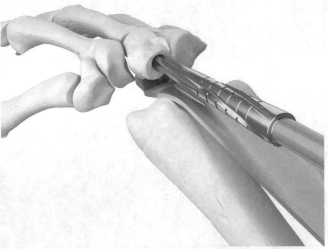

Fig. 34.12 Insertion of metacarpal reamer

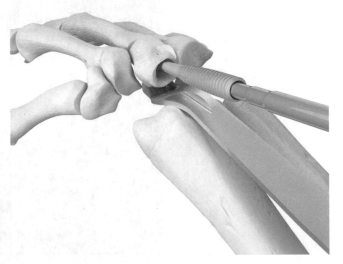

Fig. 34.13 Insertion of metacarpal screw

that the depth is as long as possible and certainly beyond the isthmus, remembering that the first centimeter of the screw is unthreaded. The depth of the reaming is checked on image intensifier.

Once the position is satisfactory, the screw depth is read from the markings on the reamer and a corresponding size screw selected.

Once the appropriate screw is opened, it is inserted using the screwdriver (Fig. 34.13). When attaching the screw to the screwdriver and during insertion, it is very important to maintain a non-touch technique, including the surgeon's and scrub staff's hands and the patient's skin, in order to maintain the integrity of the Bonit$^{(TM)}$ coating, as it may be removed if in contact with these materials.

The screw is inserted to the depth that was reamed to the capitate and metacarpal as the screw has a non-threaded distal part of 1 cm; the screw should be inserted with longitudinal force initially without any rotation while reducing the third metacarpal CMC (using the other thumb); this allows compression of this joint and obviates the need for grafting (which can be used if there is still a gap). The screw is inserted to the depth of the reaming and the position checked on the image intensifier to ensure correct position and length. The screw should not be inserted too far as the tension can be adjusted by further insertion of the screw during final assembly.

Once the metacarpal screw is inserted in a satisfactory fashion, attention is turned to the radial side.

Then a double claw retractor is inserted under the volar lip of the radius and the carpus retracted volarly to ensure the screw and carpus are protected from the radial reaming (Fig. 34.14). A sharp awl is provided to enable initial penetration of the radial articular surface; however, the author's preference is to use a sharp guide wire. The entry position of the guide wire is in the middle of the radial articular surface in the AP plane directly under Lister's tubercle and just ulnar to the ridge between the scaphoid and lunate fossas of the radius if it is still discernible. Some surgeons prefer a slightly more ulnar approach, but the most important thing is not to stray too radially, because it makes entry of the guide wire into the medulla of the radius more difficult.

If the awl is used once the penetration the radial articular surface is undertaken (checked on II), the sharpe wire is used to gain entry to the radial medullary cavity. A similar method is employed if using the guide wire direct, and as with the

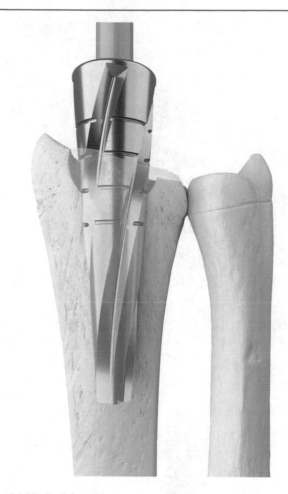

Fig. 34.15 Radial reaming

metacarpal, the guide wire is changed to the blunt or reversed and then inserted into the radius. The position of the guide wire is checked on II, and then the radius can be reamed using the radial reamer. If the radius is small or deformed, the large metacarpal reamer can be used on the radial side, because it allows fixation more proximally in the radius.

The radius is reamed using the reamer until the last marking of the reamer is reached (Fig. 34.15) or cortical chatter indicates that the reamer is of the right size. At this point, reaming should be stopped and the 15-mm cup reamer used to ream for the radial cup. This is because the cup reamer has a stop and if reamed to the stop, the correct position of the Motec articulation is chosen relative to the center of rotation of the wrist (Fig. 34.16). Once the cup reamer is used, it is removed and the radial reamer (or large metacarpal reamer if used) is reinserted and the correct-sized screw is measured from the *bottom of the cup* (Fig. 34.17). The chosen screw is then inserted into the radius and the position checked on II. If a large metacarpal screw is used, the radial reamer is used in its initial part to allow for the size of the base of the cup.

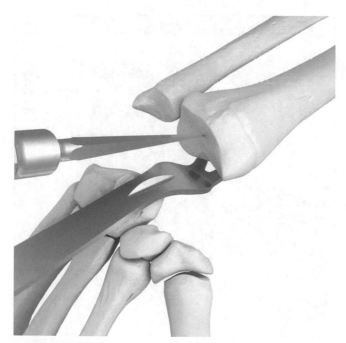

Fig. 34.14 Lifting radius with claw retractor and sharp awl

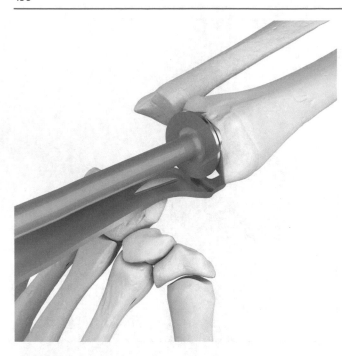

Fig. 34.16 Cup reamer

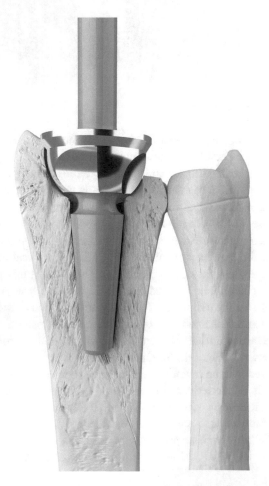

Fig. 34.17 Ideal position of cup reamer to determine correct position of radial screw

Once the radial screw has been selected, it is inserted using the screwdriver and with the same non-touch technique. It is important to ensure that the distal part of the screw is situated at the level of the base of the cup reaming. The articulation can then be trialed and inserted to complete the operation.

Prior to the insertion of the articulation, particularly if the cup trial is not used (see below), the position of the cup should be checked on the image intensifier in two planes to ensure correct depth and position.

Both trial cups and heads are available; however, the author's preference is not to trial with the trial cup because it can be difficult to remove the trial cup if it is firmly impacted on the Morse taper of the screw; therefore, the definitive cup is inserted and impacted and the trial reduction undertaken on the head alone.

Two articulations are currently available – a metal-on-metal cup (MOM) or a metal-on-PEEK cup. Both articulations have been demonstrated to be equivalent. As the articulation of the PEEK cup is thicker by approximately 2 mm, it offers an advantage in terms of the position of the center of rotation in circumstances when the wrist is tight, and in order to avoid the risk of "over stuffing" the joint, the MOM articulation increases the space available by 2 mm.

The chosen cup is inserted and impacted using the impactor from the set (Fig. 34.18); the head is then trialed using the trial heads from the set. Heads are available in the sizes of small, medium, long, and extra-long.

The head sizes differ in length by an increase in 2 mm over each size from small to extra-long. The correct ten-

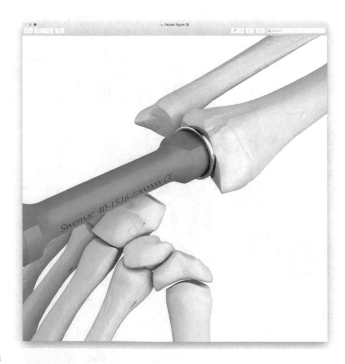

Fig. 34.18 Impaction of definitive cup

sion is an articulation that allows a full range of movement, especially dorsiflexion, without being too tight and full flexion, which can be tested by lifting the wrist from the table.

One benefit of the Motec design is that the tension on the carpal side can be finessed up until the final insertion of the articulation. Although the difference between the head sizes is 2 mm, the metacarpal screw can be rotated to provide a decrease in tension (by continuing to introduce the screw into the metacarpal, which is the reason for not over introducing the screw in the first place). Each complete rotation of the screw results in a change in length of just under one millimeter. As the screw is a cone, it should be noted that the screw cannot be reversed without loss of fixation. If it is the case that the articulation is too lax despite using an extra-long head, then the solution is to use a longer and or thicker screw to gain the length required.

Once the required head size has been determined, the trial head is removed and the definite head is inserted and impacted (Fig. 34.19). The wrist is then reduced and the stability and range of movement checked (Fig. 34.20).

The wrist is then screened using the image intensifier to ensure that the implants are correctively inserted and the range of movement assessed to ensure that there is no impingement. If a full proximal row carpectomy has been undertaken, this is unusual but on occasion as prominent radial styloid may require resection with a saw (Fig. 34.21).

The joint is washed with normal saline and the soft tissues are closed. The proximally based flap is repaired with

2/0 vicryl, the longitudinal extension allowing the joint to be tensioned correctly by lengthening or shortening the distal extension relative to the main part of the flap.

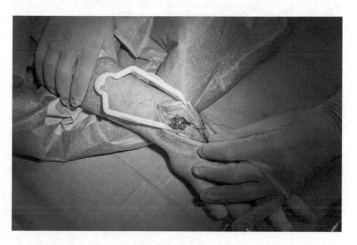

Fig. 34.20 Completion of the operation

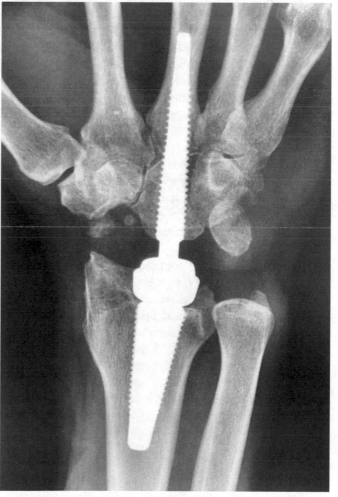

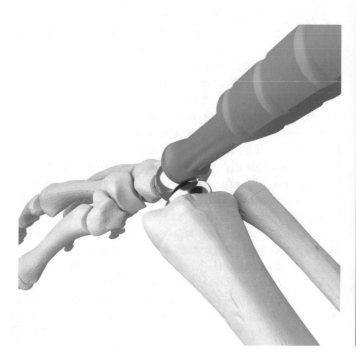

Fig. 34.19 Impaction of definitive head

Fig. 34.21 Radiograph of position of the implant

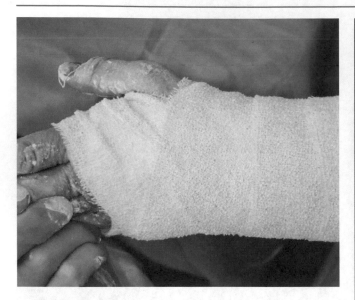

Fig. 34.22 Plaster back slab

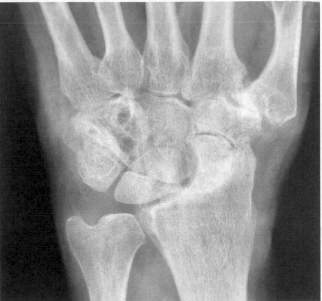

Fig. 34.23 Ideal case

The divided extensor retinaculum is repaired with interrupted 2/0 vicryl and the skin sutured with a continuous 3/0 vicryl rapide.

A Mepore dressing is applied, and after a layer of wool, the wrist is protected in a plaster of Paris back slab consisting of a dorsal slab of 12 layers and a slab around the thumb. A crepe bandage is then applied (Fig. 34.22).

Post-operatively the limb is elevated in a Bradford sling or similar device for the first 24 h and as necessary afterwards. Early active mobilization of the hand and elbow and shoulder is encouraged as well as general early mobilization. One further dose of antibiotic prophylaxis is administered.

At 10 days, the patient is reviewed and the plaster slab removed and the wound removed. Early active mobilization is encouraged at this point and no splinting is required.

Hand therapy continues, encouraging normal use and active movement with no over-pressure until 8 weeks from the date of implantation.

Patients are allowed to return to driving and normal activities from approximately 3 weeks following the operation depending upon their progress, and they are restricted from excessive weight bearing and loading and from the use of power tools until 12 weeks from the date of the operation.

Once this period has passed and a check radiograph has demonstrated integration of the implant, they are allowed to return to full activities with no restrictions in terms of the manner of use of the amount of load bearing.

Tips and Tricks

Like all operations, the Motec total wrist replacement has a learning curve, and there are certain groups of patients who may be considered relatively easy in a technical sense. The best patient to undertake a Motec on is a SLAC stage IV, because these patients tend to have good bone stock and good movement (Fig. 34.23). In addition, they tend to have very good soft tissues and are motivated to return to their activities, be it work, sport, and their social life. Similar patients who are in the same category include SNAC stage IV, Keinbock's disease, and patients with post-traumatic arthritis.

The next category of patient to consider is older patients with degenerative osteoarthritis, who are very suitable for the Motec. They generally do not provide a great technical challenge. While their bone stock may be relatively poor, this does not cause any problems, because the implant utilizes purely intra-medullary fixation. The soft tissues of these patients are generally not as good as the younger SLACs and SNACs, so the implant may require to be inserted under a little more tension than in the younger patients (as they tend to stretch up more during rehabilitation).

Revision from other operations such as radioscapholunate (RSL) fusion, four corner fusion and proximal row carpectomy are technically relatively easy and generally do not result in any intra-operative issues. Some patients who have had previous wrist surgery will tend to have a relatively stiff wrist, especially following proximal row carpectomy, and while this generally is not an issue if the wrist is very stiff, length can be gained from the carpal side and specifically by resection of the capitate, due to the fact that the Motec has no carpal plate and fixation therefore does not rely on the capitate given the fixation is from the third metacarpal. However, due to the position of the center of rotation of the wrist, it is important not to try to gain length from deeper insertion of the radial implant, because this results in soft tissue imbalance.

Any form of wrist replacement is a soft tissue procedure; therefore, the most important pre-operative assessment of these patients is to ensure that the soft tissues of the wrist are functioning satisfactorily prior to the operation being undertaken. The most common problem encountered is weakness of the extensor tendons resulting in a flexion contracture; for this reason, while the Motec is suitable for many patients with inflammatory arthritis, pre-operative assessment of the extensor tendons is essential to ensure that they are functioning sufficiently to provide dorsiflexion. If they are deficient, then another more constrained form of wrist implant may be considered or it may be prudent to consider fusion.

One unique benefit of the Motec is the ability to perform a wrist arthrodesis utilizing the proximal and distal components of the implant with an arthrodesis device instead of an articulation (Fig. 34.24). This offers the opportunity for performing a proximal row carpectomy and insertion of the proximal and distal screws, and then instead of completing the fusion with graft using the peg to provide temporary stability, the extensor tendons can then be repaired, reconstructed, or tendon transfers undertaken and allowed conversion to a total wrist by removing the arthrodesis device and converting it to a Motec articulation.

The implant may be used as a revision implant, the soft tissues are the key and if they are deficient the comments above apply. Most patients who have had a previous wrist replacement tend to have a rather distal articulation to which their soft tissues are accommodated, and it is important therefore to ensure that the Motec articulation is distal enough to reproduce this center of rotation (using the methods described above).

For conversion of total wrist fusion to Motec total wrist replacement, many provide a good result for patients who are unable to cope with a fused wrist [11]. However, it should be noted that this is a technically difficult operation and the caveats expressed above regarding the soft tissues also apply. The most important tips when converting fusion to replacement are to ensure that all adhesions of the extensor tendons are dealt with by tenolysis, to resect sufficient bone and generally more than you first think as bone tends to want to regrow to reform the fusion mass. In conversion from fusion above, all the articulation needs to be placed as distally as possible to counter the risk of a flexion contracture.

Resection of the PIN should always be undertaken, because it is a very simple procedure that helps with post-operative pain.

Fig. 34.24 Motec arthrodesis solution

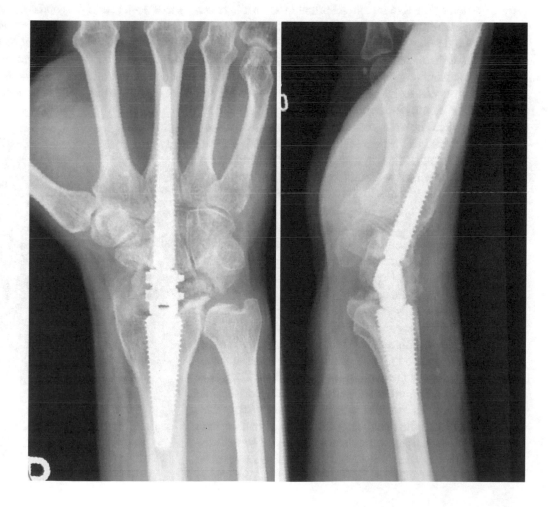

The proximally based flap allows both very good soft tissue coverage and appropriate tensioning of the flap due to the longitudinal extension of the flap to the third metacarpal. This extension provides the ability to either lengthen or shorten the repair to gain the correct tension (to lengthen, the distal arms are converted to a V from a T and to shorten, the limbs of the flap can be double-breasted).

As the flap tends to thin as it approaches the triquetrum due to the insertion of the dorsal wrist ligaments, the integrity and substance of the flap are improved by taking a sliver of bone from the dorsum of the triquetrum.

A total proximal row carpectomy should always be undertaken, because it benefits range of movement and prevents the possibility of impingement. While a PRC can prove to be a technical challenge, the use of a drill into each of the bones and insertion of a Carpalstix(TM), which is a small corkscrew device, facilitates control of the bones during removal, as does use of a curved, relatively broad, and blunt periosteal elevator introduced from dorsal to volar to sweep away the volar ligaments.

Use of the double claw retractor from the set facilitates the insertion of the wire into the capitate and metacarpal, as does placing the wrist over a kidney dish to allow the wrist to flex. Resection of a millimeter or two of the capitate facilitates insertion of the K-wire and its orientation, as it is easier to insert the wire into cancellous bone and to reference the 90-degree angle required from a flat surface.

Fixation of the metacarpal screw into the third metacarpal is the key to distal fixation of the Motec; therefore, the metacarpal screw needs to be as long and thin as possible, the threads of the screw obtaining good purchase into the third metacarpal where it flares from cancellous to cortical bone.

Because there is a 15-degree angle between the metacarpal and the capitate, a closing wedge osteotomy of this is key to obtaining length as it results in straight passage of the screw. A 1-mm resection of each edge of the third CMC joint consistently allows this as long as the prominent ridge that projects into the joint from the radial side arising from the second metacarpal is removed, and this is the key to obtaining the correction required. While not wanting to resect too much of the joint, it is important not to proceed with insertion of the wire until the correction has been obtained.

Once the osteotomy has been undertaken and the ridge removed, the capitate can be lifted up with the double claw retractor to provide alignment. Downward pressure from the surgeon's thumb onto the base of the third metacarpal countered by the lifting of the capitate by the assistant allows both alignment and direction as the wire can then be driven into the capitate directed toward the thumb. Once the sharp wire has passed through the distal part of the capitate and the base of the third metacarpal, which are experienced as two distinct points of resistance, the wire can then be reversed or changed to a blunt wire to allow the wire to find its way to the center of the metacarpal and prevent penetration of the cortices.

When the metacarpal screw is inserted, it should be initially compressed, because this closes the osteotomy, then rotated until inserted to the correct depth. It is important to get the balance between good fixation and correct depth (which can be checked on the image intensifier) and the desire not to over-insert the screw, given that it is a cone and cannot be reversed without losing fixation. One of the unique features of the Motec system, unlike other implants that rely on a carpal plate, is that the tension on the carpal side can be finessed up until the moment of insertion of the articulation by advancing the metacarpal screw, hence the need to allow approximately 1 mm of prominence of the screw to facilitate the adjustment of tension (advancing the screw by one full turn equates to just under 1 mm of forward movement).

Fixation in the capitate for this system is of benefit, but not essential, and given that in many Motec total wrists, stress shedding is seen around the capitate in time, if a fracture of the capitate should occur, it does not require any change in post-operative routine or concern about the strength of the fixation on the carpal side.

The optimal position of the metacarpal screw is with the tip of the screw well past the isthmus and the threads of the screw engaged in the good cortical bone where the metacarpal flares from cancellous to cortical bone (Fig. 34.25).

One of the most important technical tips is ensuring the position of the radial screw and hence the position of the cup, which of course then decides the center of rotation of the wrist replacement. The commonest mistake seen in cadav-

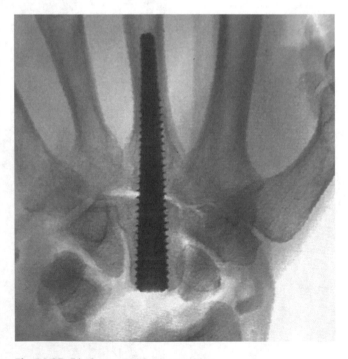

Fig. 34.25 Ideal metacarpal screw position

eric laboratory training and early cases is to impact the radial screw too proximally; this results in a wrist that is too slack even for an extra-long head and more importantly is a mechanical disadvantage for the extensor tendons. It is therefore very important not to over-ream the radius. This is why the technique of initially reaming the radius until cortical chatter or until the longest mark on the reamer is achieved is important. Once this reaming has been undertaken, the cup reamer is used; this reams the articular surface of the radius to create the space and position for the cup. More importantly, it has flange that automatically stops the reaming at the level of the rim of the distal radius, which ensures that the articulation is at the correct level in the wrist. The radial reamer is then reintroduced to ream further if necessary but more importantly the correct screw length for the radius is measured from the bottom of the cup. This method ensures that the screw is positioned correctly and the articulation is therefore at the correct level.

While most radii are suitable for the standard sizes of radial screws, larger screws are available (for special order) to cope with capacious or porotic radii. As indicated in the surgical technique above, the large metacarpal screw is also suitable for use in the radius. This is useful where the integrity of the distal radius is damaged by fracture or disease or in revision cases where the radius is damaged in the removal of the old implant. The large metacarpal screw is also useful where the radius is deformed by previous surgery or by disease, especially in rheumatoid arthritis where the radius is often smaller than usual. As this implant is available up to 70 mm, it allows fixation in the proximal, that is, cortical radius and bypasses the distal radius entirely.

Currently two articulations are available for the Motec total wrist: the original metal-on-metal (MOM) articulation and the metal-on-PEEK articulation. While long-term studies have been undertaken that demonstrate the safety and efficacy of the MOM [10], due to the concerns associated with MOM hips, it may not be suitable for all patients, surgeons, or markets and therefore it is worth noting that equivalence of PEEK articulation has been demonstrated [12]. In addition, as the PEEK articulation is thicker than the MOM by approximately 2 mm, anecdotal evidence suggests there is a mechanical advantage to the PEEK cup in terms of rehabilitation.

The author's current practice is to use the PEEK articulation as the standard prosthesis, reserving the MOM in cases where the joint is very tight and the thinness of the MOM articulation is an advantage.

The range of movement possible with the Motec total rise wrist is considerable being equivalent and possibly greater than the usual wrist as it is a ball and socket design. As result of this, when considering head length it is important to realize that when the short head is used it is possible that if a large range of movement is achieved it is possible for the screw, when in full dorsiflexion, to impinge on the dorsal rim of the cup, resulting in metalosis due to contact of the titanium of the screw on the cobalt chrome of the cup. This has been the subject of a case report [13]. In order to avoid this, a short neck should be avoided, if possible, and in this system using the method described above, if a medium neck is too tight, the solution is not to convert to a short neck but to advance the metacarpal screw to gain the necessary length and tension. The short neck remains available for those occasions where the wrist is so tight that no other possibility is available and, of course, in these occasions the resulting range of movement is unlikely to be sufficient for the impingement to occur; however, the short neck should be used with caution.

A big advantage of this system is the ability to finesse the tension right up until the insertion of the definitive implants, and the tension is adjusted by use of different head lengths and especially by use of the advancement of the metacarpal screw technique. This provides very precise and multiple adjustments prior to insertion of the definitive implants. In terms of deciding the correct tension, the wrist should achieve full dorsiflexion and some radial deviation. If the patient's wrist is lifted from the table and it fully flexes without the implant levering out then this is the best way to assess that the tension is correct.

Prior to closure, the wrist should be screened under radiographic control using the mini C-arm to assess movement and stability and especially to ensure that there is no impingement. If a full proximal row carpectomy is performed, impingement is unlikely and usually arises from a prominent radial styloid osteophyte, which can be removed with a saw.

The use of the proximally based flap allows adjustment of the tension of the repair due to the presence of the distal extension to access the third metacarpal. It can be lengthened or shortened to obtain the correct tension.

The implant is extremely stable; therefore, the period of post-operative should be as short as possible. The plaster of Paris splint is for comfort only and should be removed and active range of movement started as soon as pain and swelling allow; this is generally around 10 days post-operatively. This may be extended for the occasional case where the patient has poor healing and soft tissues, such as in patients with rheumatoid arthritis, but it should not be more than 2–3 weeks.

Because the Motec is an un-cemented implant, weight-bearing activities and the use of power tools should be restricted for the first 3 months until a radiograph indicates that the implant has incorporated. At this stage, a staged return to all normal activities with no restriction can be undertaken.

Conclusion

The human wrist has evolved over a long period to provide the movement and strength that we as a species require for the activities that we take for granted in our normal work, social and personal care requirements. Advances in wrist arthroplasty, now that we have reached the fourth generation of wrist implants, have reached the point where replacement of the wrist is a viable mainstream option for patients with end-stage arthritis of the wrist.

References

1. Tang JB. General concepts of wrist biomechanics and a view from other species. J Hand Surg Eur Vol. 2008;33(4):519–25.
2. Wolfe SW, Crisco JJ, Caley M, Orr MA, Marzke MW. The dart throwing motion of the wrist: is it unique to humans. J Hand Surg Am Vol. 2006;31(9):1429–37.
3. Charnley J. Total hip replacement by low friction arthroplasty. Clin Orthop. 1970;72:7–21.
4. Adams BD. Wrist arthroplasty: partial and total. Hand Clin. 2013;29:79–89.
5. Cooney IWP, Beckenbaugh RD, Linschied RL. Total wrist arthroplasty. Problems with implant failures. Clin Orthop Rel Res. 1984;187:121–8.
6. Weiss AP, Kamal RN, Shultz P. Total wrist arthroplasty. J Am Acad Orthop Surg. 2013;21:140–8.
7. Anneberg M, Packer G, Crisco JJ, Wolfe S. Four-year outcomes of midcarpal hema-arthroplasty for wrist arthritis. J Hand Surg Am. 2017;42(11):894–903.
8. Boeckstyns ME, Herzberg G, Messer S. Favourable results after total wrist arthroplasty. Acta Orthop. 2013;84:415–9.
9. Reigstad O, Hom-Glad T, Bolstas B, Grimsgaard C, Thorkildsen R, Rokkum M. Five to ten years prospective follow up of wrist arthroplasty in 56 non-rheumatoid patients. J Hand Surg Am. 2017;42(10):788–96.
10. Giwa L, Siddiqui A, Packer G. Motec wrist arthroplasty: 4 years of promising results. J Hand Surg Asian Pac. 2018;23(3):364–8.
11. Reigstad O, Rokkum M. Wrist arthroplasty using prosthesis as an alternative to arthrodesis: design outcomes and future. J Hand Surg Eur Vol. 2018;43(7):689–99.
12. Raja S, Cooper F, Estfan R, Packer G. Total wrist replacement: metal on PEEK articulation outcomes. Podium presentation, 14th IFSSH Berlin, June.
13. Karjalainen T, Pamilo K, Reito A. Implant failure after Motec wrist joint prosthesis due to failure of ball and socket-type articulation – two patients with adverse reaction to metal debris and polyether ether ketone. J Hand Surg Am. 2018;43(11):1044.

Volar Plating of Distal Radius Fractures

Stephanie Catherine Spence, Benjamin Hope,
and Mark Ross

Introduction

Distal radius fractures are the most common upper extremity fracture and their incidence only continues to increase. The first decision in the management of these injuries is whether the patient would benefit from operative management. This generally falls into two broad categories: closed reduction and percutaneous pinning (CRPP) and open reduction and internal fixation. Although CRPP has been practised for a century, with the advent of volar locking plates more than 20 years ago, there has been a significant shift in practice towards volar plates, which are now being favoured in certain parts of the world [1]. Their main goals include anatomic reduction with a rigid fixation, allowing for early range of motion rehabilitation.

As the use of volar plates increases, so does our understanding of the anatomy of these fractures as well as the techniques available. For some time, we have had an understanding of sagittal plane alignment correction with the aid of these plates; however, they do not intrinsically aid the surgeon with the correction of coronal plane translation. This can lead to postoperative problems secondary to a mal-reduced sigmoid notch leading to problems with the distal radioulnar joint. This will be discussed further in this chapter [2].

In more recent times with the evolution of volar locking plates, in appropriately selected fractures, a minimally invasive technique can be utilized by the surgeon. This can allow for a pronator quadratus (PQ) sparing approach with less scarring and soft tissue disruption. It has been suggested that this gives the patient a better range of motion and faster recovery postoperatively and is increasing in popularity.

Evolution of Volar Locking Plates

Third-generation volar locking plates, the implants we are familiar with today, brought with them variable angle screws that maintain angular stability. The benefit of having variable angle screws is that they allow for specific fragments to be addressed individually through the single volar plate. These screws allow for not only adjustment in a proximal to distal but also a radial to ulnar plane, allowing support of the articular surface as well as the radial column. Newer plate designs also incorporate radial column targeting screws to ensure the radial column fragment is adequately stabilized. Finally, variable angle screws also help avoid perforation of the screws into the radiocarpal and distal radioulnar joints as the ability to angle away from the articular surfaces is possible while not compromising fragment fixation.

Current Plate Designs

Key design points in modern plates include:

- Angle stable variable angle screws with anatomic distribution of polyaxial arcs
- Low profile plates with flush screw heads to minimize tendon rupture risk
- Anatomic watershed designs allowing for distal placement of the plate, especially to control the difficult lunate facet fragment, without increasing tendon irritation

S. C. Spence · B. Hope
Brisbane Hand and Upper Limb Research Institute,
Brisbane, QLD, Australia

Orthopaedic Department, Princess Alexandra Hospital,
Woolloongabba, QLD, Australia

M. Ross (✉)
Brisbane Hand and Upper Limb Research Institute,
Brisbane, QLD, Australia

Orthopaedic Department, Princess Alexandra Hospital,
Woolloongabba, QLD, Australia

The University of Queensland, St. Lucia, QLD, Australia
e-mail: research@upperlimb.com

© Springer Nature Switzerland AG 2022
W. B. Geissler (ed.), *Wrist and Elbow Arthroscopy with Selected Open Procedures*,
https://doi.org/10.1007/978-3-030-78881-0_35

It is also worth mentioning that there is a distinct difference between fixed and variable angle plates. In the fixed angle setting, the screw position is dictated by the plate itself. This is often adequate when the plate position is optimal to its anatomic design and is adequate for extra-articular fractures. In the case of more complex fractures, where the surgeon relies on the flexibly of the plate position to control key fragments, we then rely on the use of multidirectional screws. Currently, three fundamental groups of plate design that accommodate the variable angle screws are in clinical use.

Material Hardness Mismatch

This is the most common design which most commonly has a higher-grade metal screw, for instance, titanium 4, which taps into a softer grade metal plate such a titanium 2. This allows for an arc of 15 degrees of variation in all directions and can be repeated up to 3 times.

Mobile Expansion Bearing

In this setting, a mobile, spherical, expandable bearing sits within the plate. As the conical screw head engages with this bearing, it expands in the screw hole creating an interference fit. This bearing mechanism may be disengaged and reengaged multiple times.

Interference Fit

The third group of plates uses an interference fit between the threads on the screw head and those on the plate. There are a number of proprietary variations on this type.

Indications

The use of a volar plate is currently the authors' preferred technique to treat a distal radius fracture when operative management has been chosen and is technically feasible (contraindications discussed below).

There has been great discussion in the literature regarding what specifically constitutes an unstable distal radius fracture requiring fixation, but an absolute definition is not possible. There are certain principals that should be respected that will help guide the treating surgeon in their practice. Simple radiographic measurements are commonly quoted but it is important to adjust the management when taking into account the co-morbidities, physiological age and the functional demands of each individual patient. It is also important to consider that with the increased use of these plates and the

modern techniques available, such as minimally invasive fixation, coupled with the decrease in the complication profile, the relative indications for the use of volar locking plates are expanding, particularly when early mobilization and return to function is paramount.

There is a general consensus that the following parameters, based on pre-reduction injury films, require careful consideration to define an unstable fracture that may benefit from internal fixation due to increased risk of loss of position with closed management. These are based on the criteria of La Fontaine, which have stood the test of time [3]:

- Dorsal tilt >20°
- Dorsal comminution
- Intra-articular fracture
- Distal ulnar fracture
- Age greater than 60 years

The following criteria should also be reviewed on subsequent radiographs and clinical assessment if a closed reduction has been undertaken as they may indicate a developing problem:

- Articular step off/gap >1–2 mm
- Dorsal tilt >5–20 degrees (high vs. low demand patient)
- Radial shortening >2–5 mm
- Radial translation of the distal fragment with widening at the distal radioulnar joint
- Progressively worsening position of the fracture on serial radiographs particularly in the setting of a previously manipulated fracture
- Poor supination with the plaster in situ at the 1- to 2-week follow-up appointment

Relative Contraindications

One of the main benefits of volar plating systems is that they can address many fracture patterns, and their indications are broadening as the designs progress and evolve; however, there are certain circumstances where their use may not be indicated.

Highly Comminuted Intra-articular Fractures

In this situation, despite having modern implants, it may be very difficult to gain adequate hold and control of multiple small fragments. It is key to achieve anatomic reduction and fixation of the articular surface. Although with the advent of variable angle designs a large proportion of intra-articular fractures can be managed with volar locking plates, fragment-specific designs may be more suitable for highly comminuted fractures with very distal, small, or thin fragments.

Small Radial Column Fragment

Often this fracture pattern is associated with a highly comminuted fracture. Although some modern volar plates have specific radial column targeting screws, even with appropriate direction of these, it can pose a significant challenge to control and support this fragment. There has been recent innovation with the development of plates designed with radial targeting screws. These plates allow for screws to be directed directly towards the tip of the styloid unlike traditional plates. This may increase indications for the use of volar plates on smaller styloid fractures; however, preoperative insight into this and the availability of radial styloid targeting plates is required. Some radial column fragments may still require the addition of anatomic-specific radial column fixation when fragments cannot be adequately stabilized with volar plating.

Extremely Distal Volar Fracture Lines

With a distal volar fracture line, the surgeon may require the plate to place more distal on the volar surface in an attempt to control the fracture. This can be extremely hazardous. New plate designs have options that do allow for a more distal positioning of the plate, which makes this a relative contraindication; however, these fractures do still pose a problem. In situations with a dorsal shear fracture or where there is no visible volar fracture line, volar plates are not practically or biomechanically suited for stabilizing the fracture.

Fracture Dislocations

These injuries involve a wide spectrum of radiocarpal dislocations, and although they can be purely ligamentous, they are often associated with a fracture dislocation usually involving a large radial styloid fragment and volar avulsion type injuries with significant dorsal instability. In this setting, an anatomic/fragment-specific technique would be more appropriate.

Surgical Technique

Approach

The surgical approach for inserting a volar plate is through the bed of the flexor carpi radialis (FCR) tendon. This is *not* the classic Henry's approach that utilizes the interval between

the radial artery and the superficial radial nerve and is in fact ulna to the artery. A skin incision is made directly over the FCR tendon. Distal extension beyond the wrist crease is rarely necessary but has been described if a more extensive approach is required. Once the tendon is identified, the sheath is opened and the tendon is retracted ulna-wards reducing the chance of injury to the palmer cutaneous branch of the median nerve, although it is still at risk with excessive ulnar retraction of the FCR. The floor of the FCR tendon sheath is then incised allowing for entry into a plane between the flexor pollicis longus (FPL)/digital flexor tendons on the ulna side and the radial artery on the radial aspect. A plane is then established between the flexor tendons and the pronator quadratus (PQ) deep to them.

The surgeon should pay careful attention to the PQ muscle. Most commonly, PQ is elevated from the distal radius in an "L-type" fashion with the longitudinal limb along the radial border of the radius at the brachioradialis insertion and the transverse part parallel and just proximal to the watershed line. Normally, this is defined as the colour change from red muscle belly proximally to the well-defined, white tendinous portion distally. The cut should be made 1–2 mm into this tendinous portion to allow a good cuff to be created on both sides to facilitate repair at the end of the procedure (Fig. 35.1).

We advocate repairing the PQ muscle to allow for coverage of the plate. With the development of more distal plates, using them to manage more complex fractures, plates may sit in a problematic part of the distal radius. Even with adequate positioning, there remains a risk of irritation of the flexor tendons from the volar rim of the plate. We aim to reattach the PQ to its distal attachment as we find it more reliable than attaching it to the brachioradialis as previously described by other authors, with better plate coverage at the critical distal edge.

Of note, on the small percentage of occasions when we have removed the plate after fracture union, we have found the repaired PQ to be completely intact and covering the plate. We do not restrict the range of motion postoperatively to protect this repair, yet it heals. We believe with careful elevation and dissection of the PQ muscle and anatomic repair; we have observed no incidences of flexor tendon erosion secondary to the plate.

Another deep structure that is worth discussing is the brachioradialis tendon. In most cases, it is beneficial to release this tendon distal to the fracture line. It is accepted that the brachioradialis tendon is a deforming force in almost all fractures and this effect increases the longer after injury. It can contribute to difficulty with correction of radial height and inclination. As it has such an extensive attachment to the distal radial border of the radius, it can be safely released from its bony insertion distal to the fracture without proximal retraction of the tendon. This includes that portion which forms the floor of the 1st extensor compartment.

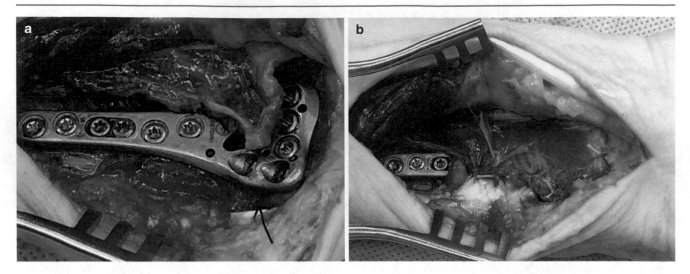

Fig. 35.1 (a) Clinical picture of the PQ elevation with the cuff of tendinous tissue distally. (b) Complete coverage of distal plate by careful elevation and repair of PQ

In our practice, we have found it uncommon to require the use of the more extensive Orbay and Fernandez approach [4, 5]. They describe the release of the radial septum with pronation of the proximal diaphyseal radius to give more access to the fracture line as well as the dorsal fragments. Although not commonly required, it is advisable to be familiar with this approach and we do utilize it on occasion. In cases where more extensive access to the dorsal fragments is required from the front, or if the surgeon is managing a delayed fracture with dorsal callus preventing the fracture from mobilizing, this approach can be very beneficial. We have particularly utilized this approach when performing corrective osteotomy for radius malunion with a volar plate and have described the technique in detail [6].

Gross Fracture Reduction

There are many techniques to address fracture reduction and a combination of these techniques may be required. The most straightforward is the classic technique of traction and manipulation. This can of course be combined with direct fracture manipulation, which on the majority of occasions can be achieved through the standard volar approach. It is also possible to access individual fragments through fracture lines and intervals. With the distal release of brachioradialis, frequently a "soft spot" of the fracture line on the border of the radius can be identified immediately deep to the tendon. It is often possible to elevate intra-articular fragments from this area using an instrument such as a Freer elevator or insert bone graft if required without the need for a separate dorsal incision. This is particularly useful when performing arthroscopic-assisted internal fixation.

As discussed previously, we have found it uncommon to require the use of the extended Orbay and Fernadez approach [4, 5]. The dorsal fragments that are most problematic are the dorsal ulnar fragments. These may also be associated with a coronal splint involving the distal radioulnar joint. These fragments are extremely important as our aim is for an early, pain free movement in particular with restoration of pronation and supination. In our experience, we only make a separate limited dorsal incision over these fragments when it is not possible to achieve a satisfactory reduction of them through the initial volar approach. In most instances, an approach between the 4th and 5th compartments through a 2-cm incision is adequate. Once the majority of the fracture complex has been reduced, this incision allows for the important dorsal ulna fragments to be reduced. Temporary hold with a Kirschner (K) wire can be helpful. The drill can then be used from the volar plate with direct visualization that the drill adequately targets the fragment. In addition, this approach also allows for the optimal screw length with adequate hold of the fragment without excessive dorsal penetration and irritation of the extensor tendons. We have found that these limited incisions for positioning of ulna screws from the volar side do *not* compromise flexion range as may be seen with formal dorsal approaches to place dorsal implants. On very rare occasions, when the fragment is too small to be held by a screw from the volar plate, a supplementary anatomic-specific plate for the dorsoulnar corner may be used.

We have utilized the aforementioned Orbay and Fernadez approaches to reduced dorsal intra-articular fragments; however, we are very satisfied with the safety and efficacy offered by the supplementary dorsal approach. Of note the majority of the exposure occurs proximal to the main part of the extensor retinaculum. An arthrotomy of the wrist is always avoided as it increases stiffness. If difficulty with articular reduction is expected, we prefer arthroscopic assistance.

Another key point to consider is the use of the image intensifier and the positioning of the arm on the arm table. We recommend that the surgeon sits cephalad to the extremity, with the assistant sitting at the end of the arm table. This allows fluoroscopy to approach parallel to the patient from the foot of the bed without obstruction. The use of the 15-degree inclination lateral brings the articular surface of the lunate fossa into view and aids with the assessment of reduction.

A major area at risk of mal-reduction, possibly due to the indirect assessment of reduction as well as the difficulty of assessment using the image intensifier, is the radial column and scaphoid facet in the sagittal plane. Malrotation of the scaphoid facet may occur and may be difficult to assess on fluoroscopy. An index of suspicion is vital. This occurs frequently when the radial column fracture line passes between the radial origins of the radioscaphocapitate ligament and the long and short radiolunate ligaments. In this setting, very careful radiographic assessment of the reduction is required in the pronated and supinated views. Reduction may look satisfactory on one view, but an indication of mal-reduction is when it looks unsatisfactory on the opposite view. Again, arthroscopy can assess this more effectively than fluoroscopy. We prefer dry/ moist arthroscopy as described by Pinal [7].

Intraoperative Techniques

Distal Volar Fracture Line

This can pose a problem if the plate is required to be placed distally to accommodate the fracture; there is a risk the screws may penetrate the joint. If the plate is placed proximally to allow for correct positioning of the distal screws then there is a risk the fracture may not be covered by the plate, leading to a biomechanically inferior construct with possible escape of volar fragments, especially on the ulnar side.

With the use of a variable angle plate, the surgeon has the option to position the plate more distally. The ulna screws can be directed perpendicular or even angled slightly proximally relative to the plate. This ensures there is no joint perforation from the screws, but at the same time the radial screws can still be adjusted to support the radial column.

Volar Ulna Fracture Line

It is vitally important to capture the volar ulna fragment to prevent secondary loss of reduction, which could result in

carpal subluxation, which is well described within the literature. When a sagittal plane fracture line exists on the ulna aspect of the distal radius, there is also a risk of screw perforation in the distal radioulna joint if a fixed angle screw is used.

With a variable angle plate, as was the case above, the plate can be deliberately placed more ulnarly past the fracture line and the screws directed away from the distal radioulnar joint.

Radial Column Support

By truly capturing the radial column and supporting it, fixation has a biomechanical advantage with more stability, particularly in the intra-articular setting. The aim with volar plating is to achieve a stable radial column similar to what can be achieved with fragment specific plates. The radial column is important due to its tricortical nature meaning that even if it a small fragment, it usually remains strong and can carry a significant portion of the scaphoid facet and volar radial ligaments. With modern variable angle designs, the radial one or two screws can be directed towards the tip of the styloid. This stabilizes the column from inside, and as we have previously described, it does so in a form that is somewhat analogous to the central pole of a marquee tent (Fig. 35.2) [8].

Residual Radial Translation of the Distal Fragment

Instability of the distal radioulna joint is a well-recognized sequelae of distal radius fractures. There are various factors that contribute to the stability of the distal radioulna joint including its osseous anatomy, joint capsule, radioulnar ligaments, triangular fibrocartilage complex, ulnocarpal ligaments, interosseous membrane and muscles. The extent to which each of these structures contributes to stability is not quantified; however, it is accepted that disruption of them can lead to instability of the distal radioulna joint. There are salvage procedures to address this; however, the preferred method is prevention of instability after distal radius fractures.

Our authors first made the observation of the radiographic parameter of "radial translation" when using fragment-specific radial column plates, as it was noted that patients fixed in this way have a lower incidence of distal radioulna joint instability [9]. By its design, the radial column plate automatically corrects any coronal plane radial translation but the volar locking plate does not. The residual radial translation contributes to instability at the distal radioulna joint due to loss of tension at the distal portion of the interosseous membrane, PQ and any remaining intact radioulnar liga-

Fig. 35.2 (**a**) Radial column support analogous to marquee tent pole. (**b**) Dual screw support of radial column

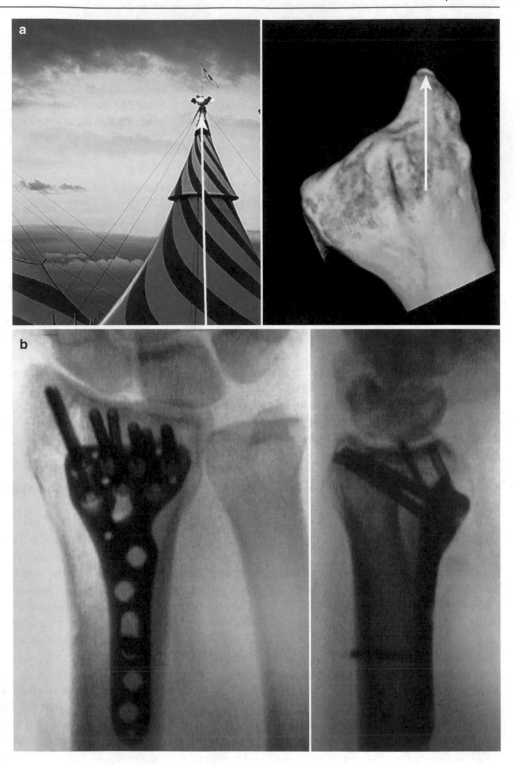

ments (Fig. 35.3). Consequently, even if the sigmoid notch is well positioned in all other respects, the ulna head may not be held firmly into the concavity, possibly contributing to instability. Wolfe et al. confirmed this with a cadaveric study showing instability resulting from the detensioning of the distal radioulnar joint from radial translation [10].

We developed a radiographic parameter to assess this. A line is drawn on the posteroanterior (PA) radiograph along the ulna aspect of the radius before the metaphyseal flare. A second line is drawn along the lunate parallel with the distal radial articulation. The proportion of the lunate on the radial side is expressed as a percentage, the mean of which

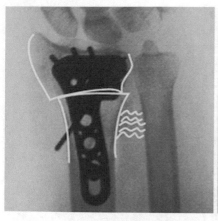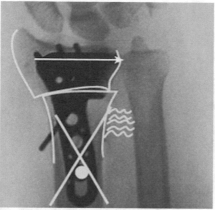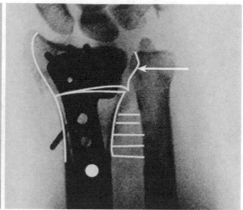

Fig. 35.3 Detensioning of interosseous membrane due to residual radial translation

was 45% in a series of uninjured wrists (Figs. 35.4 and 35.5) [9].

In the majority of fractures, this correction can be achieved using a volar locking plate as long as the surgeon is aware of the possibility of radial translation and is capable of assessing and correcting this intraoperatively. Routinely, we fix the distal fragment/s first. The distal part is then fixed to the shaft with a single diaphyseal screw placed in the distal end of the sliding hole. Radial length may then be adjusted by sliding the plate distally. Radial translation is the final parameter to be corrected, with the single screw acting as a fulcrum as follows (Fig. 35.6) [2]:

- A "crab claw" bone clamp is used. One tip of the clamp is placed distal to the shaft screw on the radial border of the plate.
- The other tip of the crab claw is placed on the ulna border of the radial shaft proximal to the fracture line.
- Once the clamp is in place and holding tension, the screw in the sliding plate hole is loosened just enough to allow the plate to translate on the radial shaft, using the shaft screw as a fulcrum.
- The crab claw is then closed progressively to translate the distal portion of the plate along with the distal fragment of the radius in an ulnar direction relative to the radial shaft in the coronal plane.
- The surgeon may simultaneously slightly rotate the clamp in a clockwise direction for the left wrist and a counter clockwise direction for the right wrist.
- Temporary K-wires through the plate can then be used to allow the assessment of the distal radioulnar joint stability through a range of motion, before committing to final plate position with the other shaft screws. Commonly increased "piano keying" when balloting the ulna head in mid rotation is seen, especially when there is an ulna styloid fragment. This does not equal the instability of the DRUJ under functional load and should not be used as a

justification for ulnar sided repairs. The key goal is to assess if the radius tracks smoothly around the ulnar head from a fully supinated position through to full pronation.
- Once satisfactory reduction and DRUJ stability has been obtained, the plate is secured to the shaft with the remaining screw holes.

It is possible to over-reduce the residual radial translation, which can lead to stiffness and limitation of forearm rotation due to over-tensioning of the interosseous membrane. Over-reduction is easily corrected, but this relies on the surgeon identifying this intraoperatively.

Minimally Invasive Distal Radius Plating

Minimally invasive surgery is a worldwide tendency in every surgical specialty including distal radius fixation. As mentioned above, the FCR approach offers excellent visualization and access to the fracture; however, it is not without its complications which have been reported widely in the literature. Minimally invasive techniques were first mentioned as far back as the early 2000s [11, 12]. These authors used K-wires combined with nonlocking mini plates to achieve fixation, sometimes alongside arthroscopic assistance. This then evolved with the advent of volar locking plates. Some surgeons advocated a double incision approach to spare the PQ muscle followed by the development of the standard FCR approach. Along with these minimally invasive approaches, new plate designs have become available to facilitate this technique.

The main indication for a minimally invasive technique is the unstable, extra-articular, or simple articular distal radius fracture, primarily for two reasons. Firstly, they are generally amenable to gross reduction by closed methods; secondly, they have a low probability of associated injuries. This technique offers patients an operation that has equivalent mor-

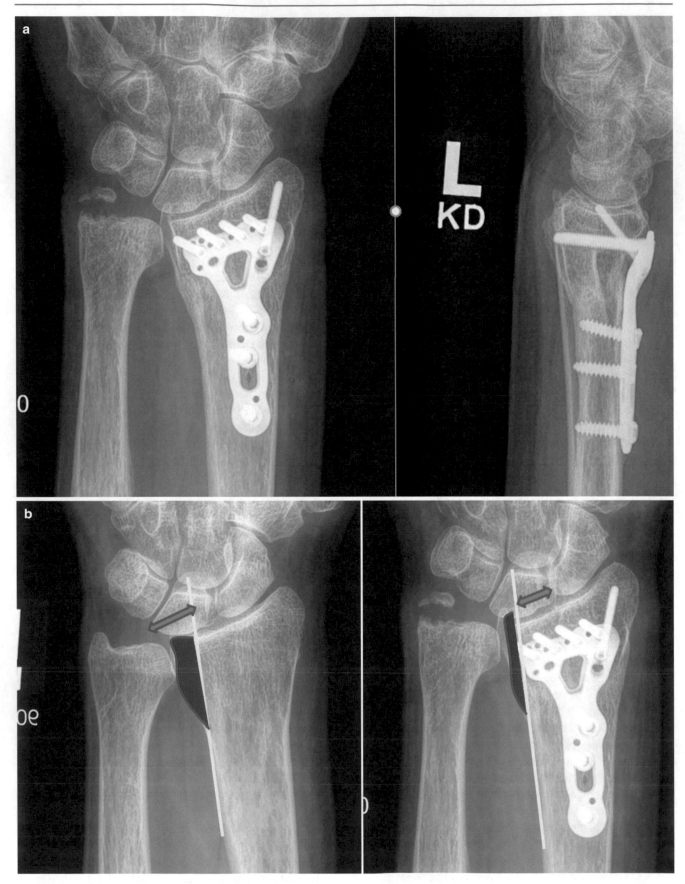

Fig. 35.4 (a) A 55-year-old female with symptomatic instability postfixation. Radial height, length and tilt are satisfactory. (b) Comparison to the other side confirms radial translation

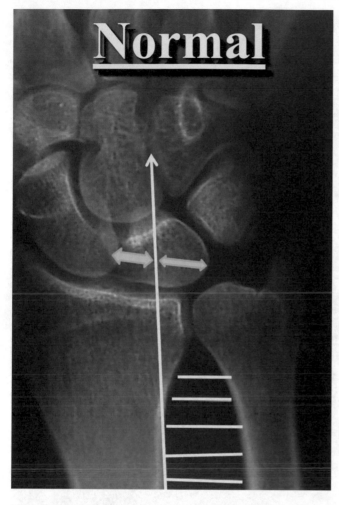

Fig. 35.5 Radiographic parameter for residual radial translation, a/ (a + b) × 100 [5]

bidity and risks to K-wire fixation but can offer patients a cast-free rehabilitation and early range of motion. There may also be an indication to treat stable extra-articular fractures in the young patient group with minimally invasive surgery when cast immobilization for a length of time is not feasible due to work commitments in a variety of occupations. As this technique evolves, the indications are being pushed with more complex fractures being fixed with this method, particularly in the setting of arthroscopic-assisted surgery. There is a steep learning curve and only the surgeon with experience in minimally invasive techniques should be considering its use in complex fracture patterns.

Surgical Technique

The group from Strasbourg in France promote a single longitudinal incision [13]. They recommend an incision over the FCR tendon 15–20 mm in size, centred over the final position of the plate. The approach incises the FCR sheath and uses the skin at a "mobile window" relying on its elasticity to access the radius. The PQ is identified, and a transverse incision is made at the watershed line. A periosteal elevator is then used to create a pocket for the plate to be inserted. Either closed methods of reduction can be used with classic K-wires to hold the fracture temporarily or the plate can be used as a reduction tool, fixing it distally first and then securing it onto the shaft to correct the dorsal tilt. Fluoroscopy use is essential. The proximal screws are placed using small incisions in the PQ inline with its fibres.

A transverse incision has also been described. The first to describe this was a group from Japan in 2011 [14].

Although the two aforementioned approaches are well established in the literature, we have developed a variation of Livernaux's longitudinal incision technique that we believe is a true PQ-sparing approach. It has been shown that to keep the PQ muscle functional, the distal tendinous attachment is vitally important and should be protected. We recommend a skin incision about 2 cm in length over the FCR tendon inline with the middle portion of the plate. The usual interval is developed through the FCR subsheath and the PQ is identified. The distal attachment of the PQ is left intact, and the radial border only is cut. A periosteal elevator is used to create a pocket under PQ to allow a mini-plate be inserted under the muscle with a specific jig attached that accommodates the PQ between it and the plate (Figs. 35.7, 35.8, and 35.9). The jig acts as a soft tissue retractor, plate holder, drill guide and reduction device. The proximal screws can be easily inserted without any disruption to the proximal PQ and the drill guides that insert into the jig allows for insertion of the distal screws with minimal damage to the PQ. Again, the fracture can be reduced using various techniques. If there is a difficulty in restoring the volar tilt, a locking screw can be placed in the most proximal shaft hole as a kickstand screw to elevate the plate from the shaft recreating the required angle of correction. The plate can then be fixed distally first and reduced onto the shaft after removing the kickstand style locking screw. If there is residual radial translation, then this can be addressed and reduced as described previously, but this can be slightly more technically demanding than with the standard plate due to the length and pivot point on the short plate and the intact PQ. Once the fracture is fixed, the PQ muscle should be repaired along its radial border to the brachioradialis tendon.

Overview of Overall Surgical Strategy for Distal Radius Fixation

The surgical plan will vary depending on the complexity of the fracture, what fragments are present, and whether it is intra- or extra-articular. There is a generic order for addressing the problems the surgeon may encounter with these fractures.

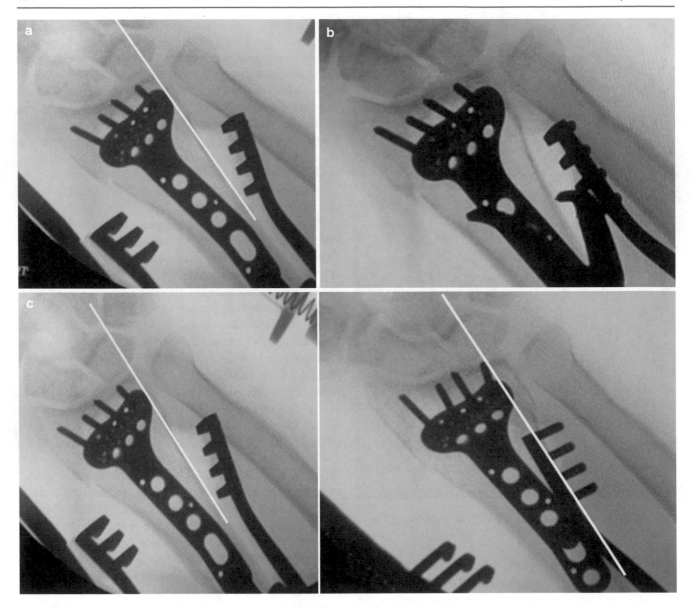

Fig. 35.6 (**a**) Intraoperative residual radial translation. (**b**) Crab claw in situ. (**c**) Pre- and postcorrection of radial translation

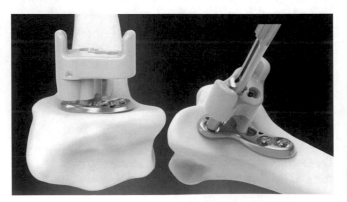

Fig. 35.7 An example of a PQ-sparing MIS guide with a mini-plate

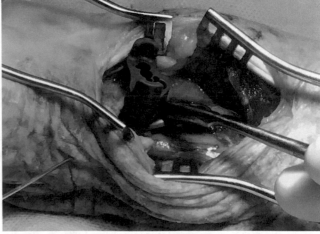

Fig. 35.8 PQ-sparing approach with normal skin incision to demonstrate use of guide to place plate deep to PQ

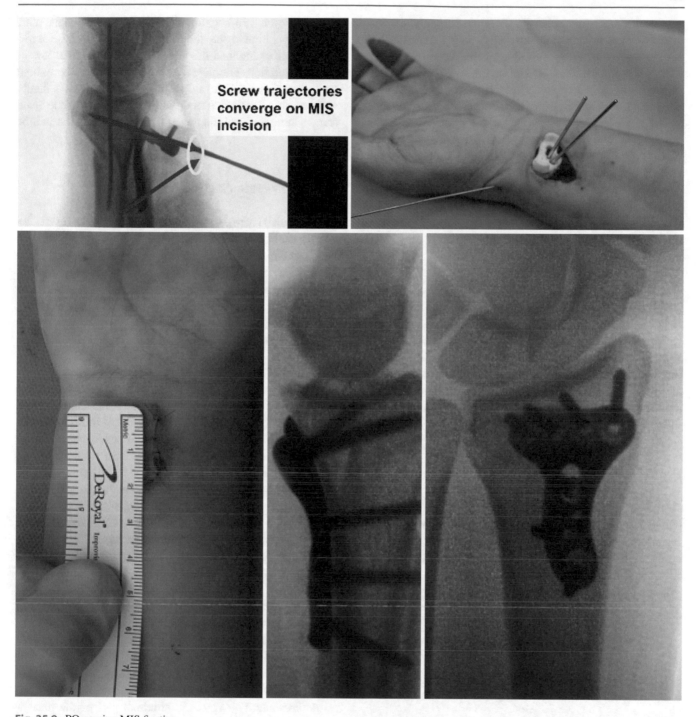

Screw trajectories converge on MIS incision

Fig. 35.9 PQ-sparing MIS fixation

Gross Reduction Through Indirect Manual Traction

There should be an attempt at restoring the general alignment and length of the radius with manual traction whenever possible. If this achieves a near acceptable reduction then the fracture can be temporarily pinned with K-wires. Fine-tuning of the reduction can then be achieved using the plate and screws as a reduction device.

Articular Surface Reduction and Arthroscopic-Assisted Reduction

The next stage should address the articular surface of the sigmoid notch and the distal articular surface. This can be employed with a variety of direct and indirect techniques. Once the surface is reduced, it can be held with multiple small K-wires as a temporary measure. It is important that these wires are positioned in such a fashion that they do not inhibit the subsequent plate application. It is very reasonable to use percutaneous wires during this stage. It can be helpful to place wires into the styloid between the first and second extensor compartments as well as through the dorsal aspect of the radius in the region of the 4th and 5th extensor compartments. It is important to reconstruct the articular surface with the wires prior to addressing the relationship between the articular and metaphyseal region and the diaphysis. If the plate is preset to the shaft (PART technique of Abe), modern arthroscopic-assisted fixation systems allow placement of temporary angle stable K-wires through guides in the plate which can be sequentially placed as arthroscopic-assisted reduction (AARIF) is fine-tuned, then replaced with cannulated pegs without loss of position (Fig. 35.10) [15].

Distal Locking Screw Placement

It is important that the locking screws address two things. The first is that screws be distributed to achieve maximal subchondral support. The second is that the screws should be directed to address specific fragments. As mentioned before, as the screws are variable angle, they can be placed safely avoiding articular penetrations at the radiocarpal joint and the distal radioulna joint.

Provisional Plate Fixation

At this stage, if the reduction appears adequate then the plate can be fixed to the shaft provisionally with K-wires. If ongoing mal-alignment is present, all aspects of this need to be considered when determining the position of the plate in

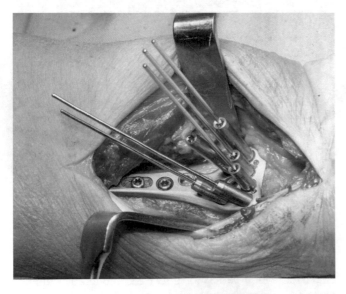

Fig. 35.10 Stepwise AARIF system (Newclip Technics, Nantes, France)

both the coronal and sagittal planes, such that when the plate is finally positioned onto the shaft, it will reduce these deformities. One example of this is when there is residual loss of radial angulation. The plate may be applied with its proximal end directed more ulnaward so that when the plate is finally reduced onto the shaft after definitive placement of the distal screws into the distal fragment, the radial angulation will be corrected.

Definitive Plate Fixation

Once the distal screws have been placed and there is satisfactory control of distal articular surface resulting in the articular surface mobilizing as one fragment, the implant can then be used as a reduction tool fine-tuning the relationship between the articular surface and the shaft.

Other Considerations

- *Sagittal plane deformity* – In extra-articular fractures prior to definitive fixation of the plate to the shaft, it is still possible to correct residual dorsal tilt of the fracture. To achieve this, the distal screws should be loosened then the proximal end of the plate is lifted off of the shaft to increase the angulation between the distal screws and the plate. In more complex intra-articular fractures, there is a risk of loss of position if the distal screws are holding individual fragments. In a similar fashion, the so-called "distal first technique" can be enrolled from the beginning of the procedure if there is difficulty reducing the dorsal tilt. The plate is applied to the distal fragment or fragments and secured with K-wires and screws with the shaft of the plate sitting off the shaft recreating the angle of dorsal tilt that requires correction. This can be facilitated by using a "kickstand" screw locked into the proximal plate to hold the desired angulation (Fig. 35.11).
- *Coronal plane deformity* – Correction of residual coronal plane translation is discussed above.
- *Radial length* – When the proximal part of the plate is initially applied to the shaft, the oblong or "sliding" hole should be utilized with a single screw. If increased radial height is required, then this screw should be loosened and either the plate is pushed from its proximal end to translate it distally or traction is applied to achieve the same result. Once restoration of the height has been restored, the screw may then be tightened again.
- *The use of bone graft* – Union with deformity is commonly a complication from distal radius volar plating particularly in the osteoporotic and elderly. If there is a large metaphyseal defect, our authors recommend the use of a

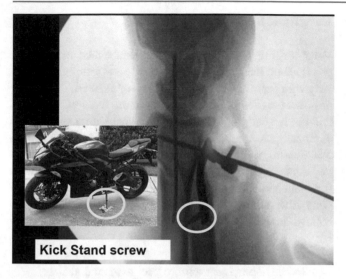

Kick Stand screw

Fig. 35.11 Kickstand screw to facilitate correction of volar tilt during distal fragment first technique

structural bone graft that has compressive strength such as an injectable calcium phosphate bone substitute. We have found that using synthetic bone graft as an adjunct, we have had less than reported loss of reduction of our fixation [16]. It is vitally important that the cavity for the graft is properly prepared. All haematoma and fibrous tissue should be removed with a curette. Once the void is free from tissue, any loose cancellous bone should be carefully packed into the surrounding walls prior to the graft insertion. Only once due care to the preparation has taken place can the bone graft be injected in a controlled manner under fluoroscopic guidance if required.

Fractures in the Elderly

There is varying literature on the utility of volar plate fixation in the elderly. With an arbitrary definition of 65 years and over, a recent randomized trial by Saving et al. showed a significant benefit with fixation versus closed management [17].

Common Errors in Distal Radius Plating

The treatment of distal radius fractures has changed dramatically since the introduction of volar locking plates and along with this the complication profile has also changed. Many of these complications are avoidable. Below is a summary of the common errors associated with distal radius plating that surgeons should be aware of. It is hoped that this chapter has equipped the surgeon with the knowledge to avoid these.

- Errors of surgical approach
  - Inadequate exposure
  - Nerve injury – especially the palmar branch of the median nerve
- Flexor tendinopathy/rupture
  - Plate design
  - Plate position close to the volar rim
  - Protruding hardware
  - Failure to restore volar tilt
- Protruding screw tips
  - Attempts to lag dorsal fragment
  - Incorrect screw length
  - Improper interpretation of intraoperative x-rays
  - Failure to utilize skyline/dorsal horizon view [18]
- Complex, distal, multiarticular fractures
  - Pattern not amenable to volar plate fixation
  - Very distal fracture lines with inadequate buttress by volar plate
  - Failure to stabilize the critical corner (volar ulnar) fragment
- Excessive or inadequate plate width
- Inadequate reduction
  - Intra-articular incongruity
  - Radial shortening
  - Coronal translation
- Inadequate plate length and placement
  - Subchondral screws/pegs too far from subchondral bone
  - Insufficient length of plate

Rehabilitation

We recommend that patients be evaluated on the first postoperative day by a hand therapist. All bulky dressings are removed and a simple dressing is applied. A thermoplastic volar forearm static splint with 15 degrees of wrist extension is fabricated for the patient. The splint should be removed when performing exercises and non-weight-bearing activities during the first six postoperative weeks. Range of motion exercises should focus on finger movements, forearm rotation, dart throwers motion and functional wrist movement. We aim to achieve 90% pronosupination by week two. If pronation and supination are not on track by week four then we apply a gentle tension rotational orthosis as long as fracture fixation allows for stress across the wrist joint. All orthotics are discarded at 6 weeks and functional tolerances are increased beginning with grip and wrist strengthening.

Tips and Tricks

The normal range of values for radial translation can vary quite significantly. It may be worthwhile considering using radiographs of the other wrist to establish a normal for your patient. This is particularly important when performing a corrective radial osteotomy.

It cannot be ignored that there is undoubtedly some potential for soft tissue problems with volar plating, particularly if care is not taken with the surgical technique. The greatest risk is inadvertent perforation of the dorsal cortex by distal locking screws. The length of the locking screws may be difficult to judge using a depth gauge because of osteoporosis and dorsal comminution. In addition, due to the trapezoidal cross section of the distal radius, screws may appear in bone on fluoroscopy but are actually too long. The third compartment is particularly at risk. It is worth noting that the engagement of the dorsal cortex is only occasionally necessary in complex intra-articular fractures. If there is any concern regarding screw length when it is necessary to engage the dorsal cortex then a small dorsal incision can allow direct visualization of the screw with low morbidity and no compromise over the screw length.

We have already discussed the importance of careful dissection of the PQ muscle so it can be repaired over the plate at the end of the procedure. If this is not done, there is a risk of late flexor tendon rupture, particularly the flexor pollicis longus that sits immediately over the plate.

Finally, an extremely devastating yet often insidious complication of volar plating is related to the volar ulnar corner fragment (Fig. 35.12). Even if all other aspects of the fracture are reduced and well fixed, if this fragment is not stabilized, then it may translate in a volar and ulna direction in association with volar ulnar subluxation of the carpus. It is essential that the plate be positioned over this fragment so it stabilizes the fragment.

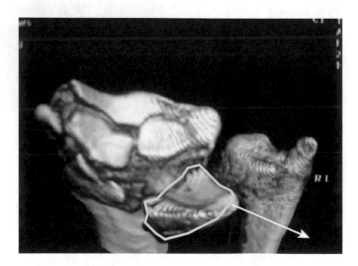

Fig. 35.12 Volar ulnar corner fragment

Conclusion

Volar locking plates are now well established in common practice and their indications for use are expanding, particularly with the availability of variable angle screws. Reviewing our own practice of distal radius fracture fixation, we found that the largest group, 85%, were treated with a single FCR approach and a volar locking plate. The next largest group, 5% of cases, was treated as above with the addition of a limited dorsal approach to aid in the reduction of the dorsal ulna fragment and optimal positioning of a screw in this fragment. Only 10% required the use of anatomic-specific fixation. We believe the benefits of a volar variable angle stable plate to be:

- Flexible deployment with respect to the radial size
- Flexibility with the positioning of the plate proximally and distally
- Accommodation of fracture line variations
- Ability to direct screws to specific fracture fragments
- Added bonuses of variable angle plates include
  - Gross adjustment of reduction
  - In situ fine tuning
  - In situ adjustment of reduction including the articular fragment
  - Screw preloading

References

1. Nellans KW, Kowalski E, Chung KC. The epidemiology of distal radius fractures. Hand Clin. 2012;28(2):113–25. https://doi.org/10.1016/j.hcl.2012.02.001. PubMed PMID: 22554654; PubMed Central PMCID: PMCPMC3345129.
2. Ross M, Allen L, Couzens GB. Correction of residual radial translation of the distal fragment in distal radius fracture open reduction. J Hand Surg Am. 2015;40(12):2465–70. https://doi.org/10.1016/j.jhsa.2015.09.008. PubMed PMID: 26489900.
3. Lafontaine M, Hardy D, Delince P. Stability assessment of distal radius fractures. Injury. 1989;20(4):208–10. https://doi.org/10.1016/0020-1383(89)90113-7. PubMed PMID: 2592094.
4. Orbay JL, Badia A, Indriago IR, Infante A, Khouri RK, Gonzalez E, et al. The extended flexor carpi radialis approach: a new perspective for the distal radius fracture. Tech Hand Up Extrem Surg. 2001;5(4):204–11. https://doi.org/10.1097/00130911-200112000-00004. PubMed PMID: 16520583.
5. Orbay JL, Fernandez DL. Volar fixation for dorsally displaced fractures of the distal radius: a preliminary report. J Hand Surg Am. 2002;27(2):205–15. https://doi.org/10.1053/jhsu.2002.32081. PubMed PMID: 11901379.
6. Potter JA, Ross M. The dorsal periosteal curtain for distal radius osteotomy via the volar approach. Tech Hand Up Extrem Surg. 2020; https://doi.org/10.1097/bth.0000000000000329. PubMed PMID: 33264258.
7. Fd P, Luchetti R, Mathoulin C. Arthroscopic management of distal radius fractures. 1st ed. Berlin, Heidelberg: Springer Berlin Heidelberg; 2010.

8. Ross M, Heiss-Dunlop W. Chapter 10 – volar angle stable plating for distal radius fractures. In: Slutsky DJ, editor. Principles and practice of wrist surgery. Philadelphia: W.B. Saunders; 2010. p. 126–39.

9. Ross M, Di Mascio L, Peters S, Cockfield A, Taylor F, Couzens G. Defining residual radial translation of distal radius fractures: a potential cause of distal radioulnar joint instability. J Wrist Surg. 2014;3(1):22–9. https://doi.org/10.1055/s-0033-1357758. PubMed PMID: 24533242; PubMed Central PMCID: PMCPMC3922865.

10. Dy CJ, Jang E, Taylor SA, Meyers KN, Wolfe SW. The impact of coronal alignment on distal radioulnar joint stability following distal radius fracture. J Hand Surg Am. 2014;39(7):1264–72. https://doi.org/10.1016/j.jhsa.2014.03.041. PubMed PMID: 24857823.

11. Geissler WB, Fernandes D. Percutaneous and limited open reduction of intra-articular distal radial fractures. Hand Surg. 2000;5(2):85–92. https://doi.org/10.1142/s0218810400000193. PubMed PMID: 11301501.

12. Duncan SF, Weiland AJ. Minimally invasive reduction and osteosynthesis of articular fractures of the distal radius. Injury. 2001;32(Suppl 1):Sa14–24. https://doi.org/10.1016/s0020-1383(01)00057-2. PubMed PMID: 11521702.

13. Zemirline A, Naito K, Lebailly F, Facca S, Liverneaux P. Distal radius fixation through a mini-invasive approach of 15 mm. Part 1: feasibility study. Eur J Orthop Surg Traumatol. 2014;24(6):1031–7. https://doi.org/10.1007/s00590-013-1364-1. PubMed PMID: 24253958.

14. Zenke Y, Sakai A, Oshige T, Moritani S, Fuse Y, Maehara T, et al. Clinical results of volar locking plate for distal radius fractures: conventional versus minimally invasive plate osteosynthesis. J Orthop Trauma. 2011;25(7):425–31. https://doi.org/10.1097/BOT.0b013e3182008c83. PubMed PMID: 21464735.

15. Abe Y, Yoshida K, Tominaga Y. Less invasive surgery with wrist arthroscopy for distal radius fracture. J Orthop Sci. 2013;18(3):398–404. https://doi.org/10.1007/s00776-013-0371-8. PubMed PMID: 23463123.

16. Saw N, Roberts C, Cutbush K, Hodder M, Couzens G, Ross M. Early experience with the TriMed fragment-specific fracture fixation system in intraarticular distal radius fractures. J Hand Surg Eur Vol. 2008;33(1):53–8. https://doi.org/10.1177/1753193407087887. PubMed PMID: 18332021.

17. Saving J, Severin Wahlgren S, Olsson K, Enocson A, Ponzer S, Sköldenberg O, et al. Nonoperative treatment compared with volar locking plate fixation for dorsally displaced distal radial fractures in the elderly: a randomized controlled trial. J Bone Joint Surg Am. 2019;101(11):961–9. https://doi.org/10.2106/jbjs.18.00768. PubMed PMID: 31169572.

18. Joseph SJ, Harvey JN. The dorsal horizon view: detecting screw protrusion at the distal radius. J Hand Surg Am. 2011;36(10):1691–3. https://doi.org/10.1016/j.jhsa.2011.07.020. PubMed PMID: 21864994.

Pronator-Sparing Distal Radius Volar Plating

36

Stephanie S. Pearce and Randall W. Viola

Introduction

Distal radius fractures are commonly treated with volar plate fixation. Traditionally, the surgical techniques for plate fixation require division of the pronator quadratus. While this provides optimal exposure of the fracture and facilitates plate positioning, the trauma incurred by pronator division and repair interferes with postoperative forearm rotation [1, 2]. Patients often require months of therapy to regain supination. Some patients never regain full supination due to pronator contracture [1, 3]. The loss of forearm rotation caused by pronator division and repair also makes it difficult to discriminate the patient with loss of rotation due to pronator division and the patient with distal radioulnar joint instability [1, 2].

Distal radius fractures treated with a pronator-sparing technique typically recover forearm rotation very quickly, often achieving full supination within 2 weeks. Those patients that do not quickly recover supination likely have distal radioulnar joint instability (DRUJ) and/or other DRUJ pathology and are treated accordingly. Acute DRUJ instability is reliably treated with long arm supination splinting, closed reduction and pinning, and/or open reduction and internal fixation with or without triangular fibrocartilage repair. Early detection of DRUJ instability is critical for achieving a good outcome. Chronic DRUJ instability is extremely difficult to manage and outcomes are often suboptimal.

Indications

- Extra-articular distal radius fractures
- Intra-articular distal radius fractures

Contraindications

- Initial treatment of grossly contaminated distal radius fractures or volar compartment syndrome requiring management with an external fixator instead of internal fixation
- Radial shaft fractures, not captured by the length of the plate
- Distal radius fractures in skeletally immature patients in which the distal fragment includes or passes distal to the physis and thus a smooth wire construct is preferred
- Non-displaced distal radius fractures amenable to closed reduction and splinting/casting

Surgical Technique

Exposure

The volar distal radius is exposed using a 7-cm incision over the volar distal forearm in the superficial interval between the flexor carpi radialis (FCR) and the radial artery (Fig. 36.1). The deep interval is between the flexor pollicis longus and the radial artery (Fig. 36.2). Dissection ulnar to the FCR tendon may injure the palmar cutaneous branch of the median nerve. The fascia along the proximal and distal aspects of the pronator quadratus is incised (Fig. 36.3a, b). Elevate the periosteum adjacent to the fracture (Fig. 36.4). The pronator may need to be retracted proximally to expose the fracture. For complex fractures that involve comminution of the metadiaphysis, where additional exposure is necessary to achieve a satisfactory reduction, the pronator is incised

S. S. Pearce
The Steadman Clinic and Steadman Philippon Research Institute, Vail, CO, USA

R. W. Viola (✉)
Department of Hand, Wrist, Elbow, and Microvascular Surgery, The Steadman Clinic and Steadman Philippon Research Institute, Vail, CO, USA
e-mail: RV@thesteadmanclinic.com

© Springer Nature Switzerland AG 2022
W. B. Geissler (ed.), *Wrist and Elbow Arthroscopy with Selected Open Procedures*,
https://doi.org/10.1007/978-3-030-78881-0_36

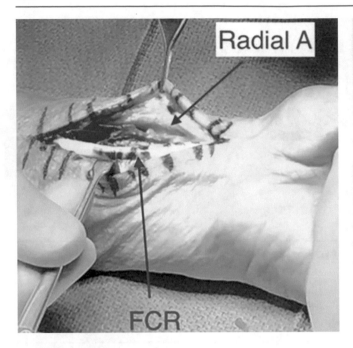

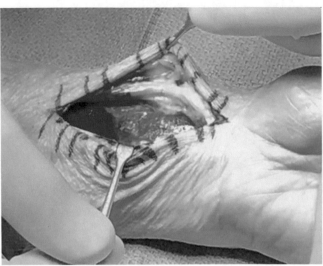

Fig. 36.1 The volar distal radius is exposed in the interval between the flexor carpi radialis (FCR) and the radial artery interval

Fig. 36.2 The deep interval between the flexor pollicis longus (FPL) and the radial artery is opened to expose the pronator quadratus

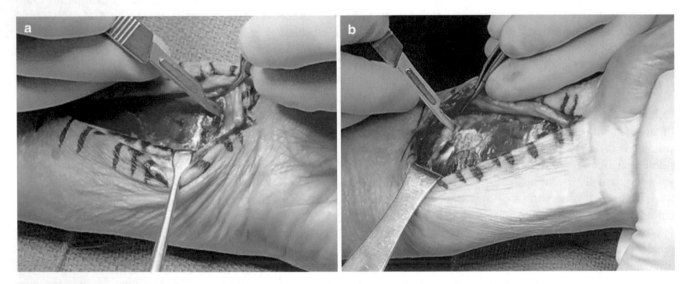

Fig. 36.3 (**a**) Incise the fascia of the distal aspect of the pronator quadratus (PQ) to expose the distal radius fracture. (**b**) Incise the fascia of the proximal aspect of the PQ to allow the distal radius plate to slide under the PQ

longitudinally along its radial margin, and it is retracted ulnarly. The volar aspect of the distal radius fracture may be visualized by retracting the pronator proximally with Ragnell retractors.

Reduction

If the fracture is amenable to closed reduction, a closed reduction is performed and provisionally stabilized with 1.6 mm (0.062″) Kirschner wires (K-wires) (Fig. 36.5). Single-ended K-wires are safest. When placing these wires, oscillating mode is recommended to minimize soft tissue injury.

1. The first K-wire is placed in the dorsal radial aspect of the fracture. The wire is hinged distally and ulnarly and drilled into the volar ulnar cortex of the radial metadiaphysis. Advancing the wire through the volar cortex is avoided as this may interfere with plate positioning.
2. If the distal radius fragment is displaced radially, a second K-wire is placed in the fracture along the volar radial aspect, anterior to the radial sensory nerve, and hinged distally to reduce the radial displacement (Fig. 36.6). This wire is then drilled into the ulnar aspect of the radial metadiaphysis.
3. If there is significant dorsal displacement, additional K-wires may be placed dorsally and hinged distally to reduce the dorsal displacement and correct the volar tilt (Fig. 36.7a, b).

Fluoroscopy is used to confirm anatomic reduction.

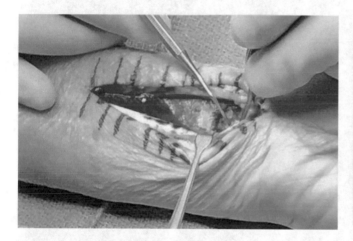

Fig. 36.4 Elevate periosteum adjacent to fracture to facilitate anatomic reduction

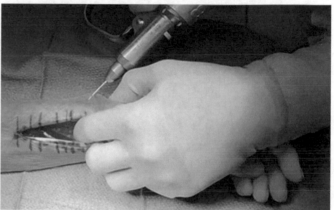

Fig. 36.6 A K-wire is placed in the radial aspect of the fracture to reduce radial displacement and restore radial inclination

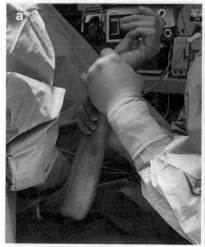
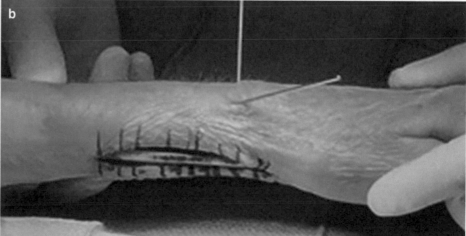

Fig. 36.5 (a) Closed reduction of distal radius. (b) K-wire provisional fixation

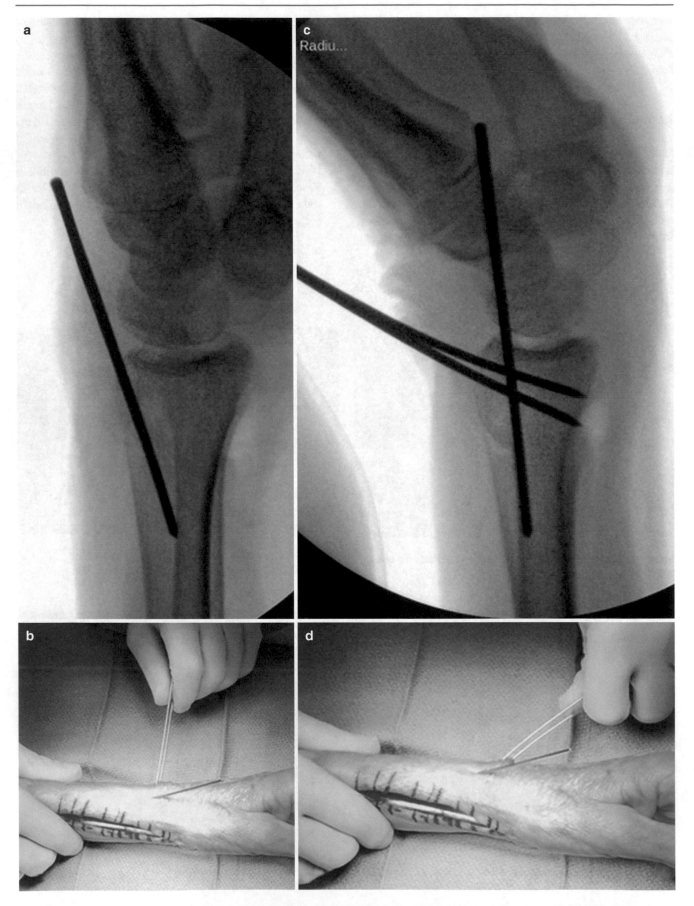

Fig. 36.7 (a) Fluoroscopic image after closed reduction and placement of the first dorsal-radial K-wire. (b) Two dorsal K-wires in distal radius at neutral position. (c) Fluoroscopic image of dorsal K-wires hinged distally restoring volar tilt. (d) K-wires hinged distally to restore volar tilt

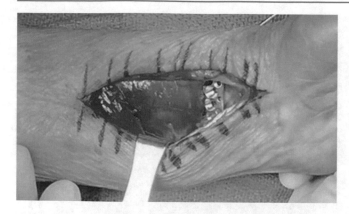

Fig. 36.8 Plate provisionally positioned under PQ

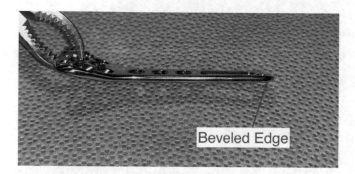

Fig. 36.9 Pronator-sparing volar distal radius plate with proximal beveled edge to be used as an elevator during plate placement

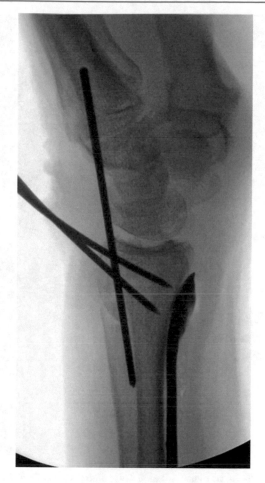

Fig. 36.10 Lateral fluoroscopic image showing plate placement proximal to watershed line

Plate Application

The appropriately sized pronator-sparing distal radius plate is chosen and is slid under the pronator from distal to proximal (Fig. 36.8). The proximal aspect of the plate is beveled and may be used as an elevator to facilitate plate placement (Fig. 36.9). The distal radius plate slides easily under the pronator from distal to proximal. The plate is provisionally positioned under direct visualization and fluoroscopic guidance. This plate is designed to sit proximal to the watershed line with the distal screws aiming more distal in order to prevent tendon injury [4] (Fig. 36.10). Once the plate is in an acceptable provisional position, the plate-centering drill guide (PCDG) is used to place the most proximal screw and center the plate on the radius (Fig. 36.11a, b). This unique patented clamp centers the most proximal screw in the radial shaft in a radioulnar direction preventing eccentric plate placement. The most proximal hole in the plate has an extended slot allowing for simple proximal-distal positioning of the plate. This technique simplifies plate placement. Once the plate is positioned using direct visualization and fluoroscopic images, the proximal-most screw hole is drilled with a 2.0 mm drill (Fig. 36.12). With position confirmed,

the non-locking 2.7-mm screw is placed and tightened (Fig. 36.13). The cleats on the deep surface of the plate maintain the position of the plate (Fig. 36.14).

Fracture Fixation

The pronator-sparing drill guide (PSDG) then attaches to the plate overlaying the pronator quadratus via pegs on the proximal and distal aspects of the plate (Fig. 36.15a–c). Once this drill guide is seated in the plate, the triple drill sleeve may be inserted into it and used to place three additional 2.7-mm locking or nonlocking screws in the proximal shaft portion of the plate using a 2.0-mm drill (Fig. 36.16). A 1.8-mm drill is used in the distal portion of the PSDG to drill the distal holes (Fig. 36.17). Once these holes have been drilled, the pronator-sparing drill guide is removed (Fig. 36.18). The holes in the distal plate may be filled with non-locking screws, locking screws, locking pegs, and/or terminally threaded cannulated locking screws (Fig. 36.19). Final fluoroscopic images are reviewed to ensure appropriate screw

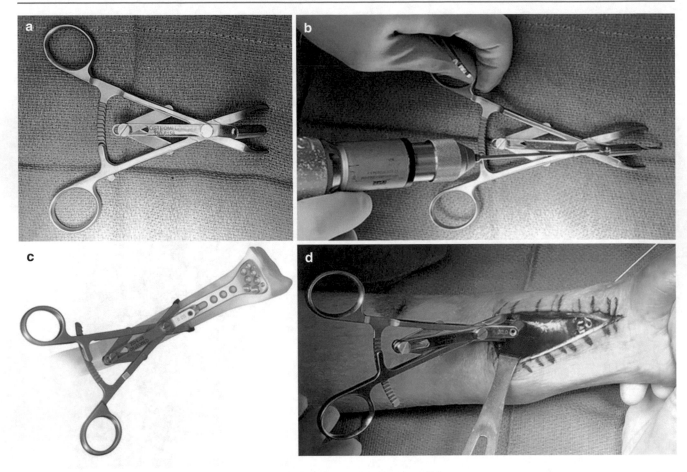

Fig. 36.11 (**a, b**) Plate-centering drill guide (PCDG). (**c, d**) PCDG centering plate on radius

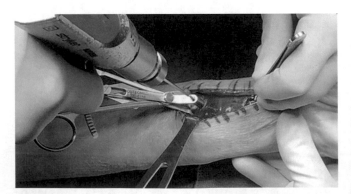

Fig. 36.12 The proximal-most hole is drilled in the slotted plate hole with aid of the PCDG

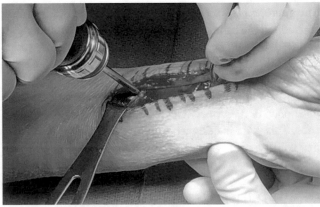

Fig. 36.13 Proximal screw tightened with plate underlying pronator

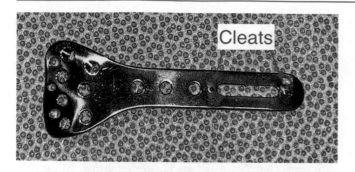

Fig. 36.14 Cleats on plate preventing rotation

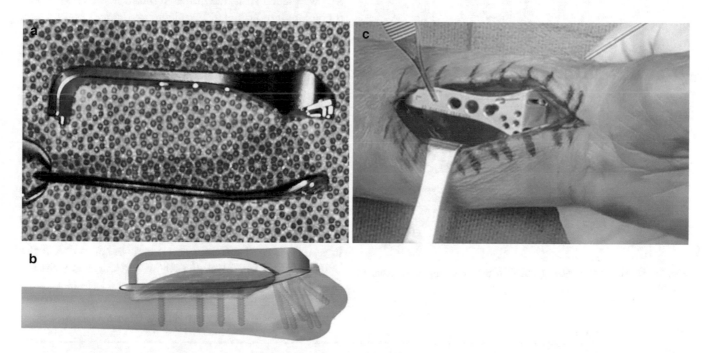

Fig. 36.15 (**a**, **b**) Pronator-sparing drill guide (PSDG) locking into plate. (**c**) PSDG placed on top of pronator in vivo

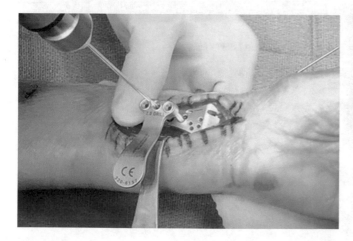

Fig. 36.16 Drilling through triple-sleeve drill guide placed in PSDG

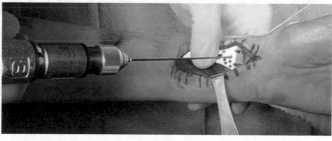

Fig. 36.17 The distal holes in the distal plate are drilled using the PSDG

placement and length (Fig. 36.20a, b). The images are evaluated for:

1. Radial inclination
2. Volar tilt
3. Distal radius articular congruity
4. Sigmoid notch articular incongruity
5. Radius length
6. Hardware position and screw length

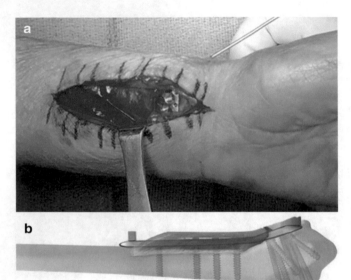

Fig. 36.18 (**a**, **b**) Removal of PSDG with underlying intact pronator and plate

Additional Treatments and Associated Procedures

After completing distal radius fixation, the distal radioulnar joint is compressed and the forearm is rotated. The forearm should rotate smoothly. If mechanical irregularity is detected with this clinical assessment of the DRUJ, the DRUJ should be inspected for pathology. A longitudinal incision is made over the DRUJ and the sigmoid notch articular congruity is assessed by direct visualization. Any articular incongruity is corrected by revision fixation. Screws placed from the dorsal sigmoid notch fragment to the volar sigmoid notch fragment may be necessary. Once sigmoid notch articular surface congruity is confirmed, DRUJ stability is assessed in pronation, supination, and neutral and compared to the contralateral side. If DRUJ instability is detected, it must be treated with long arm supination immobilization, DRUJ CRIF, DRUJ ORIF, or open repair of the TFCC.

Postoperative Rehabilitation

If the DRUJ is stable, the patient is allowed full AROM and PROM of the elbow, forearm, wrist, and digits. A wrist split is provided for comfort; however, the patient is encouraged to resume normal activities and minimize splint use. If the DRUJ requires treatment, the elbow, forearm, and wrist are immobilized accordingly.

SCREW OPTIONS

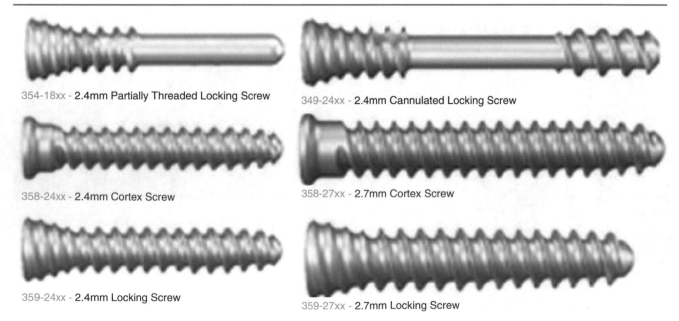

354-18xx - **2.4mm Partially Threaded Locking Screw**

349-24xx - **2.4mm Cannulated Locking Screw**

358-24xx - **2.4mm Cortex Screw**

358-27xx - **2.7mm Cortex Screw**

359-24xx - **2.4mm Locking Screw**

359-27xx - **2.7mm Locking Screw**

Fig. 36.19 OsteoMed ExtremiLock screw and peg options

Fig. 36.20 Final fluoroscopy images of plate and fixation in place. (**a**) Antero-posterior view, (**b**) lateral view

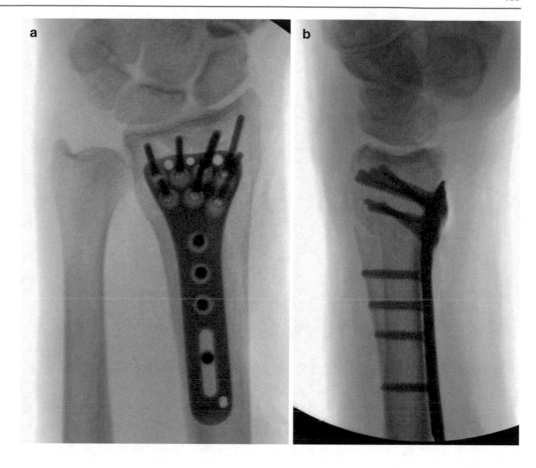

Tips and Tricks

- K-wires may be placed through the plate from the volar aspect of the distal radius to aid in reduction of volar tilt.
- The pronator-sparing distal radius plate extends proximally; therefore, it may need to be bent to accommodate the curve of the radial shaft, especially in smaller individuals.
- The distal holes of the plate are designed to aim more distal than most plates, allowing position below the watershed line to decrease tendon injury and potential delayed rupture.
- Place the initial screw hole in the center of the proximal slotted screw hole to allow for later proximal-distal adjustment, if necessary.
- Most screw sizes for this plate are available in 1-mm increments.

Conclusion

The pronator-sparing volar distal radius plate allows anatomic fixation of both intra- and extra-articular distal radius fractures using a pronator quadratus-sparing technique. This technique allows for decreased soft tissue damage and rehabilitation time since the pronator remains intact. Additionally, it permits increased efficiency for the surgeon with the use of the plate-centering drill guide and the pronator-sparing drill guide, allowing decreased plate application and dissection time, respectively.

References

1. Johnson RK, Shrewsbury MM. The pronator quadratus in motions and stabilization of the radius and ulna at the distal radioulnar joint. J Hand Surg Am. 1976;1(3):205–9.
2. Berglund LM, Messer TM. Complications of volar plate fixation for managing distal radius fractures. J Am Acad Orthop Surg. 2009;17:369–77.
3. Ploegmakers J, The B, Wang A, Brutty M, Ackland T. Supination and pronation strength deficits persist at 2-4 years after treatment of distal radius fractures. Hand Surg. 2015;20(3):430–4.
4. Imatani J, Akita K. Volar distal radius anatomy applied to the treatment of distal radius fracture. J Wrist Surg. 2017;6:174–7.

Pablo De Carli

Introduction

Fractures of the distal end of the radius are very common injuries, accounting for one-sixth of the fractures attending the Emergency Departments in the USA [1].

Many different patterns have been described. There is a huge difference between them with different prognosis and treatment. Therapeutic management included fracture reduction and immobilization with a cast, fixation with pins and plaster, external fixation and internal fixation with plates and screws. Among them, volar locking plates are the gold standard when treating the majority of these fractures today [2–4].

But before these plates were described in 2002, a generation of dorsal plates was reported by Ring and coauthors [5]; the fixation principle followed Rikli and Regazzoni Columnar Theory where they considered three columns in the wrist: an ulnar column (the ulna), a radial column (the radial half of the radius, containing the scaphoid fossa), and an intermediate column (the ulnar half of the radius, containing the lunate fossa) [6].

The first described exclusively dorsal plates—Pi plates—produced a bi-columnar fixation. Ring et al's results were satisfying, but the complication rate was not that good: 23% tendinitis, 4 out of 22 plates required removal, and 15 among 22 patients had some degree of residual pain [5]. Successive publications reported unacceptable rates of complications using these initial dorsal plates. These included nerve irritation, fragment displacement, complex regional pain syndrome (CRPS), and extensor tendon irritation and even extensor tendon rupture [2, 5, 7–14]. To prevent these complications, some authors even recommend plate elective removal in all patients [7, 8, 11].

This high complication rate led many hand surgeons to avoid the use of dorsal plates, particularly those plates of more than 2.0 or 2.4 mm thickness.

With technological improvement, dorsal plates were designed with lower profile, smoother screw heads, and the complication rate descended significantly. Kamath et al. evaluated 30 cases of stainless steel dorsal low-profile plates: they had no tendinitis nor tendon rupture, or plate removal reported. They concluded the dorsal plate complications may be caused by specific plates used rather than for the technique itself [15].

Simic et al. reported a prospective study including 60 fractures treated with dorsal low-profile plates with a minimum follow-up of 1 year. They had no tendinitis, no tendon rupture, and good and excellent clinical outcomes [16].

Rozental et al. compared functional outcome and complications of two types of dorsal plates: Pi plates and low-profile dorsal plates. Although they retrospectively evaluated only 28 patients, they report 9 reoperations for plate removal and for tendon reconstruction. The 9 re-operations were on cases treated initially with Pi plates [10].

Recent papers go further and compare results and complications between fractures treated with low profile dorsal plates and volar locking plates. They conclude that both clinical results and complication rates are not significantly different between both devices.

Yu et al. compared complication rate between 57 dorsal low-profile plates (1.2 and 1.5 mm) and 47 volar locking plates. They found no significant difference in complication rate – requiring secondary operation, in tendon irritation or in tendon rupture [17]. Disseldorp et al. compared 123 low-profile dorsal plates versus 91 volar plates. They report no difference in complication rate between both groups [18].

Yoshihiro et al. reported a prospective nonrandomized group of 112 distal radius articular fractures treated either with dorsal low-profile plate or with volar locking plates.

P. De Carli (✉)
Orthopaedic and Traumatology Department, and Hand and Upper Extremity Section, Hospital Italiano, Buenos Aires, Argentina

Clinical Surgery, Instituto Universitario Hospital Italiano de Buenos Aires, Buenos Aires, Argentina

Buenos Aires, Argentina

© Springer Nature Switzerland AG 2022
W. B. Geissler (ed.), *Wrist and Elbow Arthroscopy with Selected Open Procedures*,
https://doi.org/10.1007/978-3-030-78881-0_37

They report the same clinical results, same complication rate, and similar – although high – plate removal rate (30 of 38 dorsal and 59 of 68 volar locking plates) [19].

For these findings, we agree with Lutsky and Yoshihiro [19, 20] that there are certain patterns of distal radius fractures that have precise indication for dorsal surgical approach and dorsal plate fixation. The goal of this chapter is to present the surgical technique for the dorsal approach and plating of distal radial fractures, and to highlight some tips and tricks that arise from frequently asked questions. Current indications and contraindications are listed.

Advantages of Dorsal Approach

The concepts of "dorsal approach" and "dorsal plating" for distal radial fractures are often confused to be necessarily associated. Dorsal plating always needs a dorsal approach, certainly. But dorsal approach can be combined with volar plating or pinning, or any other configuration for fracture fixation, not necessarily followed by a dorsal implant.

The dorsal approach itself allows the surgeon:

- To assess the articular surface without arthroscopy (dorsal half of distal radius articular surface) (Fig. 37.1)
- To evaluate and manage carpal intrinsic ligament injuries or scaphoid fractures associated to distal radius (Fig. 37.2)

When treating a dorsal displaced distal radial fracture, the use of a dorsal plate adds a buttress effect for direct reduction of the fracture, neutralizing the displacing forces that the fracture suffers.

Indications [19, 20]

Even when nowadays volar locking plates are the gold standard for distal radius fractures, we consider some specific primary indications for not only dorsal approach but for dorsal fracture fixation.

These indications are:

- Dorsal shear fracture (dorsal Barton) or any fracture of the distal radius with the volar cortex intact (Fig. 37.3) [20]
- Dorsal die punch fragment (Fig. 37.4) [20]
- Fracture patterns with a volar fracture line too distal for volar fixation (Fig. 37.5).
- Fractures associated with scapholunate ligament associated lesion (Fig. 37.6) [20]
- Central depressed fragment (Fig. 37.7)
- Dorsal metaphyseal bone loss with indication of bone grafting (Figs. 37.7 and 37.8)
- Reoperation of a fracture previously fixed with a palmar plate that failed and distal radius needs to be fixed again (Fig. 37.9)

Contraindications

We do not recommend using a dorsal plate in the presence of

- Active infection
- Dorsal soft tissue, extensor tendons or dorsal skin coverage loss or severe damage

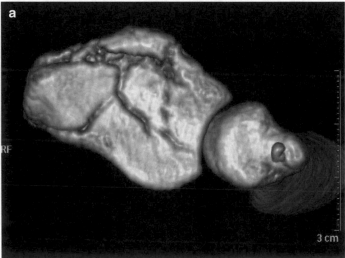
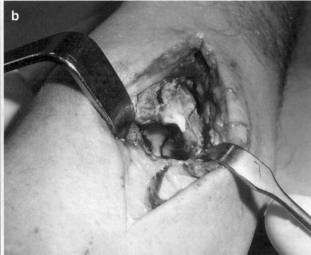

Fig. 37.1 Dorsal approach allows assessment of the radial articular surface without arthroscopy (dorsal half). (**a**) CT scan articular fracture. (**b**) The same fracture as seen through a dorsal approach

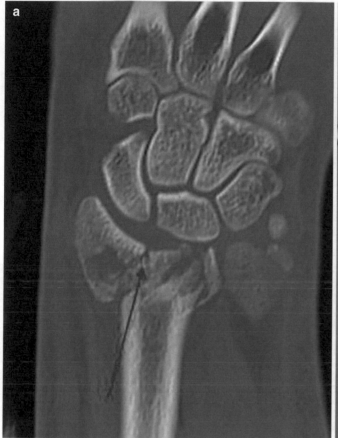
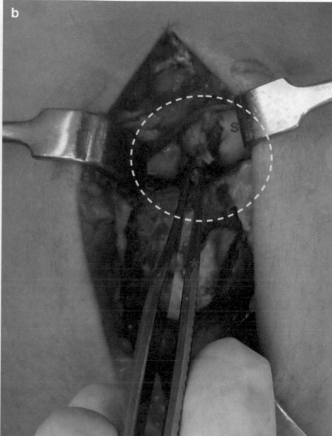

Fig. 37.2 Dorsal approach allows evaluation and management of carpal intrinsic ligament injuries. (a) The distal radius fracture line in a young man ends in scapholunate junction following a high energy trauma (arrow). (b) Dorsal approach extended to wrist joint allows direct inspection and palpation of scapholunate ligament (* forceps in the scapholunate interval; S, scaphoid; L, lunate)

- Volar shear fracture/Barton fracture/dorsal cortex and dorsal rim indemnity
- Volar displaced fractures

Technique [5, 10, 15, 18, 20, 21]

Preparation, Anesthesia, and Tourniquet

The patient is placed in a supine position with the arm abducted and extended on a radiolucent hand table. We prefer using regional anesthesia, but in some selected cases general anesthesia or wide-awake local anesthesia with no tourniquet (WALANT) may be used as well.

Prophylactic antibiotics are routinely administered preoperatively. An initial non-sterile cleansing is made of the full arm from fingers to the elbow. A non-sterile pneumatic tourniquet is used on the upper arm. The arm is prepared sterilely and draped in a standard fashion. After arm exsanguination, the tourniquet is inflated 100 mm Hg over the patient's systolic pressure. The forearm is positioned in full pronation.

We prefer the surgeon in the cephalic side and the assistant in the axillar side of the upper extremity.

Dorsal Approach (Fig. 37.10)

Depending on the radial fracture specific fragments and the preoperative fixation planning the surgeon can choose between three dorsal approaches to the distal radius.

Mid-longitudinal Approach—Global Dorsal Approach [20]

It is the most used and versatile dorsal approach. It allows reaching both dorsal radial and intermediate columns covered each one by the second and fourth extensor compartment floor [6].

A longitudinal incision is made over the Lister's tubercle, 4 to 5 cm long.

Full-thickness skin flaps are elevated from the extensor retinaculum and dorsal forearm fascia. The superficial radial nerve can be visualized distally crossing the extensor pollicis longus (EPL) tendon and should be identified, elevated,

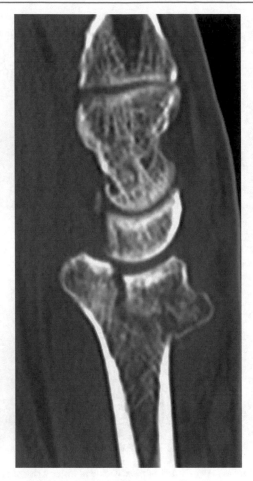

Fig. 37.3 Dorsal shear fracture, with palmar cortex intact

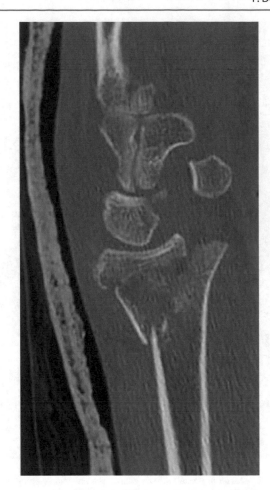

Fig. 37.5 Fracture pattern with a volar fracture line too distal for volar fixation

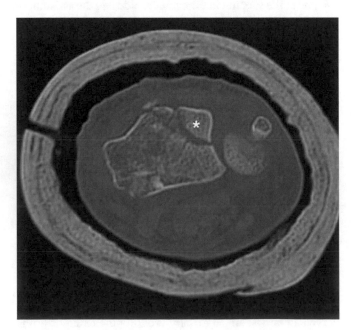

Fig. 37.4 Dorsal die punch or dorsal ulnar fragment

and protected in the skin flaps. With a moist gauze the subcutaneous tissue is gently elevated from the extensor retinaculum of the second, third, and fourth compartments. The third compartment is identified and fully opened, exposing the EPL tendon and retracting it radially. It is important to fully open the compartment to allow a better approach and to avoid postoperative EPL stenosing tenosynovitis (Fig. 37.11).

The septum between second and fourth extensor compartment is incised down to the bone trying not to enter any of the tendon compartments. Both compartments are sharply subperiosteally elevated from the dorsal radius in radial and ulnar directions, respectively. The extensor retinaculum deep layer is confluent with the dorsal periosteum; both are elevated sharply from the bone together in a single surgical plane. The second compartment deep portion or floor is thin and is quite usual to enter the compartment or finding it lacerated by the fracture. The floor of the fourth compartment, on the other hand, is thicker and stronger. Both tendon compartments are completely elevated from the dorsal radius

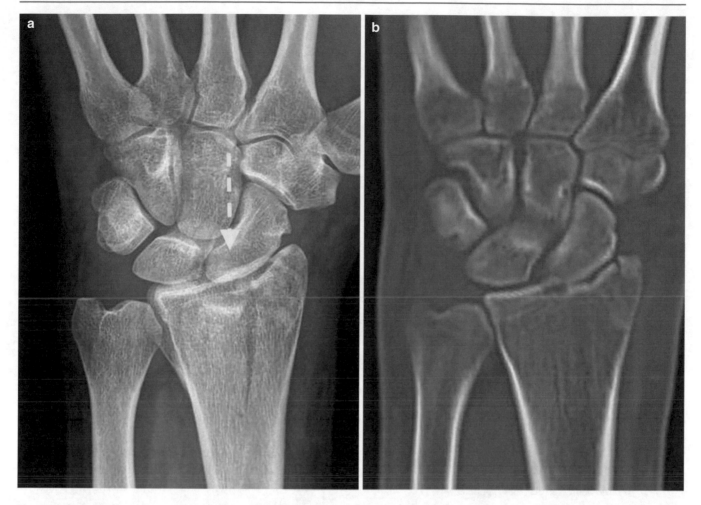

Fig. 37.6 Fractures associated with suspected scapholunate ligament associated lesion. (**a**) X-ray with scaphoid "sunken" in the radius depressed fragment. (**b**) CT scan confirms Gilula proximal carpal line broken between scaphoid and lunate proximal articular surface

until reaching the 4-5 septum ulnarly and the brachioradialis tendon radially (Fig. 37.12).

To explore the radiocarpal joint and to control the joint fragments reduction, a capsulotomy is made longitudinally distal to the dorsal rim of the radius (see Figs. 37.1b and 37.2b).

This mid-longitudinal approach is primarily indicated when both radial and intermediate columns need to be exposed. If the surgeon needs only to expose the dorsal radial column by this approach, only the second compartment shall be elevated. Conversely, if the intermediate column shall be exposed, just the fourth compartment is elevated.

Radial—Longitudinal Dorsal Approach
(See Fig. 37.10)

It is used for exposing the radial styloid and the radial column from the 1-2 retinacular septum. It is usually used for an anatomic radial lateral plate.

The anatomic snuffbox between the EPL and the extensor pollicis brevis (EPB) with the tip of the radial styloid form-

ing the floor is the landmark for beginning the skin incision, and extending it proximally as needed (see Fig. 37.10). Superficial branches of the radial nerve should be carefully protected and gently separated. The radial artery crosses the snuffbox distal to the radial styloid and should be protected as well. By blunt dissection, the deep fascia and the extensor retinaculum are reached. The radial styloid is approached by sharp dissection between the first and second extensor compartments. These are subperiosteally elevated as necessary. The Brachioradialis tendon can be released as well if needed to reduce the radial column.

The radial approach is indicated when radial styloid is going to be specifically fixated, or for fixing the radial column with a lateral radial plate.

Ulnar—Longitudinal Dorsal Approach
(See Fig. 37.10)

It is indicated when the surgeon needs to approach the dorsal ulnar corner of the radius or the intermediate column. For this last indication we prefer the mid-longitudinal approach

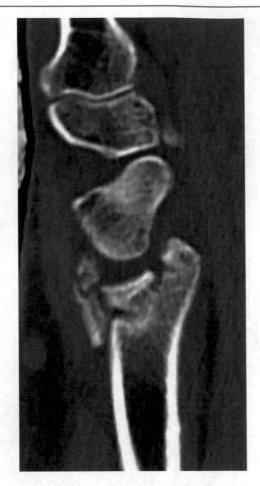

Fig. 37.7 Central depressed articular fragment

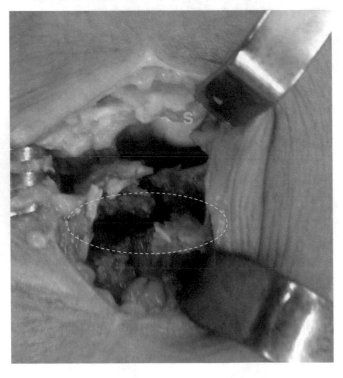

Fig. 37.8 Dorsal metaphyseal bone loss with indication of bone grafting (dotted circle, metaphyseal bone loss; S, scaphoid; L, lunate)

as the fourth compartment is easier to elevate from this approach than from the ulnar longitudinal that will be described next.

The skin longitudinal incision is made 5 mm radial to the distal radioulnar joint (see Figs. 37.10 and 37.13a).

Blunt dissection is made taking care to protect the dorsal sensory branch of the ulnar nerve. Once identified and protected, the septum between fourth and fifth extensor compartments is sharply and longitudinally sectioned (see Fig. 37.13b, c). The fourth compartment is radially elevated subperiosteally. Special care must be taken to protect the dorsal radioulnar ligament insertion in the ulnar distal corner of the radius. Its section could cause a residual distal radioulnar instability (see Fig. 37.13d).

This approach is indicated for dorsal die punch fragment's specific reduction and fixation (see Fig. 37.13e, f).

Fracture Reduction and Fixation Through Dorsal Approach

Once the selected approach is done, radial, intermediate, or both columns are clearly exposed and the fracture pattern can be directly addressed. The scapholunate ligament is explored by direct vision and palpated for injury (see Fig. 37.2b).

Lister's tubercle might be resected or not depending on the fracture and the plate that will be used for fixation.

Metaphyseal comminution and bone loss are evaluated (Fig. 37.14).

If a central articular fragment is depressed and has to be identified and reduced, a dorsal cortical fragment can be separated to open the cancellous part of the bone, identify the depressed fragment, and reduce it (Fig. 37.15a–e). Once this is done under direct vision, the fragment can be temporarily maintained with a K-wire (Fig. 37.15f) or by bone graft to keep it in place. Lister's tubercle might be useful for this purpose.

The preoperative planned method of fixation is reevaluated under direct vision of the fracture and confirmed as the most adequate way to fix it (Fig. 37.15g).

Depending on the individual fracture pattern, we can choose the most adequate fixation plate: bi-columnar 1, low-profile Pi plates, 2.0 T or L plates either locking screws. One or two plates can be needed depending on if one or the two radial columns are fractured.

A configuration described by Rikli and Regazzoni fix the fracture with one radial plate for the radial column and another with a dorsal ulnar plate at 50–70 degrees for the intermediate column [6] (Fig. 37.16).

Some of these plates are anatomic. Others have to be bended distally 10 degrees to restore normal radial volar tilt (Fig. 37.17).

Fig. 37.9 Reoperation of a fracture previously fixed with a palmar plate. (**a, b**) Failed volar plate, with radius epiphyseal fragment dorsally displaced after suffering cut off the plate and screws. (**c, d**) Volar plate removed, radius reduction and dorsal low-profile plates on untouched dorsal cortex

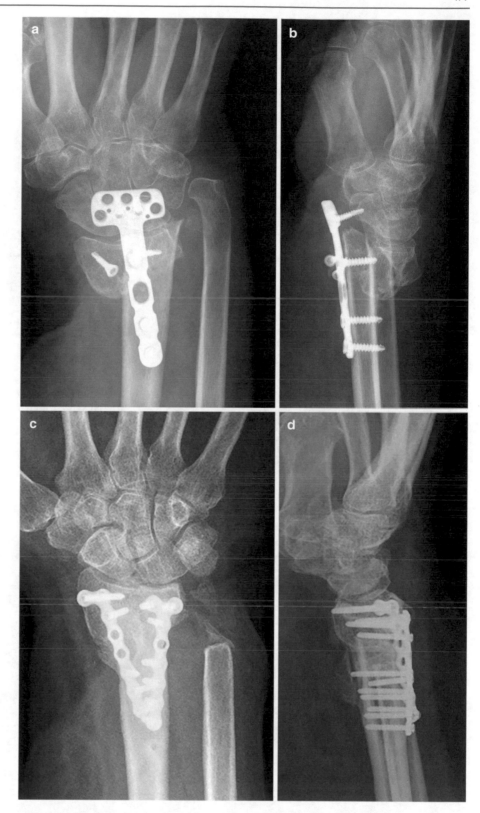

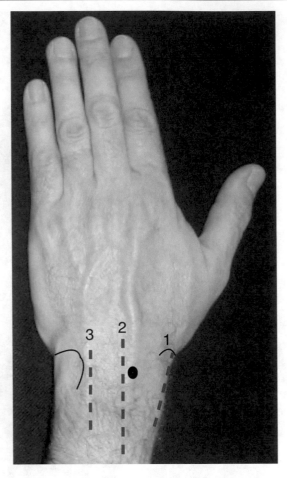

Fig. 37.10 Dorsal longitudinal approaches: 1. Radial longitudinal; 2. Mid-longitudinal; 3. Ulnar longitudinal. Landmarks: ulnar styloid, radial styloid, and Lister's tubercle

Fig. 37.12 Second and fourth extensor compartments have been sharply and subperiosteally elevated from the dorsal radius and the fracture is exposed. Second compartment is retracted to the right and fourth is retracted to the left

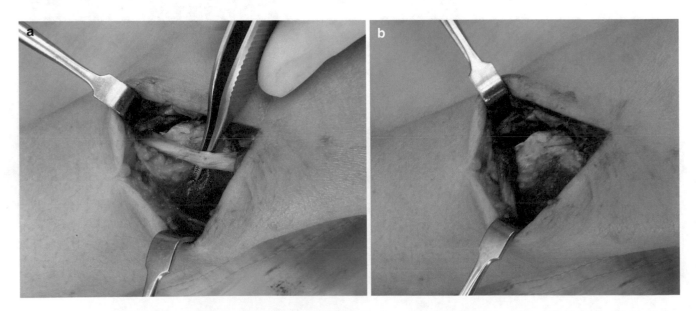

Fig. 37.11 Dorsal mid-longitudinal global approach. (**a**) Extensor pollicis longus tendon (EPL) fully liberated from its third extensor retinaculum compartment and (**b**) separated radially

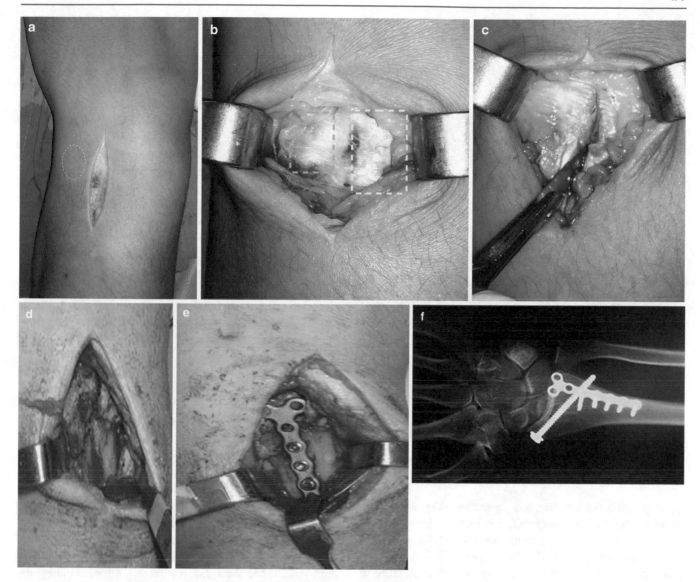

Fig. 37.13 Dorsal ulnar-longitudinal approach. (**a**) Skin incision. Ulnar head is marked with a yellow circle. (**b**) Extensor retinaculum superficial layer: green on the left, fifth extensor compartment. Yellow on the right, fourth extensor compartment. (**c**) Between both fifth and fourth extensor compartments the septum is incised deep to bone. (**d**) Fourth compartment is elevated subperiosteally; intermediate radius column and the die punch fracture are exposed. (**e, f**) The fracture is fixed with a buttress plate

When the articular fragments are too distal dorsally, the plates can be placed almost over the dorsal rim, buttressing the distal fragment without using distal screws (Fig. 37.18a, b).

If a central fragment is depressed and reduced, it can be kept in place both with cancellous bone graft and/or with distal locking screws, either fixing the distal fragment or holding it in place from the fracture site (Fig. 37.19). When using distal locking plates in a young patient it is usually unnecessary to bone graft the metaphyseal defect (Fig. 37.20).

An important principle to remember when choosing the implant is to use the smallest hardware as possible but strong enough to maintain fragment stability.

When the two columns must be reduced and fixated, it is recommended to begin by the one with less comminuted articular surface [20].

Once the plates have been placed the K-wires used for initial reduction are removed (see Fig. 37.15f, g). If the scapholunate ligament is disrupted—usually a Geissler 1 or 2 lesion, rarely 3–4—I prefer to treat it with the radius

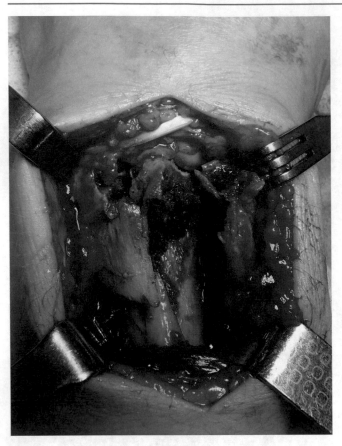

Fig. 37.14 Once the bone is approached metaphyseal bone comminution is evaluated

already fixed but in the same operation (Fig. 37.21). If a scaphoid fracture is associated, it is fixed with an antegrade cannulated screw after performning radial stabilization first.

When reduction and fixation is completed, it is usually impossible to check final joint surface reduction from the dorsal approach under direct vision if the neutral or 10 degrees volar tilt has been restored. The exception are very lax patients whose radiocarpal joints can be seen under longitudinal axis distraction.

Final fluoroscopic views including joint tilt views and obliques are performed. The wrist is taken through a range of motion to verify stable fixation. The distal radioulnar joint is assessed for dorsal ulnar instability taking the piano key sign in full pronation, supination, and neutral rotation. The wound is irrigated and closed.

Wound Closure

The joint capsule is closed with 3-0 absorbable sutures. If sectioned, the dorsal radio triquetral ligament is repaired with 3-0 or 4-0 nonabsorbable suture.

The EPL is left in its subcutaneous position, closing the extensor retinaculum below.

The extensor retinaculum deep layer is the most important structure to be repaired when closing the wound. This tissue is the protection layer for the extensor tendons. It separates the plate from the tendons avoiding their irritation and potential rupture by friction with the implant. But secondary to the energy of the dorsal displacement fracture, added to the surgical aggression when the extensor retinaculum is elevated, the floor of this retinaculum is usually violated. This is much more frequent with the thin floor of the second compartment, but it frequently happens with the fourth compartment's floor as well. If this was the situation, the extensor retinaculum floor has to be reconstructed. Extensor retinaculum superficial layer can be used for taking a flap to separate extensor tendons from the plate and the dorsal most prominent epiphyseal radius. It is key not to alter the pulley effect of the retinaculum over the extensor tendons when making this flap.

Indeed, the superficial layer or roof of the extensor retinaculum restoration is essential to avoid extensor tendons bowstringing, most for EDC and EIP [21] (Fig. 37.22a–c).

After retinaculum closure, all extensor tendons should move freely in their compartments, without friction or blocking.

Subcutaneous tissue and skin are closed following the preferred technique.

A bulky, sterile dressing and a short-arm immobilization are applied for 2 weeks at least depending on how rigid the fixation was achieved. Finger motion is encouraged from the first postoperative day. Progressive wrist exercises are initiated then with the hand therapist. Between days 10 and 15, a custom short volar splint is made and used for protection until 5 to 6 weeks postoperatively. This splint is removed four times a day for exercises controlled by the therapist.

Tips and Tricks

- What landmarks can I take if Lister's tubercle is not identifiable and a mid-longitudinal incision has to be done?

Sometimes the Lister tubercle is not identifiable as it is fragmented and displaced by the fracture itself. Therefore, we have our incision landmark missing. In these cases, the 3rd metacarpal shaft is followed in its longitudinal axis and the incision is made from the projection 1 cm distal to the ulnar head and 4 to 5 cm from this landmark to proximal (Fig. 37.23).

- What can I do if dorsal cortex bone shells come with the dorsal periosteum when elevating the extensor compartment retinacular flaps?

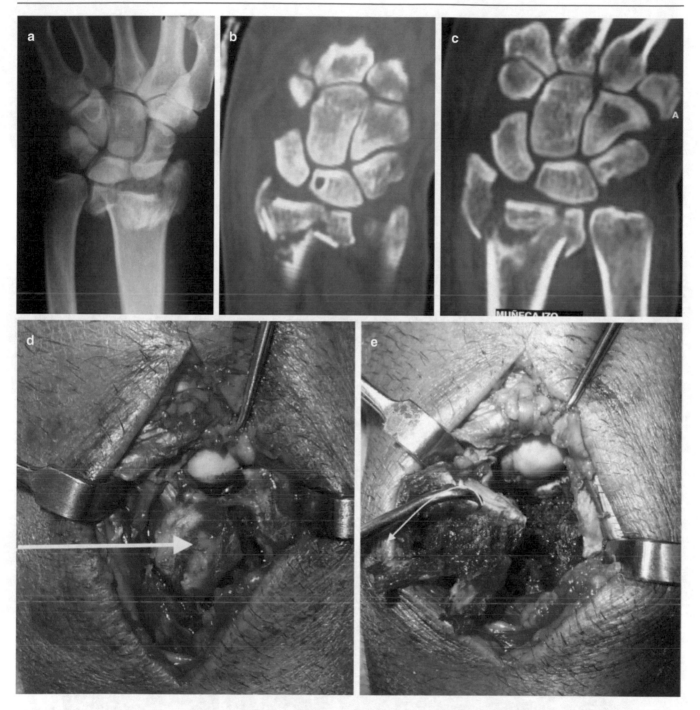

Fig. 37.15 A large articular central depressed bone fragment is identi- fied in X-rays and CT scan (**a**–**c**). (**d, e**) A dorsal cortical fragment is rotated to see and reduce the central depressed articular fragment (yel- low arrow). (**f**) The central fragment has been reduced and provisionally fixed with K-wires. (**g**) The dorsal cortical rotated fragment was reduced (yellow arrow) and the fracture fixated with a Pi plate

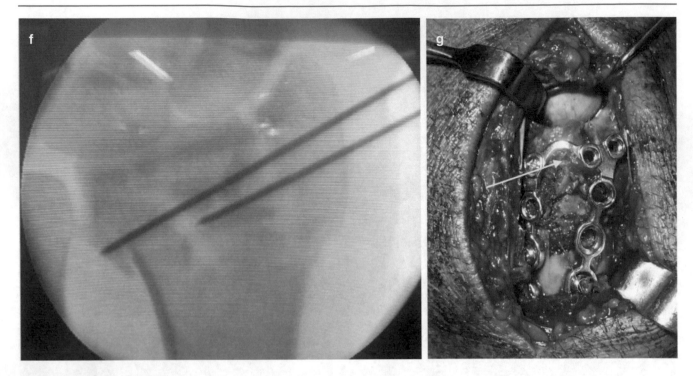

Fig. 37.15 (continued)

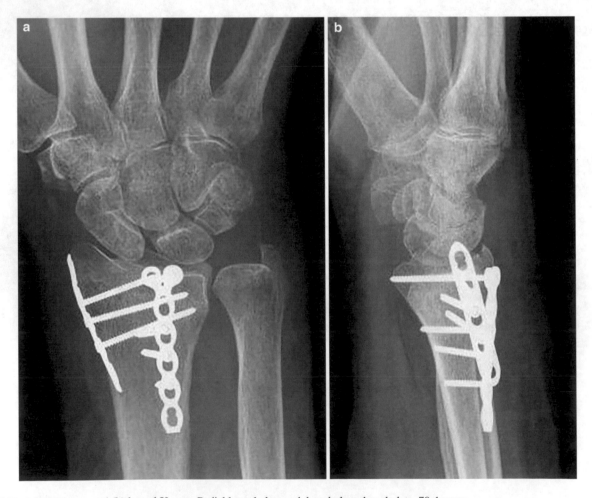

Fig. 37.16 (a) AP X-rays and (b) lateral X-rays. Radial lateral plate and dorsal ulnar dorsal plate, 70 degrees

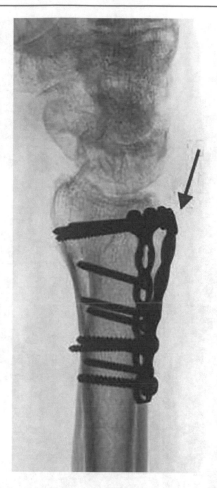

Fig. 37.17 A low-profile nonanatomic plate was bended 10 degrees to adapt to anatomy of the dorsal radius (red arrow)

In very dorsal comminuted fractures, some dorsal radial cortex bone shells can be very adherent to the dorsal periosteum and to the deep extensor tendon compartment. We do not separate them as our main goal is to protect the integrity of the extensor retinaculum floor for covering the plate and separating it from the extensor tendons when closing the wound (Fig. 37.24).

- How far can I open the dorsal capsule to see the radial joint surface?

If needed the joint capsule arthrotomy is extended in a T fashion, following the distal radius articular surface as necessary. When the small arthrotomy is not enough for joint reduction confirmation, the dorsal radio triquetral ligament can be sectioned. In this case, be sure to leave the ligament edges for final repair when closing the wound. Through this arthrotomy the dorsal half of the radius articular surface can be clearly observed. The volar half needs longitudinal traction for becoming visible and it can only be explored in a relatively lax ligament patient (Fig. 37.25).

- What landmarks can I take if I need an ulnar-longitudinal approach and the distal radioulnar joint is not clearly localized because it is hidden due to edema, hematoma, or fracture compromise?

If this landmark is difficult to identify because of the fracture deformity or secondary edema and hematoma, the longitudinal axis of the 4th metacarpal is followed (Fig. 37.26).

- Can I use the buttress effect of an anatomic dorsal plate to reduce the fracture?

If one dorsal bi-columnar plate is chosen, and the articular component of the fracture is reduced or simple, the anatomic dorsal plate can indirectly reduce the fracture displacement. The plate is dorsally placed and confirmed by fluoroscopy its correct position following the radius axis and at least 3 mm proximal to the dorsal rim. The first cortical screw is implanted in the metaphysis and progressively tightened while the assistant produces distraction of the fracture pulling gently from the index and middle fingers. As the plate is anatomic it will reduce the fracture while it is compressed to the bone by cortical screw tightening. Then locking screws complete the fixation.

- How can I avoid flexor tendon lesions by the screw tips?

When dorsal screws are drilled, do not overpass the volar cortex. The tips of the screws are risky when distal screws exceed the volar cortex. I prefer to use unicortical locking screws when fixing the distal fragments. As the radial metaphysis becomes narrower, bicortical screws are better tolerated as there is more volar muscle tissue that protects tendons from the screw tips (see Figs. 37.16b, 37.17, 37.18b, 37.19b, 37.20f).

- How can I fix a too distal dorsal fragment that contains a significant part of the articular surface?

When in spite of the buttress plate is fixated over the dorsal rim this distal fragment is still not fixated, a nonabsorbable suture from the plate to the fragment can complete its fixation (see Fig. 37.20g).

- How can I handle a volar rim fragment that might be combined with a distal radius pattern that otherwise has dorsal implant indication?

Some fracture patterns combine dorsal implant fracture patterns with a volar rim fragment that is important and contains the volar capsular and radiocarpal ligament insertions. In these cases, the drill or the screw can "push" it to volar instead of fixing

Fig. 37.18 When the dorsal fragment is too distal, a buttress locking low-profile dorsal plate can be used without distal screws. (**a**) Very distal radius fracture. (**b**) The radial styloid and the volar rim fragment were fixed with headless screws, and the dorsal fragment was buttressed with a dorsal locking plate

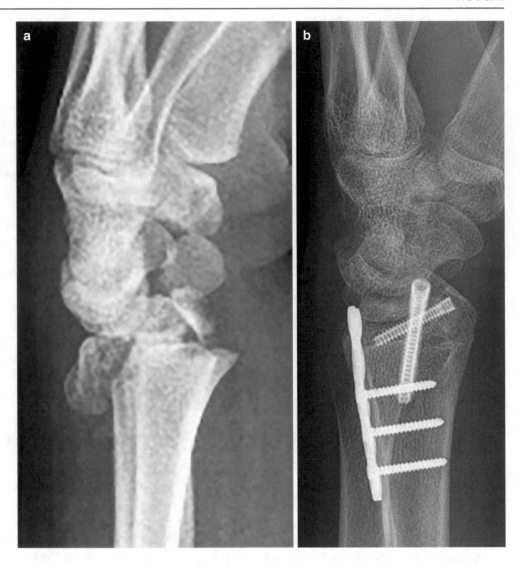

it in place. Our advice is to make a small volar incision to reduce and keep the fragment reduced while fixing it with the dorsal screw. A second chance is making a direct fixation with an interfragmentary screw from palmar to dorsal. (see Fig. 37.19b).

- In wound closure I found the extensor retinaculum floor with attrition and discontinued. How can I protect the extensor tendons from the implant friction in these cases?

This is a usual finding. It may happen deep to the second or the fourth compartment, or frequently both. Do not try to suture the extensor retinaculum floor. It is frequently useless. Rather repair it with an extensor retinaculum superficial roof flap. If the second compartment floor needs repair, take a radially based flap 10 mm wide from the superficial layer. It

must be designed at the level of the distal or transverse part of the plate, covering the distal 10 mm most prominent part of the radial dorsal epiphysis (Fig. 37.27a, b). Once the flap dissection reaches the 1-2 retinacular septum the flap is passed below ECRL and ECRB tendons, separating them from the plate and from the bone and creating a gliding surface for them (Fig. 37.27c–e).

If the floor of the 4th extensor retinaculum compartment is injured too, the same is done as described for the second compartment, but the 10 mm retinaculum superficial layer flap is elevated up to the 4-5 septum. It is passed below EDC and EIP tendons and sutured to the second compartment flap (Fig. 37.27f) [21].

If the flaps fail to reach each other, they can be sutured to the plate as close as possible.

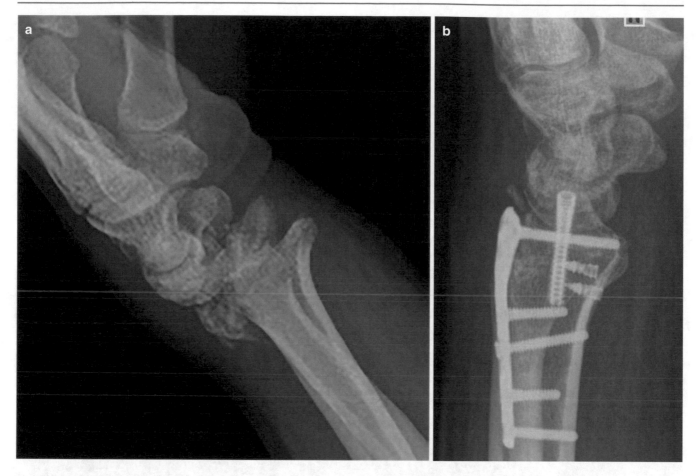

Fig. 37.19 (a) Very distal radius osteochondral fragment with dorsal rim comminution. (b) Two suture anchors hold the volar distal fragment and a dorsal low profile anatomic plate buttresses the dorsal fragment. The distal screw holds the osteochondral laminar distal fragment from the fracture line without passing through the fragment because of its very thin thickness

Warnings

- Leave at least 10 mm of extensor retinaculum roof to avoid tendon bowstringing. This is important for both second and fourth compartment tendons, but much more for EDC tendons (see Fig. 37.22b, c).
- It is quite easy to suture the superficial layer of one compartment to the floor of the other, misleading the superficial layer with the septum. Be sure there is a soft tissue layer deep to the tendons and above the implant. That is the essential of avoiding extensor tendon complications.
- When should I remove dorsal plates to avoid complications?

The literature gives a wide spectrum of removal criteria and indications. Some authors like Yoshihiro Abe et al. [19], Sanchez [11], Fitoussi [8], and Chiang [7] remove almost routinely dorsal plates. Devaux [21] recommends removal in patients younger than 70, in presence of crepitus or synovitis, screw loosening or broken plate. Surgeon should be aware that pain and crepitus may be early signs of tendon suffering from the dorsal plate (see Fig. 37.28). Plate removal rate depends on the author and on the plate profile too. Up to 76% plate removal has been reported [11]. Carter had 19% plate removal with a 2.2-mm plate [22]. However, other authors seldom had to remove the plate and had very low complication rate. All these authors used low-profile dorsal plates [15, 16]. Our advice is removing dorsal plates if there is pain, crepitus, and of course if tendinitis or tendon rupture. The best prevention for avoiding this is using low-profile plates (the less as possible for the fracture pattern that is treated), and take time and care to reconstruct the extensor retinaculum deep layer to protect tendons from the hardware and from the bone spikes (see Fig. 37.29).

Conclusion

The dorsal plates for the treatment of fractures of the distal radius have been indicated for several decades. Their initial designs—until the AO Pi plate, we could say—had rather rough screw heads and plate high profile that interfered with

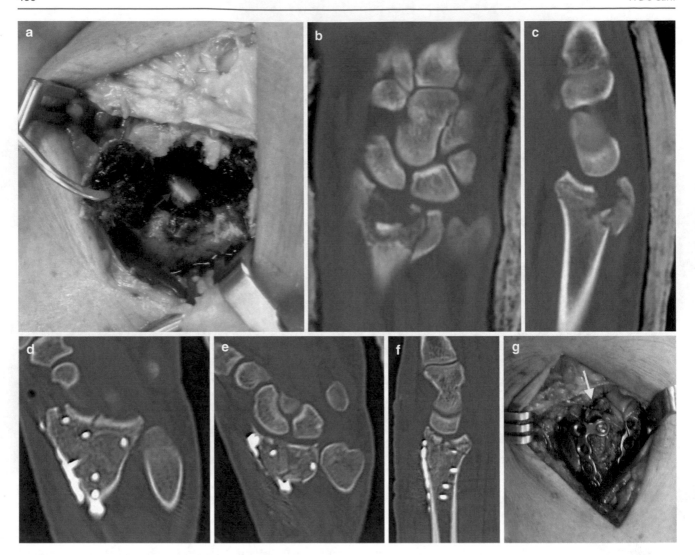

Fig. 37.20 A 30-year-old male with intra-articular comminuted distal radius fracture with a large depressed central articular fragment (**a**). (**b, c**) CT scan showing metaphyseal comminution. (**d–f**) Postoperative CT scan showing the previous depressed fragment now reduced and fixed by the locked screws from the dorsal plate. (**g**) Final fixation without need of bone graft. The arrow shows sutures from the plate to dorsal rim fragments

extensor tendons. The obvious consequence was an unacceptable frequency of irritation or extensor tendon rupture, together with a high incidence of need for plate removal. Since lower profile plates and smoother screw heads were developed, these complications became comparable to the usually used volar plates. The indications for dorsal plating were also more precise, consequence of the greater experience. We totally agree with Yoshihiro et al. [19] when they affirm: "…Certain fracture patterns are more appropriately stabilized using a dorsal plate fixation…"

Today, dorsal plates have a definitive place in the armamentarium of the surgeons for treating distal radial fractures.

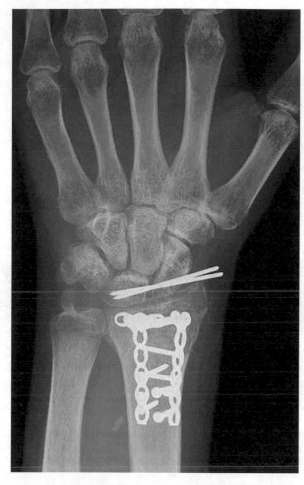

Fig. 37.21 The patient of Fig. 37.2a, b with a partial scapholunate lesion, was reduced and pinned after radial fracture fixation with two dorsal low-profile plates

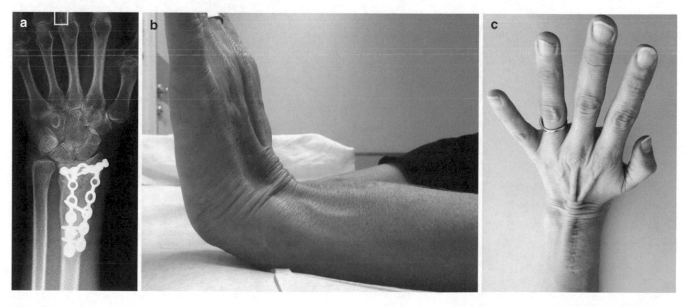

Fig. 37.22 A 45-year-old female with her articular comminuted distal radius fracture fixed by a dorsal Pi plate (**a**). A flap of the extensor retinaculum was made to separate the plate from the extensor tendons. Pulley function of the retinaculum was not preserved and she had extensor tendons bowstringing when extending her fingers with the wrist in extension (**b, c**)

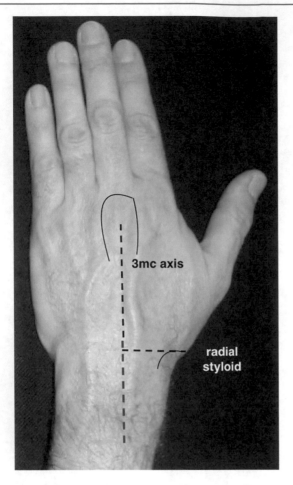

Fig. 37.23 Alternative landmarks for dorsal mid-longitudinal approach if Lister's tubercle is not identifiable. With the hand aligned with the forearm, third metacarpal axis is followed proximally

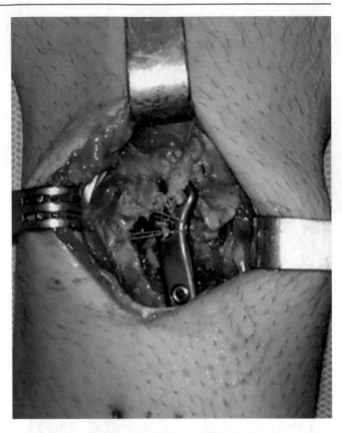

Fig. 37.24 We do not separate small cortical bone shells from periosteum when approaching the fracture dorsally. For this reason, some small bone shells can cover the distal part of the plate when closing the wound

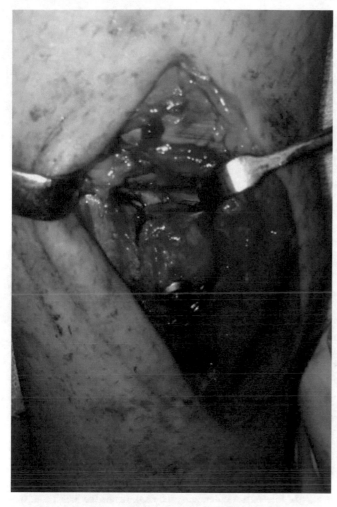

Fig. 37.25 Once the fracture is reduced and fixated, the articular surface is difficult to see, even with traction and in lax patients

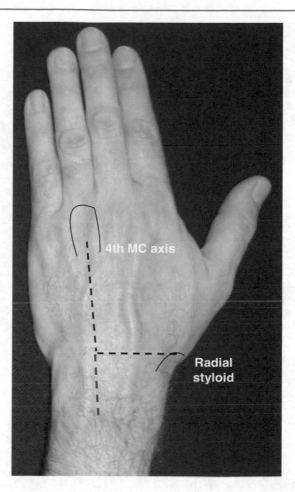

Fig. 37.26 Alternative landmarks for dorsal ulnar longitudinal approach if the ulnar head is not identifiable. With the hand aligned with the forearm, the fourth metacarpal axis is followed proximally

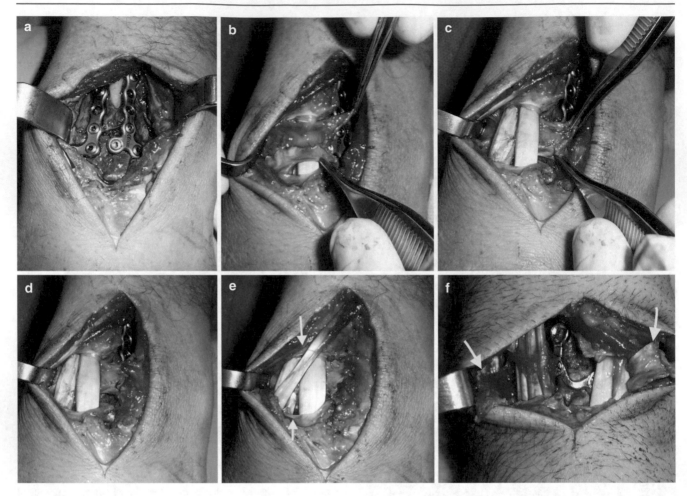

Fig. 37.27 Flap from the extensor retinaculum superficial layer to separate extensor tendons from the bone and the dorsal plate. (**a**) Fracture fixation with dorsal plates. Deep layer of extensor retinaculum is useless to cover the plate. A reconstruction must be done. (**b**) A flap is designed 10 mm wide from the second compartment, elevating the superficial layer of extensor retinaculum at the level of the distal and most prominent part of the plates (the flap is held by two forceps). (**c**) The flap is passed below the extensor tendons separating them from the plate (the forceps are still holding the flap). (**d**) As the fourth compartment is in good shape, the flap is sutured to the radial edge of the fourth retinaculum compartment. (**e**) The plate is totally separated from the extensor tendons. Arrows show the remaining superficial layer of the retinaculum essential to avoid residual tendon bowstringing. (**f**) In this case, the fourth extensor compartment needed a floor reconstruction as well. Arrows show the two flaps raised from the retinaculum superficial layer of both the second and the fourth extensor compartments

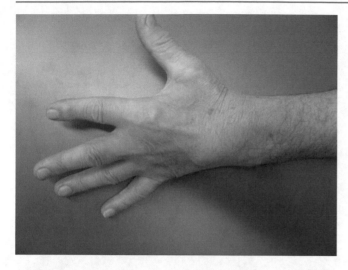

Fig. 37.28 Patient with a dorsal Pi plate and tenosynovitis. Note lack of second finger extension. The EPI tendon was ruptured when explored

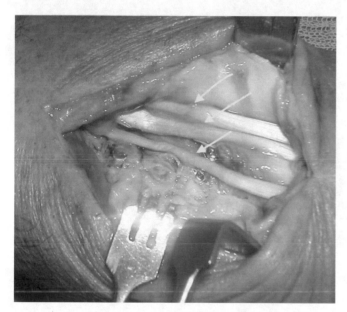

Fig. 37.29 Tendons ruptured by dorsal plate attrition. Partial rupture of three EDC tendons. The Pi plate below is uncovered and frictions with the tendons

References

1. Koval KJ, Harrast JJ, Anglen JO, Weinstein JN. Fractures of the distal part of the radius. The evolution of practice over time. Where's the evidence? J Bone Joint Surg Am. 2008;90-9:1855–1861. PMID:18762644. https://doi.org/10.2106/JBJS.G.01569.
2. Fok MW, Klausmeyer MA, Fernandez DL, Orbay JL, Bergada AL. Volar plate fixation of intrarticular radial fractures: a retrospective study. J Wrist Surg. 2013;2(3):247–54. PMID: 24436824 PMCID: PMC3764245. https://doi.org/10.1055/s-0033-1350086.
3. Jakubietz MG, Gruenert JG, Jakubietz RG. Palmar and dorsal fixed-angle plates in AO C-type fractures of the distal radius: is there an advantage of palmar plates in the long term? J Orthop Surg Res. 2012;7:8 PMID:22340861 PMCID: PMC3312832. https://doi.org/10.1186/1749-799X-7-8.
4. Orbay JL, Fernandez DL. Volar fixation for dorsally displaced fractures of the distal radius: a preliminary report. J Hand Surg Am. 2002;27(2):205–215. PMID: 11901379. https://doi.org/10.1053/jhsu.2002.32081.
5. Ring D, Jupiter JB, Brennwald J, Buchler U, Hastings H. 2nd prospective multicenter trial of a plate for dorsal fixation of distal radius fractures. J Hand Surg Am. 1997;22(5):777–784. PMID: 9330133. https://doi.org/10.1016/S0363-5023(97)80069-X.
6. Rikli DA, Regazzoni P. The double plating technique for distal radius fractures. Tech Hand Up Extrem Surg. 2000;4(2):107–114. PMID:16609399.
7. Chiang PP, Roach S, Baratz ME. Failure of a retinacular flap to prevent dorsal wrist pain after titanium Pi plate fixation of distal radius fractures. J Hand Surg Am. 2002;27(4):724–728. PMID: 12132102. https://doi.org/10.1053/jhsu.2002.33703.
8. Fitoussi F, Ip W, Chow S. Treatment of displaced intra- articular fractures of the distal end of the radius with plate. J Bone Joint Surg. 1997;79A:1303–1312. PMID: 9314392. https://doi.org/10.2106/00004623-199709000-00004.
9. Osada D, Tamai K, Iwamoto A, Fujita S, Saotome K. Dorsal plating for comminuted intra-articular fractures of the distal end of the radius. Hand Surg. 2004;9(2):181–190. PMID: 15810104. https://doi.org/10.1142/s0218810404002194.
10. Rozental TD, Beredjiklian PK, Bozentka DJ. Functional outcome and complications following two types of dorsal plating for unstable fractures of the distal part of the radius. J Bone Joint Surg Am. 2003;85(10):1956–1960. PMID:14563804. https://doi.org/10.2106/00004623-200310000-00014.
11. Sanchez T, Jakubietz M, Jakubietz R, Mayer J, Beutel FK, Grunert J. Complications after Pi plate osteosynthesis. Plast Reconstr Surg. 2005;116(1):153–158. PMID: 15988262. https://doi.org/10.1097/01.prs.0000169713.49004.7b.
12. Schnur DP, Chang B. Extensor tendon rupture after internal fixation of a distal radius fracture using a dorsally placed AO/ASIF titanium Pi plate. Ann Plast Surg. 2000;44(5):564–566. PMID: 10805309. https://doi.org/10.1097/00000637-200044050-00016.
13. Shyam Kumar AJ. Dorsal plating for displaced intra-articular fractures of the distal radius. Injury. 2005;36(1):236. PMID: 15589962. https://doi.org/10.1016/j.injury.2004.07.049.
14. Suckel A, Spies S, Munst P. Dorsal (AO/ASIF) Pi-plate osteosynthesis in the treatment of distal intraarticular radius fractures. J Hand Surg Br. 2006;31(6):673–679. PMID: 17055625. https://doi.org/10.1016/j.jhsb.2006.08.007.
15. Kamath AF, Zurakowski D, Day CS. Low-profile dorsal plating for dorsally angulated distal radius fractures: an outcomes study. J Hand Surg. 2006;31A:1061–1067. PMID:16945704. https://doi.org/10.1016/j.jhsa.2006.05.008.
16. Simic PM, Robison J, Gardner MJ, Gelberman RH, Weiland AJ, Boyer MI. Treatment of distal radius fractures with a low profile dorsal plating system: an outcomes assessment. J Hand Surg. 2006;31(3):382–386. PMID:16516731. https://doi.org/10.1016/j.jhsa.2005.10.016.
17. Yu YR, Makhni MC, Tabrizi S, Rozental TD, Mundanthanam G, Day CS. Complications of low-profile dorsal versus volar locking plates in the distal radius: a comparative study. J Hand Surg. 2011;36A:1135–1141. PMID: 21712136. https://doi.org/10.1016/j.jhsa.2011.04.004.

18. Disseldorp DJG, Hannemann PFW, Poeze M, PRG B. Dorsal or volar plate fixation of the distal radius: does the complication rate help us to choose? J Wrist Surg. 2016;5:202–10. https://doi.org/10.1055/s-0036-1571842. ISSN 2163-3916

19. Abe Y, Tokunaga S, Moriya T. Management of intra-articular distal radius fractures: volar or dorsal locking plate – which has fewer complications? Hand. 2017;12(6):561–567. PMID: 29091491 PMCID: PMC5669324. https://doi.org/10.1177/1558944716675129.

20. Lutsky K, Boyer M, Goldfarb C. Dorsal locked plate fixation of the distal radius. J Hand Surg. 2013;38A:1414–1422. PMID: 23751326. https://doi.org/10.1016/j.jhsa.2013.04.019.

21. Devaux N, Henning J, Haefeli M, Honigmann P. The retinaculum flap for dorsal fixation of distal radial fractures. J Hand Surg Am. 2018;43(4):391.e1-e7. PMID 29618418. https://doi.org/10.1016/j.jhsa.2018.01.011.

22. Carter PR, Frederick HA, Laseter GF. Open reduction and internal fixation of unstable distal radius fractures with a low-profile plate: a multicenter study of 73 fractures. J Hand Surg [Am]. 1998;23:300–7. PMID: 9556273. https://doi.org/10.1016/S0363-5023(98)80131-7.

Fragment-Specific Fixation of Distal Radius Fractures

Daniel J. Brown

Introduction

Distal radius fractures (DRF) are the commonest fractures that present to an emergency department, representing 2.5% of all injuries [1] and 15% to 18% of all fractures [2, 3]. The vast majority can be treated non-operatively with simple splints or plaster of Paris casts; however, multiple operative options exist and have been reported with good results. These traditionally include percutaneous pinning, external-fixation and open reduction and internal fixation (ORIF) with volar buttress plates [2, 4].

With the introduction of locking plate technology, at the turn of the millennium, there was a major swing to the use of volar locking plates (VLP) and the development of anatomical plates allowed this to become the standard operative treatment [5, 6].

Whilst there remains controversy as to the indications for surgery and indeed the ideal operative treatment, if any, for minimally displaced, easily reduced fractures [7]; there is less controversy that more complicated, displaced, intra-articular fractures need open anatomical reduction and rigid fixation [6, 8, 9].

Whilst VLP remains the standard treatment for the majority of fractures that require operative intervention [6, 8–10], and dorsal plating techniques certainly have a role, particularly in predominantly dorsal fracture configurations; there are certain, usually more complex, fracture configurations that may be better treated with other options and these will be discussed in this chapter. In the most complex fractures, especially in osteoporotic bone, a further option "wrist spanning plates" can be used.

This chapter discusses fragment-specific plating (FSP), a term which strictly describes the use of multiple small, anatomic plates to address individual fracture fragments. To avoid confusion, I will use the term "true FSP" to describe those techniques. This chapter will, however, discuss all uses of multiple plates in the management of DRF. These other techniques include the use of plates, screws or wires as an adjuvant to standard VLP; addressing individual fragments not controlled the VLP. Finally, a third option using a volar plate as a template and a dorsal plate as a secondary buttress plate will be described.

The concept of fragment-specific fixation was initially described by Rikli and Regazzoni in 1996 in a paper which also introduced their "3-column theory" [11]. This theory was further developed by others including Medoff who identified the specific individual fragments important in a DRF [12]. A summary of this and other relevant literature will be presented before the different techniques will be described in detail.

Three-Column Theory

There are multiple classifications of DRFs. These started with the eponymous descriptions of Colles, Smith and Barton and progressed to classifications that include various references to mechanism of injury, location of fracture lines, direction and degree of displacement, extent of articular involvement, ability to reduce, likelihood of instability and others [13]. A description of these is outside the scope of this chapter; however, a description and understanding of the important fragments that we are trying to control is essential.

The 3-column concept of DRF was first introduced by Rikli and Regazzoni in 1996 [11]. They stated that "the distal radius and distal ulna form a three-column biomechanical construction". They described a "medial column" comprising the distal ulna, triangular cartilage and the distal radio-ulnar joint; the "intermediate column" was described as the medial part of the distal radius with the lunate fossa and sigmoid notch; and the "lateral column" was described as the

D. J. Brown (✉)
Department of Trauma and Orthopaedics, Liverpool University Hospitals NHS FT and University of Liverpool, Liverpool, UK
e-mail: daniel.brown@liverpoolft.nhs.uk

© Springer Nature Switzerland AG 2022
W. B. Geissler (ed.), *Wrist and Elbow Arthroscopy with Selected Open Procedures*,
https://doi.org/10.1007/978-3-030-78881-0_38

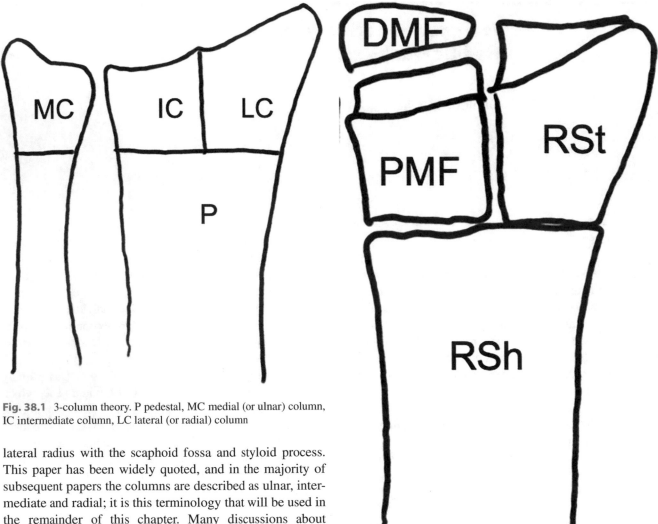

Fig. 38.1 3-column theory. P pedestal, MC medial (or ulnar) column, IC intermediate column, LC lateral (or radial) column

lateral radius with the scaphoid fossa and styloid process. This paper has been widely quoted, and in the majority of subsequent papers the columns are described as ulnar, intermediate and radial; it is this terminology that will be used in the remainder of this chapter. Many discussions about 3-column theory also use the term "pedestal" for the radial meta-diaphysis, which is usually intact [6, 7] (Fig. 38.1).

In 1984 Melone classified DRF based upon the fact that there seemed to be four basic bony fragments [14]. He described these as the radial shaft, the radial styloid, the dorsal medial fragment and the palmar medial fragment (Fig. 38.2). This description correlates well with the 3-column theory with the radial shaft corresponding to the pedestal, the radial styloid with the "radial column" and the dorsal and palmar medial fragments with the "intermediate column". Further Melone recognized that the extent and direction of displacement of these fragments were prognostic in anticipating the ability to reduce the fracture and its inherent stability. Later quantitative 3D CT scanning confirmed that these fracture fragments were the most commonly seen but noticed that the palmar intermediate column fragment is usually significantly bigger than the dorsal fragment [15].

Rikli, with Brink [16], recently expanded on his own 3-colum theory by also dividing the intermediate column into volar and dorsal "corners" and stressed that the dis-

Fig. 38.2 Fragments based upon Melone classification. RSh radial shaft, RSt radial styloid, DMF dorsal medial fragment, PMF palmar medial fragment

placed "corner" that the lunate moves with should be considered "key" and should be the first thing to be reduced and fixed. Most authors feel that the "critical corner" is the volar ulnar fragment, because it is the keystone of both the radiocarpal and radioulnar joints and displacement of this fragment can result in altered mechanics of both joints [6, 17]. Further, this fragment is the origin of the short radiolunate ligament, which is a key stabilizer of the radiolunate articulation [6, 18, 19]. This concept is not new and was discussed in Melone's 1984 paper [14] and was expanded on by Medoff below. The consequences of failing to reduce and stabilize this fragment have also been highlighted [17, 18, 20, 21], and it has been reported that this fragment is present in 13% DRFs treated operatively [17].

Medoff's seminal paper in 1995 [12] had already clarified our understanding of the intermediate column. Although Melone's and others' descriptions [14, 16] work for the more straightforward fractures, more complex fractures result in more fragments and all of these can be important to the stability of the wrist. Medoff described a dorso-ulnar corner, a volar rim, a dorsal wall and a free intra-articular fragment (Fig. 38.3). There has been much research since on the individual fragments in DRF, but this description is probably still the most useful and will be used in the remainder of this chapter.

All the discussion so far has been about the distal radius, and it is vital not to forget the medial (or ulnar) column, which, although it is usually intact, may be fractured at the level of the styloid or the neck. Many papers show that whilst the majority of ulna styloid fractures are benign and have no influence on the final prognosis of the injury [22], basal styloid fractures that disrupt the foveal attachment of the TFCC may have a significant effect on the distal radio-ulnar joint (DRUJ) [22]. Fractures of the ulnar neck, which may be benign in low-energy, osteoporotic fractures in the elderly, instead become critical in higher energy complex DRF [2, 22, 23] and their management, and also how they affect the management of the DRF, will also be discussed.

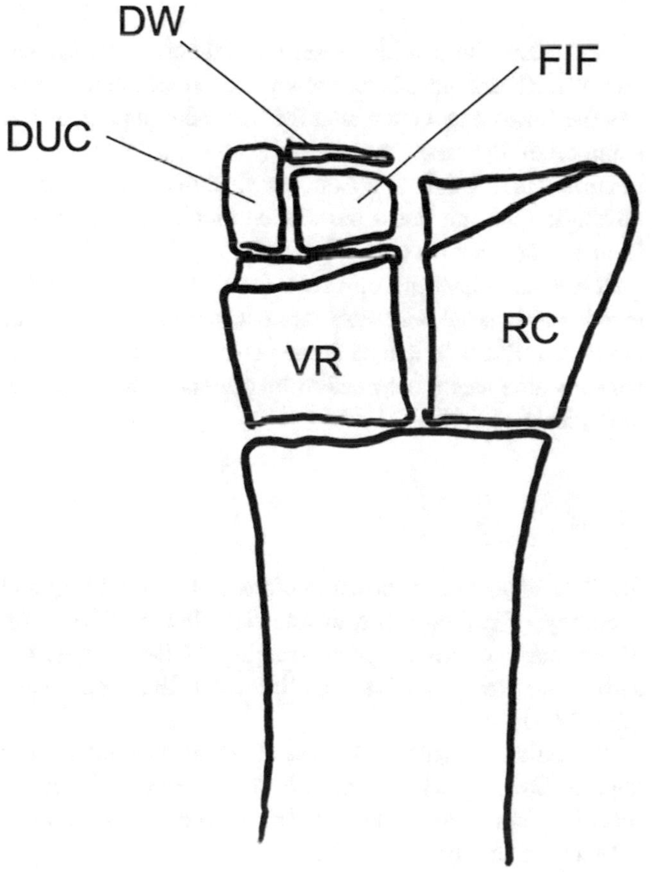

Radiographic Evaluation of DRF: Identifying the Individual Fragments

A knowledge of where the fractures lines are likely to be in a DRF and the fragments they are likely to cause makes interpretation of radiology significantly easier [12, 24].

Standard posteroanterior (PA) and lateral radiographs remain the primary assessment in DRF; however, several other projections can be used to better visualize and assess certain aspects of the bony anatomy. There is good evidence that both 2D and 3D computer tomography (CT) scans can add further information that can be vital in identifying the individual fragments when considering FSP.

The importance of Medoff's 1995 paper has already been highlighted when considering the intermediate column, but the same paper [12] also explains in detail the different radiographic views that can be utilized to better understand the fracture.

PA Radiograph

The PA projection visualizes well the radial styloid and both the volar and dorsal articular margins. On a normal wrist, the volar is proximal to the carpus, whereas dorsal is distal and overlies the carpus; this arrangement is reversed in dorsally angulated fractures. Careful correlation with the lateral allows fractures of the intermediate column to be identified as to whether they involve the dorsal or volar margins.

The PA is also essential for evaluating the amount of radial shortening by measuring the variance between the lengths of the radius and the ulna and the angle the articular surface makes to the perpendicular to the long axis of the radius (radial tilt) (Fig. 38.4). Finally, the PA is important in assessing for carpal bony and ligamentous injuries.

Lateral Radiograph

The first thing to assess on a lateral radiograph is how accurate a lateral it is. Minor degrees of forearm rotation and flexion or extension of the wrist can significantly alter measurement that may be taken from the image. A true lateral should have the wrist in a neutral position; the ulna should overlie the radius and the pisiform should lie over the distal pole of the scaphoid. It is important to note that a true lateral of the wrist is an oblique across the articular surface (due to the radial tilt).

Fig. 38.3 Medoff classification. DUC dorso-ulnar corner, VR volar rim, DW dorsal wall, FIF free intra-articular fragment

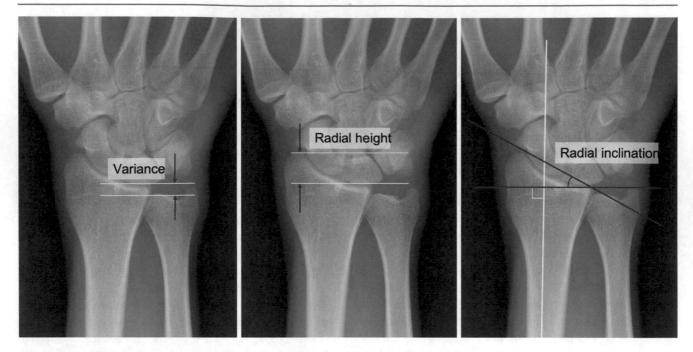

Fig. 38.4 PA radiograph demonstrating variance, radial height and radial inclination

The lateral projection is useful in assessing displacement of the extra-articular component of the fracture as well as identifying both partial and complete coronal plane fractures.

Medoff also introduced the radiographic descriptions of the vitally important volar rim fragment, describing the "teardrop" as the "volar projection of the lunate fossa," which, despite its small size ("it projects 3 mm palmarward from the flat surface of the radial diaphysis and is only 5 mm at its greatest width"), acts as "a mechanical buttress that prevents [volar] subluxation of the lunate". He also described the "teardrop angle" (Fig. 38.5), which allows assessment of its displacement.

The lateral is also useful in assessing if volar or dorsal angulation of the distal radius is likely to cause any carpal malalignment with the long axis of the radius is supposed to pass through the centre of the head of the capitate and the volar cortex of the radius through the centre of the lunate. Finally, the lateral view may identify other carpal bone fractures or signs of carpal ligament injury.

Modified PA (10° Proximally Angled) and Lateral (20° Oblique)

The aim of these projections is to give a better view of the articular surface by countering the normal volar and radial tilt. They are extremely useful intra- and post-operatively in ensuring metalwork is not within the joint (Fig. 38.6). The modified lateral is also useful in better assessing the teardrop for fractures and measuring the teardrop angle.

2D CT

2D CT scans can provide useful information in the evaluation of DRF and have been shown to more accurately classify the fracture and often alter the treatment plan [7, 24]. It is important to assess these carefully however to ensure that fracture lines are followed from one slice to another. Further no single slice can assess the whole articular surface due to its anatomic curvature.

It is essential, when using 2D CT that coronal and sagittal reconstructions are accurately referenced off the long axis of the radius. Reconstructions in the plane of the articular surface are also useful but need to be orientated to match the individual deformity.

3D CT

3D CT has also been shown to increase the reliability and accuracy of radiographic characterization of DRF [24]. 3D reconstructions (after subtraction of the carpus) are also easier to visualize and interpret than 2D scans (Fig. 38.7).

It should be noted that it is essential that slice thickness is kept as low as possible (0.6–1.0 mm) if resolution of the reconstruction is to be optimal. This is true for both 2D and 3D reconstructions.

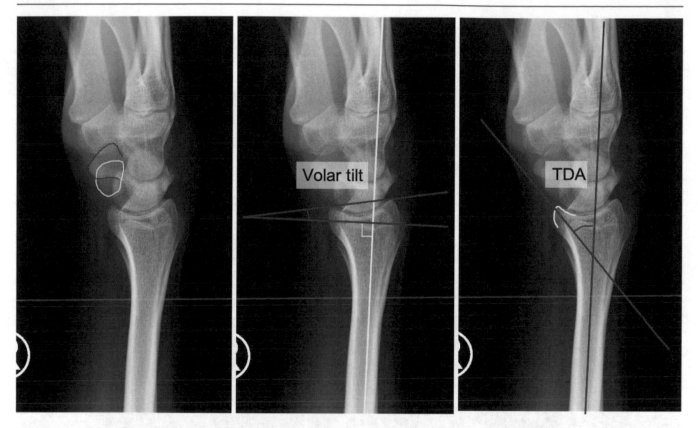

Fig. 38.5 True lateral radiograph (note pisiform overlying distal scaphoid) demonstrating volar lilt and teardrop angle

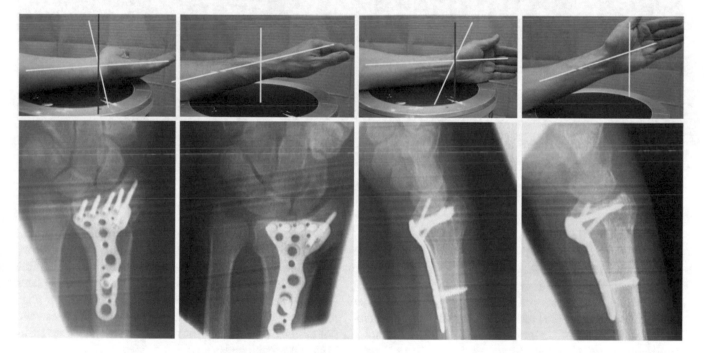

Fig. 38.6 Modified PA and lateral radiographs recommended for use intra-operatively

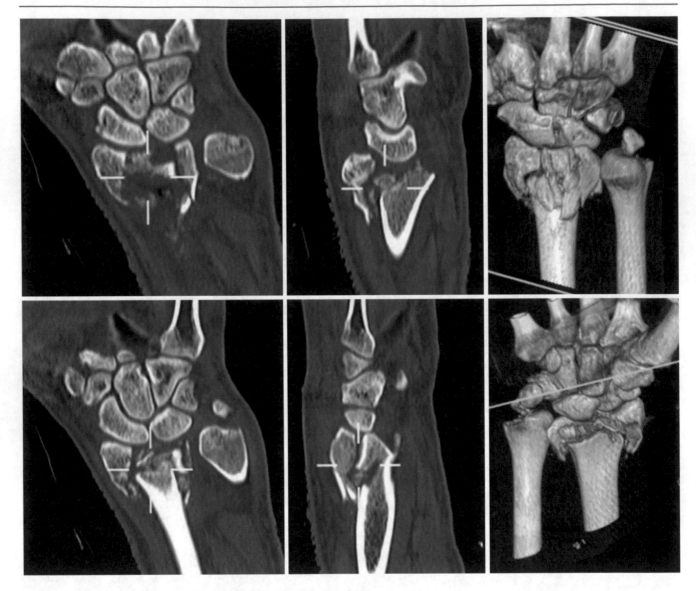

Fig. 38.7 2D (coronal and sagittal reformats) and 3D CT of the same DRF

Concepts of Fragment-Specific Plating of DRF

As mentioned previously the vast majority of DRF that require surgery can be treated with a VLP. Fragment-specific plating is only required in certain partial articular fractures (e.g., isolated radial styloid fractures [9], isolated volar lunate facet fractures [25] or isolated dorsal wall and dorso-ulnar corner fractures [25]) or, more commonly, in complex multi-column intra-articular fractures.

Three different techniques will be described

- True fragment-specific plating
- Augmented VLP
- VLP templated – dorsal buttress plating

"True" FSP

This concept was first introduced by Rikli and Regazzoni in their 1996 paper, which also introduced 3-column theory [11]. This was the first paper to advocate the use of multiple smaller lower-profile plates (in this case, AO 2.0-mm plates [Stratec Medical, Oberdorf, Switzerland]), with each plate used to control a different column. These initial plates were not designed specifically for these fractures and were traditional non-locking plates.

The term "fragment specific fixation" was introduced by Medoff and Kopylov in 1998 [26] in a paper that also introduced the TriMed Wrist Fixation System (TriMed, Valencia, CA). This system uses a combination of pin plates and wire forms which allow each fragment to be independently stabilized.

Other companies focussed more on anatomic specific locking plate technology and there are published papers on the use of fragment specific plates from AO 2.4-mm LCP Distal Radius System (DupuySynthes, West Chester, PA) [8], Acu-Loc 2 (Acumed, Hillsboro, OR) [2, 5], and others. Indeed, the majority of the major orthopaedic implant manufactures now offer fragment-specific implants for DRF.

Augmented VL Plating of DRF

An alternative approach in the management of complex DRF is to use a VLP as the main form of fixation of the DRF but augment it with other fixation devices, whether they be screws, wire forms or further plates. The aim is to insert the VLP in a standard technique and then reassess and identify any specific fragments that have not been successfully controlled [1, 21]. Secondary FSF is then performed using separate implants through separate incisions. The commonest fragments not controlled by the VLP that are suitable for this technique would be comminuted radial styloid fragments and dorsal wall and dorso-ulnar corner fragments.

VLP Templated Dorsal Buttress Plating

In this technique, a VLP is used as template for the distal fragments and a dorsal "buttress" plate (DBP) is used to reduce and hold the fragments against it.

In this technique an "anatomic" VLP is first secured to the radial diaphysis, in an ideal position, using standard technique. Once inserted the plate is used as a "template" to aid reduction of the individual fragments which are then "buttressed" against the volar plate, conferring stability without necessarily having to get screws or wires into any individual small fragment. Rigid fixation is then completed using subchondral locked screws from the volar side.

At first glance, there may not seem to be a big difference between augmented VLP and VLP templated DBP, as they both may well end up using the same implants through the same approaches. There is, however, a big difference in method that stems from a difference in thought process and planning. In the former, it is thought, pre-operatively, that the fracture and its fragments may well be controlled by the VLP alone and only, if they are not, will supplementary fixation be used. In the latter, there is a definite decision pre-operatively that the VLP will not be sufficient and that the dorsal buttress plate will definitely be used. Perhaps the former follows the "hope for the best" ideology, whereas the latter is more "plan for the worst" (as both Jack Reacher and Benjamin Disraeli would say). This distinction is, however, important, because whilst there is nothing wrong with either technique, the active decision making not only alters the implants that may be chosen but also the order in which the implants are utilized.

Approaches to the Distal Radius Utilized in FSP

Having identified the individual fragments that need to be addressed and decided on the method of fixation to be used, we next need to consider the approach used to be able to identify, reduce and fix the specific fragments.

Extended FCR Approach (Modified Henry)

Popularized by Orbay [27], this approach is the workhorse approach to the volar aspect of the radius and utilizes the internervous plane between brachioradialis and flexor capri radialis (FCR). It is usually ulnar to the radial artery. Pronator quadratus (PQ) is incised in an L-shaped fashion along its distal and radial edges and elevated. Further subperiosteal dissection under the radial remnant of PQ allows the insertion of brachioradialis to be released and allows access to the radial styloid (Figs. 38.8 and 38.9).

Volar-Ulnar Approach

For visualization of more ulna fractures, especially for "true" FSP of the critical corner a more ulnar approach can be used [6, 20]. Here the approach is in the plane between the ulna neurovascular bundle and flexor carpi ulnaris (FCU) with the flexor tendons and median nerve retracted radially. Elevation of PQ gives excellent access to the volar lunate facet. This approach can be extended distally to release the carpal tunnel (see Fig. 38.9c).

Radial

A straight radial incision allows direct access to the radial styloid. Care must be taken to identify and protect the radial sensory nerve, which will be in the centre of the surgical field [6, 9]. Brachioradialis is released from the floor of the 1st extensor compartment. Plates can either be placed on the volar aspect of the bone, the floor of the 1st extensor compartment (true lateral) or more dorsally between the 1st and 2nd extensor compartments (see Fig. 38.9d).

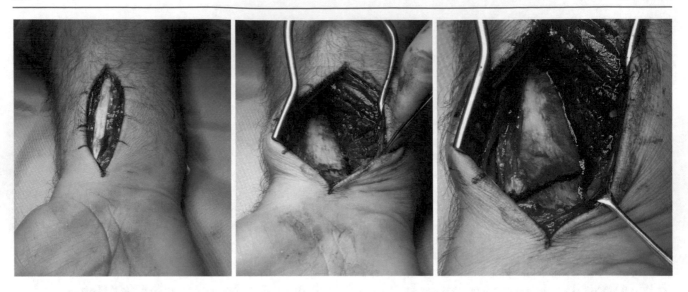

Fig. 38.8 Extended FCR approach

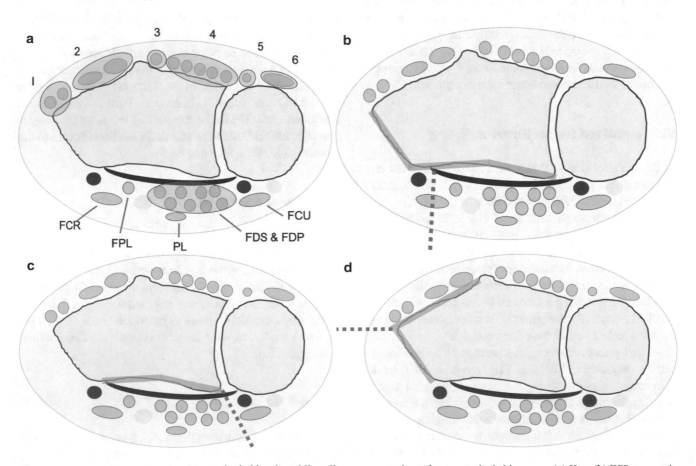

Fig. 38.9 Approaches to the wrist. Approach via blue dotted line allows access to bone fragments shaded in green. (**a**) Key. (**b**) FCR approach. (**c**) Volar-ulnar approach. (**d**) Radial approach. (**e**) Dorsal approach. (**f**) Dorso-ulnar approach. (**g**) Ulnar approach

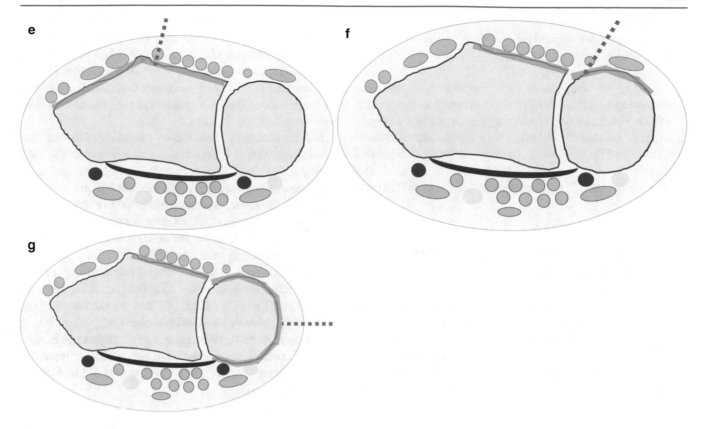

Fig. 38.9 (continued)

Dorsal

A midline dorsal incision can be used to approach either the radial column, the intermediate column or both. The approach, just ulnar to Lister's tubercle, approaches the radius through the floor of the 3rd extensor compartment after mobilising extensor pollicis longus (EPL). Subperiosteal dissection can then follow in either a radial or ulnar direction depending on the fracture. It is important to preserve the dorsal extrinsic ligaments and it is possible to use these as a hinge to allow access to the subchondral aspect of free intra-articular fragments (see Fig. 38.9e).

Dorso-Ulnar

The dorso-ulnar approach provides direct visualization of the dorso-ulnar corner (and dorsal wall) of the intermediate column [1]. A longitudinal incision over the DRUJ will allow the radius to be approached through the 5th extensor compartment after mobilizing extensor digiti minimi (EDM). Care must be taken to preserve the dorsal distal radio-ulnar ligaments (see Fig. 38.9f).

Ulnar

The ulna is most frequently approached through the interval between FCU and extensor carpi ulnaris (ECU). At this level, the bone is subcutaneous, and plates put on the medial side may be prominent; a volar placement through the same approach may be preferable [2]. At the level of the styloid, care needs to be taken to avoid damaging the ECU sub-sheath and the sensory branch of the ulna nerve [6] (see Fig. 38.9g).

Technique: How to Address Individual Fragments

In the remainder of this chapter, we will look at how to use these techniques for the various fracture configurations that one may encounter. We will specifically look at how to deal with the fragments known to be difficult to address with VLP which include [5, 7, 8, 25]

- Unstable radial styloid
- Dorsal ulna corner and dorsal wall

- Volar rim fragment
- Central free intra-articular impaction
- Fractures of the ulna

Deciding whether to use true FSF or one of the two techniques using a VLP is a fundamental, almost ideological one. It will be based as much on training and experience as on the fracture being treated. There are very few fractures that cannot be treated by both and both therefore have an important role: indeed, it is probably safe to say that if you are a master of either technique it is probably not essential to be able to do both.

True Fragment-Specific Treatment of DRF: Planning the Surgery

Having identified the individual fragments that make up the fracture, the first question to ask is which column to address first. As a general rule, it is easiest to start with the intermediate column as the fragments involving the sigmoid notch can be usefully reduced against the, usually, intact ulna head. Indeed, associated ulnar neck or head fractures (occurring in

approximately 6% of all DRF [2]) would be the only exception to this rule (see later). Another reason for addressing the intermediate column first is that, once it has been reduced and stabilized, it becomes easy to reduce the radial column to it. In contrast, it is incredibly difficult to mobilize and reduce the fragments of the intermediate column when there is an intact ulna and radial column.

Having decided to first address the intermediate column, the next question is whether to approach this from the volar or dorsal side. This decision can be aided by analysing the displacement, not only of the intermediate column fragments but also of the lunate, as seen on the initial lateral radiograph. The fragment of radius that has moved with the lunate can be considered key [16], and whilst this is usually the volar fragment, it is not always the case (Fig. 38.10). If there is any doubt, it is safer to consider the volar fragment the key as it is much more likely to cause complications if inadequately reduced and fixed [1, 17, 18, 20] than the dorsal wall fragment, which is more likely to be benign [28].

Although dorsal wall fragments are thought to be benign, displaced dorso-ulnar corner fragments need to reduced and fixed as failure to do so is one of the causes of instability of the DRUJ [1, 28].

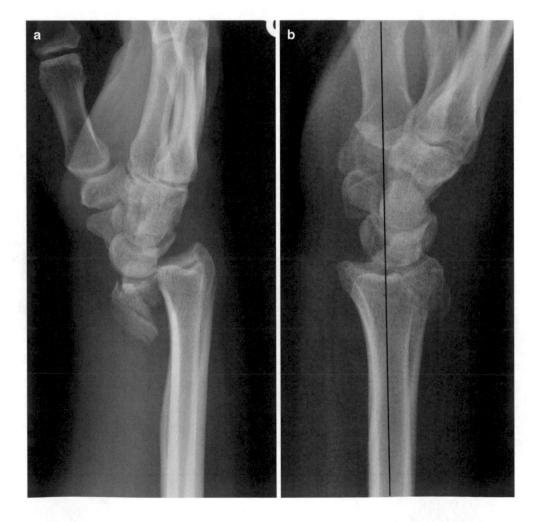

Fig. 38.10 The direction of displacement of the "lunate fragment" is key to deciding the approach to be used: (**a**) obvious volar subluxation, (**b**) subtle dorsal subluxation

Prior to reducing and fixing the intermediate column it is also essential to look for displaced free intra-articular fragments as these will need to be reduced before fixation is commenced. These fragments can be elevated and reduced through either a dorsal approach (hinging the dorsal wall out of the way on the dorsal extrinsic ligaments) or through the volar extended FCR approach by keeping the hand supinated and pronating the radial shaft allowing access to the intra-articular fragment through the meta-diaphyseal portion of the fracture [27]. Once reduced the free intra-articular fragment can be held with locked subchondral screws from a plate or being "squeezed" between two plates (one dorsally, one volar); alternatively, the defect behind it can be filled with bone graft or substitute.

The size of the fragments will decide the implant used for fixation and there are many choices available. Previous concerns about implant prominence have been addressed with much lower profile, anatomic designs and the risk of implant prominence by crossing the "watershed line" [29] are outweighed by the catastrophic consequences of not controlling the volar rim fragment [1, 17, 18]. With modern implants

even the smallest fragments can be controlled with screws [21], wire forms [25, 26], suture-plates [5], hook plates [17], or by being buttressed between the volar and separate anatomic dorsal plates [5, 8].

The radial fragment can usually be controlled by a single plate that can be applied volarly, radially or dorsally. The plate placement is chosen by a combination of the displacement and comminution of the fragments together with approach used for the fixation of the intermediate column with the former factors being key. Whilst it is possible to place a radial plate through either an extended FCR approach [30, 31] or the dorsal midline approach [8], a radial approach may be preferable for the most unstable fractures [9] (Fig. 38.11).

We return to the issue of associated ulnar neck fractures and how it alters the decision as to which column to address first. According to previously quoted literature, in the majority of fractures the radial column is comprised of a single large fragment; the intermediate column may be in several smaller fragments and the ulna may or may not be fractured at its neck (we will ignore ulna styloid fractures at this point).

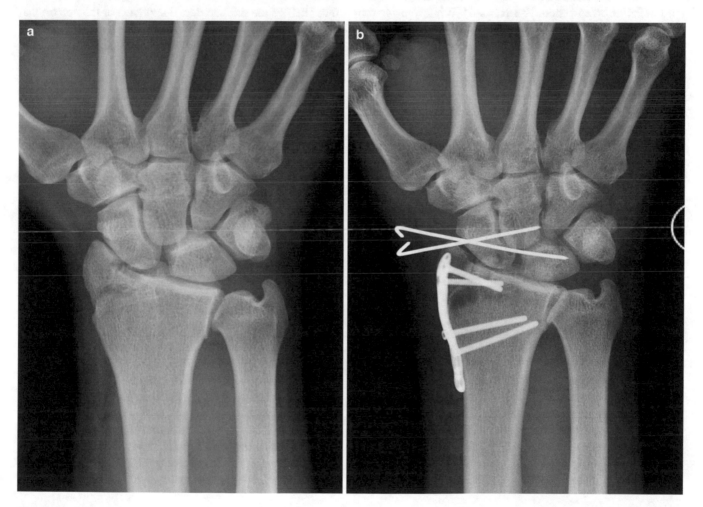

Fig. 38.11 (**a, b**) Radial styloid plate treating radial styloid fracture

As above, if the ulna is intact, it is easiest to build up the intermediate column onto the ulna and then fix the radial styloid to that. If the ulna is fractured but easily reducible and fixed (i.e., stable), it is often easiest to fix this first and then proceed with radial fixation in a standard way. If instead there is significant comminution or bone loss to the ulna, and the radius fracture is of a standard pattern, it may be easier to start the reconstruction by securing the simpler and more stable radial column first and "building" everything else on to that.

In the very unusual situation with there is comminution and instability in all three columns, it might be easier to use the technique of VLP templated DBP or even spanning wrist plating.

Augmented Volar Locking Plating

When attempting to deal with a highly complex DRF with a VLP it is essential that the VLP is anatomic and provides good distal support. Soong [29] argued that plates that crossed the "watershed line were much more likely to cause tendon irritation and should be avoided". Whilst this is probably true for the majority of fractures the consequences of not supporting the volar rim fragment outweigh this theoretical risk in the fractures we are discussing here. Indeed, certain manufacturers (e.g., Acumed, Hillsboro, OR) make two versions of the Acu-loc 2 plate for this very reason: the proximal one for simpler fractures that sit below the watershed line and a distal version for more complex fractures that sit above it. Similarly, whilst often it is safer, for soft tissue reasons, to use the narrower of two plates if there is a choice in simpler fractures, the opposite is true here, in the case of the more complex patterns.

The VLP is applied using standard methodology and the situation reassessed. There are four likely fragments that may not be adequately stabilized by a VLP alone: these are the volar rim fragment, a free intra-articular fragment, the dorsal wall or corner and an unstable radial styloid. The presence of a volar rim fragment (especially if the pre-reduction radiograph suggests volar subluxation of the lunate) and a displaced free intra-articular fragment should make you seriously question if a standard VLP (or even augmented VLP) is the correct methodology for treating this fracture.

There are specific VLPs on the market that are designed to provide adequate support for volar rim fragments; however, it should be noted that many volar lunate facet fragments are distal to the watershed line [17]. Controlling free intra-articular fragments with any single plate is very difficult. It is, however, possible to hold either fragment with wires inserted through the volar rim, parallel with the joint surface,

and then bent back through 90° and secured under the plate. It is also possible to use supplementary screws into a volar rim fragment if it is large, or to augment fixation using polyethylene or carbon-fibre braided sutures, attaching the volar extrinsic ligaments to the plate, if it is small [5]. It is also possible to use a small supplementary condylar hook plate to the VLP in certain systems. Although all of these are possible, it may be that using a true FSP solution, using a plate or wire form specifically designed for the volar lunate facet, may be easier (Fig. 38.12).

Augmentation of a VLP with a radial column plate to control an unstable radial styloid is easier, more common and widely reported. There are many suitable plates available, and they can easily be inserted through the extended FCR approach [30, 31]. Due to orthogonal positioning of the radial plate, this acts to buttress the radial column to the reduced and fixed intermediate column. As such it is not normally necessary to use many, if any, screws in the distal fragment (Fig. 38.13).

Similarly, augmented stabilization of dorsal wall and dorso-ulnar corner fragments is straightforward. A second small plate can be inserted as a buttress plate using either the ulnar half of the midline dorsal approach or the dorso-ulnar approach. Several specific plates are available. A novel way of dealing with these fractures using a minimally invasive technique is available with one of the plating systems. The Frag-loc® device with Acu-loc2 (Acumed, Hilsoboro, OR) allows a barrel to be inserted into a screw hole of the VLP and a wire passed through this to exit on the dorsal side of the wrist. A "washered" screw can then be passed over the wire from dorsal to volar, buttressing the dorsal fragment and securing it, and compressing it, when the threads of the dorsal screw engage with the internal threads of the volar barrel (Fig. 38.14) [5].

VLP Templated Dorsal Buttress Plating

Double or "sandwich" plating has been well described in the literature [4, 10, 30, 32]. There is, however, a subtle difference between the methods used in these published series and the method described here: The main difference is in the order of insertion of the various plates and screws; specifically, whether to insert any screws from the volar side before inserting the dorsal plate. Whilst the difference in technique is small, it is my opinion that the method described here may be easier, in that it uses the inherent anatomic nature of the plates to aid the reduction and fixation of fragments. This technique utilizes two plates: an anatomic and distal VLP and an anatomic low-profile dorsal plate. Although there are several manufacturers who make suitable plates (and indeed

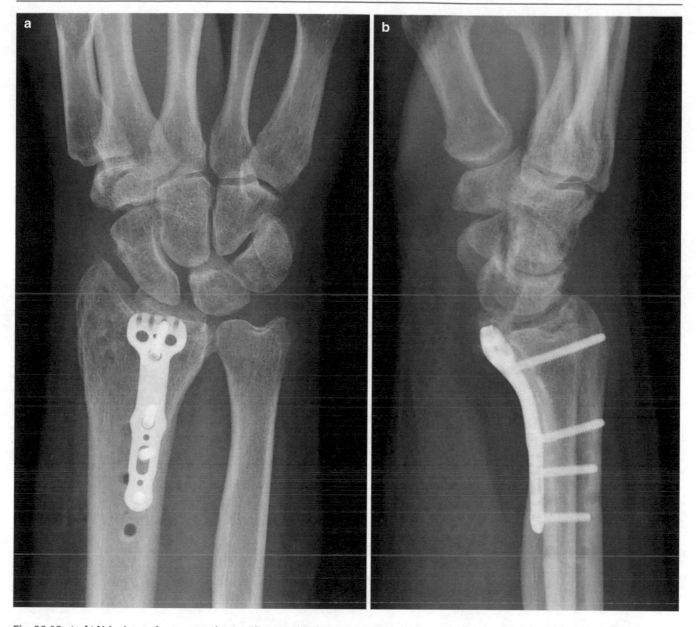

Fig. 38.12 (**a, b**) Volar lunate facet suture plate treating very distal "teardrop" fragment

the papers in the quoted literature all use Synthes 2.4 mm LCP DRP, at least dorsally), my experience is in using the distal Acu-loc2 VLP and the dorsal rim plate [2, 5] from Acumed (Hillsboro, OR) (Fig. 38.15). It is this technique that I will describe here.

The only possible contraindication to this technique would be a very small volar lunate facet fragment that could not be controlled with the VLP (although it is still possible if these fragments are controlled with the augments described in the previous section).

An extended FCR approach is utilized and a suitable plate chosen. Longer plates can be used, as required,

depending on the amount of metaphyseal or diaphyseal comminution. It is essential that the plate is applied to the flat volar aspect of the radius to enable correction of the rotational component that exists in most DRFs [11]. Care must be taken to ensure that the long axis of the plate lies along the long axis of the radius and the length adjusted so that the ulna aspect of distal end of the plate lies approximately 2 mm proximal to the distal end of the ulna head (an anatomic plate will only act as an anatomic template if applied in the correct place and orientation). In the presence of an ulna head/neck fracture, radiographs of the contralateral limb should be used as a template.

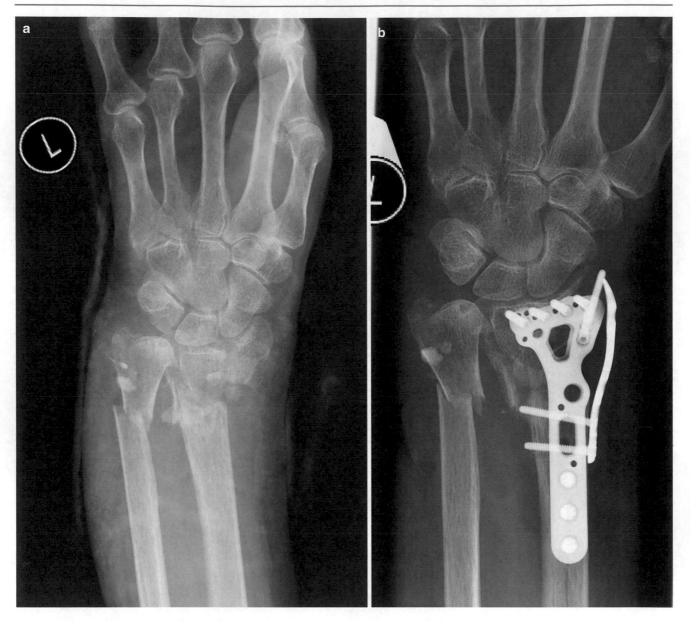

Fig. 38.13 (**a**, **b**) Volar locking plate augmented with radial plate for complex radial column fracture

Having ensured that the plate is in the correct position, the volar rim fragment is reduced with care taken to restore the "teardrop angle". Wires passed immediately distal to the plate, parallel to the articular surface, can usefully be used as joysticks by levering these around the distal edge of the plate. Further wires passed through the wire holes in the plate and guide can then provisionally secure the volar fragment. It is usual to bend all four of these wires through 90° so they are parallel with the forearm to allow the arm to be pronated to allow access to the dorsum.

A midline dorsal approach with elevation of both radial and ulnar flaps exposes the dorsal surface of the wrist. The dorsal wall is rotated distally on the extrinsic ligaments to allow any free intra-articular fragments to be elevated.

Metaphyseal defects can be packed with bone graft or substitute as required. The dorsal wall is replaced, and care is taken to ensure the dorso-ulnar corner is also reduced. The radial styloid is now reduced to the intermediate column and provisionally help with K wires. The dorsal rim plate is then positioned and used as a buttress to bring the dorsal rim and radial column down against the volar plate using non-locking screws in the metadiaphyseal segment. It is not normally necessary to put any dorsal screws in the distal fragments. Fixation is now completed by supinating the arm and placing distal screws of the volar plate into the intermediate column to support the subchondral articular surface and into the radial column and styloid (Fig. 38.16).

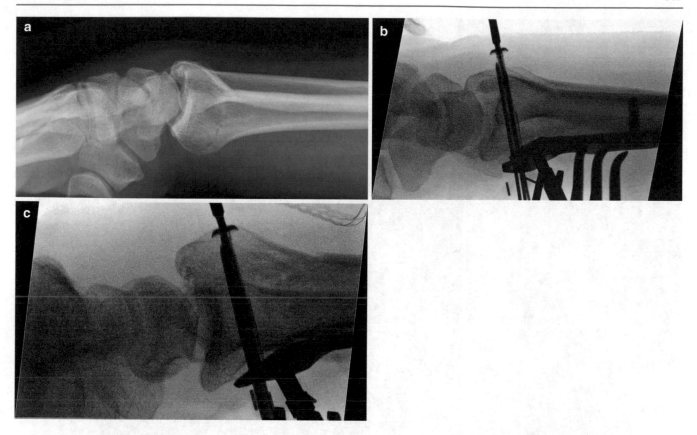

Fig. 38.14 Lateral radiographs of fracture with dorsal instability (**a**) demonstrating insertion of Frag-loc (**b**) to control large dorsal fragment (**c**)

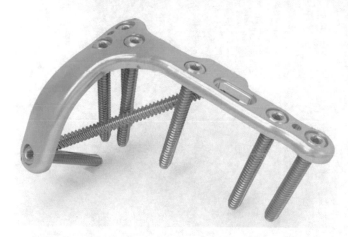

Fig. 38.15 Acumed dorsal rim plate implant (right sided)

Fractures of the Distal Ulna

The majority of fractures of the distal ulna occur with fractures of the distal radius and on the whole the clinical outcome is more determined by the radial fracture [22]. The general rule about management is to treat the DRF and only then assess and treat the ulna fracture as if it were an isolated injury. The indications for treatment are when the ulna fracture causes significant instability of the ulna column or causes instability of the DRUJ (usually due to the disruption of the foveal attachment of the triangular fibrocartilage complex (TFCC)).

When considering distal ulna fractures the management is based upon the anatomical position of the fracture

- Ulna styloid
  - Distal to foveal attachment of TFCC
  - Involving foveal attachment of TFCC
- Ulna head
- Ulna neck (and distal ulna shaft)

With regard to ulna styloid fractures, these should not alter the planned treatment of the DRF and only need to be assessed one the DRF has been stabilized. Most DRFs with concomitant ulna styloid fractures do not have any DRUJ instability, and in this case do not require treatment [23], as it has been shown that even untreated styloid non-unions do not affect surgical outcome [7]. DRUJ instability after DRF fixation, associated with a basal ulna styloid fracture, does, however, require treatment. The instability is usually the result of the intact ulna attachments of the TFCC (the foveal and superficial attachments) being displaced with the large styloid fragment. In this case, bony fixation of the styloid with wires or a single headless compression screw is appropriate. In other cases, there is disruption of the foveal attach-

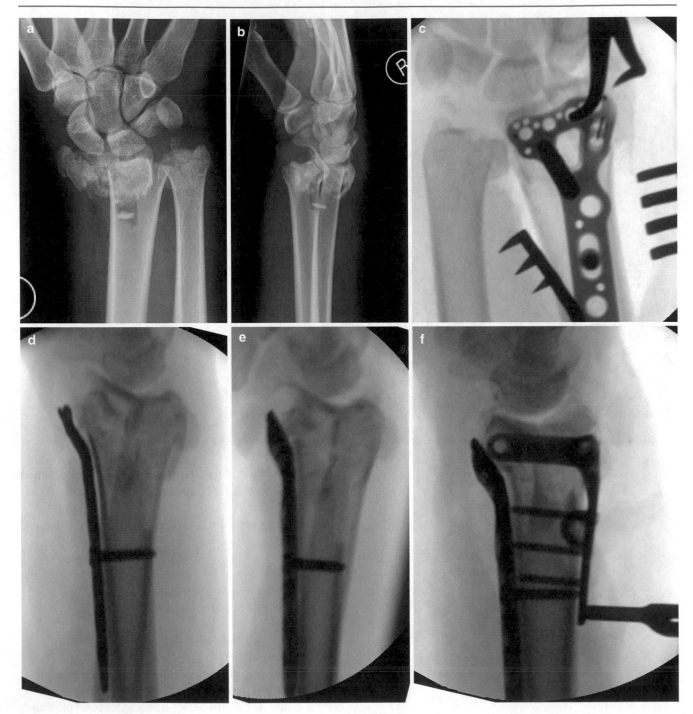

Fig. 38.16 Augmented buttress plating with volar and dorsal rim plate: (**a, b**) initial fracture, (**c, d**) insertion of volar plate as template, (**e**) reduction of volar lunate facet, (**f, g**) application of dorsal rim buttress plate, (**h**) final construct

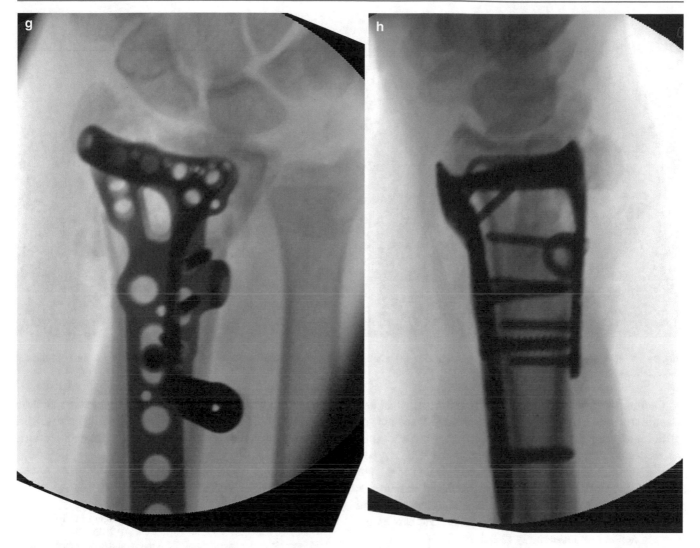

Fig. 38.16 (continued)

ment with the superficial attachment allowing the TFC to move with the styloid fragment. This will result in the DRUJ remaining unstable even after styloid fixation, and in this case this foveal attachment will need to be acutely repaired. In unusual cases, there may be DRUJ instability despite there being a small or comminuted styloid fragment that is not amenable to bony fixation. In these cases, soft tissue repair of the foveal attachment is more appropriate.

Ulna head and neck fractures usually reduce when the DRF is reduced and do not normally require specific treatment; either if the radial fracture is managed non-operatively or is operatively treated in low-energy or osteoporotic fractures [23].

In higher energy injuries, where the radius is more unstable, adding ulna column stability becomes essential. Most distal ulna fractures are simple and can be treated with an ulna plate and there are several anatomic plates available [2, 26]. These can be inserted through an ulnar approach and can be placed along the medial subcutaneous border, although volar sub-muscular placement through the same approach may result in less soft tissue irritation [2, 5].

Complex distal ulna fractures are very rare [22]. Neck fractures with excessive comminution or bone loss can be usefully treated with bridge-plating and cortico-cancellous bone grafting (Fig. 38.17).

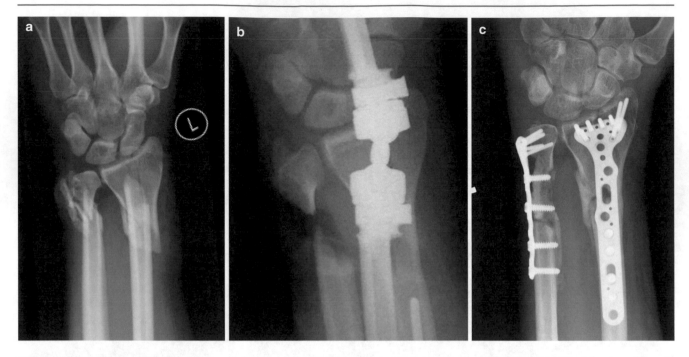

Fig. 38.17 Complex open DRF with ulna neck fractures (**a**), after debridement and temporary external fixation (**b**) and final fixation with corticocancellous bone graft (**c**)

Comminuted, unreconstructable intra-articular ulna head fractures do occur and have been described [22] and are very difficult to manage. Excision has been described but cannot be recommended in younger patients. If the DRF has been well fixed and is stable; non-operative treatment of the ulna may be appropriate in relatively undisplaced fractures. In displaced fractures a distal ulna replacement hemiarthroplasty is probably more appropriate and can be performed acutely or sub-acutely [22].

Associated Carpal Bony and Ligamentous Injuries

Complex distal radius fractures, due to their energy of injuries, may be associated with other injuries to the carpus, whether they be bony, ligamentous or a combination of the two. Although the management of these are outside the scope of this chapter, it is essential that they are not overlooked.

Conclusion

Complex fractures of the distal radius are not uncommon, are difficult to treat and have high complication rates. There is no single technique that can be used successfully; however, the techniques outlined in this chapter are extremely well suited to the management of the most complex of fractures.

It should be noted that these are not techniques to be used only rarely as they do have significant learning curves. That said, once mastered they can have very reproducible results.

References

1. Hozack BA, Tosti RJ. Fragment specific fixation in distal radius fractures. Curr Rev Musculoskelet Med. 2019;12:190–7.
2. Geissler WB. Management of distal radius and distal ulnar fractures with fragment specific plate. J Wrist Surg. 2013;2:190–4.
3. Landgren M, Abramo A, Geijer M, Kopylov P, Tagil M. Fragment specific versus Volar locking plates in primary nonreducible or secondarily redisplaced distal radius fractures: a randomised controlled trial. J Hand Surg Am. 2017;42:156–65.
4. Ring D, Prommersberger K, Jupiter JB. Combined Dorsal and Volar plate fixation of complex fractures of the distal part of the radius. J Bone Joint Surg Am. 2004;86A(8):1646–52.
5. Geissler WB, Clark SM. Fragment-specific fixation for fractures of the distal radius. J Wrist Surg. 2016;5:22–30.
6. He JJ, Blazar P. Management of high energy distal radius injuries. Curr Rev Musculoskelet Med. 2019;12:379–85.
7. Rhee RC, Medoff RJ, Shin AY. Complex distal radius fractures: an anatomic algorithm for surgical management. J Am Acad Orthop Surg. 2017;25:77–88.
8. Gavakar AS, Muthukumar S. Fragment-specific fixation for complex intra-articular fractures of the distal radius: results of a prospective single-centre trial. J Hand Surg (Eur). 2012;37E(8):765–71.
9. Hoffman JD, Stewart J, Kusnezov N, Dunn J, Pirela-Cruz M. Radial plate fixation: a novel technique for distal radius fractures. Hand. 2017;12(5):471–5.
10. Medlock G, Smith M, Johnstone AJ. Combined Volar and Dorsal approach for fixation of comminuted intra-articular distal radial fractures. J Wrist Surg. 2018;7:219–26.

11. Rikli DA, Regazzoni P. Fractures of the distal end of the radius treated by internal fixation and early function. J Bone Joint Surg. 1996;78B(4):588–92.
12. Medoff RJ. Essential radiographic evaluation for distal radius fractures. Hand Clin. 2005;21:279–88.
13. Fernandez DL, Jupiter JB. Epidemiology, mechanism, classification in fractures of the distal radius. 2nd ed. New York: Springer-Verlag; 2002. Chapter 2
14. Melone CP Jr. Articular fractures of the distal radius. Orthop Clin N Am. 1984;15(02):217–36.
15. Teunis T, Bosma NH, Lubberts B, Ter Meulen DP, Ring D. Melone's concept revisited: £D quantification of fragment displacement. J Hand Microsurg. 2016;8:27–33.
16. Brink PRG, Rikli DA. Four-corner concept: CT-based assessment of fracture patterns in distal radius. J Wrist Surg. 2016;5:147–51.
17. O'Shaughnessy MA, Shin AY, Kakar S. Stabilization of Volar ulnar rim fractures of the distal radius: current techniques and review of the literature. J Wrist Surg. 2016;5:113–9.
18. Harness NG, Jupiter JB, Orbay JL, Raskin KB, Fernandez DL. Loss of fixation of the Volar lunate facet fragment in fractures of the distal part of the radius. J Bone Joint Surg Am. 2004;86A(9):1900–8.
19. Berger RA, Landsmeer JMF. The palmar radiocarpal ligaments: a study of adult and fetal human wrist joints. J Hand Surg [Am]. 1990;15A:847–54.
20. Jupiter JB, Fernandez DL, Toh CL, Fellman T, Ring D. Operative treatment of Volar intra-articular fractures of the distal end of the radius. J Bone Joint Surg (American). 1996;78A(12):1817–28.
21. Harness NG. Fixation options for the Volar lunate facet fracture: thinking outside the box. J Wrist Surg. 2016;5:9–16.
22. Logan AJ, Lindau TR. The management of distal ulnar fractures in adults: a review of the literature and recommendations for treatment. Strategies Trauma Limb Reconstr. 2008;3:49–56.
23. Ozkan S, Fischerauer SF, Kootstra TJM, Claessen FMAP, Ring D. Ulnar neck fractures associated with distal radius fractures. J Wrist Surg. 2018;7:71–6.
24. Harness NG, Ring D, Zurakowski D, Harris G, Jupiter JB. The influence of three-dimensional computer tomography reconstructions on the characterization and treatment of distal radial fractures. J Bone Joint Surg Am. 2006;88A(6):1315–23.
25. Lam J, Wolfe SW. Distal radial fractures: what cannot be fixed with a volar plate? – the role of fragment-specific fixation in modern fracture treatment. Operative Tech Sports Med. 2010;18:181–8.
26. Leslie BM, Medoff RJ. Fracture specific fixation of distal radius fractures. Tech Orthop. 2000;15(4):336–52.
27. Orbay JL, Infante A, Khouri RK, Fernandez DL. The extended Flexor Carpi Radialis approach: a new perspective for the distal radius fracture. Tech Hand Up Extrem Surg. 2001;5(4):204–11.
28. Kim JK, Yun YH, Kim DJ. The effect of displaced dorsal rim fragment in a distal radius fracture. J Wrist Surg. 2016;5:31–5.
29. Soong M, Earp BE, Bishop G, Leung A, Blazer P. Volar locking plate implant prominence and flexor tendon rupture. J Bone Joint Surg Am. 2011;93A(4):1–8.
30. Jacobi M, Wahl P, Kohut G. Repositioning and stabilization of the radial styloid process in comminuted fractures of the distal radius using a single approach: the radio-volar double plating technique. J Orthop Surg Res. 2010;5:55–9.
31. Helmerhorst GTT, Kloen P. Orthogonal plating of intra-articular distal radial fractures with an associated radial column fracture via a single Volar approach. Injury. 2010;43:1307–12.
32. Day CS, Kamath AF, Makhni E, Jean-Gilles J, Zurakowski D. "Sandwich" plating for intra-articular distal radius fractures with Volar and Dorsal comminution. Hand. 2008;3:47–54.

Bridge Plating of Distal Radius Fractures

39

A. Jordan Grier and David S. Ruch

Introduction

Distal radius fractures are among the most commonly treated fractures of the upper extremity. The American Academy of Orthopaedic Surgeons (AAOS) reported a moderate strength recommendation for operative fixation of distal radius fractures with postreduction radial shortening >3 mm, dorsal tilt of greater than 10°, or intra-articular displacement or step-off of >2 mm [1]. A multitude of surgical treatment options have been described in the literature for those patients indicated for operative fixation. The treatment of choice for these fractures is multifactorial in nature and should be based on fracture pattern, associated injuries, status of the surrounding soft tissue envelope, and patient demographics.

The use of dorsal spanning plate fixation was first introduced in 1998 via separate reports from Burke and Singer as well as Becton, Colborn, and Goodrich as an alternative to spanning external fixation for comminuted fractures of the distal radius [2, 3]. Early reports on the use of spanning dorsal plate fixation noted good to excellent short-term functional outcomes, favorable range of motion outcomes, and excellent maintenance of fracture reduction and radiocarpal joint congruity [4–6]. Biomechanical studies comparing dorsal bridge plate fixation to external fixation also suggest that dorsal bridge plating provides for a significant increase in stiffness in axial plane loading, with the dorsal bridge plate functioning as an external fixator with a functional bone-to-bar distance of 0 [7–9]. The use of dorsal bridge plate fixation provides for a direct dorsal buttress to counteract dorsal angulation and shortening at the fracture site, while avoiding the relatively high complication rate associated with external fixation [10, 11].

A. J. Grier · D. S. Ruch (✉)
Department of Orthopaedic Surgery, Duke University Medical Center, Durham, NC, USA
e-mail: d.ruch@duke.edu

Indications and Contraindications

The primary indication for dorsal bridge plate fixation of distal radius fractures is the treatment of high-energy, comminuted fractures of the distal radius which are not amenable to fixation with standard periarticular plating systems or non-operative treatment. Becton et al. were the first to report outcomes of dorsal bridge plate fixation for this indication in their case series of 35 patients treated with a 3.5-mm internal fixator plate [2]. Ruch et al. expanded on this indication in their report of 22 patients with comminuted distal radius fractures with metadiaphyseal extension to at least 4 cm proximal to the radiocarpal articulation, all of whom went on to union at a mean of 110 days, with subsequent plate removal performed at an average of 124 days [5]. In their series neither clinical range of motion nor DASH scores were significantly correlated with duration of immobilization. Dorsal bridge plate fixation has also been indicated for use in polytraumatized patients, particularly those patients who have concomitant lower extremity injuries which require the use of the upper extremities for mobilization and rehabilitation. The use of spanning plate fixation in this setting may allow for earlier patient mobilization via the use of their injured upper extremity, while also reducing the nursing care requirements of the patient by the eliminating the need for appliance-related hygiene tasks as would be required with an external fixation construct [7]. Hanel et al. reported on their series of 62 patients treated with spanning dorsal plate fixation, of which 23 were indicated based on the presence of concomitant lower extremity injuries. Excellent radiographic outcomes were observed at final follow-up in this series including radial height within 5 mm of ulnar neutral, preserved articular congruity with no step or gap displacement at the radiocarpal joint greater than 2 mm, and preserved volar tilt to at least neutral [4]. Postoperative weightbearing following dorsal bridge plating for patients indicated for polytrauma should be tailored to the implants utilized for fixation. Huang et al. reported on the

© Springer Nature Switzerland AG 2022
W. B. Geissler (ed.), *Wrist and Elbow Arthroscopy with Selected Open Procedures*,
https://doi.org/10.1007/978-3-030-78881-0_39

biomechanical properties of dorsal bridge plates in a simulated crutch weightbearing model and noted that use of a 2.4-mm bridge plate construct resulted in consistent plate failure via wrist palmar flexion and plate bending [12]. Of note this biomechanical study utilized distal fixation to the index metacarpal only, and to date no studies have been published reporting on this testing paradigm with distal fixation to the long finger metacarpal. Given these findings, caution should be exercised in allowing patients to transition from platform weightbearing to crutch bearing in the early postoperative period. In patients treated via a bridge plate construct for the indication of polytraumatization and reliance on the upper extremities for early weightbearing, consideration should be given to the use of a plating system with an increased plate thickness (3.2 mm or 3.5 mm) to reduce the risk of implant failure via axial loading.

Favorable results have been reported following the use of dorsal bridge plate constructs for treatment of distal radius fractures in patients with osteoporotic bone and comminuted fracture patterns. Use of dorsal bridge plate fixation for this indication is particularly advantageous for those elderly patients reliant upon a gait aid, such as a cane or walker, as it may allow for an earlier return to the patient's baseline ambulatory status utilizing their injured extremity compared to what would be afforded based on postoperative restrictions following locked volar plating. Richard et al. reported on their series of 33 patients with a mean age of 70 years who were treated with dorsal bridge plating for comminuted fracture patterns [13]. Fracture union occurred in all patients, with subsequent plate removal performed at an average of 3 months from the patient's index procedure. Excellent radiographic outcomes were achieved in this cohort with a mean volar tilt of 5°, positive ulnar variance of 0.6 mm, and radial inclination of 20°. Restoration of radiocarpal articular congruity was also similar to prior reports of patients treated for high-energy fracture patterns, with an articular step-off of <2 mm in 30/33 patients.

Recently the use of dorsal bridge plate fixation has also been expanded to include management of established nonunion following operative treatment of distal radius fractures. Mithani et al. reported on their case series of eight patients who underwent operative treatment for a distal radius fracture with either dorsal locked plating, volar locked plating, external fixation, or closed reduction and percutaneous pinning who subsequently progressed to nonunion [14]. Dorsal bridge plates were removed at a mean of 148 days from placement. At final follow-up, significant improvements were observed in total arc of motion (38.8° preoperatively, 75.9° postoperatively), supination (22.5° preoperatively, 72° postoperatively), and DASH score (70.5 preoperatively, 27.6 postoperatively).

Contraindications to dorsal bridge plate fixation include distal radius fractures which are otherwise amenable to fixation with standard periarticular plating systems or nonoperative treatment, fractures with insufficient dorsal soft tissue to allow for plate coverage or this which are unable to be covered in a timely fashion, and volar shear fractures which may not be adequately reduced and controlled by dorsal fixation alone.

Surgical Technique

The patient is positioned on a standard operating table with a radiolucent hand table extension on the operative side (Fig. 39.1). Alternatively, a radiolucent stretcher-based hand table may be utilized if available. All bony prominences are well-padded to prevent iatrogenic compression-related injury. The use of intraoperative mechanical venous thromboembolism prophylaxis may be employed depending on the estimated procedure length, particularly in the setting of the polytraumatized patient undergoing concomitant operative treatment of other injuries. If desired, a non-sterile pneumatic tourniquet is applied to the operative extremity. The operative extremity is prepped and draped in standard sterile fashion according to the practices of the treating surgeon.

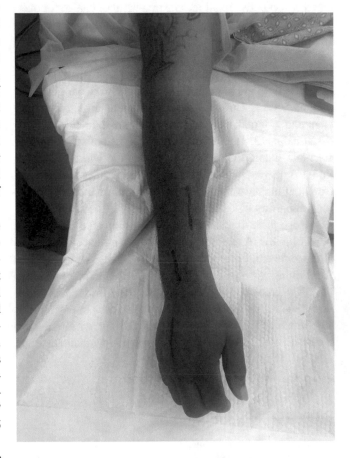

Fig. 39.1 Operating room setup with operative extremity on radiolucent hand table extension

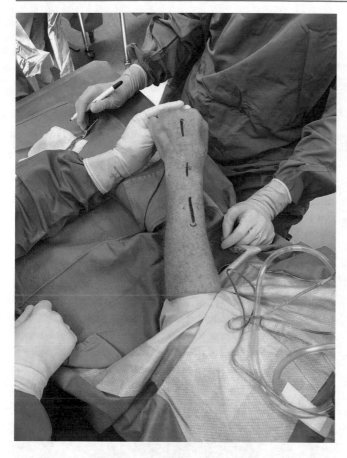

Fig. 39.2 Planned incisions (dorsal metacarpal, dorsal radiocarpal joint, distal radial diaphysis) marked with indelible surgical marker

Three incisions are marked on the dorsal surface of the operative extremity (Fig. 39.2):

1. Three-centimeter incision extending from the proximal diaphysis to the base of the long finger metacarpal.
2. Three-centimeter incision just ulnar to Lister's tubercle. This incision should additionally be centered about Lister's tubercle in cranial-caudal orientation.
3. Four-centimeter incision over the radial diaphysis. This incision should be at least 4 cm from the proximal most extent of the observed fracture comminution. Often, this incision lies just proximal to the palpable muscle bellies of the adductor pollicis longus (APL) and extensor pollicis brevis (EPB) as they traverse the distal aspect of the dorsal forearm.

Beginning with the dorsal radiocarpal incision the skin is sharply incised and dissection is carried through subcutaneous tissues with care taken to protect traversing branches of the superficial branch of the radial nerve (SBRN). Meticulous hemostasis should be maintained with bipolar electrocautery. The extensor pollicis longus (EPL) tendon is identified, and the enveloping retinaculum of the third dorsal compart-

ment is sharply incised in line with the tendon fibers. The retinacular release is extended proximally and distally, and the EPL tendon is subsequently transposed radially from the third dorsal compartment to prevent iatrogenic tendon entrapment during plate application. The extensor digitorum communis (EDC) and extensor indicis proprius (EIP) tendons are identified and carefully elevated extraperiosteally from the floor of the fourth compartment. The posterior interosseus nerve (PIN) is identified in the floor of the fourth dorsal compartment at this level, and care is taken to protect its terminal dorsal radiocarpal branches throughout the duration of the procedure. Alternatively, the treating surgeon may elect to perform a PIN neurectomy at this level prior to proceeding with spanning fixation. The fracture site is frequently identifiable in the deep layer of this incision. If identified, reduction of dorsal fracture fragments is frequently achievable via this exposure. If desired, implantation of bone graft is also possible via this incision following adequate fracture exposure and reduction.

Attention is next turned to the dorsum of the long finger metacarpal. Incision is carried through skin, and sharp dissection is carried through subcutaneous tissues over the dorsum of the proximal long finger metacarpal. Care is taken to protect any traversing branches of the SBRN. The long finger EDC tendon is identified traveling over the dorsum of the long finger metacarpal. The extensor retinaculum is sharply incised over the ulnar border of the long finger EDC tendon. Care is taken to preserve juncturae tendinum should one be encountered over the ulnar border of the long finger EDC tendon at this level. The long finger EDC tendon is carefully retracted radially to facilitate exposure of the dorsum of the long finger metacarpal.

Exposure of the radial diaphysis is accomplished via a 4-cm incision just proximal to the traversing muscle bellies of the APL and EPB. Incision is carried through skin, and sharp dissection is carried to the level of the second dorsal compartment. The lateral antebrachial cutaneous nerve (LABCN) can be encountered at this level traveling with the cephalic vein superficial to the palmar antebrachial fascia. If identified, the LABCN should be protected throughout the duration of the case. Traversing branches of the SBRN are identified and protected throughout the duration of the procedure. The SBRN can be identified in this incision exiting the interval between the brachioradialis and extensor carpi radial longus (ECRL) tendons. The interval between the ECRL and extensor carpi radialis brevis (ECRB) can be exploited to gain access to the radial diaphysis and minimize the risk of SBRN injury relative to utilizing the brachioradialis – ECRL interval for plating.

With exposure of the radial diaphysis proximally, fracture site centrally, and dorsal long finger metacarpal distally, attention is next turned to creation of a suitable corridor for plate passage. Beginning with the distal-most incision, a small key elevator (or similar sharp elevator) is used to create a potential space between the metacarpal and dorsal radio-carpal incision. The elevator is then advanced deep to the second, third, and fourth dorsal compartments into the floor of the proximal-most incision. Care is taken to avoid iatrogenic injury to either the extensor tendons or PIN (if preserved) during passage of the elevator.

The desired dorsal spanning bridge plate is then selected from the manufacturer's instrumentation set. The shortest plate which allows for a minimum of three bicortical screws to be placed proximal to the fracture site in the radial diaphysis and three bicortical screws to be placed distally in the metacarpal should be selected. The proximal portion of the plate is placed in the dorsal long finger incision and advanced in a distal-to-proximal fashion via the previously created soft tissue corridor until the proximal-most portion of the plate is visible in the proximal radial diaphysis incision. Care is taken to avoid entrapment of the dorsal extensor tendons and SBRN, and visual confirmation that the plate remains deep to the EDC, EIP, EPL, and SBRN should be performed through the dorsal radiocarpal incision. The plate can be provisionally fixed to the radial diaphysis using a small serrated bone holding forceps (Fig. 39.3).

With plate provisionally held with a small serrated bone holding forceps, a bicortical non-locking cortex screw is placed distally in the most central metacarpal hole which will allow for the addition of at least two subsequent meta-carpal screws. If a distal oblong hole is available in the selected plate, this should be utilized for placement of this preliminary distal bicortical non-locking cortex screw. With the plate in satisfactory position over the radius and metacar-pal, fracture reduction should be attempted. With the elbow in 90° of flexion, the forearm is maximally supinated, longi-tudinal traction is applied, and the previously applied ser-rated bone holding forceps is reapplied to provisionally hold the fracture reduction (Fig. 39.4). Orthogonal fluoroscopic views should be critically assessed to confirm satisfactory reduction has been achieved in both the coronal and sagittal planes prior to proceeding with plate fixation (Fig. 39.5a, b). Once fracture reduction is confirmed to be satisfactory, a bicortical non-locking cortex screw should be placed proxi-mally in the radial diaphysis via a central hole which will allow for the addition of at least two subsequent radial diaph-ysis screws. With provisional spanning fixation achieved, two additional metacarpal screws can be placed in the plate to achieve sufficient fixation. Two additional proximal

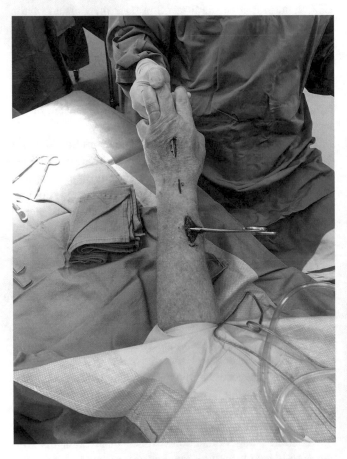

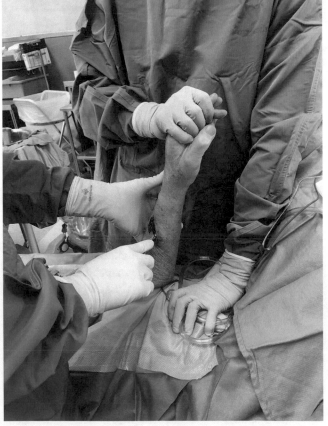

Fig. 39.3 Serrated bone holding forceps used to provisionally affix plate to radial diaphysis within wound over distal radial diaphysis

Fig. 39.4 Arm position for provisional fracture reduction −90° of elbow flexion, maximal forearm supination, longitudinal traction

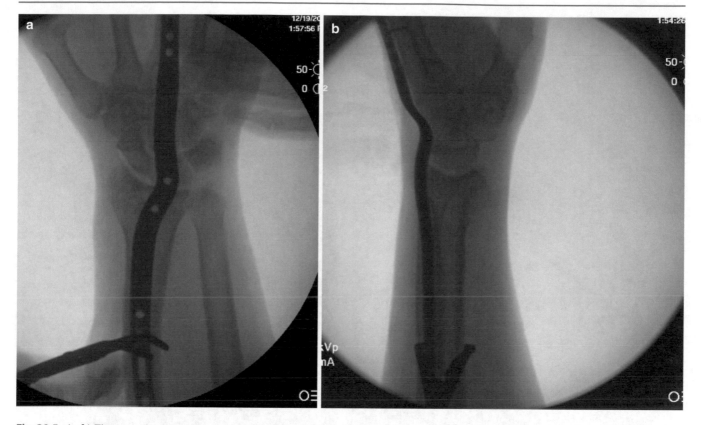

Fig. 39.5 (**a, b**) Fluoroscopic views of provisional fracture reduction with plate applied

screws in the radial diaphysis should then be placed to achieve sufficient proximal fixation.

Final fluoroscopic images should be obtained to confirm retention of satisfactory fracture reduction following the completion of instrumentation, as well as document final intraoperative implant positioning. The dorsal radiocarpal wound should be carefully inspected to ensure that no entrapment of the EDC, EIP, or EPL tendons is present (Fig. 39.6). The EPL tendon should remain transposed from its sheath, with care taken to ensure it is free of entrapment or obstruction over its entire course in the distal free. Branches of the SBRN encountered as part of the dissection should also be inspected to confirm no entrapment has occurred, and that the nerve branches do not lie directly over the plate following the completion of instrumentation. Wounds should be thoroughly irrigated with sterile irrigation fluid to remove any bone debris generated during hardware placement. Wounds should be closed either in layers or with skin closure only based on surgeon preference. Sterile soft dressings should be applied to the wounds. Postoperatively the patient should be immobilized in either a volar resting splint or removable volar forearm-based wrist orthosis based on surgeon preference.

Occupational therapy services should begin between postoperative days three and seven. Patients are generally allowed to weightbear as tolerated through their operative extremity immediately following their operation; however, this may be adjusted according to surgeon preference based on patient characteristics, fracture pattern, and fixation quality. Early emphasis on achievement of full, active composite digital flexion should be stressed to patients and their therapist. Patients are allowed to wean from their immobilization over the two weeks following their operation under the direction of their hand therapist. Clinical and radiographic follow-up should be conducted according to the surgeon's preference until fracture union is noted. Plate removal should be scheduled after clinical and radiographic fracture healing has been observed – generally no earlier than three months postoperatively. Following plate removal, patients may be placed into either a volar resting splint or forearm-based wrist orthosis and allowed to bear weight as tolerated. Patients are generally allowed to wean from immobilization over the two weeks following plate removal under the direction of their hand therapist.

Tips and Tricks

- The planned location and length of each incision may be estimated using fluoroscopic guidance by applying the plate directly over the radial diaphysis in line with the desired metacarpal to be used for fixation (index or long finger) (Fig. 39.7).

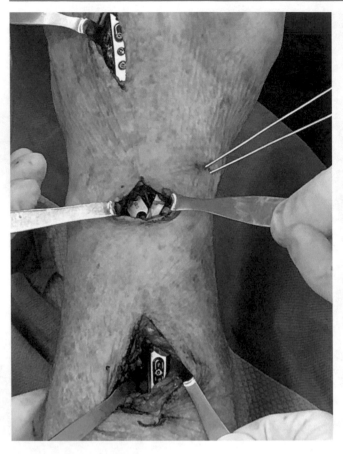

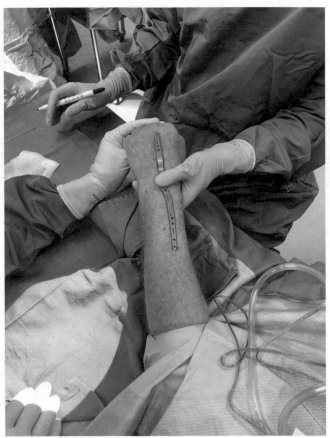

Fig. 39.6 Extensor pollicis longus (EPL) tendon visible within dorsal radiocarpal wound without evidence of tendon entrapment deep to the applied plate

Fig. 39.7 Desired dorsal spanning plate applied to the dorsal surface of the forearm and hand to estimate length and location of planned incisions

- As a result of the trauma required to produce the observed fracture, the enveloping retinaculum of the extensor pollicis longus tendon often contains a small volume of hematoma. This hematoma can often be observed from the middle incision and used to identify the underlying EPL tendon.
- Reduction of articular fragments can be performed through the dorsal radiocarpal incision using dental pick, freer, or similar elevator. Following reduction of these fracture fragments, the dorsal spanning plate is applied to provide a dorsal buttress to loss of fixation.
- Placement of an additional screw through the plate (when available based on plate manufacturer) in subchondral bone below lunate fossa provides buttress to articular reduction, which may aid in preventing collapse of this critical fragment.
- To reduce the risk of iatrogenic tendon entrapment during plate placement, a small key elevator (or similar periosteal elevator) can be inserted in an antegrade fashion deep to the digital and wrist extensors from the proximal-most incision, exiting in the distal metacarpal incision. The dorsal spanning plate is then introduced in a retrograde

fashion in direct contact with key elevator, using the unobstructed corridor created by the key elevator. The key elevator is removed from the proximal-most incision, at which time the plate will be safely placed deep to the structures at risk.
- After the completion of instrumentation, the digits should be carefully inspected to ensure normal tenodesis remains, and that full composite digital flexion can be achieved in order to confirm that the extrinsic extensor tendons have not been overlengthened. Extensor tendon overlengthening has been observed to portend unfavorable postoperative outcomes, including decreased strength, worse pain scores, and inferior functional outcomes in external fixation models which apply similar forces across the wrist to those applied in dorsal spanning plate fixation [15].
- Dorsal spanning plates may be applied as supplemental fixation to other fixation constructs. For example, in the setting of volar shear fracture patterns with extensive comminution, a volar locking plate may be utilized for fixation of the volar shear fracture with supplementary dorsal spanning plate fixation to achieve satisfactory overall length, rotation, and alignment of the remaining

fracture fragments. Once adequate fracture healing has been observed, the dorsal spanning plate can be removed, and wrist range of motion initiated with the volar locking plate still in place to reduce the risk of displacement of the volar shear fragment.

Conclusion

Dorsal spanning plate fixation provides a durable and versatile fixation construct for the treatment of distal radius fractures with metadiaphyseal fracture extension or extensive comminution unable to be adequately reconstructed using other fixation constructs. Additionally, the use of dorsal spanning plate fixation has been shown to provide favorable outcomes in elderly patients, and polytraumatized patients who require the use of their upper extremities for mobilization. Dorsal spanning plate fixation provides for an alternative treatment option for treating surgeons hoping to avoid the complications observed with wrist-spanning external fixators, while also affording the added benefit of increased resistance to axial compression. Spanning plates are now available from multiple manufacturers; however, the techniques described here are applicable to all plate designs. Treating surgeons should be familiar with the implant specifications for their plate of choice prior to its use.

References

1. Lichtman DM, Bindra RR, Boyer MI, Putnam MD, Ring D, Slutsky DJ, et al. Treatment of distal radius fractures. J Am Acad Orthop Surg. 2010;18(3):180–9.
2. Becton JL, Colborn GL, Goodrich JA. Use of an internal fixator device to treat comminuted fractures of the distal radius: report of a technique. Am J Orthop (Belle Mead NJ). 1998;27(9):619–23.
3. Burke EF, Singer RM. Treatment of comminuted distal radius with the use of an internal distraction plate. Tech Hand Up Extrem Surg. 1998;2(4):248–52.
4. Hanel DP, Lu TS, Weil WM. Bridge plating of distal radius fractures: the Harborview method. Clin Orthop Relat Res. 2006;445:91–9.
5. Ruch DS, Ginn TA, Yang CC, Smith BP, Rushing J, Hanel DP. Use of a distraction plate for distal radial fractures with metaphyseal and diaphyseal comminution. J Bone Joint Surg Am. 2005;87(5):945–54.
6. Lauder A, Agnew S, Bakri K, Allan CH, Hanel DP, Huang JI. Functional outcomes following bridge plate fixation for distal radius fractures. J Hand Surg Am. 2015;40(8):1554–62.
7. Brogan DM, Richard MJ, Ruch D, Kakar S. Management of Severely Comminuted Distal Radius Fractures. J Hand Surg Am. 2015;40(9):1905–14.
8. Chhabra A, Hale JE, Milbrandt TA, Carmines DV, Degnan GG. Biomechanical efficacy of an internal fixator for treatment of distal radius fractures. Clin Orthop Relat Res. 2001;393:318–25.
9. Wolf JC, Weil WM, Hanel DP, Trumble TE. A biomechanic comparison of an internal radiocarpal-spanning 2.4-mm locking plate and external fixation in a model of distal radius fractures. J Hand Surg Am. 2006;31(10):1578–86.
10. Hanel DP, Ruhlman SD, Katolik LI, Allan CH. Complications associated with distraction plate fixation of wrist fractures. Hand Clin. 2010;26(2):237–43.
11. Weber SC, Szabo RM. Severely comminuted distal radial fracture as an unsolved problem: complications associated with external fixation and pins and plaster techniques. J Hand Surg Am. 1986;11(2):157–65.
12. Huang JI, Peterson B, Bellevue K, Lee N, Smith S, Herfat S. Biomechanical assessment of the dorsal spanning bridge plate in distal radius fracture fixation: implications for immediate weight-bearing. Hand (N Y). 2018;13(3):336–40.
13. Richard MJ, Katolik LI, Hanel DP, Wartinbee DA, Ruch DS. Distraction plating for the treatment of highly comminuted distal radius fractures in elderly patients. J Hand Surg Am. 2012;37(5):948–56.
14. Mithani SK, Srinivasan RC, Kamal R, Richard MJ, Leversedge FJ, Ruch DS. Salvage of distal radius nonunion with a dorsal spanning distraction plate. J Hand Surg Am. 2014;39(5):981–4.
15. Kaempffe FA. External fixation for distal radius fractures: adverse effects of excess distraction. Am J Orthop (Belle Mead NJ). 1996;25(3):205–9.

Management of Distal Radius Malunions

Hermann Krimmer

Introduction

A distal radius fracture that has healed in malalignment is still a challenging complication as it leads to incongruency at the wrist joint. If the malalignment is not corrected, there is an increased risk for a painful wrist with secondary degenerative changes. The resulting discomfort ranges from pain, motion restriction, and loss of strength in the region of the wrist to a difference in external appearance. Since the consequences are sufficiently well known nowadays, the current trend is toward performing corrective surgery as early as possible. The aim of this is to reduce pain and prevent early arthrotic changes. In case of posttraumatic growth arrest with larger discrepancy of the radius and the ulna, a two-staged procedure is preferable.

Indications

The improvement in preoperative diagnosis by performing preoperative computed tomography (CT) as standard for intra-articular and complex distal radius fractures, with 3D reconstruction where necessary, has led to a better understanding of the fracture morphology. In addition, further development of osteosynthesis material with numerous fixed-angle special plates to fit the particular fracture morphology helps to enhance fixation of the fracture followed by better postoperative outcome. Nevertheless, malunion still occurs caused by insufficient primary osteosynthesis or by secondary dislocation. To reduce these problems, we regard especially for intra-articular fractures not only preoperative CT scan but also postoperative control by CT scan as a standard.

In the case of postoperative malalignment, the strategy used in the past was based on waiting for complete osseous consolidation before corrective osteotomy. Reason for that was caused by lack of stability with increased risk for dislocation. Nowadays there is no need to wait for complete healing as the fixed angle devices provide sufficient stability till bony healing is present [1]. Morbidity of the patient is shortened as it is known that a correction of alignment as early as possible leads to a rapid improvement in discomfort, while consequential damage in the form of posttraumatic arthrosis or the development of a complex regional pain syndrome (CRPS) can be avoided [2]. An existing CRPS sustained by malalignment usually improves after correction.

Malalignment following extra-articular fractures usually involves dorsopalmar and radioulnar inclination frequently in combination with radial shortening [3]. Coexisting incongruency in the region of the distal radioulnar joint (DRUJ) and an ulnar impaction syndrome resulting from radial shortening often cause ulnocarpal pain. Simple ulnar shortening is only indicated if the angulation of the articular surface of the radius is mainly preserved. In special situations due to the shape of the DRUJ, radial lengthening might be preferable. All other situations need correction osteotomy restoring shape and length of the distal radius.

For intra-articular malalignment, the indication always depends on the development of offset in the region of the articular surface. This is best assessed by CT scan and arthroscopy. However, the radiological image and arthroscopic appearance does not always have to correlate with the clinical picture. In relatively young patients, the focus is primarily on preventive effects such as the avoidance of posttraumatic arthrosis, whereas in elderly patients, on the other hand, the focus is on the discomfort. If these patients are largely pain-free, the indication for corrective osteotomy should be determined with caution. Secondary dislocation due to special fracture patterns like troublesome lunate facet should always be corrected as early as possible independent of the clinical symptoms, because severe degenerative changes with the need for salvage procedures like radiocarpal fusion rapidly occur and exclude reconstruction.

H. Krimmer (✉)
Handcenter Ravensburg, Ravensburg, Germany
e-mail: krimmer@handsurgeon.de

© Springer Nature Switzerland AG 2022
W. B. Geissler (ed.), *Wrist and Elbow Arthroscopy with Selected Open Procedures*,
https://doi.org/10.1007/978-3-030-78881-0_40

If CRPS is present following distal radius fracture malalignment, carpal tunnel syndrome must be ruled out radiologically because it can cause and sustain the clinical picture. If corresponding clinically relevant malalignment has been ascertained, after osteosynthetic management or after conservative treatment, corrective surgery should be performed as early as possible (Fig. 40.1a,b).

In posttraumatic growth disorders of the radius, considerable length deficits often occur as a result of early closure of the epiphyseal plate (Fig. 40.2a,b). Due to the soft tissue situation in such cases, it is not advisable to perform a one-stage procedure. A two-stage procedure with distraction osteotomy is preferable. When length compensation has been achieved, a change of method with internal fixed angle plate osteosynthesis is performed. This ensures good adaptation of soft tissue and avoids excessive bone grafts.

Contraindications

Furthermore, prior to performing the corrective osteotomy, it is necessary to radiologically rule out any severe arthrosis in the region of the radiocarpal articular space and in the region of the DRUJ because advanced arthrosis can represent a contraindication for corrective osteotomy. Severe degenerative changes limit reconstruction and need salvage procedures like denervation, partial wrist fusion, or prosthetic replacement. We regard slight arthritic changes not as real contraindications, but finally it's an individual decision which is additionally influenced by the preserved function. If severe restriction of hand function is present before corrective osteotomy, intensive physiotherapy is necessary.

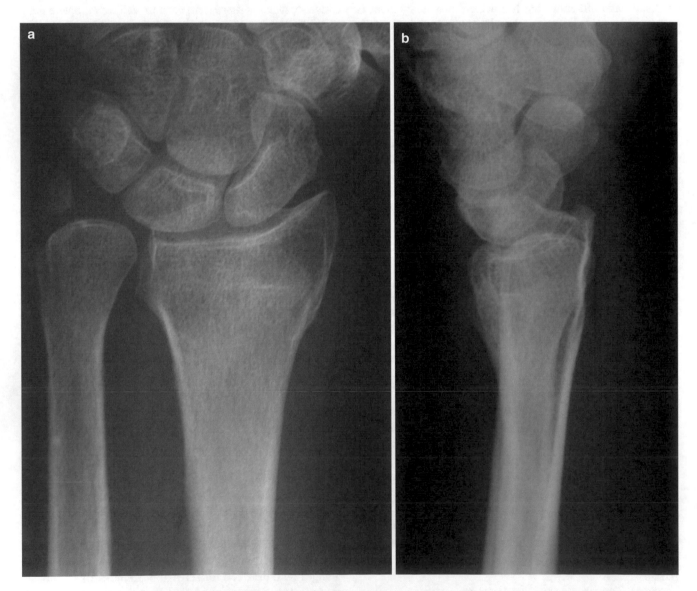

Fig. 40.1 X-ray of a wrist with a distal radius fracture that has healed in malalignment with a dorsal tilt of 30° and an ulna plus situation of 2 mm. (**a**) PA radiograph. (**b**) Lateral radiograph

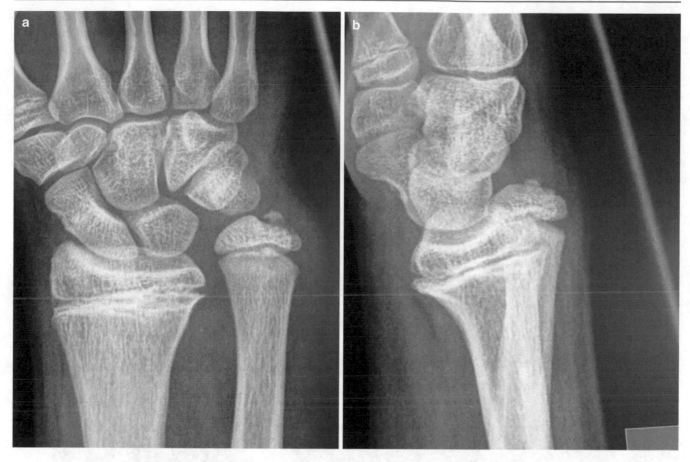

Fig. 40.2 X-ray of a 14-year-old female patient wrist ulna plus of 2 cm and increased palmar tilt of the radius to 30°. (**a**) PA radiograph. (**b**) Lateral radiograph

Diagnosis

Clinical examination with documentation of the range of motion and grip strength measurement using a dynamometer to compare sides are mandatory as well as the assessment of pain and wrist score. Prior to planning and performing corrective osteotomy, there must be not only x-ray images in PA and lateral projections available but also a current CT scan.

If there is any suspicion of additional congenital malalignment, x-ray images must be made of the opposite wrist [4].

Technique

Extra-articular Malalignment with Alteration of Shape and Length

In the past, corrective osteotomy for the more common dorsal malalignment used to be performed via a dorsal approach; for the rare palmar malalignment, it used to be performed using a palmar approach. However, through the dorsal approach it is difficult to conduct an exact adjustment of ana-

tomical positions. For that reason, the team led by Lanz preferred long before the locking plates were available the palmar approach with distal premounting of the correction plate [5, 6]. When fixed angle implants with two row distal support had been developed, this procedure became standard [7].

In Lanz's procedure, the palmar approach is extended distally in a Y shape to enhance the overview. If no significant shortening exists, the approach is performed, as for distal radius fracture, between the flexor carpi radialis (FCR) tendon and the radial artery. In the event of radial malalignment with distinct shortening, on the other hand, the approach is radial to the radial artery in order to be able to subperiosteally detach the first extensor tendon sheath and avoid obstruction of the correction by soft tissue. The third extensor tendon sheath is always opened in order to avoid secondary rupture of the extensor pollicis longus (EPL) tendon due to sharp osteotomy edges or hematoma formation (Fig. 40.3).

Following exposure of the palmar distal radial surface, the correction plate is premounted distally with four screws. The first screw to be introduced is a cortical screw, and with the other fixed angle screws, the screw head is not inserted completely. With regard to the dorsal tilt, the distal screws have to be predrilled toward proximal in order to avoid an intra-articular screw position. The distal part of the correction plate runs parallel to the articular surface of the radius. Since in the case of severe malalignment, the watershed line can often no longer be identified, plate position may have to be checked with an image intensifier. If there is loss of incli-

nation in the PA plane, the premounted plate must protrude proximally toward ulnar (Fig. 40.4a, b). To correct the dorsal tilt the plate protrudes proximally from the radial shaft after premounting. The angle between the plate and the radial shaft represents the desired correction angle. To fix the correction angle precisely the Medartis company (Medartis AG, Basel, Switzerland) offers a special instrumentation that is positioned in the plate shaft and ensures accurate angular adjustment (Fig. 40.5).

The premounted plate is removed again. Under fluoroscopic control, the osteotomy plane is now established. It can be marked with a K-wire. It usually corresponds to the former fracture plane. It is absolutely essential to make sure that the osteotomy is performed just proximal to the DRUJ, in order to avoid damaging the articular surfaces of the DRUJ During the osteotomy, the extensor tendons are protected with a Hohmann bone lever that is introduced subperiosteally. To avoid thermal necroses, a fresh saw blade should always be used. When the osteotomy has been performed, the plate is mounted in the occupied holes again and then the plate is reduced against the radial shaft proximally and centrally, resulting in accurate restoration of the articular surface angles. In the shaft region the plate can be fixed temporarily

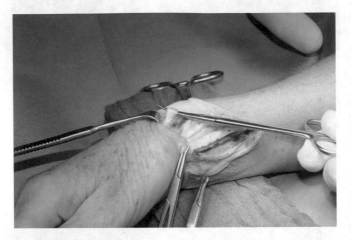

Fig. 40.3 Intraoperative opening of the third extensor tendon sheath

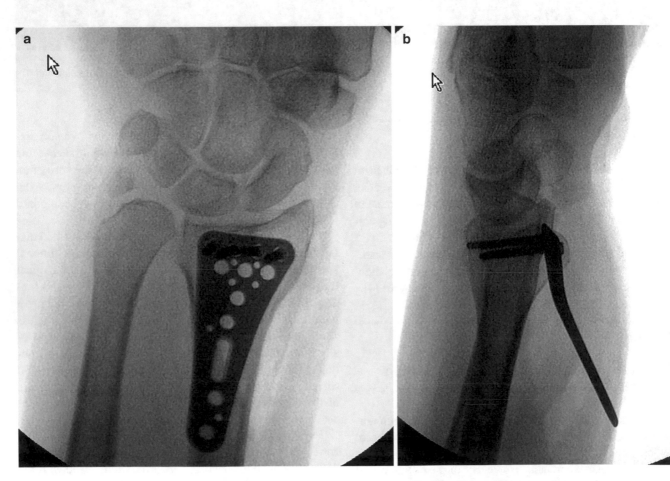

Fig. 40.4 Intraoperative plate fixation protruding at the desired correction angles. (**a**) PA view. (**b**) Lateral view

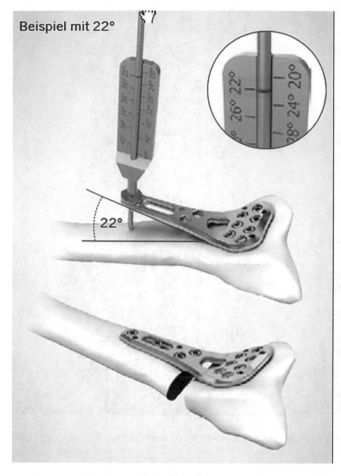

Beispiel mit 22°

22°

Fig. 40.5 Instrumentation for setting the desired correction angle. (Courtesy of Medartis AG, Basel, Switzerland)

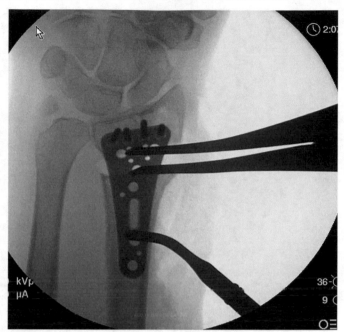

Fig. 40.6 Length compensation with nonunion retractor

using blunt reduction forceps. The correction position is now checked with fluoroscopy. Care must also be taken to ensure correct length compensation in the neutral position or a slight minus position (−1 mm) of the ulna. Introduction of a nonunion retractor to the osteotomy gap facilitates length compensation, especially in the case of relatively long distances (Fig. 40.6). Then the plate holes are filled in the shaft region (Fig. 40.7a, b).

In relatively rare cases of malalignment with increased palmar tilt of the articular surface of the radius where usually only slight radial shortening is present (Fig. 40.8a, b), it is possible in the osteotomy to leave the dorsal cortical bone alone. By palmar folding open of the osteotomy using an "open book technique," inclination and length of the radius is corrected (Fig. 40.8c, d).

Since correction nowadays is performed using a fixed-angle plate with two-row distal support as standard, an osteotomy gap of 6–8 mm can be left without any interposition of iliac crest cancellous bone, provided the bone quality is good [8]. In the case of major defects, a cancellous or corticocancellous iliac crest graft should be interposed, being held in place with a plate screw. Alternatively, bone substitute or allogenic femoral head bone can be interposed. The disadvantage of these materials is characterized by a prolonged healing time.

Extra-articular Malalignment with Simple Radial Shortening

In the case of anatomical alignment of the distal radius with correct inclination of the articular surfaces, an ulnar shortening osteotomy is a good alternative to solve the ulnar impaction, because it can be performed under control and reliably using the now standard fixed-angle ulnar shortening plates [9]. However, if special configuration of the sigmoid notch is present (Tolat type III) where there might be a risk for impingement after ulnar shortening, we prefer correction of the radius by lengthening [10, 11] (Fig. 40.9a, b).

Postoperative Regime

Following 4-week immobilization of the wrist in a thermoplastic splint, an x-ray checkup is performed and approval is given for functional follow-up treatment where applicable.

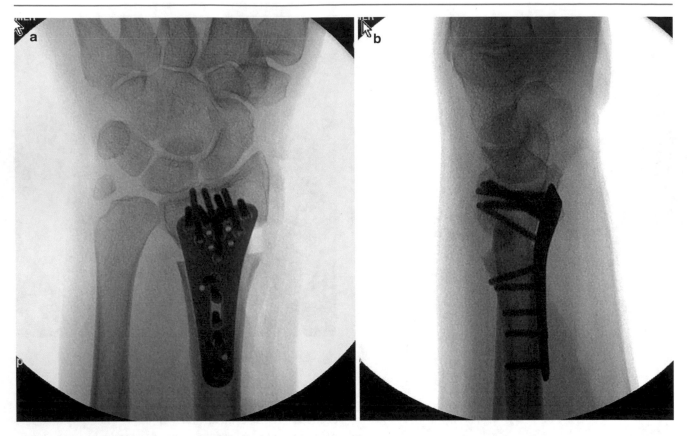

Fig. 40.7 Correction with restoration of the articular angles at the radius and length compensation of ulna −1 mm. (**a**) PA view. (**b**) Lateral view

Fig. 40.8 (**a**) PA view ulna plus 1 mm. (**b**) Lateral view with increased palmar tilt up to 40°. (**c**) PA view correction with ulna minus 1 mm. (**d**) Lateral view restoration of palmar tilt by 10°

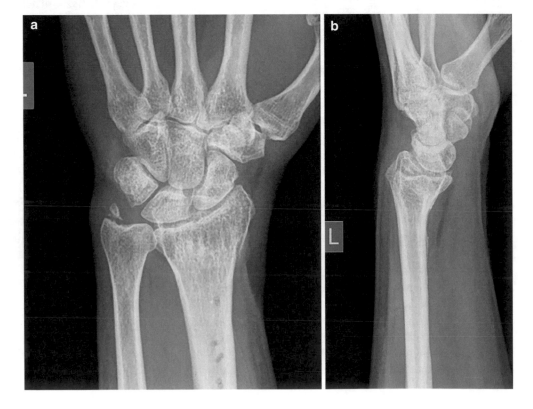

Fig. 40.8   (continued)

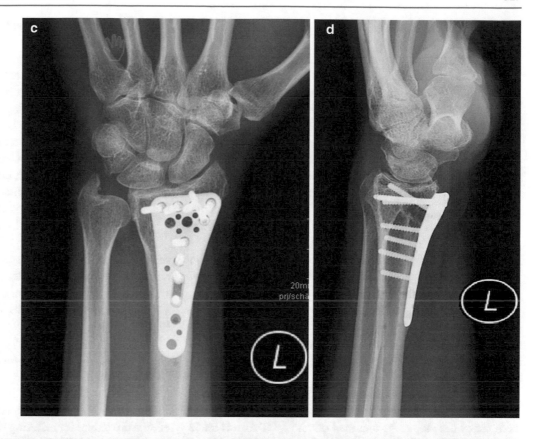

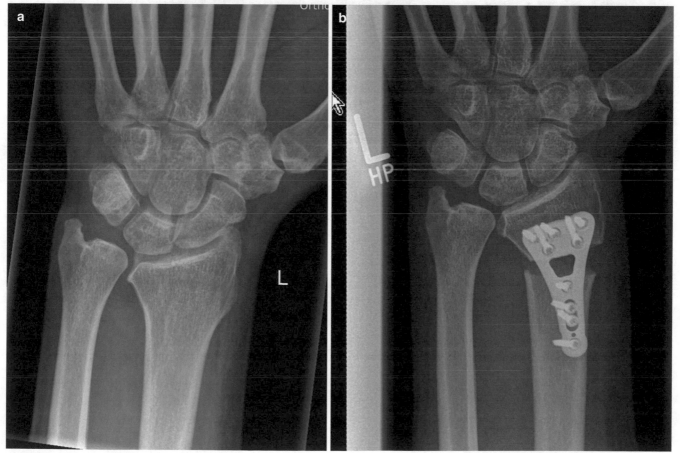

Fig. 40.9   (**a**) Ulna impaction by 3 mm ulna plus oblique shape of the sigmoid notch. (**b**) Radius lengthening up to neutral resulting in congruent DRUJ

Intra-articular Malalignment

If intra-articular malalignment requires a direct view of the articular surface, it can be achieved by performing correction from dorsal. As with dorsal fracture management, the approach is via the third extensor tendon sheath and subperiosteal exposure of the dorsal radius with a direct view of the articular surface. The osteotomy is performed in the former fracture plane under vision using a thin, sharp chisel. If the line of the osteotomy is curved, predrilling with K-wires along is helpful to break the bone in the right plane. Alternatively, it is possible to perform an arthroscopy-assisted correction [12]. When the osteotomy has been performed, K-wires can be introduced like a joystick to facilitate adjustment of the correction position. The correction outcome can then also be temporarily fixed in place with K-wires. Osteosynthesis is performed using screws or plates, depending on the fracture situation (Fig. 40.10a–d).

Preoperative 3D Planning

Preoperative 3D planning of correction osteotomy is a relatively recent development over the last few years. A CT scan is made of the side to be operated on and a CT scan is made of the opposite side for reference purposes. The malalignment is now analyzed under computer control by mirroring the injured side to the opposite healthy side. The required templates are made using a 3D printer [13]. Usually, standard plates can be chosen for fixation; in some cases, where bended and curved plate design is necessary, the required correction plates can also be custom made by 3D printer. The method is to be recommended, especially in the case of complex and intra-articular malalignments [14]. The benefit is reliable predictability of postoperative outcome.

Growth Disorders in the Region of the Radius

In the case of posttraumatic growth disorders due to premature complete or partial closure of the epiphyseal plate, often substantial longitudinal defects arise that cannot be surgically compensated in a one-stage procedure [15, 16]. In such cases, a two-stage procedure is indicated. In the first operation, a distraction fixator is mounted. Here it is crucial to mount an additional Schanz screw with a connecting rod at right angles to the distraction plane in order to prevent palmar tilting of the distal radius portion during distraction (Fig. 40.11a–c). Osteotomy is then performed proximal to the distal Schanz screws and proximal to the DRUJ. After 1 week, distraction commences with approximately 0.5 mm per day. The distraction phase can take weeks or even several months before the desired length compensation has been achieved. In a second operation, the defect zone is then bridged by plate osteosynthesis and the fixator is dismounted (Fig. 40.11d, e).

Conclusion

Correction osteotomy using a palmar approach represents a reliable procedure for restoring the articular surface and congruency of the DRUJ. The need for additional bone graft is only necessary in case of larger gaps or severe osteoporosis. Intra-articular correction is preferably performed through a dorsal approach with direct view to the articular surface or additionally assisted by arthroscopy or even 3D planning. Malunion due to growth arrest with larger length discrepancy should be preferably corrected with a two-stage procedure with the advantage of healing without bone graft and slow adaption of ligaments and soft tissue. For complex intra-articular correction, 3D planning offers a perfect solution.

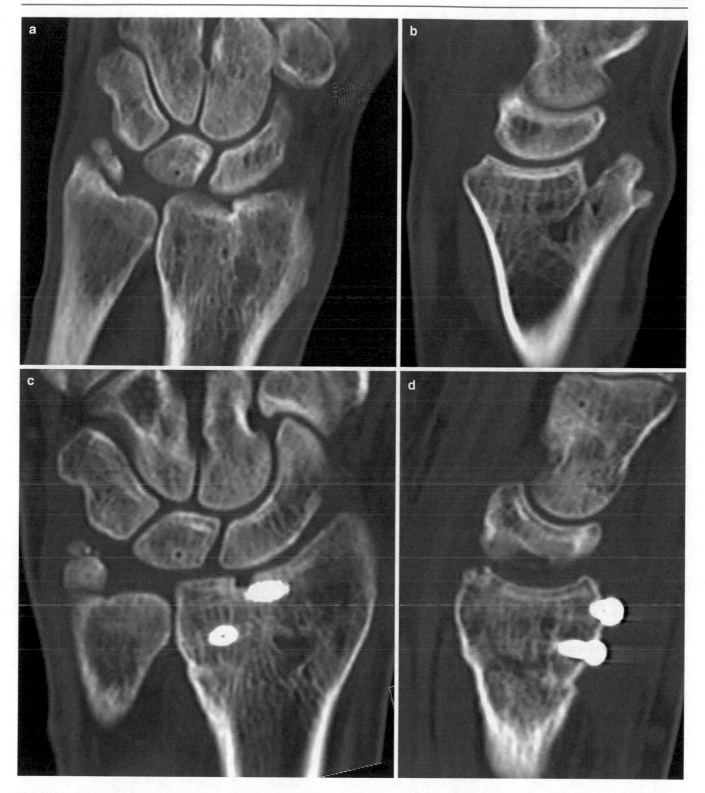

Fig. 40.10 Correction of intra-articular offset formation following distal radius fracture. (**a**) Preoperative coronal CT scan of the wrist. (**b**) Preoperative sagittal CT scan of the wrist. (**c**) Postoperative coronal and sagittal CT scan of the wrist following correction from dorsal with screw osteosynthesis. (**d**) Postoperative sagittal CT scan of the wrist following correction from dorsal with screw osteosynthesis

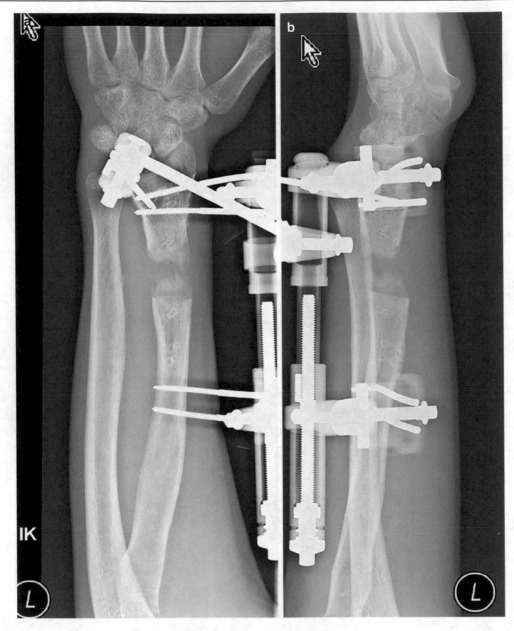

Fig. 40.11 Correction of substantial radial shortening (for preoperative, see Fig. 40.2). (**a**, **b**) PA and lateral view distraction fixator in situ. (**c**) Take note of mounting with additional transverse rod. (**d**, **e**) Procedural switch to palmar plate osteosynthesis following length compensation

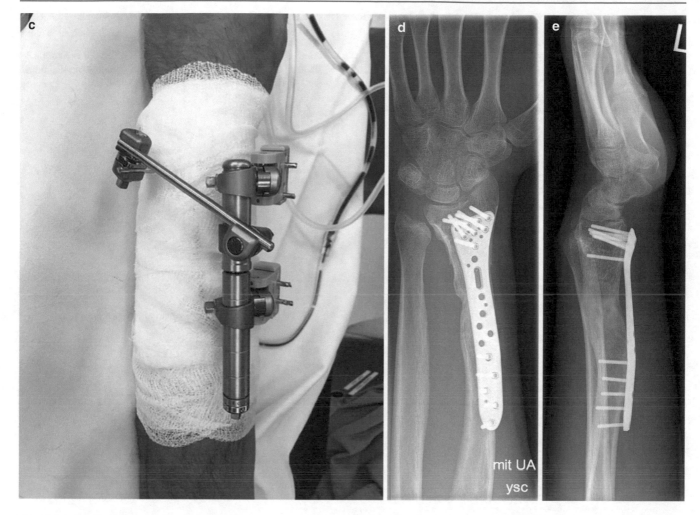

Fig. 40.11 (continued)

References

1. Krimmer H, Schandl R, Wolters R. Corrective osteotomy after malunited distal radius fractures. Arch Orthop Trauma Surg. 2020;140(5):675–80.
2. Haase SC, Chung KC. Management of malunions of the distal radius. Hand Clin. 2012;28(2):207–16.
3. Konul E, Krimmer H. Open wedge corrective osteotomy of malunited distal radius fractures through a palmar approach. A retrospective analysis. Unfallchirurg. 2012;115(7):623–8.
4. Krimmer H, Unglaub F, Langer MF, Spies CK. The distal radial decompression osteotomy for ulnar impingement syndrome. Arch Orthop Trauma Surg. 2016;136(1):143–8.
5. Prommersberger KJ, Van Schoonhoven J, Lanz UB. A radiovolar approach to dorsal malunions of the distal radius. Tech Hand Up Extrem Surg. 2000;4(4):236–43.
6. Prommersberger KJ, Van Schoonhoven J, Lanz UB. Outcome after corrective osteotomy for malunited fractures of the distal end of the radius. J Hand Surg. 2002;27(1):55–60.
7. Tarallo L, Mugnai R, Adani R, Catani F. Malunited extra-articular distal radius fractures: corrective osteotomies using volar locking plate. J Orthop Traumatol. 2014;15(4):285–90.
8. Mugnai R, Tarallo L, Lancellotti E, Zambianchi F, Di Giovine E, Catani F, et al. Corrective osteotomies of the radius: grafting or not? World J Orthop. 2016;7(2):128–35.
9. Terzis A, Koehler S, Sebald J, Sauerbier M. Ulnar shortening osteotomy as a treatment of symptomatic ulnar impaction syndrome after malunited distal radius fractures. Arch Orthop Trauma Surg. 2020;140(5):681–95.
10. Tolat AR, Stanley JK, Trail IA. A cadaveric study of the anatomy and stability of the distal radioulnar joint in the coronal and transverse planes. J Hand Surg Br. 1996;21(5):587–94.
11. Gilbert F, Jakubietz RG, Meffert RH, Jakubietz MG. Does distal radio-ulnar joint configuration affect postoperative functional results after ulnar shortening osteotomy? Plast Reconstr Surg Glob Open. 2018;6(4):e1760.
12. Del Pinal F, Clune J. Arthroscopic management of intra-articular malunion in fractures of the distal radius. Hand Clin. 2017;33(4):669–75.

13. Honigmann P, Thieringer F, Steiger R, Haefeli M, Schumacher R, Henning J. A simple 3-dimensional printed aid for a corrective palmar opening wedge osteotomy of the distal radius. J Hand Surg. 2016;41(3):464–9.

14. Shintani K, Kazuki K, Yoneda M, Uemura T, Okada M, Takamatsu K, et al. Computer-assisted three-dimensional corrective osteotomy for Malunited fractures of the distal radius using prefabricated bone graft substitute. J Hand Surg Asian Pac. 2018;23(4):479–86.

15. Gauger EM, Casnovsky LL, Gauger EJ, Bohn DC, Van Heest AE. Acquired upper extremity growth arrest. Orthopedics. 2017;40(1):e95–e103.

16. Gundes H, Buluc L, Sahin M, Alici T. Deformity correction by Ilizarov distraction osteogenesis after distal radius physeal arrest. Acta Orthop Traumatol Turc. 2011;45(6):406–11.

William B. Geissler

Introduction

The scaphoid carpal bone is the most frequently fractured bone in the carpus and accounts for nearly 70% of all carpal fractures [1]. This fracture typically occurs in young men between the ages of 15 and 30 years, and is also a common athletic injury occurring most often in contact sports [2]. It has been estimated that one in 100 college football players will sustain a fracture of the scaphoid in their career [3]. Frequently, a competitive athlete does not report his initial injury and continues to compete and eventually presents to the treating physician after the season is over with a scaphoid nonunion.

Acute nondisplaced fractures of the scaphoid have traditionally been managed with cast immobilization [4, 5]. Nondisplaced scaphoid fractures may heal in 8–12 weeks when immobilized in a short- or long-arm cast [4–6]. While cast immobilization is successful in up to 85–90% of cases, there may be significant cost to the patient with prolonged immobilization [4–6]. Prolonged immobilization may lead to muscle atrophy, joint contracture, disuse osteopenia, and financial hardship. An athlete may not be able to tolerate a lengthy course of immobilization and potentially could lose his scholarship or a worker could lose his employment.

It has been shown that the duration of cast immobilization varies dramatically according to the site of the fracture. A fracture of the scaphoid tubercle may heal within a period of 6 weeks, while a fracture of the waist of the scaphoid may require 3 months or longer. Fractures of the proximal pole may take 6 months or longer to heal with a cast because of the vascularity of the scaphoid [7]. It is frequently difficult to truly identify when a fracture of the scaphoid will heal with nonoperative management by plain radiograph alone. Frequently, a computed tomography (CT) scan may be required to thoroughly evaluate when a scaphoid is healed and treated nonoperatively.

Displaced scaphoids have a reported nonunion rate of up to 50% [2]. Factors that decrease the prognosis for healing include the amount of displacement, associated carpal instability, and delayed presentation (greater than 4–6 weeks) [1]. Traditionally, acute displaced fractures of the scaphoid, proximal pole fractures, and scaphoid nonunions are managed by open reduction and internal fixation [1, 2, 8–16]. Complications associated with open reduction and internal fixation include avascular necrosis, carpal instability, donor site pain, screw protrusion, infection, and complex regional pain syndrome [4, 17]. In one series, the biggest complication was hypertrophic scarring [2]. Multiple jigs have been designed to assist in open reduction; however, they are frequently difficult to apply and may necessitate further surgical dissection [18].

Wrist arthroscopy has revolutionized the practice of orthopedics allowing the surgeon to examine intra-articular abnormalities of the wrist under magnified and bright light conditions [19]. Whipple was one of the first surgeons to attempt arthroscopic management of scaphoid fractures [19]. His preliminary work set the stage for arthroscopic management of this common carpal fracture by many arthroscopic surgeons.

Arthroscopic stabilization provides direct visualization of the fracture reduction, particularly rotation, and the precise site for screw insertion with limited surgical dissection. This may allow for greater range of motion and early return to competition or employment. Fractures of the scaphoid are best visualized with the arthroscope in the midcarpal space. Fractures of the proximal pole are best seen with the arthroscope in the ulnar midcarpal portal, while fractures of the

Supplementary Information The online version of this chapter (https://doi.org/10.1007/978-3-030-78881-0_41) contains supplementary material, which is available to authorized users.

W. B. Geissler (✉)
Division of Hand and Upper Extremity Surgery, Section of Arthroscopic Surgery and Sports Medicine, Department of Orthopedic Surgery and Rehabilitation, University of Mississippi Medical Center, Jackson, MS, USA

waist are best visualized with the arthroscope in the radial midcarpal portal. Associated soft tissue injuries may occur with a fracture of the scaphoid and can be arthroscopically detected and managed at the same sitting.

The indications and techniques of arthroscopic management of acute scaphoid fractures and selected nonunions are described in this chapter.

Diagnostic Imaging

Posterior/anterior and lateral radiographs are mandatory to assess the amount of displacement, angulation, and alignment of a scaphoid fracture. Semisupinated and pronated views can provide additional information particularly on fractures of the proximal and distal poles of the scaphoid. It is helpful to place the wrist in ulnar deviation, thereby extending the scaphoid in a posterior/anterior view for detection of fracture displacement. A nondisplaced fracture of the scaphoid may not become apparent on radiographs for several weeks postinjury. It is important to immobilize the patient who presents with snuffbox tenderness to allow the pain to resolve or until a diagnosis has been confirmed radiographically.

Computer tomography (CT) parallel to the longitudinal axis of the scaphoid is useful to evaluate angulation, displacement, and healing. In this technique, the patient is placed prone with the arm extended overhead and the wrist radial deviated to obtain longitudinal access to the scaphoid. Coronal CT slices are obtained with supination of the forearm to a neutral position. CT evaluation which is particularly helpful to determine scaphoid healing with nonoperative management of the scaphoid fracture is chosen. It is particularly important to return a contact athlete back to sports. One advantage of operative fixation is that the screw acts as an internal splint to stabilize the fracture and the exact time to return to competition is less critical compared with nonoperative management.

Treatment

Indications

Arthroscopic fixation may be performed for acute nondisplaced fracture of the scaphoid and for acute displaced fractures which are reducible. It is important in patients who have an acute nondisplaced fracture that the risks and benefits of arthroscopic stabilization compared with cast immobilization be discussed with the patient, so that an informed decision can be made by the patient and associated family members. For acute scaphoid fractures that are reducible, the

Table 41.1 Slade–Geissler classification of scaphoid nonunions

Type	Description
I	Delayed presentation at 4–12 weeks
II	Fibrous union, minimal fracture line
III	Minimal sclerosis <1 mm
IV	Cystic formation, 1–5 mm
V	Humpback deformity with >5-mm cystic change
VI	Wrist arthrosis

fracture may reduce by a number of techniques including manipulation of the wrist in a traction tower or joysticks inserted into the proximal and distal poles of the scaphoid. The reduction is best viewed with the arthroscope in the midcarpal space.

In addition, arthroscopic visualization of selected scaphoid nonunions may be performed. Slade and Geissler published their radiographic classifications for scaphoid nonunions (Table 41.1) [20]. Type I fractures are the result of a delayed presentation (4–12 weeks) after injury. Delayed presentation has been shown with a high incidence of nonunion. In Type II injuries, a fibrous union is present. A minimal fracture line may be seen on radiographs. It is important to note that the lunate is not rotated and there is no humpback deformity. In Type III injuries, minimal sclerosis is seen at the fracture site. The sclerosis is less than 1 mm in width, and again the lunate is not rotated and no humpback deformity is seen. In Type IV injuries, cystic formation is present at the nonunion site. The cystic formation may be between 1 and 5 mm in width. No humpback deformity or rotation of the lunate is seen on plain radiographs. In Type V injuries, the cystic changes are greater than 5 mm in width, and rotation of the lunate has occurred resulting in humpback deformity. The lunate has rotated to a position of dorsal intercalated segmental instability (DISI). In Type VI injuries, secondary degenerative changes have occurred with peaking of the radial styloid with spurring along the radial border of the scaphoid.

Arthroscopic stabilization of selected scaphoid nonunions is indicated in types I–IV. After a humpback deformity has occurred, arthroscopic stabilization is not recommended and open reduction and internal fixation is required to correct the humpback deformity and DISI rotation of the lunate.

Arthroscopic Techniques

Various arthroscopic-assisted and percutaneous techniques for fractures of the scaphoid have been described in the literature [21–32]. Haddad and Goddard popularized the volar approach and the dorsal approach was popularized by Slade and colleagues [24, 26]. Geissler described his arthroscopic technique for viewing exact placement of the guide wire for eventual screw fixation [32].

Volar Percutaneous Approach

Haddad and Goddard popularized the volar percutaneous technique [24]. They recommended placing the patient supine with the thumb suspended in the Chinese finger trap. Placing the thumb under suspension allows ulnar deviation improving access to the distal pole of the scaphoid. A longitudinal 0.5-cm skin incision is made under fluoroscopic guidance over the most distal radial aspect of the scaphoid. Blunt dissection is carried down to expose the distal pole of the scaphoid. It is important to protect the cutaneous nerves as one dissects down to the distal pole of the scaphoid.

A percutaneous guide wire is then introduced into the scaphoid trapezial joint and advanced proximally and dorsally across the fracture site. The guide wire is inserted through a needle which is impaled onto the distal pole of the scaphoid. Using the needle helps to control the angulation of the guide wire. In addition, the bevel of the needle can help further direct the direction of the guide wire. The advantage of their technique by suspending the thumb in traction allows an almost 360° view of the position of the guide wire within the scaphoid. The length of the guide wire within the scaphoid is determined by placing a second guide wire next to the initial one and measuring the difference between the two. It is important when using a headless cannulated screw to use a screw 2–4 mm shorter than what is measured in the volar approach. A drill is inserted through a soft tissue protector and the scaphoid is reamed. A headless cannulated screw is placed over the guide wire. Occasionally, a second guide wire may be helpful to prevent rotation of the fracture fragments while the screw is being inserted.

Haddad and Goddard reported their initial results in a pilot study of 15 patients with acute scaphoid fractures [24]. Union was achieved in all patients in an average of 57 days (range 38–71 days). They found that the range of motion at the union was equal to that of the contralateral limb with their percutaneous technique and grip strength averaged 90% at 3 months. The patients were able to return to sedentary work within 4 days and to manual work within 5 weeks.

The advantage of their technique is that it is fairly simple and straightforward and requires minimal specialized equipment. The disadvantage of the volar approach is that the screw may be placed slightly oblique to the midwaist fracture line in the scaphoid. The scaphoid is shaped like a cone, with the widest part being distally and the smallest more proximally. It is harder to place the cannulated screw in the exact center of the scaphoid with starting at the wider distal pole of the scaphoid compared to the more narrow proximal pole.

Dorsal Percutaneous Approach

Joseph Slade was as a pioneer in the management of fractures of the scaphoid. He and his coworkers popularized the dorsal percutaneous approach [26, 27]. This technique became very popular because it involved limited surgical dissection and allowed arthroscopic evaluation and reduction of the scaphoid fracture. In his technique, the patient is placed in a supine position on the table with the arm extended. Several towels are placed under the elbow and support the forearm parallel to the floor. The wrist is then flexed and pronated under fluoroscopy, until the proximal and distal poles of the scaphoid are aligned to perform a perfect cylinder. Continuous fluoroscopy is recommended, as the wrist is flexed to obtain the true ring sign as the proximal and distal poles are aligned.

Under fluoroscopy, a 14-gauge needle is placed percutaneously in the center of the ring sign and parallel to the beam of the fluoroscopic unit. A guide wire is then inserted through the 14-gauge needle and driven across the central axis of the scaphoid from dorsal to volar, until the guide wire comes into contact with the distal scaphoid cortex. Position of the guide wire is then evaluated under fluoroscopy in the lateral, posterior/anterior, and oblique planes while the wrist is maintaining flexion. It is important not to extend the wrist at this time, as this may bend the guide wire. A second guide wire is then placed parallel to the first, so that it touches the proximal pole of the scaphoid to determine the screw length. The difference in length between the two guide wires is measured. It is of vital importance that a screw at least 4 mm shorter is chosen when utilizing Slade's dorsal technique.

Once the screw length is determined, the primary guide wire is advanced volarly through a portion of the trapezium to exit the skin on the volar aspect of the hand. The wire is continued to be advanced volarly, until it is flush with the proximal pole of the scaphoid dorsally so the wrist may now be extended.

The wrist is suspended in a traction tower and the radiocarpal and midcarpal spaces may be evaluated arthroscopically. The radiocarpal space is evaluated for any associated soft tissue injuries, and then the arthroscope is placed in the midcarpal space to evaluate the reduction of the scaphoid fracture. If the reduction of the scaphoid fracture is not determined to be satisfactory, the guide wire is continued to be advanced out volarly but yet it is still in the distal pole of the scaphoid. Joysticks may be placed at the proximal and distal poles of the scaphoid to facilitate reduction as viewed with the arthroscope in the midcarpal space. Once anatomic reduction has been obtained with the joysticks, the guide wire is then advanced proximally back into the proximal pole of the scaphoid.

The guide wire is then advanced back out dorsally with the wrist flexed, once anatomic restoration of the scaphoid fracture has been obtained. It is important that blunt dissection continues around the guide wire dorsally to minimize the risk of soft tissue impalement by the guide wire as it exits back out dorsally by the surrounding extensor tendons. A portion of the guide wire is still left out of the volar aspect of the hand, so if it breaks, easy access to the broken guide wire is possible. Through a soft tissue protector, the scaphoid is reamed over the guide wire and a headless cannulated screw is placed.

The dorsal approach has several advantages, as the screw is inserted down the central axis of the scaphoid most perpendicular to the fracture site. This allows compression directly across the fracture site, as compared to a possibly more oblique orientation with the volar approach. The concern with the dorsal percutaneous approach is that as the wrist is hyperflexed to obtain the cylinder or ring sign, it may displace the scaphoid fracture creating a humpback deformity, which may be unstable. Reduction of the scaphoid should be evaluated with the arthroscope in the midcarpal space when utilizing this technique. Frequently, it takes a surgeon and a very capable assistant with the Slade technique.

Geissler Technique

The Geissler technique has the advantage of knowing the exact starting point for the guide wire as viewed directly with the arthroscope [33] (Video 41.1). There is no guesswork concerning the insertion point and location of the headless cannulated screw. It is the author's opinion that this technique is simpler than the dorsal percutaneous approach with the ring sign. The wrist is not hyperflexed, which could distract the scaphoid fracture and cause a possible humpback deformity.

The wrist is initially suspended in a wrist traction tower (Acumed, Hillsboro, OR) (Fig. 41.1). The wrist is flexed approximately 20–30° in the tower. The arthroscope is initially placed in the 3–4 portal to evaluate any associated soft tissue injuries and the 6-R portal is made. It is important when making the initial 3–4 portal that if one is to error, error slightly ulnar and proximally. If the 3–4 portal is made too radially or too distally, placement of the guide wire would be difficult. A 14-gauge needle is inserted through the 3–4 portal and the junction of the scapholunate interosseous ligament as it inserts onto the proximal pole of the scaphoid is palpated with the needle, as viewed directly with the arthroscope in the 6-R portal (Fig. 41.2). Occasionally, some synovitis from the dorsal capsule may need to be debrided to facilitate visualization of the scapholunate interosseous ligament. It is important that as the needle is inserted through the 3–4 portal that it

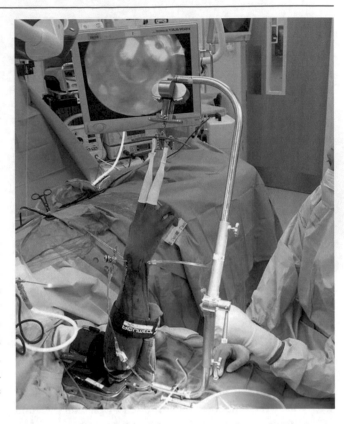

Fig. 41.1 The wrist is suspended in 10 lb of traction in the traction tower (Acumed, Hillsboro, OR). The suspension arm is out to the side, which facilitates arthroscopic and fluoroscopic reduction of fractures

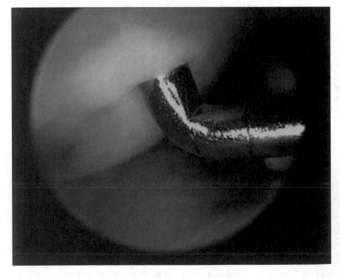

Fig. 41.2 Arthroscopic view with the arthroscope in the 6-R portal. The probe is placed in the 3–4 portal palpating the junction of the scapholunate interosseous ligament to the proximal pole of the scaphoid

passes easily into the joint and does not impale through an extensor tendon. The proximal pole of the scaphoid is impaled, once the needle is at the junction of the scapholunate interosseous ligament to the scaphoid (Fig. 41.3).

The wrist traction tower is then flexed and the starting point of the needle is confirmed under fluoroscopic visualization (Fig. 41.4). This technique allows for a consistent starting point of the very proximal pole of the scaphoid. The needle is then simply aimed toward the thumb under fluoroscopy, and a guide wire is placed through the needle down the central axis of the scaphoid to abut the distal pole (Fig. 41.5). The position of the guide wire is easily checked under fluoroscopy in the posterior/anterior, oblique, and lateral planes while rotating the forearm of the traction tower. The fluoroscopic image is not hindered by the support beam of the traction tower as it is off to the side. A second guide wire is then advanced against the proximal pole of the scaphoid and the length of the screw is determined by the difference of the two

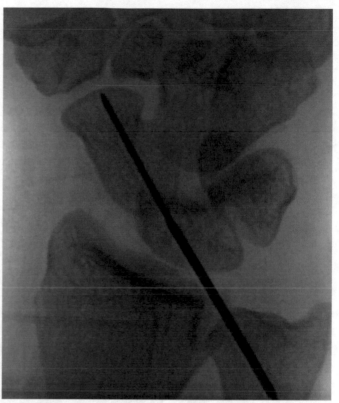

Fig. 41.5 Fluoroscopic view confirming ideal position of the starting point and guide wire through the central axis of the scaphoid fracture

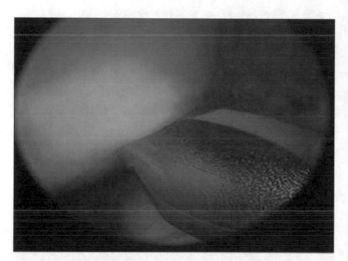

Fig. 41.3 Arthroscopic view with the arthroscope in the 6-R portal with a 14-gauge needle inserted through the 3–4 portal. The needle is palpating the junction of the scapholunate interosseous ligament to the proximal pole of the scaphoid and is impaled into the scaphoid

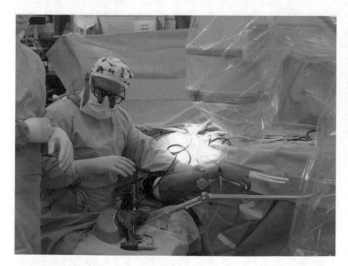

Fig. 41.4 The traction tower (Acumed, Hillsboro, OR) is flexed down to verify the starting point of the proximal pole of the scaphoid

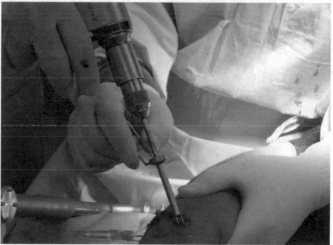

Fig. 41.6 Outside view showing reaming of the scaphoid through a soft tissue protector to protect the extensor tendons

guide wires. Just as in the Slade technique, a screw at least 4 mm shorter than what is measured is recommended.

The reduction of the scaphoid may be evaluated with the arthroscope in the midcarpal portal. If anatomic reduction is confirmed arthroscopically, the guide wire is then advanced out the volar aspect of the hand. The scaphoid is then reamed with a cannulated reamer and a screw is placed (Figs. 41.6

and 41.7). The position of the screw is then checked in the posterior/anterior, oblique, and lateral planes under fluoroscopy with the wrist stabilized by the traction tower (Fig. 41.8).

It is important to evaluate the wrist both in the radiocarpal and midcarpal spaces after placement of the screw (Fig. 41.9). It is particularly important to evaluate the radiocarpal space following screw placement because the screw may look well inserted in the scaphoid under fluoroscopy, but may still be slightly prominent proximally, which could potentially injure the articular cartilage of the scaphoid facet of the distal radius (Fig. 41.10).

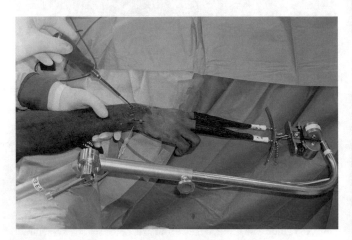

Fig. 41.7 Outside view showing a headless cannulated screw being inserted over the cannulated guide wire stabilizing the fracture of the scaphoid

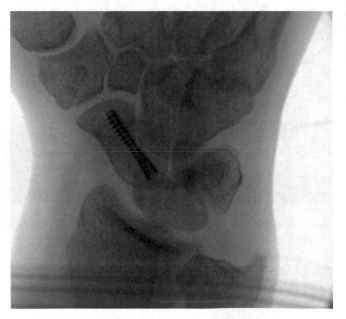

Fig. 41.8 Fluoroscopic oblique view showing ideal position of the headless cannulated screw inserted arthroscopically

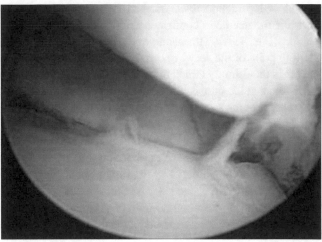

Fig. 41.9 Arthroscopic view with the arthroscope in the radial midcarpal portal demonstrating anatomic reduction to the scaphoid fracture

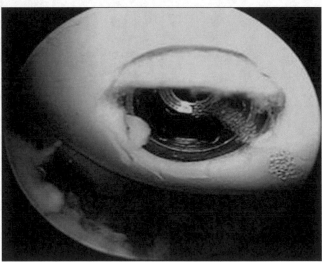

Fig. 41.10 Arthroscopic view with the arthroscope in the 3–4 portal confirming placement of the headless cannulated screw up into the scaphoid, so as not to injure the articular cartilage of the distal radius

Scaphoid Nonunions

Geissler and Slade described their use of Slade's dorsal percutaneous technique in 15 patients with a stable fibrous nonunion of the scaphoid [32]. There were 12 horizontal oblique fractures, two proximal pole fractures, and one transverse fracture in their series. The average time to presentation to surgery was 8 months. All patients underwent percutaneous dorsal fixation with a headless cannulated screw with no bone grafting. Eight of the 15 patients underwent CT evaluation postoperatively to evaluate healing. All patients healed their fractures in an average time of 3 months in their series without any bone grafting. The patients demonstrated excellent range of motion at their final follow-up because of minimal surgical dissection. Utilizing the Mayo modified score, there were 12 of 15 patients who had excellent results. Dorsal percutaneous fixation without bone grafting was recommended in most patients with a stable fibrous nonunion with no signs of humpback deformity of the scaphoid or rotation of the lunate into a DISI position. This study of evaluating patients with Type I through Type III scaphoid nonunions by Slade and Geissler's classification revealed a 100% success rate of union.

In patients who have a cystic scaphoid nonunion without a humpback deformity or rotation of the lunate, percutaneous cancellous bone grafting or injection of demineralized bone matrix (DBM) may be used. In Geissler's technique, the guide wire is placed, as previously described [33]. The scaphoid is reamed through a soft tissue protector. A bone biopsy needle is filled with DBM putty. The needle is placed over the guide wire from dorsal to proximal and inserted into the drill hole directly into the nonunion site. The guide wire is then retracted distally out of the proximal pole of the scaphoid while still remaining into the distal pole of the scaphoid. The DBM is injected through the bone biopsy needle directly into the central hole of the scaphoid until resistance is felt (Fig. 41.11). Following injection of the DBM, the guide wire is advanced back dorsally through the bone biopsy needle from volar to dorsal. In this manner, the guide wire is passed back through the original reamed tract of the proximal pole of the scaphoid out dorsally. The bone biopsy needle is then removed, and the headless cannulated screw is placed over the guide wire.

Geissler reported his results of using 1 cc of DBM putty for cystic scaphoid nonunions of the scaphoid [33]. There were 15 patients in his series who were classified by the Slade and Geissler classification Type IV. Fourteen of 15 patients healed their cystic scaphoid nonunions utilizing this technique. Arthroscopic evaluation of the wrist from both the radiocarpal and midcarpal spaces showed no extravasation of the DBM into the joint.

Discussion

While cast immobilization of an acute nondisplaced fracture of the scaphoid is effective, there are certain disadvantages including muscle atrophy, joint contracture, and stiffness. Fractures or the scaphoid are common athletic injuries occurring especially in young men [34, 35]. Most nondisplaced acute fractures of the scaphoid have been reported to heal with nonunion rates of 10–15%. However, union rates of 100% for acute fractures of the scaphoid managed by percutaneous arthroscopic-assisted fixation have been consistently reported in the literature [19–22].

Arthroscopic fixation of acute scaphoid fractures has several advantages. This can allow the patient to return quickly to the workforce or to competition. Arthroscopic fixation allows for secure stabilization through limited surgical dissection, which may result in improved range of motion. Recently, the author has been working on stabilization of transscaphoid perilunar dislocations all arthroscopically without Kirschner wires and starting early range of motion (Figs. 41.12, 41.13, 41.14, 41.15, and 41.16). Early results have been very encouraging. In addition, arthroscopic fixation allows for the management of associated soft tissue injuries which may occur with a fracture of the scaphoid (Figs. 41.17, 41.18, and 41.19).

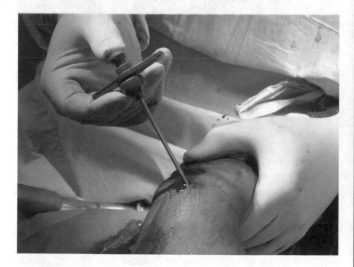

Fig. 41.11 Outside view showing the insertion of DBM putty over the cannulated guide wire through a putty pusher into the scaphoid nonunion site

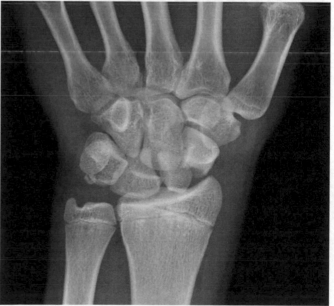

Fig. 41.12 Anterior/posterior radiograph demonstrating a transscaphoid perilunate dislocation

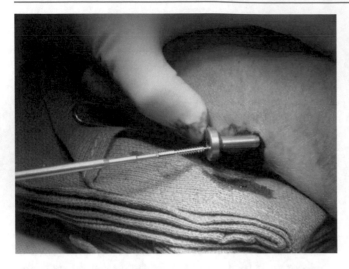

Fig. 41.13 Outside view showing placement of a scapholunate inter-carpal (SLIC) screw (Acumed, Hillsboro, OR) placement across the lunotriquetral (LT) interval for a complete tear of the lunotriquetral osseous ligament

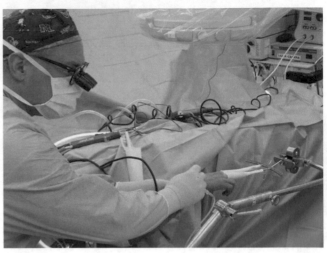

Fig. 41.15 Following stabilization of the LT interval, the traction tower (Acumed, Hillsboro, OR) is being flexed to confirm the ideal starting point of the guide wire for the scaphoid fracture

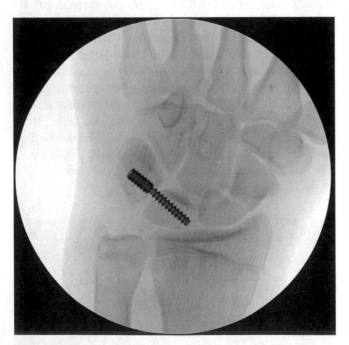

Fig. 41.14 Fluoroscopic view confirming ideal position of the SLIC screw across the injured lunotriquetral interval. Following this, the scaphoid fracture will be arthroscopically stabilized

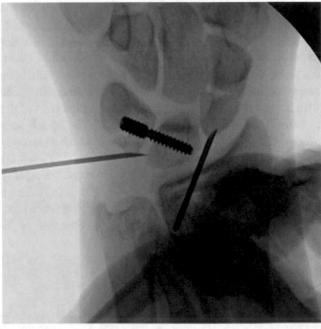

Fig. 41.16 Fluoroscopic view demonstrating the ideal starting point for the guide wire to stabilize the cannulated screw

Arthroscopic fixation has also been shown to be beneficial in treating scaphoid nonunions Type I through Type IV with the classification scheme of Slade and Geissler [36]. In patients with a stable fibrous nonunion, stabilization with a screw alone has been shown to be effective. In patients with cystic changes, arthroscopic stabilization and percutaneous injection of DBM or percutaneous cancellous bone grafting are an effective option [33].

Arthroscopic fixation limits the guesswork concerning the exact location of the starting point of a guide wire and cannulated screw, as compared to previously described percutaneous fluoroscopic techniques. The ideal starting point is at the most proximal pole of the scaphoid at the junction of the scapholunate interosseous ligament. It is very reproducible and easily confirmed under fluoroscopy without hyperflexion of the wrist causing a potential humpback deformity

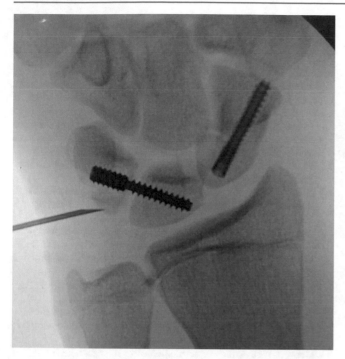

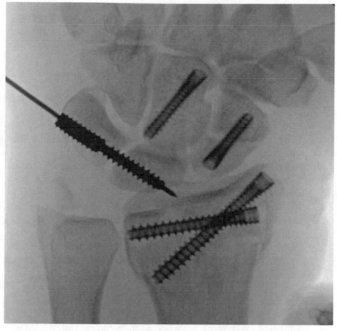

Fig. 41.17 Fluoroscopic view showing stabilization both to the LT interval and scaphoid fracture and the perilunate dislocation. This patient will be started on immediate range of motion as no Kirschner wires were utilized, which can hamper rehabilitation

Fig. 41.19 Fluoroscopic view following arthroscopic reduction of the distal radius fracture, scaphoid fracture, and SLIC screw placement (Acumed, Hillsboro, OR) of the lunotriquetral interval. The capitate fracture was stabilized percutaneously

of the scaphoid. Dorsal insertion of the screw enables central placement down the axis of the scaphoid, as compared to oblique orientation through the volar approach.

It is important to remember that these two techniques are not indicated for those patients who have severe humpback deformity, which is not correctable, or for those patients who have advanced arthrosis of the radiocarpal joint (scaphoid nonunion advanced collapse (SNAC)) [37].

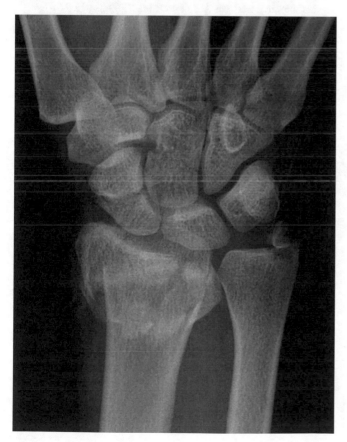

Fig. 41.18 Radiograph showing a great arc injury to the wrist involving the distal radius, scaphoid, capitate, and lunotriquetral interval

References

1. Gelberman RH, Wolock BS, Siegel DB. Current concepts review: fractures and nonunions of the carpal scaphoid. J Bone Joint Surg. 1989;71A:1560–5.
2. Cooney WP, Dobyns JH, Linscheid RL. Fractures of the scaphoid: a rational approach to management. Clin Orthop. 1980;149:90–7.
3. Rettig AC, Ryan RO, Stone JA. Epidemiology of hand injuries in sports. In: Strickland JW, Rettig AC, editors. Hand injuries in athletes. Philadelphia: WB Saunders; 1992. p. 37–48.
4. Gellman H, Caputo RJ, Carter V, et al. Comparison of short and long thumb spica casts for non-displaced fractures of the carpal scaphoid. J Bone Joint Surg. 1989;71A:354–7.
5. Kaneshiro SA, Failla JM, Tashman S. Scaphoid fracture displacement with forearm rotation in a short arm thumb spica cast. J Hand Surg. 1989;71:354–7.
6. Skirven T, Trope J. Complications of immobilization. Hand Clin. 1994;10:53–61.
7. Gelberman RH, Menon J. The vascularity of the scaphoid bone. J Hand Surg. 1980;5:508–13.
8. Rettig AC, Weidenbener EJ, Gloyeske R. Alternative management of mid-third scaphoid fractures in the athlete. Am J Sports Med. 1994;22:711–4.

9. DeMaagd RL, Engber WD. Retrograde Herbert screw fixation for treatment of proximal pole scaphoid nonunions. J Hand Surg. 1989;14:996–1003.

10. Filan SL, Herbert TJ. Herbert screw fixation of scaphoid fractures. J Bone Joint Surg. 1996;78:519–29.

11. Herbert TJ, Fisher WE. Management of the fractured scaphoid using a new bone screw. J Bone Joint Surg. 1984;66:114–23.

12. O'Brien L, Herbert TJ. Internal fixation of acute scaphoid fractures: a new approach to treatment. Aust NZ J Surg. 1985;55:387–9.

13. Rettig ME, Raskin KB. Retrograde compression screw fixation of acute proximal pole scaphoid fractures. J Hand Surg. 1999;24:1206–10.

14. Russe O. Fracture of the carpal navicular: diagnosis, nonoperative treatment and operative treatment. J Bone Joint Surg. 1960;42A:759.

15. Toby EB, Butler TE, McCormack TJ, et al. A comparison of fixation screws for the scaphoid during application of cyclic bending loads. J Bone Joint Surg. 1997;79:1190–7.

16. Trumble TE, Clarke T, Kreder HJ. Nonunion of the scaphoid: treatment with cannulated screws compared with treatment with Herbert screws. J Bone Joint Surg. 1996;78:1829–37.

17. Garcia-Elias M, Vall A, Salo JM, et al. Carpal alignment after different surgical approaches to the scaphoid: a comparative study. J Hand Surg. 1988;13:604–12.

18. Adams BD, Blair WF, Regan DS, et al. Technical factors related to Herbert screw fixation. J Bone Joint Surg. 1988;13:893–9.

19. Whipple TL. The role of arthroscopy in the treatment of intraarticular wrist fractures. Hand Clin. 1995;11:13–8.

20. Geissler WB. Arthroscopic assisted fixation of fractures of the scaphoid. Atlas Hand Clin. 2003;8:37–56.

21. Geissler WB, Hammit MD. Arthroscopic aided fixation of scaphoid fractures. Hand Clin. 2001;17:575–88.

22. Slade JF, Merrell GA, Geissler WB. Fixation of acute and selected nonunion scaphoid fractures. In: Geissler WB, editor. Wrist arthroscopy. New York: Springer; 2005. p. 112–24.

23. Cosio MQ, Camp RA. Percutaneous pinning of symptomatic scaphoid nonunions. J Hand Surg. 1986;11:350–5.

24. Haddad FS, Goddard NJ. Acute percutaneous scaphoid fixation: a pilot study. J Bone Joint Surg. 1998;80:95–9.

25. Shin A, Bond A, McBride M, et al. Acute screw fixation versus cast immobilization for stable scaphoid fractures: a prospective randomized study. Presented at American Society Surgery for the Hand, Seattle, October 5–7, 2000.

26. Slade JF III, Grauer JN, Mahoney JD. Arthroscopic reduction and percutaneous fixation of scaphoid fractures with a novel dorsal technique. Orthop Clin North Am. 2000;30:247–61.

27. Slade JF III, Jaskwhich J. Percutaneous fixation of scaphoid fractures. Hand Clin. 2001;17:553–74.

28. Taras JS, Sweet S, Shum W, et al. Percutaneous and arthroscopic screw fixation of scaphoid fractures in the athlete. Hand Clin. 1999;15:467–73.

29. Slade JF III, Grauer JN. Dorsal percutaneous repair of scaphoid fractures with arthroscopic guidance. Atlas Hand Clin. 2001;6:307–23.

30. Wozasek GE, Moser KD. Percutaneous screw fixation of fractures of the scaphoid. J Bone Joint Surg. 1991;73:138–42.

31. Kamineni S, Lavy CBD. Percutaneous fixation of scaphoid fractures: an anatomic study. J Hand Surg. 1999;24:85–8.

32. Geissler WB, Slade JF. Arthroscopic fixation of scaphoid nonunions without bone grafting. Presented American Society Surgery of the Hand, Phoenix, AZ, September 2002.

33. Geissler WB. Arthroscopic fixation of cystic scaphoid nonunions with DBM. Presented American Association Hand Surgery, Tucson, AZ, January 2006.

34. Geissler WB. Carpal fractures in athletes. Clin Sports Med. 2001;20:167–88.

35. Rettig AC, Kollias SC. Internal fixation of acute stable scaphoid fractures in the athlete. Am J Sports Med. 1996;24:182–6.

36. Geissler WB. Wrist arthroscopy. New York: Springer; 2005.

37. Fernandez DL. Anterior bone grafting and conventional lag screw fixation to treat scaphoid nonunions. J Hand Surg. 1990;15A:140–7.

M. Christian Moody, Mitchell C. Birt, and Scott Edwards

Introduction

Scaphoid plating was originally described in 1977 being designed and reported by Ender [1]. He then reported on a series of over 200 patients resulting in 99% union rate [2]. Literature regarding this fixation was generally positive. Huene et al. reported on a group of 20 patients with complicated scaphoid fractures having only one failure. Despite these promising results, the use of plating has been sparsely reported and was supplanted with the advent of the Herbert screw in 1984. Variable pitch screws were rapidly adopted, allowing for a minimally invasive technique and stable fixation.

Screw fixation provides stable bending rigidity, and the utilization of dual screw or K-wire supplementation can impart torsional stability. But difficulty with screw fixation remains with highly unstable fracture patterns, nonunion, and bone loss demanding more rigid fixation. Clinical and biomechanical studies have favored the rotational stability of plate fixation [3, 4]. Recently, for these reasons, there has been a resurgence of popularity for plate fixation, especially for unstable nonunions. Volar buttress plating provides a biomechanical advantage of buttressing and resisting the flexion and pronation forces across the scaphoid which commonly result in humpback deformity, and consequently, it provides a better environment for fracture union [5]. The often low-quality bone stock present during a scaphoid nonunion case raises a problem for screw and pin fixation and can be overcome with polyaxial locking screw technology. Further,

given the higher ultimate failure loads of plates over headless screws [5], the plates offer the opportunity to utilize more biologically active bone grafts, as opposed to those with structural support that may lack the same biological advantage [6]. Plate fixation can provide both bending and torsional stability in the setting of bone loss and even proximal pole nonunion, which can oftentimes be difficult to maintain fixation with a headless compression screw.

Initially favorable reports of modern-day volar scaphoid plating come from Ghoneim [7] and Leixnering et al. [8] yielding 100% union of scaphoid nonunions treated with volar plates were followed with other studies raising concerns for hardware complications. Esteban-Feliu et al. series of scaphoid nonunions treated with plate fixation resulted in 87% union with five patients requiring repeat procedures, three for hardware impingement [9].

Locked scaphoid plating has been used in cases of scaphoid nonunion and revision cases with encouraging early results. In addition to the first report by Leixnering, Dodds et al. reported on 20 patients with scaphoid nonunions and humpback deformity. Union was achieved in 18 of 20 patients, with 11 having avascular necrosis (AVN) and five being smokers [10]. Edwards et al. published a series of 34 patients with scaphoid nonunion with segmental defects. All patients healed by 18 weeks as verified by CT scan postoperatively. DASH scores improved from 27 to 11.8 by final follow-up. Grip strength improved from 77% to 90.5% [11]. In another series, 13 scaphoid nonunions with AVN treated with volar plating and pure cancellous bone graft resulted in 100% union with good patient-reported and functional outcomes [12].

Locked volar plates allow for the healing potential to be maximized by (1) verticalizing the scaphoid and buttresses the deforming forces; (2) maintaining a space for graft insertion and supports the nonunion site while the graft incorporates; (3) maximizing the surface area available for bony healing; and (4) preserving intraosseous vascular network and the dorsal vascular entry pathways. While the authors

M. C. Moody (✉)
Department of Orthopaedic Surgery, Division of Hand and Upper Extremity, Prisma Health System, Greenville, SC, USA
e-mail: mark.moody@prismahealth.org

M. C. Birt
Hand and Upper Extremity Surgery, University of Kansas Medical Center, Kansas City, KS, USA

S. Edwards
Department of Orthopaedic Surgery, University of Arizona College of Medicine, Phoenix, AZ, USA

acknowledge that there are many acceptable variations, our preferred technique will be discussed in this chapter.

Indications

Some of the best current indications for the volar locked plating technique include persistent nonunion after screw fixation, chronic nonunion, the rare unstable comminuted or unstable oblique acute fractures, and in any situation where conditions may result in compromised or challenging screw purchase. Nonunions can result from insufficient or delayed diagnosis and/or management, inadequate immobilization, and poor patient compliance. In our practice, if a patient presents greater than 3 months out from the date of injury and shows evidence of humpback deformity with persistent pain and dysfunction, surgical management with volar locked plating is recommended. In most cases, advanced imaging is ordered for bone integrity, vascularity assessment, and surgical planning. Figure 42.1 shows a patient who presented 4 months out from injury with imaging consistent with humpback deformity. Untreated or mismanagement of nonunions can result in continued pain, osteoarthritis, and impairment.

Contraindications

Like most internal fixation, the volar locked plating technique is contraindicated in patients with acute or chronic infection or in the presence of systemic medical conditions that make the patient unfit for surgical intervention. Also in patients with advanced stages of radiocarpal or midcarpal osteoarthritis related to scaphoid nonunion advanced collapse (SNAC II–IV), the patient will likely have persistent pain after volar plating and would benefit more from a reconstructive surgical option involving a patient-specific arthrodesis or carpectomy option. Patients with dissociative or nondissociative carpal instability should have the cause for the instability addressed in addition to providing stable scaphoid fixation. Some nonunion cases also do not allow for proximal pole screw fixation either because of the extremely small size of the proximal pole or due to fragmentation. For these cases, we recommend a vascularized medial femoral trochlea flap.

Surgical Technique

Operating Room Setup

The patient should be supine on the operating table with the hand table placed on the operative side. For anesthesia, we prefer the use of a regional nerve block with either sedation or general anesthesia. The patients should have a tourniquet placed on the upper arm to accommodate for mobility needed to manipulate the limb while using fluoroscopy during the case. Depending on the selected bone graft option, the appropriate surgical sites should be prepped in a sterile fashion as usual. Our technique utilizes bone graft from the ipsilateral wrist and/or elbow, and therefore, our surgical preparation

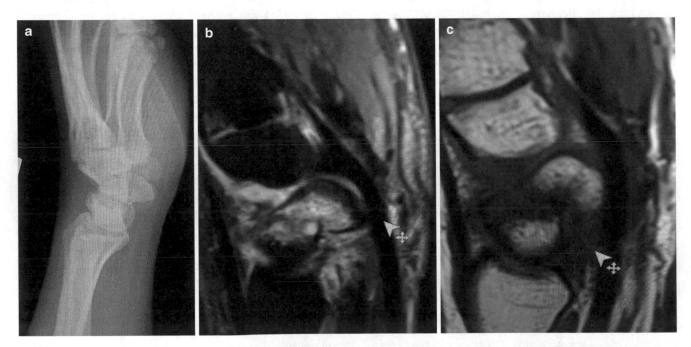

Fig. 42.1 (**a–c**) Lateral radiograph image and two sagittal MRI cuts showing a scaphoid waist fracture from a patient who presented 4 months out from injury without any immobilization. The flexion and pronation forces across the scaphoid waist fracture result in nonunion and the characteristic humpback deformity seen here

consists of scrubbing the surgical limb up to the level of the tourniquet on the upper arm. The operating surgeon should sit on the side of the patient's axilla. We prefer to have the fluoroscopy unit come in from the distal end of the hand table to allow for ease of bringing the machine in and out of the operative field when needed.

Approach

Our surgical technique utilizes a volar approach to the scaphoid following a hockey stick skin incision with the bend over the palpable distal pole of the scaphoid. The distal arm of the incision will proceed over the radial edge of the proximal thenar musculature toward the trapezium and the axis of the first metacarpal for approximately 2 cm. The proximal arm aligns with the flexor carpi radialis (FCR) for approximately 3 cm ending at the radiocarpal joint (Fig. 42.2). Once through the skin and down to the level of the FCR sheath, palpate the tubercle to maintain correct orientation. Dissection is continued through the FCR sheath exposing the FCR and underlying volar wrist capsular complex. The volar wrist capsule is clearly identified by the obliquely oriented fibers of the volar extrinsic ligaments. Distally, the thenar musculature can be incised with the muscle fibers and retracted. There is often a small arterial vessel off the volar branch of the radial artery

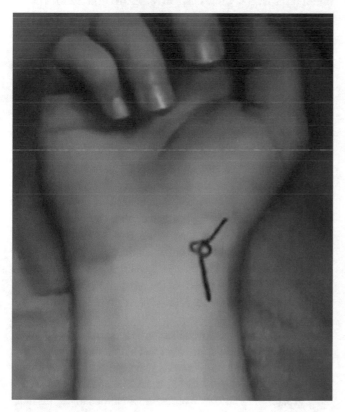

Fig. 42.2 Hockey stick incision that is centered over the distal pole of the scaphoid that is circled in the image

in this area that can be safely cauterized. Retract the FCR ulnarly. A longitudinal incision is made through the FCR subsheath and continues the incision through the capsule from the distal pole of the scaphoid toward the volar lip of the radius. Attachment of the capsule to the distal pole will require sharp removal. At this point, place the wrist on a bump to extend the wrist providing better visualization and tension of the volar capsule. Maximally ulnar deviating the wrist will extend the scaphoid further and allow full access for plating.

Good exposure is paramount to ensure the success of this procedure. For extended exposure of the proximal pole, a small portion of the capsule may be sharply elevated in a transverse manner from the volar margin of the distal radius. You may need to reflect the capsule radially and ulnarly off of the distal radius rim to achieve the necessary exposure of the proximal pole. Care must be taken not to completely detach the volar extrinsic ligaments as this potentially could allow ulnar translation of the carpus. In the authors' experiences, a minor release has not resulting in any such translation. Once exposure is completed, take a moment to clearly identify the distal pole of the scaphoid, the cartilage covered concave volar surface of the scaphoid, the nonunion site, and the entire volar surface of the proximal pole. Using a freer elevator or scalpel blade, identify and open the nonunion site and disrupt any fibrous adhesions which should be very minimal. Care should be taken to preserve the cortical rims as best as possible. Use 0.045-inch Kirschner pins as joysticks to distract across the nonunion site.

When addressing scaphoid nonunions, especially with AVN, adequate debridement is one of the most important parts of the procedure. It is critical to perform a thorough and aggressive debridement of the sclerotic and devitalized tissue from both sides of the defect. Typically white, hard, sclerotic bone should be removed, and only yellow soft healthy cancellous bone should remain. Our preferred technique utilizes a 2.0 or 3.0 mm low-speed burr for this step and/or a small curette. To reduce the risk of heat necrosis with the burr, ensure that it is on low speed and irrigate liberally. Some cases may have very thin rims of cortical bone, so careful precision with the burr or curette should be used around these delicate areas. The Kirschner pins also serve as aid in a trial reduction. Reduction is usually obtained with extension and supination of the distal fragment. We have also found that the precontoured plate helps to position the fragments into an anatomical reduction, but this cannot replace a good manual reduction by the surgeon. The surgeon should err on the side of verticalizing, or overextending the scaphoid, rather than accepting a more flexed position. Once adequate reduction of the deformity is obtained following debridement, a defect of up to 10 mm may sometimes present. Our technique calls for pure cancellous graft as it has been shown to be superior to corticocancellous grafts in terms of incorporate rate and union and has demonstrated excellent clinical results in challenging scaphoid nonunion cases with segmental bone loss and AVN [11, 12]. Pure cancellous graft is obtained from the ipsilateral distal radius and/or olecranon, and graft is not only transferred but impacted into the scaphoid defect. The choice of donor site is largely arbitrary, but occasionally, both sites are harvested in cases requiring large amounts of graft for sizable defects. The authors recommend harvesting more graft than what first appears to be required in order to make sure enough is collected to firmly pack the graft into the defect. The Kirschner pins are removed and, without distraction, the columnar forces exerted on the scaphoid's distal pole by the trapezium and trapezoid typically induce a small amount of flexion and pronation of the scaphoid, which highlights the necessity of over-reduction as stated previously. By overstuffing the defect with graft, the graft is compressed, but still helps to maintain the scaphoid height, thus stabilizing the midcarpal joint. If impacted properly, the graft only will maintain the reduction provisionally until the plate is secured. If necessary, a percutaneous retrograde Kirschner pin placed down the axis of the scaphoid can be used as temporary fixation but this is rarely necessary, and if it is, the surgeon at least should scrutinize the degree in which the graft was impacted into the defect.

A precontoured 1.5-mm locking scaphoid plate (Medartis, AG, Basel, Switzerland) is implanted by first using nonlocking, self-tapping cortical screws in the most proximal and most distal holes of the 6-hole plate. It is important to avoid positioning the proximal portion of the plate from crossing the point at which the bone's concavity becomes the convexity. This demarcation line is the point at which the nonarticulating portion of the bone becomes articulating (Fig. 42.3).

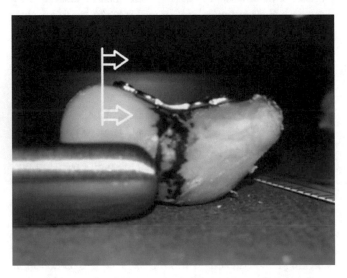

Fig. 42.3 Ideal volar plate placement distal to the "line in the sand," represented by the white line positioned over the volar aspect of the cadaver scaphoid proximal pole. The arrows demonstrate that plate placement should be distal to and not cross the scaphoid "line in the sand"

Crossing this point would result in implant impingement against the articular surface of the distal radius. This landmark varies between scaphoids and is more apparent in some patients than in others. Direct attention to plate placement relative to this "line in the sand" is mandatory for every case. It is important to begin fixation of the plate to the proximal portion of the scaphoid as there is less room for error on this proximal portion of the bone as compared to the distal portion. After compressing the plate to the bone with the cortical screws in the most proximal and distal holes, fluoroscopy is used to assess the position of the plate. There is a tendency for surgeons inexperienced with this technique to plate the plate too radial and too distal. Once proper plate placement is verified, four locking screws are placed in the remaining holes with a trajectory toward their respective poles. The two initial cortical screws are replaced with locking screws, so that each of the three proximal and three distal holes are filled with locking screws. Ideally, the locking screws should be buttressing the subchondral bone of the poles similar to how the locking screws of a distal radius volar plate buttresses the subchondral bone of the radius. For these locking screws, the bone is drilled bicortically and measured so that the screw tip engaged the subchondral bone, but does not penetrate the far cortex. Live fluoroscopy at every angle is used to confirm final plate and screw placement. Concomitant radial styloidectomy is performed for cases involving minor scaphoid nonunion arthrosis (SNAC I). Mean operative time is 40 min.

Proximal pole fractures and nonunions pose an added challenge. Usually, the fracture or nonunion site is directly at the line delineating convex from concave curvature of the proximal portion of the scaphoid; the line the plate must not pass. Consequently, the plate itself cannot play any role of buttressing the forces across the proximal pole because it should not be in contact with the pole. Rather, the burden must be placed on the locking screws directed against the subchondral bone of the proximal pole. The surgeon, however, will have difficulty sending more than one screw to abut the proximal pole subchondral bone with the plate in its current form. For proximal pole fractures and nonunions, the authors recommend modifying the plate by removing the most proximal hole, thus allowing two screws to line up adjacent to the fracture line and have the appropriate angle to abut the subchondral bone. The authors believe that this modification of the plate offers the most stable fixation of the proximal pole without added risk of plate impingement against the radius.

Although perhaps too conservative to some, it is the common practice of the authors to protect a nonunion repair with a cast postoperatively until there is plain radiographic evidence of healing and confirmed by CT scan. The authors would consider greater than 50% consolidation of callous to be "unified" and would allow patients to resume normal activity.

Tips and Tricks

- Clear visualization of the entire volar surface of the scaphoid: Reflecting a small portion of the proximal capsule off the radius will assist in visualizing the proximal pole. Care must be taken not to reflect too much capsule so as to cause ulnar translation.
- Thorough debridement: This portion of the procedure is technically demanding and requires aggressive debridement of nonviable tissue while maintaining the anatomy and bone stock of the scaphoid. The authors find a 2.0 or 3.0 mm, low-speed bur with continuous irrigation most helpful in this regard. Debridement should continue until either healthy yellow cancellous bone of the scaphoid or the remaining cortical rim of each pole. We have had successful unions even in cases in which the entire proximal pole seems to be just a cortical shell – a virtual vessel for graft.
- Verticalization of the scaphoid: The surgeon should err on the side of verticalizing, that is to over-extend and supinate the distal pole. Overstuffing the nonunion site with cancellous autograft is recommended to not only aid in reduction but maximize the osteoconductive and osteoinductive properties of the graft. It is difficult to manipulate the proximal pole to any significant degree, so it is preferable to focus attention on the distal pole.
- Pure cancellous bone graft: Multiple bone graft options are at the disposal of the surgeon. The preference of the authors is nonvascularized pure cancellous bone graft from the ipsilateral distal radius and/or olecranon given its relative ease of harvest, yet outstanding clinical performance equal to and sometimes superior to those reported for nonvascularized corticocancellous and most vascularized grafts.
- Impaction of graft: It is prudent to harvest more graft than what might seem required. Surgeons often are impressed at the amount of graft that may be impacted into the scaphoid defect. Any graft that appears to be outside the cortical boundaries of the scaphoid on intraoperative fluoroscopy usually resorbs over time with postoperative radiographs and CT scans.
- Secure the plate to the proximal portion of the scaphoid first. There is less room for error on the proximal portion, and plate positioning is more critical.
- No matter how tempting, do not cross the scaphoid "line in the sand," the delineation on the proximal portion of the scaphoid in which the concavity becomes the convexity. To do so will result in plate impingement on the radius.
- Plate modification for proximal pole fractures and nonunions. Removal of the most proximal hole in the plate allows for improved fixation and to avoid crossing the scaphoid "line in the sand" to prevent impingement on the radius. In these cases, it is even more important to direct the locking screws, so they buttress the subchondral bone of each pole, especially the proximal one.

Conclusion

The volar locked plating technique has been shown to have good patient-reported and functional outcomes in previously published studies with the use nonvascularized cancellous or corticocancellous graft and vascularized bone grafts [11]. Even in patients with AVN, volar locked plating with corticocancellous local autogenous graft has yielded reliable union rates with good patient outcomes [12].

The authors believe that the power of volar locked plating offers an opportunity to buttress deforming forces while minimizing the interosseous and extraosseous vascularity of the bone, maximizing the bony surface area of contact for healing, all the while using the most biologically active nonvascularized graft which has been shown to be pure cancellous graft.

While scaphoid screw fixation may provide stable 3-point fixation within some acute scaphoid waist fractures, this stability is lost with the absence of cortical contact, diminishing bone stock or significant deformity. Further, headless screws rely on compression to stabilize the bone. Simply put, screws are less capable of stabilizing the scaphoid if the screws have nothing to compress against, which would necessitate the use of more structural grafts and possibly compromise the ability for these types of graft to incorporate as readily as pure cancellous.

References

1. Ender HG. A new method of treating traumatic cysts and pseudoarthrosis of the scaphoid (author's transl). Unfallheilkunde. 1977;80(12):509–13. Epub 1977/12/01.
2. Bohler J, Ender HG. Pseudarthrosis of the scaphoid. Orthopade. 1986;15(2):109–20. Epub 1986/04/01.
3. Jurkowitsch J, Dall'Ara E, Quadlbauer S, Pezzei C, Jung I, Pahr D, et al. Rotational stability in screw-fixed scaphoid fractures compared to plate-fixed scaphoid fractures. Arch Orthop Trauma Surg. 2016;136(11):1623–8. Epub 2016/08/28.
4. Sander AL, Sommer K, Schaf D, Braun C, Marzi I, Pohlemann T, et al. Clinical outcome after alternative treatment of scaphoid fractures and nonunions. Eur J Trauma Emerg Surg. 2018;44(1):113–8. Epub 2017/03/01.
5. Goodwin JA, Castaneda P, Shelhamer RP, Bosch LC, Edwards SG. A comparison of plate versus screw fixation for segmental scaphoid fractures: a biomechanical study. Hand (N Y). 2019;14(2):203–8.
6. Instr Course Lecture, ASSH, 2020; Ortho Traumatol Surg Res, 2018; Clin Oral Implants Res, 2009.

7. Ghoneim A. The unstable nonunited scaphoid waist fracture: results of treatment by open reduction, anterior wedge grafting, and internal fixation by volar buttress plate. J Hand Surg Am. 2011;36(1):17–24. Epub 2011/01/05.

8. Leixnering M, Pezzei C, Weninger P, et al. First experiences with a new adjustable plate for osteosynthesis of scaphoid nonunions. J Trauma. 2011;71(4):933–8.

9. Esteban-Feliu I, Barrera-Ochoa S, Vidal-Tarrason N, Mir-Simon B, Lluch A, Mir-Bullo X. Volar plate fixation to treat scaphoid nonunion: a case series with minimum 3 years of follow-up. J Hand Surg Am. 2018;43(6):569 e1–8. Epub 2018/01/24.

10. Dodds SD, Williams JB, Seiter M, Chen C. Lessons learned from volar plate fixation of scaphoid fracture nonunions. J Hand Surg Eur Vol. 2018;43(1):57–65. Epub 2017/11/23.

11. Putnam JG, Mitchell SM, DiGiovanni RM, Stockwell EL, Edwards SG. Outcomes of unstable scaphoid nonunion with segmental defect treated with plate fixation and autogenous cancellous graft. J Hand Surg Am. 2019;44(2):160 e1–7. Epub 2018/07/01.

12. Putnam JG, DiGiovanni RM, Mitchell SM, Castaneda P, Edwards SG. Plate fixation with cancellous graft for scaphoid nonunion with avascular necrosis. J Hand Surg Am. 2019;44(4):339 e1–7. Epub 2018/08/15.

Volar Vascularized Graft for Scaphoid Nonunions

Mathilde Gras, Lorenzo Merlini,
and Christophe Mathoulin

Introduction

Scaphoid nonunion is still challenging for hand surgeons, especially at the proximal pole. Five to thirty percent of scaphoid fractures evolve toward nonunion [1, 2]. Without treatment, it leads to radiocarpal, then midcarpal arthritis, and carpal collapse with dorsal intercalated segment instability (DISI) deformity of the lunatum [3]. Nonvascularized bone graft gives nonunion in up to 20% of cases [4, 5], and in more than 50% in case of proximal pole necrosis [5]. Vascularized bone graft seems to be associated with a better rate of healing, but it is generally restricted to secondary intervention or proximal pole necrosis [5–8].

Several vascularized grafts have been described [9–18], including graft pedicled on the palmar carpal artery [19]. Mathoulin [14, 19] adopted Kuhlmann's graft harvested from the volar radius [16], vascularized by the volar carpal artery with anastomosis between the ulnar and radial arteries [20], following a cadaver study [19] (Fig. 43.1).

Indications

The indication for the volar vascular bone graft is a scaphoid nonunion without periscaphoid arthritis. Patients with radiological or clinical evidence of early radio-scaphoid arthritis may require arthroscopy or MRI of the joint surface before proceeding. In case of radio-scaphoid arthritis involving the styloid and distal scaphoid only, scaphoid nonunion advanced collapse (SNAC) wrist grade I, a radial styloidectomy, can be performed in addition to vascularized bone grafting. Age of patient is not a contraindication. A meta-analysis of treatment of scaphoid nonunion found that patient age had little

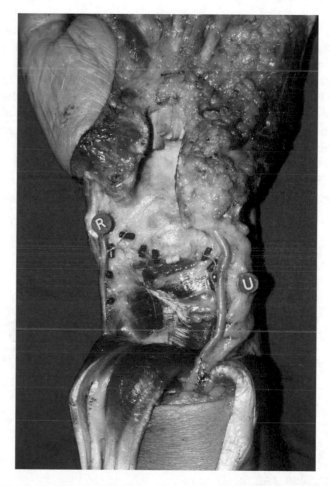

Fig. 43.1 Cadaveric dissection showing the volar carpal artery running along the distal edge of the pronator quadratus before anastomosing with the anterior interosseous artery and a branch of the ulnar artery (*R* radial artery, *U* ulnar artery). (Reprinted from Gras and Mathoulin [20] and Mathoulin and Gras [21])

effect on union rates, but that the chance of secondary nonunion increases with delay to surgery of more than 12 months from injury [5].

M. Gras (✉) · L. Merlini · C. Mathoulin
Clinique Bizet, International Wrist Center-Clinique du Poignet,
Institut de la Main, Paris, France

© Springer Nature Switzerland AG 2022
W. B. Geissler (ed.), *Wrist and Elbow Arthroscopy with Selected Open Procedures*,
https://doi.org/10.1007/978-3-030-78881-0_43

Contraindications

Absolute contraindications to volar vascularized bone grafting for scaphoid reconstruction include periscaphoid degeneration involving the entire scaphoid fossa, the scaphocapitate joint (SNAC stage II or III), and previous surgery or injury to the distal radius or radial artery resulting in disruption of the blood supply at the volar radius graft site.

A smoking patient is also a contraindication. Nicotine prevents healing.

Technique

The volar carpal artery bone graft is performed under local regional anesthesia on an outpatient basis. The arm of the patient is placed on hand table, under tourniquet control. The patient is placed in a supine position and the wrist is placed in extension and ulnar deviation. The inferior aspect of the incision is extended 2 cm proximally to allow exposure of the distal radius. The flexor carpi radialis tendon is retracted ulnarly, and the radial artery radially (Fig. 43.2).

The anterior capsule is reflected, exposing the distal radial margin and the scaphoid. Fibrous scar tissue is removed, and necrotic bone at the fracture site is curetted until healthy

bone is reached and punctate bleeding can be demonstrated. A narrow osteotome separates the scaphoid fragments. The scaphoid reduction is checked pulling on the thumb, and the bony defect is measured with intraoperative imaging.

The vascular bone graft is then harvested. The wrist is flexed to allow ulnar retraction of the flexor carpi radialis and finger flexor tendons. The pronator quadratus muscle is exposed. Parallel incisions are made, the first 1 cm proximal to the distal border of the pronator quadratus and the second few millimeters distal to it, from either side of the volar carpal artery. These incisions are made ulnar to the radial artery over the distal radius, but radial to the bone graft site. A scalpel and periosteal elevator allow detaching the strip of muscle and periosteum including the volar carpal artery, and thus mobilize the pedicle (Fig. 43.3). The bone graft, attached to the ulnar end of the pedicle, is then harvested with a 10-mm osteotome. The dimensions of the required graft are first marked on the bone. The osteotomy starts at the lateral borders. Then, the proximal and distal borders of the bone graft are osteotomized in an oblique direction to form a wedge shape followed by the medial border (Fig. 43.4). The bone graft is levered from the distal radius with a 5-mm osteotome with care to protect the pedicle. The pedicle was then dissected up to the origin of the volar carpal artery (Fig. 43.5a, b). The scaphoid fragments are then stabilized with a K-wire

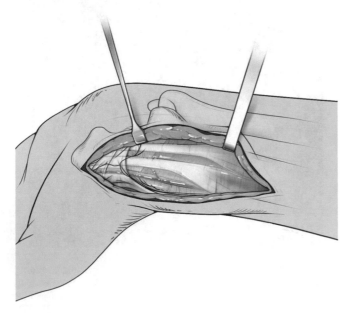

Fig. 43.2 Drawing showing the volar "Henry" approach, merely extended toward the distal tubercle of scaphoid. The passage is between the flexor carpi radialis and the radial pedicle. (Reprinted from Gras and Mathoulin [20] and Mathoulin and Gras [21])

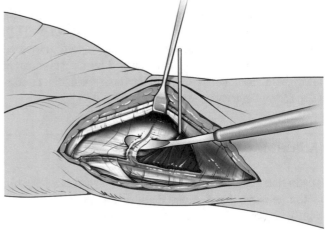

Fig. 43.3 Drawing showing the subperiosteal dissection of the lateral part of the pedicle. The wrist is in flexion with retraction of flexor pollicis longus and flexor carpi radialis tendons. The volar carpal artery is located in front of the superficial aponeurosis of pronator quadratus, running along the distal edge of the pronator quadratus. (Reprinted from Gras and Mathoulin [20] and Mathoulin and Gras [21])

inserted volarly in a distal to proximal direction, then a cannulated Herbert screw. The graft is introduced in the scaphoid defect (Fig. 43.6a, b), and if required can be secured through further screw tightening. A K-wire can be inserted through the scaphoid fragments and graft, in a direction parallel to the screw to avoid damaging the pedicle. Any bone gaps may be filled with additional cancellous bone graft har-

vested from the distal radius if needed. The position of the screw and fragments is checked with intraoperative X-rays (Fig. 43.7). Joint capsule and ligaments are sutured, with particular care to reconstitute the radioscaphocapitate ligament, and protecting the pedicle. The pronator quadratus muscle is sutured back into position. A suction drain is placed over the distal radius.

Immobilization of the wrist is maintained until radiological and clinical union. The average delay of union is about 10 weeks (Fig. 43.8a, b). The pin is removed at 3 weeks. Physiotherapy is gradually increased.

Tips and Tricks

- In case of smoking patient, the patient has to stop before the surgery and until union.
- In case of dorsal intercalated segmental instability (DISI), a temporary K-wire from radius to lunate can fix the reduction.
- A temporary K-wire can retract the distal fibers of pronator quadratus.
- The pedicle has to be dissected as far as possible, until the radial artery.
- Fracture of radius articular surface had been reported. The osteotome has to take an oblique direction to avoid this damage.
- Take care not to separate periosteum from the graft.
- The position of the screw is introduced in the scaphoid from distal to proximal by a volar approach, but as dor-

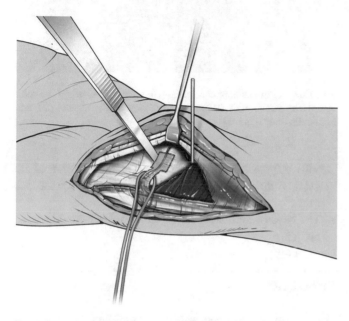

Fig. 43.4 Drawing showing the harvesting of the graft, using osteotome in oblique way, in order to avoid periosteal detachment from the graft and because the volar bone loss is classically in a pyramidal shape. (Reprinted from Gras and Mathoulin [20] and Mathoulin and Gras [21])

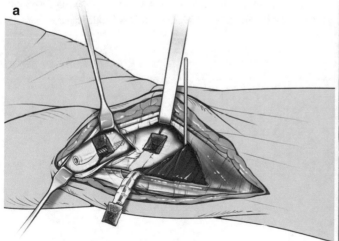
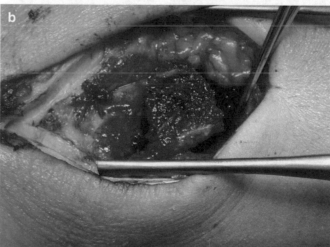

Fig. 43.5 (**a**) Drawing showing the graft harvested, with complete lateral dissection of the pedicle, in order to have a sufficient length. (**b**) Operating view showing in our presentation case, the important size of

vascularized bone graft. (Reprinted from Gras and Mathoulin [20] and Mathoulin and Gras [21])

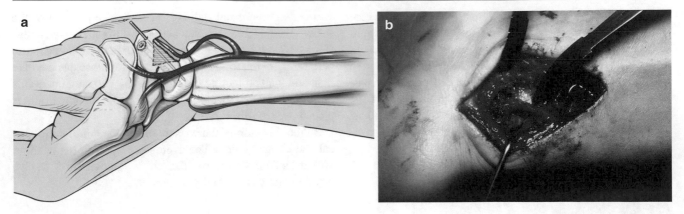

Fig. 43.6 (a) Drawing showing the vascularized bone graft put inside the volar bone defect of scaphoid. The scaphoid is fixed with a screw, and the graft is temporarily stabilized with a volar K-wire. (b) Operating view showing in our presentation case, the scaphoid filled by the volar vascularized bone graft. (Reprinted from Gras and Mathoulin [20] and Mathoulin and Gras [21])

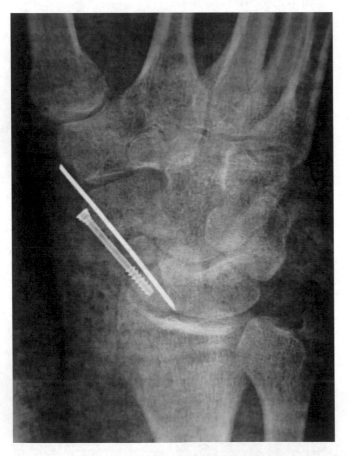

Fig. 43.7 Immediate postoperative frontal X-ray of our presentation case, with the graft perfectly in place into the scaphoid. We can check that the scaphoid humpback deformity is reduced and carpal height restored. (Reprinted from Gras and Mathoulin [20] and Mathoulin and Gras [21])

sally as possible in order to allow the introduction of the graft volarly. Too volar, the screw could expulse the graft.

- The capsule suture over the graft shouldn't compress the pedicle.

Conclusion

Volar vascularized bone graft is a good and reliable technique for scaphoid nonunion without periscaphoid arthritis. A retrospective study [20] showed better results (union rate, pain, and range of motion) in cases of primary than secondary vascularized graft.

According to the size of the defect, arthroscopic bone graft may be another alternative to this treatment.

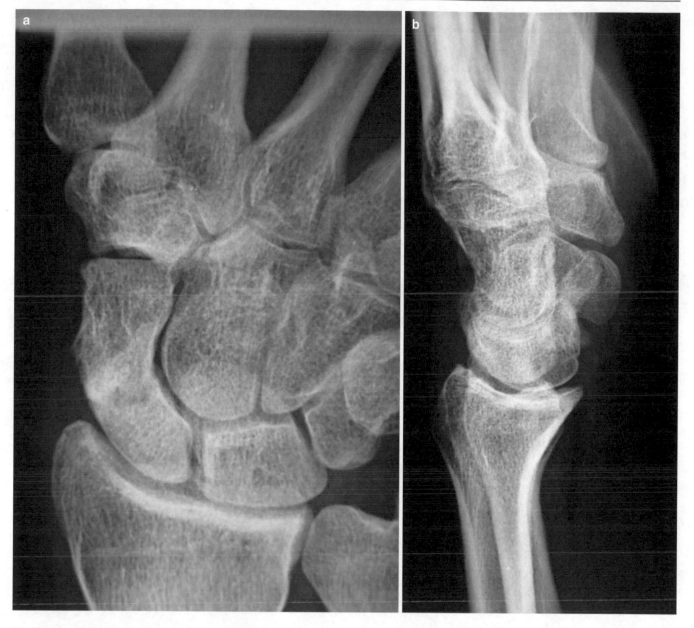

Fig. 43.8 (**a**) Frontal X-ray of our case presentation showing a perfect union at 6 months. (**b**) Lateral X-ray of our presentation case showing good reduction of preoperative adaptive DISI. (Reprinted from Gras and Mathoulin [20] and Mathoulin and Gras [21])

References

1. Kawamura K, Chung KC. Treatment of scaphoid fractures and nonunions. J Hand Surg Am. 2008;33(6):988–97.
2. Larson AN, Bishop AT, Shin AY. Dorsal distal radius vascularized pedicled bone grafts for scaphoid nonunions. Tech Hand Up Extrem Surg. 2006;10(4):212–23.
3. Ruby LK, Stinson J, Belsky MR. The natural history of scaphoid nonunion. A review of fifty-five cases. J Bone Joint Surg Am. 1985;67(3):428–32.
4. Megerle K, Keutgen X, Müller M, Germann G, Sauerbier M. Treatment of scaphoid nonunions of the proximal third with conventional bone grafting and mini-Herbert screws: an analysis of clinical and radiological results. J Hand Surg [Eur]. 2008;33(2):179–85.
5. Merrell GA, Wolfe SW, Slade JF 3rd. Treatment of scaphoid nonunions: quantitative meta-analysis of the literature. J Hand Surg Am. 2002;27(4):685–91.
6. Waitayawinyu T, Pfaeffle J, McCallister W, Nemechek N, Trumble T. Management of scaphoid nonunions. Hand Clin. 2010;26(1):105–17.
7. Borges CS, Ruschel PH, Pignataro MB. Scaphoid reconstruction. Orthop Clin North Am. 2020;51(1):65–76.
8. Sgromolo NM, Rhee PC. The role of vascularized bone grafting in scaphoid nonunion. Hand Clin. 2019;35(3):315–22.

9. Roy-Camille R. Fractures et pseudarthroses du scaphoïde carpien. Utilisation d'un greffon pédiculé. Actualité en chirurgie orthopédique. 1965;4:197–214.

10. Kawai H, Yamamoto K. Pronator quadratus pedicled bone graft for old scaphoid fractures. J Bone Joint Surg. 1988;70B:829–31.

11. Kuhlmann JN, Mimoun M, Boabighi A, Baux S. Vascularized bone graft pedicled on the volar carpal artery for nonunion of the scaphoid. J Hand Surg [Am]. 1987;12B:203–10.

12. Guimberteau JC, Panconi B. Recalcitrant nonunion of the scaphoid treated with a vascularized bone graft based on the ulnar artery. J Bone Joint Surg. 1990;72A:88–97.

13. Zaidemberg C, Siebert JW, Angrigiani C. A new vascularized bone graft for scaphoid nonunion. J Hand Surg [Am]. 1991;16A:474–8.

14. Mathoulin C, Haerle M, Vandeputte G. Greffon osseux vascularisé dans la reconstruction des os du carpe [Vascularized bone graft in carpal bone reconstruction]. Ann Chir Plast Esthet. 2005;50(1):43–8. French

15. Yuceturk A, Isiklar ZU, Tuncay C, Tandogan R. Treatment of scaphoid nonunions with a vascularized bone graft based on the first dorsal metacarpal artery. J Hand Surg [Am]. 1997;22B:425–7.

16. Brunelli F, Mathoulin C, Saffar P. Description d'un greffon osseux vascularisé prélevé au niveau de la tête du deuxième métacarpien [Description of a vascularized bone graft taken from the head of the 2nd metacarpal bone]. Ann Chir Main Memb Super. 1992;11(1):40–5. French

17. Pistré V, Réau AF, Pélissier P, Martin D, Baudet J. Les greffons osseux vascularisés pédiculés prélevés sur la main et le poignet: revue de la littérature et nouveau site donneur [Vascularized bone pedicle grafts of the hand and wrist: literature review and new donor sites]. Chir Main. 2001;20(4):263–71. French

18. Arora R, Lutz M, Zimmermann R, Pechlaner S, Gabl M. Free vascularised iliac bone graft for avascular scaphoid non-unions and Kienböck's disease. J Hand Surg Eur Vol. 2007;32(Supplement 1):75.

19. Mathoulin C, Haerle M. Vascularized bone graft from the palmar carpal artery for treatment of scaphoid non-union. J Hand Surg [Am]. 1998;23B:318–23.

20. Gras M, Mathoulin C. Vascularized bone graft pedicled on the volar carpal artery from the volar distal radius as primary procedure for scaphoid non-union. Orthop Traumatol Surg Res. 2011;97(8):800–6.

21. Mathoulin C, Gras M. Vascularized bone graft. In: Builze G, Jupiter J, editors. Scaphoid fractures: evidence-based management. Philadelphia: Elsevier; 2017.

Hamate to Scaphoid Transfer for Nonreconstructable Proximal Pole Scaphoid Fractures

44

Joshua A. Gillis, Bassem T. Elhassan, and Sanjeev Kakar

Introduction

Proximal pole scaphoid nonunions are difficult to reconstruct due to limited blood supply, fragmentation, and the need to reconstruct the scapholunate interosseous ligament (SLIL) [1]. If the articular cartilage remains viable with intact subchondral bone, bone graft can be used to attempt to achieve union [2]. The use of nonvascular bone graft with internal fixation is the most common treatment method for scaphoid nonunions [3]. This can be in the form of cancellous or corticocancellous graft and can be approached open or arthroscopically [4]. If there is evidence of avascular necrosis of the proximal pole, then a vascularized bone graft can be used to improve union rates such as the 1,2 intercompartmental suprarctinacular artery (1,2-ICSRA) flap [5–7], the volar distal radius based on the volar carpal artery [8], and the medial femoral condyle (MFC) flap [9]. If the proximal pole is fragmented or deemed nonreconstructable, non-vascularized and vascularized bone grafts have been described to replace the proximal pole, such as the proximal scaphoid allograft [10], rib (costo-osteochondral) autograft [2, 3, 11], medial femoral trochlear (MFT) bone flap [12, 13], and the proximal hamate autograft [1, 2].

The proximal hamate autograft treatment method limits the donor site to the same operative field, avoids incisions and morbidity associated with rib and knee autografts while also avoiding the use of microsurgery needed for free vascularized osteocartilaginous flaps. Due to the autologous nature of this graft, there is no risk of disease transmission or rejection as seen with osteocartilaginous allografts. Recent bio-mechanical studies have shown minimal effects upon midcarpal kinematics with harvest of the hamate up to the hook of the hamate [14]. In a majority of cases, the proximal hamate morphology is similar to the scaphoid and thus minimal contouring is needed to reconstruct the defect [1, 15]. Kakar et al. analyzed CT scans of 10 patients without carpal abnormalities and found that 60% of hamate autografts had over 90% surface correspondence to the scaphoid of less than 1 mm difference in the surfaces [15]. Wu et al. also performed an anthropometric assessment of proximal hamate autografts to proximal scaphoids in cadavers and found that 9 of 29 grafts had a poor match [16]. Of these 9 poor-fit cadavers, the hamate fragment was typically larger than the scaphoid and caused impaction on the dorsoradial aspect of the distal radius. The authors noted that hamates with smaller volar-dorsal (<10 mm) and radio-ulnar measurements would yield a better fit. Type I versus type II lunate morphology did not affect the fit of the graft [16].

During harvest of the proximal hamate, the volar capito-hamate (CH) ligament is taken with the graft, which is then used to reconstruct the dorsal SLIL by rotating the graft 180°. Biomechanically, the volar CH ligament is stronger than the dorsal CH ligament and thus can be used to reconstruct the more important dorsal SLIL [17, 18]. This can help to prevent dorsal intercalated segment instability (DISI) of the lunate after reconstruction. Other procedures such as the MFT may "overstuff" the scaphoid length and prevent the formation of a DISI deformity. In addition, with the use of the rib autograft, the SLIL is fixated to the perichondrium of the graft only, as opposed to the bone-ligament interface that exists with the volar CH ligament attachment to the hamate.

Indications

The proximal pole hamate autograft may be used to resurface the loss of the proximal osteochondral surface of the scaphoid due to nonunion and avascular necrosis. This is

J. A. Gillis
St. Joseph's Hospital, Roth McFarlane Hand and Upper Limb Centre, London, ON, Canada
e-mail: jgillis@DAL.CA

B. T. Elhassan · S. Kakar (✉)
Department of Orthopedic Surgery, Mayo Clinic, Rochester, MN, USA
e-mail: belhassan@partners.org; kakar.sanjeev@mayo.edu

© Springer Nature Switzerland AG 2022
W. B. Geissler (ed.), *Wrist and Elbow Arthroscopy with Selected Open Procedures*,
https://doi.org/10.1007/978-3-030-78881-0_44

most commonly used when there is significant fragmentation, necrosis, or degeneration of the proximal pole articular surface of the scaphoid with loss of the subchondral bone support that leads to cartilaginous collapse. In particular, it is useful when the fragments are sufficiently small to preclude reconstruction or conventional bone grafting. It can also be used when there has been a previous failed attempt at reconstruction with bone grafting, vascular or nonvascular, with or without internal fixation.

Contraindications

1. Radiocarpal arthritis (scaphoid nonunion advanced collapse [SNAC]).
2. Carpal collapse or significant intercalated instability.
3. Associated hamate arthrosis lunotriquetral ligament tear (HALT) or proximal arthrosis of the hamate (increased in type II lunates).
4. Preexisting midcarpal instability.

Technique

A preoperative CT scan with 3D reconstructions can assist analyzing the degree of proximal pole fragmentation, necrosis, and possibility of reconstruction or need for salvage. The CT can be used to determine if the proximal hamate segment would be an appropriate fit for the proximal scaphoid. 3D printing of the carpal bones may further help to determine the proper fit (Fig. 44.1). In addition, contraindications to the use of the proximal hamate autograft can be assessed.

The patient is placed supine on the operative table with the arm extended on an arm board with an upper arm tourniquet. A regional or general anesthetic is used. The arm is prepped and draped in sterile fashion.

Under tourniquet control, a dorsal longitudinal wrist incision is performed. The third extensor compartment is opened, and the extensor pollicis longus (EPL) tendon is retracted radially, along with the radial wrist extensors. The fourth extensor compartment is entered, and an ulnarly based retinacular flap is raised. A PIN neurectomy can be performed if there is any evidence of a PIN neuroma. A ligament-sparing capsulotomy is performed with the ulnar limb extended vertically from the triquetrum to the distal hamate to ensure appropriate exposure of the carpus [19]. The proximal scaphoid and lunate are visualized. If there is fragmentation, necrosis, or loss of the subchondral support, without any evidence of arthritis, then the proximal pole of the scaphoid is removed. The remaining portion of the scapholunate ligament is freed off the scaphoid, leaving it attached to the

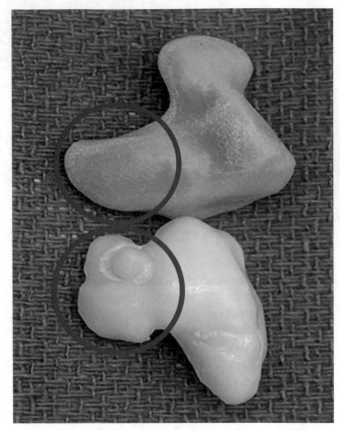

Fig. 44.1 3D-printed hamate (*top*) and scaphoid (*bottom*) bones where the hamate (pink) has been rotated 180°. Note similar morphology of the proximal poles of the hamate and scaphoid (red circles)

lunate. A limited radial styloidectomy can be performed as needed. Care is taken to not injure the volar radioscaphocapitate (RSC) and radiolunate ligaments during preparation of the scaphoid to prevent further carpal collapse or ulnar translocation. The proximal surface of the distal scaphoid is prepared to healthy corticocancellous bone using a sagittal saw or osteotome, while the tourniquet is deflated to identify punctate bleeding. The length, width, and depth of the scaphoid defect are measured.

The ipsilateral proximal hamate is harvested through the same capsular dissection. The osteotomy site is marked at the same height of the scaphoid defect, approximately 10 mm distal to the proximal tip of the hamate (Fig. 44.2) and should be proximal to the hook of the hamate. A retractor is placed under the hamate to protect underlying structures such as the ulnar neurovascular bundle and flexor tendons. Care is taken to protect the volar CH ligament during the osteotomy by placing an elevator in the triquetrohamate joint to visualize the osteotome during osteotomy (Fig. 44.2). Once excised, the autograft is rotated 180° horizontally so that the CH articular surface is now the scapholunate articular surface (Fig. 44.3). The proximal hamate

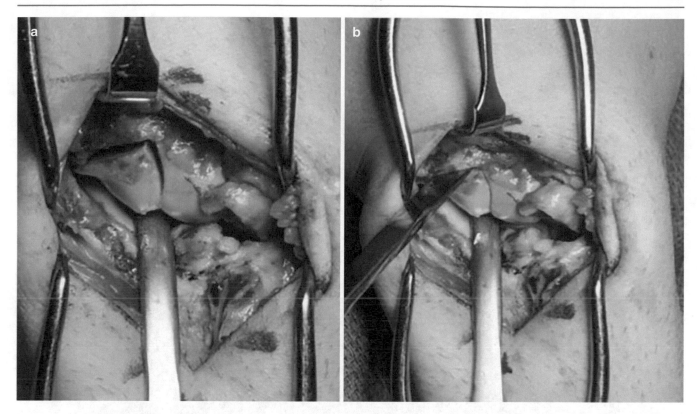

Fig. 44.2 Harvesting of the proximal hamate. (**a**) Placement of the osteotome 10 mm distal to the proximal tip of the hamate. (**b**) After osteotomy has been performed. Note the placement of a retractor underneath the hamate to prevent injury to underlying structures

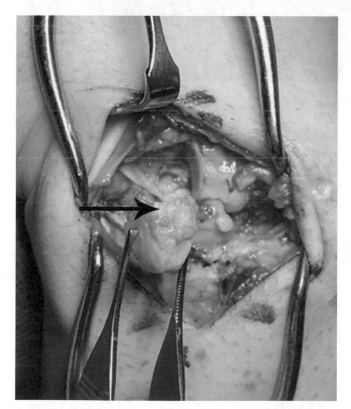

Fig. 44.3 Proximal hamate is rotated 180° such that the CH ligament (arrow) is sitting dorsally that will be repaired to the native scapholunate ligament (attached to the lunate)

becomes the proximal scaphoid, and the triquetrohamate articulation becomes the radioscaphoid articulation. The graft is trimmed to fit the defect and reduced with a temporary K-wire. The scapholunate, scaphocapitate, and radioscaphoid joints are checked to ensure proper geometry, and placement is adjusted as necessary. A derotational K-wire is placed, and the graft is fixated to the residual scaphoid using a headless compression screw (Fig. 44.4).

To reconstruct the SLIL, the lunate is reduced to neutral and stabilized with a K-wire through the capitolunate or radiolunate joints [20]. The scapholunate joint is then reduced, and the volar CH ligament, which is now dorsal, is repaired to the remnant of the SLIL on the dorsal lunate with a 2–0 nonabsorbable suture. A dorsal capsulodesis can be used to augment the repair using a distally based strip of the dorsal intercarpal ligament attached to the SLIL reconstruction, as needed. It is important to repair the capsular flap including the DIC and DRC ligaments. The capsule, retinaculum, and skin are sequentially closed.

Postoperative Care

A thumb spica splint is applied for 2 weeks, after which the patient is changed to a thumb spica cast for a further 6–8 weeks, or until a CT scan confirms union. The capitolu-

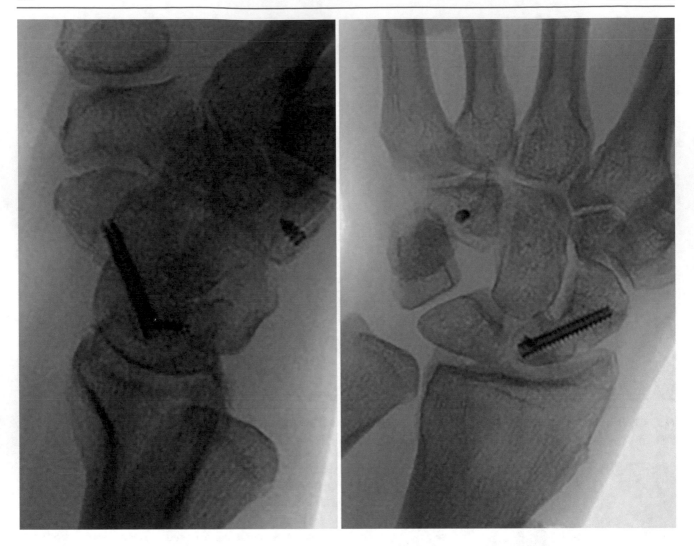

Fig. 44.4 Fluoroscopic views showing proximal hamate to scaphoid transfer after fixation

nate/radiolunate pin is then removed, and patient is placed in a removable wrist splint with progressive increase in motion and activities.

Outcomes

Options for reconstruction of the proximal scaphoid, when the articular surface cannot be repaired, include the proximal scaphoid allograft [10], rib costo-chondral autograft [2, 3, 11], MFT flap [12, 13], and the proximal hamate autograft. Carter et al. [10] described the use of a matched proximal scaphoid allograft in eight patients, four with true avascular necrosis, with a mean 8-month follow-up. All allografts achieved union between 6 and 12 months; however, two patients had persistent pain at final follow-up, one of which underwent a subsequent wrist arthrodesis [10].

Sandow [2] (2001) performed the rib costo-chondral autograft to resurface the proximal scaphoid in 47 patients

with a mean of 15-months follow-up. None of the patients were converted to a salvage procedure, with 85% of patients having good or excellent outcomes based on the Green and O'Brien Wrist Function Score [2]. They did not demonstrate any nonunion or graft displacement or DISI deformity. Yao et al. [3] also reported three cases of proximal scaphoid reconstruction using the rib autograft at a mean 58 months. All three patients improved, with minimal pain, no evidence of nonunion or DID, and a mean QuickDASH score of 17 [3].

Bürger et al. [12, 13] performed an osteochondral MFT reconstruction on 16 patients with proximal pole scaphoid nonunions with a mean of 14-months follow-up. All patients had improvement in their pain, with complete relief in 12 patients. There was no development of DISI, and union was achieved in 15 patients based on computed tomography (CT) scans [12].

Elhassan et al. [1] reported an 18-year-old male with previous ORIF of a proximal pole scaphoid fracture 12 months prior that progressed to a painful nonunion. The proximal hamate autograft was used to reconstruct the proximal scaphoid. At 3.5 years postreconstruction, the patient was pain free and working as a carpenter. His wrist motion improved from a 30° flexion/extension arc preoperatively to 60° of both flexion and extension with full forearm rotation at final follow-up. His grip strength was 110 kg on the operative side and 120 kg on the contralateral normal extremity postoperatively. His Mayo Wrist Score was 90, consistent with an excellent outcome. Radiographs demonstrated union with maintenance of the scapholunate alignment.

Complications

Potential complications of this procedure include but are not limited to malunion, nonunion, delayed union, carpal instability, and arthritis.

Tips and Tricks

- This procedure is designed for the treatment of the nonreconstructable proximal pole without evidence of arthritis. It is not intended for scaphoid waist nonunions.
- Use of the preoperative CT scan with 3D reconstructions will help determine if the morphology of the proximal hamate is a suitable donor.
- Ensure protection of the volar CH ligament during osteotomy of the hamate and protect the radiolunate and radioscaphocapitate ligaments when preparing the scaphoid to prevent ulnar translocation of the carpus.
- Preset a K-wire in the distal scaphoid which will help capture of the hamate graft when inset.
- Ensure appropriate contouring of the graft with the lunate in a reduced, neutral position.
- Repair the scapholunate ligament to the CH ligament after which a stout capsular closure including the DIC and DRC ligaments is advocated.
- Immobilize the wrist until CT confirmation of union.

Conclusion

The proximal hamate autograft is a feasible technique to reconstruct the proximal osteocartilaginous surface of the scaphoid in proximal pole nonunions not amenable to salvage of the cartilage shell. The proximal hamate autograft allows reconstruction of the proximal scaphoid and SLIL with minimal donor site morbidity, is within the same operative field and without the need for microsurgical reconstruction. Long-term follow-up studies are needed to monitor the outcomes of these patients.

References

1. Elhassan B, Noureldin M, Kakar S. Proximal scaphoid pole reconstruction utilizing Ipsilateral proximal hamate autograft. Hand. 2016;11(4):495–9.
2. Sandow MJ. Costo-osteochondral grafts in the wrist. Tech Hand Up Extrem Surg. 2001;5(3):165–72.
3. Yao J, Read B, Hentz VR. The fragmented proximal pole scaphoid nonunion treated with rib autograft: case series and review of the literature. J Hand Surg Am. 2013;38(11):2188–92.
4. Luchetti TJ, Rao AJ, Fernandez JJ, Cohen MS, Wysocki RW. Fixation of proximal pole scaphoid nonunion with nonvascularized cancellous autograft. J Hand Surg Eur Vol. 2018;43(1):66–72.
5. Steinmann SP, Bishop AT, Berger RA. Use of the 1,2 intercompartmental supraretinacular artery as a vascularized pedicle bone graft for difficult scaphoid nonunion. J Hand Surg Am. 2002;27(3):391–401.
6. Larson AN, Bishop AT, Shin AY. Dorsal distal radius vascularized pedicled bone grafts for scaphoid nonunions. Tech Hand Up Extrem Surg. 2006;10(4):212–23.
7. Shin AY, Bishop AT. Pedicled vascularized bone grafts for disorders of the carpus: scaphoid nonunion and Kienbock's disease. J Am Acad Orthop Surg. 2002;10(3):210–6.
8. Gras M, Mathoulin C. Vascularized bone graft pedicled on the volar carpal artery from the volar distal radius as primary procedure for scaphoid non-union. Orthop Traumatol Surg Res. 2011;97(8):800–6.
9. Larson AN, Bishop AT, Shin AY. Free medial femoral condyle bone grafting for scaphoid nonunions with humpback deformity and proximal pole avascular necrosis. Tech Hand Up Extrem Surg. 2007;11(4):246–58.
10. Carter PR, Malinin TI, Abbey PA, Sommerkamp TG. The scaphoid allograft: a new operation for treatment of the very proximal scaphoid nonunion or for the necrotic, fragmented scaphoid proximal pole. J Hand Surg Am. 1989;14(1):1–12.
11. Sandow MJ. Proximal scaphoid costo-osteochondral replacement arthroplasty. J Hand Surg Br. 1998;23(2):201–8.
12. Burger HK, Windhofer C, Gaggl AJ, Higgins JP. Vascularized medial femoral trochlea osteocartilaginous flap reconstruction of proximal pole scaphoid nonunions. J Hand Surg Am. 2013;38(4):690–700.
13. Higgins JP, Burger HK. Proximal scaphoid arthroplasty using the medial femoral trochlea flap. J Wrist Surg. 2013;2(3):228–33.
14. Kakar S, Greene RM, Hewett T, Thoreson AR, Hooke AW, Elhassan BT. The effect of proximal hamate osteotomy on carpal kinematics for reconstruction of proximal pole scaphoid nonunion with avascular necrosis. Hand (N Y). 2020;15(3):371–7. https://doi.org/10.1177/1558944718793175.
15. Kakar S, Greene RM, Elhassan BT, Holmes DR 3rd. Topographical analysis of the hamate for proximal pole scaphoid nonunion reconstruction. J Hand Surg Am. 2020;45(1):69.e1–7.
16. Wu K, Padmore C, Lalone E, Suh N. An anthropometric assessment of the proximal hamate autograft for scaphoid proximal pole reconstruction. J Hand Surg Am. 2019;44(1):60.e61–8.
17. Ritt MJ, Berger RA, Kauer JM. The gross and histologic anatomy of the ligaments of the capitohamate joint. J Hand Surg Am. 1996;21(6):1022–8.
18. Ritt MJ, Berger RA, Bishop AT, An KN. The capitohamate ligaments. A comparison of biomechanical properties. J Hand Surg Br. 1996;21(4):451–4.
19. Berger RA, Bishop AT, Bettinger PC. New dorsal capsulotomy for the surgical exposure of the wrist. Ann Plast Surg. 1995;35(1):54–9.
20. Linscheid RL, Rettig ME. The treatment of displaced scaphoid nonunion with trapezoidal bone graft. In: Masters techniques in orthopaedic surgery: the wrist. New York: Lippincott Williams & Wilkins; 1994. p. 119–31.

Proximal Pole Scaphoid Nonunion: Capsular-Based Vascularized Distal Radius Graft

Loukia K. Papatheodorou and Dean G. Sotereanos

Introduction

Several surgical techniques have been described for the management of scaphoid proximal pole nonunion; however, the treatment of proximal pole scaphoid nonunion especially with avascular necrosis represents a reconstructive challenge [1]. Vascularized bone grafts (VBGs) for the treatment of scaphoid proximal pole nonunion have demonstrated a more favorable union rate than the conventional bone grafts likely due to superior biologic and mechanical properties [1–3].

Many pedicled VBGs from the dorsal and volar aspect of the distal radius have been described for the treatment of scaphoid nonunion, including the VBG from distal radius based on the 1,2 intercompartmental supraretinacular artery (1,2-ICSRA) [4] and the VBG based on the palmar carpal artery [5] or the ulnar artery [6]. To avoid the need for dissection of small-caliber vessels or microsurgical anastomoses, Sotereanos et al. have described a dorsal capsular-based VBG from the distal radius for proximal pole scaphoid nonunions [7–9]. This graft is nourished by the fourth extensor compartmental artery (4 ECA) (Fig. 45.1), and it is harvested from a position that allows easy access to the proximal scaphoid pole [10].

Indications and Contraindications

The dorsal capsular-based VBG from the distal radius can be used for the management of symptomatic proximal pole scaphoid nonunion. It is also indicated for patients with avascular necrosis of the scaphoid proximal pole. This technique can be used for displaced proximal pole scaphoid fracture or scaphoid nonunions that have failed traditional bone grafting.

This graft is contraindicated in patients with scaphoid collapse with a humpback deformity or with advanced arthrosis (scaphoid nonunion advanced collapse (SNAC) wrist, stage II or greater). This technique is relative contraindicated in children and adolescents with remaining growth potential from the distal radial physis. A relative contraindication of this VBG is previous surgery or injury to the dorsal aspect of the wrist or distal radius which might damage the blood supply to the dorsal capsule.

Surgical Technique

The procedure is performed under general or regional anesthesia, tourniquet control, and loupe magnification. The patient is positioned supine with the affected arm placed on an arm table. After prepping and sterile draping, the extremity is exsanguinated with a sterile bandage and the tourniquet is inflated at 250 mm Hg. A 4-cm straight dorsal incision centered just ulnar to the Lister tubercle is performed. Dissection is carried through the subcutaneous tissues. The extensor retinaculum of the fourth dorsal compartment is partially released to expose the wrist capsule and the distal radius. The extensor pollicis longus tendon is identified and retracted radially, and the extensor digitorum communis tendons are retracted ulnarly.

The capsular-based vascularized distal radius graft is outlined with a skin marker on the dorsal wrist capsule. The flap is trapezoidal in shape with length of approximately 2 cm, and it widens from 1 cm at the radial bone block (proximal) to 1.5 cm at its base (distal) (Fig. 45.2a). Then, the capsular flap is outlined sharply with a knife. The bone graft is harvested from the distal aspect of the dorsal radius just ulnar and distal to Lister tubercle in a size approximately 1 cm × 1 cm, including the dorsal ridge of the distal radius

L. K. Papatheodorou
Department of Orthopaedic Surgery, University of Pittsburgh School of Medicine, Pittsburgh, PA, USA

D. G. Sotereanos (✉)
Department of Orthopaedic Surgery, University of Pittsburgh School of Medicine, Pittsburgh, PA, USA

University of Pittsburgh Medical Center, Pittsburgh, PA, USA

© Springer Nature Switzerland AG 2022
W. B. Geissler (ed.), *Wrist and Elbow Arthroscopy with Selected Open Procedures*,
https://doi.org/10.1007/978-3-030-78881-0_45

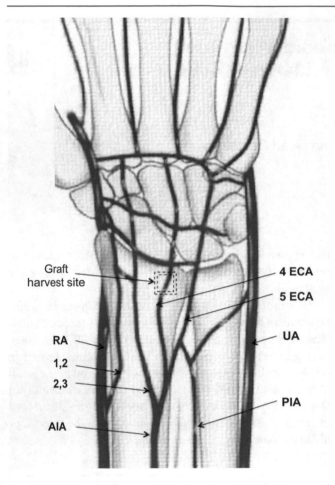

Fig. 45.1 Schematic diagram of the dorsal capsular-based bone graft harvest site and the vascular supply of the dorsal wrist. *4 ECA* fourth extensor compartment artery, *5 ECA* fifth extensor compartment artery, *1,2* 1,2 intercompartmental supraretinacular artery, *2,3* 2,3 intercompartmental supraretinacular artery, *UA* ulnar artery, *AIA* anterior interosseous artery, *PIA* posterior interosseous artery

(see Fig. 45.2a, b). The depth of the bone block is approximately 7 mm. The bone graft is outlined on the distal radius cortex with multiple drill holes using a 1.0-mm side-cutting drill bit. Using a thin osteotome, the bone graft is elevated with care to maintain 2–3 mm of the distal radius cortex intact to minimize the risk of propagation onto the articular cartilage of the radiocarpal joint. The bone graft with its capsular attachment is elevated from the underlying tissues in a proximal-to-distal direction with care to prevent detachment of the dorsal scapholunate ligament (see Fig. 45.2b).

Once the flap is elevated, attention is directed toward the scaphoid. The scaphoid proximal pole nonunion site is exposed by flexing the wrist. If a pseudarthrosis is present with disruption of the cartilage shell, the nonunion is cleaned with a dental pick and small curettes. It is important not to destabilize the nonunion site before scaphoid fixation; destabilization makes fixation extremely challenging. A small cannulated screw is used for the fixation of the scaphoid

proximal pole nonunion. With the wrist in extreme flexion, two 1-mm smooth Kirschner wires are inserted from the proximal pole of the scaphoid oriented toward the base of the thumb under fluoroscopic control. One Kirschner wire serves as a guidewire for a cannulated screw and the other serves as an anti-rotational wire. Care is taken to place the guidewire for the screw perpendicular to the fracture site and as volar as possible to enable dorsal placement of the graft. The length of the cannulated screw is determined, and the screw is inserted and buried underneath the articular surface by approximately 2 mm. Then, the anti-rotational wire is removed.

Once the fracture nonunion is secured, a dorsal trough is created across the scaphoid nonunion site in a nonarticular location using a side-cutting burr (Fig. 45.3). A micro suture anchor is placed at the floor of the trough to prevent dislodgement of the graft (see Fig. 45.3). Then, the capsular bone graft is gently inserted press-fit into the scaphoid trough with minimal rotation (10–30°) due to the close proximity of the graft donor site (Figs. 45.4 and 45.5). The graft is secured into the trough with a mattress stitch, from the suture anchor, which is passed through the perimeter of the graft periosteum. Care is taken to tie this stitch over the graft without compressing the pedicle. Hemostasis is obtained, and the wound is irrigated followed by routine closure in layers.

At the completion of the procedure, a short-arm thumb spica splint is applied with the wrist in neutral position for the first 2 weeks. At that time, the short-arm thumb spica splint is converted to a short-arm thumb spica cast for another 4 weeks. Then, a removable forearm-based thumb spica splint is used until solid union occurred. Radiographs are obtained with the cast removed 6 weeks postoperatively and monthly thereafter to assess union progression (Fig. 45.6). Return to full activities is permitted only after solid union occurs.

Outcomes

The dorsal capsular-based vascularized distal radius graft was designed to overcome the difficulties with graft harvesting and to avoid the need for microsurgical anastomoses. It is harvested from a position that allows easy access to the proximal scaphoid pole, and the short arc of rotation reduces the risk of vascular impairment caused by kinking of the nutrient vessel. Since 2000, we have used the capsular-based vascularized distal radius graft in more than 90 patients with proximal pole scaphoid nonunion with avascular necrosis in the majority of them [7–9]. Our results compare favorably to those of pedicled or free VBGs reported in the literature [1–4, 11, 12]. In our series, the overall union rate was 86%, and no patient developed donor site morbidity. Radiographic

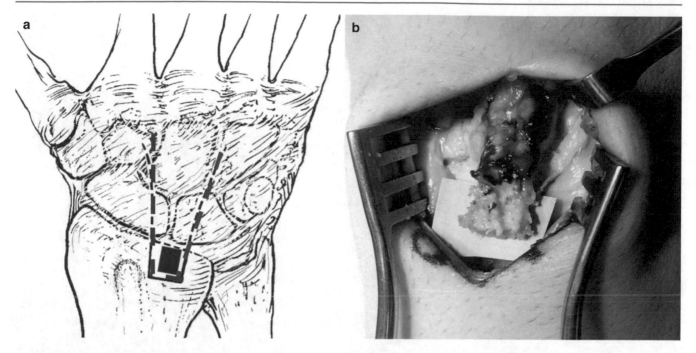

Fig. 45.2 (a) Schematic and intraoperative view of the dorsal capsular-based vascularized distal radius graft. (b) The capsular graft is outlined with red dotted line, and the bone graft is marked in blue

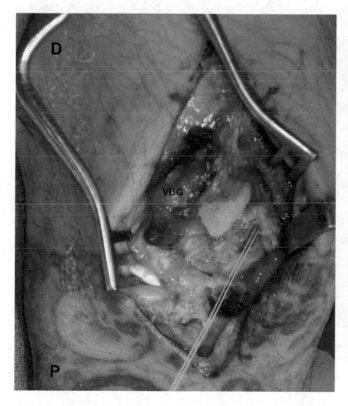

Fig. 45.3 A dorsal trough (blue dotted circle) is created across the scaphoid nonunion site, and a micro suture bone anchor (loaded with two nonabsorbable sutures) is placed deep into the scaphoid trough. *VBG* dorsal capsular-based vascularized distal radius graft, *P* proximal, *D* distal

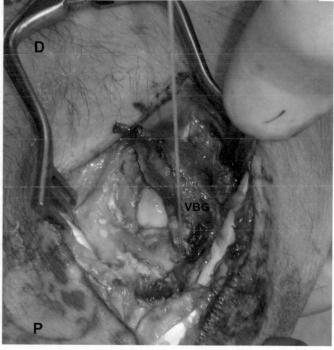

Fig. 45.4 The dorsal capsular-based vascularized distal radius graft (VBG) has been inserted into the scaphoid trough. *P* proximal, *D* distal

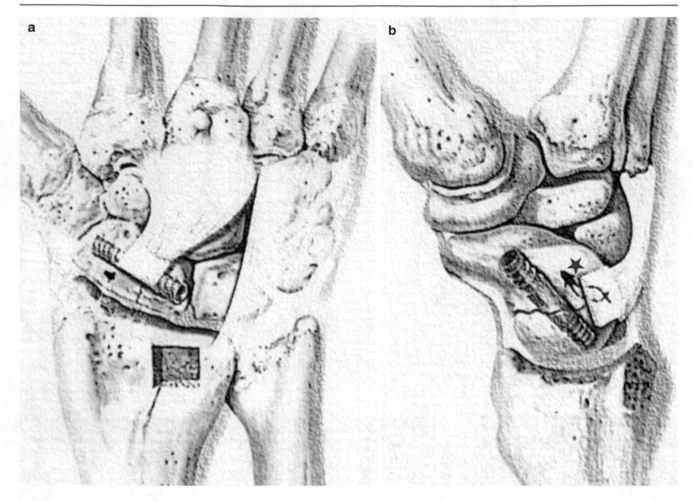

Fig. 45.5 Schematic diagram of the completed dorsal capsular-based vascularized distal radius graft. The microsuture bone anchor is marked with red asterisk. (**a**) Anteroposterior plane. (**b**) Lateral plane

evaluation revealed no arthritic changes at the dorsal ridge of the radius.

Tips and Tricks

- Leave intact 2–3 mm of the distal radius cortex to minimize the risk of an intra-articular fracture.
- Elevate the capsular flap gently, with care to prevent detachment of the dorsal scapholunate ligament.
- Full wrist flexion facilitates scaphoid proximal pole exposure.

- Insert 2 Kirschner wires from the scaphoid proximal pole toward the base of the thumb. One serves as an antirotational wire.
- Place a screw that is 6 mm shorter than measured to prevent penetration of the distal articular surface.
- Secure the graft with a micro suture anchor to avoid dislodgment in the early postoperative period.
- This technique is contraindicated for scaphoid nonunion with humpback deformity or scaphoid nonunion advance collapse wrist stage II or greater.

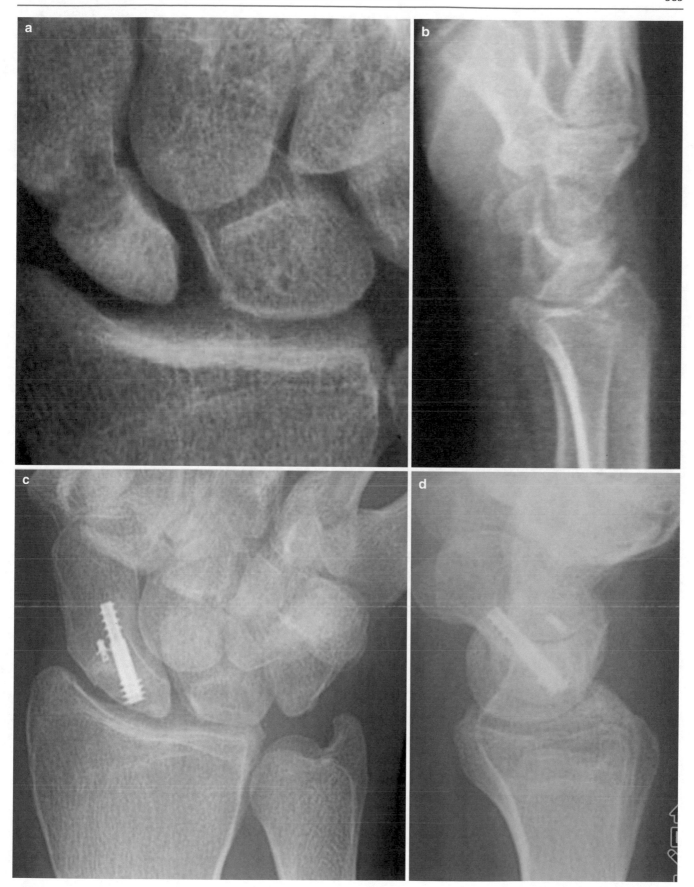

Fig. 45.6 (**a, b**) Anteroposterior and lateral radiographs of the wrist show a proximal pole scaphoid nonunion. (**c, d**) Anteroposterior and lateral radiographs at 6 months postoperatively show healing at the proximal pole scaphoid nonunion. Note the bone suture anchor next to the cannulated screw

Conclusion

Based on our experience, the dorsal capsular-based vascularized distal radius graft provides successful clinical outcomes in patients with proximal pole scaphoid nonunion. It is a simple technique and permits expedient harvesting without the need for dissection of small-caliber vessels or microsurgical anastomoses.

References

1. Pinder RM, Brkljac M, Rix L, Muir L, Brewster M. Treatment of scaphoid nonunion: a systematic review of the existing evidence. J Hand Surg Am. 2015;40(9):1797–1805.e3.
2. Merrell GA, Wolfe SW, Slade JF 3rd. Treatment of scaphoid nonunions: quantitative meta-analysis of the literature. J Hand Surg Am. 2002;27(4):685–91.
3. Munk B, Larsen CF. Bone grafting the scaphoid nonunion: a systematic review of 147 publications including 5,246 cases of scaphoid nonunion. Acta Orthop Scand. 2004;75(5):618–29.
4. Zaidemberg C, Siebert JW, Angrigiani C. A new vascularized bone graft for scaphoid nonunion. J Hand Surg Am. 1991;16(3):474–8.
5. Mathoulin C, Haerle M. Vascularized bone graft from the palmar carpal artery for treatment of scaphoid nonunion. J Hand Surg Br. 1998;23(3):318–23.
6. Guimberteau JC, Panconi B. Recalcitrant non-union of the scaphoid treated with a vascularized bone graft based on the ulnar artery. J Bone Joint Surg Am. 1990;72(1):88–97.
7. Sotereanos DG, Darlis NA, Dailiana ZH, Sarris IK, Malizos KN. A capsular-based vascularized distal radius graft for proximal pole scaphoid pseudarthrosis. J Hand Surg Am. 2006;31(4):580–7.
8. Venouziou AI, Sotereanos DG. Supplemental graft fixation for distal radius vascularized bone graft. J Hand Surg Am. 2012;37(7):1475–9.
9. Papatheodorou LK, Sotereanos DG. Treatment for proximal pole scaphoid nonunion with capsular-based vascularized distal radius graft. Eur J Orthop Surg Traumatol. 2019;29(2):337–42.
10. Dailiana ZH, Malizos KN, Urbaniak JR. Vascularized periosteal flaps of distal forearm and hand. J Trauma. 2005;58(1):76–82.
11. Chang MA, Bishop AT, Moran SL, Shin AY. The outcomes and complications of 1,2-intercompartmental supraretinacular artery pedicled vascularized bone grafting of scaphoid nonunions. J Hand Surg Am. 2006;31(3):387–96.
12. Waitayawinyu T, McCallister WV, Katolik LI, Schlenker JD, Trumble TE. Outcome after vascularized bone grafting of scaphoid nonunions with avascular necrosis. J Hand Surg Am. 2009;34(3):387–94.

Arthroscopic Assessment and Management of Kienböck's Disease

46

Duncan Thomas McGuire and Gregory Ian Bain

Introduction

Kienböck's disease is a debilitating condition resulting in avascular necrosis of the lunate. First described over 100 years ago by Robert Kienböck, the disease was initially thought to be caused by repetitive trauma to the wrist [1]. To this day, the precise etiology remains uncertain, although the theory that it is caused by a disruption of the blood supply to the lunate is well accepted. The exact cause of this disruption is unknown, although there are certain associated factors that have been identified.

Cadaveric studies have brought attention to the variable blood supply to the lunate [2]. The lunate receives its blood supply from vessels entering dorsally and volarly. In certain instances, the number of vessels entering the lunate may be fewer, possibly predisposing certain individuals to avascular necrosis of the lunate. Another theory postulates that increased venous pressure and disruption of venous outflow may be an etiological factor [3]. It is not clear, however, if this increased pressure contributes to the disease or is a secondary result of the disease.

The disease is more common in males, between the ages of 20 and 40 years. It often affects the dominant hand and is associated with negative ulnar variance. Patients typically present with wrist pain, swelling, restricted range of motion, and difficulty performing activities of daily living. For those patients who fail to improve with nonoperative modalities, surgical treatment is offered.

Historically, the radiological classification of Kienböck's disease developed by Lichtman et al. [4] has been used to classify the disease (Table 46.1), although its reliability has

Table 46.1 Lichtman classification of Kienböck's disease

Stage 1	Normal radiographs. Signal intensity changes on MRI scan
Stage 2	Sclerosis of the lunate on radiographs; fracture lines may be seen, but no collapse
Stage 3	Collapse of the lunate articular surface
Stage 3A	Normal carpal alignment and height
Stage 3B	Abnormal carpal alignment. Fixed scaphoid rotation, proximal capitate migration, and loss of carpal height
Stage 4	Collapse of the lunate associated with radiocarpal or midcarpal arthritis

been shown to be poor [5]. To improve the reliability of the classification, Goldfarb et al. proposed a modification to the classification system in which stage 3B was defined as a radioscaphoid angle greater than 60° [5]. This classification system is based on radiographic assessment and so does not take into consideration the condition of the cartilaginous articular surface.

Arthroscopy provides direct visualization of the articular cartilage and allows assessment of the radiocarpal and midcarpal joints. The disparity between radiographic and arthroscopic assessment has been highlighted by Ribak, who reported that plain radiographs correlated poorly with arthroscopic findings [6]. This was reinforced by Bain and Begg, who reported that it was not uncommon for plain radiographs to underscore the severity of the articular involvement identified with arthroscopy [7].

The Role of Wrist Arthroscopy

In 1999 Menth-Chiari et al. first described the use of wrist arthroscopy for the treatment of Kienböck's disease [8]. Their model was to use arthroscopy to assess the articular surfaces, to debride the necrotic lunate, and to perform a limited synovectomy. In their study, all patients were either

D. T. McGuire (✉)
Department of Orthopaedic Surgery, Groote Schuur Hospital, Cape Town, South Africa

G. I. Bain
Department of Orthopaedic Surgery, Flinders University of South Australia, Adelaide, SA, Australia
e-mail: greg@gregbain.com.au

© Springer Nature Switzerland AG 2022
W. B. Geissler (ed.), *Wrist and Elbow Arthroscopy with Selected Open Procedures*,
https://doi.org/10.1007/978-3-030-78881-0_46

Lichtman grade IIIA or IIIB, and all experienced relief of their painful mechanical symptoms.

Wrist arthroscopy has become a valuable assessment and primary treatment tool in the treatment of Kienböck's disease. The authors use arthroscopy to perform the initial debridement and to identify the nonfunctional joints to tailor the surgical reconstruction to the anatomic findings [7]. This system uses direct visual assessment of the articulations of the lunate and a probe to assess the degree of softening of the articular surfaces. Correlating this arthroscopic assessment with traditional investigations helps the clinician make better-informed management decisions. The advantage is that functional joint surfaces determine treatment.

Arthroscopic Technique

Wrist arthroscopy is performed using the standard technique. The patient is placed supine with their arm on an arm board. A tourniquet is used. Traction is applied from a tower mounted on the opposite side of the bed, and the arm is suspended using finger traps. A counter traction weight of 4 kg is attached to a sling and draped over the tourniquet on the patient's upper arm. Standard 3/4, 6R, and midcarpal portals are used.

The articular surface of the lunate is examined from the radiocarpal and the midcarpal joint. The articular surface is probed. If there is a subchondral fracture, then the cartilage will be soft, indicating a floating articular surface. The articular surfaces of the lunate facet of the distal radius and the head of the capitate are also inspected and probed. Fracture of the lunate may be identified and any loose bodies are removed. Synovitis is identified. If no further surgery is planned the joint is debrided.

Pathological Phases of Kienböck's Disease

Avascular necrosis of the lunate consists of three pathological phases: vascular (early), osseous (intermediate), and chondral (late) [9] (Fig. 46.1).

Early Vascular

Changes in the lunate commence with ischemia, subsequent necrosis, and revascularization. Magnetic resonance imaging (MRI) and bone scan are of value in interpreting the vascular changes.

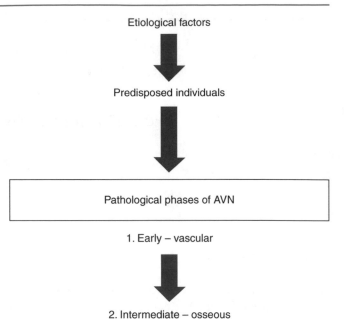

Fig. 46.1 The pathological phases of Kienböck's disease showing the association between the vascular, osseous, and chondral phases. (Reprinted from Bain and Durrant [9]. With permission of Wolters Kluwer Health)

Intermediate Osseous

Lichtman has described this phase well over the last 36 years. Computed tomography (CT) scan is of value and it demonstrates well the detail of the osseous changes [10]. The initial radiological changes are of sclerosis, followed by subchondral collapse. Multiple faults or plates occur in the trabeculae and when the formation of these outstrips the repair, the blood supply may be disrupted and result in bone necrosis [11]. It has been shown that the trabecular structure of lunates affected by Kienböck's disease is different from that of normal lunates. The trabeculations are denser and thicker, whereas the surface area and volume are lower [12] (Fig. 46.2a).

It is the authors' opinion that the subchondral bone plate is likely to be the critical part of the process of avascular necrosis, and that its survival is the key to the prognosis of articular cartilage, lunate, and the wrist. The normal lunate has longitudinal trabeculae that give axial support and prevent collapse of the bone during loading. As a result of the avascular necrosis, the trabeculae collapse and this leads to loss of height of the lunate and shortening of the carpus. In

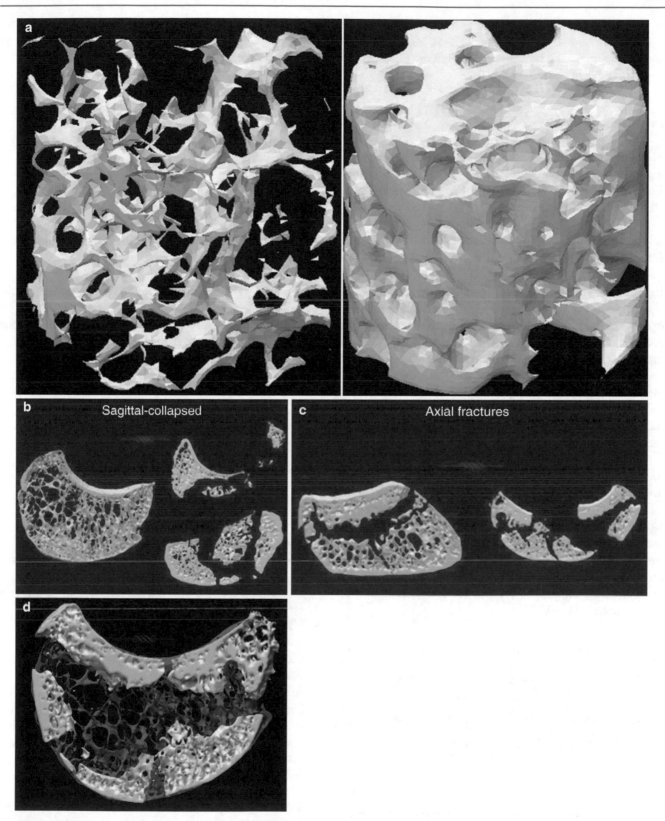

Fig. 46.2 (**a**) Micro CT scan of normal bone on the *left* and bone from a lunate affected by Kienböck's disease on the *right*. Note how the avascular, necrotic bone has larger, thicker trabeculae and is denser. (**b**) Sagittal micro CT images showing a normal lunate on the *left* and necrotic, collapsed lunates with multiple fractures on the *right*. (**c**) Sagittal micro CT images of avascular lunates with multiple fractures. The lunate on the *left* has a shear fracture in the axial plane. The fracture line has occurred at the junction between the hard bone of the subchondral bone plate and the weakened cancellous bone in the center. (**d**) Micro CT scan of the fragmented avascular lunate superimposed on a micro CT of a normal lunate. The bone of the hard subchondral bone plate is still present but there is loss of the longitudinal trabeculae, which leads to collapse and carpal shortening. (Courtesy of Dr. Gregory Ian Bain)

addition to the longitudinal collapse, shear fractures may occur with normal physiological loads, and with more advanced disease fractures occur through the proximal subchondral bone plate (Fig. 46.2b–d).

Late Chondral

The articular cartilage is often soft and can be indented, giving the impression that the articular surface has a false floor. The chondral changes will be described in more detail in the classification below.

Arthroscopic Classification

Bain and Begg first described their arthroscopic classification in 2006 [7]. This is based on the number of nonfunctional articular surfaces. The authors defined a normal articular surface as having a normal glistening appearance or minor fibrillation, with normal hard subchondral bone on probing. A nonfunctional articular surface is defined as having any one of the following: extensive fibrillation, fissuring, localized or extensive articular loss, a floating articular surface, or fracture. The number of nonfunctional articular surfaces determines the grade.

The authors observed a consistent pattern of changes in the lunate. This was based on MRI, plain radiographs, and arthroscopy. The changes always first occurred on the proximal articular surface of the lunate. The more severe cases would develop a subchondral fracture and these would have secondary chondral changes in the lunate facet of the radius. Involvement of the distal articular surface of the lunate was rare, except if a coronal fracture extended through to the surface, or in late cases. The classification was based on these observations (Fig. 46.3).

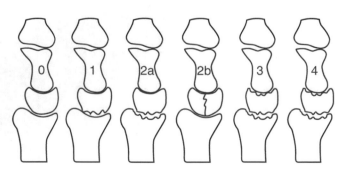

Fig. 46.3 The Bain and Begg arthroscopic classification of Kienböck's disease. The number of nonfunctional articular surfaces determines the grade. The grading system assists the surgeon to determine the best surgical option, based on the pathoanatomical findings. Although the classification was established based on arthroscopic findings, the grading can be determined based on imaging modalities. (Reprinted from Bain and Durrant [9]. With permission of Wolters Kluwer Health)

Grade 0

All articular surfaces are functional.

Grade 1

One nonfunctional articular surface—usually the proximal articular surface of the lunate.

Grade 2

Two nonfunctional articular surfaces. Divided into types A and B.

- Grade 2A: The proximal lunate and the lunate facet of the radius.
- Grade 2B: Proximal articular surface of the lunate and distal articular surface of the lunate.

Grade 3

Three nonfunctional articular surfaces—the lunate facet of the radius, proximal, and distal articular surfaces of the lunate, with a preserved head of capitate.

Grade 4

All four articular surfaces are nonfunctional.
The authors have noted the following observations [9]:

- The degree of synovitis correlates with the degree of articular damage.
- The severity of articular changes is underestimated by plain radiographs.
- Findings at arthroscopy commonly change the initial treatment plan.
- In certain cases, the articular cartilage envelope remains intact with collapse of the subchondral bone plate. This is an important subgroup where the lunate has probably revascularized. In these patients, particularly if they are young, conservative treatment may be considered, as there is potential to heal and stabilize.

Tatebe et al. performed a retrospective review of 57 patients with Kienböck's disease who had undergone wrist arthroscopy [13]. Each case was classified using the Bain and Begg classification and the number of cases of each grade is summarized in Table 46.2. They found that the number of articular surfaces involved did not correlate with

Table 46.2 Patient summary from Tatebe et al. [13]

Bain and Begg classification	
Grade	Number of cases
Grade 0	2
Grade 1	14
Grade 2	22
Grade 2A	9
Grade 2B	13
Grade 3	18
Grade 4	1

Adapted from Tatebe et al. [13]. With permission from Springer Verlag

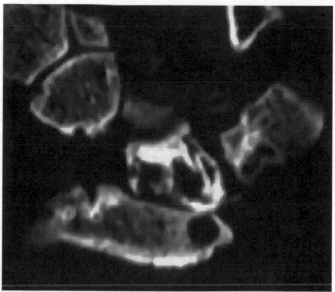

Fig. 46.5 CT scan of the wrist showing sclerosis and fragmentation of the lunate. The bone-on-bone appearance with complete loss of joint space indicates that there must be full thickness loss of the articular cartilage of the lunate and lunate facet. Arthroscopy will be of value to assess the midcarpal joint involvement before determining the best surgical reconstructive procedure. (Reprinted from Bain and Durrant [9]. With permission of Wolters Kluwer Health)

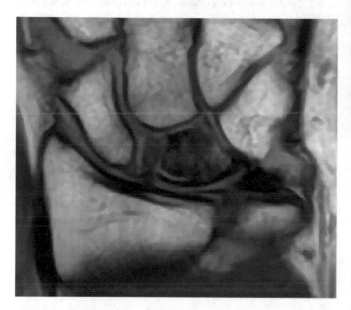

Fig. 46.4 MRI scan showing the lunate with fragmentation and a subchondral fracture extending distally. The articular cartilage has some irregularity. At this stage, the resolution of the articular cartilage is not really sufficient to recommend treatment and therefore, arthroscopy is essential to identify the integrity of the articular surface. (Reprinted from Bain and Durrant [9]. With permission of Wolters Kluwer Health)

either the Lichtman radiographic stage or the duration from onset to surgery. They did note a correlation between the number of nonfunctional articular surfaces and older age of the patient. Their conclusions were that the proximal articular surface of the lunate is usually affected, and that older patients had more nonfunctional articular surfaces.

Imaging modalities other than arthroscopy may be used to assess the articular cartilage. As the resolution of MRI continues to improve it may become a suitable standard to assess the articular surfaces prior to reconstructive surgery (Fig. 46.4). CT scans may demonstrate bone-on-bone articulations, which implies loss of cartilage and a nonfunctional articular surface (Fig. 46.5).

Articular-Based Approach to Treatment

Traditionally, Kienböck's disease has been managed based on the radiological osseous findings as defined by the Lichtman classification. However, the extent of the disease may be better understood after arthroscopy, and so the authors have used an articular-based approach to determine surgical treatment. At arthroscopy, functional and nonfunctional articular surfaces are identified and the Bain and Begg Classification determined. The principles of surgical treatment are to remove the nonfunctional surfaces and to leave the carpus articulating with functional articular surfaces, while maintaining a functional range of motion.

When discussing treatment options with the patient, the options of operative and nonoperative management should be offered. It would be common to start with conservative treatment using a wrist splint and activity modification. If the patient elects to proceed with surgery the authors obtain informed consent for the arthroscopy and the reconstruction procedure. The option of an arthroscopy without a reconstructive procedure is also discussed. An isolated arthroscopy and debridement are usually performed in those patients with Grade 0 or in patients with very advanced disease who do not want a full wrist fusion (Grade 4).

Grade 0

All articular surfaces are functional. An arthroscopic debridement and synovectomy are performed. Further treatment may involve an unloading procedure, revascularization, core decompression, or bone grafting.

An unloading procedure is performed extraarticularly. In the presence of negative ulnar variance, a radial shortening osteotomy is performed. For neutral or positive ulnar variance, a capitate shortening procedure can be performed.

A revascularization procedure or an arthroscopic decompression may also be considered. Arthroscopic core decompression has been described for this phase of the disease [14]. It is recommended only for patients with neutral or positive ulnar variance, who have grade 0 disease (Fig. 46.6).

Bone grafting of the necrotic lunate may be performed and this may be done as an arthroscopic procedure. In a technique described by Pegoli et al., the lunate is drilled at a site near the dorsal insertion of the lunotriquetral ligament after it has been confirmed that the articular cartilage is uninvolved [15]. The necrotic lunate is debrided with a motorized shaver. Osteoscopy is then performed by inserting the scope into the lunate bone to confirm adequate debridement [7]. Cancellous bone graft is harvested from the volar surface of the distal radius and inserted into the lunate through a trocar.

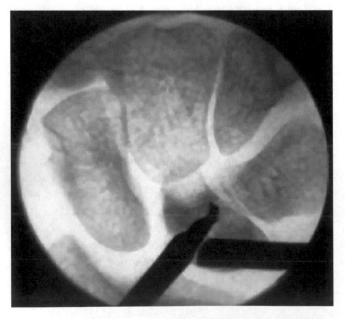

Fig. 46.6 Arthroscopic core decompression of the lunate under fluoroscopic guidance in a patient with an arthroscopic grade 0 Kienböck's disease. (Reprinted from Bain and Durrant [9]. With permission of Wolters Kluwer Health)

Grade 1

These patients have a nonfunctional proximal lunate articular surface. Treatment involves either a proximal row carpectomy (PRC) or a radioscapholunate (RSL) fusion.

Grade 2A

The proximal articular surface of the lunate and the lunate fossa are both nonfunctional. A RSL fusion removes both nonfunctional articular surfaces and enables the wrist to articulate through the normal midcarpal joint. The head of the capitate and distal lunate articular surface are uninvolved.

Grade 2B

The proximal and distal articular surfaces of the lunate are nonfunctional. This usually occurs when there is a coronal or sagittal fracture of the lunate extending between the radiocarpal and midcarpal joints. The articular surfaces of the lunate fossa of the radius and the head of the capitate are normal. A PRC is the treatment of choice. More complex procedures such as internal fixation or vascularized bone grafting tend to have poor results [7, 16].

Grade 3

Three articular surfaces are nonfunctional. Most likely it will be the capitate articular surface, which remains functional. This usually requires a salvage procedure such as a total wrist fusion or arthroplasty. An alternative option is a resurfacing hemi-arthroplasty of the distal radius that would articulate with the head of the capitate. However, the results of this procedure are not yet established (Fig. 46.7).

Grade 4

All four articular surfaces are nonfunctional. A total wrist fusion or arthroplasty is indicated.

PRC and RSL fusions are the preferred motion preserving, reconstructive procedures because they maintain the stability of the wrist, and allow a functional range of motion to be maintained [17]. If the head of the capitate is pointed, then a PRC may not be a good option, as the articulation with the lunate fossa of the distal radius may then not be congruent, and result in loading over a smaller area. This may occur in patients with a type 2 lunate, which has two distal facets, one

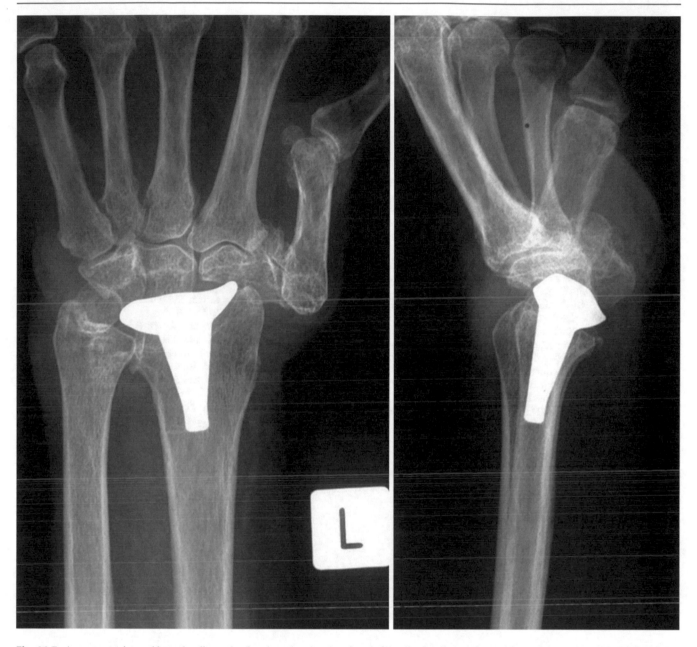

Fig. 46.7 Anteroposterior and lateral radiographs showing a hemi-arthroplasty of the distal radius performed for a patient with grade 3 Kienböck's disease

for the capitate and the other for the hamate [18]. In this case a RSL fusion may be preferred.

A RSL fusion provides a congruent articulation, but requires arthrodesis of the distal radius to the necrotic proximal lunate, which may result in a non-union. For this reason, the authors excise the proximal half of the lunate so that the fusion is from the radius to the viable distal half of the lunate [19]. This is more challenging than a conventional RSL fusion. The surgery is performed using two 1.1-mm Kirschner wires to stabilize the lunate to the scaphoid. The scapholunate unit is then fixed to the radius using Kirschner wires, small inter-fragmentary screws or staples. The triquetrum

and the distal half of the scaphoid are excised to increase the range of movement (ROM), which has been confirmed by cadaver studies [19].

Scapho-trapezoid-trapezium and scaphocapitate fusions have not been included in the treatment options because these fusions compromise the loading and kinematics of the radioscaphoid facet and have a high complication rate [20].

The approach that is presented in this paper respects the articular cartilage in patients with Kienböck's disease. It places at the front of the decision making process the patho-anatomical aspects of the articular cartilage. Regardless of the method of assessment of the articular cartilage, what is important is to assess the articular surfaces involved and to design the most appropriate procedure, taking into account the individual's pathoanatomical findings.

Although this approach was developed for vascular necrosis of the lunate, it does in principle apply to other joints in which avascular necrosis occurs.

References

1. Irisarri C. Aetiology of Kienböck's disease. J Hand Surg Br. 2004;29(3):281–7.
2. Lutsky K, Beredjiklian PK. Kienböck disease. J Hand Surg Am. 2012;37(9):1942–52.
3. Beredjiklian PK. Kienbock's disease. J Hand Surg Am. 2009;34(1):167–75.
4. Lichtman DM, Mack GR, MacDonald RI, Gunther SF, Wilson JN. Kienbock's disease: the role of silicone replacement arthroplasty. J Bone Joint Surg Am. 1977;59(7):899–908.
5. Goldfarb CA, Hsu J, Gelberman RH, Boyer MI. The Lichtman classification for Kienbock's disease: an assessment of reliability. J Hand Surg Am. 2003;28(1):74–80.
6. Ribak S. The importance of wrist arthroscopy for staging and treatment of Kienbock's disease. Presented at the 10th Triennial Congress of the International Federation of Societies for Surgery of the Hand, Sydney; March 2007.
7. Bain GI, Begg M. Arthroscopic assessment and classification of Kienbock's disease. Tech Hand Up Extrem Surg. 2006;10:8–13.
8. Menth-Chiari WA, Poehling GG, Wiesler ER, Ruch DS. Arthroscopic debridement for the treatment of Kienbock's disease. Arthroscopy. 1999;15:12–9.
9. Bain GI, Durrant A. An articular-based approach to Kienböck avascular necrosis of the lunate. Tech Hand Up Extrem Surg. 2011;15(1):41–7.
10. Quenzer DE, Linscheid RL, Vidal MA, Dobyns JH, Beckenbaugh RD, Cooney WP. Trispiral tomographic staging of Kienbock's disease. J Hand Surg Am. 1997;22(3):396–403.
11. Watson HK, Guidera PM. Aetiology of Kienbock's disease. J Hand Surg Br. 1997;22:5–7.
12. Han KJ, Kim YJ, Chung NS, Lee HR, Lee YS. Trabecular microstructure of the human lunate in Kienböck's disease. J Hand Surg Eur. 2012;37:336–41.
13. Tatebe M, Hirata H, Shinohara T, Yamamoto M, Okui N, Kurimoto S, Imaeda T. Arthroscopic findings of Kienböck's disease. J Orthop Sci. 2011;16(6):745–8.
14. Bain GI, Smith ML, Watts AC. Arthroscopic core decompression of the lunate in early stage Kienböck disease of the lunate. Tech Hand Up Extrem Surg. 2011;15:66–9.
15. Pegoli L, Ghezzi A, Cavalli E, Luchetti R, Pajardi G. Arthroscopic assisted bone grafting for early stages of Kienböck's disease. Hand Surg. 2011;16(2):127–31.
16. Lichtman DM. A classification-based treatment algorithm for Kienböck's disease - current and future considerations. Tech Hand Up Extrem Surg. 2011;15:41–7.
17. Palmer AK, Werner FW, Murphy D, Glisson R. Functional wrist motion: a biomechanical study. J Hand Surg Am. 1985;10(1):39–46.
18. Viegas SF. The lunatohamate articulation of the midcarpal joint. Arthroscopy. 1990;6(1):5–10.
19. Bain GI, Ondimu P, Hallam P, Ashwood N. Radioscapholunate arthrodesis – a prospective study. Hand Surg. 2009;14:73–82.
20. McAuliffe JA, Dell PC, Jaffe R. Complications of intercarpal arthrodesis. J Hand Surg Am. 1993;18(6):1121–8.

Pyrocarbon Lunate Replacement in Advanced Keinbock's Disease

William B. Geissler and Jarrad A. Barber

Introduction

Once met with poor outcomes, advances in implant material technology, such as the use of pyrocarbon, have allowed lunate arthroplasty to be a valuable tool in the armamentarium of treatment options for late-stage Kienbock's disease.

Historical Perspective

Early results for silicon replacement arthroplasty of the lunate were quite promising as Lichtman demonstrated in 1977 and 1982 [1, 2]. As more long-term results accrued, this early optimism has since been abandoned, chiefly because of long-term particulate synovitis [3]. At present, silicone replacement arthroplasty is not recommended.

Since that time, a number of options for late stage treatment (Stage IIIA, IIIB, and IV) have been developed. Among these, radial shortening osteotomy with or without vascularized bone graft, lunate excision with interposition allograft, capitate lengthening, isolated proximal row carpectomy, and lunate arthroplasty have all shown to improve outcomes.

For the purpose of this chapter, we will discuss modern pyrocarbon lunate arthroplasty and recent results, as well the author's preferred technique and pearls.

Modern Lunate Arthroplasty

Initially in 1997, Swanson and his colleagues tried to improve upon the shortcomings of silicon arthroplasty when they published their results on titanium implant arthroplasty. In their cohort of 21 patients, with follow-up ranging from 1 to 9 years, 19 obtained excellent pain relief and were able to return to their pre-operative level of activities. Postoperative grip strength was shown to improve significantly, increasing by 66% compared to pre-operative values [4].

Along with these positive values, this group demonstrated maintenance of carpal height and congruity along with none of the adverse bone or soft tissue changes that had been seen previously in the silicon replacement arthroplasty patients.

Recently, Viljakka, Tallroth, and Vastamäki published their promising outcomes on 11 patients who underwent titanium lunate arthroplasty with an average follow-up of 11 years [5]. Six of their patients were Lichtman stage IIIA and the remaining five were IIIB. They demonstrated quite low visual analog score at rest (0.5), night (0.3), and exertion (2.7) with an average Disabilities of the Arm, Shoulder, and Hand (DASH) score of 9.6. In their study, two patients were qualified as a failure due to dorsal dislocation. Interestingly, one of these patients continued working at his same position at his final follow-up, while the other retired due to old age, leading one to question the clinical significance of these failures.

Indications

Indications for pyrocarbon lunate arthroplasty are pain with wrist exertion accompanied by moderate-to-severe collapse of the lunate as seen on pre-operative imaging. This can apply to both Lichtman stage IIIB lunates and stage IIIA in patients with neutral or positive ulnar variance, limiting the ability to perform a radial shortening osteotomy.

W. B. Geissler
Division of Hand and Upper Extremity Surgery, Section of Arthroscopic Surgery and Sports Medicine, Department of Orthopedic Surgery and Rehabilitation, University of Mississippi Medical Center, Jackson, MS, USA

J. A. Barber (✉)
Department of Orthopaedics, Harbin Clinic, Rome, GA, USA

© Springer Nature Switzerland AG 2022
W. B. Geissler (ed.), *Wrist and Elbow Arthroscopy with Selected Open Procedures*,
https://doi.org/10.1007/978-3-030-78881-0_47

Contraindications

Contraindications to surgery are active infection of any kind; stage IV Kienbock's; muscular, neurologic, tendon disorder, or vascular diseases compromising the affected extremity; poor skin quality at the site of surgery secondary to, for instance, poorly controlled psoriasis; radial scaphoid arthritis; and gross carpal instability.

Surgical Technique

Recently, the author has begun performing pyrocarbon lunate arthroplasty for end-stage Kienbock's with good unpublished outcomes (Figs. 47.1, 47.2, 47.3). The advantage of this procedure is the replication of normal anatomy and preservation of options if salvage operations are later required.

The operation is carried out under tourniquet control and begins with a 10-cm skin incision on the dorsum of the wrist. Sharp dissection is carried down to the fascia and the skin flaps are elevated. The extensor pollicis longus is identified and released from the third compartment. The second and fourth dorsal compartments are then elevated. The extensor digitorum quinti is identified and released in the fifth compartment. A radial-based dorsal capsular flap is made exposing the lunate, which often can be quite necrotic and in multiple fragments (Figs. 47.4 and 47.5). The lunate is then removed. The articular cartilage of the capitate and the lunate fossa are inspected to ensure that there are no defects. The tendon of the extensor carpi radialis longus (ECRL) is released off the base of the index metacarpal, approximately 10 cm of the ulnar half of that tendon is harvested. The remaining tendon of the ECRL is preserved and 2–0 FiberWire (Arthrex, Naples, FL) is used in a modified Krakow fashion in preparation for dynamic transfer to the scaphoid. A burr hole is then made in the distal pole scaphoid for tendon transfer of the ECRL of the remaining intact ECRL.

The lunate is then sized and drill holes are made in the volar and dorsal part of the scaphoid and triquetrum for passage of the graft and suture. A #2 FiberWire is placed in the volar holes of the scaphoid through the implant into the volar hole of the triquetrum (Fig. 47.6). The harvested graft from

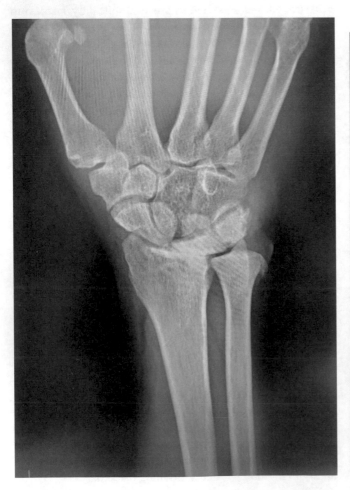

Fig. 47.1 Anterior–posterior radiograph demonstrating complete collapse of the lunate

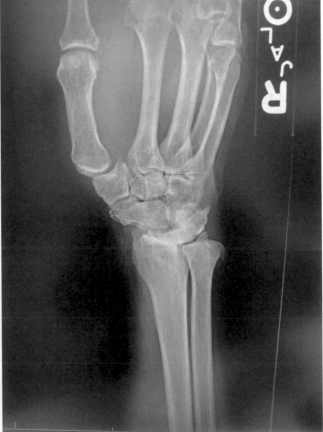

Fig. 47.2 Oblique radiograph demonstrating complete collapse of the lunate

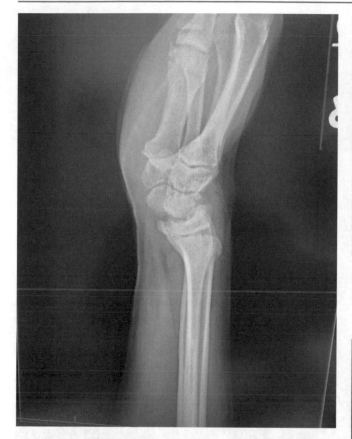

Fig. 47.3 Lateral photograph showing flattening and fragmentation of the lunate

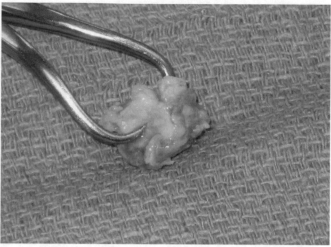

Fig. 47.5 Intra-operative photograph showing advanced collapse of the lunate due to advanced Kienbock's disease following the excision

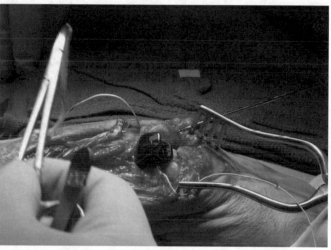

Fig. 47.6 Intra-operative photograph showing provisional position of the pyrocarbon lunate with the FiberWire passed through the volar aspect of the scaphoid, lunate prosthesis, and the triquetrum

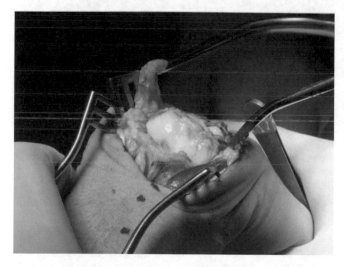

Fig. 47.4 Intra-operative photograph showing smooth articular cartilage of the lunate fossa following excision of the degenerated lunate

the ECRL is then passed through the implant and through the dorsal holes of the scaphoid and the triquetrum (Figs. 47.7, 47.8, 47.9 and 47.10). With the wrist held reduced, the graft is tied to itself with 2–0 FiberWire (Figs. 47.11, 47.12 and 47.13). Next, the tendon of the ECRL is transferred into the

distal pole of the scaphoid to act as a dynamic stabilizer (Figs. 47.14 and 47.15). The wounds are copiously irrigated and the #2 FiberWire is then passed through the dorsal capsule, secured enough to maintain the gapping between the implant in the scaphoid and triquetrum (Fig. 47.16). The dorsal and ulnar portions of the capsule are closed with 3–0 Vicryl. The retinaculum of the second compartment is closed with 3–0 Vicryl. Hemostasis then is achieved following release of the tourniquet and skin closed with 4–0 nylon (Figs. 47.17, 47.18 and 47.19). The patient is placed in a volar splint in extension following the operation.

At 2 weeks, sutures are removed and range of motion is begun at 6 weeks.

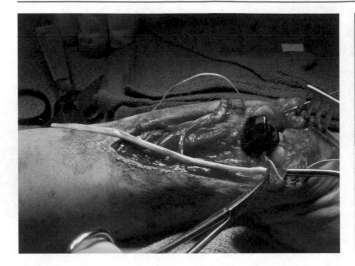

Fig. 47.7 Positioning of the tendon graft of the extensor carpi radialis longus to be passed through the carpus and the pyrocarbon lunate prosthesis

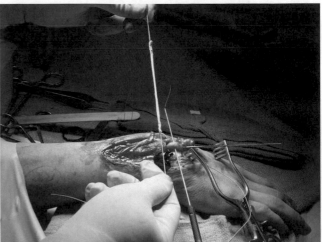

Fig. 47.9 Intra-operative photograph demonstrating placement of the tendon graft of the extensor carpi radialis longus as it is passed through the interosseous drill hole of the scaphoid. The graft in the #2 FiberWire has been passed through the remaining triquetrum, scaphoid, and the pyrocarbon lunate prosthesis

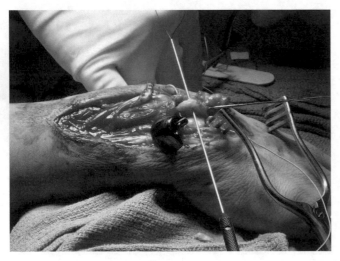

Fig. 47.8 A Hewson suture passer is passed through the mid-axis drill hole though the scaphoid to pass the tendon graft

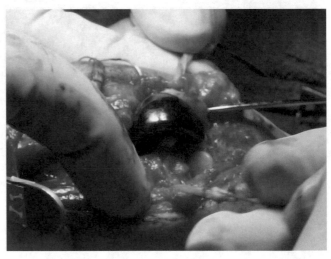

Fig. 47.10 Intra-operative photograph showing reduction of the pyrocarbon lunate in relation to the triquetrum and scaphoid

Tips and Tricks

- A standard dorsal approach is made to the radius. An approximately 10-cm half-slip of the extensor carpi radialis longus tendon is harvested. It is important not to harvest too short of the tendon for reconstruction.
- When sizing the pyrocarbon lunate arthroplasty, use a size smaller than the larger of the options. In this manner, it will decrease stiffness to the wrist with flexion and extension.
- Pass the volar suture before the dorsal tendon slip through the lunate arthroplasty to reduce to carpus.
- The free tendon graft of the extensor carpi radialis is passed through the dorsal holes of the scaphoid and lunate

prosthesis and triquetrum. It is then tied to itself to secure the prosthesis.
- Transfer the remaining portion of the extensor carpi radialis longus tendon into the distal pole of the scaphoid. Following this, the dorsal capsule can then be repaired over the implant for further stability.
- The #2 FiberWire sutures that have been passed through the volar carpus are then passed through the dorsal capsule and tied for further reinforcement and stability of the lunate pyrocarbon implant.
- The dorsal capsule is closed only along the ulnar aspect and left open in the proximal and distal aspects to improve range in motion to the carpus.

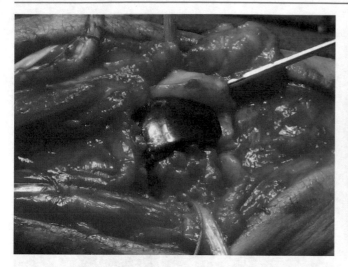

Fig. 47.11 Intra-operative photograph showing reduction of the pyrocarbon lunate to the proximal carpal now

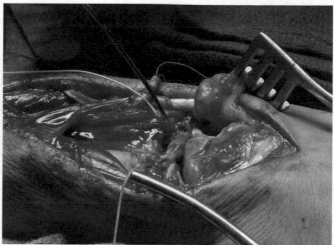

Fig. 47.13 Intra-operative photograph showing repair of the tendon slips of the extensor carpi radialis longus through the prosthesis in the dorsal aspect of the carpus

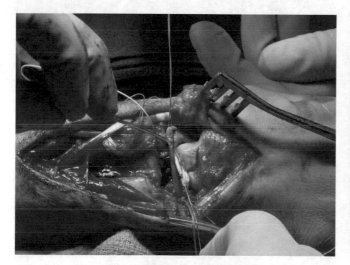

Fig. 47.12 Intra-operative photograph showing repair of the tails of the extensor carpi radialis longus tendon to themselves following passing through the carpus and the lunate pyrocarbon arthroplasty

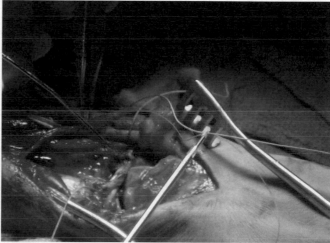

Fig. 47.14 The remaining sutures through the extensor carpi radialis tendon are then passed into the anchor of the push lock (Arthrex, Naples, FL) anchor and inserted into the distal pole of the scaphoid

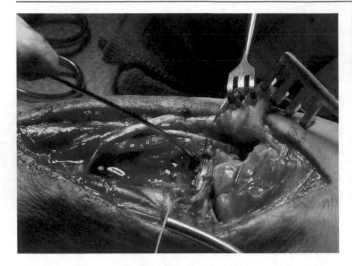

Fig. 47.15 Intra-operative photograph showing complete closure of the carpus with the pyrocarbon lunate with transfer of the remaining portion of the extensor carpi radialis longus tendon into the distal pole of the scaphoid

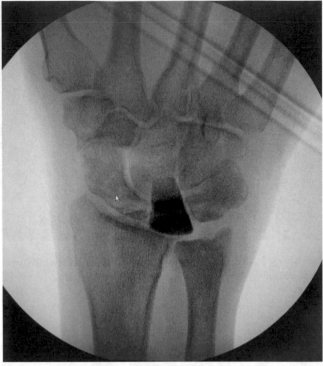

Fig. 47.17 Anterior–posterior fluoroscopy showing ideal placement and orientation of the pyrocarbon lunate

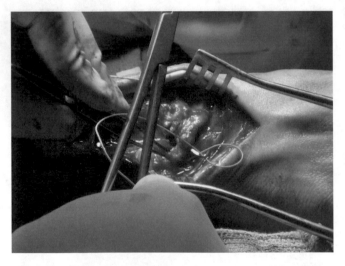

Fig. 47.16 Following reconstruction, a dorsal capsulodesis is performed for further stability following insertion of the pyrocarbon lunate arthroplasty. The #2 FiberWires (Arthrex, Naples, FL) that were passed through the volar holes of the scaphoid, pyrocarbon lunate, and the triquetrum are passed through the dorsal capsule for further reinforcement

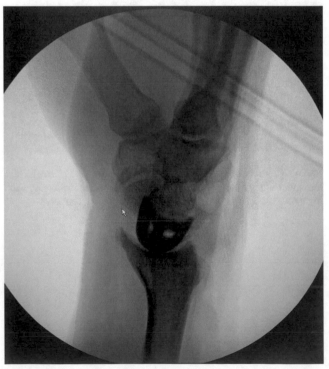

Fig. 47.18 Lateral fluoroscopy showing neutral orientation of the pyrocarbon lunate

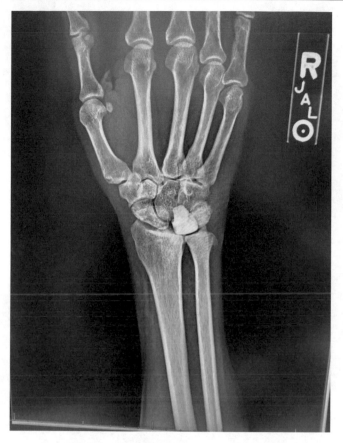

Fig. 47.19 Anterior–posterior radiograph demonstrating ideal placement for the pyrocarbon lunate

Conclusion

There are numerous options for the hand surgeon when treating end-stage Kienbock's disease. Modern lunate arthroplasty with pyrocarbon can be a useful tool for the treatment of stages IIIA and IIIB Kienbock's that does not burn any bridges regarding salvage options.

References

1. Lichtman DM, Mack GR, MacDonald RI, Gunther SF, Wilson JN. Kienbock's disease: the role of silicone replacement arthroplasty. J Bone Joint Surg. 1977;59A:899–908.
2. Lichtman DM, Alexander AH, Mack GR, Gunther SF. Kienbock's disease-update on silicone replacement arthroplasty. J Hand Surg Am. 1982;7:343–7.
3. Lichtman D, Alexander H, Turner M, Alexander C. Lunate silicone replacement arthroplasty in Kienbock's disease: a long term followup. J Hand Surg Am. 1990;15A:401–7.
4. Swanson A, deGroot Swanson G, DH DH, Pierce TD, Randall K, Smith JM, et al. Carpal bone titanium implant arthroplasty. 10 years' experience. Clin Orthop Relat Res. 1997;342:46e58.
5. Viljakka T, Tallroth K, Vastamaki M. Long-term clinical outcome after titanium lunate arthroplasty for Kienbock disease. J Hand Surg Am. 2018;43(10):945.

Arthroscopic Excision of Dorsal Ganglions

48

Meredith N. Osterman, Joshua M. Abzug, and A. Lee Osterman

Ganglion cysts about the wrist are a common pathology that present to hand surgeons and are more common in females [1]. Treatment options for these masses include observation, aspiration, or surgical excision. Historically, open surgical excision has been the gold standard of treatment. The initial description of arthroscopic ganglion excision in 1995, by Osterman and Raphael [2], has led to an increased interest in this treatment technique, given its minimally invasive nature. However, no clear distinction exists regarding the indications for performing open versus arthroscopic excision. Proposed advantages for arthroscopic excision include improved recovery with earlier return to work, better joint visualization, the ability to identify and treat other intraarticular pathology, and more satisfying cosmetic results [2–6]. However, concerns exist regarding limited visualization, specifically of the ganglion stalk. Additional concerns include the applicability of arthroscopic excision for volar and recurrent ganglions.

Anatomy

A vast majority of wrist ganglion cysts, 60–70%, occur on the dorsal aspect of the wrist [7]. Often these, ganglions communicate directly with the wrist joint via a pedicle or stalk, which most commonly originates from the membranous portion of the scapholunate ligament [7]. The importance of removing this pedicle during surgical excision is debated in the literature. Angelides attributes his 1% recurrence rate after open surgical excision to excising the stalk [8]. His dissection of the stalk under magnification showed a one-way valve-like system between the scapholunate joint and the ganglion [8]. This implies that without removal of the stalk, the ganglion cyst would re-occur. However, other studies have shown similar recurrence rates without completely visualizing, and thus clearly excising, the stalk during ganglion removal. Osterman reported no recurrence after arthroscopic excision yet only visualized and excised 61% of ganglion stalks [2]. Luchetti reported a recurrence of only 2 of 34 ganglions after arthroscopic surgical excision and only visualized and excised 27 stalks [3]. If the stalk is not clearly visualized, the area of capsular attachment to the scapholunate ligament is excised empirically during ganglion resection and thought to be equivalent to excising the stalk itself.

Volar ganglions represent 20% of all wrist ganglia and frequently present in the proximal wrist crease between the flexor carpi radialis tendon and the radial artery [9]. The mass is often fixed and painful, with symptoms directly related to wrist motion [10]. The anatomic origin is commonly from the radioscaphoid or scaphotrapezial joint [10]. Occult ganglia, volar or dorsal, present without visible or palpable deformity but may contribute to wrist pain (Figs. 48.1 and 48.2).

Patient Evaluation

History and Physical Examination

The majority of patients who present for evaluation of a dorsal wrist ganglion do so secondary to concerns regarding cosmesis. Ganglions are also associated with pain particularly on wrist extension activities and forceful grip. The volar ganglion may irritate the radial artery and the median

Supplementary Information The online version of this chapter (https://doi.org/10.1007/978-3-030-78881-0_48) contains supplementary material, which is available to authorized users.

M. N. Osterman
Philadelphia Hand to Shoulder Center, Department of Orthopedics, Thomas Jefferson University Hospital, Philadelphia, PA, USA

J. M. Abzug
Department of Orthopaedics, University of Maryland School of Medicine, Timonium, MD, USA

A. L. Osterman (✉)
The Philadelphia Hand to Shoulder Center, P.C., King of Prussia, PA, USA

© Springer Nature Switzerland AG 2022
W. B. Geissler (ed.), *Wrist and Elbow Arthroscopy with Selected Open Procedures*, https://doi.org/10.1007/978-3-030-78881-0_48

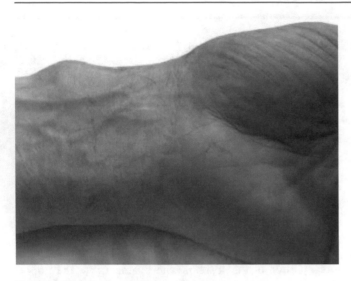

Fig. 48.1 Volar wrist ganglion cyst

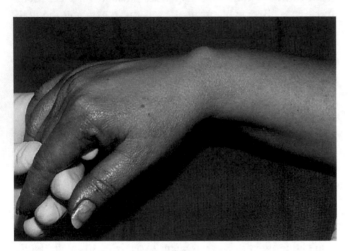

Fig. 48.2 Dorsal wrist ganglion cyst

nerve along with its palmar cutaneous branch. Occult ganglions are those that present without a palpable mass yet patients report symptoms of wrist pain. These patients present with nontraumatic, nonsystemic inflammatory wrist pain. Often these patients go undiagnosed for a period of time because clinically and radiographically there is no evidence of pathology. Ultrasound or magnetic resonance imaging (MRI) can aid in the diagnosis. A study that evaluated patients with chronic wrist pain (at least 3 months) using ultrasonographic examination found that 58% of patients had an occult ganglion as the source of their pain [11]. Westbrook looked at the reason patients present to hand clinics with dorsal wrist ganglions and found that 38% are concerned with the cosmetic appearance, 28% are concerned that the cyst is cancerous, and 26% present with pain [12]. A discussion of the etiology, natural history, and benign nature of the mass is often enough to alleviate patient fears and the desire for surgical intervention.

When diagnosing a dorsal ganglion cyst, it is imperative to ensure that the mass is truly a ganglion cyst. Many elements of the history and physical examination are not conclusive. Occurrence, progression, size, shape, texture, presence or absence of pain, and association with traumatic or repetitive activities provide little information regarding the true diagnosis. One element of history, however, can be quite helpful in determining whether the lesion is cystic. While ganglion cysts and other tumors get larger, only ganglion cysts decrease in size as well. Exceptions to this include some vascular tumors than involute over a period of months to years; however, ganglion cysts can decrease in size as quickly as overnight. On physical examination, transillumination can be helpful to differentiate a ganglion cyst from an alternative tumor. This is performed by holding a penlight to the lesion and observing the light transmit through its fluid medium, whereas a solid tissue tumor will prevent any propagation of the light.

Occasionally, ganglion cysts may herald underlying pathology, such as a scapholunate ligament injury. The history and physical examination should focus on any recent or remote trauma. Often, patients have incompetent scapholunate ligaments that remain clinically unapparent until the manifestation of an associated dorsal ganglion cyst. One study reported on 19 wrists with painful dorsal ganglia, a positive Watson scaphoid shift test, and negative radiographs that underwent ganglion excision. Postoperatively, all patients had decreased pain and 17 of the wrists had a postoperative negative Watson shift test [13]. Tenderness during palpation of the dorsal portion of the scapholunate ligament, a positive radial scaphoid shift test, or a positive straight finger resistance test may suggest scapholunate ligament pathology. Furthermore, ganglion cysts may resemble other pathologies, such as a gouty tophus, tenosynovitis, or rheumatoid pannus. A careful history and physical examination should suffice to differentiate these conditions.

Diagnostic Imaging

Magnetic resonance imaging (MRI) and ultrasonography remain the imaging modalities most commonly utilized to differentiate fluid-filled cysts from solid tumors. A study comparing the diagnostic abilities of ultrasound versus magnetic resonance imaging to detect occult wrist ganglions showed they are equally effective [14]. Nevertheless, there has been a shift toward ultrasonography as the preferred technique, given its ready availability, quickness, and lower cost. Very small ganglion cysts, known as occult ganglion cysts, although clinically significant, can be easily missed by either imaging modality. Surgeons should keep a high index of suspicion for occult ganglion cysts, even in the face of a negative reading by the radiologist. With intraoperative arthroscopic diagnosis of occult ganglia as the standard, the sensitivity of MRI scanning was found to be only 83% and the specificity only 50% [15].

Treatment

Nonoperative Management

The initial treatment of choice is a trial of nonoperative management, including splinting for comfort, prior to proceeding to operative intervention. However, the results of conservative treatment are unpredictable with success rates ranging from 30% to 85% [7]. Attempted aspiration can safely be performed on the dorsum of the wrist but attempts to aspirate volar ganglion cysts may cause injury to neurovascular structures, such as the radial artery and palmar cutaneous nerve. Adjunctive measures, such as steroid injections, sclerosing injections, and multiple cyst punctures, have been reported but show results no better than expectant management and, furthermore, carry up to a 5% complication rate [7].

Operative Management

Surgical excision remains the treatment of choice for carpal ganglion cysts refractory to conservative measures. Prior to the recognition of the ganglion stalk, recurrence rates rivaled those of expectant management but now are reported to be as low as 1% [8]. However, surgical intervention is not without risk and complications, which although rare, include recurrence, infection, neuroma, keloid, scar hypersensitivity, postoperative stiffness, grip weakness, and scapholunate instability.

Indications for surgical intervention include symptomatic ganglia that produce pain, weakness, or limitations in wrist function/range of motion. Unacceptable cosmesis is also an indication, but typically additional symptoms are necessary for us to recommend proceeding to operative intervention.

Many patients seek excision of their ganglion for cosmetic reasons or concern that the mass is malignant. Although an open incision across the dorsum of the wrist may not seem excessive to a surgeon, the patient may have another perspective. One study reported a very high postoperative satisfaction rate after arthroscopic excision, despite the fact that 17% of the patients were asymptomatic preoperatively and opted for surgery for cosmetic reasons [6]. The implication is that offering arthroscopic ganglion resections for patients primarily interested in the cosmetic appearance of their hands is reasonable. However, while surgical excision of the cyst will remove the "bump," a scar will replace the "bump." Arthroscopic excision of the cyst has the potential to remove the "bump" with minimal scarring.

Arthroscopic Technique

The patient is placed supine on the operating room table and a nonsterile pneumatic tourniquet is applied to the upper arm (Fig. 48.3) (Video 48.1). Subsequently, the remainder of the upper extremity is prepped and draped in the usual sterile fashion and the patient is placed in the standard wrist arthroscopy tower. Prior to suspension in the traction tower, it is useful to do a wrist exam under anesthesia. While the patient's arm is suspended in a traction tower, a 6-R portal is created as a visualization portal, by first placing an 18G needle to ensure appropriate placement of the portal. Once the needle confirmed the correct location, a stab incision is made through the skin only. Blunt dissection is carried out with a hemostat and a capsulotomy is made with the blunt trocar. The arthroscope is now inserted into the joint and directed radially to visualize the stalk of the ganglion at the junction of the fibrous and membranous portion of the scapholunate ligament. The typical initial visualization portal, the 3–4 portal, is avoided as the primary portal to prevent inadvertent decompression of the cyst.

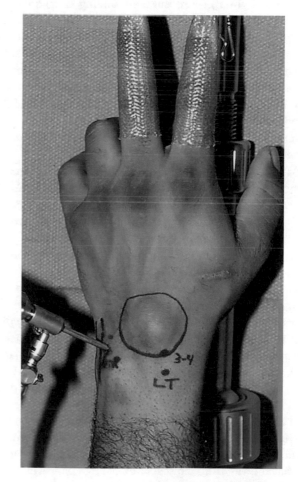

Fig. 48.3 Arthroscopic set up for dorsal ganglion cyst excision

In contrast, with volar ganglion excision, the 3–4 portal is established first, as this provides good visualization of the radial wrist ligaments, the common origin of the volar ganglion. The scope is then introduced through the 4–5 or 1–2 portal for visualization during resection of the ganglion through the 3–4 portal. The radial artery and sensory branch of the radial nerve need to be protecting with use of the 1–2 portal [16].

After the 2.7-mm arthroscopic camera is directed toward the dorsal compartment of the wrist, the capsule adjacent to the scapholunate ligament can be visualized. Occasionally, a sessile or pedunculated protrusion into the joint can be seen in the area where the extrinsic capsule joins the distal portion of the dorsal scapholunate ligament. This capsular reflection serves as part of the barrier between the radiocarpal and mid-carpal joints, and the protrusion located here has been termed the cystic stalk. More often, the surgeon may be impressed with the amount of synovitis and redundant capsule in this area instead of an actual stalk.

Once the stalk and cyst are visualized, a full radius shaver is placed through the cystic sac using the 3–4 portal. This action decompresses the cyst and may obscure any presence of an intraarticular stalk. If visualization is difficult to establish the 3–4 portal, we recommend finding Lister's tubercle and moving approximately 1 cm distal to locate the radiocarpal joint. The aforementioned technique of ensuring accurate placement is followed by utilization of an 18G needle followed by making the stab incision, utilization of a hemostat for blunt dissection, and finally inserting the trocar to perform the capsulotomy. A 2.9-mm, full-radius shaver is introduced through this portal, and every effort is made to avoid decompressing the cyst with simple introduction of the shaver.

Although the procedure implies that the cyst is removed by the arthroscope, this is often not the case. The arthroscopy procedure disrupts the communication between the cyst and the joint by excising the stalk of the cyst, while leaving behind a deflated sac that cannot re-inflate. Eventually, the empty sac is re-absorbed. Recurrences can happen only if another cyst is generated (Fig. 48.4).

The focus of the resection begins at the site of the ganglion stalk or redundant capsular material, if identified. This billowing, redundant material appears different from typical reactive synovitis. Although its exact significance is unclear, it seems to be continuous with the capsule that lies adjacent to the cyst. With this landmark, surgeons may confidently begin the capsulotomy. If neither structure is identified, the debridement begins adjacent to the dorsal scapholunate ligament and distal capsular reflection. Commonly, the cyst travels within the capsular reflection as it communicates with the scapholunate joint. Care should be taken to keep the blade of the shaver away from the scapholunate ligament at all times.

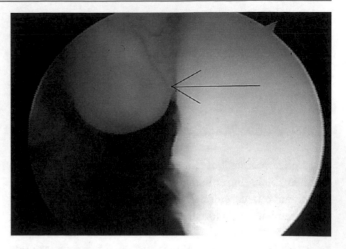

Fig. 48.4 Intraoperative arthroscopic view of ganglion stalk (*arrow*). Note the scapholunate ligament on the *right side* of the picture

On initial debridement of the capsular reflection, occasionally a flash of viscous cystic fluid may be visualized escaping into the joint. Debridement continues until approximately 1–1.5 cm of capsule has been removed.

A common mistake is to make the capsulotomy too small. The 2.9-mm shaver is helpful as a reference in gauging the size of the capsulotomy. Another common mistake is to create an incomplete capsulotomy that fails to communicate with the extra-articular space. We used to advise direct visualization of the extensor tendons to verify that a complete capsulotomy has been performed, but no longer feel this is necessary as long as the stalk and/or redundant capsule is resected. Removal of the cystic sac is not necessary, because it often resorbs over time after it is detached from its origin at the joint. If the cyst is particularly large, resorption may take some time, and patients may complain about residual prominence on the dorsum of the hand/wrist. Removal of the truncated sac may be performed by pulling it out of the 3–4 portal with a hemostat. Some dorsal ganglions may have a dual origin, from both radiocarpal and midcarpal joints (Fig. 48.5). One study showed that 74% of cysts communicated with the midcarpal joint, thus we always recommend that midcarpal arthroscopy, through standard portals, be performed [6].

Some surgeons close each arthroscopic portal with one simple nonabsorbable suture, but others leave them open or place Steri-Strip with no cosmetic detriment. Open arthroscopic wounds can rarely form sinus tracts, as reported in other joint arthroscopy. Therefore, we prefer to close these wounds with one stitch. A sterile wrist dressing comprised of 4 × 4 s and sterile webril is used in all cases and patients are placed in a volar splint for 1 week. Then a neoprene or soft support is used for comfort and as a reminder not to do forceful grip and wrist extension, such as pushups, for 6 weeks.

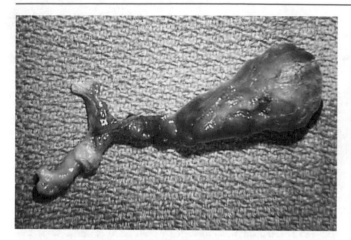

Fig. 48.5 Excised ganglion cyst with stalk

Adjuvant Options to the Arthroscopic Technique

A proposed disadvantage of arthroscopic ganglion excision is the inability to fully visualize, and thus excise, the ganglion stalk. Recent reports have proposed methods to help visualize the stalk.

A technique of injecting methylene blue into the ganglion prior to arthroscopic excision has been reported to aid in stalk visualization [17]. The dye is injected into the ganglion and the surgeon can track the methylene blue into the ganglion stalk, either in the radiocarpal or midcarpal joint. This aids in the debridement of pathologic tissue and prevents unnecessary removal of uninvolved tissues. With better visualization of the stalk, less capsular tissue is debrided and the incidence of iatrogenic scapholunate instability is theoretically decreased. This method is contraindicated in patients with methylene blue allergy or glucose-6-phosphate dehydrogenase (G6PD) deficiency. In these instances, alternative contrast agents, such as indigo carmine, can be used instead. Yao and Trindade report no ganglion recurrences using the technique of injecting indigo carmine into all ganglions undergoing arthroscopic excision. They attribute the success to improved stalk visualization and complete excision [18].

Sonography-guided arthroscopy for ganglion excision has also been reported. Yamamoto et al. used sonography to aid in the assessment of ganglion size, relationship to adjacent structures and arthroscopic excision [19]. Twenty-two patients with symptomatic dorsal ganglions underwent arthroscopic excision with color Doppler sonography. Only four stalks were completely visualized with arthroscopy alone. All 22 ganglion stalks were visualized with the aid of sonography [19].

Results/Recurrence

Recurrence of the ganglion cyst is the ultimate outcome measure for a successful surgical excision. Rates following arthroscopic excision of dorsal ganglions have been low (0–10%) in virtually every report, which is markedly lower than the recurrence rates for open excision [2, 5, 20, 21]. Recurrence rates for open excision have been reported as high as 8–40% [4, 22, 23]. However, one prospective series comparing arthroscopic and open resection found no statistical difference in recurrence rates (10.7% vs. 8.7%, respectively) [4]. Open volar ganglionectomy has similar recurrence rates of 28%, with additional complications of palmar cutaneous nerve injury and unsatisfactory scar formation [24]. In contrast, reported recurrence with arthroscopic excision is 0% [17].

Complications

Despite arthroscopy being a minimally invasive operative intervention, it still poses risks to the patient. Potential complications inherent to the surgery include infection, damage to articular cartilage or neurovascular structures, hypertrophic scar formation, and postoperative wrist stiffness or chronic regional pain syndrome. Proper establishment of portals and thorough understanding of the anatomy is imperative to help minimize these risks, particularly in recurrent ganglion excision where the scar may have abnormally displaced the extensor tendons. A systematic review performed in 2012 looked at the incidence of complications after wrist arthroscopy and found huge variations in the literature, ranging from 1% to 20% [25]. Most of the complications related to the use of concomitant pin fixation for fracture treatment and very few related to diagnostic arthroscopy or ganglionectomy. Compiling the results of all the studies yielded an overall complication rate of 4.8% [25].

Conclusion

Arthroscopic resection of dorsal, volar, or occult ganglions is a safe and effective alternative to open gangliectomy. Studies have shown that the recurrence rate is markedly lower and without increased risks of surgical complications. Concerns regarding appropriate visualization of the ganglia and/or stalk during arthroscopic excision are being addressed with newer techniques. In addition, arthroscopic excision allows for the surgeon to evaluate and/or treat co-existing intraarticular pathology, such as scapholunate or triangular fibrocartilage complex (TFCC) tears.

References

1. Janzon L, Niechajev IA. Wrist ganglia. Incidence and recurrence rate after operation. Scand J Plast Reconstr Surg. 1981;15:53–6.

2. Osterman AL, Raphael J. Arthroscopic resection of dorsal ganglion of the wrist. Hand Clin. 1995;11:7–12.

3. Luchetti R, Badia A, Alfarano M, Orbay J, Indriago I, Mustapha B. Arthroscopic resection of dorsal wrist ganglia and treatment of recurrences. J Hand Surg Br. 2000;25:38–40.

4. Kang L, Akelman E, Weiss A. Arthroscopic versus open dorsal ganglion excision: a prospective, randomized comparison of rates of recurrence and of residual pain. J Hand Surg Am. 2008;33(4):471–5.

5. Rizzo M, Berger R, Steinmann S, Bishop A. Arthroscopic resection in the management of dorsal wrist ganglions: results with a minimum 2-year follow-up period. J Hand Surg Am. 2004;29:59–62.

6. Edwards SG, Johansen JA. Prospective outcomes and associations of wrist ganglion cysts resected arthroscopically. J Hand Surg Am. 2009;34:395–400.

7. Gude W, Morelli V. Ganglion cysts of the wrist: pathophysiology, clinical picture, and management. Curr Rev Musculoskelet Med. 2008;1:205–11.

8. Angelides AC, Wallace PF. The dorsal ganglion of the wrist: its pathogenesis, gross and microscopic anatomy, and surgical treatment. J Hand Surg Am. 1976;1:228–35.

9. Greenberg JA. Arthroscopic treatment of volar carpal ganglion cysts. In: Slutsky DJ, Nagle DJ, editors. Techniques in wrist and hand arthroscopy. Philadelphia: Churchill Livingstone, Inc. (Elsevier); 2007. p. 188–90.

10. Greendyke SD, Wilson M, Shepler TR. Anterior wrist ganglia from the scaphotrapezial joint. J Hand Surg Am. 1992;17:487–90.

11. Chen HS, Chen MY, Lee CY, et al. Ultrasonographic examination on patients with chronic wrist pain: a retrospective study. Am J Phys Med Rehabil. 2007;89(11):907–11.

12. Westbrook A, Stephen A, Oni J, Davis T. Ganglia: the patient's perception. J Hand Surg Br. 2000;25(6):566–7.

13. Hwangg JJ, Goldfarb CA, Gelberman RH, Boyer MI. The effect of dorsal carpal ganglion excision on the scaphoid shift test. J Hand Surg Br. 1999;24(1):106–8.

14. Cardinal E, Buckwalter KA, Braunstein EM, et al. Occult dorsal carpal ganglion: comparison of US and MR imaging. Radiology. 1994;193(1):259–62.

15. Goldsmith S, Yang SS. Magnetic resonance imaging in the diagnosis of occult dorsal wrist ganglions. J Hand Surg Eur. 2008;33(5):595–9.

16. Ho PC, Lo WN, Hung LK. Resection of volar ganglion of the wrist: a new technique. J Arthroscop Relat Surg. 2003;19(2):218–21.

17. Lee B, Sawyer G, DaSilva M. Methylene blue-enhanced arthroscopic resection of dorsal wrist ganglions. Tech Hand Up Extrem Surg. 2011;15(4):243–6.

18. Yao J, Trindade M. Color-aided visualization of dorsal wrist ganglion stalks aids in complete arthroscopic excision. Arthroscopy. 2011;27(3):425–9.

19. Yamamoto M, Kurimoto S, Okui N, et al. Sonography-guided arthroscopy for wrist ganglion. J Hand Surg Am. 2012;37:1411–5.

20. Ho PC, Griffiths J, Lo WN, Yen CH, Hung LK. Current treatment of ganglion at the wrist. Hand Surg. 2001;6:49–58.

21. Mathoulin C, Hoyos A, Pelaez J. Arthroscopic resection of wrist ganglia. Hand Surg. 2004;9:159–64.

22. Thronburg LE. Ganglions of the hand and wrist. J Am Acad Orthop Surg. 1999;7:231–8.

23. Clay NR, Clement DA. The treatment of dorsal wrist ganglia by radical excision. J Hand Surg Br. 1998;13:187–91.

24. Jacobs LG, Govaers KJ. The volar wrist ganglion: just a simple cyst? J Hand Surg Br. 1990;15:342–6.

25. Ahsan ZS, Yao J. Complications of wrist arthroscopy. Arthroscopy. 2012;28(6):855–9.

Arthroscopic Management of Volar Ganglions

49

Carlos Henrique Fernandes
and Cesar Dario Oliveira Miranda

Introduction

Ganglia are the most common soft tissue tumors of the hand [1]. They are mucin-filled cysts which may be uni- or multi-lobulated and are closely associated with either the wrist joint or tendon sheath. It is now widely accepted that dorsal and volar wrist ganglions have similar path mechanisms and arise from mucinous degeneration of the capsular and ligament structures around the joint [2, 3]. Volar wrist ganglion is the second most common mass in the wrist, arising via a pedicle from the radio scaphoid/scapholunate interval, scaphotrapezial joint, or the metacarpotrapezial joint, in that order of frequency [4]. They usually appear between the flexor carpi radialis tendon and the flexor pollicis longus tendon. Microscopically, the pedicle contains a tortuous lumen, connecting the cyst to the underlying joint [5]. The presence of this connection is supported by the intraoperative and arthrographic findings that demonstrated movement of intra-articular contrast from the radiocarpal joint into the ganglia in 85% of patients with a volar wrist ganglion. As contrast does not appear to travel from the cyst into the joint, a one-way valve mechanism has been postulated [6].

Frequently, they are benign, well characterized, and easily diagnosed.

In the last 20 years, the wrist arthroscopy has advanced, since diagnosing the therapeutic procedures in the treatment of disease in the joint. The arthroscope makes it easy to visualize the small structures and allows evaluating the locals where through open technique would be more difficult and would cause more lesions. However, it is a less invasive with less morbidity. The video surgery started to be a gold tool to diagnose and treat intra-articular pathologies.

About two decades ago, Osterman and Raphael [7] described the technique for the treatment of the dorsal carpal ganglion. In the beginning, there was a lot of skepticism with this technique; however, it has become a routine procedure. Throughout the last few years, the arthroscopic treatment of volar carpal ganglion cyst has become more popular.

Clinical Picture

The most common reason for referral is a lump that appears on the palm side of the wrist in the wrist crease just below the thumb. Some patients may be concerned about potential malignancy. Usually, the symptoms include pain in the wrist, poor activity or palpation of the mass, decreased range of motion, and decreased grip strength.

Sometimes, they may change in size over time but are usually 1–2 cm. The skin above the cyst is unchanged, and there is no associated warmth or erythema (Fig. 49.1). Sometimes occur paresthesias from compression of the ulnar or median nerves or their branches [8]. The mass itself is compressible. It will be "rubbery" in consistency and generally movable. Transillumination of a lump in the usual anatomical location will confirm a fluid-filled cyst.

Routinely a wrist X-ray evaluation is indicated to rule out preexisting osseous lesions. An ultrasound imaging study of the wrist is also examined to confirm the diagnosis, as well as to localize the ganglion (Fig. 49.2).

The MRI of soft tissue masses of the wrist is useful to differentiate them. Ulnar volar ganglions are associated with tears of triangular fibrocartilage complex. An MRI in some circumstances helps to locate the stalk, other lesions, and in the diagnosis of occult ganglia.

Supplementary Information The online version of this chapter (https://doi.org/10.1007/978-3-030-78881-0_49) contains supplementary material, which is available to authorized users.

C. H. Fernandes
Department of Orthopedic Surgery, Universidade Federal de São Paulo, São Paulo, Brazil

C. D. O. Miranda (✉)
Department of Hand Surgery, Hand Surgery Institute Salvador, Salvador, Bahia, Brazil

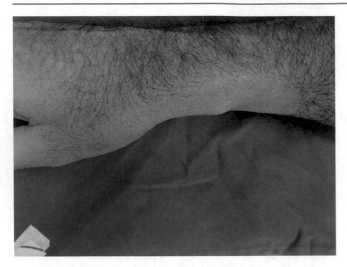

Fig. 49.1 Clinical photo of volar ganglion

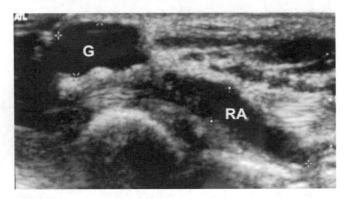

Fig. 49.2 Ultrasound appearance of volar cyst

Revision of Literature

There is a real deficit of studies of higher methodological quality, and there is a necessity for more studies to ensure the best prediction of outcomes in wrist arthroscopy [9].

We reviewed the literature on arthroscopic resection of volar wrist ganglion [28]. The publication dates ranged from 2001 to 2012 (Table 49.1). Only one was a prospective randomized study; the authors compared the open resection and arthroscopic resection. All of the other studies were level IV of evidence [10–17]. A total of 232 wrists were submitted to an arthroscopic resection. The same operative technique described by Ho et al. [18, 19] was used by all authors. One author included an intrafocal cystic portal [13].

The mean age of patients described in eight articles was 40.45 years. All reported a major incidence in women with a female: male ratio of 3:1. Of nine articles, the follow-up ranged from 12 to 56 months with a mean of 23.82 months.

There were 14 recurrences. The recurrence rate ranged from 0% to 20% with mean of 6.03%.

There were 16 (6.89%) related complications. No connection of the complication with the ganglion was described in six wrists [18, 19]. Volar hematoma was described in three patients [20, 21]. Partial lesions of the median nerve were reported in two articles [12, 21], two lesions of a branch of the radial artery [10, 11], and neuropraxis of the superficial radial nerve [10, 13, 19]. Osterman (in the 65th Annual Meeting of the American Society for Surgery of the Hand 2010) and Langner et al. [14] did not report any complications. No patient had loss of arc range of motion.

In a study of five patients of Rocchi et al. [10], the recurrence and complications were higher for midcarpal ganglions.

Recently, Langner et al. reported that patients with volar painful ganglions of the wrist and a positive ulnocarpal stress test are highly associated with TFCC abnormalities [14].

Treatment

Indications and Contraindications

Despite a natural history of spontaneous regression [15], volar ganglion cyst of the wrist can sometimes require a surgical excision. Both surgical and nonsurgical treatments are available. Although aspiration and percutaneous sclerotherapy using 75% hypertonic glucose have been used for dorsal ganglion treatment, there isn't report of its for volar ganglion [29]. Recent series have documented enhanced treatment success using various aspiration techniques after three separate treatments. However, recurrence rates exceeding 40% can still be expected. The most definitive management remains excision [22].

The literature with regard to recurrence rates demonstrates that open volar ganglion surgery is challenging. In principal, complete removal of the ganglion base is required to avoid recurrence. The cases of recurrence are often due to incomplete ganglion stalk resection, which is greater on the volar aspect due to the more complex volar anatomy. The risks of complication are also common, reaching rates >20% in some studies [16, 17]. The causes are proximity of the superficial palmar branch of the radial artery, the terminal branches of the superficial radial nerve, and the palmar cutaneous branch of the median nerve [10, 11]. Contraindications for arthroscopic management of volar ganglions are a history of wrist trauma with deformity, stiff joint, and advanced instability degenerative disease of the wrist.

Table 49.1 Studies reporting recurrence rates and complications of arthroscopic resection of a volar wrist ganglion

	Authors	Title	Year	Study design	Evidence	Wrist operated	Average age	Gender	Follow-up (months)	Recurrence	Complications
1	Ho et al.	Current treatment of ganglion of the wrist	2001	Case series	IV	6	38		16.4	0 (0%)	01 no connection with the ganglion was found (16.66%)
2	Mathoulin et al.	Arthroscopic resection of wrist ganglia	2004	Case series	IV	32	46	27W 05M	26	0 (0%)	01 volar hematoma (3.12%)
3	Rocchi et al.	Resezione artroscopica delle cisti artrogene dorsali e volari del polso. Nostra esperienza e evalutazioni cliniche	2005	Case series	IV	7	–	–	18	0 (0%)	01 neuropraxia dorsal radial nerve (14.28%)
4	Ho et al.	Arthroscopic volar wrist gangliorectomy	2006	Case series	IV	21	48.6	11W 10M	56	2 (9.52%)	05 no connection with the ganglion was found (23.80%)
5	Mathoulin and Massarella	Therapeutic interest of wrist arthroscopy about 1000 cases	2006	Case series	IV	66	42	53W 13M	32	0 (0%)	02 volar hematoma and 01 partial lesion of median nerve (4.54%)
6	Rocchi et al.	Results and complications in dorsal and volar wrist ganglia arthroscopic resection	2006	Case series	IV	17	–	–	15	1 (5.88%)	01 lesion radial artery (5.88%)
7	Rocchi et al.	Articular ganglia of the volar aspect of the wrist: Arthroscopic resection compared with open excision. A prospective randomized study	2008	Prospective randomized study	I	25	37	18W 07M	24	3 (12%)	01 neuropraxia dorsal radial nerve and 01 lesion radial artery (8.00%)
8	Rhyou et al.	Arthroscopic resection of volar ganglion of the wrist joint	2010	Case series	IV	9	43	07W 2M	15	0 (0%)	01 partial lesion of median nerve (11.11%)
9	Chen et al.	Arthroscopic ganglionectomy through an intrafocal cystic portal for wrist ganglia	2010	Case series	IV	3	30	03W 00M	–	0 (0%)	01 transient paresthesia radial nerve, resolution 1 month (33.33%)
10	Ostermann	Symposium 4—Excellence in wrist arthroscopy: extending our horizons. Arthroscopic volar ganglionectomy	2010	Case series	IV	26	37	–	–	4 (15.38)	No
11	Langner et al.	Ganglions of the wrist and associated triangular fibrocartilage lesions: A prospective study in arthroscopically treated patients	2012	Case series	IV	20	40	–	12	4 (20%)	No

Arthroscopic Technique

Because of the volar tilt of the distal radius, the volar capsule and ligaments of the radiocarpal joint are more accessible to arthroscopic instrumentation than the dorsal structures. Arthroscopic gangliectomy has the advantage of avoiding extensive dissection, scarring, and potential damage to structures. Other advantages are reduced postoperative pain and the time of return of function compared with open resection [11].

The results of the arthroscopic management of volar ganglions were originally presented in 2001 [23] by Ho et al. [9]. However, Ho et al. only described the detailed technique in 2003 [18].

Some surgeons perform the procedure by block anesthesia, but in general, we use sedation or local anesthesia in the portal and joint. The patient lies supine.

A tourniquet is applied to the arm and inflated after exsanguinations with an esmarch rubber.

The arm is fixed to an arm table and the elbow flexed to 90° with the wrist in vertical traction using double disposable plastic finger traps placed in the second and fourth or second and third fingers.

Portal sites are palpated and marked. The portal sites used for the radiocarpal joint are routinely 3–4, 4–5, and 1–2 (Fig. 49.3).

Using a syringe with a 25 × 7 mm needle, the radiocarpal joint is initially distended. Approximately, 5 ml of Bupivacaine is injected through the skin and subcutaneous tissues into the joint through 3–4 portals. We use a 40 × 8 mm needle with an outflow in portal 6U, in all cases.

Over the portals, a short skin is made, and the spreading of soft tissue with a hemostat exposes the joint capsule. This maneuver provokes extraversion of anesthetic from outside

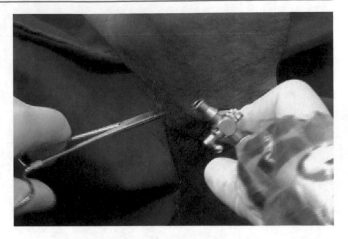

Fig. 49.4 The 2.7-mm arthroscope is introduced into the 3–4 portals. Blunt dissection is performed with a hemostat in the 1–2 portal

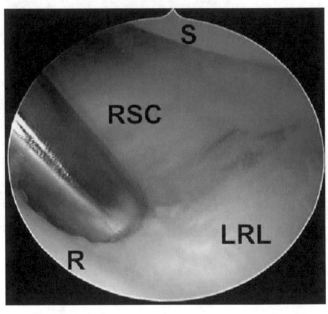

Fig. 49.5 Arthroscopic image showing the volar extrinsic wrist ligaments and the interval between the radioscaphocapitate (RSC) and long radiolunate ligament (LRL). Through this interval the cyst is resected

of joint. This maneuver is particularly important when the 1–2 portal is being created, to avoid injury to the radial artery and the radial nerve (Fig. 49.4).

We use a 2.4 mm arthroscope with a 30° visual angle, with irrigation fluid instilled by pump infusion.

The 3–4 portals give a better view. Through the 3–4 portals, the scope allows inspection of the volar radial side wrist ligaments, where the volar ganglion usually has its stalk. Frequently, synovial and capsular abnormalities were seen at the interval between the radioscaphocapitate (RSC) and long radiolunate (LRL) ligaments or between LRL and short radiolunate (SRL) ligaments [24] (Fig. 49.5).

The 1–2 portal is also the best for instrumentation, although it has been associated with a higher risk of damag-

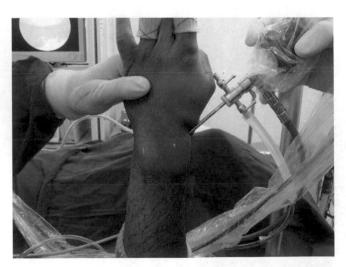

Fig. 49.3 The portal used 3–4, 4–5 and the arthroscope is placed in the 1–2 portal

ing the radial artery and sensory branch of the radial nerve [12, 21].

A 2.0- to 2.9-mm arthroscopic shaver is then introduced through 1–2 portal to deride the region. However, ganglia or their stalks cannot be observed arthroscopically in most cases. When this situation occurs, a fingertip gentle external pressure is maintained over the ganglion (Fig. 49.6). This maneuver will result in synovial and capsular bulging at the site. The shaving is performed until a hole of about 1 cm is observed in the interligamental interval. Do not use too much suction to prevent blistering and to be able to observe the mucinous liquid outlet into the radiocarpal joint (Fig. 49.7, Videos 49.1 and 49.2). Be careful that the shaver

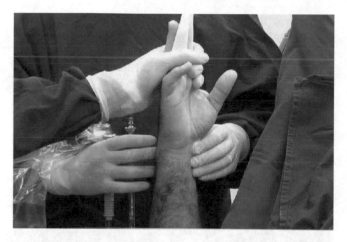

Fig. 49.6 Palpation of the volar cyst during the surgery. This maneuver helps to locate the interligamental interval where the shaver will debride

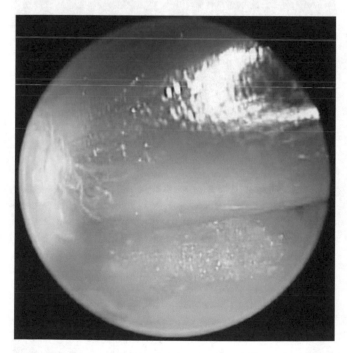

Fig. 49.7 Arthroscopic image showing mucinous liquid outlet into the radiocarpal joint

must not be advanced too anteriorly into the volar aspect of the wrist joint. A maneuver untimely could damage the important structures volar to the joint. We did not attempt to remove the ganglion wall or more of the joint capsule than was necessary to induce the gush of mucinous content. A small palmar capsulectomy defect resulted at the RSC-LRL or LRL-SRL interligamental interval after the operation, enable the flexor pollicis longus tendon can be seen, and care must be taken not to damage it with the shaver (Fig. 49.8, Videos 49.3 and 49.4).

Sometimes, we can see the mucinous liquid leakage through the portal and running down in the skin (Fig. 49.9).

The shaver was also used for trimming capsular lesion, partial tear of the scapholunate ligament, lunotriquetral ligament, volar radioscaphocapitate ligament, and triangular fibrocartilage complex (TFCC).

The ganglions that arise from the distal wrist crease are likely to originate in the scaphotrapezium-trapezoid (STT) joint or other component of the midcarpal joint (Fig. 49.10). In these situations, a finger trap applied an extra-distraction on thumb. Two extra portals are performed. The first, the radial midcarpal portal (RMC), which is located 1 cm distal to the 3–4 portals and in line with the radial margin of the third metacarpal, is performed. The second, the STT portal, is located just to the ulnar side of the extensor pollicis longus tendon, at the level of the articular surface on the distal pole of the scaphoid (Fig. 49.11). The ganglia resection is difficult because of the narrow space. Two cases of arthroscopic resection of scaphotrapeziotrapezoidal (STT) joint ganglia utilizing the STT-U and STT-R portals were described with no recurence observed after 50 months of follow-up [30].

In 2012, Yamamoto et al. reported sonography-assisted arthroscopy. With this technique, they can identify ganglia, vessels, nerves, tendons, and the blade shavers can be identified and guided to the lesion. The advantage is to avoid vascular, nerve, and tendon injuries. Unfortunately, they did not report the number of patients and if they have less complications [25].

Chen et al. [13] described a volar ganglia resection through an intrafocal cystic portal. They performed an additional puncture wound with guidance from the light source of the arthroscopy, which was introduced through the 3–4 portals, over the ganglion cyst, followed by a gentle introduction of the oscillating shaver. The objective is to remove all the residual ganglionic tissue, as well as the connecting stalk. In our opinion, because of the proximity of median nerve and radial artery, this is a very dangerous procedure.

In all cases, the tourniquet is deflated before ending the intervention to check for any potential vascular injury.

During the procedure, if a TFCC lesion is identified, this will be graded according to the Palmer classification [26] and the treatment will be made according to what can be found in another specific chapter in this book.

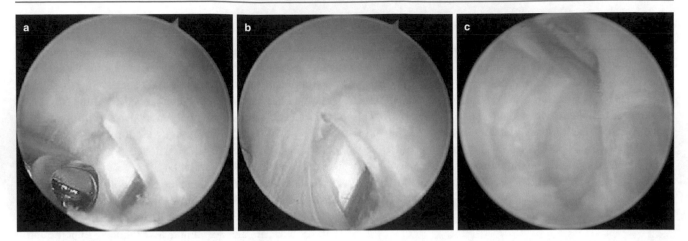

Fig. 49.8 (**a**) Arthroscopic image showing interligamental interval after the operation permit the flexor pollicis longus tendon can be seen. (**b**) Arthroscopic image showing interligamental interval after the oper- ation permit the flexor pollicis longus tendon can be seen. (**c**) Arthroscopic image showing interligamental interval after the operation permit the flexor pollicis longus tendon can be seen

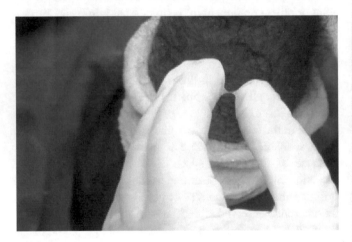

Fig. 49.9 Mucinous liquid leakage through the portal and running down in the skin

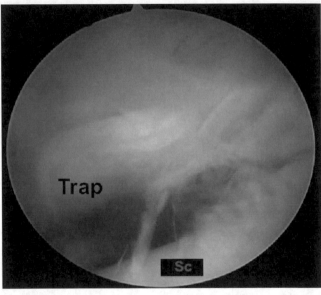

Fig. 49.11 Arthroscopic image showing the scaphotrapezium-trapezoid (STT) joint

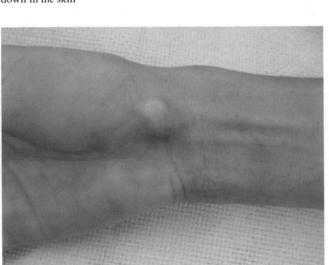

Fig. 49.10 Clinical photo of volar cyst that arises from the distal wrist crease is likely to originate in the scaphotrapezium-trapezoid (STT) joint or other component of the midcarpal joint

At completion of the procedure, single stitches are made to close the portal sites, and the wrist is protected with a bandaging. Patients are advised to move their wrists when the pain permits. The stitches are removed within 1 week. Sports and heavy manual activity should be avoided for 3 months.

Our Experience

Between 2007 and 2012, we performed 31 surgeries of arthroscopic resection of volar wrist ganglion. There were 23 female and 8 male patients. The average age was 38 years.

Two patients have a volar intra-osseous ganglion of lunate bone. In these cases, we also used a volar radial portal.

As complications, we observed transient paresthesia of superficial radial nerve with spontaneous regression in one patient, two volar hematomas, and one recurrence. We used the Allen test in postoperative period and we did not observe failure of blood to diffuse into the hand.

One patient had a volar radiocarpal ganglion confirmed by ultrasound testing, but the procedure was converted to open surgery because the mass was a lipoma.

We never used a needle passing through the ganglion into the joint to identify the interval between the ligaments because of the proximity of the radial artery.

We insert the scope through the 3–4 portals for inspection of the stalk. Therefore, the scope is changed to be introduced through an additional 4–5 portals and volar ganglion was debrided through the radioscaphocapitate (RSC) ligament and long radiolunate (LRL) ligament using a resector inserted from the 3–4 portals. The 1–2 portal is created only when we cannot remove the ganglion through 3–4 and 4–5 portals.

Because of the proximity of the gates 3–4 and 1–2 can have difficulties performing the triangulation technique with optical and blade shaver in the first procedures.

Sometimes, we introduce a Kelly clamp inside the wrist through the 3–4 portals until the palmar capsular defects. The clamp is open and we can observe the mucinous fluid entering inside of the radiocarpal joint.

After the end of procedure, fragments of synovial tissues were collected on the occasion of an endoscopic procedure and were sent to histologic study with the purpose of proving the resection of the ganglion. Our good results were confirmed by others authors that concluded the athroscopic resection is a safe and useful technique [31].

Postoperative Rehabilitation

At completion of the procedure, single stitches are made to close the portal sites, and the wrist was protected with a bandaging.

Patients are advised to move their wrists when the pain permits. The stitches are removed within 1–2 weeks. If the patient shows stiffness or swelling during this time, a therapy program should be started. Heavy manual activity should be avoided for 2 months.

Complications

Wrist arthroscopy is a fairly safe procedure with a low rate of complications. The main complication would be recurrence. One pseudoaneurysm of radial artery was described in a patient with history of hemophilia [32]. Other complications described in the literature [27] include wrist stiffness, carti-

lage injury, thermal burn, reflex sympathetic dystrophy, infection, tendon, nerve, and vessel injury.

References

1. Nelson CL, Sawmiller S, Phalen GS. Ganglions of the wrist and hand. J Bone Joint Surg. 1972;54(7):1459–64.
2. Angelides AC. Ganglions of the hand and wrist. In: Green DP, Hotchkiss RN, Pederson WC, editors. Green's operative hand surgery. 4th ed. New York: Churchill Livingstone; 1999. p. 2171–83.
3. Watson HK, Rogers WD, Ashmead D IV. Reevaluation of the cause of the wrist ganglion. J Hand Surg Am. 1989;14:812–7.
4. Greendyke SD, Wilson M, Shepler TR. Anterior wrist ganglia from the scaphotrapezial joint. J Hand Surg Am. 1992;17(3):487–90.
5. Tophoj K, Henriques U. Ganglion of the wrist—a structure developed from the joint. Acta Orthop Scand. 1971;42(3):244–50.
6. Andren L, Eiken O. Arthrographic studies of wrist ganglions. J Bone Joint Surg Am. 1971;53(2):299–302.
7. Osterman AL, Raphael J. Arthroscopic resection of dorsal ganglion of the wrist. Hand Clin. 1995;11:7–12.
8. Thornburg LE. Ganglions of the hand and wrist. J Am Acad Orthop Surg. 1999;7(4):231–8.
9. Fernandes CH, Meirelles LM, Raduan Neto J, Santos JBG, Faloppa F, Albertoni WM. Characteristics of global publications about wrist arthroscopy: a bibliometric analysis. Hand Surg. 2012;17(3):311–5.
10. Rocchi L, Canal R, Pelaez J, et al. Results and complications in dorsal and volar wrist ganglia arthroscopic resection. Hand Surg. 2006;11:21–61.
11. Rocchi L, Canal A, Fanfani F, Catalano F. Articular ganglia of the volar aspect of the wrist: arthroscopic resection compared with open excision. A prospective randomised study. Scand J Plast Reconstr Surg Hand Surg. 2008;42:253–9.
12. Rhyou I, Kim HJ, Suh BG, Chung C, Kim KC. Arthroscopic resection of volar ganglion of the wrist joint. J Korean Soc Surg Hand. 2010;15(3):136–42.
13. Chen ACY, Lee WC, Hsu KY, Chan YS, Yuan LJ, Chang CH. Arthroscopic ganglionectomy through an intrafocal cystic portal for wrist ganglia. Arthroscopy. 2010;26(5):617–22.
14. Langner I, Krueger PC, Merk HR, Ekkernkamp A, Zach A. Ganglions of the wrist and associated triangular fibrocartilage lesions: a prospective study in arthroscopically-treated patients. J Hand Surg Am. 2012;37:1561–7.
15. Rosson JW, Walker G. The natural history of ganglia in children. J Bone Joint Surg. 1989;71(4):707–8.
16. Jacobs LGH, Govaers KHM. The volar wrist ganglion: just a simple cyst? J Hand Surg Br. 1990;15(3):342–6.
17. Dias J, Buch K. Palmar wrist ganglion: does intervention improve outcome? A prospective study of natural history and patient reported treatment outcomes. J Hand Surg Br. 2003;28:172–6.
18. Ho PC, Lo WN, Hung LK. Arthroscopic resection of volar ganglion of the wrist: a new technique. Arthroscopy. 2003;19(2):218–22.
19. Ho PC, Law BKY, Hung LK. Arthroscopic volar wrist ganglionectomy. Chir Main. 2006;25:221–30.
20. Mathoulin C, Hoyos A, Pelaez J. Arthroscopic resection of wrist ganglia. Hand Surg. 2004;9(2):159–64.
21. Mathoulin C, Massarella M. Therapeutic interest of wrist arthroscopy about 1000 cases. Chir Main. 2006;25:145–60.
22. Chung KC, Murray PM. Hand surgery update V. Rosemont: American Society for Surgery of the Hand; 2011. p. 791.
23. Ho PC, Griffiths J, Lo WN, Yen CH, Hung LK. Current treatment of ganglion of the wrist. Hand Surg. 2001;6(1):49–58.
24. Mathoulin C. Resection of volar ganglia. In: Geissler WB, editor. Wrist arthroscopy, vol. 215. New York: Springer; 2005. p. 182–4.

25. Yamamoto M, Kurimoto S, Okui N, Tatebe M, Shinohara T, Hirata H. Sonography-assisted arthroscopic resection of volar wrist ganglia: a new technique. Arthrosc Tech. 2012;1(1):31–5.

26. Palmer AK. Triangular fibrocartilage complex lesions: a classification. J Hand Surg Am. 1989;14:594–606.

27. Wolfe SW, Pederson WC, Hotchkiss RN, Kozin SH. Wrist arthroscopy. In: Green's operative hand surgery. 6th ed. Philadelphia: Churchill Livingstone; 2010. p. 738–9.

28. Fernandes CH, Miranda CD, Dos Santos JB, Faloppa F. A systematic review of complications and recurrence rate of arthroscopic resection of volar wrist ganglion. Hand Surg. 2014;19(3):475–80.

29. Pires FA, Santos JBGD, Fernandes CH, Nakashima LR, Faloppa F. Sclerotherapy With 75% Hypertonic Glucose to Treat Dorsal Synovial Cysts of The Wrist. Acta Ortop Bras. 2021 Mar-Apr;29(2):101–04.

30. Ho LC, Cabello ÁP, Wai PFY, Pak CH, (2020) Arthroscopic Resection of Wrist Scaphotrapeziotrapezoidal (STT) Joint Ganglia. Journal of Wrist Surgery 09 (05):440–45 .

31. Oliveira RK, Brunelli JPF, Bayer LR, Aita M, Mantovani G, Delgado PJ, (2019) Artrhoscopic Resection of Volar Wrist Ganglion: Surgical Technique and Case Series. Revista Brasileira de Ortopedia 54 (06):721–30.

32. C. Clerico, M. Benatar, C. Dumontier, (2014) Radial artery pseudoaneurysm: A rare complication after arthroscopic treatment of a volar wrist ganglion in a hemophilia patient. Chirurgie de la Main 33 (5):361–63.

Dry Arthroscopy and Its Applications

50

Francisco del Piñal

Introduction

Traditionally, arthroscopy has been carried out using water to create a working cavity ("wet" arthroscopy). Distending the joint with fluid, however, is not nuisance-free. Water infiltrates tissues, escapes through the portals, and might cause serious problems such as compartment syndrome. Water enormously hampers any concomitant surgery after the arthroscopic exploration due to loss of definition of anatomic planes. Finally, the use of water makes it impossible to combine arthroscopy with semi-open procedures—such as intra-articular osteotomies, TFC reinsertions, and so on—as massive seepage of water will cause constant loss of vision.

Extrapolating that in other "scopies" in the human body, such as laparoscopy or thoracoscopy, water was not used to maintain the optic cavity, we realized that traction through the fingers was sufficient to keep the wrist cavity open, making the use of fluid unnecessary. As a matter of fact, all the inconveniences referred to above could be circumvented, without modifying the visual properties, if water were not infused inside the joint ("dry" arthroscopy) [1]. Large portals/mini incisions can be created for the passage of large instruments or the extraction of large bony fragments, without fear of losing watertightness. Open and semi-open arthroscopic-assisted procedures can hence be easily combined. Finally, traditional open surgery can be carried out immediately after the arthroscopy exploration leaving tissue in pristine conditions, as there has been no extravasation of fluid outside the capsule (Fig. 50.1).

Not using fluid, on the other hand, engenders a new set of problems secondary to loss of vision caused by splashes on the tip of the scope or blood and debris in the joint. This may induce the novice to give up at the first difficulty met, but the advantages of the dry technique far outweigh the difficulties encountered on the learning curve. In this work, the technical tips to carry out an uneventful operation are presented in detail.

Surgical Technique

The "dry" arthroscopy technique is similar to a standard wrist arthroscopy ("wet"), except for the fact that water is not used to maintain the optic cavity. As stated, the main shortcoming comes from the fact that if one is not able to get rid of the blood and splashes that obscure vision in an expeditious manner, surgery will become a nightmare and one will give up the dry technique.

Intuitively, one would think that removing the scope and wiping off the lens with a wet sponge is a good way of having clear vision. Although effective, this maneuver is time-consuming, and in a fracture or other complex procedures described in this chapter, there may be so much blood or debris that the maneuver may need to be repeated an exasperating number of times. Based on our experience with more than 1000 dry wrist arthroscopies, but more important seeing how others in the laboratory and surgery struggle with the same difficulties over and over again, I can recommend the following tips that are critical for a smooth procedure, some of which are improvements on our previous publications [1, 2]:

- The valve of the sheath of the scope should be kept open at all times to allow the air to circulate freely inside the joint. Otherwise, either the suction of the shaver will not function properly or the capsule will collapse inwards due to the power of the suction, resulting in blocked vision. This is critical and cannot be overemphasized (Fig. 50.2).
- Suction is necessary to clear the field, but paradoxically, suction might also blur the vision by stirring up the contents of the joint (debris, blood, or remaining saline) that may stick to the tip of the scope. It is critical, therefore, to

F. del Piñal (✉)
Unit of Hand-Wrist and Plastic Surgery, Private Practice and Hospital Mutua Montañesa, Santander, Spain
e-mail: drpinal@drpinal.com

© Springer Nature Switzerland AG 2022
W. B. Geissler (ed.), *Wrist and Elbow Arthroscopy with Selected Open Procedures*,
https://doi.org/10.1007/978-3-030-78881-0_50

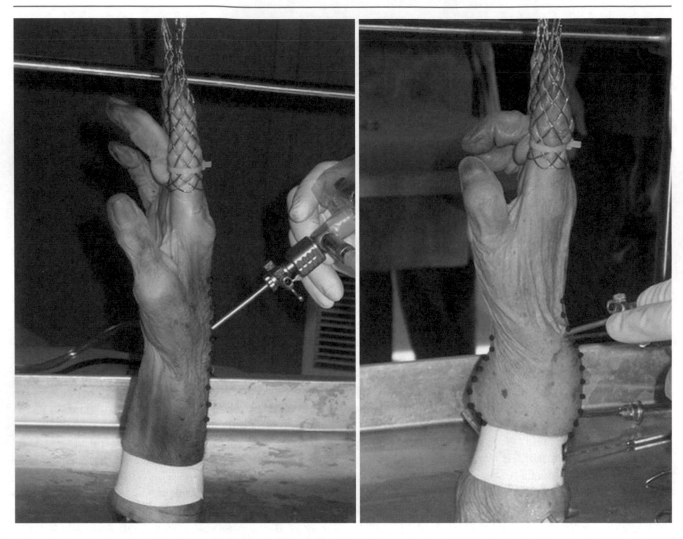

Fig. 50.1 The deformity of the wrist due to fluid extravasation after 1 h of wet arthroscopy (*right*) as compared to the *left* which was operated for the same amount of time but under the dry technique. Pictures were taken during a teaching course with cadavers in Strasbourg. Both were operated by students simultaneously in different working posts. (Copyright Dr. Francisco del Piñal, 2010)

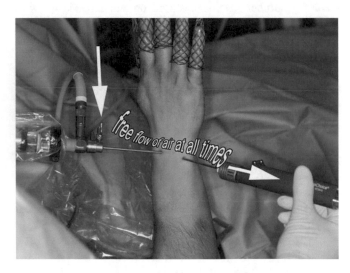

Fig. 50.2 The valve of the scope should be open at all times so as to allow air to circulate freely. (Reprinted from del Piñal [7]. With permission from Sage Publications)

open the suction of the shaver or burr only when there is the need to aspirate something. Suction power should be locked when not needed. *To sum up, the valve of the sheath of the scope should be open at all times, but suction power should only be working when needed.*

- Avoid getting too close with the tip of the scope when working with burrs or osteotomes in order to avert splashes that might block your vision. Minor splashes can be removed by gently rubbing the tip of scope on the local soft tissue (capsule, fat, etc.).

- When a clear field is needed, so as to see a gap or a step-off, we *used to* recommend drying out the joint with neurosurgical patties [1]. However, we rarely resort to this technique now and prefer to connect a syringe with 5–10 cc of saline to the side valve of the scope and then aspirate it with the synoviotome, in order to get rid of blood and debris. Pressure on the plunger of the syringe is unnecessary, as the negative pressure exerted by the

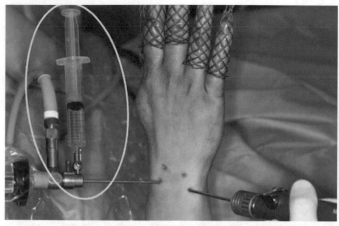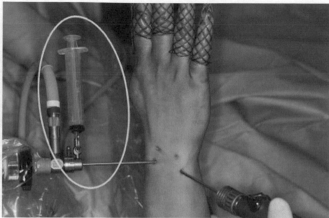

Fig. 50.3 Method used to wash out the joint and clear it of blood. Notice that the negative pressure exerted by the shaver is sufficient to aspirate the saline without extravasation of water. (Reprinted from del Piñal [7]. With permission from Sage Publications)

shaver will suck the saline into the joint, thus preventing any extravasation (Fig. 50.3). Once all the water has been aspirated, the syringe is removed, and again the suction power of the shaver is enough to dry out the joint sufficiently, thus allowing the surgeon to work. *This maneuver should be repeated as necessary throughout the procedure*, as it is much quicker than struggling with blood in the joint, or trying to dry it out with the patties.

- An important waste of time occurs when the synoviotome, burr, or any other instruments connected to a suction machine clog because the aspirated debris dries out. When this happens the operation has to be stopped in order to dismount and irrigate the synoviotome for dislodging the debris. This is to be avoided at all costs by clearing the tubing with periodic saline aspiration from an external basin by the OR nurse, or by the surgeon through joint irrigation. Joint flushing should also be done in a systematic fashion in some procedures, such as intercarpal arthrodesis or arthroscopic proximal carpectomy, in which prolonged use of the synoviotomes and burrs may cause heating of the instrument itself causing local burns (see below).
- Finally, one must understand that at most times, vision will never be completely clear but still sufficient to safely accomplish the goals of the procedure. Having a completely dried field except for specific times during the procedure is unnecessary and wastes valuable time, and we rely more on the irrigation-suction just explained above.

The technique can be summarized in these three fundamental tips:

- The valve of the scope should be open at all times.
- The suction should be closed except when needed.
- The joint should be irrigated as needed in order to remove debris and blood.

Contraindications

The dry technique is contraindicated when using vaporizers, lasers, etc., as the heat generated will not dissipate, risking widespread cartilage damage. The problem is solved easily, however, by swapping to the "wet" technique during the specific moment those kind of instruments are being used. Once the "vaporizer step" is terminated, the saline is disconnected and air is allowed to flow in the joint. The remaining water is sucked out with the synoviotome and the procedure continues "dry." In very special scenarios where running water is paramount, such as in septic arthritis, the use of the dry technique will offer no advantage and is not advised.

Risk of compartment syndrome has been considered a contraindication for arthroscopy, particularly after severe fractures, but this is not a problem when using the dry technique. Furthermore, I cannot see open wounds as a contraindication of the dry arthroscopy either, provided debridement of the portal is carried out and thorough irrigation of the joint is performed at the end of the procedure.

One concern many surgeons have about the dry arthroscopy is the possibility of burning inside the joint by the tip of the scope. This has never occurred in our experience, as the tip of the scope never warms up to that point. I should warn the reader, however, that we have experienced minor contact burns at the portals and the dorsal skin, by the synoviotome and burr. The rotating mechanism of these instruments heats up, as a result of friction, when used for very long periods of time. This is easily overcome by flushing the joint with saline that will cool down the synoviotome, and also will improve vision.

Clinical Applications

I use the dry technique in all my arthroscopic explorations, as I personally have not found it necessary to use vaporizers. However, there are four common pathologies where not using water makes an enormous difference, namely, distal radius fractures and (distal radius) malunions, arthroscopic arthrodeses, and perilunate fractures and dislocations.

Distal Radius Fractures

Despite the existence in the literature of well-performed Level 1 studies [3–5] supporting the use of the arthroscope when dealing with articular distal radius fractures, there is general resistance in the Hand Surgery community to admit so. This is sometimes justified as being due to a(-n infinitesimal) risk of compartment syndrome, and more so to the massive swelling that accompanies the wet arthroscopy which makes the open part of the procedure more awkward. Although the latter reason is true, the unvoiced reason lies in the technical difficulties of the arthroscopic part itself. This is more so the more comminuted the fracture is, which, paradoxically, is the one that benefits most from having an arthroscopic-assisted reduction [6]. Yet, there is no other single field in wrist arthroscopy where the dry technique can make such a huge difference and ease the procedure, as when dealing with articular fractures of the wrist. The dry arthroscopy allows an unimpeded combination between the open fixation part and the ability to watch the cartilaginous reduction and assess ligamentous and TFC injuries.

Our current technique [7–9] includes the use of volar locking plates in combination with arthroscopy, except in some specific fractures such as radial styloid, where cannulated screws through a transverse incision in the styloid is the preferred fixation method. For the typical three- or four-part fracture, the radius is approached between the FCR and the radial artery. After a preliminary reduction by ordinary maneuvers, a volar locking plate is applied and stabilized by inserting only the screw into the elliptical hole on the stem of the plate. The articular fragments are reduced to the plate that act as a mold, and once the "best" reduction is obtained as judged by fluoroscopic views, the articular fragments are secured to the plate by inserting Kirschner wires (K-wire) through the auxiliary holes of the transverse component of the plate. It should be underscored that definitive fixation (screws or pegs) should not yet be used, as any change will not be possible later.

The hand is suspended from a bow, the fingers pointing to the ceiling, with a customized system that allows easy connection and disconnection from the bow without losing sterility, as fluoroscopic checkups are needed [10]. Traction is carried out on all fingers with counter-traction of 7–10 kg. A small transverse incision is made just distal to Lister's tubercle, and after dilating the portal with a straight mosquito, the scope (2.7 mm; 30° angle) is introduced and directed ulnarly. In the swollen wrist, it may be very difficult to establish 6-R portal, more so because the TFC may be detached from the fovea acting as a lid blocking the entrance into the radiocarpal joint. I overcome this eventuality by establishing this portal by going blindly with a hemostat in a radial direction immediately radial to the ECU just brushing past the proximal triquetrum.

The blood and debris are aspirated by a 2.9-mm shaver inserted in 6R. Flushing and debridement are carried out until the joint is completely clean. Once the elements that need to be mobilized are identified, the scope is swapped to 6R, where it will stay until the entire fixation is done. In this position, on top of the ulnar head, the scope will have a steady point to rest upon, and will not impede reduction or displace reduced fragments (Fig. 50.4).

In simpler cases where only a single fragment remains unreduced, the fragment is freed by backing out the specific K-wire that kept it secured to the plate. Depressed fragments are lifted by hooking them with the tip of a shoulder or knee arthroscopy probe introduced from the 3 to 4 (Fig. 50.5).

Elevated fragments nearly always correspond to rim fragments that due to the effect of traction are overdistracted. They are easily repositioned by the assistant decreasing traction while the surgeon levels them with the probe or a Freer elevator. Once the fragment is reduced, it is held in position with a bone tenaculum, and stabilized by pushing the corresponding K-wire in the plate again. Free osteochondral fragments are extremely unstable and when repositioned, sink into the metaphyseal void. To avoid this, we create a supporting hammock where they can lie. This is done by inserting the distal layer of pegs in the plate, while keeping these fragments slightly overreduced. Then, they are impacted by using a Freer elevator or by releasing the traction and using the corresponding carpal bone as a mold. A grasper can be useful to grab and twist a severely displaced fragment [7].

Still under arthroscopic control, locking pegs are inserted in the plate by the other surgeon in critical spots, so as to make the articular surface stable to probe palpation. This part of the operation is quite awkward as the flexor tendons are in tension blocking the vision of the plate. Retracting ulnarly the tendons with a Farabeuf, and reducing the traction to release the flexor tendons may ease the task. As soon as the major articular fragments are stabilized, the hand is put flat on the operating table, as in this position, the remaining pegs and screws can be inserted expeditiously (Fig. 50.6).

Only in the most comminuted cases will several fragments continue to be displaced after the fluoroscopic part of the operation. Backing out all the K-wires, and attempting to reduce and fix all fragments at the same time, is an impossible endeavor in our hands. We recommend a step-by-step procedure beginning preferably from the ulnar part of the radius, advancing in a radial direction. The mechanics of the procedure is similar as for a single fragment: the corresponding K-wire is backed out, the fragment reduced, and the K-wire

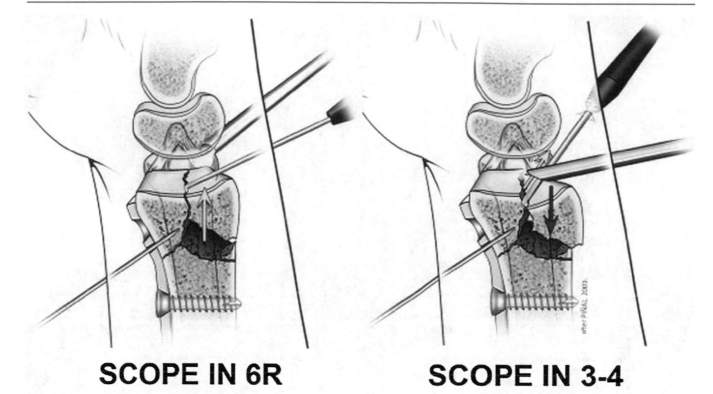

SCOPE IN 6R

SCOPE IN 3-4

Fig. 50.4 If the scope is placed in 6R it will rest on top of the ulnar head providing a stable platform from which to work, thus avoiding conflict with the reduction (*left*). Instability of the scope and conflict of space during the reduction (*yellow and red arrows*) are inevitable when the scope is placed in any other portal (*right*). (Copyright Dr. Francisco del Piñal, 2009)

pushed in, building up the rest of the articular surface to this foundation.

Once the radius fixation is over, the hand is again placed on traction and distal radioulnar joint and the midcarpal joints are assessed for instability or ligament damage.

Arthroscopic Guided Osteotomy for Distal Radius Malunion

Arthroscopy can be invaluable to locate step-offs and see the personality of the malunited fragment, to cut the bone exactly at the cartilage fracture line, and to assess the reduction (Fig. 50.7). This is more so as fluoroscopy has not proved very reliable even in the setting of acute fractures [11, 12], and because a blind osteotomy can cut in an undesired spot [13].

The technique of osteotomy has been described previously [10, 13], and the early results reported [14]. Briefly, the procedure is started by preparing the proposed site of plate fixation with the arm lying on the hand table. In order to facilitate the separation of the fragments, when later doing the intra-articular osteotomy, the external callus is removed with a rongeur and the outer callus is weakened with an osteotome. No attempt is made to go all the way to the joint or to do any rough bending or prying open of the fragment

with the osteotome, as this may break the cartilage at the incorrect place. A plate, when needed, is preplaced at this stage and held in position with a single screw through its stem as explained for acute fractures. The hand is then placed on traction. An arthroscopic arthrolysis is first carried out to create working space, as the joint is scarred and unyielding. For cutting the bone we used a shoulder periosteal elevator (of 15 and 30° angle) (Arthrex® AR-1342-30° and AR-1342-15°, Arthrex, Naples, FL, USA), and also straight and curved osteotomes (Arthrex® AR-1770 and AR-1771). Instruments with different angles are required in order to avoid damaging the cartilage, and laceration of the extensor tendons is to be avoided by the appropriate technique [13]. The osteotomes also have to be inserted through different portals in order to adapt to the different configurations of the fracture (Fig. 50.8). Stabilization of the fragments is carried out with volar locking plates when several fragments are mobilized; screws or buttressing plates are used when only one fragment needs to be addressed.

Arthroscopic Arthrodesis

The feasibility of performing intercarpal or radiocarpal arthrodesis arthroscopically was presented by Ho in a pioneering work [15]. It may be considered by the skeptical as

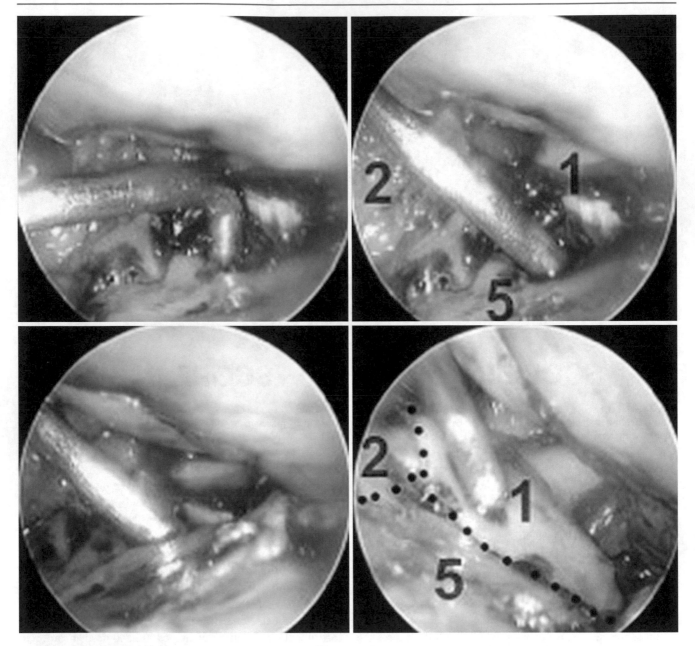

Fig. 50.5 Reduction of a depressed fragment in the scaphoid fossa. From *left* to *right*: The shoulder probe is gauging the step-off (3 mm), hooking the depressed fragment, elevating it, and leveling it to the rest of the joint. Scope in 6R, viewing radially in a right wrist. 1: volar rim of the scaphoid fossa, 2: dorsal rim; 5: scaphoid fossa. (Copyright Dr. Francisco del Piñal, 2009)

just another arthroscopic filigree. However, the procedure is sound, not only because there will be a cosmetic benefit, but above all, in my view, because the degree of insult to the ligaments will be minimized. Ligament preservation will keep the blood supply to the bones intact and with less scarring to the capsule. This, in turn, promotes bone healing and less stiffness respectively. Furthermore, the proprioception of the wrist will be undisturbed providing (in theory) some extra protection to the joint.

Although the idea of minimizing surgical insult to the wrist is appealing, the technical difficulties of the operation as presented by Ho—including more than 3 h operative time—make implementation of the technique challenging. Some of the procedural struggles come from the infusion of saline. As a matter of fact, most of the difficulties mentioned for the wet A-4CA (Arthroscopic Four Corner Arthrodesis) as described by Ho [15] are circumvented when using the dry technique. Specifically, bone graft can be accurately placed, and the swelling does not mask the bony landmarks. Furthermore, we have been increasingly employing rongeurs to remove the carpals and minimizing the use of burrs, speeding up the procedure enormously.

Fig. 50.6 Summary of the author's technique to reduce and stabilize the common scenario of a posterior depressed fragment that remains unreduced. Notice that the K-wire is backed out sufficiently enough to release this malpositioned fragment, while the rest of the reduction remains unaffected during the whole maneuver. (Copyright Dr. Francisco del Piñal, 2009)

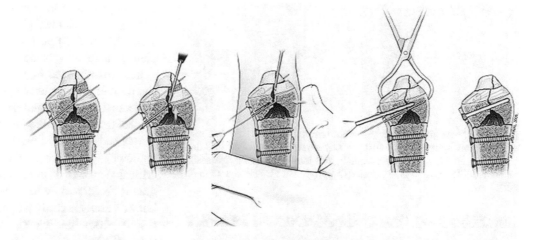

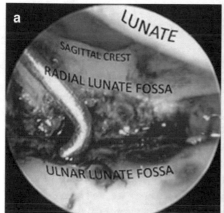
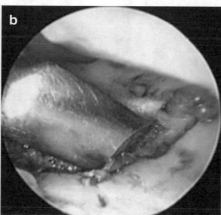
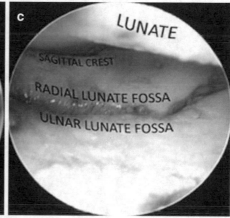

Fig. 50.7 (a) Correction of a 4-mm step-off on the lunate fossa (right wrist scope in 6R). (b) The osteotome (entering the joint through a dorsal portal) is separating the malunited fragments. (c) Corresponding view after reduction. (Copyright Dr. Francisco del Piñal, 2010)

The dry A-4CA [16] can be completed in less than 2 h (i.e., in less than 1 tourniquet time). It can be summarized in the following crucial steps:

1. Creation of a (large) scapholunate (S-L) portal: The procedure commences by creating the portals, which are easily made ulnarly (6R and UMC), but in advanced SLAC or SNAC, are not so easily made radially. This is due to architectural derangement of the carpus and often scarring from previous surgery. My preference is to create a large (1.5 cm) transverse "scapholunate portal" (midway between 3 and 4 and radial midcarpal (RMC)) corresponding to the location of the scapholunate gap or the scaphoid nonunion (Fig. 50.9). From there, work can be performed in both radiocarpal and midcarpal directions.

2. Scaphoid excision with rongeurs: The previous description of A-4CA and A-PRC [15, 17] resected the bone with a burr, but as stated, it is time-consuming and the scaphoid cannot be reused as bone graft. Conversely, using pituitary rongeurs, the scaphoid can be excised expedi-

tiously and the cancellous bone graft reused later (Fig. 50.10).

3. Midcarpal joint preparation: The cartilage and subchondral bone at the site of the 4CA are removed with a burr. A 3.0-mm pineapple burr is preferred because it tends not to get caught on bone and produces a more even surface of bone as opposed to pits created by the round burr. During burring, the suction of the instrument is maintained in the off position. Otherwise, the suction stirs up the contents of the joint and obscures the visual field. To remove debris and prevent the burr from clogging, aliquots of 5–10 mL saline are flushed through the scope's side valve with a syringe. The suction is turned on at that specific time, and once the debris is removed, the suction is again turned off.

4. Lunate reduction: After the joint surfaces are appropriately prepared, the hand is removed from the traction device to reduce the lunate. To correct the extended and ulnar translated lunate, the wrist is maximally flexed and radially translated. The lunate reduction is maintained

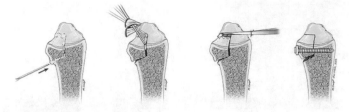

Fig. 50.8 Most malunions require multiple accesses and combinations of osteotomy types. Notice that the osteotome is introduced into the cleft between the radioscaphocapitate and long radiolunate ligaments when using the volar-radial portal. (Copyright Dr. Francisco del Piñal, 2009)

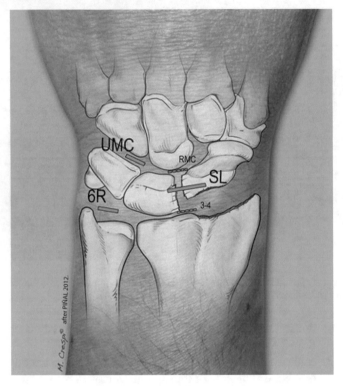

Fig. 50.9 The SL portal is located midway between the 3 and 4 and radial midcarpal portals. *SL* scapholunate portal, *RMC* radial midcarpal, *UMC* ulnar midcarpal. (Reprinted from del Piñal et al. [16]. With permission from Elsevier)

with a K-wire (1.25 mm), which is inserted about 2 cm proximal to the 4–5 portal and directed slightly radially.

5. Bone grafting: With the lunate reduced, the hand is again placed on traction to allow for the placement of bone graft under arthroscopic guidance. The cavity during traction is large, but we focus on filling the anterior aspects of the lunocapitate and triquetrohamate joints as well as the most distal aspect of the lunotriquetral joint only. For the other surfaces, bone graft is not needed because cancellous bone will contact cancellous bone once the joint is reduced. After trying several devices and methods, the technique we now employ to deliver the bone graft inside the joint is a 3.5-mm (or even 4.5 mm) drill guide. The

cancellous bone is loaded into the guide outside the wrist, and the guide is then placed into the joint through the scapholunate (SL) portal. A shoulder probe, acting as a plunger, then delivers the bone into the joint, and the bone graft is manipulated into the appropriate position with a small Freer elevator or the probe itself (Fig. 50.11).

6. Midcarpal reduction and fixation: After the bone graft is placed, the hand is taken off traction, the midcarpal joint is reduced (translocating the capitate ulnarly), and the guidewires for the cannulated screws are inserted. This critical step, one of the trickiest part of the operation, is greatly facilitated by the dry arthroscopic technique; the bony anatomy is easily palpated because the swelling that results from the classic wet technique is avoided (Fig. 50.12).

The guidewires are placed in such a fashion as to maximize purchase and avoid screw collision: The capitolunate screw is directed from the dorsal distal aspect of the capitate to the volar proximal aspect of the lunate, the triquetrolunate screw is directed from the volar triquetrum to the dorsal lunate, and the triquetrocapitate screw is directed from the dorsal distal triquetrum to the volar distal capitate. This technique avoids the problem of one screw interfering with placement of the next (Fig. 50.13).

A small transverse incision is made at the base of the long finger metacarpal for guidewire insertion and later drilling of the capitate. This allows for protection of the extensor tendon of the third finger. The surgeon's hand must be oriented nearly parallel to the patient's wrist during insertion of this guidewire; otherwise, the lunate is missed. Presently, I favor another small transverse incision over the triquetrum to insert the ulnar screws, as I fear that the dorsal branch of the ulnar nerve, the ECU, and the EDM may be at risk if done percutaneously as I used to recommend previously [16].

Correct placement of the guidewires is confirmed on fluoroscopy. Screws of appropriate length and size (presently I use 3-mm titanium AutoFIX™ [Small Bone Innovations, New York, NY]) are inserted after predrilling the port of entrance only. The radiolunate Kirschner wire is removed and a final fluoroscopic check is performed. Although the carpal height is restored by repositioning the capitate on the lunate, the radial styloid may continue to abut the carpus. In this case, the styloid should be resected. This actually takes little time to complete with the rongeur. Care should be taken to preserve intact the RSC ligament origins on the radius. Finally, the SL portal incision is closed with intradermal sutures and the other portals are dressed with nonadherent gauze. Protected range of motion is commenced at about 2–3 weeks.

To date (February 2013), I have done nine cases of dry A-4CA without complications and with fusion in all cases (Fig. 50.14). I have experience in several types of arthrode-

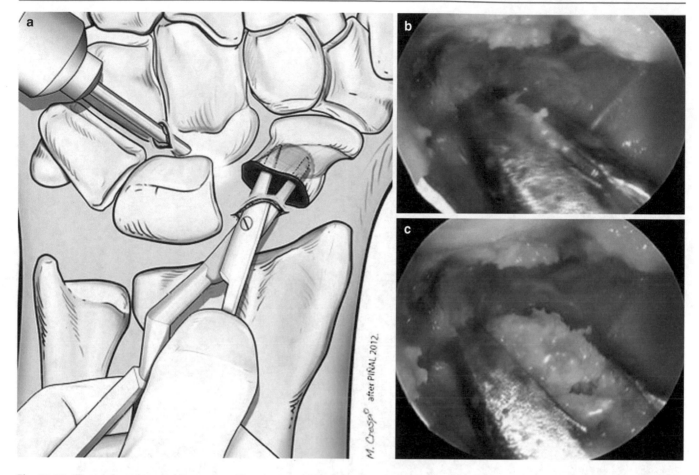

Fig. 50.10 The process of scaphoid resection with a rongeur. (**a**) With the scope in UMC the surgeon scoops out the middle third of the scaphoid with the rongeur. (**b** and **c**) Corresponding arthroscopic view. (Reprinted from del Piñal et al. [16]. With permission from Elsevier)

ses under the dry technique, including the most useful radioscapholunate (Fig. 50.15). It is too early to prove that the results are any better than open, however. Nevertheless, the possibility of achieving complex fixations through minimally invasive surgery represents the future of wrist surgery and the direction in which we should head.

Perilunate Fractures and Fracture-Dislocations

Although the benefit of treating major carpal injuries without adding further damage is self-evident, very few surgeons have experience in the technique [18–20]. Many of the difficulties of the operation come again from the need to infuse saline, as the capsular rents are massive and the fluid extravasates immediately out of the joint. Apart from a theoretical risk of compartment syndrome, the insertion of K-wires and guidewires needed to achieve carpal fixation is complicated enormously by the lack of palpable bony landmarks. Doing the arthroscopy dry reduces the difficulties.

In our practice, we schedule the surgery as soon as feasible. Usually, traction will reduce spontaneously the lunate

but if not, after establishing RMC and ulnar midcarpal (UMC) portals, the lunate is pulled and reduced with the shoulder probe with minimal difficulties. After assessment of the injured structures the hand is taken off traction and placed on the hand table. Two K-wires in the scaphoid and 1 (or 2) in the triquetrum are preset under fluoroscopic control. An additional 1.5 mm K-wire is inserted into the lunate to be used as a joystick, as this bone is uncontrollable by external maneuvers. The importance of the advantageous lack of swelling at the time of inserting these K-wires cannot be overemphasized (Fig. 50.16).

The hand is placed on traction again to reduce and stabilize the proximal carpal row under arthroscopic control. This maneuver is extremely complicated and is facilitated if the surgeon can "feel" the bony architecture. The surgeon needs to push the proximal pole of the scaphoid down with a shoulder probe (or a Freer elevator) while the lunate is kept aligned to the scaphoid (using the 1.5 mm K-wire to do so). At the same time, the S-L space is closed by compressing the scaphoid and the triquetrum (Fig. 50.17). The K-wires are driven into the lunate. An optional distal scaphoid-distal capitate can be inserted to block the midcarpal joint.

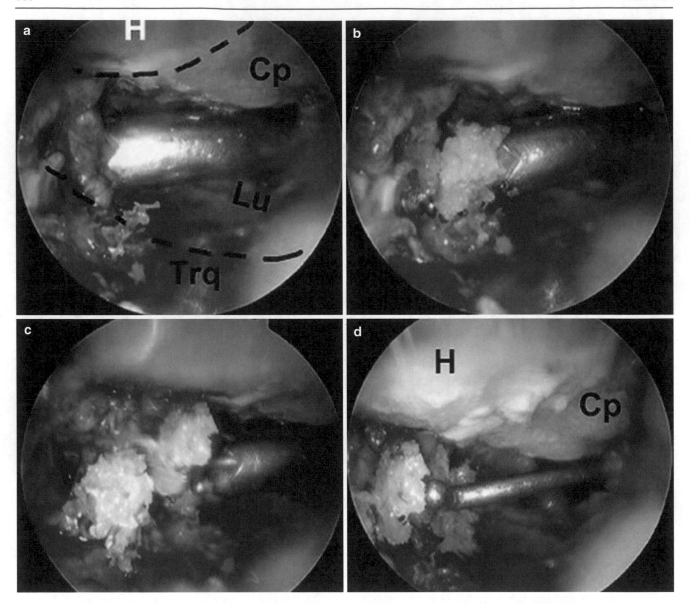

Fig. 50.11 The process of introducing the bone graft into the midcarpal space is shown. (**a**) A 3.5-mm drill guide, fully loaded of cancellous bone graft introduced from SL portal is facing the volar aspect of the lunate and triquetrum (*Lu* lunate, *Trq* triquetrum). (**b**) The plunger (the shoulder hook in this case) is starting to push the bone graft into the joint space. (**c**) All the bone graft has been delivered in the joint. (**d**) The shoulder probe or a small Freer elevator is used to compress the bone against the palmar ligaments (*H* hamate, *Cp* capitate). (Reprinted from del Piñal et al. [16]. With permission from Elsevier)

When the scaphoid is fractured, the technique is slightly modified. After prereducing the wrist, under fluoroscopic control, 2 K-wires (of 1 mm diameter to serve as guidewire) are driven in through the distal pole of the scaphoid only; another K-wire is driven into the triquetrum (directed to the lunate). Reduction of the scaphoid under arthroscopic guidance is then carried out and both K-wires are inserted into the proximal pole. In general, a distal to proximal screw is inserted using the best-placed K-wire of the 2, as the guidewire. If the fracture involves the proximal pole of the scaphoid, the wrist is slightly flexed and Slade's technique is followed to insert a proximal to distal screw.

The aftercare is similar to an open procedure (6–8 weeks of immobilization or as needed for the scaphoid to heal).

Kim et al. [19] in the largest case series published to date presented slightly better results as compared to open techniques, with maintenance of the carpal angles despite the fact that no ligament was sutured. Most importantly, they showed no case of midterm joint degeneration, inferring that arthroscopy allowed a better reduction and less blood supply disturbance on the carpals. My experience is limited to seven cases and my results endorse Park's experience [18, 19].

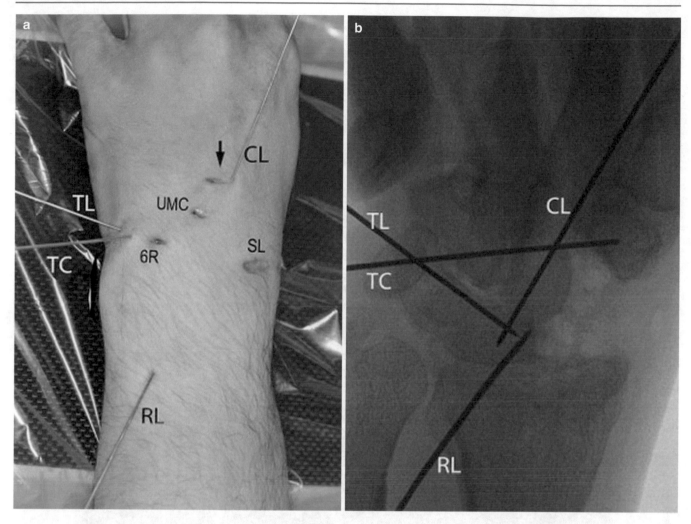

Fig. 50.12 View of the hand (**a**) and corresponding fluoroscopic view (**b**) at the end of the insertion of the guidewires. Notice that the hand is not swollen even at this late stage of the operation. *TC* triquetrocapitate, *TL* triquetrolunate, *RL* radiolunate, *CL* capitolunate, *SL* scapholunate portal, *UMC* ulnar midcarpal portal. *Arrow* points to the incision needed for the insertion of the capitolunate screw. (Reprinted from del Piñal et al. [16]. With permission from Elsevier)

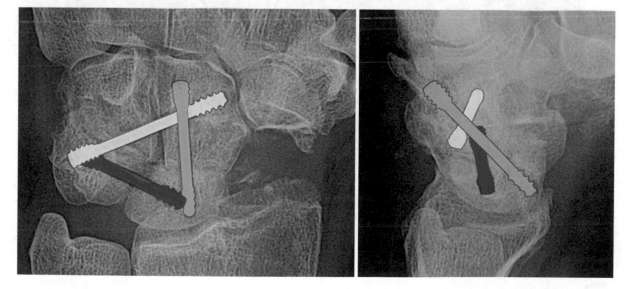

Fig. 50.13 Ideally the screws should be placed to avoid collision and provide maximal purchase as explained in the text. (Reprinted from del Piñal et al. [16]. With permission from Elsevier)

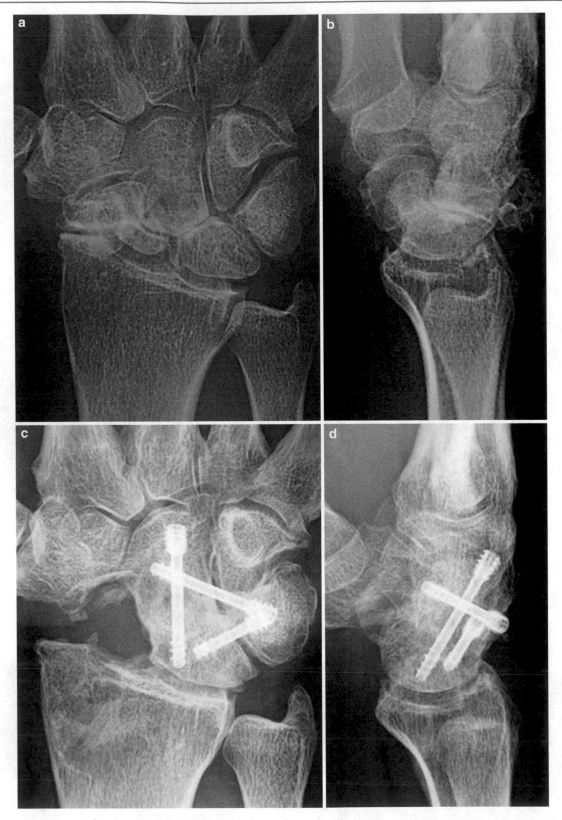

Fig. 50.14 SNAC III. (**a**, **b**) Preoperative plain X-rays. (**c**, **d**) X-rays at 15 months. (Reprinted from del Piñal et al. [16]. With permission from Elsevier)

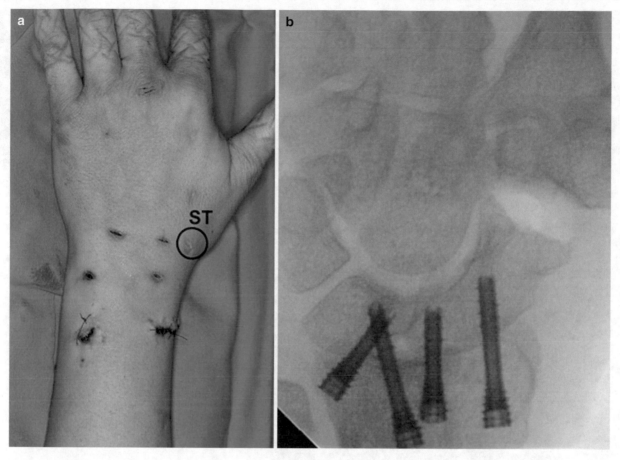

Fig. 50.15 (a) Notice minimal swelling at the end of the operation in a case of an R-S-L arthrodesis, resection of the distal pole of the scaphoid was also carried out through the ST portal. Cannulated screws were inserted through the proximal incisions (*arrows*). (b) Radiographic healing. (Copyright Dr. Francisco del Piñal, 2013)

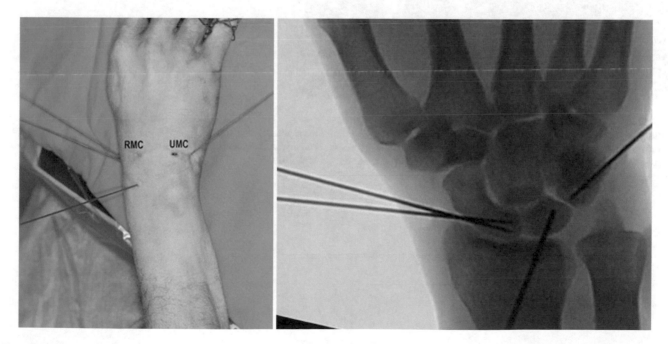

Fig. 50.16 Presetting of K-wires is done with the hand on the surgical table and under fluoroscopic guidance. Notice absence of swelling at the wrist, despite the fact that the joint has already been cleared of debris and the lunate reduced arthroscopically. Corresponding fluoroscopic view (*right*). (Copyright Dr. Francisco del Piñal, 2013)

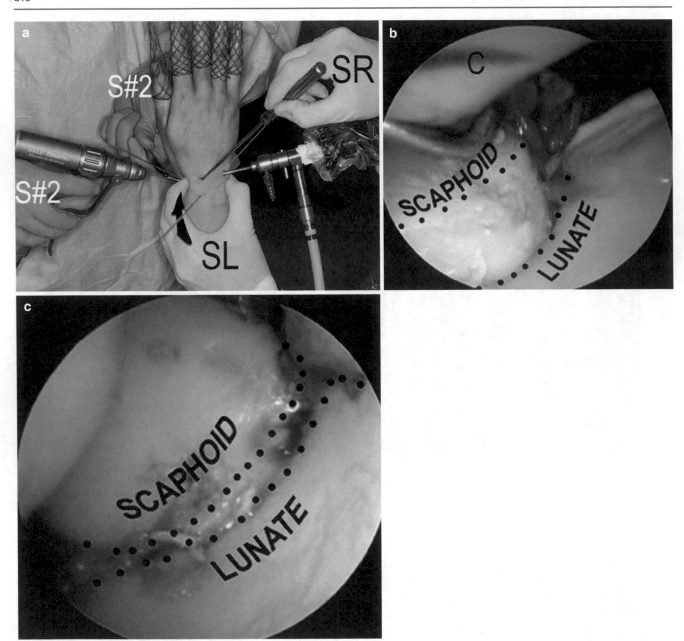

Fig. 50.17 Reduction of a perilunate dislocation. (**a**) As a one-man band, the surgeon reduces the scaphoid with the probe (Surgeon's Right hand) while with the other hand, the carpals are compressed (SLeft) and with the dorsum of the index, the lunate's K-wire is flipped volarly (*arrow*). The Assistant (S#2) then drives the K-wires in. (**b**) Corresponding arthroscopic view to (**a**), and after the K-wires have been driven in reducing the S-L space (**c**). (Copyright Dr. Francisco del Piñal, 2013)

Summary

Wrist arthroscopy can be carried out without infusing water to maintain the optical cavity, as simple traction suffices. The lack of tissue infiltration by fluid keeps soft tissues in pristine condition in the event that open surgery is needed after the arthroscopic exploration. The fact that the dry technique makes watertightness irrelevant opens a new set of possibilities by combining arthroscopy with moderate-sized incisions. Despite the fact that any modification of a technique with which one is familiar can be regarded with major reticence, the advantages of the dry technique well merit giving it a try. As a matter of fact, although in simpler arthroscopic procedures there are probably no differences, the complex ones are much simplified by doing them dry. Sooner or later, even the most reluctant wet arthroscopists will have to swap to the dry technique to get the most out of what arthroscopy might offer. On the other hand, any accomplished wrist arthroscopist will have minimal problems to swap from wet to dry and vice versa.

I should underscore that the procedures described in this chapter have a steep learning curve even for skilled arthroscopists and require the surgeon to have precise spatial orientation at the time of guidewire or osteotome placement.

References

1. del Piñal F, García-Bernal FJ, Pisani D, Regalado J, Ayala H, Studer A. Dry arthroscopy of the wrist: surgical technique. J Hand Surg Am. 2007;32:119–23.
2. Piñal D. Dry arthroscopy and its applications. Hand Clin. 2011;27:335–45.
3. Doi K, Hattori Y, Otsuka K, Abe Y, Yamamoto H. Intra-articular fractures of the distal aspect of the radius: arthroscopically assisted reduction compared with open reduction and internal fixation. J Bone Joint Surg. 1999;81:1093–110.
4. Ruch DS, Vallee J, Poehling GG, Smith BP, Kuzma GR. Arthroscopic reduction versus fluoroscopic reduction in the management of intra-articular distal radius fractures. Arthroscopy. 2004;20:225–30.
5. Varitimidis SE, Basdekis GK, Dailiana ZH, Hantes ME, Bargiotas K, Malizos K. Treatment of intra-articular fractures of the distal radius: fluoroscopic or arthroscopic reduction? J Bone Joint Surg Br. 2008;90:778–85.
6. del Pinal F, Garcia-Bernal FG, Studer A, et al. Explosion type articular distal radius fractures: technique and results of volar locking plate under dry arthroscopy guidance. Presented at the FESSH Meeting in Poznan (Poland). 2009. Book of Abstracts A0180.
7. del Piñal F. Dry arthroscopy of the wrist: its role in the management of articular distal radius fractures. Scand J Surg. 2008;97:298–304.
8. del Piñal F. Treatment of explosion-type distal radius fractures. In: del Piñal F, Mathoulin C, Luchetti C, editors. Arthroscopic management of distal radius fractures. Berlin: Springer; 2010. p. 41–65.
9. del Piñal F. Technical tips for (dry) arthroscopic reduction and internal fixation of distal radius fractures. J Hand Surg Am. 2011;36:1694–705.
10. del Piñal F, García-Bernal FJ, Delgado J, Sanmartín M, Regalado J, Cerezal L. Correction of malunited intra-articular distal radius fractures with an inside-out osteotomy technique. J Hand Surg Am. 2006;31:1029–34.
11. Edwards CC III, Harasztic J, McGillivary GR, Gutow AP. Intra-articular distal radius fractures: arthroscopic assessment of radiographically assisted reduction. J Hand Surg Am. 2001;26:1036–41.
12. Lutsky K, Boyer MI, Steffen JA, Goldfarb CA. Arthroscopic assessment of intra-articular distal radius fractures after open reduction and internal fixation from a volar approach. J Hand Surg Am. 2008;33:476–84.
13. del Piñal F. Arthroscopic-assisted osteotomy for intraarticular malunion of the distal radius. In: del Piñal F, Mathoulin C, Luchetti C, editors. Arthroscopic management of distal radius fractures. Berlin: Springer; 2010. p. 191–209.
14. del Piñal F, Cagigal L, García-Bernal FJ, Studer A, Regalado J, Thams C. Arthroscopically guided osteotomy for management of intra-articular distal radius malunions. J Hand Surg Am. 2010;35:392–7.
15. Ho PC. Arthroscopic partial wrist fusion. Tech Hand Up Extrem Surg. 2008;12:242–65.
16. del Piñal F, Klausmeyer M, Thams C, Moraleda E, Galindo C. Early experience with (dry) arthroscopic 4-corner arthrodesis: from a 4-hour operation to a tourniquet time. J Hand Surg Am. 2012;37:2389–99.
17. Weiss ND, Molina RA, Gwin S. Arthroscopic proximal row carpectomy. J Hand Surg Am. 2011;36:577–82.
18. Park MJ, Ahn JH. Arthroscopically assisted reduction and percutaneous fixation of dorsal perilunate dislocations and fracture-dislocations. Arthroscopy. 2005;21:1153e1–8.
19. Kim JP, Lee JS, Park MJ. Arthroscopic reduction and percutaneous fixation of perilunate dislocations and fracture-dislocations. Arthroscopy. 2012;28:196–203.
20. Weil WM, Slade JF 3rd, Trumble TE. Open and arthroscopic treatment of perilunate injuries. Clin Orthop Relat Res. 2006;445:120–32.

Thumb CMC Arthroscopic Electrothermal Stabilization (Without Trapeziectomy)

John M. Stephenson and Randall W. Culp

Introduction

Factors leading to degeneration of the carpometacarpal (CMC) joint of the thumb have been a major focus in the hand surgery literature. Strong association between laxity of the ligamentous and capsular structures and degenerative basal joint changes has been described [1]. A considerable amount of attention has been paid to the salvage of the already degenerated basal thumb joint, but much less focus has been paid to early intervention to prevent or delay the need for a salvage procedure. Historically, treatment of a lax basal thumb joint without degenerative changes has required a large arthrotomy which further destabilized the joint and was uncommonly performed. With recent advances in small joint arthroscopy, specifically arthroscopic evaluation and intervention of the thumb CMC joint, it is possible to treat early basal joint laxity in a minimally invasive fashion without further joint destabilization [2].

Thermal stabilization of capsular and ligamentous structures has been used with success in other areas of hand and wrist arthroscopy. Much of our understanding of this process has come from research into its application in larger joints such as the knee and shoulder [3–6]. At the time of surgery, the capsular tissue undergoes shrinkage which may persist for months after surgery as the tissue undergoes a thickening process. Histologic and ultrastructural alterations of the treated tissues have been noted. It has also been postulated that afferent sensory fibers in the capsular tissue are also interrupted through this process, which may result in a decrease in pain.

Most frequently, a radiofrequency probe (available through several manufacturers) is used. This type of technology uses electromagnetic energy to cause rapid movement of charged particles within the tissues to generate heat. Two types of radiofrequency probes are available, monopolar and bipolar. A monopolar probe generates energy that flows from the tip to a grounding pad on the body of the patient. Questions about the depth of heat penetration have been raised regarding monopolar probes, and care must be taken due to the proximity of neurovascular structures. Bipolar probes will take a path of least resistance through a conducting irrigating solution. There is greater control of depth of heating, but more potential concerns with the amount of heat generated within the joint through indirectly heating the irrigation fluid.

Thermal stabilization exploits the heat-labile intramolecular bonds that hold the triple helical structure in type I collagen. Heat-stable intermolecular bonds between chains are unaffected. Optimal temperatures for thermal stabilization have been described between 60 and 67 °C. Higher temperatures have been associated with thermal damage and necrosis of tissues. Thermal shrinkage occurs until a plateau is reached, beyond which further shrinkage cannot occur. As the tissue cools, up to 10% of initial shrinkage may be lost as some of the bonds renature. Repair through fibroblast migration begins within 1 week after injury and continues for 3 months.

Clinical Presentation

Patients with laxity of the thumb CMC joint will initially present with pain especially with pinching or grasping type activities. There may be a history of associated trauma which brought this pain to the patient's attention. Tenderness may be elicited by palpation of the CMC joint especially on the volar aspect of the joint. An effusion may be noticeable around the joint when compared to the contralateral side.

J. M. Stephenson
Department of Orthopaedic Surgery, University of Arkansas for Medical Sciences, Little Rock, AK, USA

R. W. Culp (✉)
Department of Orthopaedic Surgery, Thomas Jefferson University Hospitals, Philadelphia Hand to Shoulder Center, King of Prussia, PA, USA

© Springer Nature Switzerland AG 2022
W. B. Geissler (ed.), *Wrist and Elbow Arthroscopy with Selected Open Procedures*,
https://doi.org/10.1007/978-3-030-78881-0_51

The so-called "CMC grind test" may be positive with pain and/or crepitus when loading and translating the metacarpal on the trapezium. Laxity may be noted with subluxation of the joint, and dynamic fluoroscopic examination may aid in this determination. Differential diagnoses to consider include De Quervain's tenosynovitis, neuropathy of the superficial radial nerve, occult scaphoid fracture, isolated scaphotrapeziotrapezoid (STT), or radiocarpal arthritis. Patient will often demonstrate pain and reduced key pinch strength testing. Radiographs should be obtained to rule out other significant degenerative changes of the CMC joint and other surrounding bony pathology.

A useful radiographic technique is a stress radiograph, which is a posterior-to-anterior (PA) view of both thumbs positioned parallel to the X-ray plate with the distal phalanges pressed firmly together along their radial border. This position forces the metacarpal base laterally, and in the presence of a CMC ligament tear or laxity, radial shift of the metacarpal on the trapezium occurs.

Nonsurgical Management

Options for conservative management for the patient with a painful basal thumb joint are limited. Activity modifications specifically avoidance of grasping and key pinch may provide some temporary relief. There is a role for a trial of splinting of the joint with a hand-based thumb spica splint to see if immobilization will help with an acute pain flare. Both hard and soft thumb spica splints may be utilized by the patient in an alternating fashion depending upon their preference. An intra-articular injection of a corticosteroid can be useful in a diagnostic and therapeutic manner. Oral nonsteroidal anti-inflammatory drugs (NSAIDs) and topical anti-inflammatory gel can help with any of the above nonsurgical modalities.

Surgical Management

Diagnostic arthroscopy is a tool that can be used when there is a question of the clinical and radiographic findings, or when conservative management has failed. The degree of laxity of the CMC joint can be better quantified and arthritic changes can be documented. Findings of synovitis, loose bodies, and chondromalacia can be noted even in the presence of normal radiographs. Contraindications include generalized connective tissue disorders or excessive thumb metacarpophalangeal (MP) hyperextension. This technique can also be utilized with joint debridement to help with painful subluxation in stage I or II CMC arthritis [7].

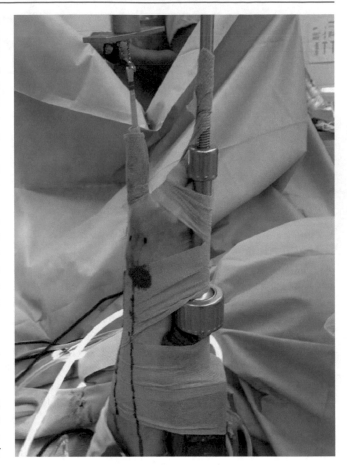

Fig. 51.1 Traction tower setup

Preparation

General or regional anesthesia may be used for this procedure. The patient is positioned supine on an operating table with an arm table on the operative side. A tourniquet may be used if desired on the upper arm. The arm should be positioned so that it is in the center of the table to facilitate the use of a traction apparatus. Once the extremity has undergone sterile prep and drape, the traction tower is assembled. A sterile finger trap is placed on the thumb past the interphalangeal (IP) joint. It is often helpful to wrap a small coban tape around the thumb to the level of the MP joint to further secure the thumb in the finger trap (Figs. 51.1 and 51.2). The elbow is bent 90° so that the ulna is parallel to the long axis of the traction tower. A couple of folded towels should be placed below the elbow and between the ulnar border of the forearm and the traction tower. The wrist should be in slight ulnar deviation at this point. A larger coban wrap may then be used in a circular fashion to wrap the fingers together first, then to the upper traction tower and then running down from the wrist to the lower forearm. This helps to hold the arm in the most desirable position for arthroscopy of the thumb

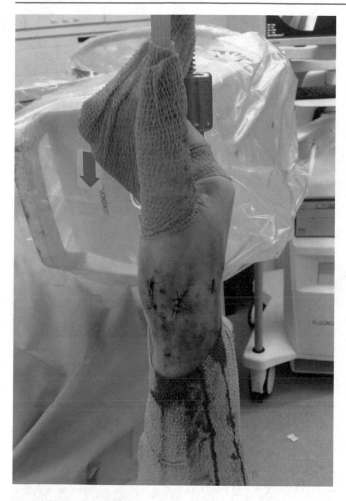

Fig. 51.2 Traction tower setup

CMC joint and prevents unwanted movement of the arm during surgery. Once satisfied with the position and stability of the setup, traction of 5–10 lb is applied to the joint. The tourniquet may be inflated to 200–250 mmHg if desired.

Often it is helpful to have a mini C-arm fluoroscope available during these procedures. This should be draped and brought into the surgical field at a 90° angle so that the "C" is oriented in a dorsal-to-volar direction with the image intensifier at the dorsum of the wrist.

Landmarks and Portals

Standard radial (1R) and ulnar (1U) portals have been described for CMC joint arthroscopy; however, it is necessary to be familiar with the surrounding anatomy. The thumb metacarpal should be palpated and marked along with the joint line. The abductor pollicis longus (APL), extensor pollicis brevis (EPB), and extensor pollicis longus (EPL) tendons should be marked. The radial artery has been described as lying ulnar to the EPB at an average distance of 11 mm

(range 4–17 mm) in a cadaveric study. However, the average distance from the EPL is within 1 mm in greater than 70% of specimens studied [8].

The 1R portal is located at the joint line directly radial to the APL (volar), and the 1U portal is located directly ulnar to the EPB (dorsal). Approximately, 1 cm will separate the two portals from one another.

An 18-gauge needle should be used to confirm the location and determine the appropriate entry angle to the joint. The needle should be directed into the joint slightly proximal to the mark for the portal. The joint should be insufflated with 1–2 mL of normal saline and the distension of the capsule should be visible. A number 11 blade should be used to cut skin only. A small mosquito type hemostat should be used to bluntly dissect the soft tissues until the capsule can be palpated with the tip of the instrument. The surgeon should be mindful of the branches of the superficial radial nerve; thus careful blunt dissection is necessary to avoid injury. Cadaveric studies have shown that of eleven specimens at least one branch of the superficial radial nerve was lying over the EPB tendon in seven specimens, the APL tendon in six specimens, and over the EPL in all eleven specimens.

After careful dissection, a blunt trocar with its surrounding sheath is then gently introduced into the joint. The inclination is slightly distal at a 10–20° angle. The 1U portal is typically the first portal established. The 1U portal is in the area of the dorsal radial ligament (DRL; volar) and the posterior oblique ligament (POL; dorsal). Sweeping the trocar to find the natural division between these two ligaments can help to preserve their integrity and make entry into the joint less traumatic. Trocar placement can be confirmed with fluoroscopy, since it is easy to fall erroneously into the STT joint. For the 1R portal, the capsule is immediately deep to the APL tendon since there is no ligamentous reinforcement in this area. This portal is usually made under direct visualization and will serve as the primary working portal. Switching portals is commonly done and should be used to obtain complete visualization of the entire joint.

Diagnostic Arthroscopy Technique

Often the initial view of the joint is obscured with hypertrophic synovium. This may be resected under visualization using a small joint arthroscopic shaver or thermal device according to the surgeon's preference. It is quite common with these small shavers to have to clear debris from them several times during the case. Continuous inflow is encouraged to clear as much debris as possible to maximize visualization and inspection of the surrounding ligaments. Irrigation fluid will also help to dissipate the heat generated by these devices.

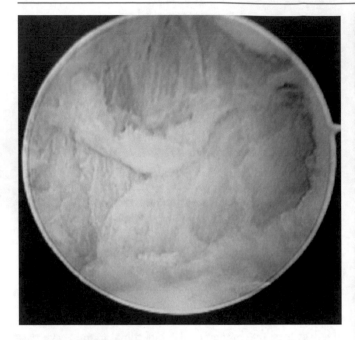

Fig. 51.3 Anterior oblique ligament

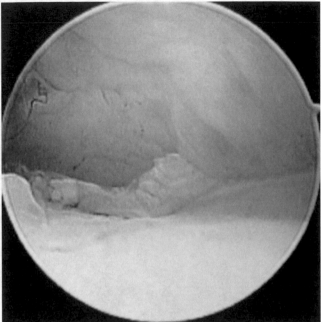

Fig. 51.4 Ulnar collateral ligament

General inspection of the joint should be done systematically, looking for osteophytes, loose bodies, and damage to the articular surface. With the camera in the 1U portal, the superficial and deep portions of the anterior oblique ligament can be identified and inspected (Fig. 51.3). Moving the camera in a more dorsal direction, the ulnar collateral ligament (UCL) can be visualized (Fig. 51.4).

At this point, the camera should be switched so that it is in the 1R portal. Again, the ulnar collateral ligament can be identified, and continuing to sweep dorsal, the posterior oblique ligament will come into view, followed by the dorso-radial ligament. After careful identification and examination of the ligaments, arthroscopic intervention may commence.

Thermal Capsular Shrinkage Technique

With the camera in the 1U portal, the thermal probe is introduced into the 1R portal. The probe should be passed over the capsular and ligamentous structures in a controlled, systematic manner. Passing the probe too rapidly will result in inefficient shrinkage; conversely, passing too slowly may result in extensive thermal damage. To proceed in a systematic manner, stabilization should start with the anterior oblique ligament and progress toward the ulnar collateral ligament. At this point, the portals should be switched. The remaining UCL and posterior oblique ligament, as well as the dorso-radial ligament, may be stabilized (Fig. 51.5). As the tissue is heated, a color change or "caramelization" of the tissue will occur along with visible shrinkage. If further

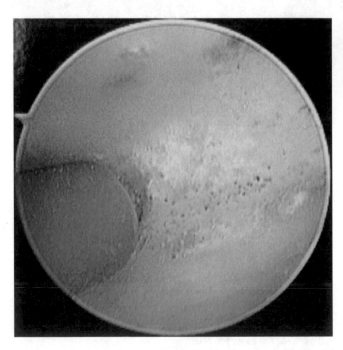

Fig. 51.5 Posterior oblique ligament after electrothermal treatment

shrinkage is deemed to be necessary, a "stripe" method should be used leaving a band of healthy tissue between treated tissues to allow for the reparative process rather than heating the entire capsule-ligamentous surface (Fig. 51.6). For proper tensioning, it should be anticipated that up to 10% of the initial shrinkage will be lost upon cooling.

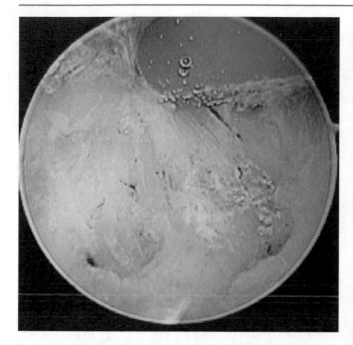

Fig. 51.6 Anterior oblique ligament-stripe technique. Notice the "caramelization" of the tissue on the inferior stripe separated from the second stripe by an untreated area of tissue

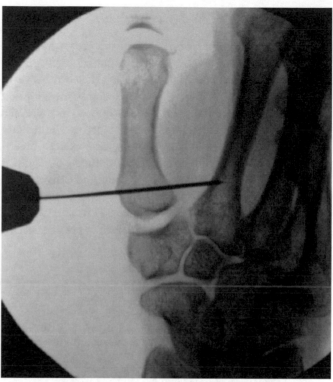

Fig. 51.8 Tight-rope trajectory

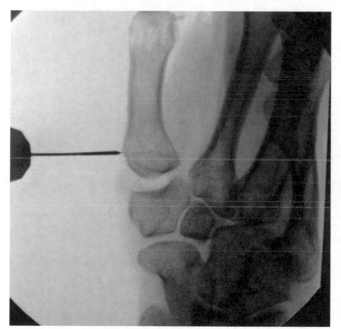

Fig. 51.7 Starting point for tightrope placement

If desired, a pin may be used to stabilize the joint. Under C-arm visualization the joint should be reduced and a 0.045-in. Kirschner wire should be inserted from the thumb metacarpal into the trapezium on the radial side. The joint can also be stabilized with a newer technique called a "tight-rope." This is a suture-button complex running from the base of the thumb to the base of the index metacarpal (Figs. 51.7, 51.8, and 51.9).

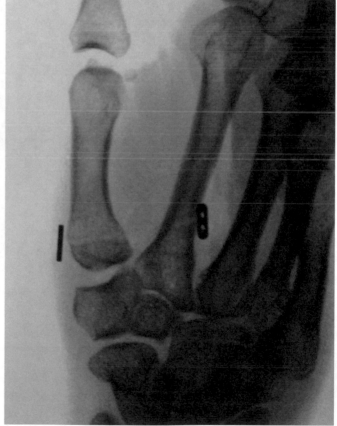

Fig. 51.9 Final placement of tightrope for stabilization

Postoperative Care

The wounds are closed according to the surgeon's preference and a well-padded thumb spica splint is then placed. Elevation is encouraged as well as early active range of motion of the remaining digits to decrease swelling. At 7–10 days postoperatively, the sutures may be removed and the patient may be placed into a thumb spica cast or custom-molded removable splint according to the surgeon's preference. The splint should be worn at all times. The pin, if placed, may be removed at 3–4 weeks and early motion started. Strengthening exercises may begin at 6 weeks postoperatively. The splint may be weaned starting in week 10 and after 3 months, the patient may return to previous activities with minimal restrictions.

References

1. Eaton RG, Lane LB, Littler JW, et al. Ligament reconstruction for the painful thumb carpometacarpal joint: a long-term assessment. J Hand Surg Am. 1984;9:692–9.
2. Berger RA. A technique for arthroscopic evaluation of the first carpometacarpal joint. J Hand Surg Am. 1997;22:1077–80.
3. Arnoczky SP, Aksan A. Thermal modification of connective tissues: basic science consideration and clinical implications. J Am Acad Orthop Surg. 2000;8:305–13.
4. Hayashi K, Markel M. Thermal modification of joint capsule and ligamentous tissues. Tech Sports Med. 1998;6:120–5.
5. Hayashi K, Peters D, Thabit G, et al. The mechanism of joint capsule thermal modification in an invitro sheep model. Clin Orthop Relat Res. 2000;370:236–49.
6. Osmond C, Hecht P, Hayashi K, et al. Comparative effects of laser and radiofrequency on joint capsule. Clin Orthop Relat Res. 2000;375:286–94.
7. Culp RW, Rekant MS. The role of arthroscopy in evaluating and treating trapeziometacarpal disease. Hand Clin. 2001;17(2):315–9.
8. Gonzalez MH, Kemmler J, Weinzweig N, et al. Portals for arthroscopy of the trapeziometacarpal joint. J Hand Surg Br. 1997;22(5):574–5.

Partial Trapeziectomy and Soft Tissue Interposition

52

Tyson K. Cobb

Introduction

Almost 20 years have passed since the early description of carpometacarpal (CMC) arthroscopy [1–3]. Since this time, improvement in equipment and surgical technique has allowed advancement of therapeutic options to allow the entire spectrum of CMC degenerative joint disease to be addressed arthroscopically. The most recent change in the treatment algorithm [4, 5] of CMC degenerative joint disease is the treatment of pantrapezial arthrosis by arthroscopic means [6]. As a result of the positive outcomes and ability to perform hemitrapeziectomy surgery through a minimally invasive arthroscopic technique, open trapeziectomy is no longer mandated for patients with degenerative arthritis of the scaphotrapeziotrapezoid (STT) joint.

Indications and Patient Selection

Patients presenting with pain or dysfunction in the area of the CMC joint are evaluated to rule out other potential causes of pain such as de Quervain's, radial-sided wrist pain associated with scaphoid nonunion advanced collapse (SNAC) or scapholunate advanced collapse (SLAC), isolated STT arthritis, ganglion cyst, other painful masses, and neurogenic pain. Following appropriate diagnosis of basal joint arthrosis, patients undergo a period of conservative treatment including nonsteroidal anti-inflammatory drugs, splints, and cortisone injections. Cortisone injections are being used less frequently in the author's practice due to potential side effects, including accelerated cartilage loss and capsular attenuation, and an increasing frequency of patients declining cortisone injections. While the frequency of multiple cortisone injections has drastically diminished over time,

one-time injections of cortisone for CMC and/or STT arthrosis continue to be utilized for many patients.

Patients who do not respond to conservative treatment and demonstrate significant disabilities on subjective and objective assessment are offered surgical intervention. Patients are counseled with respect to minimally invasive arthroscopic resection arthroplasty versus open techniques and risks and benefits of each. They are told that the minimally invasive procedure may not provide sufficient relief and that they may require a revision open surgery at a later date.

Surgical decision-making is directed by specific patient variables. While there are numerous patient-related variables that impact decision-making for the surgical treatment of basal joint arthritis, four are critical to the success and patient satisfaction following the procedure (Fig. 52.1): (1) CMC cartilage status, (2) CMC stability, (3) STT cartilage status, and (4) metacarpophalangeal (MP) pathology.

CMC Cartilage Evaluation

Patients with minimal radiographic findings who remain persistently symptomatic despite conservative treatment are candidates for diagnostic arthroscopy [7]. The extent of the cartilage loss is usually worse than the radiograph suggests. Accurate arthritis staging requires arthroscopy [4, 5]. If the cartilage is intact (Badia Stage 1), synovectomy and capsular shrinkage may provide satisfactory results. If the cartilage loss is focal (Badia Stage 2), synovectomy and first metacarpal osteotomy is an option [8, 9]. In the author's practice, it is uncommon to see patients or operate at Stage 1 or 2 because patients have been treated conservatively elsewhere prior to referral. Patients considering the less invasive procedures described above should be well aware of the potential for progression of the pathology and potential need for arthroplasty in the future. Patients who prefer to minimize the likelihood of additional procedures in the future can be effectively treated with sequential cortisone injections until

T. K. Cobb (✉)
Shoulder Elbow Wrist and Hand Center of Excellence, Davenport, IA, USA

© Springer Nature Switzerland AG 2022
W. B. Geissler (ed.), *Wrist and Elbow Arthroscopy with Selected Open Procedures*,
https://doi.org/10.1007/978-3-030-78881-0_52

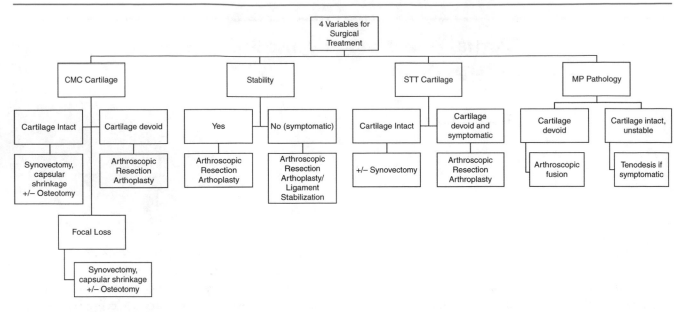

Fig. 52.1 Algorithm for surgical treatment of thumb basal joint arthritis

the arthrosis progresses sufficiently to warrant arthroplasty. While it may be true that intervening at an earlier stage with less aggressive surgical options may provide better ultimate outcome and function, evidence is lacking in the literature.

Many radiographic Eaton Stage 2 [10] cases will be found to have widespread cartilage loss (Badia Stage 3) at the time of arthroscopy. Badia Stage 3 cases are treated with arthroscopic resection arthroplasty as outlined below.

Carpometacarpal Stability

Patients with symptomatic CMC instability are counseled with respect to open and arthroscopic stabilization procedures. Many patients, especially older patients, are primarily concerned with pain relief and are less interested in stabilizing procedures. Clear benefits for this have not been demonstrated in the literature. Patients with CMC instability who desire stabilization are offered arthroscopic ligament stabilization at the time of arthroscopic resection arthroplasty. The procedure is outlined below in the section "Surgical Technique: CMC Stabilization."

Scaphotrapeziotrapezoid Cartilage Evaluation

Just as the CMC cartilage loss observed at the time of arthroscopy is usually worse than radiographs suggest, the same is true for cartilage loss involving the STT joint. Diagnostic arthroscopy of the STT joint can be helpful in establishing which radiographic Stage 3 cases are actually arthroscopic Stage 4. (Note: Badia's classification did not include Stage 4,

but it seems a logical addition.) while careful physical exam can determine the pain contribution of the STT joint, at times, it may be difficult to determine the significance of the STT arthrosis. Diagnostic injections are occasionally used to help identify the pain contributions of CMC versus STT when the significance of STT arthrosis is in question. Diagnostic injections are performed by first injecting the CMC with 1 ml of 1% lidocaine under fluoroscopic or ultrasound control to determine the amount of pain relief and improvement in pinch strength. Ten to 15 min after the CMC injection and after assessment of the amount of pain relief and strength improvement, the STT is then injected under fluoroscopic control. Ten to 15 min later, the amount of pain relief and improvement in pinch and grip strength is again evaluated. Patients who demonstrate substantial benefit from both injections are considered candidates for pantrapezial arthroscopic resection arthroplasty.

Metacarpophalangeal Joint Pathology

Metacarpophalangeal (MP) hyperextension and arthrosis should be addressed prior to surgical treatment of the CMC. Symptomatic, unstable MP joints can be stabilized with MP tenodesis. Fusion should be considered if the MP joint is symptomatic and arthritic. The author has performed many MP tenodesis for MP hyperextension (>30°) over the years. Long-term follow-up has revealed gradual return of the MP hyperextension in a number of cases. Even with return of the hyperextension, however, patients tend to remain very happy with the results provided pain relief is good. It is important to discuss the options concerning the MP joint with the patient. If the MP is unstable but asymptomatic, counsel the patient concerning the possible need for future procedures for the MP joint (if MP pathology is not addressed at the time of the index procedure). If simultaneous MP tenodesis is performed, the disadvantage discussed with the patient includes the risk of loss of correction over time, risk of converting an asymptomatic unstable joint to a symptomatic joint, and increasing the postoperative recovery time.

Surgical Technique: Arthroscopic Resection Arthroplasty of CMC and STT Joint

The procedure can be performed with general or regional anesthesia with or without a tourniquet. When a tourniquet is not used, an anesthetic with epinephrine is infiltrated preoperatively allowing sufficient time for vasoconstriction [11, 12]. The patient is placed on an operating room table with the shoulder abducted and externally rotated. The arm is placed on an arm table with a well-padded nonsterile tourniquet placed on the brachium (if used). The brachium is taped to the arm table. The arm is suspended using 5–10 pounds of finger-trap traction through the thumb (Fig. 52.2). Routine arthroscopy is performed using a 1.9 mm, a 2.3 mm, or a 2.7 mm 30° arthroscope. The smaller scopes are used on the smaller joints and in joints considered potential candidates for joint-sparing procedures such as synovectomy and metacarpal osteotomy. Most resection arthroplasties are performed with a 2.7 mm arthroscope for better field of view.

Skin incisions are made with a #15 scalpel just through the skin. A blunt hemostat is used to gently dissect through the soft tissue and through the capsule. The radial artery, superficial branches of the radial nerve, and extensor tendons are all at potential risk. These structures are protected through proper technique of blunt dissection. However, even with appropriate technique, they may be injured. These risks should be discussed with the patients preoperatively.

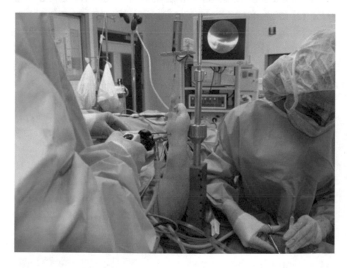

Fig. 52.2 Operating room setup

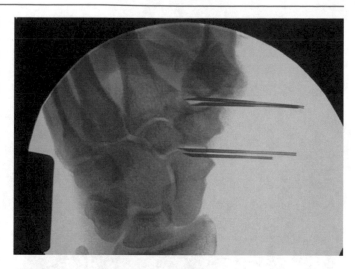

Fig. 52.3 Fluoroscopic view of portal placement. Note needles are placed parallel to the CMC and STT joints. (Reprinted with permission from Cobb et al. [6]. With permission from Elsevier)

The 1-radial (1R, volar) and 1-ulnar (1U, dorsal) portals are used for CMC arthroscopy. STT arthroscopy is performed using 1R (volar) and 1U (dorsal) portals placed approximately 1 cm proximal to the 1R (volar) and 1U (dorsal) portals as described for CMC arthroplasty. The portals are localized with hypodermic needles with the aid of fluoroscopy (Fig. 52.3). Needles are placed into the joints and confirmed to be parallel on fluoroscopy. These portals lay on either side of the first dorsal compartment. A second dorsal portal is utilized as necessary. The second dorsal portal (dorsal ulnar portal) is placed using inside-out technique by placing a blunt probe through the 1R portal across the CMC or the STT joint and exiting the dorsum of the hand (Fig. 52.4). A cannula is placed retrograde over the probe and inserted into the joint.

A full-radius mechanical shaver (typically a 3.5 mm) with suction is used to perform synovectomy and clean the joint of debris for better visualization. Radiofrequency ablation (Serfas 3.5 mm, Stryker, Santa Clara, CA) is used to perform thermal capsulorrhaphy and to perform intra-articular joint denervation. High outflow is utilized to prevent overheating during the use of radiofrequency ablation. A 4.0 mm barrel bur is used to resect 2–3 mm of bone from the distal aspect of the trapezium and proximal aspect of the first metacarpal. The STT resection arthroplasty is performed by removing 2–3 mm of bone from the distal aspect of the scaphoid and from the proximal aspect of the trapezium and trapezoid (Fig. 52.5). A 4.0 mm barrel bur (Stryker, Santa Clara, CA) is used preferentially in joints large enough to accept the larger size bur.

The author's preferred interposition material (when interposition material is used) is the Graftjacket (Wright Medical Technology, Inc., Arlington, TN). This interposition material tends to adhere effectively to the joint and

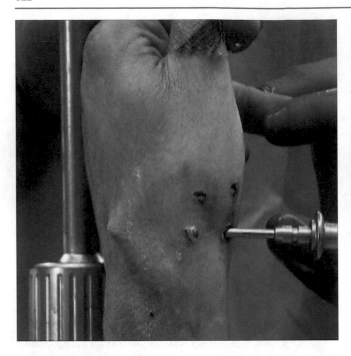

Fig. 52.4 Inside-out technique for establishing the ulnar dorsal portal for CMC or STT

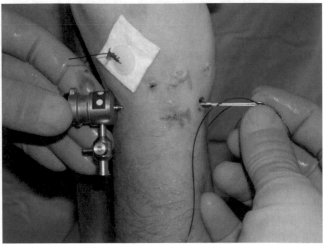

Fig. 52.6 Keith needles are shown passing through cannula in volar portal

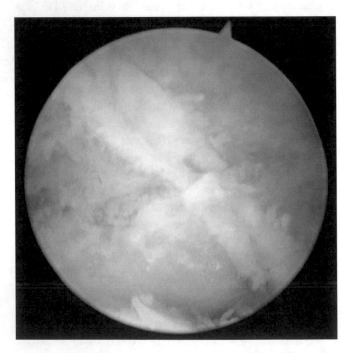

Fig. 52.5 Arthroscopic view of resected STT joint showing resection of proximal surface of the trapezium and trapezoid. The cartilage of the trapezio-trapezoid joint is shown separating the trapezium (*left*) and the trapezoid (*right*). (Reprinted with permission from Cobb et al. [6]. With permission from Elsevier)

seems to create less inflammatory response than other commercially available products. Early in the author's series, no graft fixation was utilized. However, a number of grafts were extruded from the joint, requiring removal at a later

date. Because of these experiences, the author devised two methods of fixation. The most commonly used fixation involves tying sutures over buttons external to the skin on the volar and dorsal aspects of the joint thereby securing the interposition material within the joint. This is performed by passing absorbable sutures on Keith needles through the volar portal, across the resected joint, and out the dorsum of the hand (Figs. 52.6 and 52.7). The suture is used to pull the interposition material into the resected joint (Fig. 52.8). A second suture is placed on the opposite side of the interposition material before pulling the interposition material through the joint. The interposition material is centered in the joint under arthroscopic visualization. The sutures are then tied over felt and buttons on the volar and dorsal sides of the joint. Since the volar sutures are exiting through the portal, they are passed through the skin adjacent to the portal. This minimizes any potential portal healing issues. The same method of fixation can be utilized for both CMC and STT joints. Alternatively, the interposition material can be secured in the joint using standard arthroscopic knot-tying techniques (Fig. 52.9). This is performed by passing a suture through any stable soft tissue attachment including the capsule or ligament. The interposition material is then pushed into the joint on the suture with a standard knot pusher which is then utilized to tie the sutures arthroscopically. Arthroscopic suture cutters are used to remove the excess suture.

The resected joint is infiltrated with approximately 30–60 cc of 0.25% Marcaine with epinephrine (if not contraindicated) to provide hemostasis and postoperative pain control. Hemostasis is best obtained if a portion of the Marcaine with epinephrine is placed preoperatively. This is performed by placing some of the Marcaine within the joint but more importantly infiltrating just external to the capsule volarly,

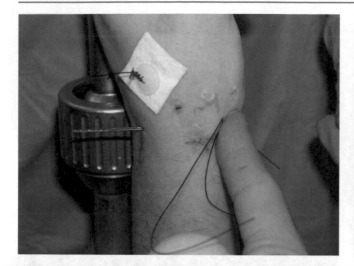

Fig. 52.7 Keith needles exiting dorsal surface of the hand

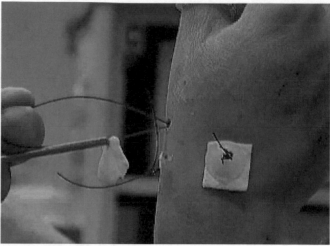

Fig. 52.9 Interposition of CMC has been tied over buttons. The STT interposition graft is being pulled into the resected STT space on PDS sutures

Postoperative Care

The portals are closed with Steri-Strips. A well-padded thumb spica splint is applied with a compressive Ace. Patients are instructed to keep their extremities elevated, apply ice, and begin gentle range of motion of the digits as soon as possible. Patients are instructed to come to the clinic for a postoperative pain block the first postoperative day if they are uncomfortable. Patients very infrequently utilize a second block. Patients are scheduled to see a hand therapist on postoperative day 5–7 for application of a hand-based arthroplast splint. They are instructed for a home program of gentle range of motion of the CMC joint in all planes. This allows the surgeon to see the patient after the patient has initiated range of motion and allows for more complete assessment without the anxiety often associated with removal of the postoperative dressing. If interposition has been fixed with felt and buttons, the pullout sutures are removed at 2 weeks (Fig. 52.10). It's the author's belief that early range of motion provides for better overall outcome. Postoperative blocks and continued therapy visits can be helpful to facilitate early range of motion in patients who are having difficulty.

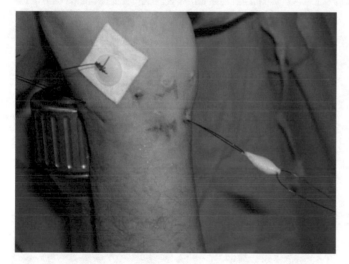

Fig. 52.8 Interposition material is pulled into the joint with sutures previously passed with Keith needles

dorsally, and medially. Following the resection arthroplasty, the assistant simply holds their fingertips over the portals to prevent the Marcaine from leaking while the surgeon infiltrates the resected joint with the remaining portion of the Marcaine. The total amount should be calculated based on patient's weight and coordinated with the anesthesia provider. There have been a few cases where we needed additional epinephrine for hemostasis purposes after we had maxed out the total amount of anesthetic which could be given. In these cases, we simply mix some epinephrine with saline to infiltrate the region, thereby providing hemostasis. On one occasion, the portal had to be extended sufficiently to allow visualization and cauterization of a bleeding branch of the radial artery.

Surgical Technique: CMC Stabilization

Arthroscopic stabilization procedures may be performed with commercially available devices (Mini TightRope™, Arthrex or CMC CableFix™, Instratek) or with a tendon graft fixed with tenodesis screws in the first and second

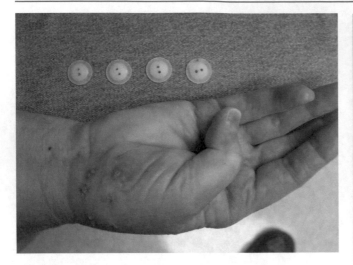

Fig. 52.10 Thumb motion at the time of button removal (2 weeks)

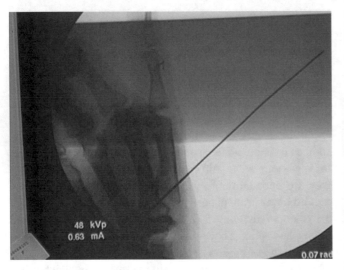

Fig. 52.11 Fluoroscopic view of guidewire placed through first metacarpal

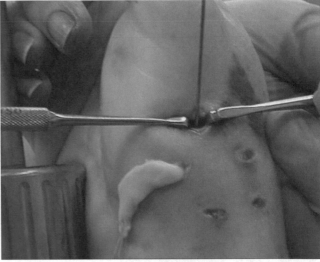

Fig. 52.12 Graph has been arthroscopically secured in the base of the second metacarpal with tenodesis screw. The graft exits the CMC volar portal. Guidewire is shown placed in the first metacarpal. Graft will be retrieved through the resected CMC space and pulled through the first metacarpal tunnel

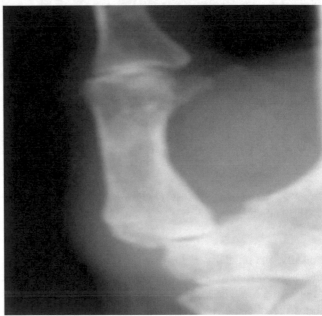

Fig. 52.13 Pre-operative film showing subluxation of CMC joint

metacarpals. The stabilization procedures are performed after arthroscopic resection arthroplasty of the CMC joint. The technique of tendon graft fixation involves placement of a guidewire through the CMC volar portal across the resected CMC space and into the base of the second metacarpal. A tunnel is drilled into the second metacarpal with a 4 mm cannulated drill. A tendon graft (usually palmaris longus) is fixed in the base of the second metacarpal with a tenodesis screw (Arthrex, Naples, FL). A guidewire is then placed through the dorsal radial border of the first metacarpal approximately 1 cm distal to the proximal end (Fig. 52.11). It is driven obliquely into the resected CMC space. A 4 mm tunnel is drilled with the cannulated drill over the guidewire (Fig. 52.12). The graft is retrieved from the CMC-resected space through the first metacarpal tunnel

with a suture passer. The first metacarpal is reduced, and the tendon graft is tensioned. Care must be taken not to overtighten the fixation which can lead to painful impingement between the first and second metacarpals. A tenodesis screw is then placed into the first metacarpal tunnel securing the palmaris longus tendon (Figs. 52.13 and 52.14). The 1–2 metacarpal space is pinned with a .062 K-wire for 4–6 weeks.

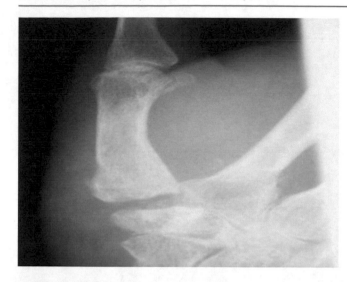

Fig. 52.14 Post-op film showing reduction after arthroscopic ligament stabilization

Results of Arthroscopic Resection Arthroplasty for Pantrapezial Arthritis (Stage 4)

We reviewed 35 cases of arthroscopic resection arthroplasty of the CMC and STT joints performed in 34 patients for pantrapezial arthrosis with minimum 1-year follow-up [6]. The average pain score improved from 7 preoperatively to 1 postoperatively ($p < 0.001$) at 1 year (Fig. 52.15). Disabilities of the arm, shoulder and hand (DASH) scores improved from 46 preoperatively to 19 at 1 year ($p < 0.001$) (Fig. 52.16). Grip strength improved 4.3 kg ($p = 0.02$) (Fig. 52.17), and key pinch improved 1.3 kg ($p < 0.001$) (Fig. 52.18). All but one patient could reach the proximal digital crease of the small finger by 1 year postoperatively. Early studies comparing open ligament reconstruction tendon interposition arthroplasty to arthroscopic resection arthroplasty of the CMC demonstrated a reduction in return-to-work time of more than 50% (Fig. 52.19). A total of 32 of the 34 patients stated that they would have the surgery again. Satisfaction was rated at the highest level of 5 for 25 patients. The average satisfaction at follow-up was 4 (range, 2–5).

Failures and Complications

Carpal tunnel syndrome frequently co-exists with CMC degenerative joint disease. Swelling associated with arthroscopic resection arthroplasty of the CMC can exacerbate a subclinical carpal tunnel syndrome necessitating urgent return to the operating room for acute carpal tunnel release. Concurrent carpal tunnel release should be discussed with patients who have a positive Tinel's over the median nerve at the wrist even if classic symptoms are absent.

Four patients in our series required additional surgery. Reasons for reoperation included deep infection in one, flexor carpi radialis tendinitis in one, and persistent pain in two. Five patients reported paresthesias in the distribution of the superficial branch of the radial nerve, all of which resolved by 3 months following surgery (The author has had patients with sustained and presumably permanent superficial branch paresthesias in cases which were not part of the published series.). Three patients developed flexor carpi radialis tendinitis, two of which responded to cortisone injection and one required surgical release.

When the author started performing arthroscopic resection arthroplasty of the CMC joint for degenerative joint disease in 2004, the longevity of this procedure was in question. However, the long-term follow-up has shown durable lasting results. The author has performed over 300 cases of arthroscopic resection arthroplasty of CMC joint. The author currently has an ongoing prospective study and joint registry with follow-up in excess of 15 years. Neither the need for revision nor the outcome appears to change with time.

The chance of revision surgery may always be slightly higher in minimally invasive procedures because those patients who do not do well have a good option, that is, open revision surgery. However, once open surgery such as ligament reconstruction tendon interposition arthroplasty has been performed, surgeons are much less likely to offer revision surgery because the options are few. Therefore, in high-risk patients (such as patients with secondary gain), it may be wise to do the last procedure first.

Need for Interposition

The indication for interposition is not well established. The author has had very good results with use of Graftjacket. However, early studies showed very good results with resection arthroplasty without interposition [13, 14]. There have been two cases of spontaneous arthrodesis (not part of the above published study) in patients who underwent resection arthroplasty without interposition. While arthrodesis is an accepted treatment for CMC degenerative joint disease, neither of these two patients was happy with their results. This complication has not occurred to my knowledge in patients receiving interposition. Placing interposition does increase surgical time and expense for the procedure. Furthermore, there is a potential higher risk of infection, disease transmission, and inflammation. We have not been able to show any true differences in outcome between arthroscopic resection arthroplasty with and without interposition [15].

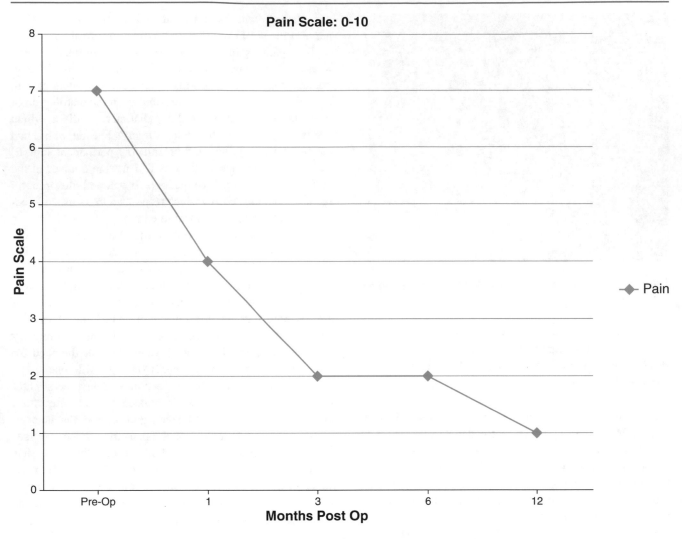

Fig. 52.15 Graph of pain scale (0–10) for pre-operative and each postoperative time interval

Comparison to the Literature

Cobb et al. [6] results seem to be similar to those reported by Ashwood et al. [16], who reported good-to-excellent results in 9 of 10 patients following arthroscopic debridement (without resection arthroplasty) of the STT joint. Rin and Mathoulin [17] reported good results in 13 cases of arthroscopic resection arthroplasty of the distal polar scaphoid for STT arthritis. Twenty-six percent improvement in grip strength and 40% improvement in pinch were reported by Garcia-Elias et al. [18], following the open resection of the distal polar scaphoid in 21 patients. Improvement in

Cobb et al.'s [6] grip and pinch was 31% and 44%, respectively.

Comparing the author's results to ligament reconstruction interposition arthroplasty and open hematoma distraction arthroplasty (HDA), the increased grip strength in the present study (31%) was better than that reported by Tomaino et al. [19], (21%) and Yang and Weiland [20] (9%) for ligament reconstruction and interposition arthroplasty but less than that reported for HDA (47%) by Kuhns et al. [21]. Improvement in key pinch for the present study (44%) was better than that reported by all three studies, 8%, 17%, and 33%, respectively.

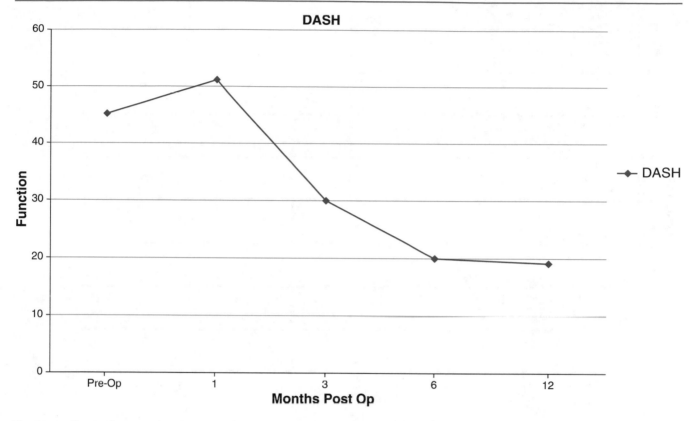

Fig. 52.16 Graph of DASH scores for pre-operative and each postoperative time interval

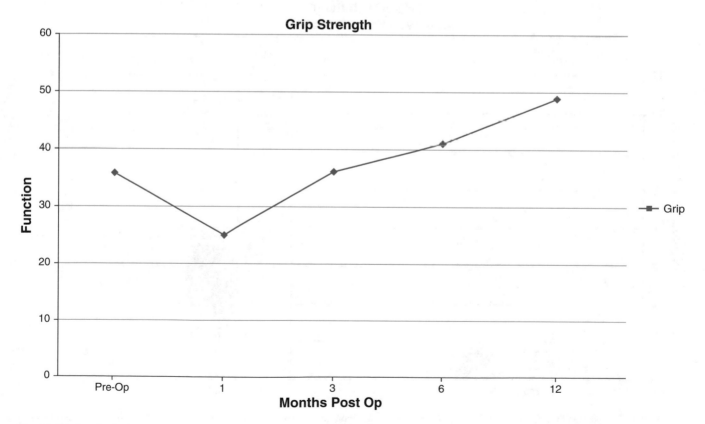

Fig. 52.17 Graph of grip strength for pre-operative and each postoperative time interval

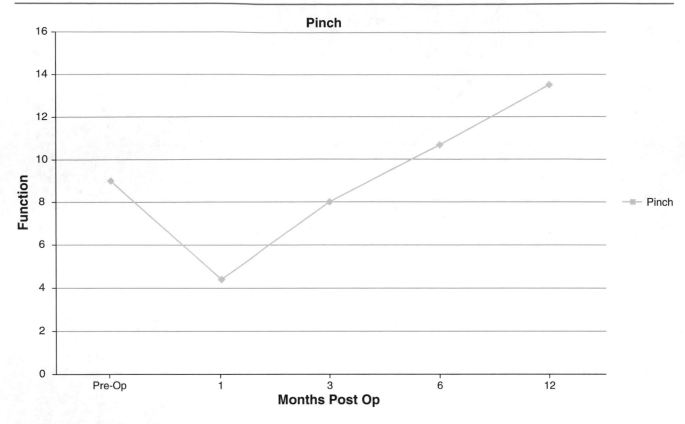

Fig. 52.18 Graph of key pinch for pre-operative and each postoperative time interval

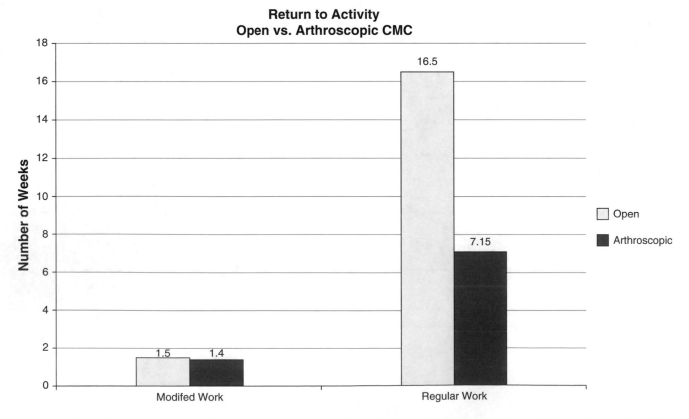

Fig. 52.19 Comparison of return to work for open ligament reconstruction tendon interposition arthroplasty versus arthroscopic resection arthroplasty of CMC

References

1. Menon J. Arthroscopic management of trapeziometacarpal joint arthritis of the thumb. Arthroscopy. 1996;12(5):581–7.
2. Berger RA. A technique for arthroscopic evaluation of the first carpometacarpal joint. J Hand Surg Am. 1997;22(6):1077–80.
3. Osterman AL, Culp R, Bednar J. Arthroscopy of the thumb carpometacarpal joint. Arthroscopy. 1997;13:3.
4. Badia A. Trapeziometacarpal arthroscopy: a classification and treatment algorithm. Hand Clin. 2006;22(2):153–63.
5. Badia A. Arthroscopy of the trapeziometacarpal and metacarpophalangeal joints. J Hand Surg Am. 2006;32(5):707–24.
6. Cobb T, Sterbank P, Lemke J. Arthroscopic resection arthroplasty for the treatment of combined carpometacarpal and scaphotrapeziotrapezoid (pantrapezial) arthritis. J Hand Surg Am. 2011;36:413–9.
7. Culp RW, Rekant MS. The role of arthroscopy in evaluating and treating trapeziometacarpal disease. Hand Clin. 2001;17(2):315–9.
8. Tomaino MM. Treatment of stage 1 trapeziometacarpal disease. Hand Clin. 2001;17:197–205.
9. Wilson J. Basal osteotomy of the first metacarpal in the treatment of arthritis of the carpometacarpal joint of the thumb. Br J Surg. 1973;60:854–8.
10. Eaton RG, Glickel SZ. Trapeziometacarpal osteoarthritis staging as a rationale for treatment. Hand Clin. 1987;3:455–71.
11. Farhangkhoee H, Lalonde J, Lalonde DH. Wide-awake trapeziectomy: video detailing local anesthetic injection and surgery. Hand. 2011;6(4):466–7.
12. Davidson PG, Cobb T, Lalonde DH. Patient perspective on carpal tunnel surgery related to the type of anesthesia: a prospective cohort study. Hand. 2013;8(1):47–53.
13. Edwards SG, Ramsey PN. Prospective outcomes of stage 3 thumb CMC arthritis. J Hand Surg. 2010;35:566–71.
14. Hofmeister EP, Leak RS, Culp RW, Osterman AL. Arthroscopic hemitrapeziectomy for the first metacarpal arthritis: results at seven-year follow-up. Hand. 2009;4(1):24–8.
15. Cobb TK, Waldon AL, Cao Y: Long term outcome of arthoscopic resection arthoplasty with or without interposition for thumb basal joint arthritis. J Hand Surg Am. 2015;40(9):1844–51.
16. Ashwood N, Bain G, Fogg Q. Results of arthroscopic debridement for isolated scaphotrapeziotrapezoid arthritis. J Hand Surg Am. 2003;28:729–32.
17. Da Rin F, Mathoulin C. Arthroscopic treatment of osteoarthritis of scaphotrapeziotrapezoid joint. Chir Main. 2006;25:S254–8.
18. Garcia-Elias M, Lluch A, Farreres A, Castillo F, Saffar P. Resection of the distal scaphoid for scaphotrapeziotrapezoid osteoarthritis. J Hand Surg Br. 1999;24:448–52.
19. Tomaino MM, Pellegrini VD Jr, Burton RI. Arthroplasty of the basal joint of the thumb. Long-term follow-up after ligament reconstruction with tendon interposition. J Bone Joint Surg Am. 1995;77:346–55.
20. Yang SS, Weiland AJ. First metacarpal subsidence during pinch after ligament reconstruction and tendon interposition basal joint arthroplasty of the thumb. J Hand Surg Am. 1998;23:879–83.
21. Kuhns C, Emerson E, Meals R. Hematoma and distraction arthroplasty for thumb basal joint osteoarthritis: a prospective, single-surgeon study including outcomes measures. J Hand Surg Am. 2003;28:381–9.

Suture-Button Suspensionplasty for the Treatment of Thumb Carpometacarpal Joint Arthritis

John R. Talley and Jeffrey Yao

Introduction

Osteoarthritis causes significant disability wherever it occurs in the body. However, when it occurs in the thumb, it may quickly become a career and lifestyle-altering problem. The thumb carpometacarpal (CMC) joint is a uniquely shaped biconcave joint containing two saddle-shaped bones that articulate perpendicularly to each other. This allows the thumb to move into a number of different positions, which provides the thumb significant range of motion and function. However, with this considerable utility, the thumb is susceptible to overuse. For reasons that are not entirely clear at this time, but thought to be due to a joint that is inherently lacking in stability, the thumb CMC joint is prone to osteoarthritis [1, 2]. A combination of overuse and a large amount of force distributed over this joint is currently the proposed etiology. As Chou et al. have shown us, 1 kg pinch at the thumb tip causes a 13 kg load at the base of the thumb [3]. It is the second most common site of osteoarthritis of upper extremity with the finger distal interphalangeal joint (DIP) joint being the most common [4].

Thumb CMC osteoarthritis is treated initially with non-surgical measures, such as splinting, medications, activity modifications, hand therapy, and intra-articular injections. However, when conservative methods are exhausted, surgical options are proposed to the patient. The surgical options are extensive, and the one selected by the surgeon is often based upon preference, comfort level, and previous training. These methods include volar ligament reconstruction [5], first metacarpal osteotomy [6–9], CMC joint arthrodesis [10, 11], total joint arthroplasty [12], and trapeziectomy [13].

Partial or complete trapeziectomy is performed with or without ligament reconstruction, tendon interposition alone, or ligament reconstruction in addition to tendon interposition [14–19]. In general, an open technique is used but some of these techniques employ arthroscopy [20–22]. Studies comparing these different techniques have not demonstrated any significant long-term differences in outcomes [1, 14, 15, 23–25]. However, trapeziectomy alone does appear to have the shortest intraoperative time and the lowest rate of complications [1, 15, 23].

Consequently, given the lack of difference in long-term outcomes, there has been a focus on improving short-term outcomes and facilitating shorter postoperative recovery times.

In general, at the time of the trapeziectomy, either partial or complete, the first metacarpal is stabilized in order to maintain the space that was previously occupied by the trapezium. This is done in order to prevent collapse of the metacarpal into that space during the time of hematoma and subsequent scar formation. The method usually consists of placing a K-wire from the first metacarpal into the second metacarpal for 4 weeks postoperatively [13, 26, 27]. During this period of time, the thumb is completely immobilized.

Given this considerable period of immobility, a new technique has been devised to decrease the amount of postoperative immobilization while still maintaining support. This technique involves suspending the thumb metacarpal from the second metacarpal to prevent subsidence into the newly created trapeziectomy space by utilizing a suture button (SB) [28]. This utilizes a device called the Mini Tightrope (Arthrex, Naples, FL). This device has been used in a number of other applications in the field of orthopedic surgery including treatment of hallux varus deformity, acromioclavicular joint dislocations, transtibial amputations, and ankle syndesmosis stabilization [29–32]. The device consists of braided polyester sutures looped between two steel buttons with one button affixed to the first metacarpal and the other to the second metacarpal. This suspends the thumb from the

J. R. Talley
Division of Plastic Surgery, Department of Surgery, Stanford University Medical Center, Palo Alto, CA, USA

J. Yao (✉)
Department of Orthopaedic Surgery, Stanford University Medical Center, Redwood City, CA, USA
e-mail: jyao@stanford.edu

© Springer Nature Switzerland AG 2022
W. B. Geissler (ed.), *Wrist and Elbow Arthroscopy with Selected Open Procedures*,
https://doi.org/10.1007/978-3-030-78881-0_53

second metacarpal eliminating the need for a K-wire to prevent subsidence. This new technique has been compared to K-wire fixation and has been shown to create similar stability [33]. The key outcome difference in this technique is the ability to begin early mobilization at 5–10 days postoperatively instead of the standard 4 weeks.

This early return of thumb movement will potentially lead to improved rates of recovery and function. The ultimate goal is to return patients back to their jobs and daily functions as quickly as possible.

Indications for Surgery

When operative management is indicated for the management of CMC arthritis, surgeons generally make these decisions based on the radiographic classifications described by Eaton and Glickel [34]. The suture-button suspensionplasty technique in conjunction with arthroscopically assisted hemitrapeziectomy is indicated for patients with Eaton stage II or III (Fig. 53.1). Stage IV requires open complete trapeziectomy. Our operative preferences and surgical approach based on Eaton stage are delineated below.

Eaton Stage I

This stage is characterized by mild widening of the trapeziometacarpal (TM) joint. Some patients are symptomatic at stage I and do not respond to nonoperative management. They are possibly indicated for arthroscopic debridement, synovectomy, and/or electrothermal capsulorrhaphy [35, 36].

Eaton Stages II and III

These stages are characterized by loss of joint space, osteophytes, and bony sclerosis. Many surgical techniques are used to treat these stages. Our previous preference was arthroscopic hemitrapeziectomy followed by K-wire pinning

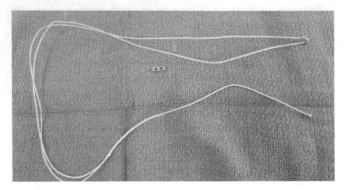

Fig. 53.1 Photo demonstrating the second-generation SB device used for thumb CMC suspensionplasty

across the CMC joint. However, as discussed previously, the immobilization that this causes may lead to patient dissatisfaction in the early postoperative period. The technique described in this chapter is designed to allow earlier range of motion while still preventing subsidence of the first metacarpal into the CMC space.

Eaton Stage IV

This stage is defined by pantrapezial osteoarthritic changes including the scaphotrapeziotrapezoid joint. When these findings are present, complete trapeziectomy is required through a standard open technique. Although the CMC space may be maintained with various techniques, our preferred technique has been to utilize suture-button suspensionplasty after open full trapeziectomy for stage IV disease.

Surgical Technique

Arthroscopic Setup and Establishment of Portals

Thumb arthroscopy is performed under either regional or general anesthesia. Regional anesthesia has the added benefit of providing postoperative analgesia. A standard wrist arthroscopy tower and 2.3 mm arthroscope are used. The operative field is set up by first placing the thumb in the finger trap, which is suspended from the arthroscopy tower (Linvatec, Largo, FL) at 12–15 lbs of traction. The finger trap and hand are then wrapped with sterile Coban (3M, St. Paul, MN) to stabilize it in the operative field (Fig. 53.2). A tourniquet is placed proximally near the axilla and inflated to 250 mmHg.

Next, the thumb CMC joint is located by palpating at the proximal end of the thumb metacarpal and feeling for the soft spot proximal to the base of the metacarpal. The 1U portal is located directly ulnar to extensor pollicis brevis tendon. Normal saline is injected into the thumb CMC space and the visualized expansion of the joint space confirms the correct location and angle of entry. A #11 blade scalpel is used to incise the skin over the 1U portal. Using a mosquito clamp, the soft tissue is bluntly dissected to avoid injury to the abductor pollicis longus, extensor pollicis brevis, extensor pollicis longus, the dorsal radial sensory nerve, and the radial artery, which are all in the vicinity. Dissection is continued down to the CMC joint capsule. The capsule is entered and the previously injected fluid elutes from the portal, again confirming successful placement. The 2.3 mm arthroscope is then inserted into the joint space, and position is confirmed on fluoroscopy. Saline is constantly infused through the arthroscopy pump, which is set to 30 mmHg to create proper joint distention, good visualization, and an adequate working space.

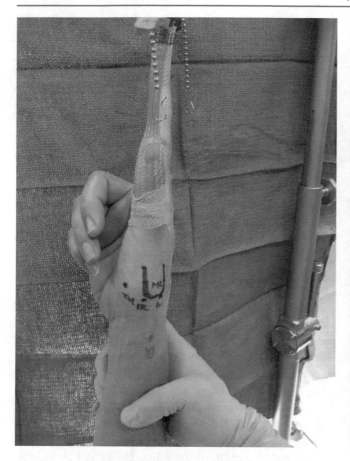

Fig. 53.2 Setup for arthroscopic hemitrapeziectomy

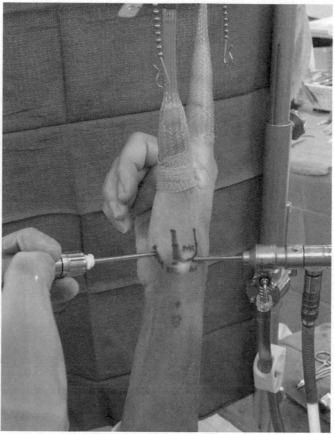

Fig. 53.3 The arthroscope is in the 1-U portal. The shaver is in the thenar portal

The next portal created is considered the "working portal." This may be placed into one of two locations: the 1R or thenar portals. The 1R portal is found radial to the abductor pollicus longus (APL) at the same level as the 1U portal. The thenar portal is approximately 90° and 1 cm volar to the 1R portal. We prefer the thenar portal as it located further from structures such as branches of the dorsal radial sensory nerve. Also, the thenar and 1U portals are perpendicular to each other, which allows the instruments to approach at angles that are favorable for visualization during arthroscopy and partial trapeziectomy (Fig. 53.3).

The thenar portal is created by placing an 18-gauge needle through the thenar musculature into the CMC joint under direct arthroscopic visualization. Once the correct position is established, the portal is finalized in the same manner as the 1U portal.

Arthroscopic Hemitrapeziectomy

The working portal is used to pass a full-radius 3.5 mm shaver into the joint. This is used to debride the joint space of degenerative articular cartilage, synovitis, articular debris, and loose bodies. After completion of debridement, the shaver is retracted and a 2.9-mm burr (Linvatec, Largo, FL)

with a 3.5 mm sheath is positioned to perform the hemitrapeziectomy. Placing a smaller burr within a larger sheath decreases the incidence of clogging by creating more space around the burr. Approximately 3–5 mm of the distal aspect of the trapezium should be removed in order to treat Eaton stage II or III. In order to improve visualization and excision, the shaver and the arthroscope should be alternated between the two portals. Fluoroscopy can also be used to confirm that the hemitrapezium has been resected appropriately.

At this stage of the procedure, the baseline subsidence of the thumb metacarpal is determined using a ballottement test. This is done under spot or live fluoroscopy and the thumb is alternatively pulled and compressed to visualize the amount of subsidence present. This subsidence is noted and later compared to the level of subsidence found following suture-button suspensionplasty (Fig. 53.4).

Open Trapeziectomy

There are two approaches to an open trapeziectomy: dorsoradial or volar (Wagner). We prefer the dorsoradial approach. This is done via a 2.5-cm incision made longitudinally over the tendons of the first dorsal extensor compartment. APL and

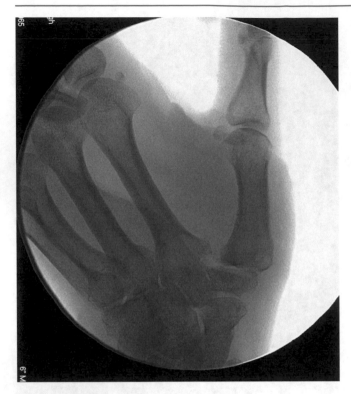

Fig. 53.4 Ballottement test shows complete subsidence of the thumb metacarpal with an axial load following hemitrapeziectomy

extensor pollicus brevis (EPB) tendons are retracted and a longitudinal capsulotomy is made over the CMC joint. The capsule is then elevated off the joint as full thickness flaps both radially and ulnarly. The trapezium is then dissected free from its attachments. It is removed with the help of osteotomes and rongeurs in a piecemeal fashion. The flexor carpi radialis tendon is preserved. Once the trapezium is removed, the space may be palpated for any additional osteophytes, which are also removed. A ballottement test, as conducted in the arthroscopic technique, to establish a baseline level of subsidence, is performed prior to suture-button suspensionplasty.

Suture-Button Technique of Suspensionplasty

An incision is made at the 1R portal site, which is volar to the APL tendon. The tissues are bluntly dissected down to the dorsal radial base of the first metacarpal. The positioning of the suture button in this location accomplishes two functions: it minimizes the chance of hardware prominence as the SB may be placed under a part of the abductor pollicis longus tendon and it promotes pronation of the thumb. If this stage of the technique is done via an open approach, the suture-button device is placed on the dorsoradial aspect of the first metacarpal. At this point, the next step is to drill a guidewire from the first metacarpal base obliquely to the

proximal diaphysis of the second metacarpal. Originally, this was done with a 1.1-mm suture-lasso guidewire (Arthrex, Naples, FL) and then a 2.7 mm drill was placed over the guidewire to make a path for the suture button. There was concern for fracture of the second metacarpal with this large drill and therefore a new guidewire was engineered. The newer guidewire has a Nitinol lasso at the proximal tip, so it acts as the suture passer. A second incision is made ulnar to the metacarpal and the tissues are bluntly dissected down to the bone. There is always a branch of the dorsal radial sensory nerve in this wound and it should be identified and protected. The second dorsal interosseous muscle is dissected from the dorsal ulnar side of the second metacarpal to allow exposure of the ulnar aspect of the bone. In general, the guidewire is directed to the metadiaphyseal junction; however, precise orientation of the guidewire has been determined to be less important [37]. The proximal and distal trajectories have been studied and a similar thumb range of motion was found. The main difference is that the suture-button device with a proximal trajectory is located further away from the nerve to the first dorsal interosseous muscle. It is clear that there is no ideal trajectory. This cadaveric study found an equivalent and full range of motion regardless of a distal trajectory through the diaphysis or a proximal trajectory through the metaphyseal region of the second metacarpal. Based on these findings, it appears that the trajectory and placement of the suture button can be variable and does not negatively impact the joint range of motion.

The guidewire is placed bicortically through the first metacarpal into the second metacarpal. It may be helpful to place a C-clamp targeting guide at the entry and exit sites to help direct the angle of the guidewire. The guidewire is then pulled through the bones out of the exit site (Figs. 53.5 and 53.6). The suture-button device is consequently pulled through the

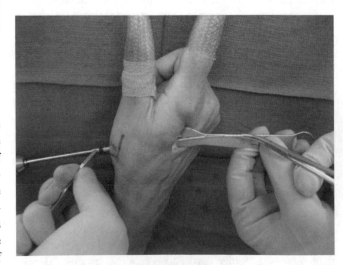

Fig. 53.5 Placement of the 1.1 mm guidewire from the thumb metacarpal to the diaphysis of the second metacarpal

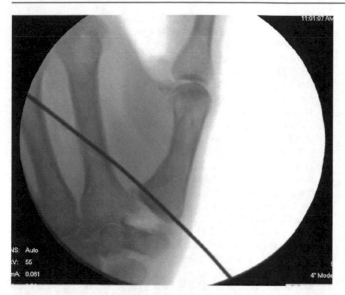

Fig. 53.6 Fluoroscopic view of the appropriate position of the guidewire

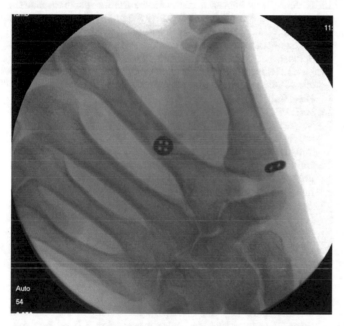

Fig. 53.7 Ballottement test shows subsidence resistance of the thumb metacarpal with an axial load following SB suspensionplasty

drilled holes as it follows the guidewire. It is then pulled flush against the thumb metacarpal where it is anchored. The second button is fitted over the sutures and placed against the dorsoulnar cortex of the second metacarpal.

The next step in the procedure is to set the tension correctly. The suture-button device should be neither too tight such that the first metacarpal impinges on the base of the second metacarpal, nor too loose that subsidence occurs. Once a provisional knot is placed temporarily, a ballottement test is conducted under fluoroscopy to confirm proper positioning (Fig. 53.7). The thumb is then taken through the full range of motion to confirm adequate motion. Adjustments are made to the suture knot as needed and once the surgeon is satisfied with the tension based on radiographic and tactile evidence, the suture is tied down. Suture ends are cut and the incisions are closed. A short-arm thumb spica splint is applied.

Postoperative Care

Surgery is performed in the outpatient setting and patient returns to clinic in 1–2 weeks for suture removal and radiographs. The films are examined for evidence of a preserved CMC joint space and then the patient is immediately enrolled in hand therapy for range of motion exercises. The patient is given a removable thermoplastic short-arm thumb spica splint to be used for comfort only.

Discussion

The above-described technique demonstrates an arthroscopic technique combined with suture-button suspensionplasty, which is minimally invasive, provides effective stabilization, and allows for early range of motion. It avoids the need for K-wire stabilization of the first metacarpal for the standard 4–5 weeks. The arthroscopic hemitrapeziectomy with suture-button placement is indicated for Eaton stage II and III, whereas open trapeziectomy and suture-button suspensionplasty are our preferred techniques for Eaton stage IV. Preliminary results have been excellent.

We have performed the suture-button suspensionplasty procedure on more than 40 patients. Several of these patients have a greater than 3-year follow-up (Fig. 53.8), and the results of which are being prepared for publication. We have had two complications that occur after this procedure and both were in the same patient. The first complication was the development of chronic regional pain syndrome 6 weeks postoperatively with related disuse osteopenia. The second complication was a fracture of the second metacarpal in that same patient. Another second metacarpal fracture complication has also been reported in the literature [38]. In addition, there have been complications noted in other areas of orthopedic surgery with the suture-button device [39–42]. The complications that occurred after trapeziectomy and suture-button suspensionplasty all happened with the first-generation device, and there have been no reports of complications in the second-generation SB device.

CMC arthritis is treated operatively with a number of different techniques, and based on the current literature, the long-term results are equivalent. The possible advantage of suture-button suspensionplasty following hemi- or complete trapeziectomy would be found in the short-term postopera-

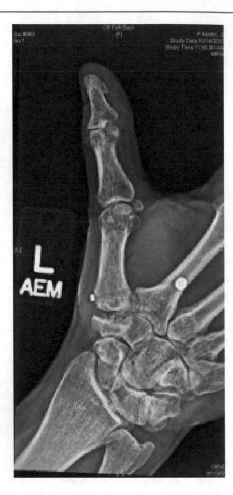

Fig. 53.8 Radiograph of a thumb 2 years following SB suspension-plasty. Note some subsidence has occurred, but the hemitrapeziectomy space is maintained

tively. We feel that the use of the SB suspensionplasty technique permits the patient to start thumb range of motion exercises earlier than with K-wire fixation and prevents the complications that can occur with K-wires, such as pin site infections, pin migration, and skin irritation. If patients undergoing this procedure ultimately have a decreased recovery time, we expect these patients to have improved satisfaction and quality of life in the short term. Long-term studies will need to be conducted to evaluate outcomes such as strength and range of motion but current results are very promising.

References

1. Wajon A, Carr E, Edmunds I, Ada L. Surgery for thumb (trapeziometacarpal joint) osteoarthritis. Cochrane Database Syst Rev. 2009;4:CD004631.
2. Yao J, Park MJ. Early treatment of degenerative arthritis of the thumb carpometacarpal joint. Hand Clin. 2008;24(3):251–61. v–vi.
3. Cooney WP 3rd, Chao EY. Biomechanical analysis of static forces in the thumb during hand function. J Bone Joint Surg Am. 1977;59(1):27–36.
4. Kaufmann RA, Logters TT, Verbruggen G, Windolf J, Goitz RJ. Osteoarthritis of the distal interphalangeal joint. J Hand Surg Am. 2010;35(12):2117–25.
5. Glickel SZ, Gupta S. Ligament reconstruction. Hand Clin. 2006;22(2):143–51.
6. Hobby JL, Lyall HA, Meggitt BF. First metacarpal osteotomy for trapeziometacarpal osteoarthritis. J Bone Joint Surg Br. 1998;80(3):508–12.
7. Wilson JN. Basal osteotomy of the first metacarpal in the treatment of arthritis of the carpometacarpal joint of the thumb. Br J Surg. 1973;60(11):854–8.
8. Parker WL, Linscheid RL, Amadio PC. Long-term outcomes of first metacarpal extension osteotomy in the treatment of carpal-metacarpal osteoarthritis. J Hand Surg Am. 2008;33(10):1737–43.
9. Tomaino MM. Basal metacarpal osteotomy for osteoarthritis of the thumb. J Hand Surg Am. 2011;36(6):1076–9.
10. Hartigan BJ, Stern PJ, Kiefhaber TR. Thumb carpometacarpal osteoarthritis: arthrodesis compared with ligament reconstruction and tendon interposition. J Bone Joint Surg Am. 2001;83-A(10):1470–8.
11. Schroder J, Kerkhoffs GM, Voerman HJ, Marti RK. Surgical treatment of basal joint disease of the thumb: comparison between resection-interposition arthroplasty and trapezio-metacarpal arthrodesis. Arch Orthop Trauma Surg. 2002;122(1):35–8.
12. Badia A. Total joint arthroplasty for the arthritic thumb carpometacarpal joint. Am J Orthop. 2008;37(8 Suppl 1):4–7.
13. Gervis WH. Excision of the trapezium for osteoarthritis of the trapezio-metacarpal joint. J Bone Joint Surg Br. 1949;31B(4):537–9. illust.
14. Davis TR, Brady O, Barton NJ, Lunn PG, Burke FD. Trapeziectomy alone, with tendon interposition or with ligament reconstruction? J Hand Surg Br. 1997;22(6):689–94.
15. Park MJ, Lichtman G, Christian JB, Weintraub J, Chang J, Hentz VR, et al. Surgical treatment of thumb carpometacarpal joint arthritis: a single institution experience from 1995-2005. Hand. 2008;3(4):304–10.
16. Burton RI, Pellegrini VD Jr. Surgical management of basal joint arthritis of the thumb. Part II. Ligament reconstruction with tendon interposition arthroplasty. J Hand Surg Am. 1986;11(3):324–32.
17. Gerwin M, Griffith A, Weiland AJ, Hotchkiss RN, McCormack RR. Ligament reconstruction basal joint arthroplasty without tendon interposition. Clin Orthop Relat Res. 1997;342:42–5.
18. Muermans S, Coenen L. Interpositional arthroplasty with Gore-Tex, Marlex or tendon for osteoarthritis of the trapeziometacarpal joint. A retrospective comparative study. J Hand Surg Br. 1998;23(1):64–8.
19. Davis TR, Brady O, Dias JJ. Excision of the trapezium for osteoarthritis of the trapeziometacarpal joint: a study of the benefit of ligament reconstruction or tendon interposition. J Hand Surg Am. 2004;29(6):1069–77.
20. Adams JE, Merten SM, Steinmann SP. Arthroscopic interposition arthroplasty of the first carpometacarpal joint. J Hand Surg Eur Vol. 2007;32(3):268–74.
21. Earp BE, Leung AC, Blazar PE, Simmons BP. Arthroscopic hemitrapeziectomy with tendon interposition for arthritis at the first carpometacarpal joint. Tech Hand Up Extrem Surg. 2008;12(1):38–42.
22. Sammer DM, Amadio PC. Description and outcomes of a new technique for thumb basal joint arthroplasty. J Hand Surg Am. 2010;35(7):1198–205.
23. Wajon A, Ada L, Edmunds I. Surgery for thumb (trapeziometacarpal joint) osteoarthritis. Cochrane Database Syst Rev. 2005;(4):CD004631.
24. Martou G, Veltri K, Thoma A. Surgical treatment of osteoarthritis of the carpometacarpal joint of the thumb: a systematic review. Plast Reconstr Surg. 2004;114(2):421–32.

25. Vermeulen GM, Slijper H, Feitz R, Hovius SE, Moojen TM, Selles RW. Surgical management of primary thumb carpometacarpal osteoarthritis: a systematic review. J Hand Surg Am. 2011;36(1):157–69.

26. Kuhns CA, Emerson ET, Meals RA. Hematoma and distraction arthroplasty for thumb basal joint osteoarthritis: a prospective, single-surgeon study including outcomes measures. J Hand Surg Am. 2003;28(3):381–9.

27. Kuhns CA, Meals RA. Hematoma and distraction arthroplasty for basal thumb osteoarthritis. Tech Hand Up Extrem Surg. 2004;8(1):2–6.

28. Cox CA, Zlotolow DA, Yao J. Suture button suspensionplasty after arthroscopic hemitrapeziectomy for treatment of thumb carpometacarpal arthritis. Arthroscopy. 2010;26(10):1395–403.

29. Gerbert J, Traynor C, Blue K, Kim K. Use of the Mini TightRope(R) for correction of hallux varus deformity. J Foot Ankle Surg. 2011;50(2):245–51.

30. Motta P, Maderni A, Bruno L, Mariotti U. Suture rupture in acromio-clavicular joint dislocations treated with flip buttons. Arthroscopy. 2011;27(2):294–8.

31. Ng VY, Berlet GC. Improving function in transtibial amputation: the distal tibiofibular bone-bridge with Arthrex Tightrope fixation. Am J Orthop (Belle Mead NJ). 2011;40(4):E57–60.

32. Storey P, Gadd RJ, Blundell C. Complications of suture button ankle syndesmosis stabilization with modifications of surgical technique. Foot Ankle Int. 2012;33(9):717–21.

33. Yao J, Zlotolow DA, Murdock R, Christian M. Suture button compared with K-wire fixation for maintenance of posttrapeziectomy space height in a cadaver model of lateral pinch. J Hand Surg Am. 2010;35(12):2061–5.

34. Eaton RG, Glickel SZ. Trapeziometacarpal osteoarthritis. Staging as a rationale for treatment. Hand Clin. 1987;3(4):455–71.

35. Culp RW, Rekant MS. The role of arthroscopy in evaluating and treating trapeziometacarpal disease. Hand Clin. 2001;17(2):315–9. x–xi.

36. Furia JP. Arthroscopic debridement and synovectomy for treating basal joint arthritis. Arthroscopy. 2010;26(1):34–40.

37. Song Y, Cox CA, Yao J. Suture button suspension following trapeziectomy in a cadaver model. Hand. 2013;8(2):195–200.

38. Khalid M, Jones ML. Index metacarpal fracture after tightrope suspension following trapeziectomy: case report. J Hand Surg Am. 2012;37(3):418–22.

39. Willmott HJ, Singh B, David LA. Outcome and complications of treatment of ankle diastasis with tightrope fixation. Injury. 2009;40(11):1204–6.

40. Kim ES, Lee KT, Park JS, Lee YK. Arthroscopic anterior talofibular ligament repair for chronic ankle instability with a suture anchor technique. Orthopedics. 2011;34(4):273.

41. Forsythe K, Freedman KB, Stover MD, Patwardhan AG. Comparison of a novel FiberWire-button construct versus metallic screw fixation in a syndesmotic injury model. Foot Ankle Int. 2008;29(1):49–54.

42. Teramoto A, Suzuki D, Kamiya T, Chikenji T, Watanabe K, Yamashita T. Comparison of different fixation methods of the suture-button implant for tibiofibular syndesmosis injuries. Am J Sports Med. 2011;39(10):2226–32.

Osteoarthritis of the Carpometacarpal Joint of the Thumb: Suture Suspensionplasty Technique Using the Internal Brace™

54

Isaac D. Gammal and David V. Tuckman

Introduction

Osteoarthritis of the hand and thumb is an exceedingly common symptomatic condition, particularly in the elderly patient. In patients older than age 75 years, thumb carpometacarpal (CMC) osteoarthritis has a radiographic prevalence of 25% in men and 40% in women [1]. It is especially prevalent in postmenopausal women. Armstrong and colleagues [2] studied the prevalence of thumb CMC arthritis in a consecutive series of 143 postmenopausal women. They found the radiological prevalences of isolated carpometacarpal and scaphotrapezial osteoarthritis were 25% and 2%, respectively. The prevalence of combined carpometacarpal and scaphotrapezial osteoarthritis was 8%; 28% of women with isolated carpometacarpal osteoarthritis and 55% with combined carpometacarpal and scaphotrapezial osteoarthritis complained of basal thumb pain.

Although the exact cause of osteoarthritis of the hand and thumb is not known, it is widely believed that mechanical stresses are to blame. The Framingham longitudinal study of radiographic hand osteoarthritis (OA) [3] examined the association between incident OA at different hand joints and maximal grip strength, which is a major determinant of forces at the proximal hand joints. Men with high maximal grip strength are at increased risk for the development of OA in the proximal interphalangeal and metacarpophalangeal (PIP), (MCP), and thumb base joints.

Reconstruction of the thumb CMC joint is among the most commonly performed hand surgery procedures. The impacts of thumb CMC arthritis on U.S. healthcare expenditures will likely increase as the number of people over 60 years of age doubles to approximately 112 million by 2050 [4]. A number of successful procedures have been employed for reconstruction of the arthritic thumb CMC joint.

Epidemiologic Findings

The prevalence of osteoarthritis of the thumb CMC joint is astounding, with the condition affecting up to approximately 1 in 4 women and 1 in 12 men [5]. Postmortem studies in Caucasians show a 50% rate of severe arthritis at the trapeziometacarpal joint. [6]. Female sex has consistently been shown to be a risk factor for the development of thumb CMC arthritis, with up to a six-fold increased incidence in women compared to men. This may be associated with an increased risk of ligamentous laxity [7]. The condition is a major cause of disability in the aging population. The prevalence of thumb CMC arthritis increases precipitously with age, with radiographic evidence rising from 9.0% in men aged 40–49 years to 31.5% in men aged ≥80 years, and 5.7% in women aged 40–49 years to 39.3% in women aged ≥80 years [8].

Numerous occupational risk factors have also been identified. Individuals in occupations believed to be at risk for thumb CMC arthritis (e.g., tailors, administrative assistants, domestic workers) have a four-fold increased risk of developing this condition. Patients whose occupations involve repetitive thumb use and heavy manual labor also have a 12-fold increased risk for thumb CMC arthritis [9]. Exposure to mechanical stress alone, however, is insufficient to fully explain the development of CMC arthritis. Other contributing factors are also involved, such as genetic and environmental factors, female gender, and comorbid predisposing influences.

Posttraumatic degeneration after intra-articular fractures may infrequently play a role in the development of thumb CMC arthritis, whereas traumatic or atraumatic ligamentous instability may hasten the process.

I. D. Gammal
Department of Orthopedic Surgery, North Shore-LIJ Medical Center, New Hyde Park, NY, USA

D. V. Tuckman (✉)
Orthopedic Associates of Manhasset, Great Neck, NY, USA
e-mail: dtuckmanmd@gmail.com

© Springer Nature Switzerland AG 2022
W. B. Geissler (ed.), *Wrist and Elbow Arthroscopy with Selected Open Procedures*,
https://doi.org/10.1007/978-3-030-78881-0_54

Anatomy and Biomechanics

The thumb is pronated and flexed approximately 80° relative to the plane of the palm at rest. This position permits opposition to the fingertips and more complex motions. The trapezium forms the base of the thumb mechanical axis [10].

The trapezium has a complex three-dimensional reciprocating saddle shape, imparting a high degree of motion and necessitating extensive secondary soft tissue stabilization [7]. The pantrapezial basal joint of the thumb is composed of five individual articulations: trapeziometacarpal (TM), trapeziotrapezoid, scaphotrapezial, scaphotrapezoidal, and trapezial-index metacarpal. The geometry of the TM joint is that of a bi-concavo-convex universal joint, both concave and convex on each side of the joint, meaning that there are two reciprocally interlocking saddle shapes that oppose each other. This unique geometry and partial constraint permits multiplanar motions, such as abduction, adduction, flexion, extension, hitchhiker, circumduction, and opposition, including screw-home torque rotation at the end phase of opposition [10]. The trapezial and metacarpal articular surfaces have different radii of curvature that become congruous only at the extremes of motion. The shallow concavity of each articular surface affords little intrinsic skeletal stability [11]. Therefore, the ligaments and muscles play varying and important roles in stability, laxity, and proprioception of this complex joint. The volar beak of the thumb metacarpal articulates with the recess in the volar trapezium, which is adjacent to the insertion of the anterior oblique "beak" ligament on the trapezium, locking into the trapezium recess pivot area during screw-home torque rotation. The complex interplay between bony and soft tissue stabilizers allows for screw-home torque rotation in the final phase of opposition, which provides the stability needed for power pinch and grasp (Fig. 54.1).

Because of the minimal bony stability of the thumb CMC joint and its lax and subluxatable nature in the resting position, it has numerous soft tissue stabilizers. As many as 16 ligaments have been identified, but six ligaments have been consistently found to confer joint stability [10, 12]. The deep anterior oblique "beak" ligament originates just ulnar to the volar styloid process at the base of the first metacarpal (beak) and inserts onto the volar central apex of the trapezium just ulnar to the ulnar edge of the trapezial ridge. Owing to its static nature and intra-articular location, the beak ligament serves as a pivot point for rotation, specifically for pronation, to produce opposition, and it becomes taut in wide abduction or extension [13].

Hand surgeons were traditionally taught that degeneration of this ligament primarily contributed to disease progression. Recent studies have disputed this assertion [11] and suggest that this is primarily a thin, capsular structure, with a mean

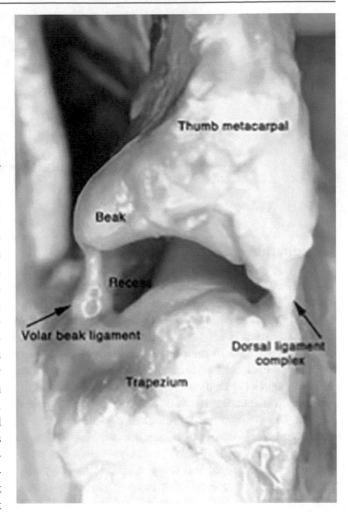

Fig. 54.1 Trapeziometacarpal joint in its resting position. (Reprinted from Edmunds [32]. With permission from Elsevier)

thickness of just 0.71 mm and variable width. Histomorphometric staining to determine morphology and cellularity also support the notion that it is primarily a capsular structure consisting of disorganized connective tissue and lacking mechanoreceptors for mechanical feedback [12].

The dorsal ligament complex of the thumb CMC joint consists of the dorsoradial ligament and posterior oblique ligament. These are the largest, thickest and strongest ligaments of the TM joint, and are generally regarded as its most important soft tissue stabilizers. It originates from the dorsoradial tubercle of the trapezium and fans out to insert broadly onto the dorsal edge of the base of the first metacarpal. The dorsal ligament complex is the key force coupler that stabilizes the TM joint in power grip or pinch during the screw-home torque rotation final phase of opposition, which tightly compresses the volar beak of the thumb metacarpal into its recess area in the trapezium [12, 13]. The dorsoradial ligament becomes taut with a dorsal or dorsoradial subluxating force in all positions of the TM joint except full extension, and tightens in supination, regardless of joint position. It also tightens in pronation when the CMC joint is flexed [13].

Strauch et al. [14] conducted cadaveric serial sectioning of the thumb CMC ligaments with the metacarpal in neutral, flexion, and extension. The authors found that the primary restraint to dorsal dislocation was the dorsoradial ligament, with the anterior oblique ligament allowing dislocation by subperiosteal stripping from the base of the first metacarpal. While the volar ligaments are lacking in normal ligamentous structure and mechanoreceptor innervation, the dorsal ligamentous complex is composed of stout collagen in an organized fashion and has proprioceptive mechanoreceptors known as Ruffini endings present close to ligamentous attachments [15].

The ulnar ligamentous complex, consisting of the volar and dorsal trapeziometacarpal ligaments, forms a conjoined attachment—the ulnar collateral ligament—and provides a checkrein effect. The multitude of ligamentous structures surrounding the thumb CMC joint leads many to conclude that it is likely stabilized by the coordinated effects of all ligaments, and our understanding of the anatomy continues to evolve [16].

The complex movement and dynamic stabilization of the thumb CMC joint depends on the extrinsic, intrinsic, and thenar musculotendinous anatomy. The abductor pollicis longus, extensor pollicis longus, extensor pollicis brevis, and flexor pollicis longus tendons provide the extrinsic support via their insertions onto the thumb metacarpal and phalanges. The intrinsic muscles affecting the thumb include the abductor pollicis brevis, adductor pollicis, flexor pollicis brevis, and opponens pollicis. There is a complex interplay between static and dynamic stabilizers during screw-home torque rotation. The intrinsic abductor pollicis brevis muscle abducts the thumb at the TM joint. The opponens pollicis then rotates the thumb, allowing flexor pollicis brevis, adductor pollicis longus, and flexor pollicis longus to further compress the TM joint. These coordinated motions allow the TM joint to gain articular congruence and rigid stability for power pinch and grasp during the final phase of opposition [11]. An additional intrinsic dynamic stabilizer has also been suggested [17]. In a radiographic analysis of 32 thumbs, activation of the first dorsal interosseous muscle appeared to reduce radial subluxation of the thumb CMC joint by an average of 4 mm.

Pathoanatomy and Altered Biomechanics

During the process of degeneration, the thumb metacarpal is pulled into adduction, with a compensatory metacarpophalangeal (MCP) hyperextension deformity. A series of studies provided compelling evidence to support the hypothesis that the degeneration of the deep anterior oblique ligament is the precursor to basal joint degenerative disease. In a cadaver study by Pellegrini et al. [18], postmortem material demonstrated eburnated lesions in the volar compartment of the TM joint in association with degenerative disruption of the adjacent deep anterior oblique ligament. The authors concluded that such a pattern would be expected in the setting of incompetent volar capsuloligamentous structures [19].

More recent studies have called these findings into question. In particular, analysis of normal anatomy has demonstrated that the volar ligaments are thin, disorganized capsular structures lacking in mechanoreceptors, which are responsible for joint proprioception [12]. In contrast, mechanoreceptors are abundant in the ligamentous attachments of the dorsal ligamentous complex, which are also stouter in structure. In addition, several cadaveric studies support the importance of the dorsoradial ligament in preventing dorsoradial displacement of the thumb metacarpal shaft relative to the trapezium [14, 20].

High compressive forces occur across the thumb CMC during pinch. They reach in excess of 12 times the applied load and may approach 20 times the applied load during maximum grasp. Cantilever bending occurs with these applied forces such that shear forces are created that are highest at the volar half of the joint's articular surface. In an analysis of articular wear patterns [19], Pelligrini found that eburnation occurred only on TM surfaces in contact areas of the volar compartment. Furthermore, metacarpal degeneration began at the volar joint margin adjacent to the beak ligament and progressed dorsally, while trapezial degeneration originated on the central palmar slope and spread centrifugally with more advanced disease. Eburnation patterns were asymmetric, involving a greater surface area on the trapezium than on the metacarpal in a ratio of nearly 3–1. These observations suggest that progressive translation of the thumb metacarpal on the trapezium is responsible for the production of arthritic surface lesions, and support the hypothesis of pathologic joint instability as the cause of CMC arthritis. Although the arthritic pattern most frequently involves the TM joint, some patients present with concomitant scaphotrapeziotrapezoid (STT) arthritis. Whether the development of STT arthritis is regulated by an alternative mechanism or is the result of further progression is currently unknown [7].

Physical Examination

Patients with osteoarthritis of the thumb CMC joint present with either varied complaints of pain localized to that area, or more vague complaints of throbbing and/or burning in the radial aspect of the hand. A thorough physical examination of the joint begins with inspection. Patients with more advanced stages of joint degeneration will often present with a thumb adduction contracture and a compensatory thumb MCP joint hyperextension deformity and laxity.

After inspection, the CMC joint is palpated and evaluated using the grind test and joint subluxation test. The CMC grind test is performed with the examiner facing the patient. With the patient's hand on a hand-examining table, the wrist is stabilized with one hand, and an axial load applied to the thumb axis with the examiner's other hand. Pain, as well as crepitus, may be elicited as the degenerative articular surfaces are compressed and rotated. The CMC subluxation test is performed in a similar fashion, although the maneuver aims to gently force the CMC joint to subluxate and the examiner determines whether this elicits pain. Crepitus may also be apparent with this maneuver. Pinch strength testing, such as the two-point key pinch test or the three-point chuck pinch test using a dynamometer, may be assessed and compared to the contralateral side. Many patients with CMC arthritis will also present with ipsilateral carpal tunnel syndrome, with rates as high as 43% [21]. The examiner should ask about numbness in the distribution of the median nerve and nocturnal symptoms, and should inspect for thenar muscle atrophy. Diagnostic maneuvers, such as Durkan's compression test, Phalen's test, and median nerve percussion, may also be performed. EMG and nerve conduction studies may be considered if clinical suspicion is equivocal.

Imaging

Standard radiographs to profile the thumb CMC joint include PA, lateral, and oblique views of the hand or wrist. A true AP view of the thumb, or Robert's view, and true lateral view of the thumb are also helpful. Robert's view is obtained with the forearm in maximum pronation and a combination of positions, including shoulder flexion and internal rotation, so that the dorsal surface of the thumb can be placed directly on the radiograph cassette. A true lateral view of the thumb is obtained with the forearm flat on the table, the hand pronated approximately 20°, the thumb flat on the cassette, and the X-ray tube angled 10° from the vertical in distal to proximal projection. Advanced imaging studies such as MRI or CT scanning are rarely necessary for diagnosis or surgical decision-making.

Eaton and Littler [22] described four progressive radiographic stages of thumb CMC arthritis to guide management, which were later modified to include STT arthritis. This modified Eaton-Littler classification is now the most commonly used radiographic classification system for thumb CMC arthritis:

- *Stage I:* Subtle carpometacarpal joint space widening
- *Stage II:* Slight carpometacarpal joint space narrowing, sclerosis, and cystic changes with osteophytes or loose bodies <2 mm

- *Stage III:* Advanced carpometacarpal joint space narrowing, sclerosis, and cystic changes with osteophytes or loose bodies >2 mm
- *Stage IV:* Arthritic changes in the carpometacarpal joint as in Stage III with STT arthritis

Nonoperative Management

Many patients with thumb basal joint arthritis can be managed successfully with nonoperative management. The aim of conservative treatment is to restore thumb functionality, including pain relief, stability, motion, and strength. A recent systematic review [23] of randomized controlled trials (RCTs) found only a few high-quality studies addressing the conservative treatment of thumb CMC arthritis. Medications have a role in the treatment of thumb CMC arthritis. Traditionally, NSAIDs form the first line of medical treatment; however, there are no RCTs on the effects of analgesics, or superiority of one analgesic over another. Hand therapy was found to be beneficial in elderly patients with severe CMC arthritis. There is evidence that both steroid and hyaluronic acid (HA) intra-articular injections can reduce pain in patients with thumb CMC arthritis, although HA is not FDA approved for injection into the thumb. The effects of steroids are achieved faster, but are short-lived compared to HA, which seems to have a longer lasting effect after a slow start. Interestingly, in a study by Wolf and Delaronde [24], surveying active members of the American Society for Surgery of the Hand, 89% of surgeons favored the use of steroid injections for conservative management of thumb CMC arthritis.

Present evidence suggests that orthoses can give some pain reduction in patients with thumb CMC arthritis for up to 1 year, but do not influence hand function or strength. There is no strong evidence showing that a custom-made orthosis was superior to a prefabricated orthosis, that the length of one orthosis was superior to another, or that a patient should constantly wear the orthosis [23].

Because it is one of the most commonly seen hand surgery diagnoses, there is a pressing need for higher quality RCTs investigating the different conservative treatment modalities for thumb CMC arthritis. Ideally, future studies should include more patients, have longer follow-up times, and subgroup analyses regarding grade of OA; they should include pain scores, strength measurements, and patient-reported outcome measures [23].

Surgical Management

There are many types of surgery for thumb CMC arthritis, all having the same aim: to reduce pain and increase function. Root treatment for thumb CMC arthritis is most often trapeziectomy, either performed alone or in combination with various other modifications to achieve durable long-term outcomes. However, for early-stage arthritis (Eaton I and II), several joint-preserving surgical options are described. First metacarpal extension osteotomy, although not commonly performed, may benefit patients with mild-to-moderate thumb CMC arthritis [25]. A closing wedge osteotomy places the thumb metacarpal base in 30° of extension without the need for soft tissue reconstruction.

Arthroscopic treatment of thumb CMC arthritis is a relatively newer option and indicated for assessment of cartilage integrity, synovectomy, and loose body removal. Partial or total trapeziectomy performed arthroscopically is also possible [25]. A recent systematic review of arthroscopic debridement or partial trapeziectomy for thumb CMC arthritis suggested reduced pain and improved patient satisfaction similar to improvements documented in open studies, with durable results up to 7.6 years out [26].

Isolated soft tissue reconstruction was proposed by Eaton and Littler in 1973 [27]. The anterior oblique ligament reconstruction was achieved by routing a portion of the flexor carpi radialis through the base of the thumb metacarpal. They noted good or excellent long-term results in 95% of patients with no or minimal articular changes (Eaton I and II). By restoring stability, they were able to reduce pain and possibly even retard joint degeneration [28]. Some authors advocate isolated imbrication of the dorsoradial capsule for early arthritis and subluxation, which may improve stability [7].

Open trapeziectomy, first described by Gervis in 1949, has long been the surgical mainstay for more severe disease (Eaton III and IV). Later adjuncts included gelatin-sponge interposition, K-wire metacarpal support and soft tissue interposition that were added because of concerns about long-term subsidence; however, no statistical association between the amount of first metacarpal subsidence and follow-up key pinch, tip pinch, or grip strength was found [29]. One of the most widely used techniques today is the ligament reconstruction and tendon interposition (LRTI), which is the preferred method of 62% of active American Society for Surgery of the Hand members [24]. Through either a dorsal or volar radial incision, the joint capsule is incised and a trapeziectomy performed. An oval window is created on the dorsal surface of the first metacarpal, and its articular surface is removed. The flexor carpi radialis (FCR) tendon is harvested at its myotendinous junction and delivered into the wrist incision. Either part or all of the FCR tendon is then passed through the oval window in the first metacarpal and sutured to itself as a soft tissue interpositional autograft. Alternatively, the abductor pollicis longus (APL) or extensor carpi radialis longus may be used. If residual MP hyperextension remains, a volar capsulodesis or MCP arthrodesis may also be performed. Despite the popularity of the LRTI,

there is only low-quality evidence supporting trapeziectomy with LRTI over trapeziectomy alone, with regard to pain, function, and adverse effects.

Aside from ligament reconstruction and interposition, there are other surgical options. Some authors prefer using a distraction hematoma arthroplasty by placing a K-wire from the first to the second metacarpal base, without a ligamentous interposition; this method has been shown to be effective in relieving pain and restoring function, despite evidence of late radiographic subsidence [30].

A simple reconstructive method for treating thumb CMC arthritis is the suture suspension arthroplasty (SSA) [31]. The SSA technique for thumb CMC arthritis reconstruction consists of trapeziectomy and a four-strand nonabsorbable suspension sling, creating a "hammock" between the distalmost insertions of the APL and the FCR. Pulling this construct tethers the base of the thumb toward the base of the index metacarpal, correcting the subluxation deformity and maintaining arthroplasty space. Additional options include the use of prostheses as spacers or trapezial replacements, although they have been only intermittently successful, and CMC arthrodesis.

Trapeziectomy and Suture Suspensionplasty Using the Internal Brace™

Exposure

Under light sedation, a nerve block of the median and terminal branches of the radial and lateral antebrachial cutaneous nerves is performed with 1% Lidocaine and 0.25% Marcaine. A 3- to 4-cm incision is made on the dorsal aspect of the CMC joint and trapezium, between the extensor pollicis longus and brevis tendons (Fig. 54.2).

The dissection is taken down to expose the abductor pollicis longus and the extensor pollicis brevis. After the ten-

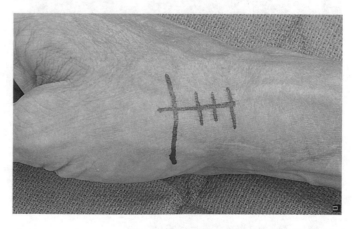

Fig. 54.2 A 3- to 4-cm dorsal skin incision over the dorsal aspect of the CMC joint

dons are exposed, a self-retaining retractor is placed between them. Next, the dissection is taken through the fatty tissue to expose the deep branch of the radial artery. The artery is mobilized dorsally and proximally and a longitudinal dorsal capsulotomy is performed.

Trapeziectomy

Subperiosteal dissection of the trapezium is taken ulnar, with the exposure of the trapeziotrapezoidal joint. The dissection is also taken radial and volar, to expose the entirety of the dorsal trapezium. It is critical to visualize the entire dorsal surface of the trapezium, including its articulations with the scaphoid, trapezoid, and first metacarpal. A freer elevator may be placed into the CMC joint to provide distraction and to aid in exposure of the dorsal surface of the trapezium and in its removal. A 9-mm McGlamry metatarsal elevator (Fig. 54.3) works extremely well for trapezium removal (at our institution, the McGlamry elevator is available in the podiatry trays). The advantage of the McGlamry elevator is its matching contour with the volar trapezial surface, allowing it to pass easily around its volar aspect and elevate the volar capsule.

It is best to remove the trapezium in three sequential steps:

1. Starting from the radial aspect of the trapezium, the McGlamry is passed around the volar aspect to elevate the volar capsule.
2. Next, the McGlamry is passed into the trapeziotrapezoidal joint to lever the trapezium out the radial side.
3. Finally, the McGlamry is passed into the CMC joint and the trapezium is levered out dorsally.

Internal Brace™ Placement

The articular surface of the first metacarpal base is exposed. This is easily achieved by inserting a small Hohmann retractor under its volar edge and flexing the first ray. The guide pin from the Arthrex 3.5 DX SwiveLock® SL anchor (Arthrex, Inc., Naples, FL) (Fig. 54.4) is drilled into the radial corner of the first metacarpal, midline between the volar and dorsal edges.

The wire is drilled until the black laser line is flush with bone (Fig. 54.5). The guidewire is overdrilled with a 3.0-mm cannulated drill. The drill guide has a depth stop at 1 cm.

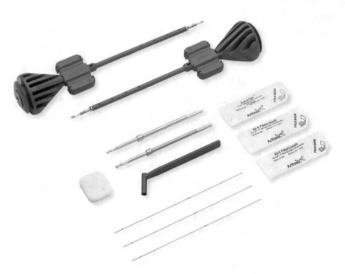

Fig. 54.4 The Arthrex 3.5 DX SwiveLock® SL anchor (Arthrex, Inc., Naples, FL) Included in the kit are two 3.5 × 8.5 mm anchors with forked eyelets, 3.0-mm cannulated drill bit (for all-suture constructs), 3.5-mm cannulated drill bit (for graft constructs), 1.35-mm guide wires, tendon sizer, and fiberwire suture

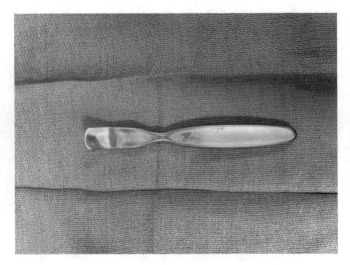

Fig. 54.3 The McGlamry metatarsal elevator

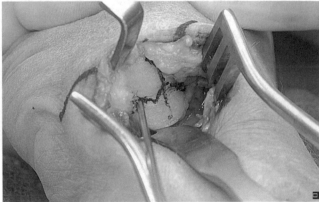

Fig. 54.5 The base of the first metacarpal is exposed with a small Hohmann retractor under its volar edge and flexing the first ray. The guide pin is drilled into the radial corner of the 1st metacarpal, midline between the volar and dorsal edges

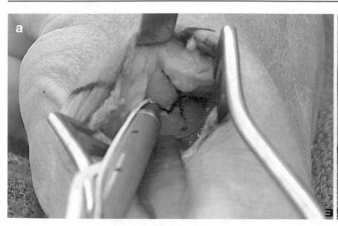
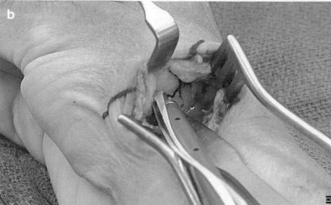

Fig. 54.6 (**a**, **b**) The preloaded anchor is inserted into the drilled hole until the laser line is flush with bone

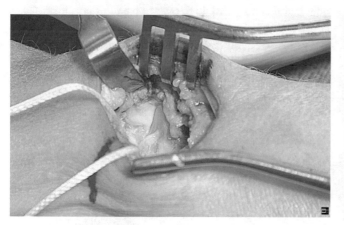
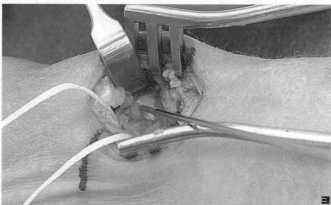

Fig. 54.7 The articular surface of the base of the second metacarpal is exposed

Fig. 54.8 The guide pin is inserted into the base of the index metacarpal 5 mm distal to the CMC joint

LabralTape™ (Arthrex, Inc., Naples, FL) is preloaded onto the forked eyelet of the first anchor. The preloaded anchor is then inserted into the drilled hole until the laser line is flush with bone (Fig. 54.6).

The articular surface at the base of the second metacarpal is identified (Fig. 54.7).

The guide pin is inserted approximately 5 mm distal to the CMC joint and then overdrilled with the 3.0-mm cannulated drill (Fig. 54.8).

Both limbs of the LabralTape™ (Arthrex, Inc., Naples, FL) are preloaded onto the forked eyelet of the second anchor. The thumb is positioned in full adduction with just enough traction to visualize the hole in the second metacarpal (Fig. 54.9).

The second anchor is then seated until the laser line is flush with bone. It is important not to over or under distract the thumb when seating the second anchor. The excess LabralTape™ (Arthrex, Inc., Naples, FL) is trimmed with a scalpel (Fig. 54.10).

Axial compression is placed on the thumb to test for any evidence of subsidence and maintenance of the arthroplasty

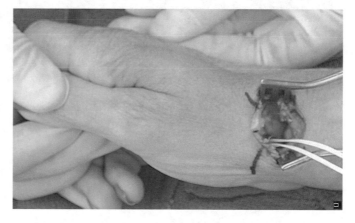

Fig. 54.9 The thumb is positioned in full adduction with just enough traction to visualize the hole in the second metacarpal

space. The thumb is then brought through a gentle range of motion (Fig. 54.11).

The capsulotomy is closed with 3-0 vicryl sutures and skin with interrupted buried 5-0 monocryl. The patient is placed in a forearm-based thumb spica splint. At 1 week, the patient is transitioned to a custom molded forearm-based thumb spica splint, which may be removed to shower. At week 4, the patient begins occupational therapy with active range of motion and begins weaning off the splint. At week 6, the splint is discontinued fully and light strengthening is

begun. The patient may resume full activity at 12 weeks postoperatively.

Surgical Tips and Tricks

It is critical to fully expose the entirety of the dorsal trapezium. The capsule is dissected off its radial and volar aspects. The dissection is continued ulnarly into the trapeziotrapezoidal joint. Next, the dissection is taken proximally into the scaphotrapezial joint and then distally into the CMC joint. This extensive dissection aids tremendously in excising the entire trapezium using the McGlamry elevator.

It is also important to tighten the Labral Tape™ as much as possible when inserting the second anchor. It is important to note that it is not possible to over-tighten this construct. Over-compressing the first and second intermetacarpal space, leading to loss of abduction and persistent pain, is possible with other techniques. With the *Internal* Brace™, when inserting the second anchor, the thumb is held in adduction and once the anchor is seated and thumb adduction released, the first metacarpal will naturally settle into a looser position.

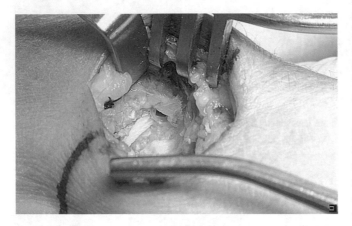

Fig. 54.10 The second anchor is then seated until the laser line is flush with bone and excess labral tape trimmed

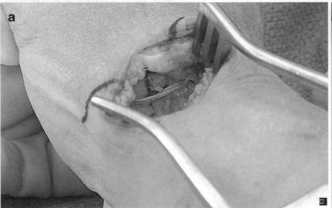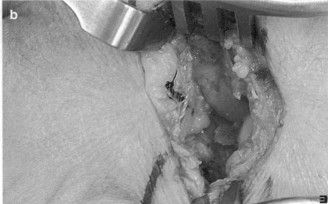

Fig. 54.11 (**a**, **b**) Axial compression is placed on the thumb to test for any evidence of subsidence and maintenance of the arthroplasty space

Conclusion

From joint sparing techniques to simple trapeziectomy, LRTI and prosthetic arthroplasty, the treatment options for moderate-to-severe thumb CMC arthritis seem innumerable. We detailed a simple, efficient and reproducible technique for open trapeziectomy augmented with the *Internal* Brace™. This is an excellent option for pain relief, functional restoration, and prevention of long-term subsidence in patients with advanced thumb CMC arthritis.

References

1. Sodha S, Ring D, Zurakowski D, Jupiter JB. Prevalence of osteoarthrosis of the trapeziometacarpal joint. J Bone Joint Surg Ser A. 2005;87(12 I):2614–8.
2. Armstrong AL, Hunter JB, Davis TRC. The prevalence of degenerative arthritis of the base of the thumb in post-menopausal women. J Hand Surg Am. 1994;19(3):340–1.
3. Chaisson CE, Zhang Y, Sharma L, Kannel W, Felson DT. Grip strength and the risk of developing radiographic hand osteoarthritis: results from the Framingham study. Arthritis Rheum. 1999;42(1):33–8.
4. Yuan F, Aliu O, Chung KC, Mahmoudi E. Evidence-based practice in the surgical treatment of thumb carpometacarpal joint arthritis. J Hand Surg Am. 2017;42(2):104–112.e1.
5. Swigart CR. Arthritis of the base of the thumb. Curr Rev Musculoskelet Med. 2008;1(2):142–6.
6. Cooney WP, Chao EYS. Biomechanical analysis of static forces in the thumb during hand function. J Bone Joint Surg Ser A. 1977;59(1):27–36.
7. Weiss A-PC, Goodman AD. Thumb basal joint arthritis. J Am Acad Orthop Surg [Internet]. 2018 [cited 2019 Dec 14];26(16):562–71. Available from: http://insights.ovid.com/crossref?an=00124635-201808150-00002.
8. Wilder FV, Barrett JP, Farina EJ. Joint-specific prevalence of osteoarthritis of the hand. Osteoarthr Cartil. 2006;14(9):953–7.
9. Fontana L, Neel S, Claise JM, Ughetto S, Catilina P. Osteoarthritis of the thumb carpometacarpal joint in women and occupational risk factors: a case-control study. J Hand Surg Am. 2007;32(4):459–65.
10. Leversedge FJ. Anatomy and pathomechanics of the thumb. Hand Clin. 2008;24:219–29.
11. Edmunds JO. Current concepts of the anatomy of the thumb trapeziometacarpal joint. J Hand Surg. 2011;36:170–82.
12. Ladd AL, Weiss APC, Crisco JJ, Hagert E, Wolf JM, Glickel SZ, et al. The thumb carpometacarpal joint: anatomy, hormones, and biomechanics. Instr Course Lect. 2013;62:165–79.
13. Bettinger PC, Linscheid RL, Berger RA, Cooney WP, An KN. An anatomic study of the stabilizing ligaments of the trapezium and trapeziometacarpal joint. J Hand Surg Am. 1999;24(4):786–98.
14. Strauch RJ, Behrman MJ, Rosenwasser MP. Acute dislocation of the carpometacarpal joint of the thumb: An anatomic and cadaver study. J Hand Surg Am. 1994;19(1):93–8.
15. Ladd AL, Crisco JJ, Hagert E, Rose J, Weiss APC. The 2014 ABJS Nicolas Andry Award: the puzzle of the thumb: mobil-

ity, stability, and demands in opposition. Clin Orthop Relat Res. 2014;472:3605–22.
16. Lin JD, Karl JW, Strauch RJ. Trapeziometacarpal joint stability: the evolving importance of the dorsal ligaments. In: Clinical orthopaedics and related research. New York: Springer; 2014. p. 1138–45.
17. McGee C, O'Brien V, Van Nortwick S, Adams J, Van Heest A. The first dorsal interosseus: a dynamic stabilizer of the radially subluxed thumb carpometacarpal joint? J Hand Ther [Internet]. 2016 [cited 2019 Dec 14];29(3):368–9. Available from: https://linkinghub.elsevier.com/retrieve/pii/S0894113014001057.
18. Pellegrini VD. Osteoarthritis of the trapeziometacarpal joint: the pathophysiology of articular cartilage degeneration. I. Anatomy and pathology of the aging joint. J Hand Surg Am. 1991;16(6):967–74.
19. Pellegrini VD. Osteoarthritis of the trapeziometacarpal joint: the pathophysiology of articular cartilage degeneration. II. Articular wear patterns in the osteoarthritic joint. J Hand Surg Am. 1991;16(6):975–82.
20. Van Brenk B, Richards RR, Mackay MB, Boynton EL. A biomechanical assessment of ligaments preventing dorsoradial subluxation of the trapeziometacarpal joint. J Hand Surg Am [Internet]. 1998 [cited 2019 Dec 14];23(4):607–11. Available from: http://www.ncbi.nlm.nih.gov/pubmed/9708373.
21. Florack TM, Miller RJ, Pellegrini VD, Burton RI, Dunn MG. The prevalence of carpal tunnel syndrome in patients with basal joint arthritis of the thumb. J Hand Surg Am. 1992;17(4):624–30.
22. Kennedy CD, Manske MC, Huang JI. Classifications in brief: the Eaton-Littler classification of thumb carpometacarpal joint arthrosis. Clin Orthop Relat Res. 2016;474(12):2729–33.
23. Spaans AJ, Van Minnen LP, Kon M, Schuurman AH, Schreuders AR, Vermeulen GM. Conservative treatment of thumb base osteoarthritis: a systematic review. J Hand Surg Am. 2015;40(1):16–21.e6.
24. Wolf JM, Delaronde S. Current trends in nonoperative and operative treatment of trapeziometacarpal osteoarthritis: a survey of US hand surgeons. J Hand Surg Am. 2012;37(1):77–82.
25. Berger AJ, Meals RA. Management of osteoarthrosis of the thumb joints. J Hand Surg. 2015;40:843–50.
26. Adams JE. Does arthroscopic débridement with or without interposition material address carpometacarpal arthritis? In: Clinical orthopaedics and related research. New York: Springer; 2014. p. 1166–72.
27. Eaton RG, Littler JW. Ligament reconstruction for the painful thumb carpometacarpal joint. J Bone Joint Surg Ser A. 1973;55(8):1655–66.
28. Eaton RG, Lane LB, Littler JW, Keyser JJ. Ligament reconstruction for the painful thumb carpometacarpal joint: a long-term assessment. J Hand Surg Am. 1984;9(5):692–9.
29. Yang SS, Weiland AJ. First metacarpal subsidence during pinch after ligament reconstruction and tendon interposition basal joint arthroplasty of the thumb. J Hand Surg Am. 1998;23(5):879–83.
30. Gray KV, Meals RA. Hematoma and distraction arthroplasty for thumb basal joint osteoarthritis: minimum 6.5-year follow-up evaluation. J Hand Surg Am. 2007;32(1):23–9.
31. DelSignore JL, Zambito-Accardi KL, Ballatori SE. Suture suspension arthroplasty for thumb carpometacarpal arthritis reconstruction: long-term outcome. J Hand Surg Am. 2015;40(9):e29–30.
32. Edmunds JO. Traumatic dislocations and instability of the trapeziometacarpal joint of the thumb. Hand Clin. 2006;22:365–92.

Alejandro Badia

Introduction

Advances in fiberoptic technology and small joint instrumentation have opened up a new world in the area of arthroscopy. However, indications for small joint arthroscopy in the hand remain poorly understood and underutilized. This is mainly due to a scarcity of papers utilizing this technique in the literature, as well as scarce hands-on training in the technical aspects of small joint arthroscopy. Despite the fact that these small joint arthroscopes have been readily available for decades, hand surgeons have been slow to adopt this methodology within their treatment protocols of both traumatic and degenerative conditions involving small joints.

Small joints to be discussed include the trapeziometacarpal, scaphotrapezial-trapezoidal, metacarpophalangeal, fifth carpometacarpal (CMC), proximal (PIP), and even distal (DIP) interphalangeal joints. Similar instrumentation is used in the temporomandibular joints and small foot articulations, but it is beyond the "scope" of this chapter.

Perhaps, the most common indication for small joint arthroscopy is its use in the thumb trapeziometacarpal or first CMC joint and is simply due to the ubiquitous nature of thumb basal joint arthritis and the myriad of treatment options that continue to be offered. Small joint arthroscopy offers a minimally invasive manner to achieve similar treatment goals and a previously described arthroscopic classification for basal joint osteoarthritis helps direct specific treatment depending on the stage of disease. This chapter will also review the brief history of trapeziometacarpal arthroscopy and provide insight as to how this technique can be incorporated into a treatment algorithm in managing this extremely common condition.

Metacarpophalangeal joint arthroscopy is even less commonly used, while traumatic and overuse injuries are frequently seen in the thumb and present an ideal indication in certain scenarios. Painful conditions affecting the metacarpophalangeal joints of the fingers are less commonly seen, yet the small joint arthroscope presents a much clearer picture of the present pathology compared to other imaging techniques or even open, and potentially harmful, surgery due to excess capsular scarring.

Proximal interphalangeal arthroscopy remains a novel technique and few papers have outlined the indications or utilization of this technique in PIP pathology. Rheumatoid arthritis (RA) may be the best indication, as the soft tissue pathology itself permits introduction of the scope into a small space due to capsular laxity. Treatment is best suited for earlier stages.

Distal interphalangeal arthroscopy remains anecdotal as does that of the fifth carpometacarpal joint, only possible since it is quite mobile.

The application of this technology to the smaller joints will soon make the treating surgeon realize that a myriad of pathologies are readily visible and can augment treatment as well as diagnosis. Similar to the wrist, small joint arthroscopy may one day supplant imaging techniques such as magnetic resonance imaging (MRI) or computed tomography (CT) in establishing an accurate diagnosis.

Thumb First Carpometacarpal (CMC) Arthroscopy

Osteoarthritis of the thumb trapeziometacarpal (TM) joint remains the most common indication for small joint arthroscopy and perhaps the only small joint technique that is now consistently mentioned in academic symposia and scientific articles. There are a plethora of different surgical options for the basal joint suggesting that none of them has an optimal success rate, or conversely, it may be that many treatment options lead to satisfactory results; therefore, the clinician continues to use his favorite technique. However, this "one

A. Badia (✉)
Badia Hand to Shoulder Center, OrthoNOW Orthopedic Urgent Care Centers, Doral, FL, USA
e-mail: Alejandro@drbadia.com

© Springer Nature Switzerland AG 2022
W. B. Geissler (ed.), *Wrist and Elbow Arthroscopy with Selected Open Procedures*,
https://doi.org/10.1007/978-3-030-78881-0_55

operation fits all" approach may not be optimal since different stages of basal joint arthritis are clearly recognized. Furthermore, first CMC osteoarthritis of the thumb has many different clinical presentations and one technique cannot be used for all of the different stages and a patient's individual needs. When conservative treatment has failed, there are many surgical options and should be individualized to the particular patient.

The early stages of basal joint osteoarthritis are frequently seen in middle-aged women and can be frustrating since current open surgical options may be deemed too aggressive for this patient population. These patients often fail conservative treatment and are searching for a solution to provide definitive pain relief while allowing them to be active. The use of anti-inflammatories, splinting, corticosteroids, and even hyaluronic injections serves only as palliative measures, with none of them affecting a permanent change in the joint pathophysiology or mechanics. Furthermore, the use of injectable corticosteroids can hasten cartilage degradation and lead to further capsular attenuation/instability. The rare cases of transient synovitis may experience some relief, but the inevitable progressive loss of cartilage demands a more aggressive intervention. Second to the DIP joint, the thumb basal joint remains the most common, but most symptomatic location for osteoarthritis in the hand. Ironically, it is also the most critical for hand function and perhaps the increased motion and demands this joint experiences lead to the condition itself. The ascent of mankind has been largely attributed to the unique function of the human thumb basal joint and likely led to the progression of tool use in hominid evolution. Treatment of this functionally important joint remains a priority for the hand surgeon, and it is important to utilize the wide variety of surgical techniques to optimally manage this condition.

Traditionally, the basal joint has been treated by surgical means only when conservative options have been exhausted and the patient demands a more aggressive treatment. The primary option has been, and still remains, some type of open trapezial resection arthroplasty. This explains why the procedure is not often offered to younger patients, and why high-demand patients will forego operative treatment, even when symptoms are quite severe. While the literature demonstrates good results in a multitude of studies and using a variety of techniques, it nevertheless is a surgically aggressive procedure since removal of a complete carpal bone is required in order to achieve pain relief. This is understandable in the most advanced cases where the trapezium is typically flattened, has pan-trapezial disease, or has severe deformity including marginal osteophytes. However, earlier stages warrant a more conservative option that allows for future interventions if the primary treatment is not successful. Other options, perhaps less aggressive, include arthrodesis, which can provide an excellent pain relief but has the

obvious limitation of loss of motion or joint replacement. Joint arthroplasty, like in any other joint in the body, has the added risk of failure of the implant, whether this be silicone or of metallic and plastic components and is still not accepted by many clinicians. This is also not a good alternative for the younger, high-demand patients.

Evolution of Basal Joint Arthroscopy

The refinement of fiberoptic technology has allowed us to apply the ideals of minimally invasive surgery to small joints including the wrist, foot, temporomandibular, and now the small joints of the foot and hand. Yung-Cheng Chen's classic treatise on arthroscopy of the wrist and finger joints in 1979 reviewed the technique and indication of performing small joint arthroscopic procedures using the Watanabe No. 24 arthroscope as early as in 1970 [1]. Surprisingly, within that paper there was no mention of arthroscopy of the thumb trapeziometacarpal joint, perhaps the small joint arthroscope's broadest clinical indication. In his review, there was a detailed description of arthroscopy of the wrist, metacarpophalangeal joints, and the proximal interphalangeal joints. While wrist arthroscopy has been universally accepted [2] as a critical tool for management of pathology in this small joint, the smaller joints remain underutilized regarding this methodology. This author reviewed the extensive clinical applications of both MCP and first CMC joint arthroscopy 7 years ago [3] but only recently has the latter gained acceptance and even been discussed in academic presentations as yet another option for treatment of thumb arthritis.

Jay Menon published the first important clinical paper on basal joint arthroscopy in the *Journal of Arthroscopic and Related Surgery* in 1996 [4]. This clinical series, "Arthroscopic Management of Trapeziometacarpal Joint Arthritis of the Thumb," reviewed patients undergoing arthroscopic hemitrapeziectomy and interpositional arthroplasty using either autogenous tendon graft, Gortex, or fascia lata allograft. It was not clear as to what extent of arthritis was involved in the series, but it appeared the technique was reserved for more advanced stages. This early paper did not present the possibility of performing arthroscopy on less advanced stages but rather avoided destabilizing the basal joint by not performing an open arthrotomy on advanced cases which otherwise would have had an open complete trapeziectomy. More than 80% of the patients had complete pain relief in his series of 25 patients, perhaps akin to results utilizing the open technique. However, he clearly outlined the advantages of doing this arthroscopically including the minimally invasive nature with less risk of injuring the radial sensory nerve coupled with less post-op pain. He did not comment on one obvious advantage, namely that arthroscopy of the trapeziometacarpal joint can assess the true articular changes providing a more accurate joint assessment than routine radiographs. This encourages us to treat basal joint osteoarthritis in much earlier stages and the clinical indication for surgery could be the failure of conservative treatment, not simply patients with advanced X-ray changes. Herein lies the major advantage of small joint arthroscopy, as it provides a new option for treating patients with the earliest stages of basal joint arthritis.

One year after Menon's clinical study paper, Berger from the Mayo Clinic presented a technical discussion of first carpometacarpal joint arthroscopy as a technique paper in the *Journal of Hand Surgery* (JHS American) in 1997 [5]. The clear advantages of arthroscopy in assessing the anatomy, as opposed to a standard open arthrotomy, were presented. He reasoned that open joint visualization would be difficult due to the depth and constraint of the joint, while the arthroscope could avoid disruption of the multiple ligaments that he described with Bettinger in a separate anatomic review [6]. Berger's paper also reviewed 12 cases that he had performed from 1994 in diverse clinical indications including several Bennett fractures of the metacarpal base. He further commented that there was excellent visualization and no complication with this procedure, yet clear indications for first CMC joint arthroscopy were not outlined, but this did present a viable alternative to the more invasive open surgery. This paper was followed by an interesting barrage of letters to the editor arguing over whether Berger or Menon had presented the index article on this new technique for the thumb. The next clinical paper on thumb arthroscopy was not until 1997, by Osterman and Culp in the journal *Arthroscopy*, wherein two groups of patients were described: traumatic and degenerative [7]. Their paper validated the use of arthroscopy for the thumb carpometacarpal joint, also suggesting that arthroscopy may determine the degree of trapezial surface involvement and even promoted its usage in younger patients. This led this author to use arthroscopy of the thumb carpometacarpal joint to accurately stage the degree of cartilage wear and determine specific treatment based upon this information [8]. While Jay Menon and others may have introduced the use of arthroscopy to limit the invasive nature of partial trapezial excision, I believe the technique may be uniquely suited to manage those patients who, until now, were not candidates for any surgical option.

Like any other joint, arthroscopy of the thumb carpometacarpal joint is only helpful, if the operating surgeon clearly understands the anatomy, particularly the functional ligaments so critical to function and perhaps implicated in the development of arthrosis. The first description of the trapeziometacarpal ligaments occurred in 1742 in a treatise by Weitbrecht, entitled Syndesmology, where these ligaments were mentioned in a cursory manner [9]. A variety of authors have since further described the details of this anatomy with the pinnacle, as mentioned, coming from Bettinger, Berger,

and others from the Mayo Clinic in 1999 [6]. They described a total of 16 ligaments including ligaments between the metacarpal and trapezium and two ligaments attaching the trapezium to the second metacarpal, apart from separate stabilizers for the scaphotrapezial and trapezoidal joints. They determined that this complex of ligaments acts as tension bands to prevent instability from cantilever bending forces exerted on the trapezium by the mechanics of pinch. This was a very important concept since large loads are transferred to the trapezium, and there is no fixed base of support since the underlying scaphoid is a mobile carpal bone. Therefore, it is the dysfunction and weakening of these key ligaments that may lead to the condition of basal joint arthritis. It was later surmised by van Brenk that the dorsoradial collateral ligament was the critical ligament preventing trapeziometacarpal subluxation [10]. He calculated this based upon a cadaveric study where serial sectioning of four key ligaments ultimately determined that the radial collateral ligament (RCL) was the key structure in preventing dorsoradial subluxation. Furthermore, Zancolli, known for his thorough knowledge of functional hand anatomy, also supported this concept, although he added a controversial theory that aberrant, redundant slips of the abductor pollicis longus (APL) may cause a compressive force of the dorsoradial aspect of trapeziometacarpal joint possibly leading to arthrosis [11]. He surmised that the underlying ligamentous laxity is due to underlying variations in an individual person's ligamentous laxity or a hormonal predilection that could perhaps explain the increased prevalence among women. My personal discussions with him ultimately led to my developing an arthroscopic classification, since the articular findings may help determine which ligaments are most commonly afflicted in the arthritic process. An intrinsic cause for basal joint arthritis was suggested by Xu and Strauch, who indicated that the trapeziometacarpal joint is smaller and less congruous in women and might also have a thinner layer of hyaline cartilage, adding an additional etiology to explain the increased incidence of basal joint osteoarthritis in women [12]. This, too, is my experience and suggests that the greatest applicability of arthroscopy may be in younger women who present with this disease at a much earlier age and have, implicitly, less surgical treatment options.

In 1979, Pellegrini in *Hand Clinics* reaffirmed the functional role that the volar beak ligament plays in limiting dorsal translation of the metacarpal during pinch function [13]. The volar oblique ligament and the dorsoradial ligament (DRL) are well visualized during arthroscopy and can allow for therapeutic intervention as well. Pellegrini proposed that the attritional changes in the volar oblique ligament seen at its metacarpal insertion site may be related to increased estrogen receptors at this site. This is consistent with a gender predilection for this affliction. I have indeed noted consistent full thickness cartilage loss at the insertion of the volar beak ligament on the deep metacarpal base, while the rest of the metacarpal appears normal via arthroscopic evaluation. More detailed anatomic, clinical, and even biomechanical concepts have been described by Bettinger and Berger in their study emphasizing the functional ligamentous anatomy of this joint [14]. It was noted that the arthroscopic anatomy is less complicated due to limited number of structures seen from an intra-articular vantage point. It was a pioneering technique article as well, outlining which of the two main portals provides visualization of which corresponding ligaments. Further portals were later described to further define the surface anatomy of this joint but predominantly to assist in performing triangulation during arthroscopic interventions. For example, Orellana and Chow described a radial portal which they suggested was safer due to its position relative to the radial artery and branches of the superficial radial nerve [15]. Later, Walsh and Akelman described the thenar portal, which was much more palmar, passing through the thenar musculature, allowing for improved triangulation and more "birds eye" visualization of the joint [16]. Slutsky later described a more distal portal, at the first webspace, allowing better examination of the dorsal structures and better access to the deep trapezial osteophyte typically seen [17]. These newer portals confirm that thumb CMC arthroscopic surgery is now in a state of evolution and hopefully will allow us to better understand arthritis at this level. Arthroscopic assessment of these structures over time may allow us to elucidate the cause of dorsal subluxation as a factor in basal joint arthritis.

An early clinical series by Culp and Rekant first suggested that arthroscopic evaluation, debridement, and synovectomy "offer an exciting alternative for patients with Eaton and Littler stages I and II arthritis" [18]. They were the first to discuss radiofrequency (RF) at the basal joint, describing radiofrequency "painting" of the volar capsule of the trapeziometacarpal joint, in order to stabilize the critical palmar ligaments that may cause dorsal subluxation and subsequent basal joint arthrosis. They recommended that if the majority of the trapezial surface is arthritic, then at least one-half of the distal trapezium should be resected via arthroscopic burr. The short-term results described in this paper followed arthroscopic hemi- or complete trapeziectomy in conjunction with electrothermal shrinkage reporting nearly 90% excellent or good results in 22 patients with a relatively short follow-up. They were the first to indicate that no "bridges had been burned," since patients who have the arthroscopic procedure can always undergo a more aggressive open and complete excisional trapezial arthroplasty. They conclude that debridement and thermal capsular shrinkage is a good treatment option for early arthritis of the basal joint, although the paper does seem to focus on a more advanced stage.

It is important to understand the role of RF in this new indication, since orthopedic surgeons have benefited from the use of radiofrequency in multiple joints during the past two decades. In recent years, we are realizing that it may have some detrimental effects, and it is important to look at this technology more critically. As with any new technique, selective use of this technology and careful adherence to certain principles may allow for a safe use of RF in a variety of clinical scenarios. Shoulder instability had been commonly treated using radiofrequency to stabilize the joint, particularly in those patients with global instability who traditionally had not been considered good operative candidates [19]. More recently, this technique has been largely abandoned in shoulder capsulorrhaphy due to poor results and even potential complications [20]. One must scrutinize the literature, as perhaps the technology was applied in an overaggressive manner or even poor patient selection. While it has also been used in the knee and some other joints, there has been minimal mention in the literature of its application to the wrist, let alone small joints of the hand. This is largely due to the fact that arthroscopy of the small joints has had only cursory discussion in the literature.

Radiofrequency has had many medical applications since the late nineteenth century including creating lesions in brain tissue and has been used in cardiology, oncology, and colorectal surgery. Markel and colleagues first demonstrated the effect of radiofrequency energy on the ultrastructure histology of the joint capsular collagen in a basic science study [21]. They noted that similar clinical applications had been performed with a nonablative laser in orthopedics but offered an alternative that radiofrequency provided several advantages over the use of a laser. RF is less expensive and safer than laser technology, while the devices are much smaller and easily maneuverable in their application to arthroscopic techniques. Early basic science studies on a sheep joint first demonstrated that the thermal effect was characterized by the fusion of collagen fibers without tissue ablation, charring, or even crater formation. They described a linear relationship between the degree of collagen fiber fusion and increasing treatment temperature. This indicates that the technology must be judiciously utilized with avoidance of aggressive use. It was determined that the coagulated tissue mediates a mild inflammatory reaction leading to the degradation and replacement of the affected capsule with stronger, fibrous tissue. This could potentially help to stabilize a joint and might have specific application in the trapeziometacarpal joint since instability is part of the clinical spectrum in many cases. Later, Markel and Hecht looked specifically at monopolar radiofrequency energy on the joint capsular properties and determined that monopolar radiofrequency caused an increased capsular damage in the immediate area and depth correlating with the wattage used [22]. Of note was that heat production increased linearly with the duration of application. Arthroscopic lavage could protect the synovial layer from permanent damage, as demonstrated in sheep.

These findings all indicate that radiofrequency probes must be used with adequate fluid lavage as well as for short durations and with the minimal wattage necessary to achieve the desired effect. We are referring here to monopolar radiofrequency, since it is commonly accepted among orthopedic surgeons that monopolar radiofrequency causes lesser heat production than bipolar modalities. This is critical to the hand surgeon, since small joints have correspondingly thinner capsules and are in close continuity to neurovascular structures. This is a completely different scenario, as compared to the knee or shoulder. Future studies might specifically compare monopolar versus bipolar radiofrequency treatments in these small joints.

Based upon the early clinical papers, while taking full advantage of the technologies available, it soon became clear that a thorough staging system would be beneficial, utilizing these arthroscopic findings to actually dictate treatment. First, the clinical studies discussed have primarily focused upon more advanced osteoarthritis, discussing results after some manner of arthroscopic-assisted hemitrapeziectomy. Second, there was little mention of the degrees of arthritis noted during arthroscopy and how that might influence treatment. Furthermore, it is likely that the patient whose joint is less affected might benefit most from an arthroscopic treatment method. This author therefore developed an arthroscopic classification which could dictate treatment for the respective stages herein delineated (Table 55.1).

The arthroscopic staging was gradually developed as a result of nearly 20 years of performing an arthroscopic assessment for recalcitrant basal joint arthritis which did not improve after an often extensive conservative treatment. The condition is, of course, staged radiographically as per Eaton's criteria [23]. Obvious exceptions were inpatients with advanced (Eaton stage IV) arthritis with significant scaphotrapezial-trapezoidal (STT) arthrosis or trapezial collapse who then underwent a trapezial excisional suspension-plasty using a slip of abductor pollicis longus similar to Thompson's description [24]. The advanced stage of disease really required excision of the entire trapezium, while stage IV patients with mild STT changes were still often treated via arthroscopy. Cobb describes a technique where both trapeziometacarpal and STT joints can simultaneously undergo arthroscopic treatment, although I did not consider that in my treatment algorithm here described [25]. An additional exception was for older, low-demand patients who did well

using a cemented total joint arthroplasty, as this required almost no immobilization and minimal therapy [26, 27]. This open surgery also allowed me to correct z-deformities by performing intrinsic releases of the adduction contracture coupled with an MCP volar capsulodesis. The last exception to arthroscopic management was the occasional young, usually male laborer who underwent a trapeziometacarpal joint fusion in good position of function for heavy pinch and grip. This indication for arthrodesis has been amply described in the literature and remains a good option, although arthroscopic hemitrapeziectomies may soon obviate even that procedure in some cases [28].

Except in clear-cut radiographic stages, where one can predict the arthroscopic stage, one performs the procedure with understanding that several therapeutic options are available once the arthroscopic stage is defined. These stages will later be delineated. The arthroscopic surgery is performed under wrist block regional anesthesia, usually only requiring several cc's of lidocaine at median and radial sensory nerves of the wrist, 2–3 cm proximal to volar wrist crease. It is performed with tourniquet control and the upper arm is secured to arm board over this tourniquet via either a wide tape or a Velcro strap. A single large Chinese finger trap is used on the thumb with 5–8 lbs. of longitudinal traction using a shoulder holder directly in line with the elbow flexed at 90°, so that the thumb tip points to the ceiling. One can utilize the specialized wrist arthroscopy traction tower but it is superfluous and more costly, since an easy unencumbered access to the thumb is later necessary to drive a K-wire and fluoroscopy can be more easily introduced into the field. The trapeziometacarpal (TM) joint is then identified by palpating the more prominent metacarpal base. The joint is best localized by using an 18-gauge needle on a small syringe containing either lidocaine or lactated ringer's solution, so that the joint can be insufflated and distended. The needle needs to be introduced a bit more distally than expected and aimed cephalad, since the metacarpal dorsal flare/lip needs to be cleared (Fig. 55.1). One can usually only introduce 1–2 cc due to small nature of the joint and the degree of laxity and joint swelling will influence this. Caution must be used to ensure the STT joint is not actually distended and less experienced surgeons should use fluoroscopy when the needle is in the joint to both confirm the precise location and help determine the trajectory of the soon-to-be-placed trochar/sheath assembly. The location for this initial distention will often vary based upon which hand (left or right) and the location of occasionally large, interfering prominent osteophytes. The longitudinal portal stab wound incision is then made in line with the needle penetration and will likely be at either the 1-R (radial) or the 1-U (ulnar) portal, as described by Berger [5]. The incision for the 1-R (radial) portal is placed just volar to the abductor pollicis longus (APL) tendon and is typically used for a clear assessment of the dorsoradial

Table 55.1 Badia arthroscopic classification for thumb CMC arthritis

Stage I	Diffuse synovitis, intact articular cartilage, and volar capsular laxity
Stage II	Central focal articular cartilage loss of trapezium, deep metacarpal base loss, and synovitis
Stage III	Widespread articular cartilage loss, deep osteophyte on trapezium

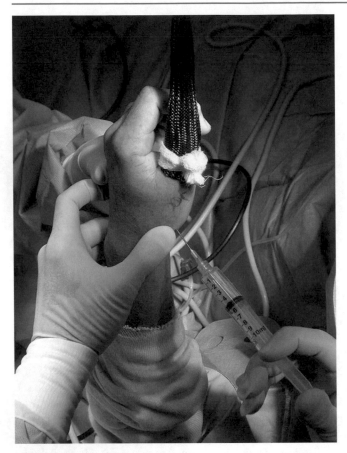

Fig. 55.1 Joint insufflation of the thumb basal joint in preparation for arthroscopic exploration. Note the needle trajectory which follows the course of thumb metacarpal base flare and helps orient for a correct arthroscope insertion angle

larger 2.9-mm more aggressive shaver or cutter may be used in advanced cases where a hemitrapeziectomy is fully expected to be undertaken. The larger shavers allow for much better suction and evacuation of debrided joint material. Many cases utilize radiofrequency, for either ablation or thermal shrinkage as discussed, so it needs to be available per the surgeon's choice. Radiofrequency can also be used to perform chondroplasty in less advanced cases demonstrating focal articular cartilage wear or fibrillation. Ligamentous laxity and capsular attenuation are treated with thermal capsulorrhaphy, also using the same RF shrinkage probe. One must be careful to avoid thermal necrosis and consequently, a striping technique is used to tighten the capsule of redundant or lax joints. Ample joint irrigation fluid is necessary during this treatment in order to minimize any thermal injury. In lesser stages of arthrosis, the arthroscopic treatment is completed, once the joint synovectomy is performed, arthroscopic stage has been assigned, and the joint adequately debrided. The decision to use RF is made at this point but no further arthroscopic procedure is done in the early stages. The decision will have been made if adjunctive corrective metacarpal osteotomy is to be performed. In advanced cases, the shaver is now substituted for a mechanical shaver in order to proceed with partial trapeziectomy. A 2.9-mm long barrel-type burr is then used to remove the distal 3–5 mm of the remaining articular cartilage and subchondral bone. This is preferable to the round burrs due to the speed and ease of use, while some surgeons (Berner, Cobb, and the like) try to utilize a larger, 3.5-mm burr since this will quickly remove the necessary trapezial surface. A strategic plan of joint resection is needed in order to avoid leaving significant prominent ridges or sections of the trapezium that may cause later impingement and persistence of pain. My strategy has usually been to divide the trapezial surface into four quadrants, two dorsal and two volar, or radial and ulnar. One begins at the area of shaver entry since the bone to resection is directly afoot, and this will create space for easier approach of the other quadrants (Fig. 55.2). If the scope is in the 1-R portal of a right thumb, then the burr would be in the 1-U portal facilitating subchondral resection of the dorsoulnar quadrant first. Once that side of the joint is cleared, the arthroscope can be changed to the opposite portal allowing the resecting burr to now enter the opposite portal, namely the 1-R portal in the previous example delineated. The radial palmar/dorsal quadrants can now be better approached for resection. At this point, several options are possible in order to encourage fibrous tissue ingrowth to create a new pseudojoint. Menon described a variety of materials including Gortex, graft jacket, or tendon to interpose [4]. In my early experience, spanning nearly 10 years, I used a tendon graft which would serve as an "arthroscopic anchovy" and function as a biologic, albeit now inert, material to encourage fibrous ingrowth. This was quite successful and

ligament (DRL), posterior oblique ligament (POL), and ulnar collateral ligament (UCL). The incision for the 1-U (ulnar) portal, which allows better evaluation of the anterior oblique ligament (AOL-volar/oblique) and UCL, is made just ulnar to the extensor pollicis brevis (EPB) tendon but palmar to the extensor pollicis longus (EPL). The portals should be just distal to the dorsal branch of radial artery which lies across the ST joint and should avoid any sensory radial nerve branches, since the portals are, again, longitudinal, but one should always enter the capsule and spread with a straight small mosquito clamp. This will push the sensory nerves away from the portal sites. A short-barrel 1.9-mm 30° inclination arthroscope is usually used for complete visualization of the TM joint articular surfaces, capsule, and intrinsic ligaments. A 2.7-mm scope may be preferred when a more advanced Eaton stage is indicated, since the larger scope may scuff the articular cartilage but is irrelevant in that scenario. The larger scope will actually assist in distracting the joint and provide a better field of view, while not risking the more delicate, and costly, 1.9 scope. A 2.0-mm full radius mechanical shaver with suction is used in most cases, particularly for initial debridement and visualization. Again, the

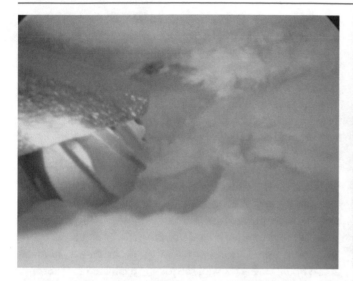

Fig. 55.2 Arthroscopic view of the thumb trapeziometacarpal joint demonstrating dorsoradial resection of trapezial surface using a 2.9-mm burr in a Badia stage III arthritic joint

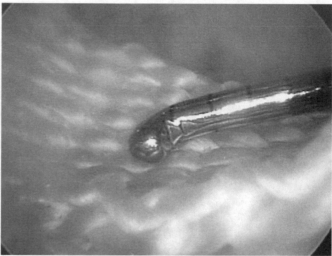

Fig. 55.3 Arthroscopic view of the Artelon polyurethane urea sheet lining the trapezium after arthroscopic limited hemiresection

was even utilized in Ehlers-Danlos patients, notoriously known for poor results in basal joint reconstruction due to their extreme underlying joint laxity, the proposed cause for the current arthritic process. Several patients did well enough to request the opposite thumb be similarly addressed, and my first experience in handling this challenging clinical scenario was published as a case report [29]. However, the dead tissue being pushed into the joint was not easily controllable via portals and I did not feel the complete joint surface was well lined by this flimsy material, despite being autogenous. Around 2004, a synthetic but biologically compatible material known as Artelon began to be used for open thumb CMC joint stabilization. This material degraded into lactic acid chains and CO_2 over time, and there were basic science studies suggesting the neoformation of fibrocartilage in animals [30]. This material demonstrated good clinical results in several early studies, particularly showing improved pinch strength recovery as opposed to classic complete trapezial resection procedures [31]. While I too utilized it in a number of open cases, it soon became apparent that the material could naturally be used for an arthroscopic interposition (Fig. 55.3). The material "wings" did not need to be secured, as the joint capsule itself would keep the material in place and it would serve as a scaffold for fibrous tissue ingrowth. This was described in a technique journal article but, after many years, was largely abandoned by this author due to cost issues and other unrelated matters [32]. It should be noted that in my experience, and that of many others, there was never an adverse reaction clinically seen. However, a recent trend to simplifying the trapezial resection procedures led me to consider not interposing any material at all. Meals gave rebirth to the simple concept that resection of the trapezium alone would suffice and he added simple k-wire pin-

ning of the joint in a distracted position soon termed "hematoma distraction arthroplasty" or HDA. He demonstrated very comparable results to much more complex procedures traditionally utilized [33]. This was simply a fancier delineation of complete trapeziectomy published by Gervin a half century ago [34]. However, it appears that the pinning provides several beneficial effects, including keeping the joint distracted so ample fibrous tissue can form within a maintained biologic cavity. The other advantage for the arthroscopic technique is that little joint stabilization is provided in this minimally invasive surgery; therefore, pinning of the metacarpal base over the trapezium keeps the joint well reduced and the metacarpal "centralized" over the functional center of the trapezium (Fig. 55.4). A thumb spica cast is typically worn for 5–6 weeks to allow for hematoma maturation and fibrous tissue ingrowth; hence, any decrease in swelling, or unopposed pull of the APL tendon, might allow for dorsal re-subluxation of the metacarpal base, possibly hindering the formation of this stabilizing tissue. New techniques, including suture/bone button stabilization devices, allow for "suspension" of the metacarpal base without the need for pinning. However, complications, such as impingement against the second metacarpal base or bone fracture at the tunnel location, must be taken into account [35].

These arthroscopic interposition arthroplasties are obviously indicated for more advanced arthritis, but a joint modification might only be needed if the joint can be debrided and stabilized; hence, a discussion on arthroscopic staging [8] is necessary to delineate when and how metacarpal base osteotomy is performed.

Staging by arthroscopy (Badia) is critical in order to indicate what further joint procedure, articular or extra-articular, is performed, once the assessment has been made after synovectomy and appropriate debridement. Arthroscopic stage I

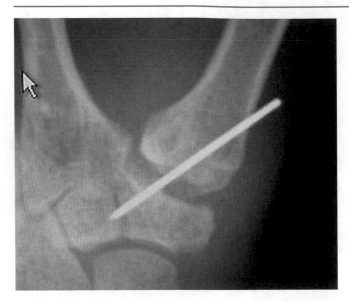

Fig. 55.4 X-ray demonstrating transfixing pin of the thumb trapezio-metacarpal joint in palmar abduction after arthroscopic hemiresection of the trapezium in a Badia stage III joint. The immobilization allows for fibrous tissue ingrowth in the new space created and now maintained by the temporary pin fixation

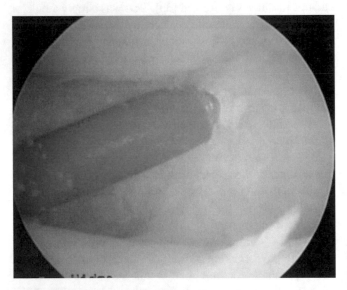

Fig. 55.5 Arthroscopic view of Badia stage I basal joint arthritis illustrating the synovitis but intact articular cartilage surface on both trapezium and metacarpal base

patients are characterized by diffuse synovitis but with minimal, or no, articular cartilage loss (Fig. 55.5). Capsular or specific ligamentous laxity is a typical finding at this stage. This arthroscopic appearance is not commonly seen, since most patients present late, having dealt with symptoms for a prolonged period, or referred at a delayed time, once conservative means have been exhausted. Primary care physicians, orthopedic surgeons, and even hand specialists typically feel there are few options available to these patients failing traditional nonoperative treatment. These patients will undergo synovectomy,

by both mechanical shaving and radiofrequency, with frequent shrinkage capsulorrhaphy performed depending on findings. The joint is then stabilized in a thumb spica cast from 1 to 4 weeks depending on the extent of capsular laxity. More unstable joints required longer immobilization in order to achieve joint stability and might also be pinned in a reduced position with thumb in palmar abduction. Stabilization of the capsule and aggressive synovectomy are hoped to slow the progression of articular cartilage degeneration.

Arthroscopic stage II patients are typified by focal articular wear on the central to dorsal aspect of the trapezium. It can be argued that this likely represents an irreversible degenerative process and demands a joint modifying procedure in order to alter joint deforming forces and progression of subluxation. Once synovectomy, debridement, and any loose bodies are removed, the joint is evaluated to determine the degree of instability and extent of capsular incompetence. A thermal shrinkage capsulorrhaphy is then often performed, with thermal chondroplasty occasionally done to anneal the cartilage borders (Fig. 55.6). The scope is then removed and an open incision usually extended from the ulnar portal is performed in order to identify the metacarpal base and metaphyseal-diaphyseal junction. A dorsoradial closing wedge osteotomy, according to Wilson's original technique [36], is then performed in order to place the thumb in a more extended and abducted position altering the joint force vector (Fig. 55.7). Usually, only a 2–3 mm wide dorsoradially based wedge of bone is excised by a combination of oscillating saw/osteotome. The idea is to minimize the tendency for metacarpal subluxation as well as change the contact points of degenerative articular cartilage. The osteotomy is stabilized usually by a single oblique Kirschner

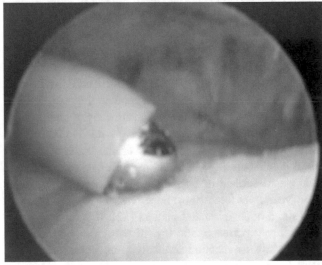

Fig. 55.6 Radiofrequency stabilization of the edge of a focal cartilage defect in a thumb Badia arthroscopic stage II. The joint contact points will subsequently be altered by a dorsoradial closing wedge osteotomy during the same procedure

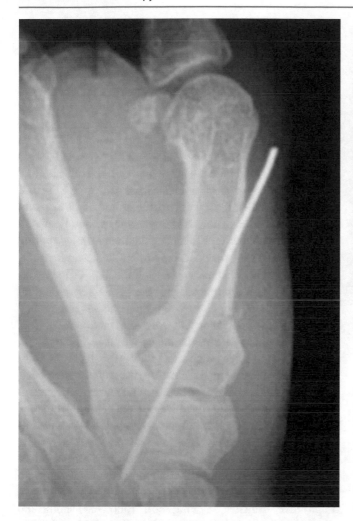

Fig. 55.7 X-ray showing centralized metacarpal base and pin fixation after dorsoradial closing wedge osteotomy in order to alter joint force vector and minimize further cartilage wear

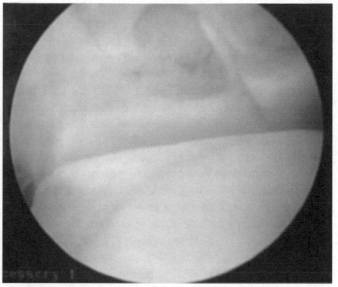

Fig. 55.8 Arthroscopic view of the scaphotrapezial-trapezoidal (STT) joint showing scaphoid distal pole to be burred down limiting painful impingement from overlying trapezium and trapezoid

wire, also placed across the TM joint in a reduced position so that the metacarpal base sits squarely over the trapezium. This fixation allows for healing of the osteotomy in the reduced position and hopefully leads to a correction of the metacarpal subluxation, typically seen in this stage. A thumb spica short arm cast is worn during osteotomy bone healing and the wire is removed at 5–6 weeks post-op. While the osteotomy has been published as solely an open surgery by multiple authors, only arthroscopy can truly determine which patients should undergo this osteotomy. This has demonstrated good results in the past, including a more recent paper by Tomaino [37], but we can surmise that perhaps any poor results achieved were due to a poor indication; namely that only patients with a moderate stage of arthritis should undergo osteotomy, and this can now be determined arthroscopically. I published a modest series of patients having undergone this technique of combined arthroscopic debridement with metacarpal osteotomy while further outlining specifics of the technique [38]. This represented only

a fraction of the potential patient series that underwent this surgery and, interestingly, even late follow-up on my patients has demonstrated that the metacarpal remains "centralized." It is frankly unclear if the capsular shrinkage played a major role versus the alteration of joint mechanics by the osteotomy but suffice it to say that I have yet to convert any of these arthroscopic-assisted joint modifying procedures into any type of trapeziectomy or salvage procedure.

Arthroscopic stage III is characterized by a nearly complete trapezial articular cartilage loss (Fig. 55.8). The metacarpal base can also demonstrate the loss of cartilage to varying degrees. Arthroscopic findings indicate that this is not an articulation that can be salvaged and a simple debridement or even joint modifying osteotomy would not provide a good result in this scenario. At this point, an arthroscopic hemitrapeziectomy, as earlier described, is performed by burring away the remaining articular cartilage and subchondral bone to achieve a bleeding surface. This acts to not only increase the joint space, but provides the key bleeding which creates the so-called hematomaplasty. Whether interposition material is placed or not, an oblique transfixing K-wire is used, coupled with a thumb spica cast in an abducted position, and maintained for about 6 weeks in order to encourage fibrous tissue ingrowth within the interposition space. This is followed by generally a minimal period of hand therapy to focus on pinch strengthening, as joint motion is rapidly restored no matter what therapy is done. While Artelon material for interposition represents a good option obviating tendon procurement, it has become increasingly apparent that generous resection of the trapezial surface without specific interposition material should suffice.

It should always be noted that arthroscopic stage III can also be treated by any traditionally open technique such as excisional arthroplasty, arthrodesis, or even total joint replacement. This will largely depend on surgeon preference as well as patient needs and wishes.

Since arthroscopy remains underutilized and joint images are not readily available to study, we must take note of the correlations between arthroscopic and radiographic staging in order to better understand the role of arthroscopy and the typical findings at each stage. The most consistent arthroscopic findings in the group of patients who displayed radiographic changes compatible with stage I of the disease included fibrillation of the articular cartilage on the ulnar third of the base of the first metacarpal, disruption of the dorsoradial ligament, and diffuse synovial hypertrophy. We also noted attenuation of the anterior oblique or beak ligament (AOL) often being able to visualize the thenar muscles below the capsule, almost as a veil. The frequent injection of steroids likely influences this factor and a future study correlating frequency/amount of corticosteroids with joint findings would be quite valuable.

Typical arthroscopic findings seen in patients determined to be stage II arthritis were significant but focal wear of the distal surface of the trapezium, loss of metacarpal base cartilage near insertion of the AOL ligament, disruption of the dorsoradial ligament, and more significant attenuation of the AOL. We typically would also see more intense synovial hypertrophy. Most of the patients with this arthroscopic stage also presented as stage II radiographically, but it is not uncommon to discover patients deemed stage I may actually have more advanced findings once the joint is accurately assessed. This represents the great advantage of this technology since there is little other way to see what the true joint status is. Only rarely did we find less cartilage wear than was supposed or predicted on the plain X-rays. Therefore, radiographic stage III is only rarely considered stage II arthroscopically, but that finding would greatly influence and expand the treatment options. Since arthroscopic findings in early disease may have the most clinical impact on our decision-making for definitive treatment, due to lack of good options for conservative treatment, it is important to review the patient outcomes for arthroscopic stage II disease.

In 2003, a retrospective assessment evaluated arthroscopic stage II patients with adequate follow-up in the prior 3-year period [38]. Forty-three patients (38 female and 5 male) had been arthroscopically diagnosed as having stage II basal joint osteoarthritis of the thumb between 1998 and 2001. All the procedures were performed by me with follow-up data generated by visiting fellows for objectivity. The average age was 51, with range of 31–69 years of age. The right thumb was involved in 23 patients and the left in 20. There was no improvement after a minimum 6 weeks of conservative treatment under my direction, although most patients had been failing conservative measures by referring doctors for over a year. The surgical procedure consisted of arthroscopic synovectomy, debridement, frequent thermal capsulorrhaphy followed by an extension-abduction closing wedge osteotomy in all cases. A .045-in. Kirschner wire provided stability to the osteotomy site, while a short arm thumb spica cast was maintained for 4–6 weeks until pin removal. The average follow-up was 43 months (range: 24–64 months).

Consistent arthroscopic findings in the selected group were frank eburnation of the articular cartilage of the ulnar third of the base of the first metacarpal and central third of the distal surface of the trapezium, disruption of the dorsoradial ligament, attenuation of the anterior oblique ligament, and synovial hypertrophy. The osteotomy healed within 4–6 weeks in all the cases. Radiographic studies at final follow-up depicted maintenance of centralization of the metacarpal base over the trapezium and no appreciable progression of arthritic changes in almost all 42 patients. Average range of thumb metacarpophalangeal (MP) joint motion was 5–50° and thumb opposition reached the base of the small finger in all cases. The average pinch strength was 9.5 lbs. (73% from nonaffected side). At final follow-up, the patients were evaluated by the Buck-Gramcko score, which takes into account both the subjective and objective outcomes [39]. The mean total Buck-Gramcko score in our series was 48.4 representing a "good outcome." The constant pain in one of the patients was due to progressive osteoarthritis after the procedure. She did not respond to steroid injections and finally had to undergo arthroscopic-assisted hemitrapeziectomy due to progressive arthritis. A long-term follow-up should be obtained in future to better assess the utility of this technique and publish these findings specifically in stage II patients after a minimum 10-year follow-up.

Arthroscopy in patients who had radiographic features of stages III and IV generally displays widespread full thickness cartilage loss with or without a peripheral rim on both articular surfaces, paradoxically less severe synovitis, although we do note more frayed volar ligaments and often less laxity. This clearly constitutes arthroscopic stage III and the treatment options here are quite varied. The arthroscope can be removed and the most appropriate open procedure performed. I prefer the arthroscopic interposition arthroplasty in most of the cases. Based on the above findings and clinical experience, I proposed the arthroscopic classification and treatment algorithm, as outlined in Table 55.1.

Trapeziometacarpal Arthroscopy: Clinical Utility

Clinical assessment and radiographic studies used to be the only tools available for the selection of treatment modalities for thumb CMC arthritis. Eaton and Glickel proposed a staging system for this disease that has been widely applied [20]. Later, Bettinger et al. [40] described the trapezial tilt as a parameter to predict further progression of the disease. They found that in advanced stages (Eaton stages III and IV), the trapezial tilt was high (50° ± 4°; normal: 42° ± 4°). Barron et al. concluded that there appears to be no indication for magnetic resonance imaging (MRI), tomography, or ultrasonography in the routine evaluation of basal joint disease [41].

While I believe that a radiographic classification is important for a stepwise interpretation of the progression of this entity, my experience has demonstrated instances when it is very difficult to make an accurate diagnosis of the extent of disease based solely on radiographic studies. Recent advances in arthroscopic technology have allowed a complete examination of smaller joints throughout the body with minimal morbidity [1]. Moreover, arthroscopy has already proved to be reliable for direct evaluation of the first carpometacarpal joint, as previously discussed [5].

In early stages of thumb basal joint arthritis, for instance, in Eaton stage I, it is very common to find essentially normal radiographic studies, despite the presence of painful limitation of the thumb. In our experience, we have found that this group of patients displays mild to moderate synovitis, which could benefit from a thorough joint debridement combined with thermal shrinkage of the ligaments to enhance the stability. This, of course, after assuming they have not responded well to conservative treatment including splinting, nonstreoidal anti-inflammatory drug (NSAID) use, and corticosteroid injection. This stage is typically seen in middle-aged women who are not suitable candidates for more aggressive procedures. Arthroscopic treatment provides a particularly good option for this ubiquitous subset of the patients.

Tomaino concluded that first metacarpal extension osteotomy is a good indication for Eaton stage I [37]. This may not be necessary in the occasional patient who undergoes arthroscopy at an early time and demonstrates no focal cartilage loss. Future studies may indicate that synovectomy, and perhaps thermal capsulorrhaphy, may avoid progression of disease and the need for a mechanical intervention. However, the arthroscopic findings that I previously described for arthroscopic stage II of the disease demand a joint modification such as osteotomy, in order to minimize the chance of further articular degeneration. My retrospective study indicates that this approach is efficacious, with only one out of 43 thumbs developing progressive arthritis requiring further surgery.

There remains little doubt that if complete articular cartilage loss is the arthroscopic scenario; the logical further step is to perform some type of trapezium excision with interposition arthroplasty. Menon described a technique demonstrating arthroscopic debridement of the trapezial articular surface and interposition of autogenous tendon, fascia lata, or Gortex patch into the CMC joint in patients with stages II

and III with excellent results [2]. I have demonstrated that this arthroscopic technique is even effective in patients with underlying severe ligamentous laxity, as in Ehrler-Danlos syndrome [33]. Newer techniques may allow the arthroscopic insertion of Artelon, which has proven successful with open techniques and confirmed histologically [30]. In either case, complete excision of the trapezium may not be desirable, particularly in younger patients. The stage III treatment needs to be further assessed by evaluating long-term clinical results.

According to the arthroscopic classification proposed, I recommend arthroscopic synovectomy and debridement of the basal joint in patients with stage I arthritis. In patients with stage II disease, synovectomy and debridement are combined with dorsoradial osteotomy of the first metacarpal. In both these stages, thermal shrinkage is used to manage ligamentous laxity. Finally, for stage III of the disease, arthroscopic interposition arthroplasty is my treatment of choice, although other factors must be considered in making this determination.

Arthroscopic assessment of the trapeziometacarpal joint allows direct visualization of all components of the joint including synovium, articular surfaces, ligaments, and the joint capsule. It also allows for the extent of joint pathology to be evaluated and staged with intraoperative management decision-making based on this information. I recommend this arthroscopic staging to ensure better judgment of this condition in order to provide the most adequate treatment option to patients who have this disabling condition.

Future studies assessing the clinical long-term results utilizing arthroscopy will likely ensure its place in the treatment armamentarium for trapeziometacarpal osteoarthritis.

STT Arthroscopy (Scaphotrapezial-Trapezoidal)

Arthroscopy of the STT joint was a natural offshoot to the thumb CMC joint, since the former is frequently involved when advanced basal joint arthritis is present. While Cobb reported simultaneous arthroscopic management of both TM and STT joints [42], the role of arthroscopy for the STT joint is likely best suited for focal disease where a minimally invasive option is sought. Ashwood and Bain described simple arthroscopic debridement for isolated STT arthritis demonstrating 90% good and excellent results in their small series [43]. Fontes also described a simple resection of the distal pole of the scaphoid as a useful technique for painful STT arthrosis [44].

The technique is relatively simple, since instability is not an issue and the goal is to increase the joint space and avoid painful impingement. The joint is localized by ascending the scaphoid from the radial midcarpal portal, followed by creat-

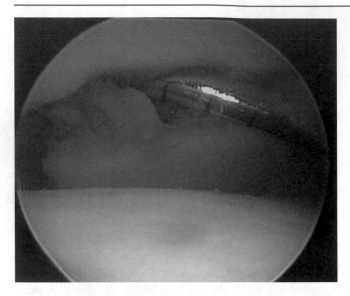

Fig. 55.9 Arthroscopic view of the thumb MCP joint illustrating how a hook probe can derotate an avulsed bony gamekeeper fragment, obviating the need for joint arthrotomy to reduce

ing a working portal that can be volar [44] or more recently, a radial portal has been described by Carro et al. [45]. Simple debridement is done using a 2.0-mm full radius shaver and then limited resection of the distal pole of the scaphoid is performed using burr (Fig. 55.9). The joint space is markedly widened but one must be careful not to resect the critical volar ST ligaments, one advantage of this procedure as opposed to open techniques.

Minimal post-op immobilization is another surgical advantage of this methodology, and pain relief is generally excellent assuming patient selection was properly performed.

A long-term study is necessary to determine the late outcomes and secure the role of STT arthroscopy among the various techniques used for treatment of this common arthritic malady.

Metacarpophalangeal Arthroscopy

While arthroscopy of the metacarpophalangeal joints of the hand was first described almost three decades ago, the clinical utility and indications remain poorly understood. Many orthopedic surgeons are unfamiliar with this possibility, hence unable to offer it to their patients as an option. Furthermore, hand surgeons rarely utilize this technology, despite the fact that both acute injury and chronic pain are commonly found in the MCP joint, thumb, and digits alike. It seems that minimal exposure within the literature as well as little hands-on training has contributed to the underutilization of what is a very useful technique to manage certain pathology in the hand.

Dr. Chen first described arthroscopy of the metacarpophalangeal (MCP) joints, among other small joints of the hand as previously mentioned, in his 1979 paper in *Orthopedic Clinics of North America* representing a paradigm shift in arthroscopy indications [1]. Despite a cursory review, this paper first described the use of the Watanabe No. 24 arthroscope within the wrist, metacarpophalangeal joints, and even interphalangeal joints of the hand. Although he described both PIP and DIP joints being scoped, there was surprisingly no mention of the trapeziometacarpal joint. However, he did first introduce the concept of placing a small arthroscope into the metacarpophalangeal joint of several digits including the thumb. He went on to describe the anatomy followed by several clinical case reports where he described the arthroscopic findings and clinical utility. Overall, he described 90 arthroscopies performed in multiple joints encompassing 34 clinical cases as well as two cadaveric arms. Despite this broad introduction to small joint arthroscopy, the idea of MCP joint treatment was not truly developed until much later.

Ironically, it was sports medicine arthroscopists, Vaupel and Andrews, who first described a report using arthroscopic treatment of the metacarpophalangeal joint about 6 years after Chen's report [46]. They described a professional golfer who was severely limited due to a 1-year history of chronic painful synovitis within the thumb MCP joint. They performed a synovectomy and also an arthroscopic burring of a small chondral defect that had been identified at the time of procedure. The patient did so well that he was able to return to his sport within a 6-month period and has remained pain free at his 2-year follow-up. While this was a tremendous clinical advance, it was published in the *American Journal of Sports Medicine* where hand surgeons would likely not take note of this paper. Furthermore, despite an excellent outcome and a positive response to a new technique, no clinical indications were recommended for future usage and this remained an isolated case report until 2 years later when Wilkes presented the first clinical series of an MCP joint problem treated with arthroscopic means [47]. He reported on 13 cases of arthroscopic rheumatoid synovectomy in five patients suffering from advanced rheumatoid arthritis. While these patients lacked the usual joint subluxation or advanced destruction, they did have marked synovitis found in the joint space and within the recesses of the collateral ligament origins. Despite an adequate follow-up of nearly 4 years, the patients did demonstrate recurrence of pain and this treatment did not seem to alter the natural history of RA at the MCP joint. This series was also published in a low-profile journal, the *Journal of the Medical Association of Georgia*, and therefore gave limited exposure to hand surgeons or even arthroscopic surgeons. A clinical paper exposed to hand surgeons was not seen until 1994 where it finally reached the *Journal of Hand Surgery—British Volume* in another case report [48]. The subject was a young male presenting with swelling and recalcitrant locking of the metacarpophalangeal joints of both index and middle fingers, bilaterally, and represents a typical presentation for hemochromatosis. Until then, the treatment of arthropathy was osteotomy and arthroplasty or even a joint arthrodesis for more advanced cases. Hemochromatosis is a rarely seen hematologic condition that is actually treated with phlebotomy and the joint manifestations are not well understood. Nevertheless, it was apparent to these surgeons that arthroscopy presented a superior alternative to open surgery with better visualization of the joint and subsequent treatment of the synovitis with faster recovery due to its minimally invasive approach. The focus, however, of the case report was on the disease itself and gave no further recommendations regarding arthroscopy, besides stating that arthroscopic surgery is "of value." Since the arthroscopic treatment was downplayed by the unusual pathology being treated, the common clinical application of this technology was not clearly apparent or yet elucidated.

In 1995, Ryu and Fagan presented a small series on the treatment of the ulnar collateral ligament Stener lesion arthroscopically, which represented the first time that we could see a common clinical application for this new minimally invasive approach [49]. They described an arthroscopic reduction of a Stener lesion in eight thumbs, with an average follow-up period of just over 3 years, showing how simple reduction of the Stener lesion into the joint can place the avulsed ligament alongside its insertion site on the debrided base of the proximal phalanx. Prior to reduction, the ligament had been sitting outside the adductor aponeurosis and could therefore not heal in the necessary position. Once the reduction was performed, the ligament insertion site was aggressively debrided and the joint pinned to immobilize and allow healing. Upon removing the cast, a brief course of therapy was introduced and at follow-up no patient reported any pain or functional limitation. There was an excellent range of motion with strength parameters equal to or often greater than the thumb on the unaffected side. The only reported complication was an isolated simple pin tract infection. These results demonstrated that an all arthroscopic reduction of a Stener lesion obviated the need for open repair and subsequent complications such as prolonged recovery and stiffness. This was a clear clinical advantage and represented the first common clinical application that could encourage arthroscopic treatment of MCP joint pathology. Surprisingly, there was no mention of bony gamekeeper's lesions, and there was no comparative study with the open method. Nevertheless, the primary triumph of this paper was that it was published in a widely read journal, first exposing hand surgeons to this minimally invasive technique and opening the door to other utilizations. In reality, this paper first introduced the concept of arthroscopic surgery in small joints to the greater hand surgery community. Nevertheless, despite the fact that this paper was published nearly 20 years

ago, the technique remains minimally utilized and there have been few clinical series since then.

About 5 years later, in 1999, Rozmaryn and Wei presented the first broad paper on the technical aspects of metacarpophalangeal arthroscopy with elaboration on the possible indications and advantages of this still unknown technique [50]. They commented that there may be a misconception that the MCP joint is too small to perform any arthroscopic procedures in a useful or relevant manner. Although no clinical series was presented, they discussed the wider indications that might be addressed with this procedure. They discussed joint synovectomies and biopsies as previously mentioned and reaffirmed the concept of collateral ligament debridement while mentioning the possibility of ligament repair. They also introduced the removal of loose bodies, treatment of osteochondral lesions, management of juxta-articular lesions, and treatment of intra-articular fractures and other possible clinical applications. They also noted that only a few case reports were presented in the literature, and they surmised why this technique perhaps was not yet expanded upon. We must be cognizant, however, that this ample review was published in the journal *Arthroscopy: The Journal of Arthroscopic and Related Surgery*, and this would have created little exposure to dedicated hand surgeons, the clinicians most apt to utilize the technique. This report discussed some technical aspects and reviewed the anatomic landmarks for the first time since Dr. Chen's simplistic description of a rudimentary arthroscope nearly 20 years before. They stated that the advantages of arthroscopic versus open techniques were similar to those enjoyed in larger joints and that over time, more indications would emerge.

During the same year of Rozmaryn and Wei's technical paper, a broad review paper was published in *Hand Clinics* and entitled, "Arthroscopy of the Metacarpophalangeal Joint," by Slade and Gutow [51]. This represented the initially thorough analysis of the technique, including detailed technical explanations followed by some representative cases, including a brief mention of the minor complications and how to avoid them. However, the mantra "triumph of technology over reason" was also mentioned, suggesting arthroscopy of this small joint may not have been seen as practical or even useful. They explained that small joint arthroscopy required not only specialized instrumentation but also a working understanding of the anatomy within these joints. Their broad review soon revealed that there were a wide variety of indications that could greatly benefit from this technology. Detailed treatment techniques were described as illustrated by case examples, particularly in the topic of intra-articular fracture treatment. A new method was also described where arthroscopy could be combined with small bone anchor application for reattachment of collateral ligament injuries. This may represent a difficult technique, but the authors clearly outlined the relative advantages of this method. In a discussion comparing arthroscopic synovectomies in rheumatoid patients with other joints treated in the same patient with open means, both surgeons and the patients alike clearly noted the decreased post-op swelling and the expedited rehab leading to faster return to activity. This represents a clear advantage of the arthroscopic technique as opposed to open means and in that same year, there was an obscure paper in the rheumatology literature that discussed the use of "mini-arthroscopy" of metacarpophalangeal joints in staging a synovitis and using this as an effective biopsy tool. The paper was written by rheumatologists in Germany and the paper focused on the scoring system of synovitis within rheumatoid patients with minimal elaboration of the operative technique [52]. They simply used this as a tool for assessing the degree of disease involvement but again emphasized its clinical utility. The authors, nonsurgeons, noted that micro-arthroscopy provided an objective technique for joint evaluation allowing visually guided synovial biopsy with improved accuracy and diminished the risk of any sampling errors. They performed this under local anesthesia, showing that general anesthesia was not necessary and, of course, could be done as an ambulatory procedure. Therefore, if the rheumatologists could see the great benefit of this technique, hand as well as arthroscopic surgeons could further develop its clinical application. In that same year Wei, who had coauthored the first technical description of metacarpophalangeal joint arthroscopy [50], presented an ample clinical series of arthroscopic synovectomies in rheumatoid arthritis describing 21 patients treated with arthroscopic synovectomy with good short-term results [52]. Although his intent was for this to be a technique article, he noted that the early results were promising and that this procedure would be useful in other types of arthritis or orthopedic maladies. He questioned the long-term outcomes and theorized what might be the ideal timing for this surgery in arthritic patients. This remains an unanswered question, although Sekiya et al. elaborated on previous surgeons' descriptions by assessing 21 patients with rheumatoid arthritis in 27 proximal interphalangeal joints and 16 metacarpophalangeal joints. This represented the first clinical use of PIP joint arthroscopy and lent further support for metacarpophalangeal joint arthroscopic synovectomy [53]. He supported the concept that arthroscopic assessment of the joint surface and synovial lining was an optimal indication for arthroscopy including diagnostic biopsies under direct visualization. He also reasoned that arthroscopy for the small joints in the hands "will become a standard procedure in the near future." Their study did not assess other pathologies. Their study, also published in an arthroscopy journal, represents the last clinical series of arthroscopic surgery within the MCP joint. It is apparent that there is a paucity of clinical papers in the literature and that further discussion regarding the indications and clinical application of this tool is necessary in order to stimulate the hand surgeon to include this option in his realm of treatment possibilities. While the arthroscopic surgeon, typically known as a "sports medicine" specialist, may consider this option, it certainly remains for the hand surgeon to develop the clinical indications since we typically assess the more complex injuries, particularly the recalcitrant few. Therefore, it is up to hand surgeons to expand the applications of this still vastly underused methodology and this might include hand specialists who commonly do not perform wrist arthroscopy since the technique is much less daunting as later to be outlined. It is important to understand the indications and what role arthroscopy has in both detecting and treating these pathologies.

MCP Arthroscopy Indications

Traumatic and degenerative problems of the metacarpophalangeal joint are commonly encountered by hand specialists. Acute injury can involve any one of these joints and the thumb is the most commonly affected due to its relatively unprotected position. The thumb MCP ulnar collateral ligament (UCL) tear is a frequently seen injury and is often erroneously termed "gamekeeper's thumb" when this should really be coined "skier's thumb," as the former refers more to a chronic attritional lesion. Acute trauma can also affect the finger MCPs with both ligamentous injuries and articular fractures presenting as a painful, swollen joint after injury. The term "overuse syndromes" may actually represent a previously occult acute injury that was not addressed or a chronic synovitis of unknown etiology. Plain X-rays will rarely shed light on chronic pain issues unless advanced degenerative disease or arthropathy is present, and imaging studies such as MRI are notoriously nonspecific in such small joints. Ultrasound presents a newer, more cost-effective modality that can determine if effusion is present, but not allow for anatomic diagnosis. Therefore, arthroscopy of the involved MCP joint will clarify the diagnosis and also allow for potential treatment in a wide variety of indications of both thumb and digit MCP joints (Table 55.2).

Surgical indications to perform MCP arthroscopy will usually involve chronic conditions as opposed to acute injury,

Table 55.2 Indications for MCP arthroscopy

Acute	Chronic
Recent thumb ulnar collateral stener	Persistent MCP pain after trauma
Bony displaced gamekeeper's thumb	MCP OA—early/moderate grade
Septic MCP joint	Rheumatoid arthritis w/o ulnar drift
Articular die-punch fracture phalangeal base	Chronic synovitis

since the latter can often be managed conservatively with appropriate immobilization. The thumb UCL avulsion is a common exception where open repair of a Stener lesion is often required and simple immobilization may not suffice. In fact, an arthroscopic repair has been described in the literature, as previously outlined [31]. With increasing familiarity of small joint arthroscopy, more acute indications may develop allowing an accurate assessment of the precise injury and subsequent specific treatment.

Acute indications generally involve an associated fracture that will need synovectomy, fracture debridement followed by articular reduction. This is likely true, since the majority of ligamentous injuries will adequately heal with conservative immobilization, or are so severe that the resultant instability will lead to open management and repair. Perhaps, the ideal acute indication for MCP arthroscopy is reduction of a collateral ligament avulsion fracture with a rotated fragment sitting within the joint. Once arthroscopic debridement at the fracture site has been performed, a small hook probe is used to simply derotate the bony fragment via arthroscopic visualization (see Fig. 55.9). Kirschner wire fixation can then be performed with a combination of arthroscopic control and fluoroscopic confirmation, as published by this author [54] (Fig. 55.10). Additionally, another acute, albeit less common, indication would be a die-punch articular fracture, usually of the proximal phalanx base, where the scope can be used to control for the best articular reduction possible while facilitating the reduction itself. Besides a thorough synovectomy, the complete removal of any floating loose osteochondral fragments can be performed. This helps to reduce the posttraumatic inflammatory process in addition to reducing the fracture more anatomically. This arthroscopic method has the intrinsic advantage of a more exact articular reduction with the minimally invasive perk of limiting capsular

adhesions, therefore faster recovery of an improved range of motion. Furthermore, like in any other arthroscopic acute indication, a thorough assessment of associated soft tissue lesions can be performed and treated as needed. This may include MCP dislocations, where the acute capsule and ligamentous avulsions can be debrided after reduction, minimizing the scarring and expediting the healing process, even without an actual soft tissue repair.

Chronic processes affecting the MCP joint, however, tend to be the most common indications for arthroscopy of these small joints. This is a welcome alternative since few options exist in a persistently painful "knuckle" joint. As discussed, most acute injuries heal with appropriate rehabilitation and/ or immobilization, with more severe trauma being managed by open repairs. Therefore, persistent pain and disability, despite prolonged conservative treatment in both thumb and finger MCP trauma, may represent the most common indication for MCP arthroscopy. It is not infrequent to encounter persistent symptoms after cast treatment for a skier's thumb or perhaps a border digit hyperabduction injury. This is likely due to a more severe ligamentous injury than originally assessed, or perhaps a concomitant articular cartilage injury associated with persistent synovitis. Oftentimes, the contralateral ligament is injured as well and was not fully addressed at the time of initial treatment. An arthroscopic evaluation, whether in an acute or a chronic setting of injury, can accurately determine the location and extent of injury and can lead to concomitant treatment, whether by simple debridement and/or by thermal radiofrequency capsulorrhaphy (Fig. 55.11). Typically, these types of ongoing complaints are managed by a prolonged course of NSAIDs, therapy, or a number of cortisone injections. In the setting of more substantial pathology, these treatments only provide temporary

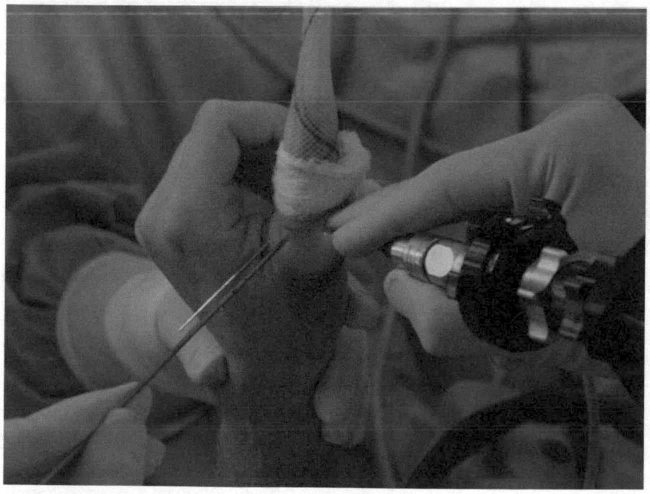

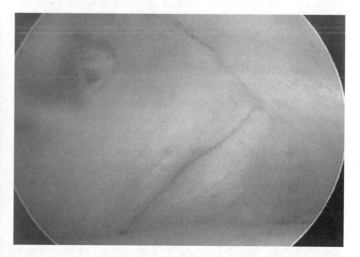

Fig. 55.10 External view of MCP arthroscopic treatment of an ulnar collateral bony avulsion where k-wire fixation will maintain reduction of the arthroscopically reduced fragment

Fig. 55.11 Thermal shrinkage capsulorrhaphy in a chronically painful MCP joint stabilizes the capsule and collateral ligament minimizing the chance of recurrent painful synovitis. A period of post-op immobilization is necessary and dictated by the severity of the collateral ligament fraying

relief, if any, and cannot be sustained indefinitely. Herein lies the optimal value of arthroscopic treatment, since it provides a relatively simple option to both make a definitive diagnosis and provide treatment based on these findings.

Persistent, occult pain, often associated with chronic swelling and stiffness, also represents a clear indication to offer arthroscopic evaluation. These symptoms may stem from an unrecognized injury, initial presentation of osteoarthritis, or even an idiopathic synovitis that is occasionally seen and remains a diagnostic and even therapeutic dilemma. Open synovectomy has been mostly indicated for rheumatoid indications, but until now, this has been the sole option for any patient presenting with a swollen, painful MCP joint that has failed conservative measures [55]. Steroid injections are frequently effective here, but can classically lead to acceleration of cartilage and capsular degeneration. These repeat injections to one joint must be recognized as a catabolic process and must be diminished. Arthroscopic debridement will avoid this complication and even possibly retard the degenerative and arthritic process. This benefit greatly outweighs the minimal complications that we might rarely see while the recovery is rapid.

Although not as common a location as other hand joints, degenerative arthritis of the MCP joints may represent a new frontier for arthroscopic assessment and treatment in managing this frustrating condition. The earliest stages of osteoarthritis are not clearly seen on plain radiographs and the diagnosis is often a clinical one. After adequate conservative treatment with NSAIDs and perhaps a course of therapy, the logical next step for treatment remains an intra-articular corticosteroid injection. If symptoms recur despite several injections, clinicians are often at a dead end since surgery is not usually offered to early stages of arthrosis or even younger patients. In this scenario, arthroscopic debridement becomes the best option short of joint replacement. Open arthrotomies with synovectomy are difficult due to limited visualization and poor access to certain regions of the joint. Furthermore, the approach itself can lead to marked post-op stiffness simply due to the arthrotomy itself. In rheumatoid disease, silicone arthroplasty remains the gold standard for MCP joints, while posttraumatic arthrosis and osteoarthritis are not typically good indications for replacement arthroplasty [56]. Arthroscopy provides a minimally invasive alternative before offering arthroplasty, which in this indication would consist of the newer metallic or pyrocarbon nonconstrained replacement options now available [57].

Inflammatory arthritides, such as rheumatoid arthritis, are typically managed with systemic pharmacotherapy, the newer disease-modifying agents, and perhaps in later stages, replacement arthroplasty for MCP involvement. Rarely, a mono- or pauci-articular form is identified and a biopsy can be taken during arthroscopic rheumatoid synovectomy, confirming the diagnosis. Therefore, early-stage involvement of these joints may warrant an arthroscopic synovectomy and capsular shrinkage, as shown by Sekiya [53]. However, this approach is best suited when only a few joints are involved, perhaps retarding the joint destruction and is impractical for severe, diffuse involvement. Furthermore, long-term results of arthroscopic rheumatoid synovectomy are necessary. Until more surgeons become adept at this technique, it will be difficult to collect sufficient data to justify its use in these advanced indications. Therefore, to break this vicious cycle, hand surgeons must learn this minimally invasive approach and begin to frequently apply it in the more ubiquitous pathologies.

MCP Arthroscopic Technique

Metacarpophalangeal arthroscopy demands the use of an arthroscope 1.9 mm in diameter or less due to the narrow, relatively constrained anatomy of these small joints. A 1.9-mm 30° arthroscope, as described by maxillofacial surgeons for temporomandibular (TMJ) pathology, is utilized [58]. While newer arthroscopes are becoming available, even as small as 1 mm, the 1.9 scope should suffice for the described indications herein. The use of a 2.0-mm shaver is critical for synovectomy and most debridements, while small radiofrequency probes, including ablation and shrinkage applications, are often useful.

Small joint arthroscopy, including MCP joints, only requires local anesthesia and light intravenous (IV) sedation. The portal sites are both injected with minimal local anesthesia, followed by several cc's of lidocaine, or similar short-acting agents, introduced into the joint once the hand is vertically suspended using a single Chinese fingertrap on the involved digit. Intravenous sedation may be needed only to control tourniquet discomfort depending on the planned time of procedure or patient's/anesthesiologist's preference. The use of lidocaine with epinephrine may even obviate the need for a tourniquet since these are typically short-lasting procedures.

Once 3–4 kg (5–8 lbs.) of traction is applied, the joint-line is typically palpable and more local anesthesia might be introduced into the joint, typically with the 18-gauge needle in order to determine the location site for the portals. Longitudinal portal small incisions (stab wounds) are made with a small scalpel in the site of visible capsular bulging. This orientation is used, since the patient's MCP joint is typically immobilized in flexion and the incision direction is oriented parallel to the plane of motion. It is crucial to introduce the trocar into the joint in an atraumatic fashion since most indications are for otherwise pristine joints and one must minimize iatrogenic injury within the narrow interval. The space between the metacarpal head and proximal phalanx base is very narrow and one should find the appropriate position and insertion angle by inserting a small curved clamp, once the joint is adequately distended with lidocaine or lactated ringer's solution. The arthroscope is then inserted at this exactly same angle and a thorough cursory joint examination is now performed. Portal anatomy is relatively simple, as radial and ulnar portals lie on either side of the visible or palpable extensor tendon. Rarely, a third portal is for outflow, or better instrument direction, and is created by palpating the capsule, identifying an area moving due to external pressure, and then inserting an 18-gauge needle to mark the area and possible portal site. A thorough synovectomy is usually performed at the outset since this allows a thorough inspection of the joint and to localize the pathology. As this is done with a small full radius shaver, the articular structures, including the capsule and collateral ligaments, will soon be more apparent. A radiofrequency ablator probe can also make this ablation process more precise and rapid. It is important to use RF judiciously, as the joint capsule is relatively thin and subcutaneous, and thermal injury can result in either capsule or articular surface. Once synovectomy is underway, the surgeon can now begin to identify any pathologic or anatomic variations and it should be done in a reproducible systematic manner in order to avoid overlooking pathology. For example, one may begin on the radial collateral ligament, then assess the volar plate, look for sesamoids, then the ulnar collateral ligament, finally followed by the dorsal capsule and extensor. The articular surface of both proximal phalanx and metacarpal head is then evaluated including the synovial recesses and the collateral ligament origins. Once specific pathology is identified and treated, the arthroscope is retired and portals are closed with benzoin and steri-strips only, obviating any stitches which is where dorsal hand scarring may result and can easily be avoided. Any pins utilized are cut underneath the skin and the thumb MCP is usually protected with a short arm thumb spica plaster intra-op splint in MCP extension and thumb palmar abduction/opposition. Conversely, arthroscopy of any of the digits will necessitate a dorsal metacarpophalangeal block splint, usually in full MCP flexion in order to allow the collateral ligaments to heal in their most taut position and to minimize any resultant loss in motion, usually flexion. The period of immobilization is determined by the type and extent of pathology found during the arthroscopic intervention and can be determined intraoperatively. Post-op therapy often plays a crucial role, although only after the appropriate period of immobilization.

MCP arthroscopy remains a vastly underutilized but very useful technique for both diagnosing and treating acute and chronic injuries afflicting that joint. While the indications expand among the few utilizers, the majority of hand surgeons would benefit from the minimal training needed to include this in their treatment armamentarium [59, 60].

Proximal Interphalangeal Arthroscopy

Arthroscopy of the proximal interphalangeal (PIP) joints should still be viewed as an emerging procedure and very little has been written in the literature. Despite this, Chen's hallmark paper in *Orthopedic Clinics of North America* did present one clinical case and eight cadaveric studies utilizing small joint arthroscopy of the PIP joint [1]. The only clinical case was in a rheumatoid patient, which foreshadowed future attempts since only RA has been studied as an indication in this rarely performed procedure.

The initial paper devoted solely to PIP joint arthroscopy was published by Thomsen et al. in a 2002 volume of the *Journal of Hand Surgery* [61]. They focused on anatomic findings, including portal anatomy, in eight cadaveric PIP joints followed by two clinical cases. The only firm conclusion was that the technique was possible, although technically demanding and limited by instrumentation, and that indications needed to be delineated while commenting that synovitis, infection, and loose body excision would be the main indications. In this early clinical description, one of the patients was rheumatoid while the other was a removal of a loose body coupled with synovectomy.

In the same year, Sekiya and his group presented a thorough analysis of both MCP and PIP arthroscopy in 21 rheumatoid patients, as previously mentioned in the MCP arthroscopy discussion [53]. Twenty-seven PIP joints and 16 MCP joints underwent rheumatoid synovectomy, although most reportedly had only "joint irrigation." They determined it was a promising procedure allowing biopsies and concluding that synovectomies led to an early clinical improvement. There was no mention of the results' longevity but it was felt that small joint arthroscopy, including PIP, could become a standard procedure in the future. They did warn that the technique was very limited, both by joint configuration/morphology and largely by the equipment utilized. The rigidity and relative size of the arthroscope would not permit exploration of the volar half of the middle phalanx base and even the proximal phalangeal condyles could only be seen by significant flexion of the joint. Therefore, this is the only hand joint where vertical traction is not utilized and the finger is held horizontally while the small scope is introduced in the interval between the central slip and lateral band in his modified portal from Thomsen's description. While this study focused on the rheumatoid disease, we must recall that the PIP joint is more commonly involved in routine osteoarthritis. No clinical study reviewing this very common pathology has been published. It should also be noted that this work was published in the journal *Arthroscopy* where, again, few hand surgeons might see a technique reviewed that likely only they would utilize. This can now be seen as a recurring theme that perhaps has slowed the advent of small joint arthroscopy of the hand.

Sekiya did publish a follow-up study, now in a hand technique journal, where he expanded modestly upon his experience in RA PIP arthroscopy but did now conclude that the results tend to be long lasting, and that no patients had required reoperation, a notable finding [62]. His follow-up study also included one thumb interphalangeal joint, perhaps the first clinical mention of arthroscopy in a distal interphalangeal joint (DIP). Actually, the true DIP joint of a digit was first scoped in order to realize an arthroscopic-assisted arthrodesis, as described by Cobb in his chapter on "Frontiers in Small Joint Arthroscopy" with coauthors, Berner, Badia, and Topper in 2011 *Hand Clinics* [60]. The topic of DIP arthroscopy is so novel and currently limited that it warrants no further discussion. Suffice it to say that when micro-arthroscopes, in the range of 1–1.2 mm, become widely available in the future, we may then see indications develop for this innovative approach. Arthroscopic debridement for early OA, truncation of mucous cysts with evacuation, and synovectomy may all be routine procedures in future as the technology emerges.

Indications do remain narrow for PIP arthroscopy largely due to the relatively large size and rigidity of the scope in this bicondylar joint, which is anything but a flat surface. Although similar to the knee in bony architecture, the small size of the joint does not permit the same visualization at the current time.

Therefore, the technique remains limited to dorsal compartment synovectomy, mainly in rheumatoid, and perhaps larger osteoarthritic patients. Removal of loose bodies, infection lavage, and now joint arthrodesis might be possible as well. Joint debridement and synovectomy should be performed solely with mechanical shaving since the joint is subcutaneous where the application of RF (radiofrequency) could be problematic.

PIP Arthroscopic Technique

The anatomic nuances of the PIP joint necessitate that this arthroscopy be performed horizontally, allowing free motion of the digit during the scope permitting visualization of most elements of the joint, although the entire volar compartment is essentially inaccessible. Traction in a vertical position would hamper that visualization and would not permit joint flexion.

The PIP joint should be insufflated with 1–2 cc of lidocaine, once adequate digital block anesthesia is achieved. This joint distention is performed dorsally allowing the dorsal recesses to become prominent and facilitate 1.9-, or perhaps 1.5-mm, arthroscope insertion. The portals are simply on either side of the central slip, easily found between that

key landmark and the lateral bands. In his initial paper, Sekiya described a more volar and lateral portal, essentially traversing the transverse retinacular ligament, about 1–2 mm dorsal to the midaxial line [53]. It must again be emphasized that the palmar aspect of the joint is not visualized sufficiently, which happens to be the predominant location for synovitis at the PIP joint, in addition to the dorsal recess, currently amenable to excision. This technical issue could be overcome if perhaps flexible micro-arthroscopes can pass over and around the proximal phalangeal condyles, hence providing more visualization. The procedure would also require smaller shavers that can also follow the contours of the joint. An additional problem is that inadequate suction power currently limits the efficacy of shavers this small in diameter. Even today's 2-mm suction shavers are somewhat limited when trying to aggressively debride and aspirate a dense amount of scarred capsule. Therefore, there are currently both optical and mechanical limitations in technically being able to realize an optimal PIP joint arthroscopic procedure. Once these issues are resolved, the indications should quickly expand, although it may be some decades before this becomes an everyday procedure for the hand surgeon.

CMC Arthroscopy of Ulnar Digits

The fourth and fifth carpometacarpal joints are also amenable to arthroscopic intervention, due to the flexible nature of these joints. Pathology, however, is relatively rare here and the indication is primarily for traumatic-related condition. It is relatively common to have posttraumatic issues at this joint, either arthrosis and/or synovitis, that would benefit from synovectomy and debridement [60]. Articular fractures of either the hamate or the corresponding metacarpal base often lead to later degenerative changes that can cause pain. Insertion of a 1.9-mm arthroscope and concomitant debridement with a shaver and/or RF probe (Fig. 55.12) can provide good pain relief and perhaps avoid fusion of the CMC joint, which is currently a necessary procedure in cases of posttraumatic arthrosis not responding to conservative treatment such as corticosteroid injection. The fusion itself might be able to be done arthroscopically, as currently seen in limited carpal fusions by colleagues such as Ho [63].

Conclusion

Small joint arthroscopy of the hand is currently limited by a combination of technical considerations that are improving continuously, and a lack of clear indications and surgeon utilization likely due to scarce arthroscopy training and scant literature on the topic. The latter reason is self-imposed, and

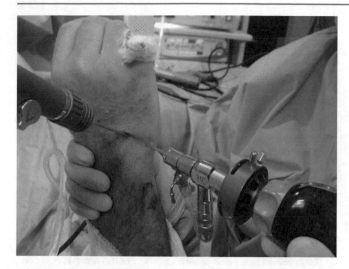

Fig. 55.12 Arthroscopic debridement of the fifth CMC joint in patient with persistent pain after an articular fracture of the small finger metacarpal base

hand surgery organizations must provide more opportunities for "hands-on" training in the usage of the small arthroscope to emerging surgeons who might not be exposed to this in their fellowship training. EWAS (European Wrist Arthroscopy Association) has made major strides in training hand surgeons to push the envelope when it comes to wrist arthroscopic procedures, even publishing entire textbooks covering a single indication for its usage [64]. There have been some courses (AANA, Miami, Strasbourg) that have covered the topic to some degree, largely in the area of the thumb basal joint, enabling colleagues to now consider this as a viable alternative for treatment in their patients. Much more needs to be done to expose surgeons to all the small joint procedures possible in the hand, ultimately to benefit their patients who are increasingly looking toward minimally invasive options.

References

1. Chen YC. Arthroscopy of the wrist and finger joints. Orthop Clin North Am. 1979;10(3):723–33.
2. Gupta R, Bozentka DJ, Osterman AL. Wrist arthroscopy: principles and clinical applications. J Am Acad Orthop Surg. 2001;9(3):200–9.
3. Badia A. Arthroscopy of the trapeziometacarpal and metacarpophalangeal joints. J Hand Surg Am. 2007;32(5):707–24.
4. Menon J. Arthroscopic management of trapeziometacarpal joint arthritis of the thumb. Arthroscopy. 1996;12:581–7.
5. Berger R. Arthroscopic evaluation of the first carpometacarpal joint. J Hand Surg Am. 1998;23:757.
6. Bettinger PC, Linscheid RL, Berger RA, Cooney WP, Kai-Nan A. An anatomic study of the stabilizing ligaments of the trapezium and trapeziometacarpal joint. J Hand Surg Am. 1999;24:786–98.
7. Osterman AL, Culp R, Bednar J. Arthroscopy of the thumb carpometacarpal joint. Arthroscopy. 1997;13:3.
8. Badia A. Trapeziometacarpal arthroscopy: a classification and treatment algorithm. Hand Clin. 2006;22:153–63.
9. Weitbrecht J. Syndesmology. Philadelphia: WB Saunders; 1969. p. 1742.
10. Van Brenk B, Richards RR, Mackay MB, Boynton EL. A biomechanical assessment of ligaments preventing dorsoradial subluxation of the trapeziometacarpal joint. J Hand Surg Am. 1998;23:607–11.
11. Zancolli EA, Cozzi EP. The trapeziometacarpal joint: anatomy and mechanics. In: Zancolli E, Cozzi EP, editors. Atlas of surgical anatomy of the hand. New York: Churchill Livingstone; 1992. p. 443–4.
12. Xu L, Strauch RJ, Ateshian GA, et al. Topography of the osteoarthritic thumb carpometacarpal joint and its variation with regard to gender, age, site, and osteoarthritic stage. J Hand Surg Am. 1998;23:454.
13. Pelligrini VD. Pathomechanics of the thumb trapeziometacarpal joint. Hand Clin. 2001;17(2):175–84.
14. Bettinger PC, Berger RA. Functional ligamentous anatomy of the trapezium and trapeziometacarpal joint (gross and arthroscopic). Hand Clin. 2001;17(2):151–69.
15. Orellana MA, Chow JC. Arthroscopic visualization of the thumb carpometacarpal joint: introduction and evaluation of a new radial portal. Arthroscopy. 2003;19(6):583–91.
16. Walsh EF, Akelman E, Fleming BC, DaSilva MF. Thumb carpometacarpal arthroscopy: a topographic, anatomic study of the thenar portal. J Hand Surg Am. 2005;30:373–9.
17. Slutsky D. The use of a dorsal-distal portal in trapeziometacarpal arthroscopy. Arthroscopy. 2007;23(11):1244.e1–4.
18. Culp RW, Rekant MS. The role of arthroscopy in evaluating and treating trapeziometacarpal disease. Hand Clin. 2001;17(2):315–9.
19. Massoud SN, Levy O, Copeland SA. Radiofrequency capsular shrinkage for voluntary shoulder dislocation. J Shoulder Elb Surg. 2007;16(1):43–8.
20. Lubowitz JH, Poehling GG. Glenohumeral thermal capsulorrhaphy is not recommended—shoulder chondrolysis requires additional research. Arthroscopy. 2007;23(7):687.
21. Lopez MJ, Hayashi K, Fanton GS, Thabit G, Markel MD. The effects of radiofrequency energy on the ultrastructure of joint capsular collagen. Arthroscopy. 1998;14(5):495–501.
22. Hecht P, Hayashi K, Cooley AJ, Lu Y, Fanton GS, Thabit G, Markel MD. The thermal effect of monopolar radiofrequency energy on the properties of joint capsule. Am J Sports Med. 1998;26(6):808–14.
23. Eaton RG, Glickel SZ. Trapeziometacarpal osteoarthritis. Staging as a rationale for treatment. Hand Clin. 1987;3:455–71.
24. Thompson JS. Suspensionplasty: trapeziometacarpal joint reconstruction using abductor pollicis longus. Operat Tech Orthop. 1996;6:98–105.
25. Cobb T, Sterbank P, Lemke J. Arthroscopic resection arthroplasty for treatment of combined carpometacarpal and scaphotrapeziotrapezoid (pantrapezial). J Hand Surg Am. 2011;36(3):413–9.
26. Braun RM. Total joint replacement at the base of the thumb—preliminary report. J Hand Surg. 1982;7:245–51.
27. Badia A, Sambandam SN. Total joint arthroplasty in the treatment of advanced stages of thumb carpometacarpal joint osteoarthritis. J Hand Surg Am. 2006;31(10):1605–14.
28. Goldfarb C, Stern P. Indications and technique for thumb carpometacarpal joint arthrodesis. Tech Hand Up Extrem Surg. 2002;6(4):178–84.
29. Badia A, Young L, Riano F. Bilateral arthroscopic tendon interposition arthroplasty of the thumb carpometacarpal joint in a patient with Ehlers-Danlos syndrome: a case report. J Hand Surg Am. 2005;30(4):673–6.
30. Gisselfält K, Edberg B, Flodin P. Synthesis and properties of degradable poly(urethane urea)s to be used for ligament reconstructions. Biomacromolecules. 2002;3:951–8.
31. Nilsson A, Liljensten E, Bergstrom C, Sollerman C. Results from a degradable TMC joint spacer (Artelon) compared with tendon arthroplasty. J Hand Surg Am. 2005;30(2):380–9.

32. Badia A. Arthroscopic indications for artelon interposition arthroplasty of the thumb trapeziometacarpal joint. Tech Hand Up Extrem Surg. 2008;12(4):1–6.

33. Kuhns CA, Meals RA. Hematoma and distraction arthroplasty for basal thumb osteoarthritis. Tech Hand Up Extrem Surg. 2004;8:2–6. Gervis simple resection.

34. Gervis HW. Excision of the trapezium for osteoarthritis of the trapeziometacarpal joint. J Bone Joint Surg Br. 1949;31:537–9.

35. Yao J. Suture-button suspensionplasty for the treatment of thumb carpometacarpal joint arthritis. Hand Clin. 2012;28(4):579–85.

36. Wilson JN. Basal osteotomy of the first metacarpal in the treatment of arthritis of the carpo-metacarpal joint of the thumb. Br J Surg. 1973;60:854–8.

37. Tomaino MM. Treatment of Eaton stage I trapeziometacarpal disease with thumb metacarpal extension osteotomy. J Hand Surg Am. 2000;25(6):1100–6.

38. Badia A, Khachandani P. Treatment of early basal joint arthritis using a combined arthroscopic debridement and metacarpal osteotomy. Tech Hand Upper Extrem Surg. 2007;11(2):168–73.

39. Buck-Gramcko D, Dietrich FE, Gogge S. Evaluation criteria in follow-up studies of flexor tendon therapy [in German]. Handchirurgie. 1976;8:65–9.

40. Bettinger PC, Linscheid RL, Cooney WP 3rd, An KN. Trapezial tilt: a radiographic correlation with advanced trapeziometacarpal joint arthritis. J Hand Surg Am. 2001;26:692–7.

41. Barron OA, Eaton RG. Save the trapezium: double interposition arthroplasty for the treatment of stage IV disease of the basal joint. J Hand Surg Am. 1998;23:196–204.

42. Cobb T. Arthroscopic STT, arthroplasty. J Hand Surg Am. 2009;34(Suppl 1):42–3.

43. Ashwood N, Bain G, Wardle N. STT scope. Results of arthroscopic debridement for isolated Scapho-trapeziotrapezoidal Arthritis. Orthop Proc JBJS (Br). 2008;90-B (Suppl I 3-4)

44. Bare J, Graham A, Tham S. Scaphotrapezial joint arthroscopy: a palmar portal. J Hand Surg Am. 2003;28:605–9.

45. Carro L, Golano P, Farinas O, Cereza L, Hidalgo C. The radial portal for scaphotrapeziotrapezoid. Arthroscopy. 2003;19(5):547–53.

46. Vaupel GL, Andrews JR. Diagnostic and operative arthroscopy of the thumb metacarpophalangeal joint. A case report. Am J Sports Med. 1985;13(2):139–41.

47. Wilkes LL. Arthroscopic synovectomy in the rheumatoid metacarpophalangeal joint. J Med Assoc Ga. 1987;76:638–9.

48. Leclercq G, Schmitgen G, Verstreken J. Arthroscopic treatment of metacarpophalangeal arthropathy in haemochromatosis. J Hand Surg Br. 1994;19:212–4.

49. Ryu J, Fagan R. Arthroscopic treatment of acute complete thumb metacarpophalangeal ulnar collateral ligament tears. J Hand Surg Am. 1995;20:1037–42.

50. Rozmaryn LM, Wei N. Metacarpophalangeal arthroscopy. Arthroscopy. 1999;15:333–7.

51. Slade JF 3rd, Gutow AP. Arthroscopy of the metacarpophalangeal joint. Hand Clin. 1999;15:501–27.

52. Wei N, Delauter SK, Erlichman MS, Rozmaryn LM, Beard SJ, Henry DL. Arthroscopic synovectomy of the metacarpophalangeal joint in refractory rheumatoid arthritis: a technique. Arthroscopy. 1999;15:265–8.

53. Sekiya I, Kobayashi M, Taneda Y, Matsui N. Arthroscopy of the proximal interphalangeal and metacarpophalangeal joints in rheumatoid hands. Arthroscopy. 2002;18:292–7. Badia bony gamekeeper

54. Badia A, Riano F. Arthroscopic reduction and internal fixation for bony gamekeeper's thumb. Orthopedics. 2006;29(8):675–8.

55. Thompson M, Douglas G, Davison EP. Synovectomy of the metacarpophalangeal joints in rheumatoid arthritis. Proc R Soc Med. 1973;66(2):197–9.

56. Swanson AB. Finger joint replacement by silicone rubber implants and the concept of implant fixation by encapsulation. Ann Rheum Dis. 1969;28(Suppl 5):47–55.

57. Parker WL, Rizzo M, Moran SL, Hormel KB, Beckenbaugh RD. Preliminary results of nonconstrained pyrolytic carbon arthroplasty for metacarpophalangeal joint arthritis. J Hand Surg Am. 2007;32(10):1496–505.

58. McCain JP, Sanders B, Koslin MG, Quinn JH, Peters PB, Indresano AT. Temporomandibular joint arthroscopy: a 6-year multicenter retrospective study of 4,831 joints. J Oral Maxillofac Surg. 1992;50(9):926–30.

59. Berner S. Metacarpophalangeal arthroscopy: indications and technique. Tech Hand Up Extrem Surg. 2008;12(4):208–15.

60. Cobb T, Berner S, Badia A. New frontiers in hand arthroscopy. Hand Clin. 2011;27(3):383–94.

61. Thomsen N, Nielsen N, Jorgensen N, Bojsen-Moller F. Arthroscopy of the proximal interphalangeal joints of the finger. J Hand Surg Br. 2002;27(3):253–5.

62. Sekiya I, Kobayashi M, Okamoto H, Iguchi H, Waguri-Nagaya Y, Goto H, Nozaki M, Tsuchiya A, Otsuka T. Arthroscopic synovectomy of the metacarpophalangeal and proximal interphalangeal joints. Tech Hand Up Extrem Surg. 2008;12(4):221–5.

63. Ho P-C. Arthroscopic partial wrist fusions. Tech Hand Up Extrem Surg. 2008;12(4):242–65.

64. DelPinal F, Luchetti R, Mathoulin C, editors. Arthroscopic management of distal radius fractures. Heidelberg: Springer Verlag; 2010.

Endoscopic Carpal Tunnel Release

56

Steven M. Topper

Introduction

The debate in the literature between open and endoscopic carpal tunnel release (ECTR) through the 1990s and into the early part of the twenty-first century was voluminous. In the end, we were left with no definitive scientific proof favoring one procedure over the other. Consequently both are still done today. While the controversy has died down, questions still remain. The Academy of Orthopedic Surgeons work group, which created clinical and diagnostic guidelines for carpal tunnel release, expressed in their 179-page report what is generally accepted as the conventional wisdom. They concluded that ECTR was favored for outcome measures of pain, pinch strength, and fewer wound complications at 12 weeks. Open carpal tunnel release was favored for the complication of reversible nerve issues (neuropraxia is less likely with OCTR). There were no differences for functional status and symptom severity at 1 year, including complications or infections [1]. In other words, both procedures are equally safe and effective, and there is a somewhat quicker recovery with the endoscopic approach in the first 3 months. Perhaps societal issues such as cost-effectiveness and quality of life will drive us to seek more definitive answers such as happened with laparoscopic cholecystectomy [2]. Until that time we are left with randomized controlled trials and meta-analyses that generally have insufficient power and inconsistent outcome measures making it hard to draw conclusions [3]. Fortunately, division of the transverse carpal ligament is an effective way to treat carpal tunnel syndrome. The application of minimally invasive (endoscopic) techniques to the most commonly performed orthopedic procedure, back in the 1980s, made sense. The hope was that it would decrease the morbidity of the procedure and yield a quicker recovery. In so doing, it may also create a societal cost saving, in light of the number of working young people that have carpal tunnel surgery. Though there is no definitive scientific proof that this has been accomplished, there is also no proof that it hasn't. Early on there were major concerns about safety because the technical aspects of the procedure required a relatively new skill set. Triangulation used in all arthroscopic and endoscopic procedures is a universal skill set among orthopedic, plastic, and general surgeons today.

Anatomy

There are several anatomic points that are important to understand in order to perform endoscopic carpal tunnel release safely and effectively.

Transverse Carpal Ligament

Incomplete release of the transverse carpal ligament (TCL) has been touted as a cause for failure of both open and endoscopic carpal tunnel release. From the endoscopic perspective, the distal aponeurotic portion of the ligament can be hidden by the fat pad. Additionally, just beyond the distal aspect of the ligament (about 4.8 mm) lies the superficial palmar arch. While striving for a complete release is important, this must be done judiciously so as not to cause neurovascular injury. The goal is to maximize volume increase in the carpal canal in order to decompress the median nerve. In a cadaver study, Cobb et al. [4] demonstrated that incomplete release of the distal 4 mm of the TCL allows carpal arch widening (volume increase) that is no different from that following complete division of the TCL (Fig. 56.1). So, while complete release is the goal, it is not necessary to fight for every last distal fiber and increase the risk of neurovascular injury.

S. M. Topper (✉)
Colorado Hand Center, Colorado Springs, CO, USA
e-mail: stopper@coloradohandcenter.com

© Springer Nature Switzerland AG 2022
W. B. Geissler (ed.), *Wrist and Elbow Arthroscopy with Selected Open Procedures*,
https://doi.org/10.1007/978-3-030-78881-0_56

INCOMPLETE CT RELEASE

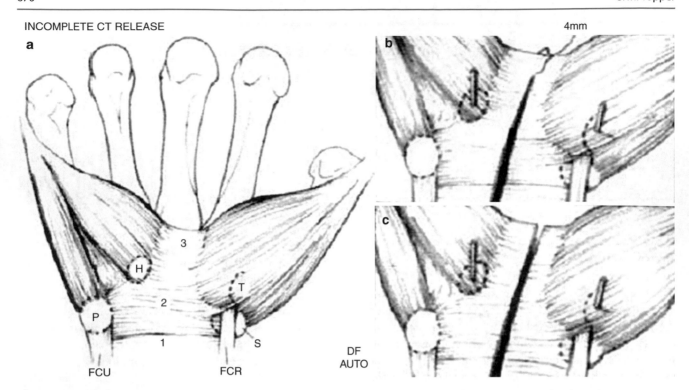

Fig. 56.1 (**a**) Three segments of flexor retinaculum. H, hamate hook; T, trapezium; P, pisiform; S, scaphoid; FCU, flexor carpi ulnaris; FCR, flexor carpi radialis. 1, proximal; 2, middle, true transverse carpal ligament; 3, distal aponeurotic portion of the flexor retinaculum. (**b**) Partial release of the flexor retinaculum. (**c**) Complete release of the flexor reti- naculum. K wires are shown in hamate hook and trapezium. Reprinted from Cobb TK, Cooney WP. Significance of Incomplete Release of the Distal Portion of the Flexor Retinaculum. J Hand Surg Br. 1994; 19: 283–285. With permission from Sage Publications

Hook of the Hamate

There is an increased risk of neuropraxia with endoscopic carpal tunnel release. This can be minimized by hugging the ulnar aspect of the carpal canal with the endoscopic instrument. In order to do this effectively and provide for a straight line of pull, it is important to place the skin incision in relation to the hook of the hamate. Unfortunately, the hook of the hamate can be difficult to palpate, and the use of Kaplan's cardinal line is unreliable. Based on an anatomic study [5], the hook of the hamate can be reliably localized with the technique demonstrated in Fig. 56.2.

Palmar Fascia

Palmar displacement of the flexor tendons after release of the transverse carpal ligament (Bowstringing) has been implicated as a cause for weakness after carpal tunnel surgery. In fact step cut lengthening of the transverse carpal ligament has been advocated to prevent this [6]. The majority of the palmar fascia is not divided with endoscopic carpal tunnel release which provides an uninjured natural tissue barrier to bowstringing.

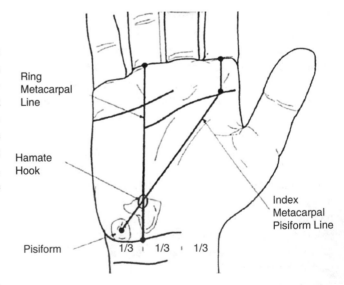

Fig. 56.2 The pisiform is palpated. A line is drawn from this point to the proximal palmar crease at the level of the central aspect of the index finger. A second line is drawn from the central portion at the base of the ring finger to the distal flexor crease of the wrist at the junction of the middle and ulnar thirds. The junction of these two lines marks the location of the hook of the hamate. Reprinted Cobb TK, Cooney WP, An K. Clinical Location of Hook of Hamate: A Technical Note for Endoscopic Carpal Tunnel Release. J Hand Surg Am. 1994; 19: 516–518. With permission from Elsevier

Transligamentous Branch of the Median Nerve

The recurrent motor branch of the median nerve passes around the distal edge of the TCL in most cases. It also can pass through the ligament in up to 23% of cases, which causes challenges with both open and endoscopic carpal tunnel release [7]. Fortunately, the nerve rarely arises from the ulnar aspect of the median nerve and is therefore rarely encountered. This underscores another important reason to hug the ulnar aspect of the canal when performing endoscopic carpal tunnel release. Anatomic variations such as a persistent median artery or aberrant muscle-tendon relationships and dimpling of the TCL should alert the surgeon to the presence of a transligamentous branch. Dealing with a transligamentous branch safely, for both open and endoscopic carpal tunnel release, is about visualization. Therefore the presence of a transligamentous branch does not necessarily preclude accomplishing the procedure (Fig. 56.3).

Glabrous Skin

Glabrous skin (palm of hands and sole of feet) is unique in that it has no hair follicles and it is highly innervated. One of the distinct advantages of the single incision approach to endoscopic carpal tunnel release is the ability to place the incision outside of the glabrous skin, avoiding the associated morbidity and potential wound complications. This advantage is lost with the two incision endoscopic techniques. Additionally the two incision technique is fraught with a higher complication rate [8].

Exposure

The patient is positioned supine on the operating room table with the arm abducted on a hand table. It is useful to place the hand palm up in a holder or over a surgical towel so that the wrist is extended 15–20° (Fig. 56.4). The hand, wrist, forearm, and arm proximal to the elbow should be completely exsanguinated using an Esmark bandage. The tourniquet is then elevated to create a bloodless field. The surgeon's

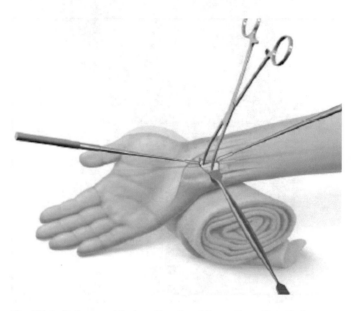

Fig. 56.4 Patient positioning. Reprinted from Centerline Endoscopic Carpal Tunnel Release: Surgical Technique. Arthrex, Inc., 2010. With permission from Arthrex, Inc.

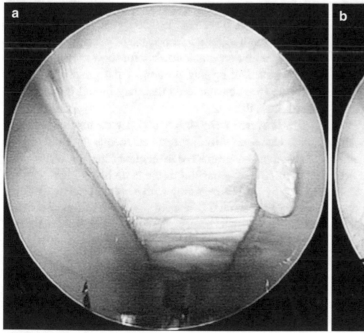
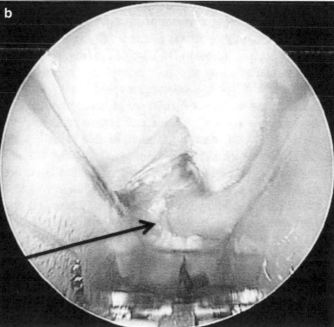

Fig. 56.3 (a) Endoscopic view showing a dimple in the distal 1/3 of the transverse carpal ligament. There is a small synovial frond on the *right*. (b) Post-division of the TCL. *Arrow* locates the transligamentous branch of the median nerve

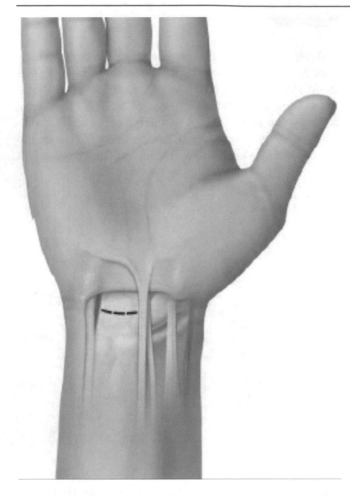

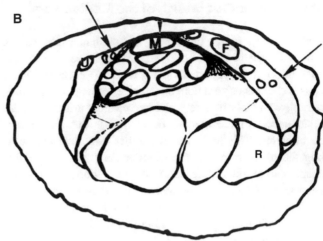

Fig. 56.6 Cross section of the wrist. The flexor retinaculum and the antebrachial fascia are closely apposed anteriorly in the middle (*arrowhead*) and split medially and laterally. *Large arrows* show antebrachial fascia. *Small arrows* show flexor retinaculum. M, median nerve; U, flexor carpi ulnaris; F, flexor carpi radialis. Reprinted from Cobb TK, Dalley BK, Posteraro RH, Lewis RC. Anatomy of the Flexor Retinaculum. J Hand Surg Am. 1993; 18: 91–99. With permission from Elsevier

Fig. 56.5 Incision. Reprinted from Centerline Endoscopic Carpal Tunnel Release: Surgical Technique. Arthrex, Inc., 2010. With permission from Arthrex, Inc.

hand, when holding the instrument, should naturally align the blade assembly so that it points axially from the ulnar side of the carpal tunnel to the base of the ring finger. This course is anatomically optimal for avoiding injury to the median nerve. Right-handed surgeons will usually prefer a position in the axilla for a right carpal tunnel release and cephalic position for a left release. It is vice versa for left-handed surgeons. The surgeon should be able to easily view the monitor over the assistant's right or left shoulder. General or regional anesthesia is advised so that visualization is not obscured by a carpal canal full of anesthetic fluid.

The surgical incision is placed transversely in or near one of the wrist flexion creases (usually the proximal) between the flexor carpi ulnaris and the palmaris longus (PL) (Fig. 56.5). If the patient does not have a PL, the radial extent of the incision should be 2 cm ulnar to the flexor carpi ulnaris. The incision is usually 2 cm in length. Veins that cross the incision are coagulated with a bipolar and divided. Placement of the skin incision and the position of the hook of

the hamate will set the trajectory of the endoscopic device. Therefore it is advisable to mark out the hook of the hamate, at least initially, as a surgeon is becoming comfortable with placement of the incision.

The soft tissue dissection is started on the radial aspect of the incision and taken directly down to the antebrachial fascia. In this location, the flexor retinaculum is closely adherent to the antebrachial fascia. As you move medial and lateral from the center, these tissues divide, and it is much easier to get out of the proper plane of dissection [9] (Fig. 56.6). This dissection is then swept in an ulnar direction. This method reveals a consistent plane that mobilizes Guyon's canal contents, allowing for their retraction out of harm's way. During this portion of the procedure, fascial bands are often encountered that may inhibit the mobilization of these tissues.

This is overcome by simply dividing the restricting fascial bands. Once mobilized, the subcutaneous fat and Guyon's canal contents are retracted in an ulnar direction with a blunt retractor. The antebrachial fascia is divided in line with the incision by simply spreading with a blunt tip scissor. It is not necessary to create a U-shaped flap as has been advocated, which creates unnecessary surgical trauma. This maneuver creates access to the carpal tunnel. A small two-prong skin retractor is placed on the leading edge of the transverse carpal ligament and used to elevate this structure. This is actually the most important step of the operation. By securing the leading edge of the TCL, the exposure is set and should be maintained until the operation is complete.

Preparation

A small Hegar dilator is then used to dilate the carpal tunnel and create a track for the endoscopic device (Fig. 56.7). The dilator is aimed at the base of the ring finger while holding the wrist in slight extension. Gently pass the dilator distally down the ulnar side of the tunnel hugging the hook of the hamate and advance distally until the tip is past the transverse carpal ligament. This is palpated by the index finger on the surgeon's non-instrument hand. When the dilator is in the carpal canal, there is a definite sense of a substantial structure (TCL) between the dilator and the skin. When the dilator is subcutaneous or in Guyon's canal, it is distinct and easily palpated. Next a small synovial elevator is used to dissect adherent synovium from the underside of the transverse carpal ligament (Fig. 56.8). This is a critical step because the safety of this procedure is directly related to clear visualization of the underside of the transverse carpal ligament. Follow the same path as the dilator and scrape the underside of the transverse carpal ligament from proximal to distal. A noticeable rough, washboard-like effect will be felt. The

carpal tunnel is now prepared for insertion of the endoscopic device; however, it is important to check for proper blade extension and retraction before insertion into the patient's hand.

Procedure

The endoscopic device is then inserted into the carpal canal (Fig. 56.9). It is important to hug the underside of the TCL and use the leading edge of the device to push synovium out of the way. This is achieved by the surgeon dropping his hand toward the patient's arm as soon as the device is inserted and prior to advancing it into the carpal canal. While aiming at the base of the ring finger, advance the instrument distally, hugging the hook of the hamate to assure an ulnar course. Use a sufficient number of proximal-to-distal passes to accurately define an ulnar "strip" of the transverse carpal ligament. Transverse fibers of the ligament should be the only thing visualized in the viewing portal of the device. It is important not to deploy the blade until this level of

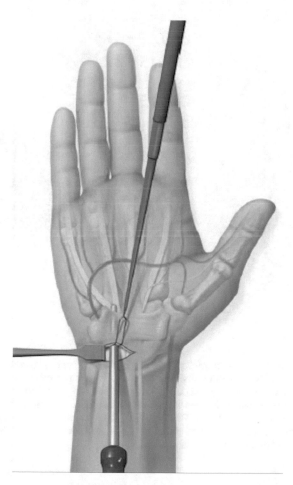

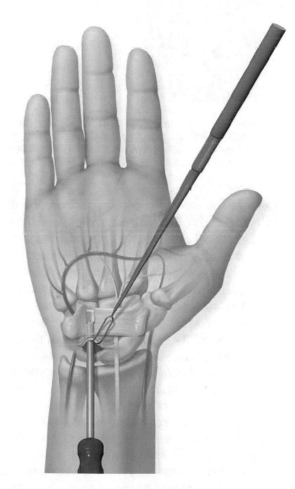

Fig. 56.7 Dilation of the carpal canal. Reprinted from Centerline Endoscopic Carpal Tunnel Release: Surgical Technique. Arthrex, Inc., 2010. With permission from Arthrex, Inc.

Fig. 56.8 Synovial elevator. Reprinted from Centerline Endoscopic Carpal Tunnel Release: Surgical Technique. Arthrex, Inc., 2010. With permission from Arthrex, Inc.

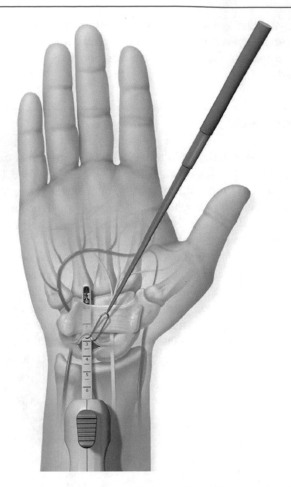

Fig. 56.9 Placement of the endoscopic device, hugging the ulnar aspect of the carpal canal and axially aligned with the ring finger. Reprinted from Centerline Endoscopic Carpal Tunnel Release: Surgical Technique. Arthrex, Inc., 2010. With permission from Arthrex, Inc.

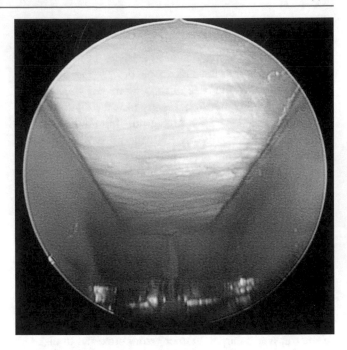

Fig. 56.10 Endoscopic view precut

visualization is achieved (Fig. 56.10). Defining the distal edge of the TCL is assisted by using a digit from the non-instrument hand to ballot in the area of the distal edge previously defined during the dilation of the canal. This demonstrates the transition between the terse TCL and the more pliable distal aponeurotic fibers. Sometimes this can be obscured by the distal fat pad, but that doesn't matter because you never deploy the blade into the fat pad! Once a clear path from the distal end of the TCL to the proximal end is confirmed, the blade is deployed distally, and the transverse carpal ligament is divided as the device is withdrawn along the previously established path. It is important to ensure that the device hugs the underside of the transverse carpal ligament during this portion of the procedure (Fig. 56.11). It is advisable not to put any downward pressure on the hand with the surgeon's non-instrument hand during this portion of the procedure. This helps avoid injury to the ulnar artery as it often takes a more oblique course from the hook of the hamate to the superficial arch than is depicted in standard anatomic textbooks [10]. The device is then reinserted to confirm complete division of the transverse carpal ligament

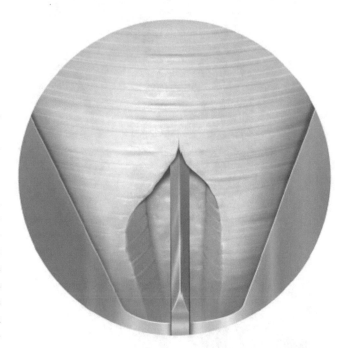

Fig. 56.11 The blade is deployed distally and withdrawn smoothly in one continuous motion dividing the TCL. It is important to hug the underside of the ligament during this motion to keep any surrounding soft tissues out of the viewing portal so that there is nothing for the blade to cut except the TCL. Reprinted from Centerline Endoscopic Carpal Tunnel Release: Surgical Technique. Arthrex, Inc., 2010. With permission from Arthrex, Inc.

(Fig. 56.12). It should be easier to insert the device after TCL division. The spread of the TCL and consequent stretching of the fat pad will often reveal a few distal fibers initially hidden by the fat pad that are divided at this time. In the past, some

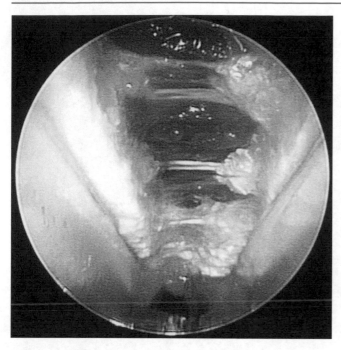

Fig. 56.12 Endoscopic view post-cuts

The wound is closed with a subcuticular suture or Steri-Strip which yields the best cosmetic results. During the initial exposure, I like to preserve the subcutaneous fat as a vascularized flap if possible. This can then be placed between the antebrachial fascia and the skin to provide for vascularized interposition that minimizes adhesions. It is a good idea to inject Marcaine without epinephrine into the carpal tunnel for immediate postoperative pain control. The wound is dressed with Xeroform, gauze sponge, and Coban, and the tourniquet is released. The Coban bandage is changed to a BAND-AID® before the patient leaves the postoperative holding area.

Aftercare

The wound is kept clean and dry for 5 days. Activity is only restricted by the patient's comfort level as there are no mandatory restrictions. The wound is checked at 2 weeks postoperatively, and a final check is performed at 6 weeks postoperatively.

have advocated a partial ligament resection of the distal portion of the TCL with the first pass. The proximal portion is then cut with a second pass. The completeness of TCL division is then refined and accessed with a third pass. I have found this approach to be unnecessary as minimizing passes with the instrument also minimizes neuropraxia. The procedure is complete when the device can be freely advanced to the mid-palm without obstruction. The device may also be rotated (blade retracted) after a complete release to allow the surgeon to inspect the cut edges of the ligament. In addition to the video monitor image, assess completeness of ligament division by several means; sensing the reduced "pressure" upon the instrument when it is reinserted in a decompressed carpal tunnel; noting the more subcutaneous course of the blade assembly after division; the scope light shining through the skin without obstruction; and inserting a small right-angle retractor and looking directly inside of the released carpal tunnel at the cut edges of the ligament. In some cases, there will be a persistent constriction of the proximal forearm fascia on carpal tunnel contents. In these cases, it may be necessary to release the proximal forearm fascia. Using tenotomy scissors, release the forearm fascia proximal to the skin incision, taking care to protect the median nerve. This prevents the forearm fascia from acting as a constricting band that could continue to compromise the median nerve function. I find this to be necessary in about 10% of cases.

References

1. CTS treatment guideline (American Academy of Orthopedic Surgeons Web site). http://www.aaos.org/Research/guidelines/CTStreatmentguide.asp Link to PDF, "CTS Treatment Guideline." 2008. Accessed 23 Jan 2009.
2. Chung KC, Walters MR, Greenfield ML, Chernew ME. Endoscopic versus open carpal tunnel release: a cost-effectiveness analysis. Plast Reconstr Surg. 1998;102:1089–99.
3. Abrams RA. Endoscopic versus open carpal tunnel release. J Hand Surg Am. 2009;34:535–9.
4. Cobb TK, Cooney WP. Significance of incomplete release of the distal portion of the flexor retinaculum. J Hand Surg Br. 1994;19(3):283–5.
5. Cobb TK, Cooney WP, An K. Clinical location of hook of hamate: a technical note for endoscopic carpal tunnel release. J Hand Surg Am. 1994;19:516–8.
6. Jakab E, Ganos D, Cook FW. Transverse carpal ligament reconstruction in surgery for carpal tunnel syndrome: a new technique. J Hand Surg Am. 1991;16:202–6.
7. Tountas CP, Bihrle DM, MacDonald CJ, Bergman RA. Variations of the median nerve in the carpal canal. J Hand Surg Am. 1987;12:708–12.
8. Palmer DH, Paulson JC, Lane-Larsen CL, Peulen VK, Olson JD. Endoscopic carpal tunnel release: a comparison of two techniques with open release. Arthroscopy. 1993;9:498–508.
9. Cobb TK, Dalley BK, Posteraro RH, Lewis RC. Anatomy of the flexor retinaculum. J Hand Surg Am. 1993;18:91–9.
10. Rotman MB, Manske PR. Anatomic relationships of an endoscopic carpal tunnel device to surrounding structures. J Hand Surg Am. 1993;18(3):442–50.

Steven Shin and Juntian Wang

Introduction

Injuries to the hand and wrist are some of the most common musculoskeletal injuries in sports, accounting for approximately 3–9% of sports-related injuries [1]. As the part of the body that grips the stick, throws the ball, or sustains impact, the hand and wrist are vulnerable to injury, whether due to acute trauma or chronic overuse. The complex anatomy and function of the hand and wrist may render the diagnosis and treatment challenging. One cannot argue that sports are playing an increasingly significant role at every level of our society, e.g., the competitive amateur athlete, the collegiate scholarship recipient, or the professional athlete. Therefore, more and more attention is being paid to getting the athlete back to play not only safely but as quickly as possible. Innovative treatments for some hand and wrist injuries are now allowing for decreased time of postoperative immobilization, early initiation of therapy, and faster return to safe and effective play. In this chapter, we will discuss three well-known hand and wrist injuries in sports: thumb ulnar collateral ligament injuries, thumb carpometacarpal dislocations, and triangular fibrocartilage complex injuries.

Thumb Ulnar Collateral Ligament Injuries

Injuries to the thumb ulnar collateral ligament (UCL) are a common athletic injury. Gerber et al. coined the term "skiers' thumb" due to the prevalence in skiing-related injuries – thought to be caused by the thumb getting caught on the ski pole or strap [2]. The proposed mechanism is forceful radial deviation at the thumb metacarpophalangeal (MP) joint. The UCL is most often torn distally from the palmar-ulnar base of the proximal phalanx; mid-substance tears and tears at the metacarpal attachment are much less common [3]. The lack of a digit radial to the thumb makes it more susceptible to injury than the radial collateral ligament (RCL). In fact, RCL injuries are reported to account for only approximately 10% of thumb collateral ligament injuries [4].

Patients generally present with nonspecific symptoms of swelling, ecchymosis, and decreased range of motion at the thumb MP joint. A palpable mass may indicate a Stener lesion, but the absence of such a mass does not rule out a lesion [3]. All patients should be evaluated for joint stability. In general, the thumb MP joint is stressed at both zero degrees (full extension) and 30 degrees of flexion. Assessing the joint in extension tests the stability of the accessory collateral ligament, while assessing in flexion tests the stability of the proper collateral ligament. In general, if radial deviation of the proximal phalanx produces laxity greater than 30 degrees, then the joint is considered to be unstable [5–8].

Indications

Not every acute tear of the thumb UCL requires operative treatment. Partial tears and even complete tears without instability do not necessarily require acute repair. The indications for acute repair are instability as described above and the presence of a Stener lesion, which is a special type of UCL tear whereby the distally torn ligament reflects proximally and is located superficial to the adductor aponeurosis [3]. In these cases, it is impossible for the UCL to heal back anatomically to the proximal phalanx, therefore requiring surgical repair.

For those tears where the patient has recalcitrant pain and evidence on imaging of a persistent tear, operative treatment is indicated if nonoperative treatment has been exhausted. In chronic cases where the distal ligament is still closely approximated to the proximal phalanx base, primary repair of the ligament can be performed. However, if the ligament is scarred and retracted and its length cannot be restored, a

S. Shin · J. Wang (✉)
Cedars-Sinai Medical Center, Department of Orthopaedics,
Cedars-Sinai Orthopaedic Center, Los Angeles, CA, USA
e-mail: steven.shin@cshs.org; juntian.wang@cshs.org

© Springer Nature Switzerland AG 2022
W. B. Geissler (ed.), *Wrist and Elbow Arthroscopy with Selected Open Procedures*,
https://doi.org/10.1007/978-3-030-78881-0_57

tendon graft reconstruction is indicated using the palmaris longus tendon (or another tendon if it is not available).

For athletes, the indications to surgically repair the acute ligament tear are similar. However, the exact treatment needs to be tailored to the individual situation. The athlete's sport, position, level of play, timing of injury, hand dominance, and pain level are important factors to consider when deciding how to treat the injury. A thorough discussion of the risks and benefits of playing or not playing with the injury is necessary.

Contraindications

Contraindications to surgical repair of the UCL tear are similar to those of other ligament injuries. These include the presence of infection, open injury, open physis, and internal joint derangement (such as osteoarthritis).

Technique: Repair with Internal Brace Augmentation

The description of this technique consists of the traditional repair augmented with a suture tape construct. The advantages of this technique, in the senior author's (SSS) experience, are less postoperative immobilization, earlier rehabilitation, and faster return to safe and effective play [9, 10].

Under regional or general anesthesia, the patient is placed supine on the operating table. A tourniquet is placed on the affected arm. The limb is prepped and draped sterilely, and the tourniquet is inflated to the appropriate setting. A curved, hockey stick incision is made at the ulnar, mid-axial aspect of the thumb MP joint. The incision curves proximally and dorsally for good exposure of the proximal ligament. The subcutaneous tissues are spread, taking care to avoid injury to sensory nerves. A longitudinal incision is made at the border of the ulnar sagittal band and the extensor pollicis longus (EPL) tendon, allowing for a cuff of tissue on the sagittal band thick enough for later repair of this interval. The ulnar sagittal band, which is continuous with the adductor aponeurosis, is reflected volarly to reveal the underlying UCL tear. If a Stener lesion is present, one should carefully separate the retracted ligament from the underlying aponeurosis and attempt to restore the full length of the ligament. If continuity of the ligament to the volar aspect of the proximal phalanx base cannot be achieved, then the surgeon should give consideration to ligament reconstruction with a tendon graft. The joint surfaces and volar plate should be inspected to document injury to those structures, although surgical repair of these structures is not usually required.

A guidewire for a 2.5-mm PushLock anchor (Arthrex, Naples, FL) is inserted into the palmar-ulnar base of the proximal phalanx, approximately 2–3 mm distal to the joint, in a slightly distal direction to avoid entering the joint. The guidewire is overdrilled with a 1.8-mm drill bit (included in the kit). After passing a 1.3-mm wide SutureTape (Arthrex, Naples, FL) and 3–0 FiberWire (Arthrex, Naples FL) through the eyelet of the anchor, the anchor eyelet is inserted into the bottom of the hole, such that the anchor body just contacts the cortex. The anchor body is then tapped into the phalanx until completely buried. The driver is removed, and the tape and suture tails are pulled on to ensure good purchase of the anchor within the phalanx. The FiberWire suture is then passed through the distal ligament as a grasping suture. A second free needle is used to pass the second suture tail through the distal ligament. A knot is then tied, drawing the ligament toward the drill hole in the phalanx base. This completes the traditional suture anchor repair of the ligament. An alternative knotless technique can be performed by first placing the grasping stitch through the distal UCL and then inserting the suture tails and SutureTape into the phalanx with the PushLock anchor.

Next, a guidewire for a 3.5 mm SwiveLock (Arthrex, Naples, FL) is inserted into the metacarpal head just proximal and dorsal to the attachment of the UCL. This avoids injury to the proximal UCL by the anchor when inserted. The guidewire is overdrilled with the 3.0 mm drill bit. The distally anchored SutureTape tails are placed onto the fork tip of a SwiveLock anchor and inserted into the bottom of the hole in the metacarpal head (Fig. 57.1). The anchor body is

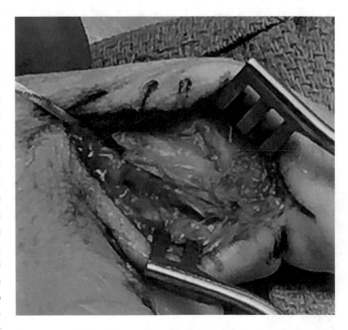

Fig. 57.1 Thumb UCL repair with internal brace augmentation. The SutureTape tails are overlying the UCL and coming out of the anchor site at the metacarpal head

inserted into the hole while maintaining steady pressure on the fork tip at the bottom of the hole; this completes the internal brace augmentation of the repair. After ensuring full motion and appropriate tension on the repair, the extraneous suture tape tails are cut and removed, and the incision is closed in layers in the standard fashion. A plaster thumb spica splint is applied with the interphalangeal (IP) joint free. The tourniquet is deflated, and brisk capillary refill to the tip of the thumb is noted.

Tips and Tricks

Having an assistant maintain the thumb MP joint in 30 degrees of flexion and neutral in the coronal plane when SwiveLock anchor is inserted into the metacarpal head is probably the most important part of this procedure. Not doing so will cause limitation in flexion and/or overtightening of the repair. Due to the noted strength of the augmented repair at time zero, the patient can begin early motion of the thumb MP joint, even as early as 2–3 days postoperatively [11]. At this time, the patient can wear a removable hand-based thumb brace for comfort but is encouraged to remove the brace as much as possible for exercises. Return to play is typically around 5–6 weeks, with the rate-limiting factor being the patient's pain tolerance.

Conclusion

Thumb UCL tears are a common injury in almost every sport. As discussed above, there are many different factors that must be considered when considering the type and timing of treatment. With the advent of internal brace augmentation of the traditional suture anchor repair, there is less postoperative immobilization, earlier rehabilitation, and therefore faster return to safe and effective play in the senior author's experience.

Thumb Carpometacarpal Dislocations

Thumb carpometacarpal (CMC) dislocations are typically caused by an axial load on a flexed thumb metacarpal, leading to dorsal displacement of the first metacarpal. Volar dislocations are uncommon. Strauch et al. reported that the dorsoradial ligament is necessarily disrupted to dislocate the first metacarpal [12]. While the anterior oblique or beak ligament was long thought to be the primary stabilizer of the thumb CMC joint, the dorsoradial ligament is now considered to be the primarily stabilizer of the thumb CMC joint. More frequently seen than the pure thumb CMC dislocation is the Bennett fracture, where the volar base of the first meta-

carpal is fractured. Unaddressed, either injury can lead to early arthritis, pain, and dysfunction at the thumb CMC joint.

Symptoms of thumb CMC dislocations include pain over the thenar eminence and inability to make a fist. Standard posteroanterior and lateral radiographs of the injured thumb as well as the uninjured hand should be obtained. A stress radiograph, where the thumbs are positioned in parallel and pressed together along their radial aspects, can show radial shifting of the first metacarpal base.

Indications

Thumb CMC dislocations can result in complete or partial tears of the ligaments stabilizing the joint. Clinical stability and lack of radiographic subluxation are indicative of partial tears; these injuries can be treated nonoperatively with immobilization. Absolute indications for operative treatment include an unstable CMC joint after initial successful closed reduction, unsuccessful closed reduction, and open injuries. A relative indication is earlier return to sport, which in the senior author's experience is possible with open reduction and repair of the dorsoradial ligament with internal brace augmentation. This technique is described below.

Contraindications

There are no well-described contraindications to treatment of thumb CMC dislocations. General orthopedic principles should be adhered to.

Technique: Open Reduction of Thumb CMC Joint and Repair of Dorsoradial Ligament with Internal Brace Augmentation

Under regional or general anesthesia, the patient is placed supine on the operating Table. A tourniquet is placed on the affected arm. The limb is prepped and draped sterilely, and the tourniquet is inflated to the appropriate setting. A longitudinal incision is made over dorsal aspect of the thumb CMC joint. The subcutaneous tissues are spread, and care is taken to avoid injury to sensory nerves. The extensor pollicis brevis (EPB) and abductor pollicis longus (APL) tendons are retracted dorsally and volarly, respectively. The underlying dorsoradial ligament (DRL) is often seen torn off distally from the thumb metacarpal base. The disruption in the capsuloligamentous complex is utilized to reveal the dislocated CMC joint. The articular surfaces are inspected, and any injury is noted.

A guidewire for a 3.5 mm SwiveLock (Arthrex, Naples, FL) is placed into the dorsal aspect of the first metacarpal

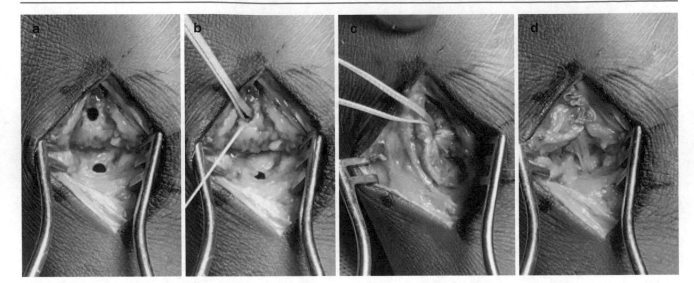

Fig. 57.2 Patient with thumb CMC dislocation undergoing surgery. Intraoperative photos demonstrate drill holes in the first metacarpal base and trapezium (**a**), FiberWire and SutureTape secured in the meta-

carpal drill hole (**b**), repair of the dorsoradial ligament (**c**), and completed internal brace (**d**)

base 2–3 mm distal to the joint. A second guidewire is placed into the dorsal trapezium (Fig. 57.2a). Both guide wires are overdrilled with a 3.0-mm drill bit. A SutureTape (Arthrex, Naples, FL) and 3–0 FiberWire (Arthrex, Naples, FL) are secured in the metacarpal base with a SwiveLock (Fig. 57.2b). The FiberWire suture is used to repair the dorsoradial ligament (Fig. 57.2c). With the joint reduced, the SutureTape tails are brought proximally and secured in the trapezium with another SwiveLock, completing the internal brace construct (Fig. 57.2d). Additional fine Vicryl sutures are used to repair the capsular disruption and augment the repair. Stability of the reduced CMC joint is confirmed. The incision is closed in layers in the standard fashion. The tourniquet is deflated, and brisk capillary refill to the thumb and fingers is noted. Finally, a plaster thumb spica splint is applied.

Tips and Tricks

With the joint reduced and prior to repair of the dorsoradial ligament, a provisional K-wire can be placed across the CMC joint or from the first to second metacarpal bases to maintain the reduction. This K-wire is removed after repair of the dorsoradial ligament and placement of the internal brace construct to assess the stability of the CMC joint.

Conclusion

Although relatively rare, pure dislocations of the thumb CMC joint are well-known injuries in sports and often require surgical treatment. In the senior author's experience,

the advent of internal brace augmentation of the dorsoradial ligament repair has allowed for the time of postoperative immobilization to be minimized and rehabilitation started sooner, allowing for faster return to safe and effective play.

Triangular Fibrocartilage Complex Injuries

The triangular fibrocartilage complex (TFCC) provides intrinsic stability to the distal radioulnar joint (DRUJ). Based on Palmer et al.'s classification, TFCC injuries are typically divided into traumatic versus degenerative injuries [13]. Acute traumatic injuries can occur when the athlete falls on an extended wrist with the arm pronated or when there is a traction injury to the ulnar side of the wrist. Patients can present with pain over the ulnocarpal joint and difficulty with rotational movements of the wrist. Exam findings include pain with radioulnar deviation or prono-supination; a positive fovea sign, i.e., point tenderness at the interval between the ECU and FCU tendons distal to the ulnar head; and perhaps a positive DRUJ shuck test denoting DRUJ instability. Although MRI is a valuable tool for the diagnosis of TFCC tears, arthroscopy is both a valuable diagnostic and therapeutic tool in the treatment of these injuries. Because this chapter is focused on open techniques, only open repair of the peripheral TFCC tear will be described; arthroscopic debridement or repair of TFCC tears will not be discussed.

TFCC injuries can be challenging to manage in athletes given their different levels of performance and expectations. These injuries can be common in gymnasts and cheerleaders who perform activities that require bearing their full body weight on their hands and wrists. Chawla et al. proposed that excess load bearing on the wrist may result in asymmetric

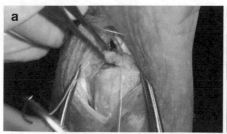 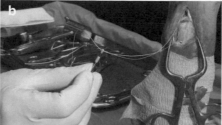 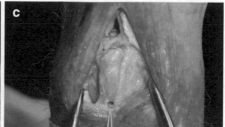

Fig. 57.3 TFCC repair showing a grasping suture passed through the peripheral TFCC (**a**), suture tails through the eyelet of a PushLock (**b**), and completed repair with suture tails coming out of a hole in the ulna (**c**)

closure of the distal radial and ulnar physes, with the radial physis closing prematurely and thereby increasing stress on the ulnar aspect of the wrist and TFCC [14].

Indications

Early repair of the peripheral TFCC tear is indicated if there is concomitant DRUJ instability and more predictable results are desired for earlier return to play. It is also indicated if nonoperative treatment, e.g., immobilization, fails to heal the tear and restore stability or resolve pain.

Contraindications

An absolute contraindication to open repair of the TFCC is infection. Relative contraindications include ulnar positive variance and an open distal ulna physis (although the technique described below does not violate the physis).

Technique: Open Repair of Peripheral TFCC Tears

Under regional or general anesthesia, the patient is placed supine on the operating table. A tourniquet is placed on the affected arm. The limb is prepped and draped sterilely, and the tourniquet is inflated to the appropriate setting. Finger traps are applied, and the hand is placed in the wrist traction tower with 10–12 lb. of traction. Dry or wet arthroscopy is performed according to surgeon preference. A diagnostic arthroscopy is performed, and the peripheral TFCC tear is confirmed. The instruments are removed from the wrist.

A longitudinal incision is made directly over the ulnar styloid. The subcutaneous tissues are spread, taking care to avoid injury to the dorsal ulnar sensory nerve, which is retracted and protected. A longitudinal incision is made in the extensor retinaculum ulnar to the ECU tendon. The ECU tendon is retracted. The capsule at the ulnocarpal joint is incised longitudinally and elevated off of the ulnocarpal joint. The detached peripheral rim of the TFCC is visualized.

The fovea is curetted, and a small drill hole is made there to stimulate bleeding and healing of the TFCC. A 3-0 FiberWire suture is passed through the peripheral rim of the TFCC (Fig. 57.3a), and both tails are brought proximally around the ulnar styloid, with one tail dorsal and the other volar to the ulnar styloid. A 1.8 mm hole is drilled into the distal ulna proximal to the ulnar head. Both suture tails are buried and secured in the hole using a 2.5-mm PushLock anchor (Fig. 57.3b). Additional fine Vicryl sutures are placed through the rim of the TFCC and adjacent capsular and periosteal tissue to augment the repair. A tight capsular repair is performed (Fig. 57.3c). Traction is released on the wrist, and improved stability of the DRUJ is confirmed. The retinaculum is also repaired tightly, and the incision is closed in layers. The tourniquet is deflated, and brisk capillary refill to the fingers is noted. Finally, a short arm ulnar plaster splint is applied.

Tips and Tricks

There are several advantages to the open TFCC repair. In cases of chronic DRUJ instability, there is often extraneous capsule, and this can be excised prior to capsular closure. There is also often concomitant pathology affecting the ECU tendon, e.g., tenosynovitis or instability, both of which can be addressed through an open approach to the TFCC. A nonunited ulnar styloid can also be excised through an open approach. The senior author (SSS) has not seen any difference in protecting his TFCC repairs postoperatively with short arm versus long arm immobilization; he therefore prefers to use short arm immobilization for 4 weeks postoperatively before the patient begins therapy. It is typically around 3–4 months before the patient can begin sports-specific activities.

Conclusion

Like thumb UCL tears, TFCC injuries are common athletic injuries, especially in stick or ball-handling sports. Depending on the location of the tear and the presence or absence of DRUJ instability, these injuries can be treated nonoperatively or operatively. Operative treatments can be arthroscopic or open. We describe an open repair technique for peripheral TFCC tears that is preferred by the senior author for the reasons described above.

References

1. Rettig AC. Athletic injuries of the wrist and hand. Part I: traumatic injuries of the wrist. Am J Sports Med. 2003;31(6):1038–48.

2. Gerber C, Senn E, Matter P. Skier's thumb. Surgical treatment of recent injuries to the ulnar collateral ligament of the thumb's metacarpophalangeal joint. Am J Sports Med. 1981;9(3):171–7.

3. Stener B. Displacement of the ruptured ulnar collateral ligament of the metacarpophalangeal joint of the thumb. J Bone Joint Surg Br [Internet]. 1962;44-B(4):869–79. Available from: https://doi.org/10.1302/0301-620X.44B4.869

4. Edelstein DM, Kardashian G, Lee SK. Radial collateral ligament injuries of the thumb. J Hand Surg Am. 2008;33(5):760–70.

5. Posner MA, Retaillaud JL. Metacarpophalangeal joint injuries of the thumb. Hand Clin. 1992;8(4):713–32.

6. Heyman P, Gelberman RH, Duncan K, Hipp JA. Injuries of the ulnar collateral ligament of the thumb metacarpophalangeal joint. Biomechanical and prospective clinical studies on the usefulness of valgus stress testing. Clin Orthop Relat Res. 1993;292:165–71.

7. Heyman P. Injuries to the ulnar collateral ligament of the thumb metacarpophalangeal joint. J Am Acad Orthop Surg. 1997;5(4):224–9.

8. Palmer AK, Louis DS. Assessing ulnar instability of the metacarpophalangeal joint of the thumb. J Hand Surg Am. 1978;3(6):542–6.

9. De Giacomo AF, Shin SS. Repair of the thumb ulnar collateral ligament with suture tape augmentation. Tech Hand Up Extrem Surg. 2017;21(4):164–6.

10. Patel NA, Lin CC, Itami Y, McGarry MH, Shin SS, Lee TQ. Kinematics of thumb ulnar collateral ligament repair with suture tape augmentation. J Hand Surg Am. 2019;45(2):117–22.

11. Shin SS, van Eck CF, Uquillas C. Suture tape augmentation of the thumb ulnar collateral ligament repair: a biomechanical study. J Hand Surg Am. 2018;43(9):868.e1–6.

12. Strauch RJ, Behrman MJ, Rosenwasser MP. Acute dislocation of the carpometacarpal joint of the thumb: an anatomic and cadaver study. J Hand Surg Am. 1994;19(1):93–8.

13. Palmer AK. Triangular fibrocartilage complex lesions: a classification. J Hand Surg Am. 1989;14(4):594–606.

14. Chawla A, Wiesler ER. Nonspecific wrist pain in gymnasts and cheerleaders. Clin Sports Med. 2015;34(1):143–9.

Bracing and Rehabilitation for Wrist and Hand Injuries in Collegiate Athletes

58

William B. Geissler, Michael Brown, and W. Cody Pannell

With 25% of all athletic injuries being wrist and hand injuries [1], athletic trainers, physical therapists, and sports-medicine physicians spend a great deal of time in prevention and care of these injuries. High-risk sports such as football, gymnastic, wrestling, and basketball athletes account for a majority of traumatic wrist and hand injuries. A Division 1A collegiate sports program will spend in the range of $25,000–$75,000 per year on preventive bracing, splinting, and taping products for injuries of the wrist and hand. Injuries to the wrist and hand may be a result of the mechanism of injury or by repetitive microtrauma to the area. Normal ROM and stability of the wrist are important in prevention of wrist and hand injuries and aid in the participation in most athletic activities. Prevention of soft tissue injuries is the most common reasons for preventative bracing and taping, whereas traumatic injuries to bony structures are the most common reasons for casting and splinting. After initial care, rehabilitation assists in restoring function. This article focuses on preventative bracing, protective padding, and rehabilitation for common wrist and hand injuries.

Common Injuries

Common injuries to the wrist and hand at the collegiate level are most prevalent with football, gymnastic, wrestling, and basketball sports. Some of the most common injuries seen in collegiate sports are collateral ligament tears, proximal and distal interphalangeal (IP) joint dislocations, wrist ligamentous injuries, metacarpal fractures, and scaphoid fractures. The type and management of the injury will depend on many factors such as time of season, the sport, and the position played [2]. Phalangeal collateral ligament tears are particularly common in contact sports. Sports such as football and basketball, in which the use of the hands and digits to fight for position on the field or court, often result in a valgus or varus stress to the proximal interphalangeal (PIP) joint. Collateral ligament sprains or complete tears occur as a result of load failure of the tissues. Baseball players often suffer from direct lever-type forces while sliding headfirst into a base, with the fingertips extended. Collateral ligament tears of the fingers are most often referred to by coaches and players as the famous "jammed finger."

Common deformities of the distal interphalangeal (DIP) joint occur in sports such as basketball and football as a result of the ball striking the tip of the finger and resulting in what is referred to as a mallet finger deformity (avulsion of the terminal extensor tendon). Injury to the volar aspect of the DIP joint can occur as a result of forced extension of a flexed digit resulting in flexor digitorum profundus (FDP) avulsion (grabbing a jersey to make a tackle and the runner forcefully pulling away). This injury is termed a jersey finger deformity [3]. When ligamentous injuries occur to the wrist, the scapholunate ligament or the triangular fibrocartilage complex is often affected. Scapholunate dissociation or TFCC injuries may occur during sport as a result of a fall or due to wrist position during a sport specific movement, such as blocking in football.

Eighty-five percent of all hand fractures that occur in sports happen while playing American football, basketball, or lacrosse. In collegiate football, hand and wrist fractures comprised 39.9% of all injuries [4] with the incidence occurring more frequently during game competition [5]. American football has the highest rate of hand fractures among sports, accounting for 50% of all hand fractures. Two-thirds of all hand fractures are metacarpal fractures. Isolated wrist sprains

W. B. Geissler
Division of Hand and Upper Extremity Surgery, Section of Arthroscopic Surgery and Sports Medicine, Department of Orthopedic Surgery and Rehabilitation, University of Mississippi Medical Center, Jackson, MS, USA

M. Brown (✉) · W. C. Pannell
School of Health-Related Professions, Department of Physical Therapy, University of Mississippi Medical Center, Jackson, MS, USA
e-mail: mbrown23@umc.edu; wpannell@umc.edu

© Springer Nature Switzerland AG 2022
W. B. Geissler (ed.), *Wrist and Elbow Arthroscopy with Selected Open Procedures*,
https://doi.org/10.1007/978-3-030-78881-0_58

are not as common; however, athletes do fall on the outstretched arm. Falls on an outstretched arm with the wrist extended greater than 90 degrees are the mechanism for scaphoid fractures. Scaphoid fractures to the wrist constitute 70% of all wrist fractures [6]. These injuries may be prevented with proper bracing and taping. However, when the injuries do occur, management through appropriate surgical interventions, rehabilitation, and return to play measures is important for successful return. These steps include proper bracing, casting, or taping with appropriate padding. Rehabilitation techniques to restore appropriate ROM, strength, and function for sport. Rehabilitation is a process that continues before returning to play and is continued until the athlete has made maximum recovery.

Prevention

Although preventing all injuries to the hand and wrist is impossible, experienced sports medicine personnel do their best to prevent the most common injuries when the athlete's sport position duties allow, such as taping the wrist. Prevention of common athletic wrist injuries is often accomplished by several bracing and taping techniques. Bracing and taping techniques are customized to the athlete's position. The fundamental principle of preventive bracing and taping is to provide support, limit excessive ROM, and allow for protection against forces that cause injury. Supplies that are used include cloth athletic tape, neoprene, and sometimes a thermoplastic material.

The wrist is often taped as a preventive measure in sports such as gymnastics and football. These two sports subject athletes to forceful loading of the wrist in an extended position. For example, offensive linemen in football must extend the wrist while applying a direct force to the body of a defensive player during pass blocking. Gymnasts often must support their body weight. In both sports, there are direct forces to the extended wrist that may result in potential injuries. Figure 58.1 shows the classic taping technique for the wrist. This technique prevents excessive wrist extension and flexion. Figure 58.2 shows an "X" technique that provides extra support to limit the appropriate excessive direction. The "X" is applied to the volar side of the hand and wrist if limiting extension is the desired objective.

The "X" is applied to the dorsum of the hand and wrist if limiting flexion is the desired objective. There are several keys to remember about this taping technique. First of all, the "X" must be anchored (secured) at both ends of the "X" as shown in the figure. Second, the tape must be long enough so that there is enough of a lever arm on both sides of the joint to actually prevent excessive motion. If the tape does not go far enough distally and proximally, forces applied to the

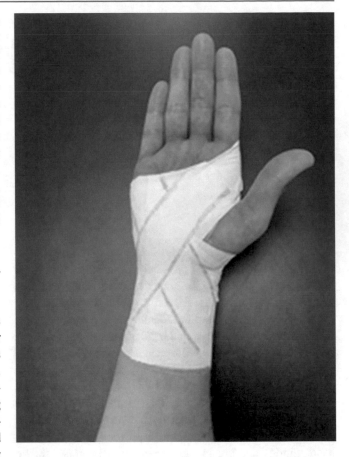

Fig. 58.1 The "X" technique prevents excessive wrist extension and flexion

wrist will not be prevented, and the athlete is more likely to injure the wrist. There are also several off-the-shelf prophylactic wrist braces that can be used to limit wrist hyperextension primarily. Although the athlete perceives prophylactic bracing as cumbersome, these braces are usually cost-efficient. By limiting hyperextension of the wrist, injuries such as scapholunate ligament tears and scaphoid fractures can be prevented.

In sports such as basketball and football, the IP joint of the thumb is also taped for injury prevention. Figure 58.3 shows how the collateral ligaments of the thumb are supported. Again, the tape is applied so that there is an opposite preventive force applied when a direct varus or valgus force is applied in the opposite direction. There has been a long-standing argument among experts as to whether cloth tape applies enough force to actually prevent injury. Research has shown that cloth athletic tape loosens up soon with athletic activity and, therefore, cannot prevent injury. However, other research has shown that applying cloth tape to joints of the body, such as the wrist, knee, ankle, or even shoulder, actually improves proprioception (kinesthetic awareness) and thus increases dynamic stability of the joint.

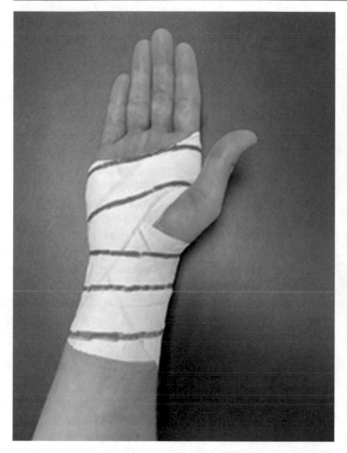

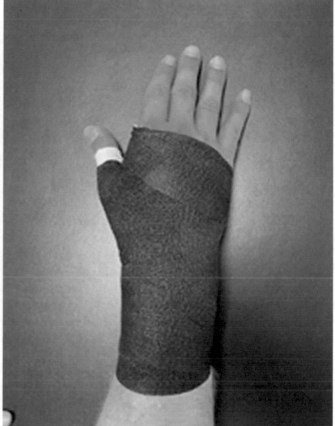

Fig. 58.2 The "X" technique provides extra support to limit the appropriate excessive direction. The "X" supplies the volar side of the hand and wrist if limiting extension is the desired objective

Fig. 58.3 The tape is applied so that the opposite preventive force resists direct varus or valgus force when applied in the opposite direction. This taping technique supports the collateral ligaments of the thumb

Rehabilitation

Rehabilitation of hand and wrist injuries in sports requires teamwork between the physician, athlete, therapist, and/or athletic trainer. The stages of rehabilitation include initial tissue healing, recovery of motion and flexibility, recovery of strength and power, recovery of endurance, and return to activities on the playing field [7].

Recovery of motion is the most important aspect of rehabilitation. It has been well documented that a few millimeters of motion prevent debilitating adhesions. The inexperienced athletic trainer or physical therapist will concentrate too early on strengthening because the patient is an athlete. Too often, basic ROM exercises are believed to be too conservative and not sport specific. Inexperienced coaches have contributed to this noncompliance by generalizing all finger injuries as being a "jammed finger." In such cases, the standard treatment protocol has always been buddy taping the injured finger to the finger next to it and returning to play. Physicians and therapists often see athletes who have been given this treatment after the season, and the athletes have

adhesions and nonfunctional ROM. The athlete is left trying to compete in a sport with a grip strength that is fair at best. For the multisport high school athlete, this means that after football season, the athlete is unable to grip a bat or stick to begin preparing for the next sport. However, gaining acceptable ROM is essential before functional strength gains can be achieved (specific exercises to gain ROM). To regain full ROM in the injured fingers, edema must be controlled. If left alone, fluid within the joints forms fibrous scar tissue that blocks the normal mechanics of the finger joints. Therapists and athletic trainers must keep in mind two kinematic characteristics of the fingers, with the exception of the thumb. First, the four metacarpophalangeal (MP) joints are condyloid with only 2 degrees of freedom. Second, IP joints (proximal and distal) have 1 degree of freedom. The primary motions of both joints are flexion [8] routine activities on the playing field. Recovery of motion is the most important and extension. Swelling that is not addressed easily blocks the primary movement that allows for gripping motions. Control or decrease of swelling to the fingers may be achieved by retrograde massage, proper elevation, compression, and icing immediately after therapy or participation in sports.

Early emphasis on controlling edema is paramount to a successful return to play. Retrograde massage should be performed by the rehabilitation professional by placing the athlete's fingers in an elevated position (above the heart), gripping the athlete's swollen digit distally, and sliding the therapist's fingers in a proximal direction to the head of the metacarpals. This gives the therapist a vision of a wave-like action to the edema. Hand or massage lotion can be used to decrease friction and allow for an easy glide. This can easily be taught to the athlete so that the athlete can perform the maneuver frequently throughout the day. Surgically repaired fingers, with healing incisions or open wounds, require care to work around the incision. Other tips to control swelling in the athlete's hand would be to wear compression gloves while he or she is not in therapy. The injured athlete should keep the hand elevated above the heart while not in therapy, to minimize swelling. Holding the injured hand in the dependent position quickly causes swelling to pool within the involved digit. Finally, when appropriate, performing active/passive ROM to the digit with hand placed in an elevated position decreases swelling and reduces the likelihood of the nonfunctional stiff joint. Synchronous wrist and digital tenodesis exercises and individual joint-blocking exercises are two excellent non-resistive exercises to begin early to regain maximum ROM in all digital joints.

Joint-blocking exercises are used in collateral ligament tears, phalangeal fractures, and, when appropriate, flexor tendon repairs. The experienced therapist and athletic trainer recognize that the wrist plays a vital role in rehabilitation of the fingers. Many times, injured patients drop their wrists into slight flexion, even while pain is controlled in the fingers. If the wrist is maintained in this position for too long, it becomes stiff. It is important that the athlete be educated to maintain ROM of the wrist and, when possible, hold the wrist in extension, especially while performing exercises. Optimal grip strength and ROM of the digits are accompanied by slight wrist extension. Also, the classic incorrect position of the hand and wrist during the healing phase includes slight wrist flexion, MP extension, and IP flexion. This is not functional in either sports or activities of daily living. This can be prevented by placing the injured hand in a wrist cock-up splint, especially at night, during the rehabilitation phase of recovery. The experienced therapist and trainer position the digit with the MP joint in flexion and the IP joint in extension to prevent ligament contracture. It is best for the hand to heal with MP joints extended and the IP joints flexed. It is also important when applying casts that the distal end of the cast or splint stops just proximal to the palmar crease of the volar surface of the hand, so that the splint does not prevent MP joint flexion and cause an extension contracture of the MP joint. Strengthening exercises may begin at different times, depending on the type of injury and/or type of fixation, if surgery is necessary. Most patients with

fractures and tendon injuries begin some form of strengthening at 4–6 weeks. To strengthen the muscle, resistance must be applied. Muscle tissue adapts to the amount of force placed upon it. There are several ways to do this in the hand and wrist. Resistive rubber bands, putty, dumbbells, and even manual resistance placed on the muscle by the therapist or athletic trainer can be used to overload the muscle. When ligaments of the wrist are injured or recovering from surgery, it is important to remember that traction forces placed upon these tissues are detrimental to tissue healing. A repaired scapholunate or lunotriquetral interosseous ligament should not have any traction forces placed upon it until about 12 weeks postoperatively. This key principle is important to the athletic trainer or sports therapist to communicate with the strength coach to initiate strengthening exercises but to limit traction to the injured hand. Routine lifts in the weight room, such as the power clean, snatch, and deadlift, are contraindicated for healing ligaments of the wrist. Other pitfalls in rehabilitation of the healing hand and wrist include allowing athletes to participate in plyometric or agility drills too soon. Box jumping and bag drills may not use the hand and wrist, but they do pose a risk for falling on the outstretched wrist, which may cause reinjury. Athletes should be given time for complete bone and soft tissue healing and to demonstrate strength that is near (within 85%) that of the uninvolved extremity. It is important to limit conditioning exercises in athletes with exposed Kirschner wires under casts, to decrease potential pin track infections.

Playing Casts and Splints

The rules governing orthoses for competitive play vary with the specific sport, the level of play, and the game official in charge of inspection and approval. Certain sports, such as swimming, wrestling, and (in some states) high school basketball, may not allow playing orthoses to be worn during competition (although they may be used during practice). A degree of uniformity for orthotic regulation has been attained in the rulebooks of the National Federation of State High School Association, the National Collegiate Athletic Association (NCAA), and the professional sports leagues. In general, firm, but soft, plastics (consistency approximately that of a pencil eraser), such as RTV 11 (General Electric, Waterford, New York), a silicone-based paste applied in several layers alternating with gauze bandage wrapping, and Soft Cast (3 M, Minneapolis, Minnesota) a pre-impregnated gel roll, are popular, approved ingredients for construction of playing orthoses. Fiberglass or Gore-Tex may be used. Gore-Tex allows the patient to shower with the cast on. Prefabricated heat-malleable Plastazote splints have become popular. A layer of closed-cell polyurethane foam may be used to cover any of these orthoses during play or practice. The NCAA Committee on

Competitive Safeguards and Medical Aspects of Sports (CSMAS) states that the padding used to immobilize and protect an injury must follow the standards of Rule 1–26.4 with the subsequent guidelines: covering should be pliable (flexible or easily bent) material, covered on all exterior sides and edges with not less than ½ inch thickness of slow-rebounding foam.

In metacarpal fractures, flexion of the MP joints relaxes the intrinsic and extrinsic flexors, neutralizing their tendency to shorten and dorsally angulate the fractured metacarpal. The wrist may be positioned in 20 degrees of extension. The MP joints may be left free or placed in 50–60 degrees of flexion at the discretion of the treating physician. The IP joints usually are left free. Buddy taping or splinting the injured finger to an adjacent finger prevents snagging and reinjury. The index finger is paired with the middle finger, the middle and ring finger are paired together (leaving the index finger free for writing and independent pinching), and the small finger is matched to the ring finger as closely as possible. For skill players (players that routinely handle the ball), the authors prefer to avoid taping across the flexor pads and finger joint creases to preserve sensation and finger flexion. For non-skill, position players, the dominant hand may be covered completely with protective splint and padding.

Return to Play

Return-to-play criteria obviously vary from injury to injury. However, basic principles do apply.

If fractures are present, the athlete should not be returned to play before callus formation has begun, and there are minimal local symptoms such as edema. If a playing cast is worn over the injury, the athlete must be able to withstand a blow to the injured area [9]. Finally, if the injury involves collateral ligaments, three parameters must be taken into consideration. First, stability to the joint should not be compromised. If complete healing has not occurred, bracing or taping the joint for stability should be considered. Second, acceptable ROM to successfully participate should be present. A lack of ROM decreases grip strength. Digits that do not have acceptable ROM will not be able to perform proper gripping, such as handling a racket, club, or bat. The inability to grab and hold onto objects does not allow the injured athlete to perform such activities such as tackling or catching. However, there are sports and positions in sports that allow for the wrist and hand to be completely covered in a cast and the athlete to still be able to participate. For example, in football, a linebacker or lineman can compete in what many athletic trainers refer to as a "club cast" (Fig. 58.4). For some fractures of the hand and wrist, the athletic trainer can position the injured wrist and/or hand so that the wrist is in slight extension, and the MP joints and IP joints are flexed, so that the hand is placed somewhat in a full-fist position (Fig. 58.5).

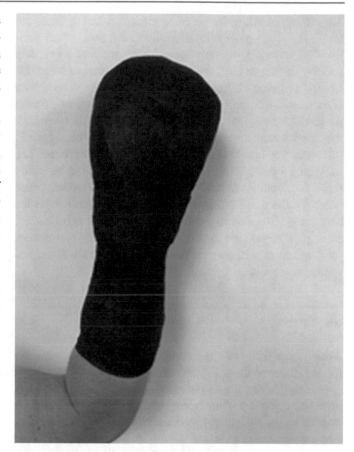

Fig. 58.4 The club cast is useful for non-skill position athletes for early return to competition. The concern is not reinjury to the athlete's original lesion but to protect the digit from the high forces of grasping as compared with those of a direct blow

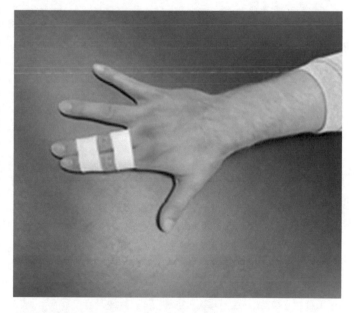

Fig. 58.5 Protective taping or bracing may be used to support fractures of the metacarpophalangeal joint. Buddy taping as pictured above may allow the athlete to return early to competition and limit reinjury to the involved digit

This does not allow for grasping objects with the digits but may allow for earlier return to play in the non-skilled positions in sports. A playing splint in the form of a properly padded short arm cast, with the MP joints free, can provide limited gripping ability and perhaps allow for more skilled activities within sports. Metacarpal fractures that are nondisplaced and stable can often be treated in a short arm cast with the injured metacarpal/finger taped to the adjacent finger. In this case, the injured finger is taped to the middle finger. The only time the index finger or the fifth finger should be buddy taped is if either of those fingers is actually injured. When possible, the middle finger should be buddy taped with the ring finger. The key to a safe return to play is to follow the principles mentioned earlier and to choose the appropriate playing cast that allows for acceptable function with appropriate protection.

Summary

Athletic injuries of the hand and wrist are common. Management of these injuries should be a multi-discipled approach. Ideally, the key to management of these injuries is prevention. Athletes are more at risk for certain injuries depending on the sport played. Previously described bracing and taping techniques are useful to prevent injury. Once injury occurs, knowledge of the injury and healing process is important. The key is to brace the hand or wrist in the position of protection but also function. Once healing of the injured hand and wrist has occurred, skilled rehabilitation of the injury is crucial. This requires close communication between all parties involved in the athlete's care. For example, the physical therapist and the strength and conditioning coach communicate to allow continuation of the athlete's strength and conditioning programming but also to limit traction to the involved extremity while healing. Finally, once the injury has been rehabilitated, protective playing casts and splints are useful to allow the athlete to return early to competition and to decrease the risk of reinjury.

References

1. Rettig AC. Athletic injuries of the wrist and hand. Part 1. Traumatic injuries of the wrist. Am J Sports Med. 2003;31:1038–48.
2. Geissler WB, Burkett JL. Ligamentous sports injuries of the hand and wrist. Sports Med Arthrosc Rev. 2014;22(1):39–44.
3. Zlotolow D, Bennett C. Athletic injuries of the hand and wrist. Curr Orthop Pract. 2008;19(2):206–11.
4. Cairns MA, Hasty EK, Herzog MM, Ostrum RF, Kerr ZY. Incidence, severity, and time loss associated with collegiate football fractures, 2004-2005 to 2013-2014. Am J Sports Med. 2018;46(4):987–94.
5. Bartels D, Hevesi M, Wyles C, Macalena JA, Kakar S, Krych AJ. Epidemiology of hand and wrist injuries in National Collegiate Athletic Association Football Players from 2009 to 2014: incidence and injury patterns…American Orthopaedic Society for Sports Medicine Annual Meeting, July 11-14, 2019, Boston, Massachusetts. Orthop J Sports Med. 2019;7:1–2.
6. Geissler WB. Arthroscopic management of scaphoid fractures in athletes. Hand Clin. 2009;25(3):359–69.
7. Freeland A. Hand fractures: repair, reconstruction, and rehabilitation. Philadelphia: Churchill Livingstone; 2000. p. 67.
8. Austin NM. The wrist and hand complex. In: Levangie PK, Norkin CC, editors. Joint structure and function: a comprehensive analysis. 5th ed. New York: McGraw-Hill; 2011.
9. Rettig M. Wrist fractures in the athlete. Distal radius and carpal fractures. Clin Sports Med. 1998;17(3):469–89.

Elbow Arthroscopy: Anatomy, Setup, Portals, and Positioning

59

Sonya M. Clark

Arthroscopy of the elbow is a technically challenging yet rewarding procedure. Elbow arthroscopy has greatly evolved since its introduction. Burman [1] initially described elbow arthroscopy in 1931, but it was not until more than 50 years later in 1985 when Andrews and Carson [2] described intra-articular elbow anatomy and the various portals used for elbow arthroscopy in the supine position. More recently, in 1989, the prone position for elbow arthroscopy was described by Poehling and colleagues [3].

Since its introduction, the indications and procedures performed with elbow arthroscopy have expanded. Elbow arthroscopy can be a safe and effective procedure, but it poses greater neurologic and technical challenges than arthroscopy of the shoulder and knee. There is potential for neurovascular injury because of the complex relationship of these structures to the joint (Fig. 59.1). To safely perform elbow arthroscopy, great familiarity of the normal elbow anatomy and surrounding neurovascular structures must be appreciated when making portals.

This chapter will provide a summary of the key anatomy, portal placement, and basic surgical setup and technique for elbow arthroscopy.

Anatomy

A comprehensive understanding of the anatomy of the elbow is essential before proceeding with elbow arthroscopy. Important bony anatomic landmarks include the medial and lateral epicondyles, the olecranon process, and the radial head. Anatomic landmarks should be palpated and marked prior to portal placement.

The soft spot, also known as the anconeus triangle, is located in the center of the triangle formed from the lateral

S. M. Clark (✉)
Upstate Hand Center, Spartanburg, SC, USA

© Springer Nature Switzerland AG 2022
W. B. Geissler (ed.), *Wrist and Elbow Arthroscopy with Selected Open Procedures*,
https://doi.org/10.1007/978-3-030-78881-0_59

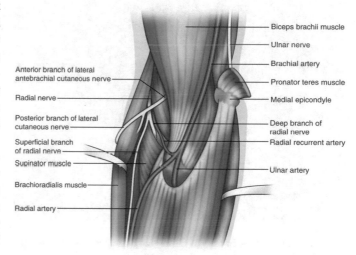

Fig. 59.1 Important neurovascular structures within the antecubital fossa

epicondyle, radial head, and olecranon process. The soft spot can be used to insufflate the joint prior to portal placements, and it can also be used as a direct lateral portal (Fig. 59.2).

Several sensory nerves surround the elbow, including the medial antebrachial cutaneous, the medial brachial cutaneous, the lateral antebrachial cutaneous, and the posterior antebrachial cutaneous nerves [4]. The medial antebrachial cutaneous nerve provides sensation to the medial aspect of the forearm and elbow. The medial brachial cutaneous nerve supplies sensation to the posteromedial aspect of the arm, to the level of the olecranon. The lateral antebrachial cutaneous nerve supplies sensation to the elbow and lateral aspect of the forearm. It is a branch of the musculocutaneous nerve and exits between the brachialis muscle and the biceps. The posterior antebrachial cutaneous nerve supplies sensation to the posterolateral elbow and posterior forearm. It is a branch of the radial nerve and courses down the lateral aspect of the arm [5].

The median, radial, and ulnar nerve and brachial artery are the main neurovascular structures around the elbow [4].

689

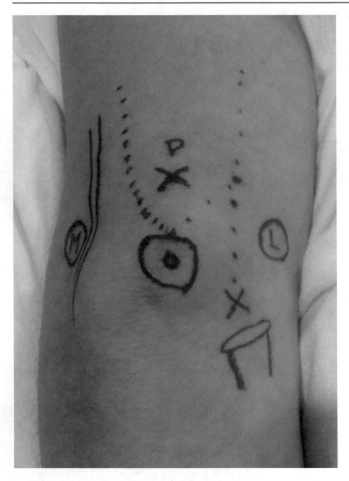

Fig. 59.2 Surface landmarks of the elbow. Posterior view. Medial epicondyle, ulnar nerve, and olecranon process are outlined in relation to elbow joint. X, soft spot portal; P, posterocentral portal

Indications and Contraindications

The indications for elbow arthroscopy are numerous and include both diagnostic and therapeutic indications. Diagnostic indications include septic arthritis, traumatic and degenerative arthritis, and intra-articular fractures [6, 7]. Therapeutic indications include the removal of loose bodies, synovectomy, capsular release, plica excision, treatment of osteochondritis dissecans, and tennis elbow release. New evolving indications include olecranon bursectomy and arthroscopic-assisted fracture management [8, 9].

Contraindications for elbow arthroscopy include any conditions that distort the normal soft tissue or normal bony anatomy, which prevents making accurate portal placement [10]. In patients with prior ulnar nerve transposition, or a subluxing ulnar nerve, the nerve should be identified prior to portal placement to prevent iatrogenic injury. Extensive heterotopic ossification, prior skin grafts or flaps, and burns preclude safe joint access and should be avoided [11].

Surgical Technique

Anesthesia

General or regional anesthesia may be used for elbow arthroscopy. Most surgeons prefer general anesthesia for elbow arthroscopy because of patient comfort and complete muscle relaxation. The use of regional anesthesia can complicate the postoperative neurologic assessment and can be compromised by the use of supraclavicular and extended axillary blocks [5].

Instrumentation

A standard 4.0-mm, 30° arthroscope provides exceptional visualization of the elbow joint. Sometimes a smaller 2.7 mm arthroscope may be useful for visualization in adolescent patients and in smaller viewing spaces, such as the direct lateral portal and in the posterior compartment [5, 8]. Cannulas are utilized to allow ease in switching working and viewing portals, without repeated joint capsule trauma. In addition, the risk of neurovascular injury is minimized when fewer portals are established. It is vital to maintain the arthroscopy portals with cannulas in order to decrease fluid extravasation into the soft tissues and swelling [5]. Maintaining capsular distention is key to successful elbow arthroscopy. If there is fluid extravasation into the soft tissues, the capsule will collapse and prevent further elbow arthroscopy.

In elbow arthroscopy, side-vented inflow cannulas should be avoided to prevent fluid extravasation into the soft tissues [12]. Only blunt-tipped and conical trocars should be used, to decrease the possibility of articular cartilage or neurovascular injury [8]. Specialized arthroscopic instruments, forceps, probes, shavers, and burrs, are utilized in elbow arthroscopy [5].

Gravity inflow or a mechanical pump can be used in elbow arthroscopy. Some surgeons think that gravity provides for enough joint distention while minimizing fluid extravasation. A mechanical pump can safely be used, but the inflow pressure should be minimized, no greater than 35 mmHg, in order to lessen fluid extravasation [5].

Patient Positioning

Supine Position
Andrews first described supine positioning for elbow arthroscopy in 1985 [2]. After adequate anesthesia has been obtained, care is taken to pad all bony prominences and place the shoulder at the edge of the operating table. The patient is positioned with the shoulder in 90° of abduction and 90° of

elbow flexion. The arm is then secured using an overhead traction device, and a non-sterile tourniquet is applied.

Supine positioning offers numerous advantages [13]. The supine setup is simple and allows for easy airway access for anesthesia. The anatomy is clearly defined and oriented in this familiar anatomic position. Furthermore, if the procedure needs to be converted to open, it's a simple task.

The weakness of the supine position includes the difficulty working in the posterior compartment and the need for an additional traction device.

Prone Position

Poehling first described the prone position for elbow arthroscopy in 1989 [3]. After adequate anesthesia has been obtained, the patient is rolled onto chest rolls. The nonoperative extremity is placed onto a well-padded arm board, with the shoulder in 90° of abduction and the elbow in 90° of flexion (Figs. 59.3 and 59.4). The operative extremity should be supported appropriately to allow the shoulder to be abducted 90° and the elbow hanging freely at 90° of flexion. This can be achieved by either a padded bolster or several rolled towels positioned on an arm board.

There are several advantages to the prone position. The posterior compartment is easily accessed without the need for traction. In addition, the arm can be effortlessly manipulated from full extension to full flexion. "Flexion of the elbow allows the neurovascular structures to sag anteriorly, providing a greater margin of error, when establishing anterior portal sites" [14].

The main disadvantage of the prone position is the general anesthesia requirement and poor airway access by anesthesia. Furthermore, conversion to an open procedure is much more difficult as compared to the supine position. Therefore, if anterior open procedures are necessary, this will require repositioning to a supine procedure.

Lateral Decubitus Position

O'Driscoll and Morrey first described the lateral decubitus position in 1993 [15].

After the patients are placed under general anesthesia on a bean bag, the patient is turned and secured in a lateral decubitus position. An axillary roll and non-sterile tourniquet is applied. The shoulder is flexed and internally rotated 90°. The arm is positioned on a padded arm holder, positioning the elbow in 90° of flexion (Fig. 59.5).

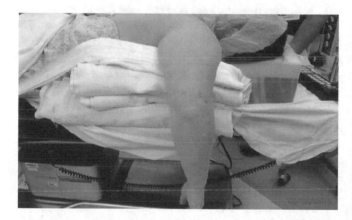

Fig. 59.3 Prone positioning with shoulder flexed and abducted 90° over a padded arm table with folded blankets

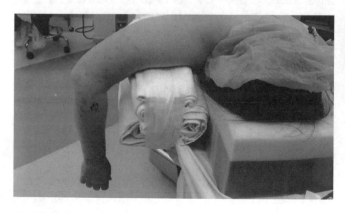

Fig. 59.4 Prone positioning for elbow arthroscopy

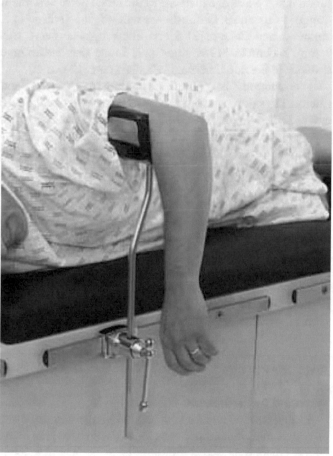

Fig. 59.5 Picture of arm holder for lateral position

The lateral decubitus position allows for the benefits of prone positioning, without the airway difficulty of the prone position. The disadvantage of the lateral decubitus position is the need for a padded arm holder and difficulty with converting to an open procedure.

Portals

Numerous portals have been described for elbow arthroscopy. The most common portals utilized are the anterolateral, proximal lateral, midlateral, anteromedial, proximal medial, and straight posterior [11].

Portal placement is key to visualization and protection of the nearby neurovascular structures. The initial portal utilized can be an area of debate but is a matter of surgeon preference. Some surgeons describe initial visualization in the posterior compartment, but most prefer to visualize the anterior compartment first [8, 16, 17]. The real debate rests in where to start anteriorly: anteromedially or anterolaterally.

Several authors have studied the distances from the portals to the various neurovascular structures. Knowledge about the distances between the portals and neurovascular structures is paramount because it helps to diminish the risk of injury. Using the anterolateral portal, Lynch et al. [18] found that the average distance to the radial nerve was 4 mm (range 3–10 mm) from the sheath of the arthroscope. Andrews and Carson [2] found that the radial nerve was 7 mm. Lidenfeld in his study [17] found that the average distance to the radial nerve was 3 mm (range, 2–5 mm).

The anteromedial portal, according to Andrews and Carson [2] study, showed the median nerve to be 10 mm away. Lynch et al. [18] found the median nerve to be 3–10 mm away, and Lidenfeld [17] measured an average distance of 11 mm to the median nerve (range, 10–12 mm).

Numerous authors have described beginning with an anteromedial approach to decrease the risk of injuring the neurovascular structures because the average distance between the median nerve and medial portals is greater than the distance between the lateral portals and the radial or posterior interosseous nerve [8, 16, 17, 19]. However, there are also many surgeons who initially create a lateral portal and then establish a medial portal either under direct visualization with a spinal needle or utilizing an inside-out technique with a switching stick [16].

Anterior Portals

Proximal Anterolateral Portal

Field and several authors [4, 20, 21] have described the proximal anterolateral portal as located 2 cm proximal to the lateral epicondyle and 2 cm anterior to the lateral epicon-

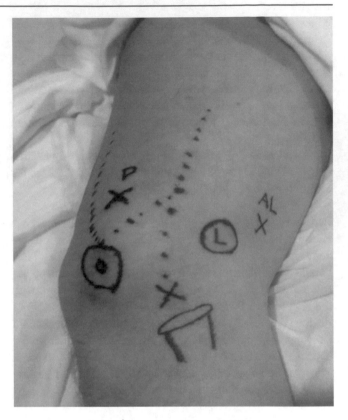

Fig. 59.6 Lateral view of bony landmarks and portals. AL, proximal anterolateral portal; X, direct lateral or soft spot portal; 0, olecranon process; P, posterocentral portal; L, lateral epicondyle

dyle or directly on the anterior humerus (Fig. 59.6). Visualization from this portal best illustrates the trochlea, tip of the coronoid the medial structures of the joint (Figs. 59.7 and 59.8). Investigators have illustrated that this portal is the safest anterolateral portal, as it is the furthest from the radial nerve [14].

Anterolateral Portal

In 1985, Carson and Andrews originally described the anterolateral portal as being located 3 cm distal and 2 cm anterior to the lateral epicondyle [2]. However, this portal places the radial nerve at risk for injury [18]. Several authors have described the radial nerve to be located an average 3–7 mm from the anterolateral portal [2, 17, 18]. In an effort to reduce iatrogenic injury, the original distal anterolateral portal should be avoided, and a more proximal anterolateral portal should be utilized. In 1994, Field and colleagues compared three lateral portals: the proximal anterolateral portal, a middle anterolateral portal, and the distal anterolateral portal. The anterolateral (distal) portal is closest to the radial nerve and should be avoided.

Middle Anterolateral Portal

Some refer to this portal as the anterior superolateral portal. This portal is described as 1–2 cm directly anterior to the

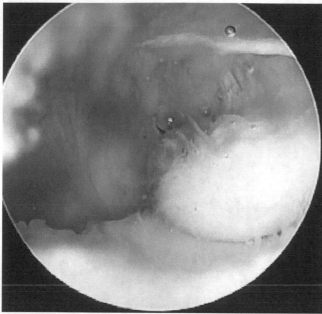

Fig. 59.7 Supine position: view from proximal anterior lateral portal

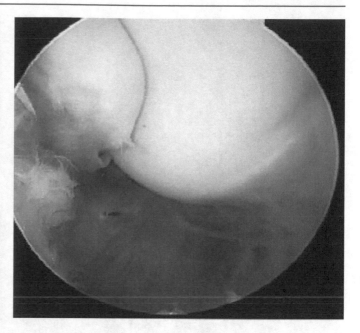

Fig. 59.9 Prone position: view from middle anterior lateral portal

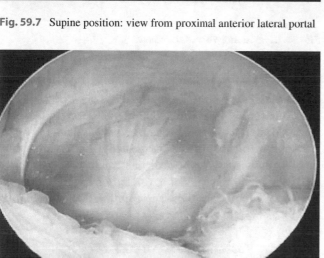

Fig. 59.8 Supine position: view from proximal anterior lateral portal, showing medial capsule

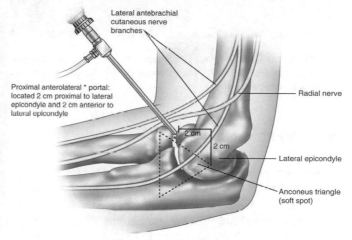

Fig. 59.10 Lateral view of the elbow in prone position

lateral epicondyle [14] (Fig. 59.9). This portal is ideal for arthroscopic lateral epicondyle release. The use of this portal increases the distance to the radial nerve, compared to the anterolateral portal (Fig. 59.10).

Proximal Anteromedial Portal

This portal is also known as the superomedial portal. Popularized by Poehling, it is located 2 cm proximal to the medial epicondyle and 2 cm anterior or just anterior to the intermuscular septum [3] (Fig. 59.11). The medial intermuscular septum should be palpated, and the portal is established anterior to the septum; this minimizes injury to the ulnar

nerve. This portal provides excellent visualization of the lateral elbow and radiocapitellar joint. The more proximal location of this portal allows the arthroscope to lie almost parallel to the median nerve when inserted and is considered safer than the anteromedial portal [5, 17].

Anteromedial Portal

This portal is located 2 cm anterior and 2 cm distal to the medial epicondyle [2]. This portal visualizes the proximal capsular insertion and lateral elbow joint. It is used primarily for instrumentation when working in the medial recess of the elbow [8]. The medial antebrachial cutaneous nerve is at risk when this portal is created.

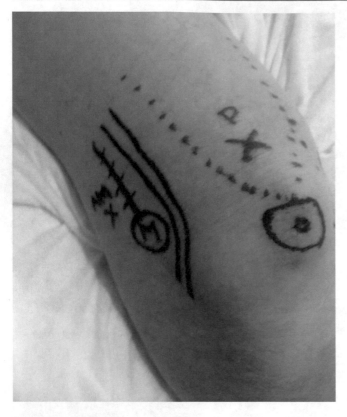

Fig. 59.11 Medial view of surface landmarks and portals. AM, proximal anteromedial portal; P, posterocentral portal. *Dashed line* marks intermuscular septum

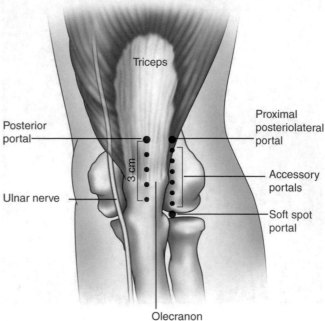

Fig. 59.12 Posterior view of the elbow

Posterior Portals

Posterocentral Portal

This portal is located 3 cm proximal to the tip of the olecranon. It passes within 23 mm of the posterior antebrachial cutaneous nerve and 25 mm within the ulnar nerve [4] (Fig. 59.12). It allows excellent visualization of the entire posterior compartment, and it pierces the triceps muscle just proximal to the musculotendinous junction [8]. To improve visualization when making this portal, the cannula and trocar are placed and maneuvered in a vigorous circular motion, to rid the soft tissues adherent in this area.

Proximal Posterolateral Portal

This portal, also known as the posterolateral portal, is located at the lateral border of the triceps tendon and 2–3 cm proximal to the tip of the olecranon. Usually, it is made under direct visualization with a spinal needle, with the arthroscope in the posterocentral portal. Once localized, a blunt trocar is placed aiming toward the olecranon fossa while passing through the triceps muscle. The olecranon tip, olecranon fossa, and posterior trochlea can be well visualized; however, initial visualization may be difficult because of synovi-

tis and fat pad hypertrophy, requiring initial debridement with a shaver. The posterior capitellum is not well visualized from this portal [4]. This portal is useful as a working portal for removal of loose bodies and osteophytes from the posterior compartment [7, 22]. The posterior and medial antebrachial cutaneous nerves average 25 mm from this portal [18]. The ulnar nerve is not at risk for injury, as long as the cannula is kept lateral to the posterior midline; it is approximately 25 mm from this portal [4].

Accessory Posterolateral Portals

Portal placement can be anywhere along a line, extending from the posterolateral portal to the soft spot portal, because of the unique posterolateral anatomy of the elbow.

Varying the portal position is useful for gaining access to the posterolateral recess and changing the orientation of the joint.

Direct Lateral Portal (Soft Spot Portal)

This portal is located at the center of the triangle formed by the lateral epicondyle, olecranon process, and radial head. Initially, it is used by many to insufflate the joint. Using a spinal needle, the portal is created under direct visualization. The posterior antebrachial cutaneous nerve passes approximately 7 mm from this portal. The portal is used as a working portal in radial head resection and osteochondritis dissecans lesions and a viewing portal for the posterior compartment [12]. Only this portal allows access and visualization of the radioulnar joint and posterior capitellum [5].

Conclusion

Arthroscopy of the elbow is an accepted surgical procedure for numerous elbow conditions [5]. In order to be successful in elbow arthroscopy, a thorough knowledge of the anatomy and portal placement is mandatory. The complexity of elbow arthroscopy procedures attempted should be determined by the individual surgeon's experience and skill level. Future advances in elbow arthroscopy will continue to emerge as clinical experience and new techniques and surgical equipment are refined.

References

1. Burman MS. Arthroscopy or the direct visualization of the joints: an experimental cadaveric study. J Bone Joint Surg. 1931;13:669–95.
2. Andrews JR, Carson WG. Arthroscopy of the elbow. Arthroscopy. 1985;1:97–107.
3. Poehling GG, Whipple TL, Sisco L, Goldman B. Elbow arthroscopy: a new technique. Arthroscopy. 1989;5:220–4.
4. Baker CL, Brooks AA. Arthroscopy of the elbow. Clin Sports Med. 1996;15:261–8.
5. Baker CL, Grant LJ. Arthroscopy of the elbow. Am J Sports Med. 1999;27:251–64.
6. Ramsey ML. Elbow arthroscopy: basic set up and treatment of arthritis. Instr Course Lect. 2002;51:69–72.
7. Savoie FH, Nunley PD, Field LD. Arthroscopic management of the arthritic elbow: indication, technique and results. J Shoulder Elb Surg. 1999;8:214–9.
8. Abboud JA, Ricchetti ET, Tjoumakaris F, Ramsey ML. Elbow arthroscopy: basic setup and portal placement. J Am Acad Orthop Surg. 2006;14:312–8.
9. Dodson CC, Nho SJ, Williams RJ, Altchek DW. Elbow arthroscopy. J Am Acad Orthop Surg. 2008;16(10):574–85.
10. O'Driscoll SW, Morrey BF. Arthroscopy of the elbow: diagnostic and therapeutic benefits and hazards. J Bone Joint Surg Am. 1992;74:84–94.
11. Walcott GD, Savoie FH, Field LD. Arthroscopy of the elbow: setup, portals and diagnostic technique. In: Altchek DW, Andrews J, editors. The athletes elbow. Philadelphia: Lippincott Williams and Wilkins; 2001. p. 249–73.
12. Ramsey ML, Naranja RJ. Diagnostic arthroscopy of the elbow. In: Baker Jr CL, Plancher DL, editors. Operative treatment of elbow injuries. New York: Springer; 2002. p. 162–9.
13. McKenzie PJ. Supine position. In: Savoie FH, Field LD, editors. Arthroscopy of the elbow. New York: Churchill Livingstone; 1996. p. 35–9.
14. Field LD, Altchek DW, Warren RF, O'Brien SJ, Skyhar MJ, Wickiewicz TL. Arthroscopic anatomy of the lateral elbow: a comparison of three portals. Arthroscopy. 1994;10:602–7.
15. Rubin CJ. Prone or lateral decubitus position. In: Savoie FH, Field LD, editors. Arthroscopy of the elbow. New York: Churchill Livingstone; 1996. p. 41–7.
16. Andrews JR, St. Pierre RK, Carson WG Jr. Arthroscopy of the elbow. Clin Sports Med. 1986;5:653–62.
17. Lindenfeld TN. Medial approach in elbow arthroscopy. Am J Sports Med. 1990;18:413–7.
18. Lynch GJ, Meyers JF, Whipple TL, Caspari RB. Neurovascular anatomy and elbow arthroscopy: inherent risks. Arthroscopy. 1986;2:191–7.
19. Verhaar J, Memeren HV, Brandsma A. Risks of neurovascular injury in elbow arthroscopy: starting anteromedially or anterolaterally? Arthroscopy. 1991;7:287–90.
20. Strothers D, Day B, Regan WR. Arthroscopy of the elbow: anatomy, portal sites, and description of the proximal lateral portal. Arthroscopy. 1995;11:449–57.
21. Savoie FH, Field LD. Anatomy. In: Savoie FH, Field LD, editors. Arthroscopy of the elbow. New York: Churchil Livingstone; 1996. p. 3–24.
22. Drabicki RR, Field LD, Savoie FH. Diagnostic elbow arthroscopy and loose body removal. In: Savoie FH, Field LD, editors. The elbow and wrist. Philadelphia: Elsevier; 2010. p. 17–24.

Arthroscopic Management of Elbow Contractures

60

Erich M. Gauger and Julie E. Adams

Introduction

The primary purpose of the elbow is to aid in the placement of the hand in space and act as a stabilizer during carrying, lifting, pushing, and pulling. The elbow must have mobility, stability, and strength and be pain-free to allow independent function [1]. The main focus of this chapter is to outline the surgical technique for arthroscopic management of elbow contracture to achieve sufficient mobility to carry out these functions.

Normal elbow range of motion in the sagittal plane (flexion-extension) is 0–145° [2]. There have been several papers addressing the functional range of motion of the elbow. Morrey et al. [3] demonstrated in 1981 that most activities of daily living can be accomplished with elbow flexion from 30° to 130° and 100° arc of pronosupination. More recent studies have utilized three-dimensional optical tracking system with results that have differed slightly [4–7]. Sardelli et al. [7] demonstrated a maximal flexion arc of 130° (23–142) for functional tasks (including cellular telephone tasks and typing on a keyboard). The definition of a stiff elbow varies by study with ranges from 30° to 40° of reduction in extension or flexion less than 105–130° [8, 9]. Davila et al. [1] point out that loss of extension can be compensated for by simply moving closer to an object while one cannot flex the wrist and neck enough to reach the face if elbow flexion is less than 105–110°.

Etiology and Classification

Causes of elbow contracture include posttraumatic issues, primary (rheumatoid arthritis, septic arthritis, osteoarthritis, hemophilic arthritis), congenital (arthrogryposis), burns, spasticity, head injury, stroke, and heterotopic ossification [1, 10]. It has been suggested that contracture types may be categorized into two types [11]. Intrinsic contractures are secondary to intra-articular pathology (incongruity, chondral defects, osteophytes, loose bodies, fracture malunion). Extrinsic causes are related to extra-articular pathology such as contracture of the ligaments and joint capsule, muscle contracture or adherence to the capsule, and heterotopic ossification. Most cases are mixed, with secondary extra-articular soft tissue contractures present in intrinsic contractures [11].

The elbow is vulnerable to stiffness for several potential reasons: (1) it possesses highly congruent articular surfaces comprising three joints (ulnotrochlear, radiocapitellar, proximal radioulnar) within a single joint capsule, which can thicken as much as 3–4 mm after injury; (2) it is vulnerable to heterotopic ossification formation after injury, possibly due to the brachialis muscle covering the anterior capsule; (3) prolonged immobilization is sometimes prescribed for complex fractures; and (4) the position of minimal intra-articular pressure and maximum compliance of the elbow is in 70° flexion—pain generation may occur with motion outside of this pressure nadir [1, 8, 12–15].

Surgical Indications and Contraindications

The main indication for arthroscopic management of elbow contracture is the loss of a functional arc of motion that persists after a period of conservative therapy consisting of physical therapy and/or splinting. During the preoperative evaluation, passive and active arc of motion should be assessed, as well as the quality of the end range of motion. A distinct block to range of motion may be due to impinging

E. M. Gauger
Orthopaedic Surgery, Allina Health, Coon Rapids and St Paul, Minneapolis, MN, USA

J. E. Adams (✉)
Department of Orthopedic Surgery, University of Tennessee College of Medicine – Chattanooga, Chattanooga, TN, USA

© Springer Nature Switzerland AG 2022
W. B. Geissler (ed.), *Wrist and Elbow Arthroscopy with Selected Open Procedures*,
https://doi.org/10.1007/978-3-030-78881-0_60

osteophytes or heterotopic ossification, whereas a more soft endpoint can be secondary to capsular contraction. Pain at the extremes of range of motion may indicate an osteophyte impinging in the olecranon fossa (extension) or the coronoid fossa (flexion). Although arthroscopic treatment can address intrinsic issues such as osteophytes, loose bodies, or contracture, the presence of arthritic pain throughout the arc of motion is suggestive of more widespread changes in the joint that may not be adequately addressed by arthroscopy. The status of the major peripheral nerves should be documented prior to surgery; specifically, many patients with elbow contracture may have concomitant ulnar neuropathy. Some patients may not specifically note ulnar nerve symptoms until they are brought to attention by specific query, examination, and provocative maneuvers. The location of the ulnar nerve is noted, and patients are examined for a subluxating ulnar nerve.

Imaging studies in general include three-view plain film radiographs of the elbow and consideration of axial imaging. CT scan particularly with three-dimensional reconstructions is specifically useful to identify bony areas of impingement which limit motion. MRI may be especially useful for assessment of chondral lesions and synovitis.

Contraindications to arthroscopic contracture release include factors that cannot be addressed by arthroscopy: severe heterotopic ossification, extrinsic disease such as contracture secondary to muscle spasticity, stroke or scar tissue (burns), and extensive widespread joint changes which may respond more appropriately to a joint resurfacing-type procedure. In addition, forearm pronation/supination can only be addressed in a limited fashion arthroscopically. Relative contraindications primarily relate to distorted anatomy such as prior ulnar nerve transposition—particularly submuscular—or the severely contracted elbow.

Surgical Technique

General anesthesia is preferred by most surgeons including the authors [16]. Patient positioning under regional anesthesia may be uncomfortable. The use of general anesthesia allows for immediate assessment and following of neurological function in the postoperative period.

Setup: Elbow arthroscopy can be performed with the patient in the supine, prone, or lateral decubitus positions [17]. The supine position was the first position described by Andrews and Carson [18]. There are several benefits to this position including ease of setup, excellent exposure of the anterior joint without viewing the anatomy "upside down," and direct access to the airway for the anesthesiologist. Unfortunately, the supine position requires the use of a traction device and an assistant to stabilize the elbow during the procedure as well as limits access to the posterior aspect of the joint. The prone position allows more freedom of movement and better access to the posterior aspect of the elbow if more invasive procedures are required including open debridement of olecranon osteophytes. Disadvantages include the difficulty in the actual positioning of the patient which requires careful attention to padding of bony prominences and the challenge of airway management. The lateral decubitus position allows for many of the advantages of the prone position without the anesthetic concerns and is the authors' preferred position. The patient can be positioned with the use of a bean bag and safety straps. After positioning, the arm is placed in an arm holder. The elbow should be slightly higher than the shoulder to prevent impingement of the arthroscopic instruments on the table [17]. The arm is inspected, insuring that there is complete access to the elbow with instruments and that it can be flexed and extended. Airplaning the bed slightly toward the surgeon allows for improved access to the elbow. A sterile or nonsterile tourniquet may be used.

Because fluid extravasation and edema can limit safety and working time, it is important to consider fluid management at the start of the procedure. Techniques to limit extravasation such as low pump pressures (25–35 mmHg) and low flow cannulas without side fenestrations as well as increased use of retractors to permit visualization instead of simply relying on joint distension may be helpful [16, 19]. In addition, early establishment of a working outflow site is critical to allow appropriate fluid control.

It is helpful to mark the anatomic landmarks on the skin before potential distortion from joint distension and edema caused by extravasation of saline [17, 20, 21]. The medial epicondyle and lateral epicondyles, radial head, olecranon medial intermuscular septum, and the path of the ulnar nerve are outlined [22]. Close attention should be paid to the location of the ulnar nerve, specifically noting if it subluxates. Intended portal sites are then marked out in relation to the anatomic landmarks.

Following inflation of the tourniquet, the elbow is insufflated with 20–30 ml of sterile saline into the joint with an 18G needle through an intended portal or via the center of a triangle bordered by the olecranon, lateral epicondyle, and radial head known as the "soft spot." Joint distension expands the joint to push the neurovascular structures away from the portal sites and facilitate entry into the joint [12, 17, 20, 21, 23]. Another step which has been suggested to decrease the risk of neurovascular injury is to place the portals with the elbow in flexion, which has been shown to increase the nerve to portal distance [24]. Gallay et al. [25] demonstrated that the stiff elbow has 15% the capsular compliance of a normal elbow and less ability for capsular distension with the volume of a normal elbow averaging 14 ml compared to 6 ml for a stiff elbow. Neurovascular structures are therefore at increased risk in the arthroscopic treatment of elbow contractures.

Portal Placement: There has been no demonstration of superiority for any given starting portal, but several points should be taken into consideration. Since the anterior compartment portals are in closer proximity to neurovascular structures, the argument is made that these portals should be placed first prior to excessive fluid extravasation. The choice between an anterior medial portal and anterior lateral portal is also based upon surgeon preference [18, 24, 26, 27]. The authors prefer starting anterolateral first. An 18G needle is placed just anterior to the radiocapitellar joint. This can be used to insufflate saline into the joint; extension of the elbow indicates intra-articular placement. The skin only is incised with a #15 blade, and blunt dissection down to the capsule proceeds with a hemostat, with a sudden egress of fluid indicating penetration of the capsule. The blunt trocar and cannula for a standard 4.0 or 4.5 mm arthroscope are placed.

The anteromedial portal, which generally lies 1 cm anterior and 1 cm medial to the medial epicondyle, is made with an inside-out technique. Once intra-articular placement of the trocar and cannula is confirmed either by bony feel or by visualization with the camera, the blunt trocar is replaced and driven over to the medial side to push out toward the skin. The portal site is made and a cannula is placed. A switching stick can be used during the procedure to switch the viewing and working portals.

Additional portals may be used for visualization or working or for retraction. The proximal anteromedial portal was described by Poehling et al. [26] 2 cm proximal to the prominence of the medial epicondyle and directly anterior to the medial intermuscular septum. This is the safest of all medial portals but offers the worst visualization of the radiocapitellar joint; it is very effective as a retractor portal [17].

The mid-anterolateral portal is placed 1 cm anterior to the prominence of the lateral epicondyle and just proximal to the radiocapitellar joint [28]. The proximal anterolateral portal is located 1–2 cm proximal and 1 cm anterior to the lateral epicondyle and penetrates the brachioradialis, brachialis, and extensor carpi radialis muscles. The proximal anterolateral portal provides excellent visualization of the radiocapitellar joint and may also be used for instrument or retractor placement. A "soft spot" portal can be used to visualize the radial head; it is made at the center of a triangle between the radial head, lateral epicondyle, and tip of the olecranon.

Once the anterolateral and anteromedial portals are made, the arthroscope is placed in the anterolateral portal and a shaver in the anteromedial portal. In general, bony work is completed prior to capsular work to limit fluid egress [19]. An arthroscopic shaver is utilized to debride intra-articular adhesions, thickened synovium, and plicae. The shaver is usually allowed to drain to the floor without suction, which could potentially pull in capsule or other tissues unintentionally. Loose bodies are removed with the shaver or appropri-

ately sized biter. The shaver should be aimed away from the capsule to prevent inadvertent injury to neurovascular structures. A burr can be used to remove osteophytes from the coronoid and radial head fossae. One key to visualization is the use of retractors in accessory portals. The capsule can be stripped off of the humerus with an elevator; if capsular resection is performed, it proceeds from a medial to lateral direction. Previous radial head fractures may distort local anatomy and create arthrofibrosis and adhesions between the capsule and radial nerve. Because of the close proximity of the radial nerve, resection of the anterior capsule within 2–3 cm of the radial head is avoided [19]. Unlike open procedures, in which capsulectomy is routinely performed, arthroscopic capsulectomy increases the risk of nerve injury and is not commonly performed; in the authors' hands, capsulotomy is typically adequate.

Posterior Compartment

Following completion of work in the anterior portion of the joint, attention is turned toward the posterior compartment. The direct posterior portal is the main working portal. It is made 2–3 cm proximal to the tip of the olecranon. Because this portal is through the thick triceps muscle, an incision is made with the blade down to the bone. This directly enters the posterior fossa and is a "potential" space. This is usually filled with fat and fibrous tissue. It is useful to use the blunt trocar to sweep the fossa to clear it and provide a space for visualization; it is usually necessary to shave the synovium to gain a view. The posterolateral portal is made level with the olecranon tip at the lateral joint line. It is most commonly used for visualization [17, 19, 29]. An additional retractor portal can be placed at any site away from the ulnar nerve [17].

After obtaining adequate visualization, facilitated by aggressive debridement of excess synovium at the olecranon fossa, bony work can proceed with removal of loose bodies and burring of osteophytes, particularly within the olecranon fossa but also along the tip and sides of the olecranon. Caution should be exercised in the posteromedial aspect of the joint, as the ulnar nerve is located directly adjacent to the capsule; the shaver should be aimed away from the capsule while facing that area. The elbow is repeatedly flexed and extended while looking for impingement of the olecranon within the fossa. Keener et al. [30] demonstrated that 12–14 mm of the olecranon tip can be resected without injuring the insertion of the triceps. Capsular release can be performed with a blunt trocar to elevate the capsule off the posterior humerus, arthroscopic biter, or sharp dissection. Capsular release is completed when the triceps is visualized at which time any adhesions between the capsule and triceps can be disrupted.

Ulnar Nerve

Special consideration must be given to the ulnar nerve when surgically managing an elbow contracture. In a cadaver study, Gelberman et al. [31] demonstrated that elbow flexion led to decreased cubital tunnel volume and increased intraneural pressure. Williams et al. [32] conducted a retrospective review of 164 consecutive patients who underwent open or arthroscopic release of a contracted elbow and found that 15.2% of patients with preoperative flexion ≤100° had new-onset post-procedure ulnar nerve symptoms compared to 3.7% patients with preoperative flexion >100°. This supports previous recommendations to decompress the ulnar nerve if there is less than 90–100° of preoperative flexion or if the patient had symptoms consistent with ulnar nerve compression at the elbow [10, 22, 33]. Typically, decompression has been accomplished through an open approach that can allow concurrent release of the posteromedial capsule [10, 33] or the posterior bundle of the medial collateral ligament [22]. Ruch et al. [34] showed that open release of the posterior and transverse bundles of the medial collateral ligament can be performed without compromise of elbow stability. Recently, there has been evidence to suggest that arthroscopic ulnar nerve decompression is possible [35]. The technique involves utilizing a posterolateral portal for viewing and a direct posterior portal for initial debridement with a shaver followed by a smooth biter to carefully resect capsule from 3 to 4 cm proximal to the medial epicondyle to the posterior edge of the medial collateral ligament [35].

Postoperative Management

At the conclusion of the procedure, the arthroscope is removed, and excess fluid is "milked" out of the joint, portals are closed with nylon sutures, and elbow range of motion is carefully assessed with a goniometer prior to applying a sterile compressive dressing. The goal of postoperative rehabilitation is to maintain or improve the range of motion measured at the completion of the procedure. There is no single protocol for the contracted elbow; depending on the severity of the contracture and patient compliance, therapy programs are individualized. Typically, each elbow is placed in a posterior slab splint in full extension with the extremity elevated and judicious use of ice for edema control. The splint is removed on the first postoperative day at which time range of motion commences. For minimal contractures and a compliant patient, instruction in a home physical therapy regimen including active and passive range of motion exercises may be all that is required; most patients are referred to physiotherapy and find it useful. For more substantial contractures, a nighttime static progressive splint may be beneficial. For severe contractures or noncompliant patients, one can con-

sider continuous passive motion (CPM) machines. However, recent evidence questions the efficacy of CPM use after open elbow contracture release [36]. If CPM is utilized, it is necessary to use the full range of motion, necessitating satisfactory pain control with narcotics, continuous regional anesthetics, or local anesthetic by continuous infusion [37]. One potential issue with CPM use under regional block is the potential for ongoing nerve irritation (i.e., the ulnar nerve), which is masked by the regional anesthesia.

Outcomes and Complications

There have been no randomized control trials evaluating arthroscopic elbow contracture release, but there does exist a substantial body of literature suggesting that arthroscopic release improves range of motion [38–51] (Table 60.1). Arthroscopic debridement has been shown to improve range of motion and pain in a cohort of 35 professional athletes with elbow osteoarthritis. All athletes returned to their sport, and 18 continued to participate in high-level competitions with 5 patients winning national or international competitions [50].

Only one study directly compared open versus arthroscopic elbow contracture release in the setting of osteoarthritis; outcomes and complication rates are comparable, and both procedures can yield reliable improvements in elbow range of motion [52]. Likewise, when examining the literature with respect to open and arthroscopic releases, the outcomes appear to be similar [53–58].

While elbow arthroscopy has been utilized for a variety of clinical problems, it remains a technically challenging procedure with the potential for serious complications given the proximity of important neurovascular structures. Injury to each of the susceptible peripheral nerves about the elbow has been reported following elbow arthroscopy; injury is probably underreported. In addition, certain diagnoses or conditions confer what appears to be an increased risk with this procedure. In a series from the Mayo Clinic, transient nerve palsies were noted in 12 of 473 elbow arthroscopies [16]. Statistically significant factors associated with injury included diagnosis of contracture and performing a capsular release [16]. Posttraumatic contractures are also subject to distortion of bony and/or soft tissue landmarks, which may make neurovascular structures more vulnerable to injury [38]. Compartment syndrome has been shown to be an infrequent, albeit devastating complication of the procedure [59]. Kim et al. [60] studied the learning curve for arthroscopic treatment for limitation of elbow range of motion and found a statistically significant decrease in operative time after the initial 15 patients and that operative time was negatively correlated with range of motion. Interestingly, increasing surgeon experience did not correlate with post-

Table 60.1 Literature regarding contracture release

Author (Year)	# pts	Surgical indication	Exclusion criteria	Mean F/U (mos)	Mean flexion (°)			Mean extension (°)			Improve arc of motion	Complications	Comments
					Pre-op	Post-op	Improve	Pre-op	Post-op	Improve			
Jones and Savoie [13]	12	Flexion contracture and failed nonoperative tx: ≥3 Mos of PT and splinting		22	106	138	32	−38	−3	35	67	1 permanent PIN palsy required surgical intervention 1 MUA 3 weeks post-op	
Timmerman and Andrews [39]	19	Posttraumatic pain and stiffness that failed conservative therapy, minimum 15° flexion contracture	Arthroscopic finding of loose bodies or osteophytes without capsular or soft tissue scarring	2	123	134	11	−29	−11	18	29	1 repeat arthroscopic procedure for debridement. 1 open arthrotomy 5 mos after arthroscopic procedure	
Byrd [40]	5	Dysfunction due to limited ROM secondary to radial head fx. No improvement with PT		24	124	138	14	−41	−11	30	44	None	
Kim et al. [41]	25	ADL disrupted due to lack of elbow ROM with no improvement after 6 mos PT	Rheumatoid arthritis, PVNS	25	113	130	17	−21	−14	7	24	2 cases transient median nerve palsy 1 arthroscopic burr breakage	
Phillips and Strasburger [42]	25	Arthrofibrosis		18	118	137	19	−31	−7	24	41	1 reoperation due to inadequate capsular release with continued stiffness/pain	
Savoie et al. [43]	24	Painful restricted motion due to arthritic process refractory to 3–6 mos nonop tx		32	90	139	49	−40	−8	32	81	1 portal site infection: Resolved with Abx, HO in 1 patient, 2 pts. with recurrent effusion with 1 requiring excision radial head	Arthroscopic modification of the open Outerbridge-Kashiwagi procedure
Kim and Shin [44]	63	ADL disrupted due to lack of elbow ROM with no improvement after 3 mos PT	Arthrofibrosis caused by inflammatory disease and tuberculous arthritis	42.5	108	131	23	−29	−9	20	43	2 cases transient median nerve palsy	
Ball et al. [45]	14	Restricted elbow ROM interfered with ADL and did not improve with nonop tx	Sig intrinsic disease, primary degenerative or inflammatory arthritis, posttraumatic HO	≥12	117.5	133	15.5	−35.4	−9.3	26.1	50	1 portal site infection: Resolved with Abx and I&D	

(continued)

Table 60.1 (continued)

Author (Year)	# pts	Surgical indication	Exclusion criteria	Mean F/U (mos)	Mean flexion (°)			Mean extension (°)			Improve arc of motion	Complications	Comments
					Pre-op	Post-op	Improve	Pre-op	Post-op	Improve			
Lapner et al. [46]	20	Undisplaced radial head fx with failure of ≥6 mos therapy and <30–130° ROM or pain		54	130	137	7	−22	−10	12	9	None	Incomplete data on 8 pts. lost to follow-up
Nguyen et al. [47]	22	Failure of nonsurgical tx for >6 mos and interference with ADL, avocation, sports, or hobbies	Insufficient nonsurgical tx, active infection, inadequate motion or skin coverage, post-op compliance, HO, poor articular surfaces	25	122	141	19	−38	−19	19	38	No major neurovascular complications Medial antebrachial cutaneous nerve neuroma 3 pts. portal tenderness	1 patient with pre-op flexion 75° developed ulnar neuropathy, resolved by 3-year follow-up
Kelly et al. [48]	24	Degenerative arthritis with impingement with an average of 56 mos nonoperative tx		67	111	132	21	−20	−9	11	32	None	
Somanchi and Funk [49]	22	Painful or stiff elbow with or without locking episodes after a period of failed nonoperative tx		25	132	138	6	−26.6	−24	2.6	18	2 ulnar neuropathy: 1 resolved spontaneously, 1 resolved after decompression	
Yan et al. [50]	35	Pain that affected their athletic training with failed conservative therapy for >3 mos		43	125	134	9	−14	−7	7	16	2 pts. with residual loose bodies with 1 pt. returning to OR. 1 transient ulnar neuropathy	All patients were professional athletes (mostly wrestling, judo, weight lifting)
Cefo and Eygendaal [51]	27	Symptomatic loss of flexion or extension >20° despite 6 mos PT	Unable to comply with post-op rehab protocol, sig intrinsic disease, HO, primary degenerative or inflammatory arthritis, previous ulnar nerve decompression, required hardware removal	3	123	133	10	−24	−7	17	26	1 portal site infection: Resolved with Abx	

Tx treatment, *PT* physical therapy, *ROM* range of motion, *MUA* manipulation under anesthesia, *PIN* posterior interosseous nerve, *Tx* treatment, *fx* fracture, *ADL* activities of daily living, *mos* months, *F/U* follow-up, *PVNS* pigmented villonodular synovitis, *sig* significant, *HO* heterotopic ossification, *pts.* patients, *I&D* irrigation and debridement, *abx* antibiotics, *OR* operating room

operative motion and clinical outcomes; the authors theorize that this is related to the influence of "case mix" or the tendency for a surgeon to treat more difficult cases as they become more proficient [60].

References

1. Davila SA, Johnston-Jones K. Managing the stiff elbow: operative, nonoperative, and postoperative techniques. J Hand Ther. 2006;19(2):268–81.
2. O'Driscoll S. Arthroscopic osteocapsular arthroplasty. In: Yamaguchi K, O'Driscoll S, King G, McKee M, editors. Advanced reconstruction elbow. 1st ed. Rosemont: American Academy of Orthopaedic Surgeons; 2007.
3. Morrey BF, Askew LJ, Chao EY. A biomechanical study of normal functional elbow motion. J Bone Joint Surg Am. 1981;63(6):872–7.
4. Magermans DJ, Chadwick EK, Veeger HE, van der Helm FC. Requirements for upper extremity motions during activities of daily living. Clin Biomech (Bristol, Avon). 2005;20(6):591–9.
5. Henmi S, Yonenobu K, Masatomi T, Oda K. A biomechanical study of activities of daily living using neck and upper limbs with an optical three-dimensional motion analysis system. Mod Rheumatol. 2006;16(5):289–93.
6. Pieniazek M, Chwala W, Szczechowicz J, Pelczar-Pieniazek M. Upper limb joint mobility ranges during activities of daily living determined by three dimensional motion analysis: preliminary report. Ortop Traumatol Rehabil. 2007;9(4):413–22.
7. Sardelli M, Tashjian RZ, MacWilliams BA. Functional elbow range of motion for contemporary tasks. J Bone Joint Surg Am. 2011;93(5):471–7.
8. Hotchkiss R. Elbow contracture. In: Green D, Hotchkiss R, Pederson W, Wolfe S, editors. Green's operative hand surgery. 5th ed. New York: Churchill-Livingstone; 2005. p. 667.
9. Søjbjerg JO. The stiff elbow. Acta Orthop Scand. 1996;67(6):626–31.
10. Blonna D, Bellato E, Marini E, Scelsi M, Castoldi F. Arthroscopic treatment of stiff elbow. ISRN Surg. 2011;2011:378135.
11. Morrey BF. Post-traumatic contracture of the elbow. Operative treatment, including distraction arthroplasty. J Bone Joint Surg Am. 1990;72(4):601–18.
12. Lindenhovius AL, Linzel DS, Doornberg JN, Ring DC, Jupiter JB. Comparison of elbow contracture release in elbows with and without heterotopic ossification restricting motion. J Shoulder Elb Surg. 2007;16(5):621–5.
13. Tucker SA, Savoie FH 3rd. FH, O'Brien MJ. Arthroscopic management of the post-traumatic stiff elbow. J Shoulder Elb Surg. 2011;20(2 Suppl):S83–9.
14. Nirschl R, Morrey B. Rehabilitation. In: Morrey B, editor. The elbow and its disorders. 3rd ed. Philadelphia: Saunders; 2000. p. 141.
15. Morrey B. Splints and bracing at the elbow. In: Morrey B, editor. The elbow and its disorders. 3rd ed. Philadelphia, PA: Saunders; 2000. p. 150–4.
16. Kelly EW, Morrey BF, O'Driscoll SW. Complications of elbow arthroscopy. J Bone Joint Surg Am. 2001;83-A(1):25–34.
17. Steinmann S. Elbow arthroscopy. J Am Soc Surg Hand. 2003;3:199–207.
18. Andrews JR, Carson WG. Arthroscopy of the elbow. Arthroscopy. 1985;1(2):97–107.
19. Keener JD, Galatz LM. Arthroscopic management of the stiff elbow. J Am Acad Orthop Surg. 2011;19(5):265–74.
20. Adams JE, Steinmann SP. Nerve injuries about the elbow. J Hand Surg Am. 2006;31(2):303–13.
21. Lynch GJ, Meyers JF, Whipple TL, Caspari RB. Neurovascular anatomy and elbow arthroscopy: inherent risks. Arthroscopy. 1986;2(3):190–7.
22. Van Zeeland NL, Yamaguchi K. Arthroscopic capsular release of the elbow. J Shoulder Elb Surg. 2010;19(2 Suppl):13–9.
23. O'Driscoll SW, Morrey BF. Arthroscopy of the elbow diagnostic and therapeutic benefits and hazards. J Bone Joint Surg Am. 1992;74(1):84–94.
24. Stothers K, Day B, Regan W. Arthroscopy of the elbow: anatomy, portal sites, and a description of the proximal lateral portal. Arthroscopy. 1995;11(4):449–57.
25. Gallay SH, Richards RR, O'Driscoll SW. Intraarticular capacity and compliance of stiff and normal elbows. Arthroscopy. 1993;9(1):9–13.
26. Poehling GG, Whipple TL, Sisco L, Goldman B. Elbow arthroscopy: a new technique. Arthroscopy. 1989;5(3):222–4.
27. Lindenfeld TN. Medial approach in elbow arthroscopy. Am J Sports Med. 1990;18(4):413–7.
28. Field L, Altchek D, Warren R. Arthroscopic anatomy of the lateral elbow: a comparison of three portals. Arthroscopy. 1994;10(6):602–7.
29. Yamaguchi K, Tashjian R. Setup and portals. In: Yamaguchi K, O'Driscoll S, King G, McKee M, editors. Advanced reconstruction elbow. Rosemont: American Academy of Orthopaedic Surgery; 2007. p. 3–11.
30. Keener J, Chafik D, Kim H, Galatz L, Yamaguchi K. Insertional anatomy of the triceps brachii tendon. J Shoulder Elb Surg. 2010;19(3):399–405.
31. Gelberman RH, Yamaguchi K, Hollstien SB, Winn SS, Heidenreich FP Jr, Bindra RR, et al. Changes in interstitial pressure and cross-sectional area of the cubital tunnel and of the ulnar nerve with flexion of the elbow an experimental study in human cadavera. J Bone Joint Surg Am. 1998;80(4):492–501.
32. Williams BG, Sotereanos DG, Baratz ME, Jarrett CD, Venouziou AI, Miller MC. The contracted elbow: is ulnar nerve release necessary? J Shoulder Elb Surg. 2012;21(12):1632–6.
33. Sahajpal D, Choi T, Wright TW. Arthroscopic release of the stiff elbow. J Hand Surg Am. 2009;34(3):540–4.
34. Ruch DS, Shen J, Chloros GD, Krings E, Papadonikolakis A. Release of the medial collateral ligament to improve flexion in post-traumatic elbow stiffness. J Bone Joint Surg Br. 2008;90(5):614–8.
35. Kovachevich R, Steinmann SP. Arthroscopic ulnar nerve decompression in the setting of elbow osteoarthritis. J Hand Surg Am. 2012;37(4):663–8.
36. Lindenhovius AL, van de Luijtgaarden K, Ring D, Jupiter J. Open elbow contracture release: postoperative management with and without continuous passive motion. J Hand Surg Am. 2009;34(5):858–65.
37. O'Driscoll SW, Giori NJ. Continuous passive motion (CPM): theory and principles of clinical application. J Rehabil Res Dev. 2000;37(2):179–88.
38. Jones GS. Savoie 3rd FH. Arthroscopic capsular release of flexion contractures (arthrofibrosis) of the elbow. Arthroscopy. 1993;9(3):277–83.
39. Timmerman LA, Andrews JR. Arthroscopic treatment of posttraumatic elbow pain and stiffness. Am J Sports Med. 1994;22(2):230–5.
40. Byrd JW. Elbow arthroscopy for arthrofibrosis after type I radial head fractures. Arthroscopy. 1994;10(2):162–5.
41. Kim SJ, Kim HK, Lee JW. Arthroscopy for limitation of motion of the elbow. Arthroscopy. 1995;11(6):680–3.
42. Phillips BB, Strasburger S. Arthroscopic treatment of arthrofibrosis of the elbow joint. Arthroscopy. 1998;14(1):38–44.
43. Savoie FH 3rd, Nunley PD, Field LD. Arthroscopic management of the arthritic elbow: indications, technique, and results. J Shoulder Elb Surg. 1999;8(3):214–9.

44. Kim SJ, Shin SJ. Arthroscopic treatment for limitation of motion of the elbow. Clin Orthop Relat Res. 2000;375:140–8.

45. Ball CM, Meunier M, Galatz LM, Calfee R, Yamaguchi K. Arthroscopic treatment of post-traumatic elbow contracture. J Shoulder Elb Surg. 2002;11(6):624–9.

46. Lapner PC, Leith JM, Regan WD. Arthroscopic debridement of the elbow for arthrofibrosis resulting from nondisplaced fracture of the radial head. Arthroscopy. 2005;21(12):1492.

47. Nguyen D, Proper SI, MacDermid JC, King GJ, Faber KJ. Functional outcomes of arthroscopic capsular release of the elbow. Arthroscopy. 2006;22(8):842–9.

48. Kelly EW, Bryce R, Coghlan J, Bell S. Arthroscopic debridement without radial head excision of the osteoarthritic elbow. Arthroscopy. 2007;23(2):151–6.

49. Somanchi BV, Funk L. Evaluation of functional outcome and patient satisfaction after arthroscopic elbow arthrolysis. Acta Orthop Belg. 2008;74(1):17–23.

50. Yan H, Cui G, Wang J, Yin Y, Ao Y. Arthroscopic debridement of osteoarthritic elbow in professional athletes. Chin Med J. 2011;124(24):4223–8.

51. Cefo I, Eygendaal D. Arthroscopic arthrolysis for posttraumatic elbow stiffness. J Shoulder Elb Surg. 2011;20(3):434–9.

52. Cohen AP, Redden JF, Stanley D. Treatment of osteoarthritis of the elbow: a comparison of open and arthroscopic debridement. Arthroscopy. 2000;16(7):701–6.

53. Charalambous CP, Morrey BF. Posttraumatic elbow stiffness. J Bone Joint Surg Am. 2012;94(15):1428–37.

54. Urbaniak JR, Hansen PE, Beissinger SF, Aitken MS. Correction of post-traumatic flexion contracture of the elbow by anterior capsulotomy. J Bone Joint Surg Am. 1985;67(8):1160–4.

55. Husband JB, Hastings H 2nd. The lateral approach for operative release of post-traumatic contracture of the elbow. J Bone Joint Surg Am. 1990;72(9):1353–8.

56. Marti RK, Kerkhoffs GM, Maas M, Blankevoort L. Progressive surgical release of a posttraumatic stiff elbow. Technique and outcome after 2–18 years in 46 patients. Acta Orthop Scand. 2002;73(2):144–50.

57. Tan V, Daluiski A, Simic P, Hotchkiss RN. Outcome of open release for post-traumatic elbow stiffness. J Trauma. 2006;61(3):673–8.

58. Katolik LI, Cohen MS. Anterior interosseous nerve palsy after open capsular release for elbow stiffness: report of 2 cases. J Hand Surg Am. 2009;34(2):288–91.

59. Angelo RL. Advances in elbow arthroscopy. Orthopedics. 1993;16(9):1037–46.

60. Kim SJ, Moon HK, Chun YM, Chang JH. Arthroscopic treatment for limitation of motion of the elbow: the learning curve. Knee Surg Sports Traumatol Arthrosc. 2011;19(6):1013–8.

Radial Head Arthroplasty

Leigh-Anne Tu, Michael N. Nakashian, and Mark E. Baratz

Introduction

Radial head and neck fractures are among the most common elbow fractures and account for approximately one-third of all elbow fractures in adult patients [1]. The vast majority of patients are between 20 and 64 years of age with no gender predominance; however, the mean age of male patients is typically younger than female patients [1, 2]. The mechanism of injury that leads to a fracture is a fall onto an outstretched arm with the forearm in pronation and the elbow partially flexed. This action drives the radial head into the capitellum causing it to fracture. In 1954, Mason classified radial head fractures into three types [3]. Type I fractures are nondisplaced. Type II fractures are marginal fractures with displacement, impaction, or angulation. Type III fractures are comminuted fractures involving the entire radial head (Fig. 61.1). In 1962, a fourth type was added to this classification system by Johnston to include a fracture with dislocation. A Type IV injury involves a radial head fracture with a concomitant ulnohumeral (UH) dislocation (Fig. 61.2). In 1987, Broberg and Morrey added a metric definition of displacement (<2 mm or >2 mm) and an area of involvement of the articular surface (>30%) to differentiate between Mason types I and II fractures [4]. The Mason classification, however, has shown low interobserver and intraobserver reliability; hence, it is difficult to derive conclusive treatment algorithms using this classification system [5].

Although nondisplaced fractures typically occur in isolation, displaced fractures commonly occur with associated injuries. In fact, radial head fractures have been reported to occur with associated lesions in almost one-third of cases [6, 7]. Injuries to the medial and lateral collateral ligaments, interosseous ligament, olecranon, coronoid, and capitellum, as well as associated elbow dislocation, can all have a detrimental effect on elbow stability. It has been reported that injury to the medial collateral ligament is associated with comminuted radial head fractures 85–91% of the time and injury to the interosseous ligament 9% of the time [8]. Therefore, the treatment of radial head fractures must be individualized, considering both patient factors and associated injuries.

In general, nonoperative treatment with early range of motion is indicated for nondisplaced or minimally displaced fractures. These fractures are associated with good or excellent results, and many studies have demonstrated most patients achieving full function and recovery of range of motion of the elbow after injury [9–11]. In contrast, there is more variability with treatment of displaced or comminuted radial head and neck fractures. Radial head resection for comminuted fractures has been described for the treatment in the absence of valgus instability of the elbow or axial instability of the forearm [12, 13]. We cannot recommend head resection in the face of acute radial head fractures for two reasons: the degree of associated injury to the soft tissue stabilizers of the elbow may not be immediately quantifiable; the radial head tensions the lateral complex augmenting a primary stabilizer of the elbow and, of course, functions as an important secondary stabilizer [14, 15]. Radial head excision is more widely used as a delayed procedure, particularly when head deformity leads to loss of rotation or when there is post-traumatic arthritis of the radiocapitellar joint. Even in the best circumstance, radial head resection leads to several millimeters of proximal radial migration, mild cubitus valgus, and increased load across the ulnohumeral joint with a concomitant increase in the incidence of ulnohumeral arthritis [16].

L.-A. Tu (✉)
Department of Orthopedics, University of Pittsburgh Medical Center, Bethel Park, PA, USA

M. N. Nakashian
Brielle Orthopaedics at Rothman Institute, Brick Township, NJ, USA

M. E. Baratz
Department of Orthopedic Surgery, University of Pittsburgh Medical Center, Bethel Park, PA, USA

© Springer Nature Switzerland AG 2022
W. B. Geissler (ed.), *Wrist and Elbow Arthroscopy with Selected Open Procedures*,
https://doi.org/10.1007/978-3-030-78881-0_61

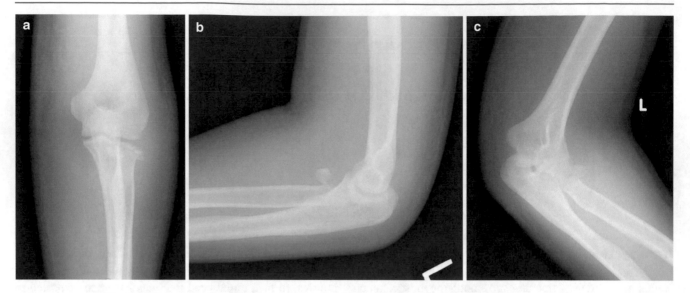

Fig. 61.1 Type III radial head fracture with complete articular comminution and displacement. AP (**a**), lateral (**b**), and oblique radiocapitellar views (**c**)

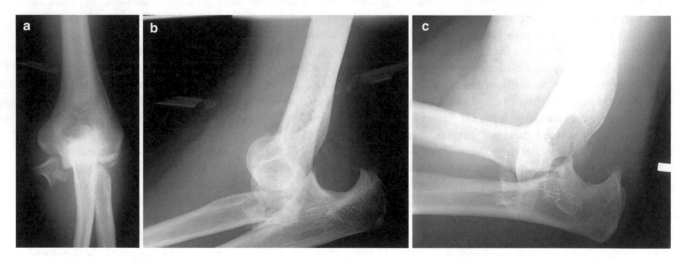

Fig. 61.2 Type IV radial head fracture demonstrates a comminuted radial head fracture with an ulnohumeral dislocation. AP (**a**), lateral (**b**), and oblique radiocapitellar views (**c**)

The design of new implants has changed treatment. Headless screws, small headed screws, and smaller, low profile plates have improved our ability to repair comminuted fractures [17]. Improved results have been reported with open reduction internal fixation (ORIF) of simple partially displaced radial head fractures. However, results from repairing comminuted fractures and especially those with more than three fragments are less reproducible [18]. Ultimately, the goal of ORIF is to achieve an acceptable reduction with a stable construct that allows protected forearm rotation and elbow motion in the first 5–7 days following surgery. If this cannot be reliably achieved, then arthroplasty should be considered.

Indications

Radial head arthroplasty (RHA) is a valuable addition to the surgeon's armamentarium for complex, comminuted radial head fractures with associated elbow instability. Normally the radiocapitellar (RC) joint bears 57% of the axial load across the elbow joint [19] and 88% of the load with valgus stress [20]. These facts underscore the importance of retaining or replacing the radial head in order to maintain normal joint reactive forces.

In those instances, where a fracture of the radial head is not repairable and excision is not considered to be optimal due to potential instability, RHA is a reliable method to reestablish radiocarpal mechanics. Injury to the lateral ulnar collateral ligament (LUCL) complex and ulnar collateral ligament (UCL) will lead to greater elbow instability if the radial head is not replaced and the ligaments are not repaired. Similarly, injury to the interosseous membrane will lead to longitudinal forearm instability without restoration of the radial head. The majority of these associated ligamentous injuries occur with Mason type III radial head fractures [7].

Nonunion or malunion after radial head or neck fracture can be troublesome for a patient and lead to articular incongruity. RHA can also be used in cases of nonunion or malunion to restore the anatomy and biomechanics of the elbow. The results of using RHA for chronic post-traumatic elbow disorders have proven safe and durable with a functional range of motion [21].

Contraindications

Contraindications to radial head arthroplasty include local or regional infection and inadequate bone stock. A simple, repairable fracture should be a contraindication to RHA as these fractures should be treated with open reduction internal fixation to preserve the native radial head.

Relative contraindications include severe ulnohumeral and radiocapitellar arthritis. In fractures that extend beyond the bicipital tuberosity, attempts to use a radial head implant may result in mismatch of the rotational axis of the implant and capitellum. Patient factors should also be considered, including skeletally immature patients, and patients who are cognitively incapable of following the postoperative protocol may not be candidates for radial head arthroplasty.

Preoperative Planning: Implant Choice

The current radial head implants used today are metal, consisting of either cobalt-chromium or titanium. These metallic implants are thought to be superior to the earlier silicone designs because of their ability to restore axial and valgus stability. There are a few options when considering implant choice including loose-fitting stems (smooth) and fixed stems (press-fit or cemented) as well as monopolar vs. bipolar designs.

A loose-fitting stem generally allows the implant to settle into a position that best recreates the native head-neck relationship. During pronation, the proximal radius moves anterior and medial with respect to the capitellum. During supination, the radius moves posterior and lateral. With a loose-fitting stem, the radial head engages the capitellum, while the proximal radius translates with respect to stem. Given that these implants are intentionally loose, the devel-

opment of lucency around the stem is unavoidable. However, good short- and intermediate-term results have been reported with this stem design [22, 23].

Fixed stems achieve a tight fit within the intramedullary canal; therefore correct positioning is mandatory. The heads are designed to replicate the concavity and eccentricity of the native radial head. If the head design or placement does not match the native state, the head will edge-load on the capitellum. This leads to premature wear. Press-fit stems rely on bony ingrowth. Intraoperative radial shaft fractures can occur as a result of the large hoop stresses created due to oversizing of the stem [24]. In comparison to loose-fitting stems, press-fit stems have shown increased loosening over time that requires implant removal [25].

A bipolar prosthesis allows articulation in the head-neck junction of the implant, which in turn allows centering of the radiocapitellar joint. This theoretically allows for more congruent contact with the capitellum throughout elbow range of motion. Good mid- to long-term results have been reported with these implants [26]; however, dislocation of the prosthesis is a unique complication that has been reported in the literature [27].

The author's preferred technique for radial head arthroplasty as described below is based on the use of the Katalyst (Integra, Austin, TX) implant which is a modular bipolar prosthesis. It has a cobalt-chrome telescoping shaft and ball that links to the head with a polyethylene lining. The polyethylene lining allows the head to be coupled to the shaft in the elbow without releasing the lateral ligament complex. The telescoping shaft allows adjustment of implant length in situ to adjust to different neck cuts and fracture patterns. A minimum of 1 mm of distraction via the telescoping shaft is necessary for the head to function as a bipolar implant.

Technique in Detail

We find that the easiest approach to the radial head is with the patient supine, the affected arm on a radiolucent hand table, and the shoulder internally rotated to provide access to the lateral aspect of the elbow. This positioning also allows access to the medial side if necessary with external rotation of the shoulder. The arm can also be brought across the chest easily for exposure to the olecranon if needed. The radiolucent hand table provides easy visualization and manipulation using intraoperative fluoroscopy. A non-sterile tourniquet placed on the upper arm usually allows adequate room for exposure, but a sterile tourniquet can be used if necessary. After anesthesia is induced, and prior to preparation, intraoperative fluoroscopy is used to document valgus, varus, posteromedial, or posterolateral instability. Instability is evidenced by widening of the medial or lateral ulnohumeral joint space.

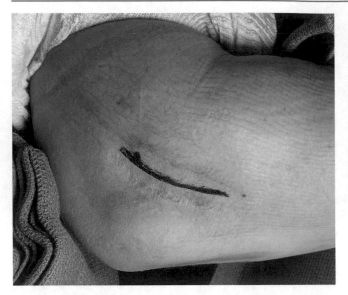

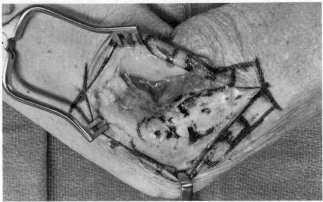

Fig. 61.4 After skin incision, the lateral condylar ridge and center of the proximal radial shaft are marked with a marking pen and connected with a curvilinear incision

Fig. 61.3 The lateral skin incision is marked from the lateral epicondyle to the center of the radial head and neck

For isolated radial head fractures, we prefer the lateral ligament sparing approach to the elbow. This is a curvilinear, lateral incision drawn from the lateral epicondyle of the humerus to the midaxial line of the radial neck (Fig. 61.3). Most coronoid fractures, with the exception of the anteromedial facet fractures, can also be approached through this lateral side with the radial head excised. Following skin incision, the radial head can be approached through either the traditional Kocher interval between extensor carpi ulnaris and anconeus or by splitting the extensors in line with the midaxial line of the radius. The Kocher interval tends to lie posteriorly over the lateral ulnar collateral ligament, and thus care must be taken not to disrupt the ligament if it is still attached. If the Kocher interval is used, the capsular incision must be brought anteriorly to avoid the lateral ulnar collateral ligament.

We prefer the extensor splitting approach (Fig. 61.4). Once the extensor fascia is exposed, the deep bony landmarks are identified. The lateral condylar ridge, lateral epicondyle, and center of the proximal radial shaft are marked and connected with a curvilinear incision. The extensor origin and capsule are elevated off the anterior aspect of the lateral condylar ridge and the capitellum. Fascia of the common extensor origin is split along with the annular ligament exposing the radial head and neck. It is important to make this incision sharply to preserve the annular ligament for repair during closure (Fig. 61.5). This incision is kept in the midline, bisecting the radial head and shaft to protect the lateral collateral ligament complex. If necessary, the muscle of the common extensor origin can be split exposing the oblique fibers of the supinator. Dividing the proximal edge of the supinator exposes the proximal radial

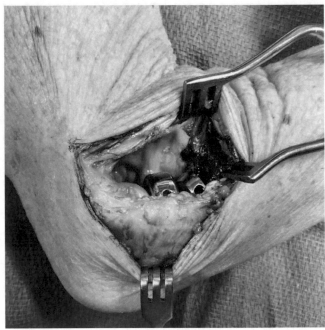

Fig. 61.5 The annular ligament is sharply incised and preserved for later closure

diaphysis. This portion of the procedure is performed with the forearm in pronation to move the posterior interosseous nerve (PIN) away from the field distally and medially to protect it from damage. Because the nerve lies 5–6 cm from the radiocapitellar joint, it is rare for the nerve to be in harm's way (Fig. 61.6). It is also important to limit the use of reverse retractors such as small Hohmann or Bennett retractors placed anterior on the proximal radial shaft. These retractors can put direct pressure on the PIN. If more joint exposure is needed, the incision can be carried more proximally, and the origin of the brachioradialis can be elevated.

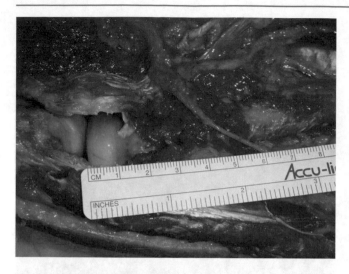

Fig. 61.6 The posterior interosseous nerve pierces the supinator muscle and lies 5–6 cm from the radiocapitellar joint

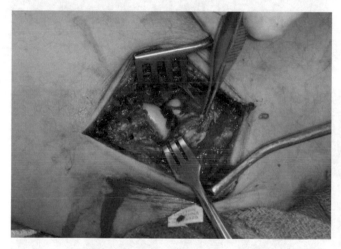

Fig. 61.7 Elbow is extended, and common extensor fascia is retracted to reveal torn lateral ulnar collateral ligament complex beneath it

The lateral ulnar collateral ligament should be inspected. The competency of the lateral ligament complex is not always apparent on first glance. With elbow dislocation, the lateral complex is stripped "inside out" from the humerus. The extent of lateral instability is clear when the lateral complex and common extensor are stripped and the lateral epicondyle is left bare. In other cases, the injury can be more subtle. Because the soft tissue injuries of elbow dislocations propagate from the inside of the elbow out, the capsule with the LUCL may be disrupted, while the extensor origin is intact. This is the "intact extensor origin head fake" that disguises instability from a "naked capitellum" [28]. To assess this, extend the elbow and retract the posterior limb of the extensor origin (Fig. 61.7). The capsule and associated LUCL origin are normally adjacent the articular cartilage. If the lateral wall of the capitellum is "naked," the

LUCL origin is ruptured, and the elbow is in the early stages of PLRI [28].

The fractured radial head is then inspected with the goal of reconstructing the native head through open reduction and internal fixation. We define a "reconstructable" head fracture as one that can be fixed with sufficient stability to begin motion within 1–2 weeks and has a reasonable chance to heal. Oftentimes, the degree of comminution is greater than anticipated based on preoperative imaging. When the head is dissociated from the shaft and there are no soft tissues attached, the prospects for healing are diminished. If the head is not repairable, the loose fragments are removed. Refer to the lateral radiograph of the injured elbow; it will often direct you to remote fragments that are displaced anteromedially into the brachialis or posterolaterally beneath the lateral complex.

Using a microsagittal saw, the neck is cut perpendicular to the shaft at the metaphyseal-diaphyseal junction. This cut will usually be just distal to the distal margin of the lesser sigmoid notch of the ulna. An understanding of the implant system and head sizes used is essential as the goal of this cut is to replace the amount of removed bone with the implant. A cutting guide in the Katalyst system allows you to estimate the location of the cut for an implant positioned with 1 or 3 mm of distraction between the head and stem collar (Fig. 61.8). Either degree of distraction is acceptable. We generally make the cut to accommodate 3 mm of distraction. When there is significant fracture comminution extending into the proximal shaft, we preserve as much bone stock as possible and will

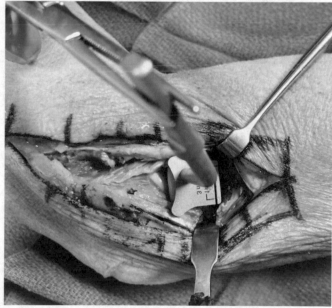

Fig. 61.8 Cutting guides can be used to estimate the neck cut which will usually be at the metaphyseal-diaphyseal junction

cement the stem to ensure stability. Once the remaining head has been excised, the capitellum, coronoid process, and the sigmoid notch are examined. Fractures and articular damage of these structures are addressed and documented to maximize joint congruity and stability and to assign prognosis. Oftentimes, the sigmoid notch will be noted to have impaction or shear injury. Loose bodies are removed and the joint is irrigated.

Injury to the interosseous membrane and distal radioulnar joint is assessed by the "radius pull test" [29]. The proximal radius is grasped with a towel clip, and a proximal load is applied (Fig. 61.9). With fluoroscopy at the wrist, proximal migration of the radius is estimated using "feel" and the change in ulnar variance at the wrist (Fig. 61.10). A change in variance more than 3 mm suggests rupture of the interosseous membrane. If the variance changes more than 6 mm, it is likely that both the TFCC and interosseous membrane are disrupted [29].

If radial head replacement seems to be the appropriate management for the injured elbow, the fractured head is then reassembled on the back table, and an appropriate size head is chosen (Fig. 61.11). When examining the native radial

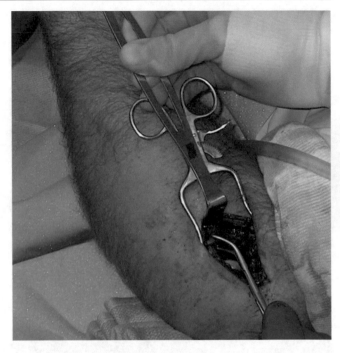

Fig. 61.9 The radius pull test: The proximal radius is grasped with a towel clip, and an axial load is applied

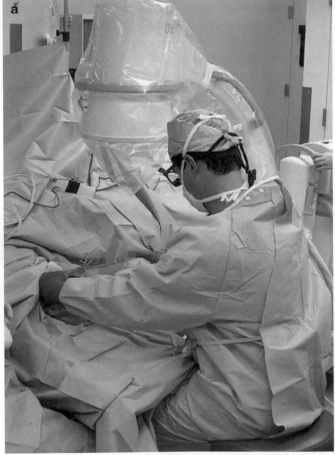

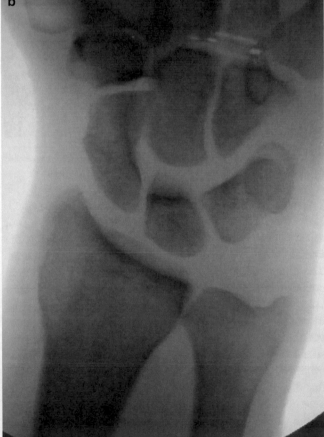

Fig. 61.10 During the radius pull test, the fluoroscopic imaging should be centered on the wrist (**a**). A normal wrist x-ray during radius pull test indicates no proximal migration of the radius. If wrist x-rays demonstrate a relative ulnar positive variance, then IOM or TFCC injury should be suspected (**b**)

head, one can see that the head is not round but instead is oval with a lesser and greater diameter. When sizing the head, choose the head that is closest to the lesser diameter.

The replication of length is a critical and often challenging step. The major downfall is "overstuffing" of the radiocapitellar joint, which may lead to premature radiocapitellar wear and erosions, as well as ulnohumeral arthritis. On the other hand, "understuffing" the head may result in residual valgus instability and increased loads at the ulnohumeral joint due to the loss of the load-sharing role of the radial head.

Studies have shown that we cannot rely on the anteroposterior radiograph of the ulnohumeral joint as a guide to radial head size. Rowland et al. characterized the appearance of the

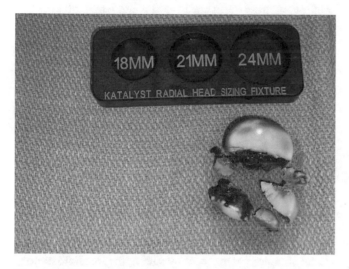

Fig. 61.11 The radial head fragments should be pieced together on the back table and sized. When in between two sizes, the smaller size is chosen

ulnohumeral joint on the anteroposterior view of the elbow joint and showed that the lateral portion of the joint may be nonparallel and wider laterally and, therefore, should not be confused with overlengthening of the elbow caused by placing a radial head implant that is too long [30]. Shors et al. also showed that standard radiographs will not reproducibly show changes in the ulnohumeral space when the implant is underlengthened by as much as 2 mm or overlengthened by as much as 4 mm [31].

If possible, radial length is judged by the length of the resected head and neck. But if comminution of the radial head prohibits accurate measurement of the length, we recommend obtaining AP radiographs of the contralateral elbow to assess the appearance of the medial and lateral ulnohumeral joint and replicate this as closely as possible.

In our opinion, judging the appropriate length of the implant can be difficult especially after the implant is placed in the elbow. This is particularly true when the elbow is destabilized by injuries to the collateral ligaments and the capsule. The Katalyst system has a wand for each head size accounting for either 1 or 3 mm of distraction and with window cutouts that allow the surgeon to see through to the ulnohumeral joint (Fig. 61.12). Place the elbow in 90° of flexion with the forearm in neutral. Make certain that the ulnohumeral joint is reduced. The wand with the anticipated head size and head-stem distraction is placed between the capitellum and cut surface of the proximal radius. While looking through the cutting guide, the ulnohumeral joint space can be assessed for distraction of the ulnohumeral joint.

The appropriate stem diameter is determined by sequential broaching of the proximal radius. Each implant manufac-

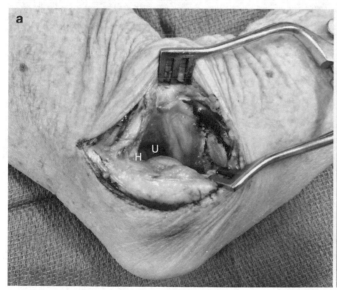
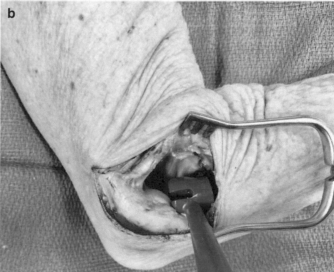

Fig. 61.12 (a) With the radial head removed, the ulnohumeral joint can be easily visualized. H, humerus; U, ulna. (b) Measuring guide with window cutouts that allow the surgeon to see through to the ulnohumeral joint

turer has determined an ideal fit of the shaft into the radius; some implants have a smooth shaft allowing rotation in the proximal radius, while some are made for cemented implantation and others for bony ingrowth. The Katalyst radial head system has 6.5 and 7.5 mm broaches. The stem is implanted into the proximal radius with the set screw removed allowing the telescoping portion of the stem set to rest in a fully collapsed position. The modular head is then coupled to the stem, in situ. The head and inner stem are then distracted from the outer stem by placing the 1 mm "first spacer" followed by a 2 mm spacer (Fig. 61.13). This affects 3 mm of

distraction between the head and outer stem. Avoid increasing the distraction.

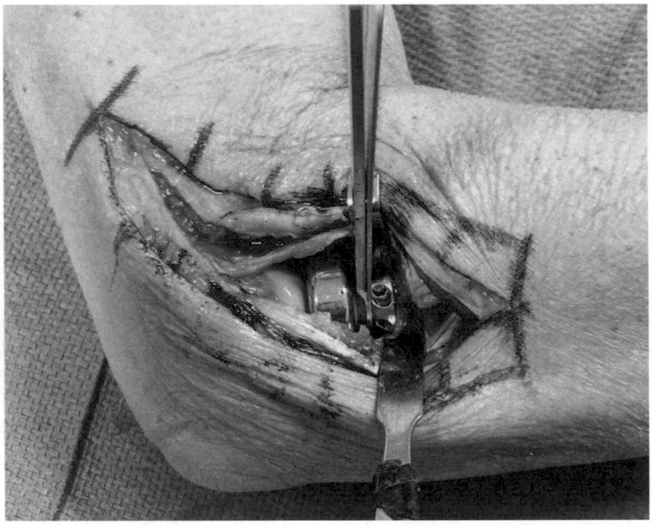

Once the implant is placed, the elbow is brought through a full range of flexion, extension, and forearm rotation. Stability can be hard to assess and may need to be postponed until after the lateral complex is repaired. The articulation of the head on the capitellum is checked to confirm smooth and centered motion. Fluoroscopic images are taken with the elbow flexed and extended with both forearm pronation and supination.

If the lateral ulnar collateral ligament is injured, then it must be repaired. Lateral ulnar collateral ligament injuries are often accompanied by injuries to the extensor origin. Given that both these elements are important for stability, we prefer to address the extensor origin and lateral ulnar collateral ligament together in our lateral complex repair. Fixation to the lateral epicondyle is obtained with a single 2.0-mm drill hole directed from anterior to posterior at the axis of elbow rotation. Divide the lateral aspect of the capitellum into four quadrants (Fig. 61.14). The tip of the drill should be just at the central edge of the antero-distal quadrant (Fig. 61.15). One end of a nonabsorbable suture is fed through this drill hole (Fig. 61.16). The posterior limb of the suture is then sewed to the lateral ulnar collateral ligament and posterior portion of the extensor tendon as one layer running-locking fashion from proximal to distal then back proximally. The lateral ligament complex starts at the lateral epicondyle and fans out posteriorly to the supinator crest (Fig. 61.17). The repair should replicate this anatomy. The lateral complex is tensioned by sliding the free limb through the bone and tying it down against the lateral epicondyle (Fig. 61.18). The radial head position and stability of the

Fig. 61.13 The head and stem are distracted in situ with spacers to set the telescoping distance

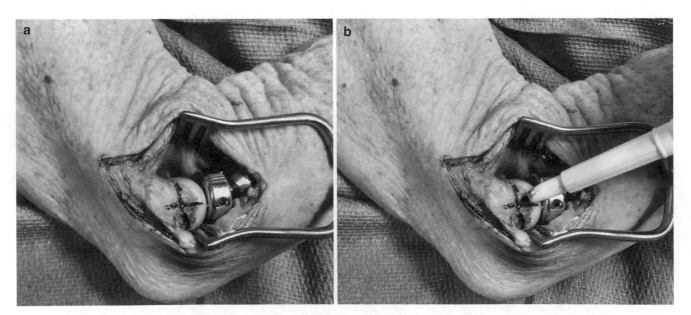

Fig. 61.14 The lateral epicondyle is divided into four quadrants (**a**). The entry point of the drill should be just at the edge of the antero-distal quadrant (**b**)

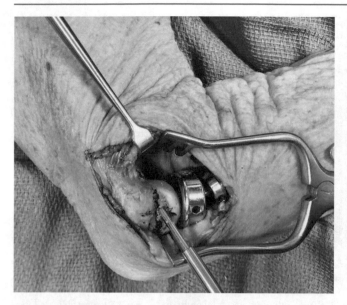

Fig. 61.15 A single drill hole directed from anterior to posterior at the tip of the lateral epicondyle

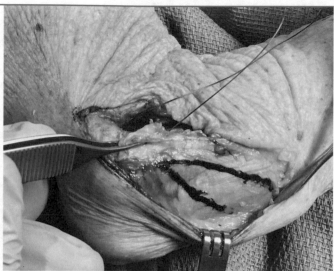

Fig. 61.17 The lateral ligament complex starts at the lateral epicondyle and fans out posteriorly to the supinator crest

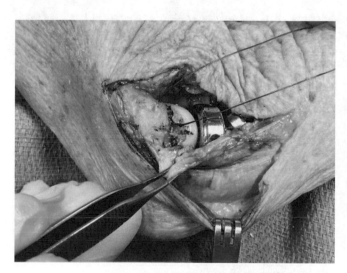

Fig. 61.16 One end of a nonabsorbable suture is then fed through this drill hole

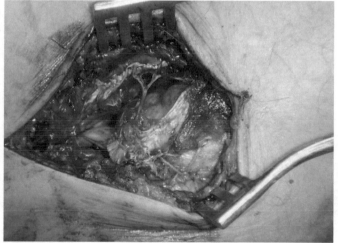

Fig. 61.18 A Krakow stich using nonabsorbable suture is placed through the lateral ulnar collateral ligament and tied over the lateral epicondyle

joint are assessed by placing the elbow and forearm through a range of motion. It is essential to reevaluate elbow stability after repair of the lateral complex (Fig. 61.19). If the elbow remains unstable, particularly with flexion of 45° or more, we favor repair of the medial collateral ligament. If repair of the medial collateral ligament does not restore adequate stability, we will place a static elbow fixator or internal joint stabilizer (Skeletal Dynamics).

The lateral wound is closed by suturing the anterior limb of the split extensor origin to the posterior limb. The previously incised annular ligament is taken together with the

extensor and repaired with a nonabsorbable suture (Fig. 61.20). The repair of the annular ligament also helps to better center the radial head on the capitellum [32].

If the lateral ulnar collateral ligament is intact at the time of surgery or the repair of the lateral ulnar collateral ligament is stout, the elbow is splinted in 90° of flexion with the forearm in supination. Forearm supination helps close the medial joint space, allowing an injured ulnar collateral ligament to heal in an anatomic position (Fig. 61.21). A lateral radiograph taken with elbow splinted while the patient is still anesthetized helps confirm that the elbow is reduced (Fig. 61.22).

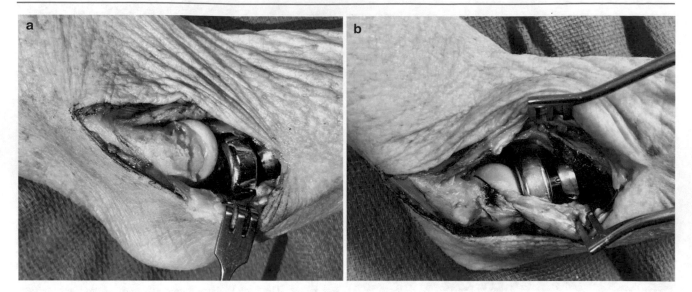

Fig. 61.19 Prior to lateral ulnar collateral ligament complex repair, the radial head subluxes posterolaterally (**a**). With lateral ulnar collateral ligament complex repair, the radial head is now centered on the capitellum (**b**)

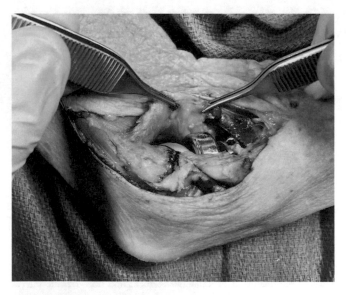

Fig. 61.20 The annular ligament is taken together with the extensor and repaired with a nonabsorbable suture

Tips and Tricks

Patient positioning and fluoroscopic imaging are critical when performing radial head arthroplasty efficiently and accurately. Variations in patient body habitus and associated ipsilateral arm pathology must be considered in the preoperative plan. For example, when placing patients in a supine position and using an arm table, it is important to examine the degree of shoulder motion capable of obtaining internal rotation prior to prepping and draping. At times, shoulder arthritis or stiffness could lead to limitations on internal range of motion, making intraoperative

imaging difficult in the supine position with radiolucent arm table. In such a case, a perfect lateral image may be difficult to obtain without placing undue varus stress on the elbow. When this occurs, placement of a bump behind the ipsilateral scapula can be helpful. Another option for positioning in this situation is to place the arm across the body, using a pneumatic arm holder on the hand and wrist. This allows positioning of the elbow in such a way as to eliminate varus stress, with the added benefit of freeing up the assistant's hands to help with holding retraction of soft tissues. In addition, a mini C-arm can be brought up horizontal to the floor and result in a fairly simple, perfect lateral view while keeping the arm in the holder. In this case, to obtain an AP view, the mini C-arm is repositioned in a vertical position, and the arm is released from the arm holder and brought into extension.

During the surgical approach, it is often difficult to discern the separate fascial planes of the extensor intervals, especially soon after a trauma when hematoma and tissue destruction can obscure normal anatomy. Often with radial head fractures, the lateral collateral complex and extensor origin are avulsed, making exposure relatively straightforward. In this case, the traumatic avulsion creates the approach interval. When no avulsion has occurred, radial head arthroplasty can be performed via either an extensor splitting or Kaplan or Kocher approach. One useful tip during the lateral approach, in order to identify the fascial intervals, is to take advantage of their respective distal insertion sites. By holding the wrist in neutral or even slight extension, this effectively immobilizes the wrist extensors. The fingers are then passively and fully flexed and extended, which creates visible and palpable motion within the EDC and allows identification and isolation of this motor group and of the interval adjacent to the

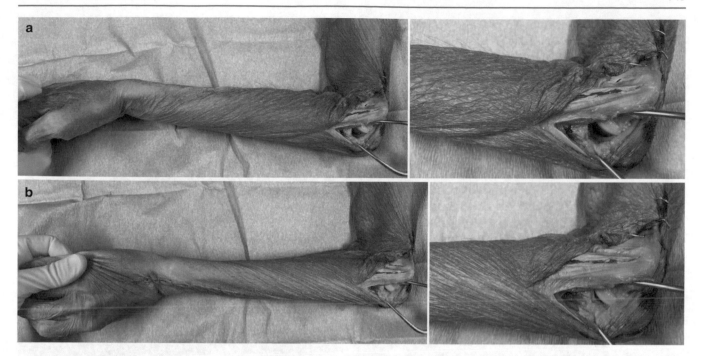

Fig. 61.21 With the lateral ulnar collateral ligament repaired, but with the ulnar collateral ligament ruptured, pronation results in a widening of the ulnohumeral joint space (**a**). Supination hinges the elbow on the intact lateral ulnar collateral ligament, thus closing down the ulnohumeral joint space. This allows the ulnar collateral ligament to heal in an anatomic position (**b**)

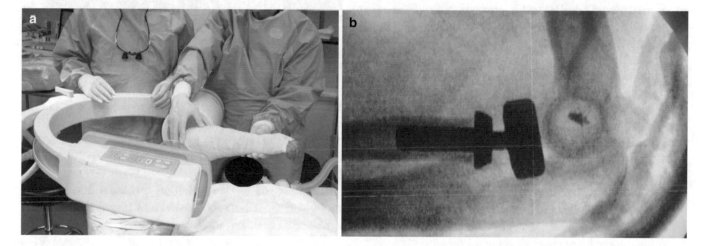

Fig. 61.22 Lateral radiograph taken with elbow splint while the patient is still anesthetized (**a**). Lateral radiograph in the splint confirms that the elbow is reduced (**b**)

immobile ECRL. This is useful in identifying this interval when the normally visible plane is obscured by hematoma, swelling, and/or tissue destruction due to the trauma itself.

On occasion, it may be difficult to displace the radial neck out into the wound. In this case, great care should be taken in not placing a hinge retractor such as a Hohmann anteriorly, as aggressive or lengthy pressure to deliver the neck out into the wound could cause compressive injury to the posterior interosseous nerve (PIN). A larger broad bone clamp such as a lobster claw can be used, placed just a few millimeters distally to the cut surface, and used to pull the radial shaft slightly outward to allow exposure of the neck for in-line broaching and stem impaction without hinging off the anterior soft tissues. It is critical not to place this clamp too distal as this could injure the PIN along its course. Alternatively, a Hohmann retractor can be safely placed posteriorly, hinging the neck out of the wound anteriorly and laterally. In addition, the use of a side-loading implant or implant that permits in situ coupling reduces the amount of exposure necessary to successfully place the implant.

One of the key elements to a successful radial head arthroplasty is correct sizing of the implant. Often radiographs can be deceiving, making accurate assessment difficult, especially in the setting of an unstable elbow since the radiocapitellar joint can subluxate until the LUCL is repaired. Both overstuffing and understuffing the radiocapitellar joint can lead to the complications of early capitellar articular wear or insufficient valgus support, respectively. A useful landmark for determining the correct neck size is the most proximal aspect of the lesser sigmoid notch. Most systems have a sizing guide for the neck cut. While the trial radial head and stem implant are typically too large to see the lesser sigmoid notch, one useful tip is to use the cut guide placed into the gap created after cutting the neck. This guide is often less bulky, and a marking pen can be used to mark the proximal extent of the notch on the guide. This can then be measured with a ruler, to give a fairly accurate measurement of length from the neck cut to the proximal edge of the notch and help in determination of optimal implant neck length. As this is a stable anatomic landmark which is not variable with motion, it creates a more accurate guide compared to placing the trial and evaluating for the space between the implant and capitellum, as this space can be altered based on forearm position, varus vs. valgus stress, and degree of instability.

Unexpected injuries to the ligament and bone are common when treating radial head fractures resulting from elbow fracture dislocations. It is useful to have the following equipment available in the operating room:

- Radiolucent hand table
- Drill
- Microsagittal saw
- Suture anchors
- 2-mm drill bit
- #5 nonabsorbable suture to repair the lateral complex to the bone
- Static external fixator—in the event that stability cannot be restored with head replacement and ligament repair
- Internal joint stabilizer (Skeletal Dynamics)
- Suture tape with anchors to augment repair

When evaluating an AP radiograph of your final radial head implant, the implant will appear to overhang the lateral edge of the capitellum (Fig. 61.23). Remember that the native radial head is surrounded by cartilage that does not appear on plain radiographs. The reason for this lateral overhang is that the radial head tensions the lateral ligament complex.

Rehabilitation

The postoperative regimen is tailored to the individual patient depending on stability and associated injuries. Traditionally, forearm rotation is customized depending on the ligamen-

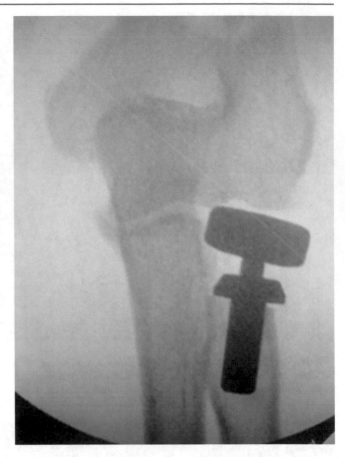

Fig. 61.23 Final AP radiograph demonstrating appropriate positioning of the radial head with lateral overhang

tous disruption. Pronation is the favored position if the lateral ligaments are deficient, and supination is the position utilized for concurrent medial instability. With a secure repair of the lateral complex, the elbow can be initially immobilized in supination.

The goal of all rehabilitation protocols is early, safe mobilization. If both the medial and lateral sides are stable, active-assisted motion is started within the first 5–7 days with intermittent bracing for 3–4 weeks. With a medial ligamentous injury and stable lateral repair, we recommend overhead flexion and extension exercises and forearm rotation with the elbow at 90°. These are begun at 5–7 days and performed three to four times/day. Between exercises, the elbow is supported with a brace with elbow at 90°. We no longer use hinged braces as the brace often slides down the arm placing the axis of rotation of the brace posterior that of the elbow joint. While in the static brace we recommend isometric contraction of the triceps, brachialis, and biceps to restore normal muscle tone. At the initial postoperative visit, we obtain a "Captain Morgan View." This is standing view performed out of the postoperative dressing with the elbow flexed and the palm of the hand placed on the abdomen. The lateral aspect of the elbow is positioned against the cassette (Fig. 61.24). If the

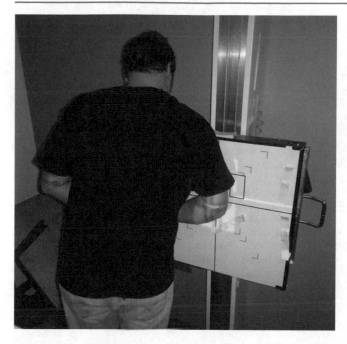

Fig. 61.24 The "Captain Morgan View" is taken with the elbow flexed and the palm of the hand placed on the abdomen

initial postoperative lateral radiograph shows a widened joint space, then the patient is re-examined with radiographs a week later and then every 2 weeks until congruency is restored. If the humerus appears centered on the olecranon fossa, we have waited as long as 8 weeks to see a truly concentric reduction. If there is residual translation, we will recommend repeat surgery with revision repair of collateral ligaments, augmentation with anchor and suture tape, application of an internal joint stabilizer, or application of a static external fixator.

If healing proceeds uneventfully and motion is progressing, we will not recommend physical therapy. If motion is limited between 6 and 8 weeks, we institute a formal physical therapy program including passive motion and static progressive splinting. Once the ligament injuries have had time to heal, strengthening of the elbow is initiated, and this is usually between 8- and 12-week status post-surgery.

Conclusion

Radial head arthroplasty has been shown to have good outcomes when used for radial head fractures. Regardless of design, radial head implants are proven to restore elbow stability, even in unstable elbow fracture dislocations. Nevertheless, there certainly are disadvantages to radial head arthroplasty. The radial head's anatomy is complex and highly variable. The currently available implants do not replicate the radial head's anatomy perfectly. Still, the results of radial head arthroplasty are far more promising than both radial head excision and ORIF in the setting of unreconstruc-

table radial head fractures. Radial head implants afford immediate stability to the elbow and allow for early range of motion of the elbow.

References

1. Van Riet RP, Glabbek F, Morrey BF. Radial head fracture. In: The elbow and its disorders. 4th ed. Philadelphia: Saunders Elsevier; 2009. p. 359–89.
2. Duckworth AD, Clement ND, Jenkins PJ, Aitken SA, Court-Brown CM, McQueen MM. The epidemiology of radial head and neck fractures. J Hand Surg Am. 2012;37(1):112–9.
3. Mason ML. Some observations on fractures of the head of the radius with a review of one hundred cases. Br J Surg. 1954;42(172):123–32.
4. Broberg MA, Morrey BF. Results of treatment of fracture-dislocations of the elbow. Clin Orthop Relat Res. 1987;216:109–19.
5. Sheps DM, Kiefer KRL, Boorman RS, Donaghy J, Lalani A, Walker R, et al. The interobserver reliability of classification systems for radial head fractures: the Hotchkiss modification of the Mason classification and the AO classification systems. Can J Surg. 2009;52(4):277–82.
6. van Riet RP, Morrey BF. Documentation of associated injuries occurring with radial head fracture. Clin Orthop Relat Res. 2008;466(1):130–4.
7. van Riet RP, Morrey BF, O'Driscoll SW, Van Glabbeek F. Associated injuries complicating radial head fractures: a demographic study. Clin Orthop Relat Res. 2005;441:351–5.
8. Davidson PA, Moseley JB, Tullos HS. Radial head fracture. A potentially complex injury. Clin Orthop Relat Res. 1993;297:224–30.
9. Duckworth AD, Watson BS, Will EM, Petrisor BA, Walmsley PJ, Court-Brown CM, et al. Radial head and neck fractures: functional results and predictors of outcome. J Trauma. 2011;71(3):643–8.
10. Duckworth AD, Wickramasinghe NR, Clement ND, Court-Brown CM, McQueen MM. Long-term outcomes of isolated stable radial head fractures. J Bone Joint Surg Am. 2014;96(20):1716–23.
11. Herbertsson P, Josefsson PO, Hasserius R, Karlsson C, Besjakov J, Karlsson MK. Displaced Mason type I fractures of the radial head and neck in adults: a fifteen- to thirty-three-year follow-up study. J Shoulder Elb Surg. 2005;14(1):73–7.
12. Antuña SA, Sánchez-Márquez JM, Barco R. Long-term results of radial head resection following isolated radial head fractures in patients younger than forty years old. J Bone Joint Surg Am. 2010;92(3):558–66.
13. Furry KL, Clinkscales CM. Comminuted fractures of the radial head. Arthroplasty versus internal fixation. Clin Orthop Relat Res. 1998;353:40–52.
14. King GJ, Zarzour ZD, Rath DA, Dunning CE, Patterson SD, Johnson JA. Metallic radial head arthroplasty improves valgus stability of the elbow. Clin Orthop Relat Res. 1999;368:114–25.
15. Johnson JA, Beingessner DM, Gordon KD, Dunning CE, Stacpoole RA, King GJW. Kinematics and stability of the fractured and implant-reconstructed radial head. J Shoulder Elbow Surg. 2005;14(1 Suppl S):195S–201S.
16. Mikić ZD, Vukadinović SM. Late results in fractures of the radial head treated by excision. Clin Orthop Relat Res. 1983;181:220–8.
17. Ikeda M, Sugiyama K, Kang C, Takagaki T, Oka Y. Comminuted fractures of the radial head. Comparison of resection and internal fixation. J Bone Joint Surg Am. 2005;87(1):76–84.
18. Ring D, Quintero J, Jupiter JB. Open reduction and internal fixation of fractures of the radial head. J Bone Joint Surg Am. 2002;84(10):1811–5.
19. Halls AA, Travill A. Transmission of pressures across the elbow joint. Anat Rec. 1964;150:243–7.

20. Markolf KL, Lamey D, Yang S, Meals R, Hotchkiss R. Radioulnar load-sharing in the forearm. A study in cadavera. J Bone Joint Surg Am. 1998;80(6):879–88.

21. Shore BJ, Mozzon JB, MacDermid JC, Faber KJ, King GJW. Chronic posttraumatic elbow disorders treated with metallic radial head arthroplasty. J Bone Joint Surg Am. 2008;90(2):271–80.

22. Grewal R, MacDermid JC, Faber KJ, Drosdowech DS, King GJW. Comminuted radial head fractures treated with a modular metallic radial head arthroplasty. Study of outcomes. J Bone Joint Surg Am. 2006;88(10):2192–200.

23. Doornberg JN, Parisien R, van Duijn PJ, Ring D. Radial head arthroplasty with a modular metal spacer to treat acute traumatic elbow instability. J Bone Joint Surg Am. 2007;89(5):1075–80.

24. Chanlalit C, Shukla DR, Fitzsimmons JS, An K-N, O'Driscoll SW. Effect of hoop stress fracture on micromotion of textured ingrowth stems for radial head replacement. J Shoulder Elb Surg. 2012;21(7):949–54.

25. Flinkkilä T, Kaisto T, Sirniö K, Hyvönen P, Leppilahti J. Short- to mid-term results of metallic press-fit radial head arthroplasty in unstable injuries of the elbow. J Bone Joint Surg Br. 2012;94(6):805–10.

26. Sershon RA, Luchetti TJ, Cohen MS, Wysocki RW. Radial head replacement with a bipolar system: an average 10-year follow-up. J Shoulder Elb Surg. 2018;27(2):e38–44.

27. Burkhart KJ, Mattyasovszky SG, Runkel M, Schwarz C, Küchle R, Hessmann MH, et al. Mid- to long-term results after bipolar radial head arthroplasty. J Shoulder Elb Surg. 2010;19(7):965–72.

28. Guss MS, Hess LK, Baratz ME. The naked capitellum: a surgeon's guide to intraoperative identification of posterolateral rotatory instability. J Shoulder Elb Surg. 2019;28(5):e150–5.

29. Smith AM, Urbanosky LR, Castle JA, Rushing JT, Ruch DS. Radius pull test: predictor of longitudinal forearm instability. J Bone Joint Surg Am. 2002;84(11):1970–6.

30. Rowland AS, Athwal GS, MacDermid JC, King GJW. Lateral ulnohumeral joint space widening is not diagnostic of radial head arthroplasty overstuffing. J Hand Surg Am. 2007;32(5):637–41.

31. Shors HC, Gannon C, Miller MC, Schmidt CC, Baratz ME. Plain radiographs are inadequate to identify overlengthening with a radial head prosthesis. J Hand Surg Am. 2008;33(3):335–9.

32. Galik K, Baratz ME, Butler AL, Dougherty J, Cohen MS, Miller MC. The effect of the annular ligament on kinematics of the radial head. J Hand Surg Am. 2007;32(8):1218–24.

Lateral Epicondylitis

Mark Steven Cohen

Introduction

Lateral epicondylitis, or tennis elbow, is the most common affliction of the elbow.

The origin of the extensor carpi radialis brevis (ECRB) has been implicated as the source of pathology in this condition [1–11]. Reported histopathologic findings in the affected tendon origin include vascular proliferation and hyaline degeneration, which are consistent with a chronic, degenerative process [6, 8, 11, 12]. Most commonly, surgical treatment is directed at excision of this pathologic tissue through an open approach or more recently arthroscopic methods [2, 9, 13–20].

This chapter covers the anatomy of the extensor tendon origins at the humeral epicondyle based on anatomic dissections [21]. The location of the ECRB tendon origin is defined relative to intra-articular landmarks. Using this data, a technique for arthroscopic lateral epicondylitis surgery is presented with early clinical results.

Anatomy

The ECRL and the ECRB have a unique relationship at the level of the elbow. The ECRL overlies the proximal portion of the ECRB such that the ECRL must be elevated anteriorly in order to visualize the superficial surface of the ECRB. A thin film of areolar connective tissue separates these two structures.

The ECRL origin is entirely muscular along the lateral supracondylar ridge of the humerus (Fig. 32.1). The muscle origin has a triangular configuration with the apex pointing proximally. In contrast, the origin of the ECRB is entirely tendinous. While it blends with the origin of the EDC, when

dissected from a distal to proximal direction and using the tendon undersurface, it can be separated from the EDC back to the humerus (Fig. 62.1). The anatomic origin of the ECRB is located just beneath the distal most tip of the lateral supracondylar ridge (Fig. 62.2). The footprint is diamond shaped measuring approximately 13 by 7 mm (Fig. 62.3). At the level of the radiocapitellar joint, the ECRB is intimate with the underlying anterior capsule of the elbow joint, but it is easily separable at this level [21]. Using this data, an arthroscopic technique was designed for lateral epicondylitis.

Technique

The patient is positioned in the lateral decubitus position with the arm supported. All bony prominences are well padded. We favor regional anesthesia. Bony landmarks are drawn out including the path of the ulnar nerve. Once the tourniquet is inflated, the elbow is insufflated with an 18 gauge needle introduced through the soft spot of the elbow (mid-lateral portal).

Next, a standard anteromedial portal is established (Fig. 62.4). This is started several centimeters proximal and anterior to the medial epicondyle and anterior to the palpable intermuscular septum. Care is taken to slide along the anterior humerus, and the joint is entered with a blunt introducer or a switching stick. This medial portal allows one to view the lateral joint including the radial head, capitellum, and the lateral capsule. It is often helpful at this point to open the inflow to allow distension of the capsule. If visualization is a problem, a retractor can be introduced through a proximal anterolateral portal 2–3 cm proximal and just anterior to the lateral supracondylar ridge. A simple freer elevator is useful for this purpose. By tensioning the capsule anteriorly, improved visualization of the lateral capsule and soft tissues can be achieved.

M. S. Cohen (✉)
Department of Orthopaedic Surgery, Rush University Medical Center, Chicago, IL, USA
e-mail: Mark_S_Cohen@rush.edu

© Springer Nature Switzerland AG 2022
W. B. Geissler (ed.), *Wrist and Elbow Arthroscopy with Selected Open Procedures*,
https://doi.org/10.1007/978-3-030-78881-0_62

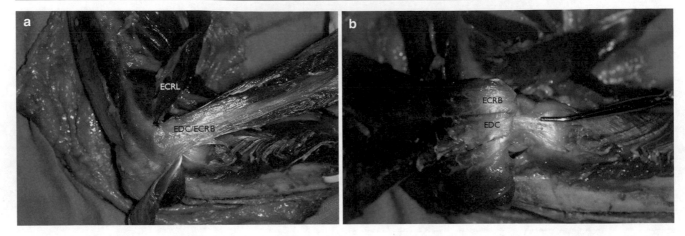

Fig. 62.1 (**a**) Lateral view of cadaveric specimen. The ECRL has been reflected anteriorly (it has a purely muscular origin) and the extensor carpi ulnaris posteriorly revealing the common extensor tendon origin of the ECRB and EDC. These are indistinguishable when viewed from the outer surface. (**b**) The muscles and tendons have been reflected proximally. The origins of the ECRB anteriorly and the EDC posteriorly are identifiable on the undersurface of the extensor origin. Note the underlying lateral collateral ligament (probe). (Courtesy of Mark S. Cohen, Chicago, IL, with permission)

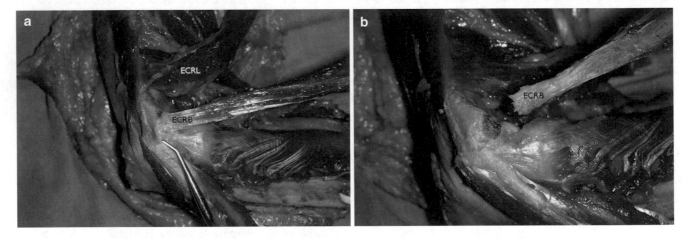

Fig. 62.2 (**a**) The EDC has been removed allowing better visualization of the bony ECRB origin on the humerus. (**b**) The ECRB footprint is identified with elevation of the tendon from the humerus. (Courtesy of Mark S. Cohen, Chicago, IL, with permission)

A modified anterolateral portal is established using an inside-out technique. This is started 2–3 cm above and anterior to the lateral epicondyle (see Fig. 62.3). The portal is slightly more proximal than a standard anterolateral portal. This allows instrumentation down to the tendon origin rather than entering the joint through the ECRB tendon itself. If lateral synovitis is present, this can be debrided with a resector.

The capsule is next released. Occasionally in epicondylitis, one can find a disruption of the underlying capsule from the humerus (Fig. 62.5). Most commonly, the capsule is intact although small linear tears can be present (Fig. 62.6). We have found it easier to release the lateral soft tissues in layers using a monopolar thermal device. In this way, the

capsule is first incised or released from the humerus. When it retracts distally, one can appreciate the ECRB tendon posteriorly and the ECRL, which is principally muscular, more anterior. As noted above, the ECRB tendon spans from the top of the capitellum to the midline of the radiocapitellar joint.

Once the capsule is adequately resected, the ECRB origin is released from the epicondyle (see Figs. 63.4 and 63.6). This is started at the top of the capitellum and carried posteriorly. The lateral collateral ligament is not at risk if the release is kept anterior to the midline of the radiocapitellar joint [18]. On average, adequate resection of the ECRB must include approximately 13 mm of tendon origin from anterior to posterior [21]. Care is taken to drive the scope in ade-

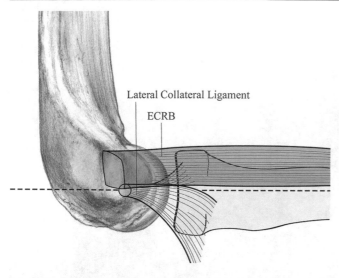

Lateral Collateral Ligament

ECRB

Fig. 62.3 Schematic diagram depicting the relationship between the ECRB origin at the humerus and bony landmarks. Note that the ECRB footprint origin is diamond shaped and located between the midline of the joint and the top of the humeral capitellum beneath the most distal extent of the supracondylar ridge. The tendon does not originate on the epicondyle specifically. Note the relationship between the ECRB origin and the underlying lateral collateral ligament. (Courtesy of Mark S. Cohen, Chicago, IL, with permission)

quately to view the release down to the midline of the radio-capitellar joint. Typically, the entire ECRB retracts distally away from the humerus.

Care is taken not to release the extensor aponeurosis, which lies behind the ECRB tendon. This can be visualized as a stripped background of transversely (longitudinally) oriented tendon and muscular fibers much less distinct than the ECRB (see Fig. 62.6). It is located posterior to the ECRL which again is principally muscular in origin. If the aponeurosis is violated, one will debride into the subcutaneous tissue about the lateral elbow.

Discussion

In recent years, there has been an interest in arthroscopic treatment of lateral epicondylitis [13–20]. A cadaveric study demonstrated that arthroscopic release of the extensor carpi radialis brevis was a safe, reliable, and reproducible procedure for refractory lateral epicondylitis [16]. However, the results of arthroscopic treatment of this condition have been variable. Tseng reported satisfactory results in 9 of 11 patients [20]. However, he also had a 33% complication rate. Stapleton and Baker compared five patients treated arthroscopically with ten patients treated by open debridement [19]. They reported similar results and complication rates between the two groups. Later, Baker et al. reported on

39 elbows treated arthroscopically with 37 reported being "better" or "much better" at follow-up [13]. Peart et al. reported on 33 arthroscopic procedures for lateral epicondylitis with 28% of patients failing to achieve good or excellent outcomes [17].

The variable results reported using various arthroscopic techniques may be related to increased difficulty in identifying the ECRB origin through the arthroscope [15]. The tendon is extra-articular, and capsular release is required to visualize its origin. The tendon footprint is diamond shaped and located between midline of the radiocapitellar joint and the top of the humeral capitellum averaging 13 by 7 mm (see Fig. 62.3). The posterior interosseous nerve should be well medial and distal to the area of dissection. The lateral collateral ligament is not compromised as long as the release does not course posterior to the midline of the radial head [18]. The ligament is not at risk if the release is kept anterior to the midline of the radiocapitellar joint. Care is taken not to release the extensor aponeurosis, which lies superficial to the ECRB tendon.

We reviewed a consecutive series of 36 patients with recalcitrant lateral epicondylitis treated with arthroscopic release using the aforementioned technique [22]. There were 24 men and 12 women with an average age of 42 years at the time of surgery. The cohort had symptoms for an average of 19 months prior to surgical intervention. Intraoperative findings revealed significant lateral intra-articular synovitis in approximately 30% of patients. Approximately 75% of cases had an intact elbow capsule or a minor linear capsular tear, while 25% had a significant proximal capsular disruption. All patients were evaluated by independent examiners for the purposes of this study at a minimum 2-year follow-up. On average, patients required 4 weeks to return to regular activities and 7 weeks to return to full work duties. No major complications were reported. One patient had a neurapraxia of the superficial radial nerve that resolved by 2 weeks postoperatively. The average functional component of the Mayo Elbow Performance Score at follow-up averaged 11.1 out of 12 (range 5–12). Grip strength averaged 91% of the opposite, uninvolved side. Subjective pain ratings as measured on a visual analog scale improved from 8.1 to 1.5 ($p < 0.01$). However, ten patients reported continued pain with strenuous activities and repetitive use of the affected arm. Two patients continued to have significant pain and were considered failures [22].

In summary, arthroscopic release of the ECRB appears to be an effective option for the surgical treatment of chronic lateral epicondylitis unresponsive to conservative modalities. Knowledge of the anatomy, including the extensor tendon origins as visualized from an intra-articular perspective, is essential for effective surgical release.

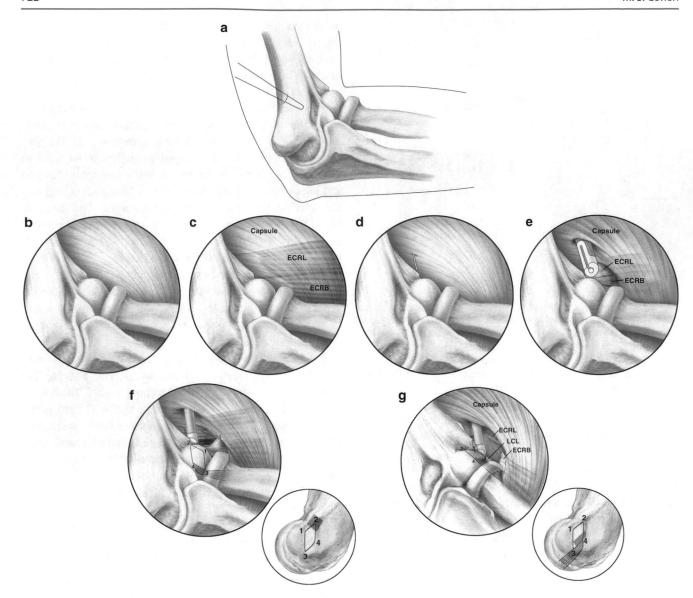

Fig. 62.4 (**a**) Diagram depicting the medial portal used in visualization for the arthroscopic lateral epicondylar release. (**b**) Field of view from the medial portal. (**c**) Diagram depicting the relationship of the extensor tendon origins when viewed intra-articularly. These are located outside (*behind*) the elbow capsule. (**d**) Needle used to help establish a modified lateral portal. Note how this is begun slightly proximal and anterior to the proximal margin of the humeral capitellum. (**e**) Release of the capsule from the lateral humeral margin allowing visualization of the tendinous origins behind. The ECRL is more anteriorly located and is muscular. The ECRB is more posterior. (**f**) The ECRB is released from the top of the capitellum to the (**g**) midline of the radiocapitellar joint. (Courtesy of Mark S. Cohen, Chicago, IL, with permission)

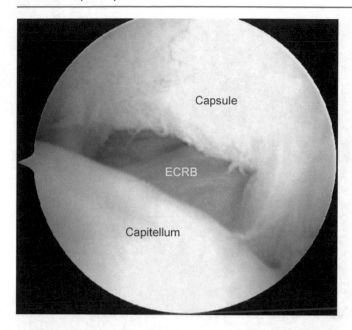

Fig. 62.5 Initial intraoperative view of a patient with recalcitrant lateral epicondylitis. Note the capsular disruption. In some cases, the capsule is noted to have torn away from its humeral origin. (Courtesy of Mark S. Cohen, Chicago, IL, with permission)

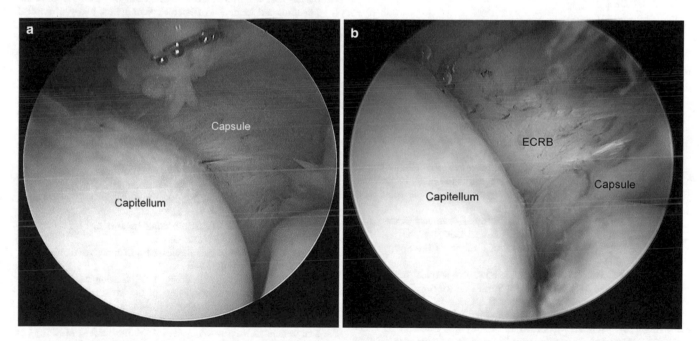

Fig. 62.6 (**a**) Initial intraoperative view of a patient treated surgically for lateral epicondylitis. The lateral capsule obstructs the view of the extensor tendon origins. Note the small longitudinal rent in the capsule. (**b**) The capsule has been released revealing the muscular ECRL anteriorly and the tendinous ECRB more posteriorly. Note the capsular layer distally which is deep to the tendon. (**c**) The ECRB has been released. Behind this, one can see the muscular ECRL anteriorly and the extensor aponeurosis which lies behind the ECRB (*asterisk*). It is characteristically composed of longitudinally stripped tendinous fibers much less distinct than the ECRB. (**d**) Final close-up view following ECRB release. One can see the thick ECRB origin which has retracted distally following release. (Courtesy of Mark S. Cohen, Chicago, IL, with permission)

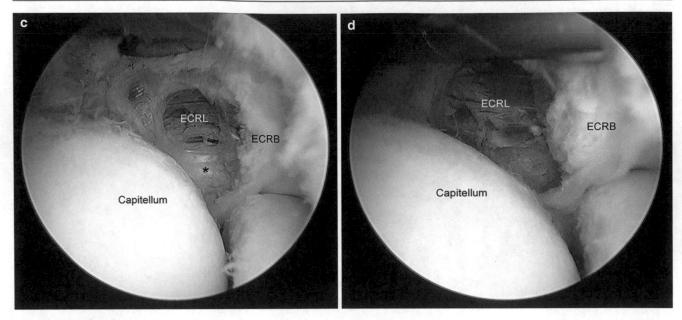

Fig. 62.6 (continued)

References

1. Bunata RE, Brown DS, Capelo R. Anatomic factors related to the cause of tennis elbow. J Bone Joint Surg. 2007;89A:1955–63.
2. Coonrad RW, Hooper WR. Tennis elbow: its course, natural history, conservative and surgical management. J Bone Joint Surg. 1973;55A:1177–82.
3. Cyriax JH. The pathology and treatment of tennis elbow. J Bone Joint Surg. 1936;18:921–40.
4. Garden RS. Tennis elbow. J Bone Joint Surg. 1961;43-B:100–6.
5. Gardner RC. Tennis elbow: diagnosis, pathology, and treatment. Clin Orthop. 1970;72:248–51.
6. Kraushaar BS, Nirschl RP. Tendinosis of the elbow (tennis elbow). Clinical features and findings of histological, immunohistochemical, and electron microscopy studies. J Bone Joint Surg. 1999;81A:259–78.
7. Morrey BF. Reoperation for failed surgical treatment of refractory lateral epicondylitis. J Shoulder Elb Surg. 1992;1:47–55.
8. Nirschl RP. Elbow tendinosis/tennis elbow. Clin Sports Med. 1992;11:851–70.
9. Nirschl RP, Pettronc FA. Tennis elbow. The surgical treatment of lateral epicondylitis. J Bone Joint Surg. 1979;61A:832–9.
10. Organ SW, Nirschl RP, Kraushaar BS, Guidi EJ. Salvage surgery for lateral tennis elbow. Am J Sports Med. 1997;25:746–50.
11. Regan W, Wold LE, Coonrad R, Morrey BF. Microscopic histopathology of chronic refractory lateral epicondylitis. Am J Sports Med. 1992;20:746–9.
12. Spencer GE, Herndon CH. Surgical treatment of epicondylitis. J Bone Joint Surg. 1953;35-A:421–4.
13. Baker CL, Murphy KP, Gottlob CA, Curd DT. Arthroscopic classification and treatment of lateral epicondylitis: two-year clinical results. J Shoulder Elb Surg. 2000;9(6):475–82.
14. Cohen MS, Romeo AA. Lateral epicondylitis: open and arthroscopic treatment. J Am Soc Surg Hand. 2001;3(1):172–6.
15. Cummins CA. Lateral epicondylitis: in vivo assessment of arthroscopic debridement and correlation with patient outcomes. Am J Sports Med. 2006;34:1486–91.
16. Kuklo TR, Taylor KF, Murphy KP, Islinger RB, Heekin RD, Baker CL Jr. Arthroscopic release for lateral epicondylitis: a cadaveric model. Arthroscopy. 1999;15:259–64.
17. Peart RE, Strickler SS, Schweitzer KM Jr. Lateral epicondylitis: a comparative study of open and arthroscopic lateral release. Am J Orthop. 2004;33:565–7.
18. Smith AM, Castle JA, Ruch DS. Arthroscopic resection of the common extensor origin: anatomic considerations. J Shoulder Elb Surg. 2003;12(4):375–9.
19. Stapleton TR, Baker CL. Arthroscopic treatment of lateral epicondylitis. Arthroscopy. 1996;10:335–6.
20. Tseng V. Arthroscopic lateral release for treatment of tennis elbow. Arthroscopy. 1994;10:335–6.
21. Cohen MS, Romeo AA, Hennigan SP, Gordon M. Lateral epicondylitis: anatomic relationships of the extensor tendon origins and implications for arthroscopic treatment. J Shoulder Elb Surg. 2008;17(6):954–60.
22. Lattermann C, Romeo AA, Anbari A, Meininger AK, McCarty LP, Cole BJ, Cohen MS. Arthroscopic debridement of the extensor carpi radialis brevis for recalcitrant lateral epicondylitis. J Shoulder Elb Surg. 2010;19(5):651–6.

Arthroscopic and Open Radial Ulnohumeral Ligament Reconstruction for Posterolateral Rotatory Instability of the Elbow

63

Michael J. O'Brien, Felix H. Savoie III, and Larry D. Field

Introduction

Elbow dislocations are rare injuries that usually respond very favorably to conservative treatment in a brace. However, persistent instability that results from an elbow dislocation can be devastating. There has been a growing interest in the diagnosis and treatment of posterolateral rotatory instability (PLRI) of the elbow since the original description by O'Driscoll in 1991 [1]. PLRI has been described as an instability pattern of the elbow that results from an incompetent radial ulnohumeral ligament complex (RULC). Anatomical studies have attempted to define the involved tissue. Dunning et al. stated that both the radial ulnohumeral ligament (RUHL) and the radial collateral ligament (RCL) must be sectioned to achieve PLRI. They also stated that they could not visually differentiate the two ligaments at their humeral origin. The authors could only distinguish the RUHL from the RCL by identifying the distal extent of the RUHL at the supinator crest of the ulna [2]. Seki et al. were able to show that sectioning just the anterior band of the lateral collateral complex induced instability. This suggests that an intact RUHL alone cannot stabilize the elbow [3]. This data demonstrates that the entity of PLRI is in fact a spectrum of injury. Although originally described as sequelae of an elbow dislocation, these anatomic studies and a report by Kalainov et al. support our own experience that there is a continuum of injury between PLRI and frank elbow dislocation [1, 4, 5].

This instability is best demonstrated clinically with the pivot shift test of the elbow. This test, as first described by O'Driscoll, in the supine position may elicit gross instability or simply pain and apprehension [1]. Two other clinical tests

described by Regan are also useful in the diagnosis of PLRI, (1) pain when pushing up from an arm chair with the palms facing inward and (2) having the patient push up from a prone or wall-leaning position first with the forearms maximally pronated and then repeating the test with the forearms supinated, reproducing either pain, instability, or both [6, 7].

We prefer to examine the elbow with the patient in the prone position and use the table as a base to stabilize the humerus. The elbow in this position mimics the exam of a flexed knee, and the findings are more easily reproduced between examiners. We begin by manually rotating the forearm with the elbow in 90° of flexion, palpating the radiocapitellar joint, and using the wrist to supinate the forearm. This movement reproduces the radial column subluxation as the forearm rotates away from the humerus. The radial head movement on the capitellum is more easily seen and felt in this position, and the elbow can be flexed and extended while maintaining the subluxation force (Fig. 63.1a, b).

Imaging studies for PLRI can be helpful. Radiographs may reveal an avulsion fragment from the posterior aspect of the humeral lateral epicondyle in acute cases. However, radiographs are often normal. A stress radiograph or fluoroscopy while performing the pivot shift test may show the radial head and proximal ulna moving together in a subluxated and posterolaterally rotated position. Magnetic resonance imaging (MRI) of the elbow has been described to identify a lesion in the RUHL [8]. MRI arthrography is the best modality to identify lesions to the medial and lateral collateral ligaments. A formal arthrogram with injection of contrast dye into the elbow joint prior to the scan can greatly enhance the effectiveness of the test.

While much has been written about the pathoanatomy and biomechanics of the lesion, little has been reported on the surgical treatment of these patients. There are no large published series on the outcomes of the surgical treatment of PLRI. The present study reviews the outcomes of the authors' experiences with arthroscopic repair, plication, and open grafting techniques previously described by the senior authors [4].

M. J. O'Brien · F. H. Savoie III (✉)
Department of Orthopaedics, Tulane University School of Medicine, New Orleans, LA, USA
e-mail: fsavoie@tulane.edu

L. D. Field
Upper Extremity, Mississippi Sports Medicine and Orthopaedic Center, Jackson, MS, USA

W. B. Geissler (ed.), *Wrist and Elbow Arthroscopy with Selected Open Procedures*,
https://doi.org/10.1007/978-3-030-78881-0_63

Fig. 63.1 Demonstration of the prone pivot shift exam, showing the elbow reduced (**a**) and subluxated (**b**) with a dimple over the dislocated radiocapitellar joint. (Courtesy of Dr. Felix H. Savoie, III)

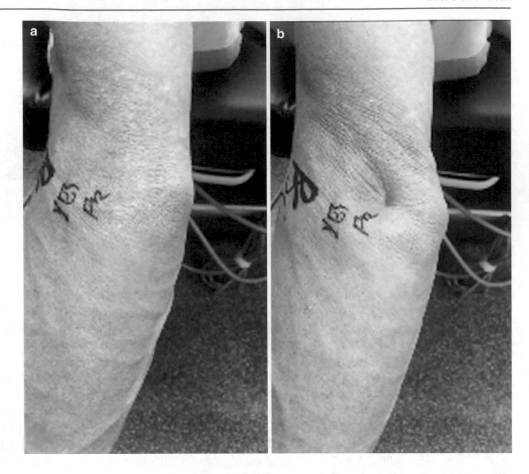

Surgical Technique

Most cases of simple dislocation respond to nonoperative management. However, return to full activities may take 3–4 months. In cases in which the instability recurs, or when initial evaluation reveals a bony avulsion of the lateral collateral ligament complex proximally off of the humerus, surgical treatment may be indicated. Acute repair of the RUHL may also be indicated in high-level athletes, who cannot afford to miss large portions of the athletic season. Arthroscopy of the acutely injured elbow demands speed and precision. A concrete preoperative plan must be formulated and followed, with adjustment made for arthroscopic findings. Patients with significant coronoid fracture, associated radial head fracture, or distal humerus fracture are not included in this report.

Arthroscopic Repair

In the elbow with an acute or chronic avulsion of the RUHL, arthroscopic repair can very effective. The procedure begins with the establishment of a proximal anterior medial portal and a diagnostic arthroscopy of the anterior compartment.

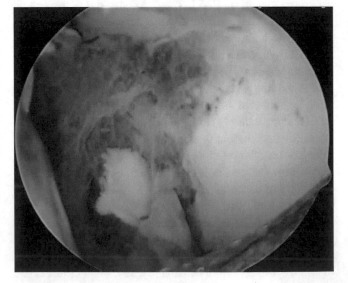

Fig. 63.2 A view from the proximal anterior medial portal of the hematoma often seen in an acute dislocation. (Courtesy of Dr. Felix H. Savoie, III)

Fractures of the radial head or coronoid can be identified. In the acute setting, abundant hematoma will be encountered in the joint (Fig. 63.2), and tearing of the anterior capsule is readily apparent. One can often also see the damage to the

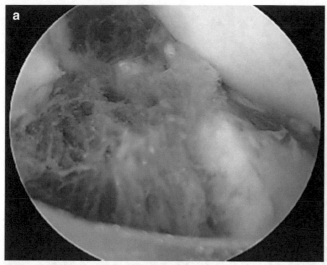
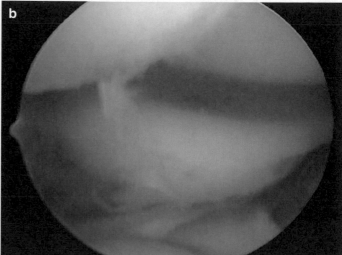

Fig. 63.3 (a) The arthroscopic view of the damaged brachialis and torn anterior capsule often noted in acute dislocations. (b) The laxity seen in the annular ligament and the displacement of the radial head from the capitellum in acute and chronic PLRI are visualized from the medial portal. (Courtesy of Dr. Felix H. Savoie, III)

brachialis muscle through the torn capsule (Fig. 63.3a, b). A proximal anterior lateral portal can be established to clean out the associated hematoma.

On the lateral side, laxity of the annular ligament and lateral collateral ligament (LCL) complex will be evident in every case. Occasionally, the LCL complex will be flipped into the radiocapitellar joint. Of importance is to view the annular ligament for damage and place a suture in it if necessary. Valgus load and forearm supination demonstrates posterolateral rotatory instability with the radial head subluxating off the capitellum, indicative of injury to the RUHL. One can also view "around the corner" of the proximal capitellum for damage to the collateral ligament part of the radial ulnohumeral ligament complex. On the medial side, an arthroscopic valgus stress test can be performed to evaluate for incompetence of the medial ulnar collateral ligament (MUCL). During evacuation of hematoma, great care is taken not to resect or damage the LCL complex.

The arthroscope is next placed into the posterior central portal, and the hematoma in the posterior compartment of the elbow is evacuated via a proximal posterior lateral portal. Both of these portals need to be relatively proximal to allow for the later repair of the ligament, usually at least 3 cm above the olecranon tip. A view of the medial gutter will show hemorrhage, and sometimes tearing of the capsule, near the posterior aspect of the medial epicondyle (Fig. 63.4).

One common finding is the ability to move an arthroscope placed down the posterolateral gutter from the posterior central portal straight across the ulnohumeral articulation into the medial gutter. This maneuver is not possible in a stable elbow and is termed the "drive through sign of the elbow" (Fig. 63.5). It is somewhat analogous to the "drive through sign" in shoulder instability. The elimination of the laxity

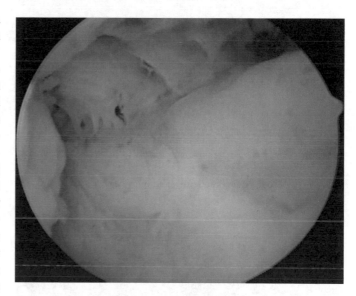

Fig. 63.4 The concomitant tearing of the capsule of the medial capsule in acute instability is visualized from a posterior portal. (Courtesy of Dr. Felix H. Savoie, III)

that allows this maneuver is one of the key aspects of confirming an adequate arthroscopic reconstruction in patients with PLRI.

The lateral gutter and capsule is evaluated next. The arthroscope is easily advanced down the lateral gutter, owing to incompetence of the LCL complex. It is very important to stay close to the ulna as the lateral gutter is evaluated and the hematoma debrided, as the avulsed ligament and bone fragments are displaced distally and may inadvertently be removed by the shaver (Fig. 63.6). The origin of the LCL complex on the posterior aspect of the lateral epicondyle can be visualized as a bare area where the ligament has avulsed

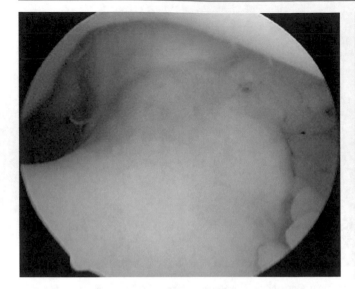

Fig. 63.5 The "drive through sign" of the elbow is performed by placing the arthroscope into the lateral gutter and moving it straight across the ulnohumeral articulation into the medial gutter. (Courtesy of Dr. Felix H. Savoie, III)

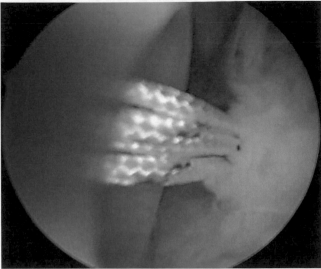

Fig. 63.7 The site of anchor placement into the humerus just lateral to the olecranon fossa of the humerus as viewed from the posterior portal. (Courtesy of Dr. Felix H. Savoie, III)

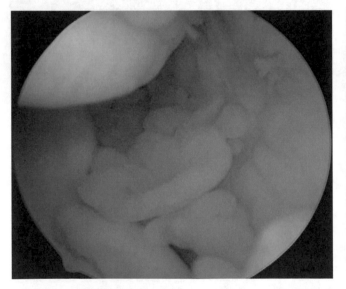

Fig. 63.6 The bone and soft tissue fragments often seen in the lateral gutter in acute dislocation. (Courtesy of Dr. Felix H. Savoie, III)

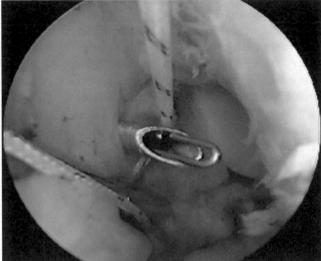

Fig. 63.8 Once an adequate anchor has been placed, the sutures are retrieved though the torn radio-ulnohumeral ligament in preparation for repair. (Courtesy of Dr. Felix H. Savoie, III)

off of the humerus. It is usually directly lateral and slightly inferior to the center of the olecranon fossa. This area on the posterior humerus should be lightly debrided with a motorized shaver.

Once the area of damage has been defined, an arthroscopic anchor may be placed into the humerus at the site of origin of the RUHL (Fig. 63.7). A percutaneous suture passer is placed through a "soft spot" portal to retrieve the sutures. The limbs of the suture are retrieved to place two horizontal mattress sutures through the non-injured part of the ligament. In the case of a bony avulsion, we place one set of sutures around

the bone fragment and the other distal to the fragment (Fig. 63.8). The sutures are tensioned while viewing with the arthroscope down the lateral gutter, which should have the effect of pushing the arthroscope out of the lateral gutter as tension is restored to the LCL complex. The elbow is extended, and the sutures are tied beneath the anconeus muscle, tightening the ligament. Motion and stability are evaluated with the arthroscope back in the anterior compartment (Fig. 63.9), confirming tension has been restored to the annular ligament.

Arthroscopic Plication

The development of an arthroscopic technique for the treatment of chronic PLRI was described by Smith et al. in 2001 [4]. Chronic posterolateral instability of the elbow is more readily seen during examination under anesthesia and on arthroscopic evaluation. While viewing from the proximal anterior medial portal, the ulna and radial head can be seen to subluxate posterolaterally during the performance of a pivot shift test. In most cases, the annular ligament is intact as the entire proximal radio-ulnar joint shifts on the humerus.

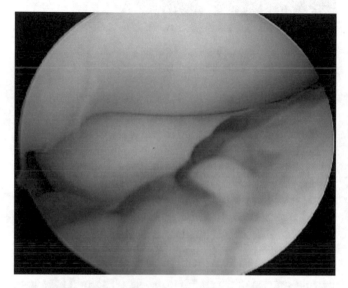

Fig. 63.9 The repaired ligament is visualized from the posterior portal. (Courtesy of Dr. Felix H. Savoie, III)

The arthroscopic technique for chronic instability has two key features: plication of the two major components of the complex and repair of the complex to the humerus. We believe both components can be managed via arthroscopic techniques if there is enough ligamentous and capsular tissue. This assessment is in part determined by the preoperative evaluation, including palpation of the structures in the area to be reconstructed, the amount of prior surgery, and the tissue present on MRI arthrography.

If adequate lateral tissue is present, the tissue in the posterolateral gutter is assessed arthroscopically and prepared with a shaver or rasp. Four to seven absorbable sutures are then placed in oblique fashion beginning at the most distal extent of the RUHL complex attachment to the ulna. The sutures are placed into the lateral gutter via an 18-gauge spinal needle that slides along the radial border of the ulna. The first suture is delivered into the joint through the mid-portion of the annular ligament (Fig. 63.10a). Subsequent sutures are brought into the joint in a progressively more proximal position. Each suture is immediately retrieved with a retrograde suture retriever that passes into the joint from the posterior lateral aspect of the lateral epicondyle (Fig. 63.10b). It is quite important that the retrograde retriever comes under the entire RUHL near its proximal attachment to the humerus.

Once all the sutures have been placed, they are retrieved one at a time percutaneously through the existing skin portals and pulled to tension the sutures and evaluate the plication. If the reconstruction has been properly performed and the tissue is adequate for plication, the arthroscope is driven out of the lateral gutter as this tensioning occurs. The arthro-

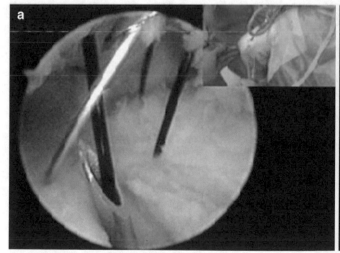
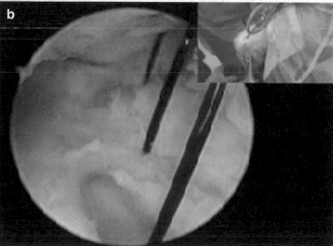

Fig. 63.10 (a) The suture is retrieved using a retrograde retriever introduced along the posterior aspect of the lateral epicondyle and under the proximal end of the RUHL complex. (b) The views of the closed radial gutter once all the sutures are placed and just before the sutures are tensioned. (Courtesy of Dr. Felix H. Savoie, III)

scope is then removed and the elbow extended, and the sutures are tied individually from distal to proximal.

The exam under anesthesia is repeated with the arthroscope placed first in the posterior central portal and then in the proximal anterior medial portal, while the pivot shift test is performed to evaluate the adequacy of the reconstruction. If there is laxity or subluxation still present after the sutures are pre-tensioned, an anchor can be placed at the isometric point of the lateral epicondyle to further tension the LCL complex to the humerus. An anchor is placed as in the acute repairs, and one limb of suture is passed under all of the loops of the plication sutures to a retriever and then retrieved back over the plicated sutures to pull the entire plicated complex back to the humerus. This is usually noted as part of the preoperative planning and is accomplished before the plication sutures are tied.

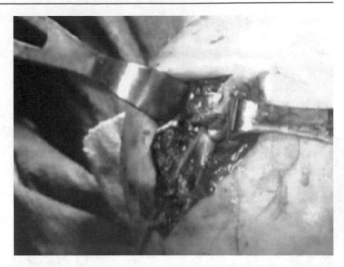

Fig. 63.11 Anatomical picture of the graft reconstruction for PLRI. (Courtesy of Dr. Felix H. Savoie, III)

Postoperative Management

In both acute and chronic cases, patients are immediately placed into a splint or hinged brace with the elbow in approximately 30° of extension to relax tension on the repair. Fluoroscopy or radiographs should be obtained to check the reduction after the splint or brace is applied, as additional flexion may be necessary to tighten the reconstruction and keep the joint reduced. The first postoperative visit usually takes place within 3–5 days of the surgery, and the patient is placed into a hinged elbow brace that allows comfortable movement, usually 0°–45°. Shoulder, peri-scapular, wrist, and hand exercises are initiated and allowed as long as they do not produce pain in the elbow.

The patient is seen at 2-week intervals and motion slowly increased as pain and swelling allow. Once the repair begins to mature, usually between 6 and 8 weeks, physical therapy is initiated to include more aggressive upper extremity and core strengthening exercises with the elbow brace in place. Full range of motion of the elbow should be obtained by 8 weeks postoperatively, if not sooner. Depending on individual progression, patients are allowed to start strengthening exercises out of brace at 10–12 weeks. They must be able to perform all strengthening exercises pain-free in the brace, prior to progression out of the brace.

Open Technique

The open technique for plication and repair is similar to that described by O'Driscoll [1]. After diagnostic arthroscopy confirms the presence of instability and the absence of associated pathology, an extensile posterolateral approach is used and the anconeus muscle split or retracted anteriorly to access the

RUHL complex. If adequate tissue is found to allow repair, the ligaments are plicated and repaired back to the humerus, as described in the above section on arthroscopic repair.

In revision surgery, or in patients with inadequate tissue for repair, a palmaris autograft or gracilis allograft may be used to reconstruct the lateral ligament complex. The supinator crest of the ulna just posterior to the radial neck is dissected free and the insertion site identified. A 4 mm bone tunnel is created at the supinator crest, at the ulnar attachment of the RUHL. A Beath pin is drilled from this point out the ulnar side of the ulna, and a passing suture is used to pull the mid-portion of the graft into the ulna. The graft is secured using an interference screw technique. The two free graft limbs are then brought proximally, pulling one under the annular ligament and one over the ligament, and attached to the isometric point on the posterior aspect of the lateral epicondyle. The graft should be slightly lax in extension and tighten with flexion (Fig. 63.11).

Patient Data Outcomes, Combined Open and Arthroscopic Reconstruction

Material and Methods

A retrospective chart review was performed on all patients with elbow instability treated surgically by the senior authors. Sixty-one patients with posterolateral elbow reconstructions were identified. Of those patients treated operatively, 54 (89%) had complete data available for review. All patients were evaluated for Andrews–Carson scores, length of follow-up, surgical technique employed (open versus arthroscopic), age, sex, and previous elbow surgery [9].

Table 63.1 Comparison of Andrews–Carson scores

Andrews–Carson scores	Subjective		Objective		Overall		Average F/U months
	Pre-op	Post-op	Pre-op	Post-op	Pre-op	Post-op	
Arthroscopic	55	83	91	93	146	176	33
Open	58	86	86	96	144	182	44
Total	57	85	88	95	145	180	41

Results

All 54 patients had a PLRI repair, plication, or graft performed. Forty-one patients (20 arthroscopic and 21 open) had a combined plication and repair, 10 patients (6 open, 4 arthroscopic) had acute or subacute repairs for recurrent elbow instability, and three patients (all open) were reconstructed with a free tendon graft. Ten of the 20 arthroscopically treated and 11 of the 21 open plication/repair patients had the addition of an anchor to supplement the arthroscopic suture plication.

The average follow-up was 41 months (range 12–103 months). Overall Andrews–Carson scores for all repairs improved from 145 to 180 ($p < 0.0001$) [9] (Table 63.1). Subjective scores improved from 57 to 85 ($p < 0.0001$), and objective scores improved from 88 to 95 ($p = 0.008$). Subdividing the technique yielded these overall results: arthroscopic repairs improved from 146 to 176 ($p = 0.0001$) and open repairs 144–182 ($p < 0.001$). Acute repairs performed the best, with nine of ten returning to normal activities and one to near normal. There was no statistically significance difference between the results of open and arthroscopic repair.

Patient Data Outcomes, All-Arthroscopic Reconstruction

Material and Methods

A separate patient cohort was identified consisting of 14 consecutive patients who underwent all-arthroscopic RUHL reconstruction utilizing the same surgical technique in the acute (less than 3 weeks) or subacute (less than 3 months) period following elbow dislocation. All patients participated in athletics and underwent RUHL repair utilizing suture anchors in the humerus. Patients were evaluated with Mayo Elbow Performance Scores (MEPS), and length of follow-up, age, sex, and return to sport were determined.

Results

All 14 patients underwent an all-arthroscopic PLRI reconstruction by repairing the RUHL to the humerus with suture anchors. Outcome scores as determined by the Mayo Elbow Performance Score were excellent in all 14 patients. All returned to sport at their previous level of activity with no resulting instability.

Discussion

The diagnosis of PLRI is made by patient history and physical examination and confirmed with radiologic findings. The diagnosis may be supplemented by arthroscopic confirmation of instability including abnormal movement of the radial head and proximal radio-ulnar joint on the humerus, varus opening, and the arthroscopic "drive through sign of the elbow." The posterolateral pivot shift test described by O'Driscoll may be performed both supine and prone and when combined with the internal rotation push-up and chair lift tests of Regan give a clear clinical picture of instability [1, 6].

Instability findings may coexist with the standard examination findings of lateral epicondylitis, radial tunnel syndrome, and posterolateral plica syndrome. Indeed, as noted by Kalainov, PLRI may actually be a cause of these other problems of the elbow [5]. It is interesting to note that 25% of patients in our study had previous surgery for chronic recurrent lateral epicondylitis. We believe that uncorrected posterolateral instability of the elbow may result in increased tension on the lateral musculature as it attempts to stabilize the elbow, thereby producing a secondary lateral epicondylitis. Other tertiary findings such as an inflamed posterolateral plica and inflammation of the posterior interosseous nerve in or near the radial tunnel may also occur with the instability. A high index of suspicion for the instability is necessary to fully evaluate the elbow of patients with all of these findings. The clinical examination recommended by O'Driscoll and by Regan certainly will assist in the determination of coexisting instability in the setting of lateral elbow pain [1, 6].

Additionally, the close proximity of the extensor carpi radialis brevis to the radial ulnohumeral ligament and lateral collateral ligament complex may potentially contribute to the iatrogenic development of PLRI during lateral epicondylitis procedures. In performing a standard ECRB release and repair for recalcitrant lateral epicondylitis, the treating surgeon must remain on the anterior aspect of the lateral epicondyle to avoid damage to the RUHL.

In most of our patients, repair and plication, whether open or arthroscopic, seemed to be an effective method of managing the instability. Although grafting was necessary in only three of the patients in the first cohort, one should always be prepared to utilize a supplemental graft. In our patients, we used a gracilis allograft with satisfactory results. We have found the number of previous surgeries and the time from the initial injury to definitive treatment to be the best predictors of the need for a graft. However, our low numbers prevent any meaningful recommendation of this technique.

Furthermore, the second patient cohort demonstrates the excellent results that may be obtained from an arthroscopic repair in the first 3 months following injury. All patients in this cohort were able to return to sport at the same level that they previously participated. Early arthroscopic repair may be indicated in young athletes following elbow dislocation to allow them faster return to play.

In summary, we have described four clinical tests for posterolateral rotatory instability of the elbow: (1) supine pivot shift, (2) prone pivot shift, (3) internal rotation wall push-up, and (4) chair push-up. We recommend MRI arthrography to assist in the preoperative evaluation. In surgical cases, arthroscopic confirmation of instability by the "drive through sign of the elbow" from the posterior portal, and the abnormal movement of the radial head on the humeral capitellum while viewing from the proximal anterior medial portal, confirms the presence of the instability. Finally, a ligament repair and a plication technique have been described that can be performed either arthroscopically or open with a high rate of success.

The current studies show that arthroscopic repair and/or plication of the RUHL complex can be as successful as open repair. This technique is technically demanding and requires speed and precision with a thorough understanding of elbow anatomy. Despite these concerns, arthroscopic repair and plication of the RUHL can effectively stabilize an elbow with acute or chronic PLRI and produce a high degree of patient satisfaction.

References

1. O'Driscoll SW, Bell DF, Morrey BF. Posterolateral rotatory instability of the elbow. J Bone Joint Surg Am. 1991;73(3):440–6.
2. Dunning CE, Zarzour ZD, Patterson SD, et al. Ligamentous stabilizers against posterolateral rotator instability of the elbow. J Bone Joint Surg Am. 2001;83A(12):1823–8.
3. Seki A, Olsen BS, Jensen SL, et al. Functional anatomy of the lateral collateral ligament complex of the elbow: configuration of Y and its role. J Shoulder Elb Surg. 2002;11(1):53–9.
4. Smith JP, Savoie FH, Field LD. Posterolateral rotatory instability of the elbow. Clin Sports Med. 2001;20(1):47–58.
5. Kalainov DM, Cohen MS. Posterolateral rotatory instability of the elbow in association with lateral epicondylitis. A report of three cases. J Bone Joint Surg Am. 2005;87(5):1120–5.
6. Regan W, Lapner PC. Prospective evaluation of two diagnostic apprehension signs for posterolateral instability of the elbow. J Shoulder Elb Surg. 2006;15(3):344–6.
7. Yadao MA, Savoie FH, Field LD. Posterolateral rotator instability of the elbow. Inst Course Lect. 2004;53:607–14.
8. Potter HG, Weiland AJ, Schatz JA, et al. Posterolateral rotator instability of the elbow: usefulness of MR imaging in diagnosis. Radiology. 1997;204(1):185–9.
9. Andrews JR, Carson WG. Arthroscopy of the elbow. Arthroscopy. 1985;1(2):97–107.

Internal Brace for Elbow Instability

64

William B. Geissler and Kevin F. Purcell

Introduction

Management of elbow instability presents a challenge to the orthopedic surgeon. Both the lateral collateral ligament (LCL) and ulnar collateral ligament (LCL) play an integral role in providing stability to the elbow joint [1–12]. Generally, UCL injuries are seen in athletes such as pitchers, javelin throwers, or other overhead athletes [12, 13]. LCL injuries are usually associated with simple or complex elbow dislocations [12, 13]. There has been a significant increase in the number of UCL injuries diagnosed among athletes [1, 4, 14]. Similarly, there has been an increase in the number of UCL reconstructions performed on athletes as well [8, 15].

UCL repair had poor functional results in athletes when compared to UCL reconstruction [16–18]. Hence, UCL reconstruction techniques such as the docking or modified Jobe technique were rendered as the gold standard for surgical management of medial elbow instability. Conversely, there are newer studies demonstrating that UCL repair is a viable option in the young adult and adolescent patients with acute UCL tears [19, 20]. Dugas et al. were the first to describe performing UCL repair with internal brace augmentation [1]. This has since increased the interest in UCL repair with suture augmentation in acute/subacute UCL injuries because of the benefits afforded to patients. UCL repair augmented with internal bracing has shown to be equally or more biomechanically stable than UCL reconstruction [1, 4, 5]. Internal bracing has an increased load to failure and greater resistance to gap formation than traditional UCL reconstruction techniques [5]. A hallmark of UCL repair

with internal bracing is earlier return to play (≈6 months) than UCL reconstruction (≈12 months) [8]. In addition, internal bracing has been shown to increase the biomechanical stability of UCL reconstruction such as the docking technique [8, 15].

There is still controversy on the preferred management of LCL insufficiency with regard to repairing or reconstructing the LCL [2, 9, 12]. However, internal bracing increases the biomechanical stability of both the repaired and reconstructed LCL. Utilizing the internal brace mitigates the need for external fixation or prolonged immobilization to protect repaired/reconstructed LCL [2, 9, 10]. It allows these patients to begin immediate range of motion exercises to help decrease incidence of postoperative stiffness.

The InternalBrace™ (Arthrex Inc.) technique is an important skill that the shoulder/elbow surgeon should have in his/her armamentarium. In this chapter, we provide the reader with a detailed technique of the InternalBrace™ with tips and tricks to ameliorate the difficult aspects of this procedure.

Indications

UCL repair is warranted after failure of a non-operative trial that includes physical therapy, non-steroidal anti-inflammatory drugs, and strengthening of the flexor/pronator mass. These patients usually have intractable medial elbow pain, and UCL injury is confirmed with magnetic resonance imaging (MRI). The UCL should be assessed for any degenerative changes because this dictates surgical management [7]. Also, the physician should inquire if patients are experiencing any ulnar nerve pathology. There is a subset of patients with medial elbow instability that have ulnar nerve pathology such as cubital tunnel syndrome or ulnar neuritis [12]. Generally, UCL reconstruction/repair is reserved for overhead athletes such as pitchers, gymnasts, javelin throwers, etc. [12]. UCL repair with internal bracing should be

W. B. Geissler (✉)
Division of Hand and Upper Extremity Surgery, Section of Arthroscopic Surgery and Sports Medicine, Department of Orthopedic Surgery and Rehabilitation, University of Mississippi Medical Center, Jackson, MS, USA

K. F. Purcell
Department of Orthopedic Surgery, University of Mississippi Medical Center, Jackson, MS, USA

© Springer Nature Switzerland AG 2022
W. B. Geissler (ed.), *Wrist and Elbow Arthroscopy with Selected Open Procedures*, https://doi.org/10.1007/978-3-030-78881-0_64

733

performed on patients with acute/subacute tears [1]. UCL reconstruction is performed on patients with chronic UCL tears [1, 7].

LCL repair is generally indicated in fracture dislocations of the elbow, namely, the terrible triad injury [12]. Also, LCL repair is warranted in symptomatic posterolateral rotatory instability (PLRI) of the elbow [11].

Contraindications

Patients who are unable to follow postoperative protocol such as non-weight bearing (NWB) or refuse to engage in physical therapy/rehabilitation.

Surgical Technique

Lateral Ulno-Humeral Ligament Reconstruction

The standard lateral approach is made to the elbow centered over the lateral epicondyle. Sharp dissection is carried down to the lateral fascia where thick skin flaps are elevated. The origin of the extensor carpi radialis longus, brevis, and comminus is elevated from the lateral epicondyle, and close attention is made not stray posterior to the affect the ulno-humeral lateral complex. Usually in patients with trauma or a fracture with lateral instability, the surgeon will fall into the defect (Fig. 64.1). The lateral ulno-humeral complex usually tears off the humeral side exposing the elbow. Dissection is continued distally and posteriorly to expose the proximal olecranon opposite of the radial head. This will be the site for insertion for the first 4.75 swivel lock anchor with fiber tape (Arthrex, Naples, FL). The ideal starting point would be mid-way anterior-posterior on the olecranon and just opposite of the radial head. If the anchor is placed too far distally, the fiber tape can snap on the radial head causing pain particularly if a radial head implant is placed. If the anchor is placed to proximately, it does not provide adequate lateral support to the elbow. It is important that the hole be drilled obliquely, so the anchor will remain within the canal of the ulnar and not protrude out the ulna aspect to affect the ulna nerve (Fig. 64.2). It is very important to tap this drill hole as this is hard cortical bone and the anchor cannot be inserted without tapping the bone (Fig. 64.3). The anchor with the fiber tape and #2 fiber wire are inserted to the hole in the olecranon (Fig. 64.4). The fiber wire from the anchor is placed through the distal aspect of the lateral ulnar humeral complex for repair.

The second 4.75 swivel lock anchor (Arthrex, Naples, FL) will then be placed on the lateral epicondyle. The most ideal location is slightly anterior to the midline of the lateral epicondyle (Fig. 64.5). This is relatively an oblique edge, and it's hard to get the most ideal stating point. It should be

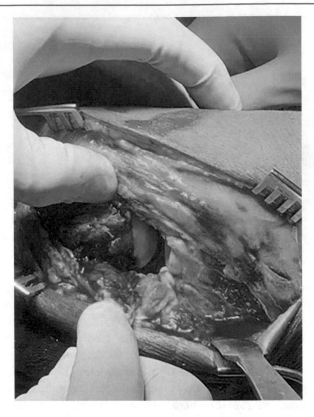

Fig. 64.1 Intraoperative photograph demonstrating the lateral approach to the elbow following elbow dislocation. The patient had complete stripping of the lateral ulnar humeral complex ligaments off the humeral epicondyle

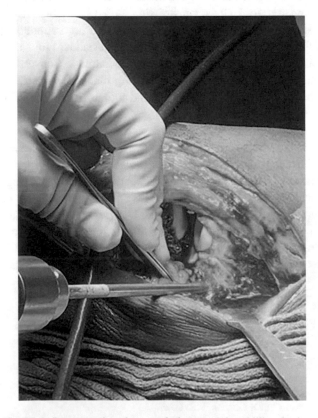

Fig. 64.2 Intraoperative photograph demonstrating drilling for insertion of the internal brace for lateral instability. The ideal landmark for the olecranon internal brace insertion is midway anterior-posterior of the olecranon opposite of the radial head

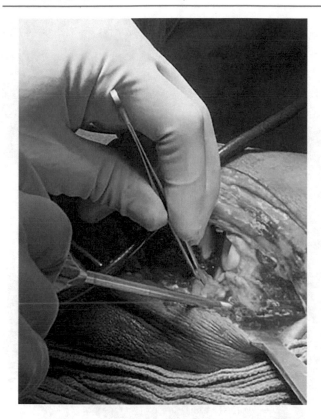

Fig. 64.3 It is vital to tap the drill hole prior to anchor insertion due to the hard cortical bone

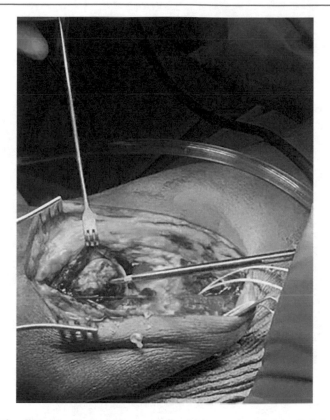

Fig. 64.5 The ideal starting point for the humeral anchor is slightly anterior to the midline

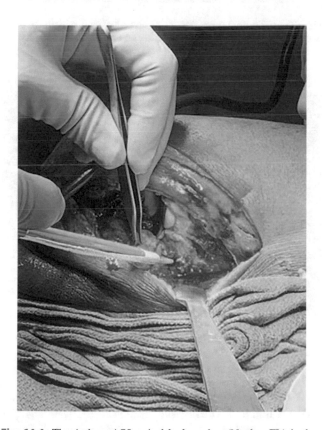

Fig. 64.4 The Arthrex 4.75 swivel lock anchor (Naples, FL) is then inserted into the drill hole

drilled obliquely, ending proximally so the anchor does not protrude into the olecranon fossa. The goal is to keep it midlined to in the humerus so it does not protrude either through the anterior or posterior aspects to the distal humerus. The humerus is drilled and tapped as again this is a hard, cortical bone and the anchor cannot be inserted unless the bone has been tapped. Fiber tape for the first anchor on the olecranon is then inserted into the second anchor, which is inserted into the humerus to form the internal brace (Fig. 64.6). The elbow is held at −30 full extension while the anchor is being placed. Usually the fiber tape self-tensions itself as anchor is being screwed into the humerus (Fig. 64.7). For localized lateral instability to the elbow, this internal brace immediately provides instability to the elbow (Figs. 64.8, 64.9, 64.10, and 64.11). The remaining #2 fiber wire is then placed in the proximal aspect of the lateral ulno-humeral complex and is tied. The remaining #2 fiber wire is placed distally and is tied, and then the two sutures are tied to themselves to further provide stability to the elbow. Lastly, the fiber tape that was inserted through the proximal anchor can be passed through the remaining part of the lateral ligament complex and is tied down. This can leave a bulky knot, and the knot is passed through the muscle, which decreases its irritability. The remaining part of the extensor muscular is then closed in a pants-over-vest fashion. The elbow is immobilized for 2 weeks and then placed in a hinge brace at −20° extension

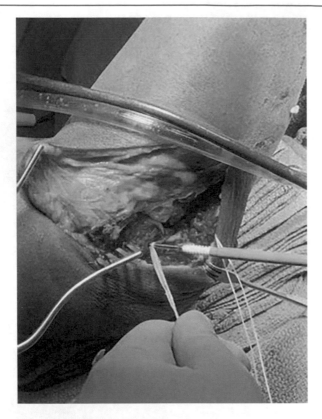

Fig. 64.6 After the drill hole has been tapped, the second Arthrex 4.75 swivel lock anchor (Naples, FL) is then inserted into the lateral epicondyle with the elbow at approximately −30° of full extension

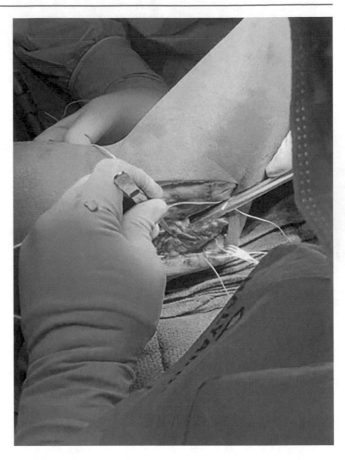

Fig. 64.8 The remaining fiber wire and fiber tape sutures from the anchors can then be inserted to the lateral ulna humeral complex for direct primary repair

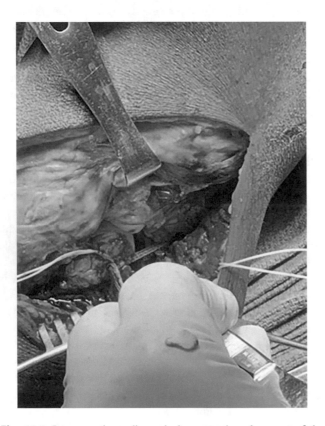

Fig. 64.7 Intraoperative radiograph demonstrating placement of the internal brace in immediate stability to the elbow

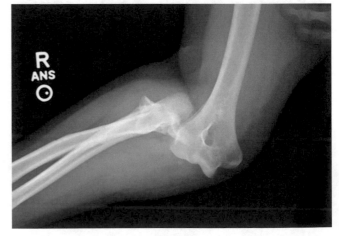

Fig. 64.9 Anterior-posterior radiograph showing a right fracture dislocation of the elbow with gross instability

for 3 weeks, and then range- and motion-strengthening exercises are initiated. The internal brace is inserted (Fig. 64.12). Again, the ideal starting point is opposite to the radial head on the olecranon so the brace does not snap in the implant (Figs. 64.13 and 64.14).

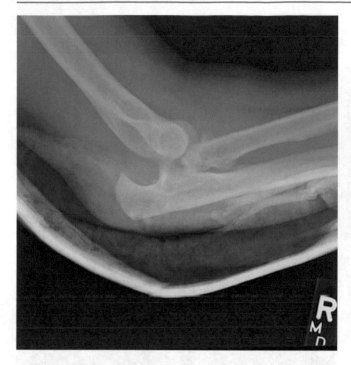

Fig. 64.10 Lateral radiograph showing a grossly unstable elbow dislocated despite cast immobilization

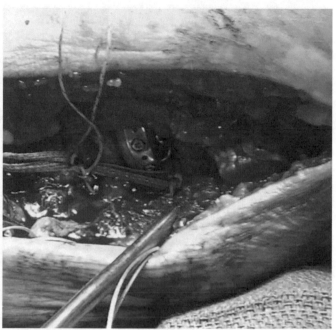

Fig. 64.12 The radial head is anatomically stabilized back to the proximal radial shaft. A lateral internal brace is performed providing immediately instability back to the grossly unstable elbow

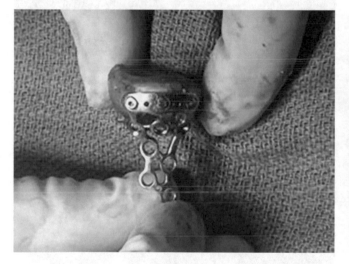

Fig. 64.11 The patient had a comminuted fracture to the radial head. The radial head is put back together on the back table and stabilized with a Medartis radial head plate (Basel, Switzerland)

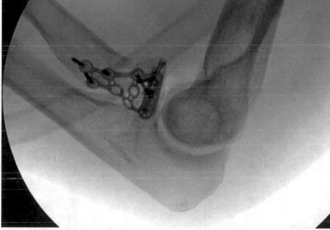

Fig. 64.13 Intraoperative fluoroscopic view demonstrating immediate stability to the elbow following open internal fixation of the radial head and lateral internal brace stabilization

Ulnar Collateral Ligament Reconstruction

The standard medial approach is made to the elbow centered about the medial epicondyle (Figs. 64.15, 64.16, and 64.17). Blunt dissection is carried down to avoid injury to branches of the medial antebrachial cutaneous nerve. These are identified distally and carefully protected. The ulnar nerves are identified and traced through the flexor carpi ulnaris. It's a surgeon's preference to continue to work around the nerve or for it to be transposed anteriorly following the procedure. The flexor carpi ulnaris is split, and the base of the coronoid and proximal olecranon is identified (Fig. 64.18). The ideal starting point for the anchor is mid-way anterior-posterior on the olecranon at the level of the coronoid process. The ulna is drilled obliquely as described before and tapped, and the 4.75 swivel lock anchor with fiber tape and fiber wire is inserted (Arthrex, Naples, FL) (Fig. 64.19). The ideal placement for the second anchor will be the base of the humeral epicondyle and slightly anterior if possible. The hole is

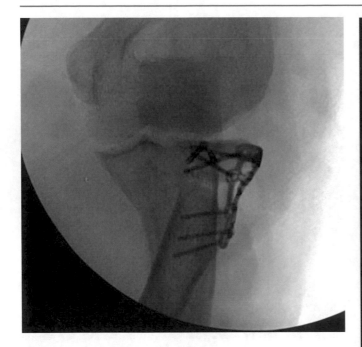

Fig. 64.14 Anterior-posterior fluoroscopic view shown anatomic reduction to the radial head and stability to the elbow following internal brace stabilization

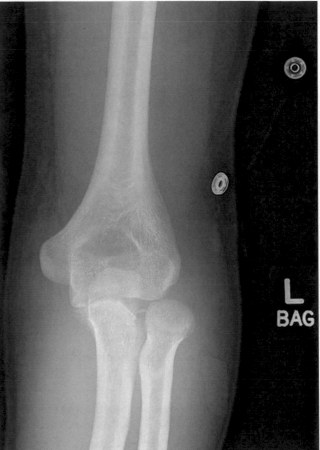

Fig. 64.16 Anterior-posterior radiograph showing gross instability to the elbow with radial translation

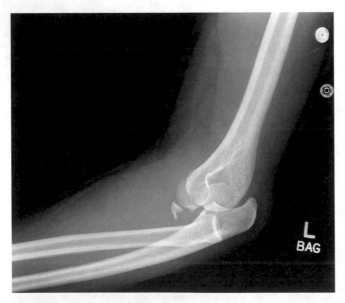

Fig. 64.15 Lateral radiograph showing a fractured dislocation to the elbow with a large coronoid fragment

drilled obliquely, so the anchor does not protrude into the olecranon fossa and stays within the confines of the distal humerus. The fiber tape from the first anchor is then passed through the second anchor after the drill hole has been tapped and inserted at the elbow −30° with full extension (Fig. 64.20). As before, the fiber tape usually self-tensions as you place the anchor (Fig. 64.21). The remaining #2 fiber wire for both anchors are passed through the medial ligament

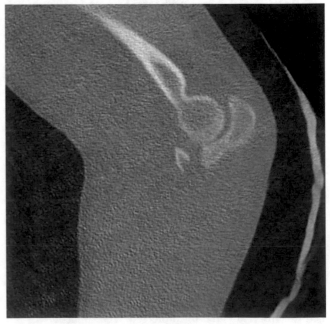

Fig. 64.17 Lateral CT evaluation demonstrating a large coronoid fragment in the grossly unstable elbow

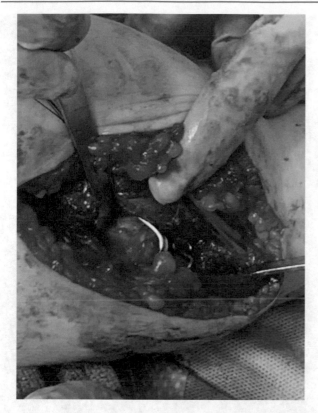

Fig. 64.18 Intraoperative photograph demonstrating medial approach to the elbow with stabilization to the coronoid fragment with a Medartis coronoid plate (Basel, Switzerland)

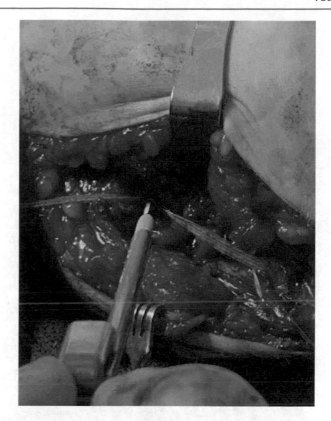

Fig. 64.20 Intraoperative photograph showing insertion of the 4.75 swivel lock anchor on the medial epicondyle with the elbow flexed at 30° (Arthrex, Naples, FL)

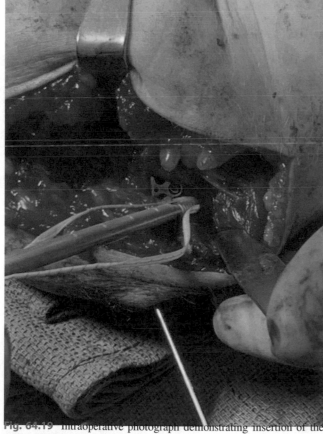

Fig. 64.19 Intraoperative photograph demonstrating insertion of the 4.75 swivel lock anchor (Arthrex, Naples, FL) on the olecranon just adjacent to the coronoid plate

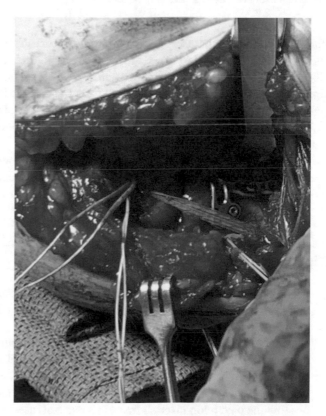

Fig. 64.21 Intraoperative photograph showing stability back to the elbow with medial internal brace over the coronoid plate

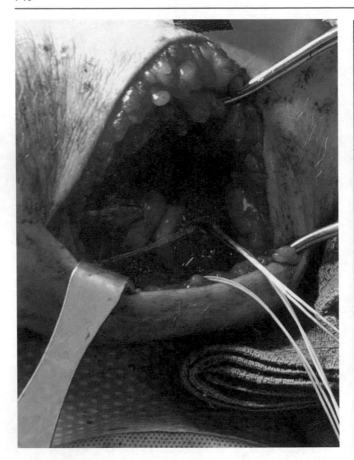

Fig. 64.22 Intraoperative radiograph showing the lateral internal brace stabilizing the lateral aspect of the elbow

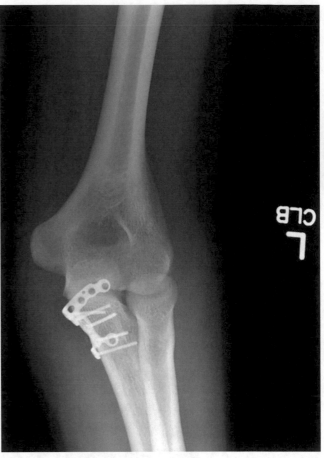

Fig. 64.23 Anterior-posterior radiograph with a coronoid plate showing restoration of stability to the elbow

complex and tied to themselves. The remaining fiber tape on the humeral anchor can be passed through the remaining portion of the ulnar collateral ligament securing this part of the ligament. The knot can be bulky so the fiber tape knot is passed through the muscle of the flexor carpi ulnaris. At this point, the ulnar nerve can be transposed depending on the surgeon's preference (Figs. 64.22, 64.23, and 64.24).

The elbow is immobilized for 2 weeks, and then a removable brace at −20° extension for 3 weeks and then regular strengthening exercises are then initiated through physical therapy (Figs. 64.25 and 64.26).

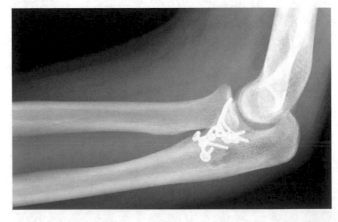

Fig. 64.24 Lateral radiograph of the elbow shoeing complete stability with no sub-locking of the joint

Tips and Tricks

- Make sure to tap the drill holes before attempting to insert the anchor. In hard cortical bone, the anchor will not advance unless it is tapped.
- Make sure to insert the anchors in an oblique fashion into the olecranon and the humerus. In this manner, the anchors will not protrude out the opposite cortex. This will decrease any irritation to the anchor and to avoid penetrating the olecranon inserted fossa in a humeral inserted anchor.

- Ideally on the humerus the starting point for the drill hole should be anterior to the midline. Elbow ligament stability is important in particular in extension, and by placing the anchor slightly anterior, will tighten up the internal brace extension as compared to elbow flexion.

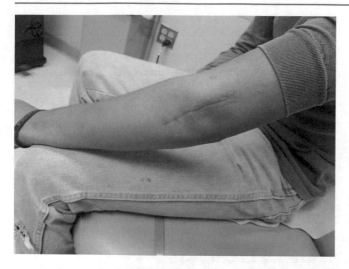

Fig. 64.25 Photograph of the patient showing approximately −10° of full extension of 3 months postoperatively

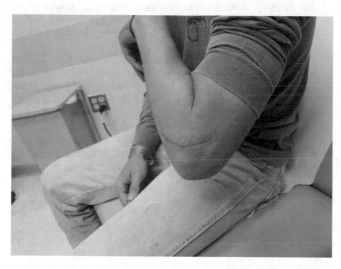

Fig. 64.26 Lateral radiograph showing complete flexion to the elbow following the devastating injury 3 months post injury

- Tighten the fiber tape with the elbow at −30° at full extension. This will provide the most stability to the internal brace reconstruction.
- Use the additional fiber wire on the anchors to further secure the collateral ligament complex, as well as the remaining fiber tape on the humeral anchor.
- Remember the fiber tape knot can be quite bulky, and it is important to pass this through the muscle to decrease soft tissue irritation.
- Pay close attention to the medial antebrachial cutaneous nerves through the medial cited approach. If these are lacerated, it can result in troublesome and problematic neuromas.
- Transposition of the ulnar nerve is surgeon dependent.

Conclusion

Ligamentous reconstruction for UCL injuries is the gold standard for the management of UCL injuries. However, several studies demonstrated UCL repair with internal bracing is more biomechanically stable than UCL reconstruction techniques such as the docking technique or modified Jobe reconstruction [1, 4, 5]. The InternalBrace™ offloads the stress from the UCL repair while it is healing. UCL repair with the internal bracing increases load to failure and torsional stiffness with less gap formation than UCL reconstruction techniques [1, 5, 21, 22] and restores valgus stability similar to that of the native ligament [4]. The main feat of UCL repair with internal bracing for the athlete is earlier return to play and being able to participate in more rigorous physical training earlier than UCL reconstruction [4, 6–8, 22].

The orthopedic surgeon must thoroughly analyze if the patient is an ideal candidate for UCL repair with internal bracing. This procedure is usually offered to younger athletes that are eager to return to sports after failed nonoperative management [7]. The UCL tissue must be healthy appearing and free of chronic degenerative changes such as fraying or fibrosis. Also, patients with large bony avulsions off the medial epicondyle or sublime tubercle are poor candidates for the procedure [7]. This bone loss associated with this procedure will compromise the ligamentous stability. Also, patients have to be committed to participating in a postoperative rehabilitation program.

The InternalBrace™ can be used to augment UCL reconstruction if primary repair cannot be performed on the patient [8, 15]. It decreases the stress placed on the allograft. Also, internal bracing is used to augment LCL repair/reconstruction as well [2, 9–11].

In summation, internal bracing is a novel procedure with several advantages and an important technique for the shoulder/elbow surgeon to understand. Future studies need to investigate the long-term functional outcomes of internal bracing, functionality of UCL repair with internal bracing in older athletes, and optimal sites for suture tape/anchor placement for LCL repair/reconstruction.

References

1. Dugas JR, Walters BL, Beason DP, Fleisig GS, Chronister JE. Biomechanical comparison of ulnar collateral ligament repair with internal bracing versus modified Jobe reconstruction. Am J Sports Med. 2016;44(3):735–41.
2. Greiner S, Koch M, Kerschbaum M, Bhide PP. Repair and augmentation of the lateral collateral ligament complex using internal bracing in dislocations and fracture dislocations of the elbow restores stability and allows early rehabilitation. Knee Surg Sports Traumatol Arthrosc. 2019;27(10):3269–75.

3. Yoo J-S, Yang E-A. Clinical results of an arthroscopic modified Brostrom operation with and without an internal brace. J Orthop Traumatol. 2016;17(4):353–60.

4. Bodendorfer BM, Looney AM, Lipkin SL, Nolton EC, Li J, Najarian RG, et al. Biomechanical comparison of ulnar collateral ligament reconstruction with the docking technique versus repair with internal bracing. Am J Sports Med. 2018;46(14):3495–501.

5. Jones CM, Beason DP, Dugas JR. Ulnar collateral ligament reconstruction versus repair with internal bracing: comparison of cyclic fatigue mechanics. Orthop J Sports Med. 2018;6(2):2325967118755991.

6. Wilk KE, Arrigo CA, Bagwell MS, Rothermich MA, Dugas JR. Repair of the ulnar collateral ligament of the elbow: rehabilitation following internal brace surgery. J Orthop Sports Phys Ther. 2019;49(4):253–61.

7. Moore AR, Fleisig GS, Dugas JR. Ulnar collateral ligament repair. Orthop Clin North Am. 2019;50(3):383–9.

8. Leasure J, Reynolds K, Thorne M, Escamilla R, Akizuki K. Biomechanical comparison of ulnar collateral ligament reconstruction with a modified docking technique with and without suture augmentation. Am J Sports Med. 2019;47(4):928–32.

9. Melbourne C, Cook JL, Della Rocca GJ, Loftis C, Konicek J, Smith MJ. Biomechanical assessment of lateral ulnar collateral ligament repair and reconstruction with or without internal brace augmentation. JSES Int. 2020;4(2):224–30.

10. Ellwein A, Füßler L, Ferle M, Smith T, Lill H, Pastor M-F. Suture tape augmentation of the lateral ulnar collateral ligament increases load to failure in simulated posterolateral rotatory instability. Knee Surg Sports Traumatol Arthrosc [Internet]. 2020. Available from: https://doi.org/10.1007/s00167-020-05918-5.

11. Scheiderer B, Imhoff FB, Kia C, Aglio J, Morikawa D, Obopilwe E, et al. LUCL internal bracing restores posterolateral rotatory stability of the elbow. Knee Surg Sports Traumatol Arthrosc. 2020;28(4):1195–201.

12. Wolfe SW, Hotchkiss RN, Pederson WC, Kozin SH, Cohen MS. Green's operative hand surgery. Philadelphia: Elsevier; 2016.

13. Savoie FH, O'Brien M. Chronic medial instability of the elbow. EFORT Open Rev. 2017;2(1):1–6.

14. Urch E, Limpisvasti O, ElAttrache NS, Itami Y, McGarry MH, Photopoulos CD, et al. Biomechanical evaluation of a modified internal brace construct for the treatment of ulnar collateral ligament injuries. Orthop J Sports Med. 2019;7(10):2325967119874135.

15. Bernholt DL, Lake SP, Castile RM, Papangelou C, Hauck O, Smith MV. Biomechanical comparison of docking ulnar collateral ligament reconstruction with and without an internal brace. J Shoulder Elb Surg. 2019;28(11):2247–52.

16. Conway JE, Jobe FW, Glousman RE, Pink M. Medial instability of the elbow in throwing athletes. Treatment by repair or reconstruction of the ulnar collateral ligament. J Bone Joint Surg Am. 1992;74(1):67–83.

17. Andrews JR, Timmerman LA. Outcome of elbow surgery in professional baseball players. Am J Sports Med. 1995;23(4):407–13.

18. Azar FM, Andrews JR, Wilk KE, Groh D. Operative treatment of ulnar collateral ligament injuries of the elbow in athletes. Am J Sports Med. 2000;28(1):16–23.

19. O'Connell RS, O'Brien M, Savoie FH. Primary repair of ulnar collateral ligament injuries of the elbow. Oper Tech Sports Med. 2020;28(2):150735.

20. Savoie FH 3rd, Trenhaile SW, Roberts J, Field LD, Ramsey JR. Primary repair of ulnar collateral ligament injuries of the elbow in young athletes: a case series of injuries to the proximal and distal ends of the ligament. Am J Sports Med. 2008;36(6):1066–72.

21. Bachmaier S, Wijdicks CA, Verma NN, Higgins LD, Greiner S. Biomechanical functional elbow restoration of acute ulnar collateral ligament tears: the role of internal bracing on gap formation and repair stabilization. Am J Sports Med. 2020;48(8):1884–92.

22. Dugas JR, Looze CA, Capogna B, Walters BL, Jones CM, Rothermich MA, et al. Ulnar collateral ligament repair with collagen-dipped FiberTape augmentation in overhead-throwing athletes. Am J Sports Med. 2019;47(5):1096–102.

Pediatric Ulnar Collateral Ligament Injuries

Timothy Luchetti, Justine S. Kim, and Mark E. Baratz

Introduction

The ulnar collateral ligament (UCL) is comprised of three portions – anterior, posterior, and transverse bundles [1, 2]. The anterior band is the most clinically significant and originates on the medial epicondyle of the distal humerus. It inserts onto the sublime tubercle of the coronoid process of the ulna. The posterior band inserts onto the posteromedial olecranon, while the transverse band connects the two insertion points on the ulna.

The UCL is the primary restraint to valgus stress when the elbow is between 20° and 120° of flexion [1]. This type of stress is consistent with throwing maneuvers as in baseball, football, javelin, and tennis. The elbow can only flex and extend without rotation, resulting in compressive forces laterally and distraction forces medially during valgus stress. Elbow UCL injury or valgus instability occurs when the elbow undergoes radially directed force that exceeds the tensile properties of the ligament or strength of the epicondyle to which the ligament is attached. Cadaveric data have demonstrated that the acceleration phase of throwing generates forces that exceed UCL tensile strength, thereby contributing to elevated injury risk with repetition [3]. UCL injuries are becoming increasingly common among athletes [4], even children [5]. The diagnosis and management of UCL injuries has continued to evolve over the years. We review operative indications, contraindications, and surgical technique for UCL injuries

and present a case of failed non-operative management due to persistent UCL stress.

Case

A 7-year-old right-hand dominant female gymnast presented to the orthopedic clinic at our children's hospital 4 days following an anterior left elbow dislocation. The patient stated she was trying to complete a vault during gymnastics practice and landed on her outstretched left arm. The injury resulted in a closed, displaced fracture of the medial epicondyle of the left humerus. This patient underwent a bedside reduction at an outside hospital in the emergency department on the day of the injury and was referred to us for follow-up evaluation and definitive management. On presentation, physical examination demonstrated a normal neurologic and vascular examination. The medial epicondyle avulsion was displaced 5.5 mm (Fig. 65.1). We initially recommended non-operative management, and immobilization in a long-arm cast was initiated for 3 weeks. The patient was seen 3 weeks later, and early controlled mobilization was initiated. She did well initially and was discharged from our care. She returned to gymnastics after completing a course of therapy. For several years, she competed without issue.

Three years later, she returned complaining of 1 year of medial elbow pain. She reported that a week prior to this presentation, she had landed a back handspring with immediate left elbow pain, exacerbating her baseline chronic pain. She noted that her greatest pain was with flexion of the elbow. She did not feel she could continue to participate in gymnastics.

On physical examination, she had tenderness with palpation over the under surface of the epicondyle at the insertion of the ulnar collateral ligament. She had laxity with a valgus stress and pain during the moving valgus stress test. She had a positive Tinel's sign over the ulnar nerve at the elbow. Based on history, clinical exam findings, and radiographic

T. Luchetti · M. E. Baratz
Department of Orthopedic Surgery, University of Pittsburgh Medical Center, Bethel Park, PA, USA
e-mail: baratzme@upmc.edu

J. S. Kim (✉)
Department of Plastic and Reconstructive Surgery, University of Pittsburgh Medical Center, Pittsburgh, PA, USA
e-mail: kimjs4@upmc.edu

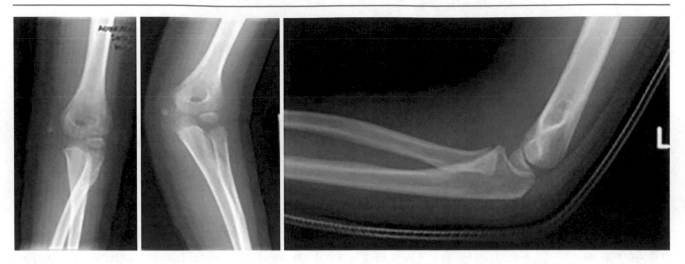

Fig. 65.1 Patient 1: Immediate post-injury left elbow radiographs. Three-view left elbow radiographs demonstrating medial epicondyle extra-articular avulsion with 5.5 mm of displacement

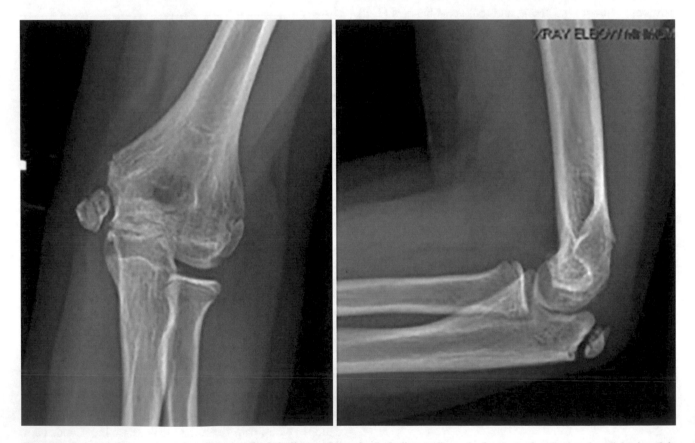

Fig. 65.2 Patient 1: 3 years post-injury, pre-operative left elbow radiographs. Left elbow radiographs demonstrating displaced medial epicondyle fracture with non-union

imaging (Fig. 65.2), the patient was diagnosed with a non-united medial epicondyle fracture and ulnar nerve compressive neuropathy.

The patient and her family elected to proceed with surgical intervention. At our recommendation, the patient underwent non-union excision with repair of the ulnar collateral ligament and in situ ulnar nerve decompression.

Technique

Surgery was conducted under general anesthesia with a left upper extremity tourniquet. An incision was made over the medial aspect of the left elbow. The ulnar nerve was identified between the two heads of the flexor carpi ulnaris muscle and released through the cubital tunnel where there were

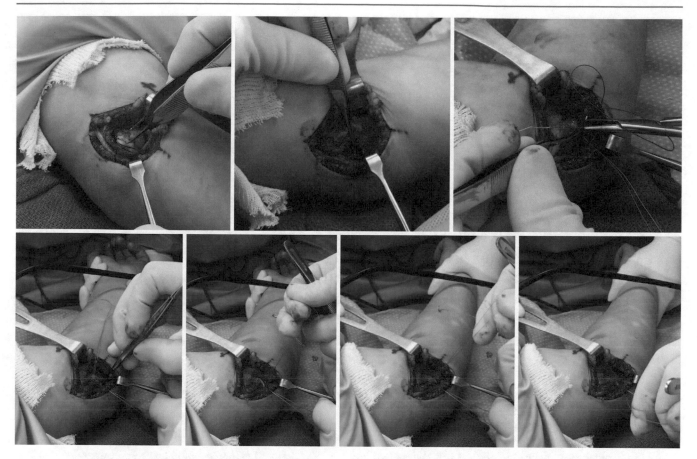

Fig. 65.3 Patient 1: Operative intervention. First row: Incision is made over the medial aspect of the left elbow. Identify the ulnar nerve between the two heads of the flexor carpi ulnaris muscle and release through the cubital tunnel. Excise the humeral epicondylar non-union. Take care to preserve the capsule and fibers of the anterior band of the UCL. Run a locking suture with 4-0 FiberLoop to grasp the anterior band of the medial collateral ligament and repair the ligament. Second row: Lock the anchor at the sublime tubercle. Approximate the medial joint line by placing the elbow in 60° of flexion, supinating the forearm, and applying a varus stress to the elbow. Bring the second limb of the suture anchor through the end of the ligament and suture tendon down to bone

signs of nerve compression. The nerve was released up to the brachium proximally until surrounded by loose areolar tissue. Distally, the nerve was decompressed until surrounded by fatty tissue. Excision of the humeral epicondylar non-union was performed by elevating the flexor pronator origin off of the epicondyle. Care was taken to preserve the capsule and fibers of the anterior band of the ulnar collateral ligament during the posterior tissue dissection.

A running locking suture with 4-0 FiberLoop (Arthrex, Inc., Naples, FL) was used to grasp the fibers of the anterior band of the medial collateral ligament and repair the ligament. A mini Mitek suture anchor (DePuy Mitek Inc., Norwood, MA) was placed near the center of the trochlea. The medial joint line was approximated by placing the elbow in 60° of flexion, supinating the forearm, and applying a varus stress to the elbow. One limb of the anchor suture was run along the fibers of the anterior band of the medial collateral ligament and back proximally. The second limb of the suture anchor was brought through the end of the ligament at the point of isometry and used to suture the tendon down to

bone. The FiberLoop was tied to the suture anchor, augmenting the ligament repair.

The fascia of the flexor pronator was repaired to the posterior capsule to create a smooth surface over the medial epicondyle. Flexion and extension of the elbow demonstrated that the ulnar nerve did not subluxate anteriorly. A sterile dressing and splint were applied with the elbow in 90° of flexion and full forearm supination (Fig. 65.3).

Post-operative Course

The long-arm splint was removed at 2 weeks. A removable brace was applied. The child was taught wrist curls with her forearm resting on her thigh. She was also permitted to exercise on a treadmill and stationary bike. At 4 weeks, she had 30–90° of elbow motion. She had normal sensation to light touch distally and a negative Tinel's. Radiographs showed a concentric joint and no residual bone in the region of the medial epicondyle (Fig. 65.4). She was instructed to prog-

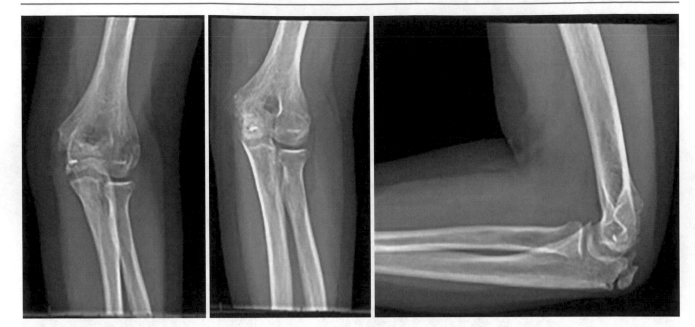

Fig. 65.4 Patient 1: 11 weeks post-operative left elbow radiographs. Left elbow radiographs demonstrating suture anchor placement in the medial epicondyle in good position

ress to range of motion exercises and to wean brace use during the day. She was allowed to return to gymnastics for conditioning, running, and jumping while in the brace.

At the 5-week post-operative clinic visit, the patient had no pain, numbness, or re-injury and resumed participation in light gymnastics. She had full elbow motion and was enrolled in occupational therapy for gentle therapy of the wrist and shoulder. Valgus loading was prohibited.

By 11 weeks post-operatively, she had no pain with valgus stress. She was permitted to perform resistive exercises and light work on the bar. Floor work was prohibited.

At 4 months, the patient was instructed to continue physical therapy and released for full return to gymnastics. The patient was seen at 6 months with no new complaints after fully participating in all gymnastics activities. On exam, she had symmetric range of motion from 0° to 145° (Fig. 65.5).

The patient returned roughly 1.5 years after surgery with recurrent left elbow pain after a particularly intense series of gymnastics events. On exam, there was no obvious deformity. She had tenderness with palpation over the medial epicondyle and flexor pronator mass. Elbow flexion, extension, supination, and pronation were symmetric with the right side with pain on extension. Sensory and vascular exams were normal. Radiographs of the left elbow demonstrated prior resection of the medial epicondyle with repair of the medial collateral ligament and no changes from prior radiographs (Fig. 65.6). She was instructed to rest for 2 weeks and start wrist curls to strengthen forearm flexor muscles. She improved with time and strengthening exercises and has continued to do well. She was last seen 2 years post-operatively.

Tips and Tricks

- Non-operative management is the recommended first-line treatment for UCL injuries with or without medial epicondyle fracture.
- Indications for surgical intervention in the acute setting include medial epicondyle fractures demonstrating displacement with entrapment of the bony fragment within the joint, intra-articular involvement, open fracture, ulnar nerve dysfunction, greater than 2 to 15 mm displacement, or greater than 2 to 5 mm displacement in athletes who throw or gymnasts.
- Indications for surgical intervention in the chronic setting include history of failed non-operative management, nonunion, persistent UCL laxity, medial elbow pain, ulnar nerve dysfunction, and patient desire to return to competitive sport.
- Contraindications include patient inability to comply with post-operative rehabilitation and ulnotrochlear or radiocapitellar arthritis.
- Be cautious and meticulous during dissection to prevent injury to the ulnar nerve or branches of the medial antebrachial cutaneous nerve.
- Release any point of compression of the ulnar nerve proximally and distally.
- Preserve the capsule and fibers of the anterior band of the ulnar collateral ligament during the posterior tissue dissection.
- Initiate early range of motion in the post-operative period, as early as 2 weeks.

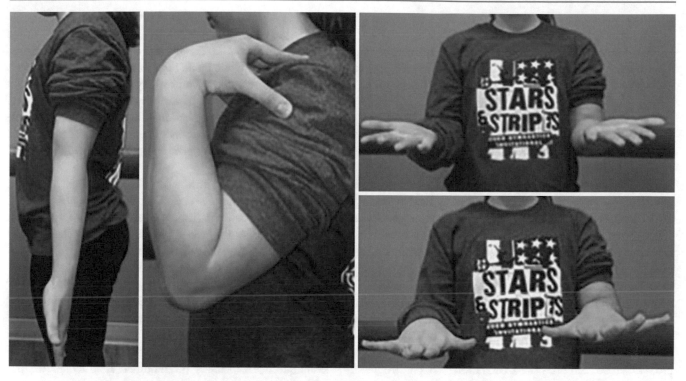

Fig. 65.5 Patient 1: 6-month follow-up clinical exam. Clinical exam demonstrating full range of motion (0–145°) and symmetry with right, un-injured side

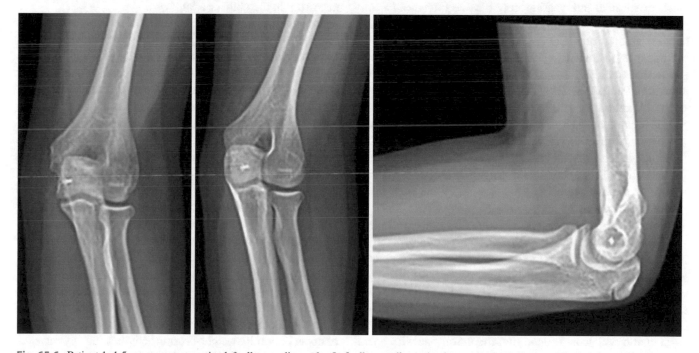

Fig. 65.6 Patient 1: 1.5-years post-operative left elbow radiographs. Left elbow radiographs demonstrating prior resection of the medial epicondyle with stable repair of the medial collateral ligament

- Allow patients to return to full activities no earlier than 4 months post-repair.
- Encourage strengthening exercises of the forearm flexor muscles to reinforce the UCL repair, stability, and function.

Considerations and Outcomes

Persistent instability after elbow dislocation in a child was first described by Albert in 1881 [6]. This typically is thought to occur in young adults with a dislocation in late adolescence prior to physeal closure [7]. This phenomenon was described as "posterolateral capsule and ligamentous complex laxity" by Osborne in 1966 [8]. Most authors recommended bracing for at least 8 weeks after reduction [9].

Virtually all of the early literature regarding surgical management of pediatric elbow dislocations focused on the posterolateral ligamentous complex [8, 10]. But UCL tears can and often do occur in acute upper extremity trauma, particularly after an acute elbow dislocation. This is frequently associated with a medial epicondyle avulsion, as was the case in our patient.

Historically, UCL injuries were difficult to diagnose, and lack of surgical intervention may have led athletes to early retirement from their sport. With heightened awareness and understanding of UCL pathoanatomy, improved physical exam, and advanced imaging, our ability to diagnose and treat these injuries has vastly improved over time. Non-operative treatment after successful closed reduction and immobilization is still advocated as first-line treatment. Some authors have argued that elbow instability can become a chronic problem even with minimally displaced medial epicondyle fractures as the anterior bundle of the UCL may be stretched [11–13] or because of pain associated with non-union of the avulsed bone. This was likely the issue in our aforementioned case report.

Operative indications for acute medial epicondyle fractures have included displacement with entrapment of the bony fragment within the joint, intra-articular involvement, open fracture, ulnar nerve dysfunction, greater than 2 to 15 mm displacement, greater than 2 to 5 mm displacement in athletes who throw or gymnasts, and history of failed non-operative management. Kamath et al. (2009) performed a systematic review and found that the union rate with operative fixation was 9.33 times better than with non-operative management; however, the two groups did not differ in terms of pain or ulnar nerve symptoms at final follow-up [14].

Our patient had minimal displacement and no ulnar nerve symptoms after reduction of her elbow dislocation and was managed appropriately with non-operative treatment. With time and continued gymnastic activity, however, she developed elbow pain associated with the non-union and valgus laxity. Erdil et al. (2012) discussed the operative management of symptomatic medial epicondyle non-union [2]. The authors recognized the controversy surrounding this topic and advocated excision of the fragment with ligamentous repair and anterior transposition of the ulnar nerve to restore normal elbow joint anatomy. They further recommended early physical therapy at post-operative day 5 with range of motion exercises.

A related entity, attritional UCL attenuation, occurs in older, overhead athletes (i.e., baseball, water polo, tennis, gymnastics, wrestling). These patients are more vulnerable because of excessive, repetitive valgus force place on the elbow during normal play [15]. This occurs particularly during late cocking and early acceleration phases of the throwing motion [15].

The original UCL reconstruction was developed by Jobe and involved detaching and reflecting the flexor-pronator mass, submuscular transposition of the ulnar nerve, and tunneling of the posterior humeral cortex. Modifications of this technique have included the modified Jobe technique, the docking technique, American Sports Medicine Institute (ASMI) modification, and the hybrid interference screw fixation technique [16, 17]. Ligament reconstruction is rarely necessary in the child or adolescent.

Recent literature suggests that the incidence of sports injuries has been increasing during the last few decades [5, 18]. Roughly 35 million children participate in sports each year in America, and over 3.5 million sports injuries occur annually [5]. In 1 recent survey of 203 healthy youth baseball players, 46% of players reported having been encouraged to keep playing despite ongoing arm pain [19]. Year-round leagues, baseball showcases, and multiple travel teams have all contributed to the epidemic of overuse injuries in the United States [20]. While the concept of year-round training was typically associated with professional sports, children and adolescents are increasingly being expected to "specialize" within a single sport in order to maintain a competitive edge for recruiting efforts [1].

In keeping with the overall trends, upper extremity sports injuries are on the rise in youth sports. Estimates suggest that between 20% and 40% of 9- to 12-year-olds and 50% to 70% of adolescent baseball players develop elbow pain annually. This trend is most obvious in those kids involved in overhead or upper extremity weight-bearing activities (i.e., gymnastics and football) [5].

Young athletes are predisposed to a unique subset of injuries that are associated with the physiological changes of growth and development. They are at particularly high risk of chronic overuse injuries due to open growth plates. Elbow growth occurs at multiple apophyses during development.

There are three distinct physes that serve as the attachment sites for key elbow stabilizers, and they are all at risk during adolescence [21]. These injuries often involve the medial aspect of the elbow. Most commonly, the patient presents with either an apophysitis or a medial epicondyle fracture [13]. Medial epicondylar fracture can involve disruption through the apophysis or off the undersurface of the epicondyle. The diagnosis of UCL tear is becoming more common, as made evident by the increasing rate of UCL reconstruction over the last two decades [1].

UCL injury in pediatric cohorts tends to be more acute in nature than what is observed in adults. For children and adolescents, we recommend initial non-operative treatment in most cases of suspected UCL injury: rest, ice, NSAIDs, and physical therapy. Return to sport is on a gradual basis. We do not recommend that overhead athletes return to full sport until pain has completely subsided and they have a normal exam. Rettig et al. observed that 42% of adult, elite throwing athletes were able to return to their previous level of competition with rehabilitation [22]. We are unaware of an equivalent study in children and adolescents.

UCL reconstruction is a common procedure in adult overhead athletes, and indications continue to expand to increasingly younger athletes [20, 23, 24]. One of the largest series of these cases demonstrated that 58 out of 60 adolescents were able to return to participate in their sport at their prior level of competition within 6 months of the procedure [13]. The existing literature has had a bias away from the pediatric population [1]. In rare instances, we have performed surgery for acute avulsion of the UCL in adolescents with irreducible elbow dislocations [25, 26]. In most cases, soft-tissue disruptions of the UCL in children have been successfully treated non-operatively. It is the child or adolescent with a symptomatic non-union that seems to develop persistent or recurrent pain. It should be noted that even this is a small percentage of all the children seen with bony avulsions at the origin of the UCL.

Surgical intervention of UCL injuries is complicated in children due to the juxtaposition of the medial epicondyle apophysis. Males have a wider ligament than females, but the location of the ligament origin appears to be consistent across genders and throughout growth and development [13]. The anatomic origin of the anterior band of the UCL is consistently 3 mm medial to the cartilaginous interface of the medial epicondyle apophysis with the main humeral bone [13].

When a patient has open elbow physes, traditional techniques for ligament reconstruction in adults can result in a number of potential complications: poor fixation through the apophyseal cartilage cap, minor growth disturbance of the apophysis, and iatrogenic medial epicondyle fracture due to disruption of the apophysis (if one does not already exist). We are unaware of any study performed specifically for UCL reconstruction in elbows with open physes. This makes it difficult to counsel patients and their parents about expected outcomes with conservative versus surgical management. In the rare instances where a ligament reconstruction has been necessary, we have anchored the proximal end of the graft in a non-anatomic location: the center of the trochlea to avoid disruption of growth plates (Figs. 65.7, 65.8, 65.9, 65.10, and 65.11).

Medial epicondyle fractures are much more common in the pediatric age group [12]. The anterior band of the UCL attaches to the apophysis of the medial epicondyle throughout childhood and adolescence [13]. This origin can be disrupted with even minimally displaced medial epicondyle fractures and may lead to persistent and symptomatic micro-instability of the elbow. In cases of medial epicondyle non-union, this micro-instability may be the culprit of ongoing medial elbow pain. As described above, this condition is managed in our hands with excision of the non-union and repair of the ligament in a non-anatomic position in the center of the trochlea. This eliminates the risk of growth arrest.

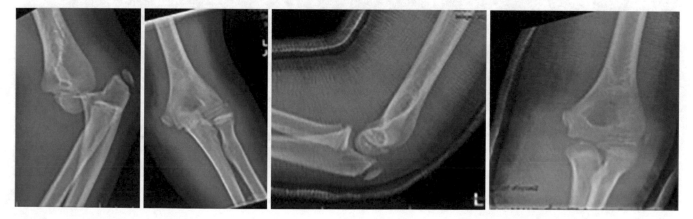

Fig. 65.7 Patient 2: Pre- and post-reduction radiographs of a 12-year-old male wrestler who had an elbow dislocation

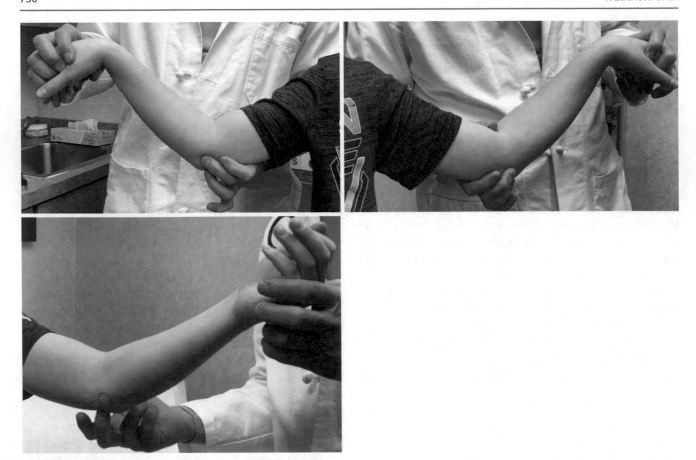

Fig. 65.8 Patient 2: Physical exam 13 months after the injury. Patient complained of pain with workouts, push-ups, and intermittent locking of the elbow. Physical exam demonstrated pain and laxity with a mov- ing valgus stress test. There was positive Tinel's sign over the ulnar nerve at the elbow

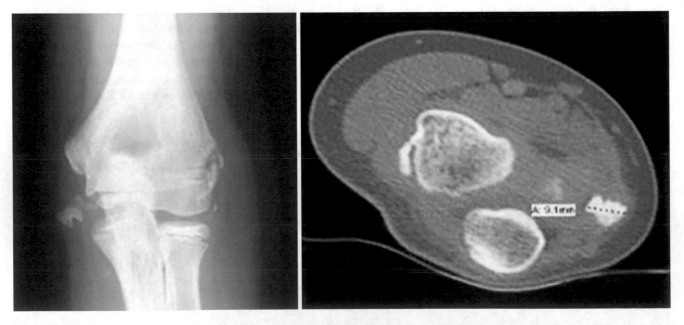

Fig. 65.9 Patient 2: PA and computed tomography of the left elbow. Demonstrates heterotopic ossification on the medial aspect of the elbow joint

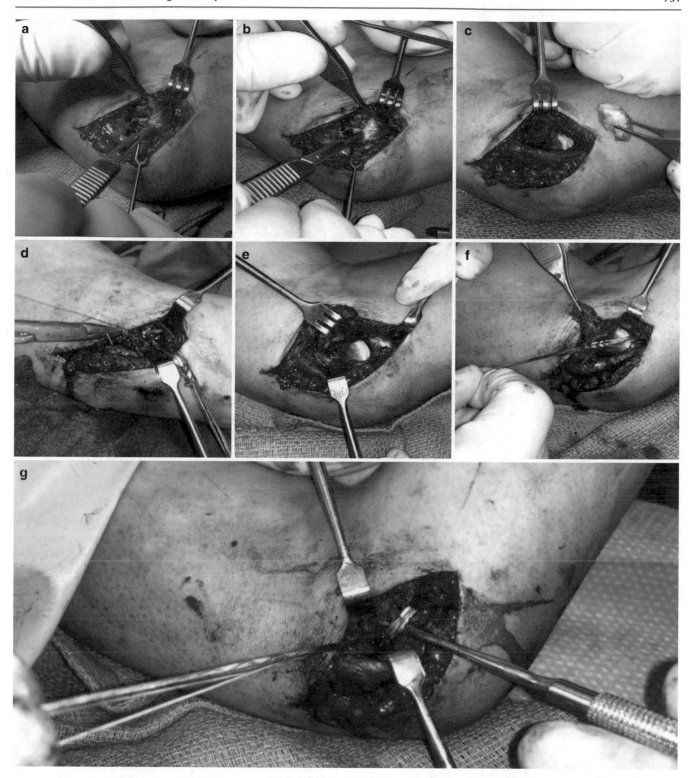

Fig. 65.10 Patient 2: Ligament reconstruction. (**a, b**) Two collections of heterotopic bone. (**c**) Removed heterotopic bone. (**d**) Absence of UCL post resection of heterotopic bone. (**e**) Distal fixation of palmaris longus (PL) graft. (**f**) Closure of capsule prior to proximal fixation of PL graft. (**g**) PL graft with internal brace tensioned with elbow at 60° of flexion and forearm in full supination with slight varus stress to fully close down the medial joint line. A freer elevator is placed beneath the graft to avoid over-tensioning. The graft and tape are fixed proximally and distally with interference screws

Fig. 65.11 Patient 2: Follow-up. At 3 months, patient demonstrated full active range of motion with flexion, extension, pronation, and supination. At this time, the patient had no pain and began weight training. At 7 months, he was able to pinch hit in the Little League World Series

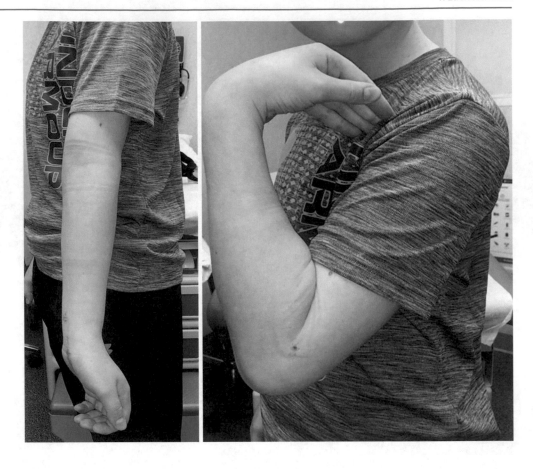

Conclusion

Our patient ultimately received surgical treatment with restoration of her function, resolution of pain, and return to gymnastics. In a normal elbow, the flexor carpi ulnaris and flexor digitorum superficialis muscles offset valgus stress during throwing motions. Preventative efforts should focus on strengthening the forearm flexors to further stabilize the medial elbow [3]. This was emphasized to our patient when she returned at nearly 1.5 years post-operatively with elbow pain.

Pediatric UCL injuries run the gamut from Little Leaguer's elbow (apophysitis) to medial epicondyle fracture to overuse UCL tears. Clinical results of UCL reconstruction in young athletes are thought to be equivalent to those in adult athletes [27]. However, this is likely due to shrewd surgical indications by the publishing authors. There are a number of important social and anatomic considerations in treating child and adolescent athletes with UCL pathology. If surgical intervention is instituted, we recommend excision of the medial epicondyle and direct ligament repair to the trochlea.

References

1. Cain EL, Andrews JR, Dugas JR, Wilk KE, McMichael CS, Walter JC, et al. Outcome of ulnar collateral ligament reconstruction of the elbow in 1281 athletes: results in 743 athletes with minimum 2-year follow-up. Am J Sports Med. 2010. https://doi.org/10.1177/0363546510378100.
2. Erdil M, Bilsel K, Ersen A, Elmadag M, Tuncer N, Sen C. Treatment of symptomatic medial epicondyle nonunion: case report and review of the literature. Int J Surg Case Rep. 2012. https://doi.org/10.1016/j.ijscr.2012.04.021.
3. Rahman RK, Levine WN, Ahmad CS. Elbow medial collateral ligament injuries. Curr Rev Musculoskelet Med. 2008. https://doi.org/10.1007/s12178-008-9026-3.
4. Li NY, Goodman AD, Lemme NJ, Owens BD. Epidemiology of elbow ulnar collateral ligament injuries in throwing versus contact athletes of the National Collegiate Athletic Association: analysis of the 2009–2010 to 2013–2014 seasons. Orthop J Sports Med. 2019. https://doi.org/10.1177/2325967119836428.
5. Greiwe RM, Saifi C, Ahmad CS. Pediatric sports elbow injuries. Clin Sports Med. 2010. https://doi.org/10.1016/j.csm.2010.06.010.
6. E A. Lehrbuch der Chirurgie and Operationsleehre, sweite Auflage. Urban Schwarz. Wien. 1881;II.
7. Trias A, Comeau Y. Recurrent dislocation of the elbow in children. Clin Orthop. 1974. https://doi.org/10.1097/00003086-197405000-00012.

8. Osborne G, Cotterill P. Recurrent dislocation of the elbow. J Bone Jt Surg Br. 1966;48:340.
9. Tachdjian MO. Pediatric orthopedics, vols. I and II. Philadelphia: WB Saunders; 1972: 766 pp. (vol. I), 1001 pp. (vol. II).
10. Kapel O. Operation for habitual dislocation of the elbow. J Bone Jt Surg. 1951;33:707.
11. Schwab GH, Bennett JB, Woods GW, Tullos HS. Biomechanics of elbow instability: the role of the medial collateral ligament. Clin Orthop Relat Res. 1980;146:42–52.
12. Woods GW, Tullos HS. Elbow instability and medial epicondyle fractures. Am J Sports Med. 1977. https://doi.org/10.1177/036354657700500105.
13. Zell M, Dwek JR, Edmonds EW. Origin of the medial ulnar collateral ligament on the pediatric elbow. J Child Orthop. 2013. https://doi.org/10.1007/s11832-013-0518-3.
14. Kamath AF, Baldwin K, Horneff J, Hosalkar HS. Operative versus non-operative management of pediatric medial epicondyle fractures: a systematic review. J Child Orthop. 2009. https://doi.org/10.1007/s11832-009-0192-7.
15. Dugas JR, Ostrander RV, Cain EL, Kingsley D, Andrews JR. Anatomy of the anterior bundle of the ulnar collateral ligament. J Shoulder Elb Surg. 2007. https://doi.org/10.1016/j.jse.2006.11.009.
16. Donohue BF, Lubitz MG, Kremchek TE. Elbow ulnar collateral ligament reconstruction using the novel docking plus technique in 324 athletes. Sports Med Open. 2019. https://doi.org/10.1186/s40798-018-0174-8.
17. Erickson BJ, Chalmers PN, Bush-Joseph CA, Verma NN, Romeo AA. Ulnar collateral ligament reconstruction of the elbow: a systematic review of the literature. Orthop J Sports Med. 2015. https://doi.org/10.1177/2325967115618914.
18. Fleisig GS, Andrews JR. Prevention of elbow injuries in youth baseball pitchers. Sports Health. 2012. https://doi.org/10.1177/1941738112454828.
19. Makhni EC, Morrow ZS, Luchetti TJ, Mishra-Kalyani PS, Gualtieri AP, Lee RW, et al. Arm pain in youth baseball players: a survey of healthy players. Am J Sports Med. 2015;43(1). https://doi.org/10.1177/0363546514555506.
20. Petty DH, Andrews JR, Fleisig GS, Cain EL. Ulnar collateral ligament reconstruction in high school baseball players: clinical results and injury risk factors. Am J Sports Med. 2004. https://doi.org/10.1177/0363546503262166.
21. Kramer DE. Elbow pain and injury in young athletes. J Pediatr Orthop. 2010. https://doi.org/10.1097/BPO.0b013e3181c9b889.
22. Rettig AC, Sherrill C, Snead DS, Mendler JC, Mieling P. Nonoperative treatment of ulnar collateral ligament injuries in throwing athletes. Am J Sports Med. 2001. https://doi.org/10.1177/03635465010290010601.
23. Olsen SJ, Fleisig GS, Dun S, Loftice J, Andrews JR. Risk factors for shoulder and elbow injuries in adolescent baseball pitchers. Am J Sports Med. 2006. https://doi.org/10.1177/0363546505284188.
24. Vitale MA, Ahmad CS. The outcome of elbow ulnar collateral ligament reconstruction in overhead athletes: a systematic review. Am J Sports Med. 2008. https://doi.org/10.1177/0363546508319053.
25. O'Brien MJ, Lee MR, Savoie FH. A preliminary report of acute and subacute arthroscopic repair of the radial ulnohumeral ligament after elbow dislocation in the high-demand patient. Arthroscopy. 2014. https://doi.org/10.1016/j.arthro.2014.02.037.
26. Savoie FH, Trenhaile SW, Roberts J, Field LD, Ramsey JR. Primary repair of ulnar collateral ligament injuries of the elbow in young athletes: a case series of injuries to the proximal and distal ends of the ligament. Am J Sports Med. 2008. https://doi.org/10.1177/0363546508315201.
27. Azar FM. Operative treatment of ulnar collateral ligament injuries of the elbow in athletes. Oper Tech Orthop. 2001. https://doi.org/10.1016/S1048-6666(01)80036-7.

Arthroscopic Management of Osteochondritis Dissecans of the Capitellum

Noah C. Marks and Larry D. Field

Osteochondritis dissecans (OCD) is an increasing cause of elbow dysfunction and pain in the adolescent athlete. The most common site of osteochondritis dissecans of the elbow is the capitellum. This condition is a potentially sport-ending injury for an athlete, with possible long-term sequelae such as degenerative arthritis. Although no single cause of capitellum osteochondritis dissecans has been universally accepted, patients with this pathology do have common findings in regard to history and physical exam. In this chapter, radiographic findings consistent with OCD of the capitellum are discussed in detail. In order to provide the reader with a base to guide both clinical and operative decision-making, the conservative and operative treatment indications and options are discussed based on a review of the literature and our personal experience. As arthroscopic technique has advanced, arthroscopic surgery has become the standard procedure for surgical treatment of capitellar osteochondritis dissecans. This procedure is technically demanding and requires a thorough understanding of elbow arthroscopy portals in order to be able to assess and treat this pathology utilizing arthroscopic technique. We will discuss in detail our preferred arthroscopic technique for the treatment of osteochondritis dissecans of the capitellum.

Osteochondritis dissecans (OCD) is an increasing cause of elbow dysfunction and pain in the adolescent athlete. It is a localized condition involving the articular surface that results in the separation of a segment of articular cartilage and subchondral bone. The most common site of osteochondritis dissecans of the elbow is the capitellum. However, lesions have also been reported in the trochlea, the radial head, as well as the olecranon and olecranon fossa [1–4].

N. C. Marks
Mississippi Sports Medicine and Orthopaedic Center, Jackson, MS, USA

L. D. Field (✉)
Upper Extremity, Mississippi Sports Medicine and Orthopaedic Center, Jackson, MS, USA
e-mail: lfield@msmoc.com

The true cause and natural history of capitellum OCD remain unknown, and the optimal treatment remains controversial. This can be attributed, in part, to the relative infrequency of the condition. Additionally, other conditions involving the immature elbow have been confused with a true OCD. These conditions include but are not limited to osteonecrosis, osteochondral fractures, hereditary epiphyseal dysplasia, little league elbow, and Panner's disease [5–7].

Osteochondritis dissecans generally occurs in athletes aged 11–21 years who report a history of overuse [5, 6]. The osteonecrotic lesion usually involves only a segment of capitellum, located primarily at a central or anterolateral position [8, 9]. This condition is a potentially sport-ending injury for an athlete, with possible long-term sequelae such as degenerative arthritis [9, 10].

Pathogenesis

No single cause of osteochondritis dissecans has been universally accepted [5]. There have been a number of hypotheses proposed put forward regarding the etiology of osteochondritis dissecans including trauma, genetics, ischemia, and disordered ossification [11, 12].

There is a relatively high prevalence of OCD among young baseball players and gymnasts [13]. The elbow is subjected to a high valgus stress during the late cocking and early acceleration phases of throwing. In gymnastics, there are high impact and shear forces applied through the elbow [14]. These mechanisms lend support for the proposed role microtrauma plays in this pathologic entity. Additionally, the blood supply to the capitellum is supplied by one or two end vessels with minimal collateral flow [15]. This likely predisposes the developing chondroepiphysis to an avascular state in the setting of repeated microtrauma [14, 16].

The actual cause of OCD of the capitellum may indeed be multifactorial. However, the most influential factors in the

W. B. Geissler (ed.), *Wrist and Elbow Arthroscopy with Selected Open Procedures*, https://doi.org/10.1007/978-3-030-78881-0_66

development of OCD seem to be related to repetitive micro-trauma and overuse to a chondroepiphysis that is vulnerable secondary to its blood supply [5, 7, 14].

Preoperative Considerations

History

Osteochondritis dissecans is primarily a disorder of the young athlete and rarely occurs in adults. The typical patient is usually between the ages of 11 and 21, with the majority developing symptoms between 12 and 14 years [5, 6, 17]. Males are more commonly affected, but this disorder is also prevalent among female gymnasts. The dominant arm is almost always involved, and bilateral involvement has been reported in some 5–20% [18]. History of overuse is often described with common sport activities such as baseball, gymnastics, weightlifting, racquet sports, and cheerleading [19]. The initial complaint is of pain and stiffness in the elbow that is often relieved by rest. There is usually no history of a specific traumatic event. Symptoms may also include catching, popping, or locking. Pain is often localized over the lateral aspect of the elbow, but it may also be poorly defined [18].

Physical Examination

The most common finding on physical examination is tenderness over the radiocapitellar joint [20]. It is also not uncommon for the patient to exhibit flexion contractures of between 5° and 30° [5, 20–23]. Clicking, catching, grinding, or locking suggests fragment instability or loose bodies. Crepitus and an effusion may be present as well [5, 6, 18, 19]. Provocative tests such as the active radiocapitellar compression test may help to confirm the diagnosis [24]. In this test, the patient actively pronates and supinates the forearm

with the elbow in full extension. The resultant muscle contraction compresses the radiocapitellar joint and elicits lateral compartment pain in a positive test. Since valgus overload can cause both capitellum OCD and tears in the medial ulnar collateral ligament (MUCL), the integrity of the MUCL should be examined as well.

Imaging

Radiographs are the initial diagnostic test of choice. Standard anteroposterior (AP) and lateral views of the elbow will usually show the classic findings associated with OCD. The addition of an AP view with the elbow in 45° of flexion may improve the ability to detect radiographic finding associated with OCD [25]. Early in the disease process, radiographs may be negative. As the condition progresses, there is capitellar flattening and radiolucency. A rim of sclerotic bone often surrounds the radiolucent crater, which is typically located in the central or anterolateral aspect of the capitellum (Fig. 66.1). Late findings can include radial head enlargement and osteophyte formation, and loose bodies may be present if the necrotic segment becomes detached.

MRI has become the standard modality for further evaluation [5, 25]. Not only can MRI assess the articular surface, but it can also define both size and extent of the lesion (Fig. 66.2). Early, stable lesions show changes on T1-weighted images, but T2-weighted images may remain normal. On the other hand, advanced lesions show changes on both T1- and T2-weighted images [5, 26]. Loose in situ lesions may demonstrate a cyst under the lesion. MR arthrography can provide further information as to the extent of the injury [25, 26]. Contrast can show separation of a detached or partially detached piece from subchondral bone. Progressive healing can also be followed via plain radiographs or MRI. If the fragment remains stable, the central sclerotic fragment gradually becomes less distinct, and the surrounding area of radiolucency slowly ossifies [5, 9].

Fig. 66.1 Anteroposterior (**a**) and lateral (**b**) radiographs demonstrating radiolucency and rarefaction typical of osteochondritis dissecans of the elbow

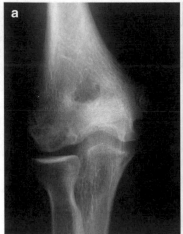
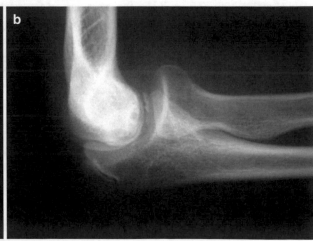

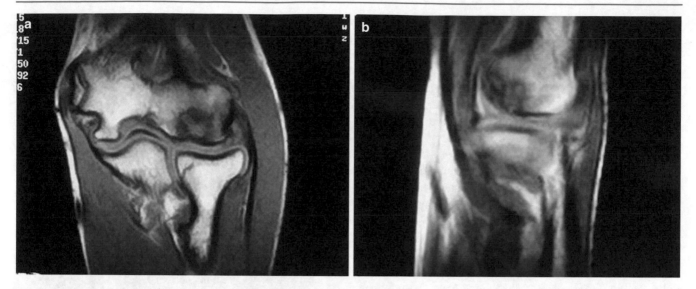

Fig. 66.2 Coronal (**a**) and sagittal (**b**) MR images of the same lesion shown in Fig. 66.1. Increased signal of the T2 image indicates disruption of the articular surface

Treatment Options

Options for the surgical management of symptomatic OCD include nonoperative measures, fragment excision, fragment fixation, and osteochondral autograft reconstruction of the lesion. Management decisions are based primarily on the integrity of the articular cartilage and status of the involved segment: whether it is stable, unstable but attached, or detached and loose. The size and location of the lesion as well as the status of the capitellar physis also affect decision-making [21, 27, 28].

Stable lesions with intact cartilage and in situ subchondral fragments are managed conservatively [5, 18, 25]. Surgical indications include persistent or worsening symptoms despite prolonged conservative care, loose bodies, or evidence of instability including violation of intact cartilage or detachment [5, 18, 29, 30].

Conservative Management

Recently, some literature suggests that radiographic information alone is not sufficient to determine if a lesion can be successfully treated nonoperatively. Specifically, Takahara et al. [28, 31] retrospectively reviewed 106 cases of capitellar OCD with an average 7-year follow-up in a level II study. They found that lesions that healed completely with nonoperative treatment had the following characteristics on initial presentation: open capitellar physis, good elbow motion, and radiographic findings of localized flattening or lucency of the subchondral bone. Lesions that fit that criteria were classified as stable.

Nonsurgical treatment is typically selected for patients with intact, nondisplaced, stable lesions, and it involves activity modification with cessation of sports participation [28, 32, 33]. Sports and other aggravating activities are avoided until symptoms subside, approximately for 3–6 weeks. We recommend protecting the elbow in a hinged elbow brace during that time. The straight hinges function to offload the capitellum by correcting the normal valgus tilt of the elbow. As symptoms decrease, physical therapy can begin. Gentle range of motion exercises followed by strengthening are instituted as symptoms dictate. The athlete can usually return to unrestricted sports activities within 3–6 months after treatment has begun [19]. Patients with intact lesions caught early and treated conservatively have the best prognosis. However, it is prudent for the clinician to inform the patient and family of possible long-term sequelae [9, 10, 14, 16, 18, 23, 25].

Surgical Treatment

Operative intervention is indicated for patients that do not improve with appropriate nonoperative treatment have, the presence of loose bodies with mechanical symptoms, or an unstable lesion [7, 13]. Takahara et al. [28, 31] found that conservative treatment failed when patients with unstable lesions had one of the following findings at presentation: a closed capitellum physis, fragmentation, or restriction of elbow motion greater than 20°.

Multiple operative procedures have been described for treating these lesions including drilling of the defect [13], fragment removal with or without curettage/drilling of the residual defect [9, 10, 13, 16, 23, 34, 35], fragment fixation by a variety of methods [13, 36–39], reconstruction with osteochondral autograft [13, 38, 40–43], autologous chondrocyte implantation [13, 44], and closing-wedge osteotomy of the lateral condyle [13, 45]. Comparisons of the results of the various operative techniques, however, are difficult because of their largely retrospective nature, different outcome measures, and the relative infrequency of osteochondritis dissecans [13].

Arthroscopic surgery is becoming the standard procedure for the surgical treatment of capitellar osteochondritis dissecans [46, 47]. Advantages include the minimally invasive nature of the procedure with the potential for early rehabilitation, access to the lesion and the entire elbow joint, and ability to identify and treat concurrent lesions including the removal of loose bodies [13]. Studies on arthroscopic debridement and abrasion arthroplasty have shown encouraging short- and mid-term results [9, 21, 22, 28, 35, 47–50]. Recently a level III review of the literature by de Graff et al. [51] suggested that both good short-term and long-term results can be achieved in a majority of patients treated arthroscopically for OCD of the capitellum. However, their review also emphasized the need for enhanced methodology and longer follow-up. Miyake et al. [52] recently retrospectively evaluated 106 patients who underwent arthroscopic debridement of a capitellar OCD lesion. They found patients with large lesions and open proximal radial physes had both poor radiographic and clinic outcomes. Excellent short-term results were obtained in the remaining patient groups.

To treat OCD lesions arthroscopically, the angle of approach through portal access is of utmost importance in order to thoroughly debride, drill, or place osteochondral plugs. Most surgeons use a variation of a six-portal approach [13, 21, 46, 53] (Fig. 66.3). These portals include standard anteromedial, anterolateral, direct posterior, posterolateral, and direct lateral portals [13, 53]. Baumgarten et al. [21] identified the use of two direct lateral portals as the key to effective arthroscopic treatment of osteochondritis dissecans of the capitellum. Davis et al. [53] performed a cadaveric study evaluating the dual direct lateral portals and found that 78% of the entire capitellar surface area was accessible through these portals. In addition, the portals remain safely proximal and posterior to the lateral ligamentous complex [53]. A distal ulnar portal (Fig. 66.4) has recently been described and is placed approximately 3–4 cm distal to the posterior aspect of the radiocapitellar joint and just lateral to the palpable posterior edge of the ulna [47]. This portal is typically used as a viewing portal, while the standard soft-spot portal is used as a working portal [47]. Some authors have described an arthroscopic-assisted drilling method, using a hole drilled through the radius shaft [54]. In this novel approach to drilling of an OCD lesion, a 1.8 mm K-wire is drilled into the radial head from approximately 3 cm distal. The OCD lesion can usually be completely accessed by altering the flexion angle in both pronation and

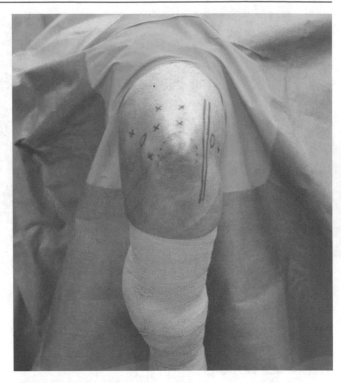

Fig. 66.3 Common arthroscopic elbow portals

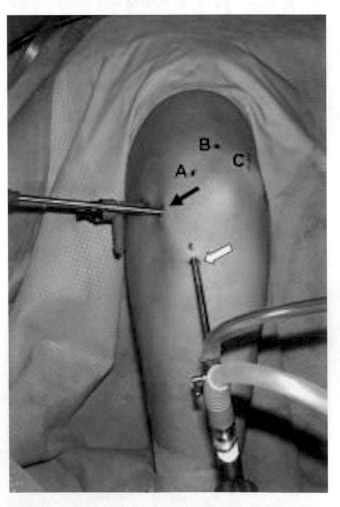

Fig. 66.4 The distal ulnar portal approximately 3–4 cm distal to radiocapitellar joint and just lateral to the palpable posterior edge of the ulna

supination [54]. The angle of approach, however, can be in close proximity to the posterior interosseous nerve. Also, this procedure requires drilling across the normal cartilage surface of the radius [47, 54].

The surgical treatment of unstable lesions depends on the size and location of the lesion. Smaller lesions can be debrided with good pain relief. There is still debate over treatment of larger lesions with debridement versus repair versus osteochondral autografts. Shimada et al. [55] suggested that lesions less than 1 cm² could be treated with debridement, chondroplasty, and possibly microfracture or drilling and lesions greater than 1 cm² should be treated with osteochondral autograft or fixation. Takahara et al. [9, 28] found lesions with defects greater than 50% of the capitellar width had a poorer prognosis after fragment removal alone.

Poor results after treatment have been noted in lesions that extend through the lateral margin of the capitellum resulting in the absence of a complete circumferential border of healthy articular cartilage and subchondral bone [13, 22, 34] (Fig. 66.5). Byrd and Jones [34] postulated that the lateral fragment noted in the study by Ruch et al. [22] is similarly associated with loss of the lateral border of the capitellum and portends a possible poor prognosis [13]. The lateral column of the capitellum supports compressive forces when the elbow undergoes either a valgus stress or an axial load. The lack of a lateral buttress impedes the formation of fibrocartilage by subjecting the defect to increased radiocapitellar forces. In a similar fashion, engagement of the radial

head into the defect compromises healing. This situation may also lead to accelerated radiocapitellar arthrosis. ElAttrache and Ahmad et al. [56] stated that more than 6–7 mm of lateral column involvement may not be best treated by microfracture alone. They did report successfully treating lesions that were an average of 1.32 cm² with microfracture alone provided there was no lateral column involvement. Interestingly, this is in contrast to the suggestion by Shimada et al. [55] that lesions >1 cm² should be treated with osteochondral autograft or fixation. Perhaps, this is demonstrates that, to an extent, involvement of the lateral column may be more important than the absolute size of the lesion when choosing treatment methods.

Osteochondral autograft transplantation has been recently introduced as another treatment option for capitellum osteochondritis dissecans [13, 38, 40–43]. Indications for this procedure have included lesions involving over 50% of the articular surface area, disruption of the lateral buttress (see Fig. 66.5), and engagement of the radial head [28, 33, 57]. Cylindrical osteochondral grafts are harvested from a donor site, typically the lateral femoral condyle. The plug is inserted perpendicular to the subchondral bone (Fig. 66.6) [31, 40]. These authors have suggested that the procedure may reduce the progression to osteoarthritis and lead to better long-term results [47]. Several reports have described success with osteochondral autograft transfer and osteochondral mosaicplasty [13, 41, 43, 55, 58–61] (Table 66.1).

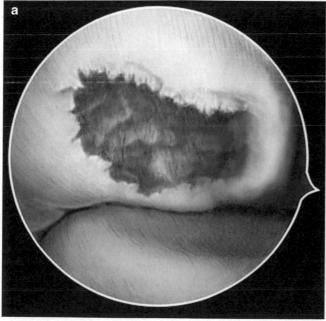
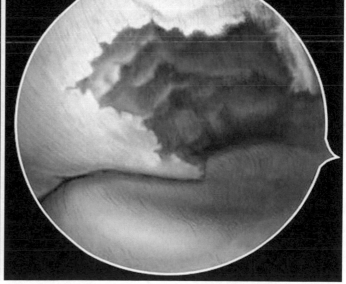

Fig. 66.5 View of osteochondritis dissecans lesion of capitellum in the right elbow of the patient in prone position viewing from posterolateral portal. Contained osteochondritis dissecans lesion (**a**) with circumfer- ential healthy cartilage present. Similar lesion with loss of lateral column support (**b**)

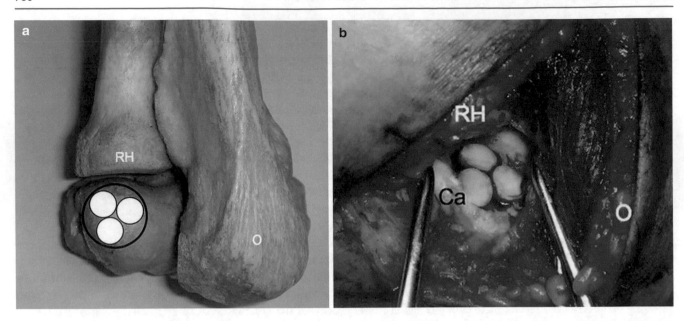

Fig. 66.6 Osteochondral autograft reconstruction of osteochondritis dissecans lesion of the capitellum: schematic drawing (**a**) and intraoperative view (**b**)

Table 66.1 Results of osteochondral autograft transfer and mosaicplasty for OCD of the capitellum

Author	Mean follow-up	Mean score (points)	Number of patients	Pain-free at final follow-up	Patients return to sport level
Tsuda et al. [58]	16 months	193 (Timmerman, 200 max)	3	3	3
Shimada et al. [55]	25.5 months	93.8 (Japanese Orthopaedic Association, 100 max)	10	8	8
Yamamoto et al. [43]	3.5 years	–	18	–	14
Iswasaki et al. [59]	24 months	183 (Timmerman, 200 max)	8	7	6
Iswasaki et al. [41]	45 months	191 (Timmerman, 200 max)	19	18	17
Ovesen et al. [60]	30 months	93.5 (Mayo, max 100) 92.5 (constant, max 100)	10	8	10
Shimada et al. [61]	36 months	180 (Timmerman, 200 max)	26	–	26

Authors' Preferred Technique

Arthroscopic Excision and Drilling

The authors utilize general anesthesia and the prone position for arthroscopic evaluation and treatment of the elbow. The patient is placed prone on the operating table over chest rolls to ensure adequate ventilation. The shoulder is abducted to 90°, and the arm is supported by an arm positioner or an arm board (Fig. 66.7). The arm board is placed parallel to the operating table, centered at the shoulder. A sandbag, foam support, or rolled blankets are placed under the upper arm to elevate the shoulder and allow the elbow to rest in 90° of flexion.

Surface landmarks are marked on the skin prior to creating portals. Important landmarks to outline are the radial head, olecranon, lateral epicondyle, medial epicondyle, and ulnar nerve (see Fig. 66.3). Prior to making portals, the joint should be distended with 20–30 ml of sterile saline. Placing an 18-gauge spinal needle in either the olecranon fossa or the soft spot bounded by the lateral epicondyle, olecranon, and radial head can provide access to the elbow joint. Neurovascular structures are displaced away from the joint with distention of the joint, which gives an additional margin of safety [20, 62].

The arthroscope is introduced through the proximal anteromedial portal. This portal is located 2 cm proximal to the medial epicondyle and just anterior to the medial intermuscular septum (Fig. 66.8). The medial intermuscular septum is identified by palpation, and the portal is made anterior to the septum so that the ulnar nerve is not injured. The blunt trocar is introduced into the portal, anterior to the septum,

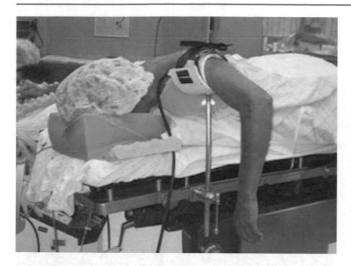

Fig. 66.7 Prone position for arthroscopic treatment of the elbow

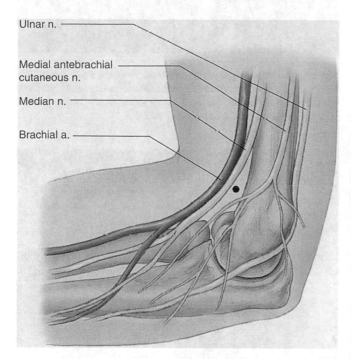

Ulnar n.

Medial antebrachial cutaneous n.

Median n.

Brachial a.

Fig. 66.8 Illustration demonstrating anatomic positioning of the proximal anteromedial portal

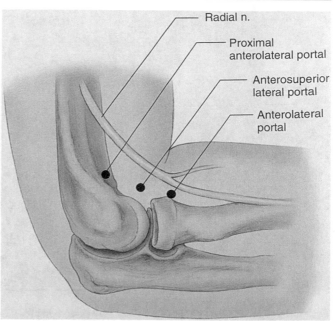

Radial n.

Proximal anterolateral portal

Anterosuperior lateral portal

Anterolateral portal

Fig. 66.9 Illustration demonstrating anatomic positioning of common lateral arthroscopic portals

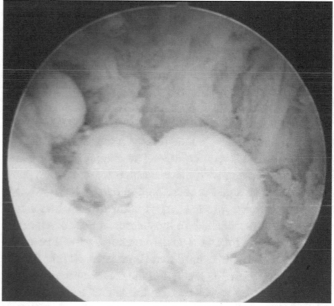

Fig. 66.10 Loose bodies found in the anterior compartment of the elbow

and aimed toward the radial head while maintaining contact with the anterior surface of the humerus. This allows the brachialis muscle to remain anterior and protect the median nerve and brachial artery. The trocar enters the elbow through the tendinous origin of the flexor-pronator group and medial capsule. Once entrance into the joint is confirmed, the anterolateral portal is established under direct visualization. The proximal anterolateral portal is positioned 2 cm proximal and 1–2 cm anterior to the lateral epicondyle (Fig. 66.9) and in some cases may be used as the initial portal in elbow arthroscopy. The blunt trocar is aimed toward the center of the joint while maintaining contact with the anterior humerus

and pierces the brachioradialis muscle, brachialis muscle, and lateral joint capsule before entering the anterior compartment. The coronoid fossa is a common place for loose bodies to be localized (Fig. 66.10). Although the osteochondritic lesion may be noted on the anterior aspect of the capitellum, it is most commonly identified at the posterior aspect of the capitellum. One should always perform a varus and valgus stress test, while the scope is in the anterior portal to

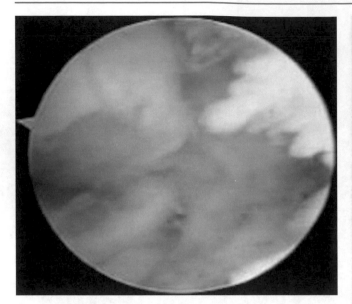

Fig. 66.11 Posterolateral gutter of a patient with osteochondritis dissecans demonstrating the synovitis and inflamed posterolateral plica

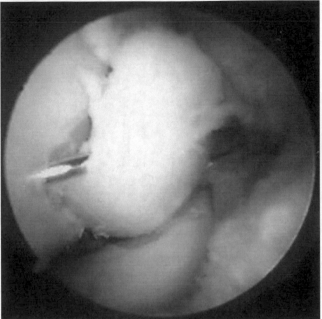

Fig. 66.12 Arthroscopic management of a detached osteochondritic lesion of the capitellum viewed from the anteromedial portal. The loose fragment is temporarily stabilized with a spinal needle before excised with a grasper from the anterolateral portal

document any concomitant instability of the elbow. Once a complete diagnostic arthroscopy of the anterior compartment of the elbow with removal of any associated loose bodies has been completed, the inflow is left in the proximal anteromedial portal, and the scope is transferred to a straight posterior portal. The straight posterior or trans-triceps portal is located 3 cm proximal to the tip of the olecranon in the midline posteriorly [34, 63] (see Fig. 66.3). This portal allows visualization of the entire posterior compartment as well as the medial and lateral gutters. The blunt trocar is advanced toward the olecranon fossa through the triceps tendon and posterior joint capsule. The medial gutter is evaluated initially along with the olecranon fossa, and any loose bodies noted in either of these are removed. The arthroscope is then continued into the lateral compartment, and a soft-spot portal is established. In most cases of osteochondritis, a relatively large, inflamed posterolateral plica will be noted, along with synovitis in this lateral compartment (Fig. 66.11). The soft-spot portal is located in the center of the triangular area bordered by the olecranon, the lateral epicondyle, and the radial head. This portal is also known as the direct lateral portal or midlateral portal (see Fig. 66.3). The blunt trocar passes through the anconeus muscle and the posterior capsule and into the joint. This inflammatory tissue is excised through a posterior soft-spot portal. At this point, the 30° arthroscope is removed, and a 70° arthroscope is substituted through the posterior central portal. Utilization of the 70° arthroscope may allow complete evaluation of the osteochondritis dissecans lesion of the capitellum (Fig. 66.12). The shaver is placed through the soft-spot portal, and any loose fragments of the osteochondritic area are debrided.

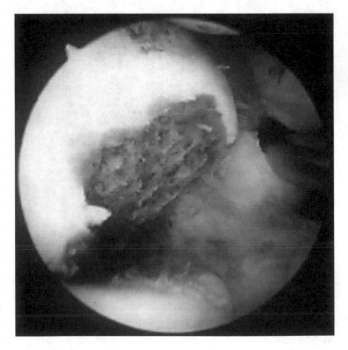

Fig. 66.13 The subchondral base after excision of the fragment and debridement with a shaver

The necrotic bone is then removed, and, in an attempt to stimulate blood flow, multiple drill holes are placed into the main body of the capitellum using either a drill or an awl (Fig. 66.13).

Postoperative Considerations

Rehabilitation

Rehabilitation following arthroscopic treatment begins within a week with the patient placed in a double-hinged elbow brace. Gentle range of motion exercises are started initially, and, as swelling and pain subside, patients are slowly allowed to resume athletic activities in the brace. The brace is gradually weaned after 8–12 weeks postoperatively as long as the patient remains free of significant pain or any mechanical symptoms. Generally, full return to activities and sports is possible after approximately 12–16 weeks.

References

1. Joji S, Murakami T, Murao T. Osteochondritis dissecans developing in the trochlea humeri: a case report. J Shoulder Elb Surg. 2001;10:295–7.
2. Patel N, Weiner SD. Osteochondritis dissecans involving the trochlea: report of two patients (three elbows) and review of the literature. J Pediatr Orthop. 2002;22:48–51.
3. Vanthournout I, Rudelli A, Valenti P, Montagne JP. Osteochondritis dissecans of the trochlea of the humerus. Pediatr Radiol. 1991;21:600–1.
4. Mitsunaga MM, Adishian DA, Bianco AJ Jr. Osteochondritis dissecans of the capitellum. J Trauma. 1982;22:53–5.
5. Bradley J, Petrie R. Osteochondritis dissecans of the humeral capitellum: diagnosis and treatment. Clin Sports Med. 2001;20:565–90.
6. Schenck RC Jr, Goodnight JM. Osteochondritis dissecans. J Bone Joint Surg Am. 1996;78:439–56.
7. Yadao MA, Field LD, Savoie FH III. Osteochondritis dissecans of the elbow. Instr Course Lect. 2004;53:599–606.
8. Konig F. Ueber freie Korper in den Gelenken. Deutsche Zeitschr Chir. 1887;27:90–109.
9. Takahara M, Ogino T, Sasaki I, et al. Long term outcome of osteochondritis dissecans of the humeral capitellum. Clin Orthop. 1999;363:108–15.
10. Bauer M, Jonsson K, Josefsson PO, et al. Osteochondritis dissecans of the elbow: a long-term follow up study. Clin Orthop. 1992;284:156–60.
11. Gardiner TB. Osteochondritis dissecans in three members of one family. J Bone Joint Surg Br. 1955;37:139–41.
12. Stougaard J. Familial occurrence of osteochondritis dissecans. J Bone Joint Surg Br. 1964;46:542–3.
13. Baker CL 3rd, Romeo AA, Baker CL Jr. Osteochondritis dissecans of the capitellum. Am J Sports Med. 2010;38(9):1917–28.
14. Singer KM, Roy SP. Osteochondrosis of the humeral capitellum. Am J Sports Med. 1984;12:351–60.
15. Haraldsson S. On osteochondrosis deformans juvenilis capituli humeri including investigation of intra-osseous vasculature in distal humerus. Acta Orthop Scand. 1959;38(suppl):1–232.
16. Jackson DW, Silvino N, Reiman P. Osteochondritis in the female gymnast's elbow. Arthroscopy. 1989;5:129–36.
17. Pappas AM. Osteochondritis dissecans. Clin Orthop. 1981;158:59–69.
18. Shaughnessy WJ. Osteochondritis dissecans. In: Morrey BF, editor. The elbow and its disorders. 3rd ed. Philadelphia: WB Saunders; 2000. p. 255–60.
19. Peterson RK, Savoie FH III, Field LD. Osteochondritis dissecans of the elbow. Instr Course Lect. 1998;48:393–8.
20. McManama GB Jr, Micheli LJ, Berry MV, et al. The surgical treatment of osteochondritis of the capitellum. Am J Sports Med. 1985;13:11–21.
21. Baumgarten T, Andrews J, Satterwhite Y. The arthroscopic classification and treatment of osteochondritis dissecans of the capitellum. Am J Sports Med. 1998;26:520–3.
22. Ruch D, Cory J, Poehling G. The arthroscopic management of osteochondritis dissecans of the adolescent elbow. Arthroscopy. 1998;14:797–803.
23. Woodward AH, Bianco AJ Jr. Osteochondritis dissecans of the elbow. Clin Orthop. 1975;110:35–41.
24. Baumgarten TE. Osteochondritis dissecans of the capitellum. Sports Med Arthr Rev. 1995;3:219–23.
25. Takahara M, Shundo M, Kondo M, et al. Early detection of osteochondritis dissecans of the capitellum in young baseball players: report of three cases. J Bone Joint Surg Am. 1998;80:892–7.
26. Fritz RC, Stoller DW. The elbow. In: Stoller DW, editor. Magnetic resonance imaging in orthopedics & sports medicine. 2nd ed. Philadelphia: Lippincott-Raven; 1997. p. 743–849.
27. Mihara K, Tsutsui H, Nishinaka N, Yamaguchi K. Nonoperative treatment for osteochondritis dissecans of the capitellum. Am J Sports Med. 2009;37(2):298–304.
28. Takahara M, Mura N, Sasaki J, Harada M, Ogino T. Classification, treatment, and outcome of osteochondritis dissecans of the humeral capitellum. J Bone Joint Surg Am. 2007;89:1205–14.
29. Chess D. Osteochondritis. In: Savoie III FH, Field LD, editors. Arthroscopy of the elbow. New York: Churchill Livingstone; 1996. p. 77–86.
30. Nagura S. The so-called osteochondritis dissecans of Konig. Clin Orthop. 1960;18:100–22.
31. Takahara M, Mura N, Sasaki J, Harada M, Ogino T. Classification, treatment, and outcome of osteochondritis dissecans of the humeral capitellum: surgical technique. J Bone Joint Surg Am. 2008;90(Suppl 2, Part 1):47–62.
32. Mihara K, Suzuki K, Makiuchi D, Nishinaka N, Yamaguchi K, Tsutsui H. Surgical treatment for osteochondritis dissecans of the humeral capitellum. J Shoulder Elb Surg. 2010;19:31–7.
33. Ruchelsman DE, Hall MP, Youm T. Osteochondritis dissecans of the capitellum: current concepts. J Am Acad Orthop Surg. 2010;18:557–67.
34. Byrd T, Jones K. Arthroscopic surgery for isolated capitellar osteochondritis dissecans in adolescent baseball players: minimum three-year follow-up. Am J Sports Med. 2002;30:474–8.
35. Tivnon MC, Anzel SH, Waugh TR. Surgical management of osteochondritis dissecans of the capitellum. Am J Sports Med. 1976;4:121–8.
36. Harada M, Ogino T, Takahara M, et al. Fragment fixation with a bone graft and dynamic staples for osteochondritis dissecans of the humeral capitellum. J Shoulder Elb Surg. 2002;11:368–72.
37. Kuwahata Y, Inoue G. Osteochondritis Dissecans of the elbow managed by Herbert screw fixation. Orthopedics. 1998;21:449–51.
38. Oka Y, Ikeda M. Treatment of severe osteochondritis dissecans of the elbow using osteochondral grafts from a rib. J Bone Joint Surg Br. 2001;83:838–9.
39. Takeda H, Watarai K, Matsushita T, et al. A surgical treatment for unstable osteochondritis dissecans lesions of the humeral capitellum in adolescent baseball players. Am J Sports Med. 2002;30:713–7.
40. Iwasaki N, Kato H, Ishikawa J, Masuko T, Funakoshi T, Minami A. Autologous osteochondral mosaicplasty for osteochondritis dissecans of the elbow in teenage athlete: surgical technique. J Bone Joint Surg Am. 2010;92(Suppl 1, Part 2):208–16.
41. Iwasaki N, Kato H, Ishikawa J, Masuko T, Funakoshi T, Minami A. Autologous osteochondral mosaicplasty for osteochondritis

dissecans of the elbow in teenage athletes. J Bone Joint Surg Am. 2009;91(10):2359–66.

42. Nakagawa Y, Matsusue Y, Ikeda N, et al. Osteochondral grafting and arthroplasty for end-stage osteochondritis dissecans of the capitellum: a case report and review of the literature. Am J Sports Med. 2001;29:650–5.

43. Yamamoto Y, Ishibashi Y, Tsuda E, Sato H, Toh S. Osteochondral autograft transplantation for osteochondritis dissecans of the elbow in juvenile baseball players: minimum 2-year follow-up. Am J Sports Med. 2006;34(5):714–20.

44. Iwasaki N, Yamane S, Nishida K, Masuko T, Funakoshi T, Kamishima T, Minami A. Transplantation of tissue-engineered cartilage for the treatment of osteochondritis dissecans in the elbow: outcomes over a four-year follow-up in two patients. J Shoulder Elb Surg. 2010;19:e1–6.

45. Kiyoshige Y, Takagi M, Yuasa K, Hamasaki M. Closed-wedge osteotomy for osteochondritis dissecans of the capitellum: a 7-to 12-year follow-up. Am J Sports Med. 2000;28(4):534–7.

46. Savoie FH. Guidelines to becoming an expert elbow arthroscopist. Arthroscopy. 2007;23:1237–40.

47. Van Den Ende KI, McIntosh A, Adams J, Steinmann S. Osteochondritis dissecans of the capitellum: a review of the literature and a distal ulnar portal. Arthroscopy. 2011;27(1):122–8.

48. Bojanic I, Ivkovic A, Boric I. Arthroscopy and microfracture technique in the treatment of osteochondritis dissecans of the humeral capitellum: report of three adolescent gymnasts. Knee Surg Sports Traumatol Arthrosc. 2006;14(5):491–6.

49. Brownlow HC, O'Connor-Read LM, Perko M. Arthroscopic treatment of osteochondritis dissecans of the capitellum. Knee Surg Sports Traumatol Arthrosc. 2006;14(2):198–202.

50. Rahusen FT, Brinkman JM, Eygendaal D. Results of arthroscopic debridement for osteochondritis dissecans of the elbow. Br J Sports Med. 2006;40(12):966–9.

51. de Graaff F, Krijnen MR, Poolman RW, Willems WJ. Arthroscopic surgery in athletes with osteochondritis dissecans of the elbow. Arthroscopy. 2011;27(7):986–93.

52. Miyake J, Masatomi T. Arthroscopic debridement of the humeral capitellum for osteochondritis dissecans: radiographic and clinical outcomes. J Hand Surg Am. 2011;36(8):133–1338.

53. Davis JT, Idjadi JA, Siskosky MJ, ElAttrache NS. Dual direct lateral portals for treatment of osteochondritis dissecans of the capitellum: an anatomic study. Arthroscopy. 2007;23:723–8.

54. Aria Y, Hara K, Fujiwara H, Minami G, Nakagawa S, Kubo T. A new arthroscopic-assisted drilling method through the radius in a distal-to-proximal direction for osteochondritis dissecans of the elbow. Arthroscopy. 2008;24:237e1–4.

55. Shimada K, Yoshida T, Nakata K, Hamada M, Akita S. Reconstruction with an osteochondral autograft for advanced osteochondritis dissecans of the elbow. Clin Orthop Relat Res. 2005;435:140–7.

56. Gonzalez-Lomas G, Ahmad C, Wanich T, ElAttrache N. Osteochondritis dissecans of the elbow. In: Ryu RKN, editor. AANA advanced arthroscopy: the elbow and wrist. 1st ed. Philadelphia: Saunders Elsevier; 2010. p. 40–54.

57. Ahmad C, ElAttrache N. Treatment of capitellar osteochondritis dissecans. Tech Should Elbow Surg. 2006;7(4):169–74.

58. Tsuda E, Ishibashi Y, Sato H, Yamamoto Y, Toh S. Osteochondral autograft transplantation for osteochondritis dissecans of the capitellum in nonthrowing athletes. Arthroscopy. 2005;21: 1270–2.

59. Iwasaki N, Kato H, Ishikawa J, Saitoh S, Minami A. Autologous osteochondral mosaicplasty for capitellar osteochondritis dissecans in teenaged patients. Am J Sports Med. 2006;34:1233–9.

60. Ovesen J, Olsen BS, Johannsen HV. The clinical outcomes of mosaicplasty in the treatment of osteochondritis dissecans of the distal humeral capitellum of young athletes. J Shoulder Elb Surg. 2011;20:813–8.

61. Shimada K, Tanaka H, Matsumoto T, Miyake J, Higuchi H, Gamo K, et al. Cylindrical costal osteochondral autograft for reconstruction of large defects of the capitellum due to osteochondritis dissecans. J Bone Joint Surg Am. 2012;95(11): 992–1002.

62. Brown R, Blazina ME, Kerlan RK, et al. Osteochondritis of the capitellum. J Sports Med. 1974;2:27–46.

63. Menche DS, Vangsness CT Jr, Pitman M, et al. The treatment of isolated articular cartilage lesions in the young individual. Instr Course Lect. 1998;47:505–15.

Arthroscopic Treatment of Elbow Fractures

Michael R. Hausman and Steven M. Koehler

Introduction

Recently there has been an increased interest in elbow arthroscopy. Yet elbow arthroscopy is not new. Burman reported the first attempt at elbow arthroscopy in 1931 in the *Journal of Bone and Joint Surgery*. He found the elbow to be "unsuitable for examination, since the joint space is so narrow for the relatively large needle" [1]. One year later, he reversed his opinion and successfully arthroscopically examined ten cadaveric elbows [2]. Yet despite early pioneering work of elbow arthroscopy, interest in elbow arthroscopy did not become widespread until relatively recently. It was not until 1985 that Andrews and Carson reported the first elbow arthroscopy in vivo and described many of the portals used today [3]. Since then, interest in elbow arthroscopy and its indications has rapidly expanded.

Trauma is a more recent application of elbow arthroscopy [4]. Intra-articular fractures of the elbow often occur in conjunction with injury of the collateral ligaments and capsule. The complex osteology of the elbow and close proximity of vital neurovascular structures make exposure challenging and, often, limited. Further complicating exposure is the need to avoid damaging ligaments, which, if sectioned, could potentially exacerbate the initial injury by increasing instability. Consequently malreduction or incomplete reduction is not uncommon, and hardware penetration of the articular surface may occur. Elbow arthroscopy may improve the visualization of the articular surface and, via magnification, facilitate accurate reduction and fixation.

Considerations

The successful application of elbow arthroscopy to trauma treatment involves several modifications of technique. First, timing is very important. Initially after fracture, there is bleeding from the fracture surfaces that can only be controlled with higher inflow pressures (greater than 35 mmHg). This results in rapid swelling making conversion to open surgery much more difficult. If possible, a delay of 24–36 h after injury allows clot to form on the fractured surfaces and allows the use of lower perfusion pressure (<25–30 mmHg) which minimizes swelling and, thus, extends working time and facilitates conversion to an open procedure, if necessary. Second, a newly fractured elbow comes pre-distended by fracture hematoma, which makes joint entry relatively easy. Third, unlike in other indications for elbow arthroscopy, prior to fracture, the joint was normal with no contractures or deformity. The capsule is supple and thin and easy to penetrate. Thus, entering the joint in a trauma case is, in many ways, easier than for a contracture, where the capsule may be thick and tough and the joint volume markedly constricted. Thus, the challenge is not entering the joint, but patiently lavaging and debriding the hematoma with a small-diameter shaver (3.5 mm) directed posteriorly toward the humerus, until good visualization is achieved.

Contraindications

The contraindications in the arthroscopic treatment of elbow arthroscopy are the same as those for all elbow arthroscopic procedures. Submuscular transposition of the ulnar nerve is a contraindication, unless the entire procedure is to be done without medial portals. Arthroscopy is also contraindicated in the event that visualization cannot be achieved and conversion to open, standard techniques would make a procedure easier or provide a more precise reduction.

M. R. Hausman · S. M. Koehler (✉)
Department of Orthopaedic Surgery, Mount Sinai Medical Center, New York, NY, USA
e-mail: Steven.Koehler@mountsinai.org

© Springer Nature Switzerland AG 2022
W. B. Geissler (ed.), *Wrist and Elbow Arthroscopy with Selected Open Procedures*,
https://doi.org/10.1007/978-3-030-78881-0_67

Technique

Timing

As mentioned previously, timing of the intervention is very important. A 24–48 h delay avoids the problem of bleeding from the fracture surface, as discussed above [5, 6]. A tourniquet is routinely used.

Positioning

The supine position, described in 1985 by Andrews and Carson, offers maximum flexibility and access for fracture fixation [3]. In our practice, we have modified this position to include an adjustable shoulder positioner, such as the McConnell arm holder (McConnell Orthopedic Manufacturing Co., Greenville, Texas) (Fig. 67.1). This allows the patient's arm to be placed either across the chest or at the patient's side, conferring multiple advantages: the ability to move the arm in space; easy access for fluoroscopy; easy elevation of the arm to minimize "breakthrough bleed-

ing"; and application of longitudinal traction of the arm, which frequently assists with reduction. The posterior compartment is accessed with the arm across the patient's chest, and the anterior compartment is accessed with the shoulder abducted 90° and the humerus parallel to the floor.

Instrumentation

Generally, a 4.0 mm arthroscope with a 30° offset is used. This typically provides excellent visualization for all procedures. Occasionally, a 70° arthroscope is useful for viewing the coronoid base or the capitellum and anterior surface of the humerus from the distal posterolateral portal. A smaller 2.7 mm scope can be used for smaller spaces or pediatric patients younger than 5–7 years.

Flow management is vital to the success of elbow arthroscopy; thus, special trocars and cannulae without fenestrations should be used to avoid the extravasation of fluid into the subcutaneous layer [1]. Therefore, we also recommend liberal use of switching sticks and cannulae once the portals are established (Fig. 67.2). This also serves to decrease the

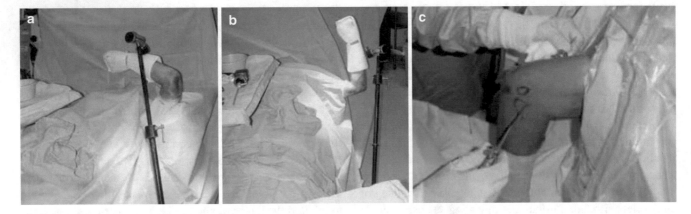

Fig. 67.1 Our preferred patient positioning for elbow arthroscopy: supine with a McConnell arm positioner. (**a**) Position for access to the posterior compartment. (**b**) Position for anterior elbow access. (**c**) Alternative lateral decubitus position demonstrating access to the anterior compartment

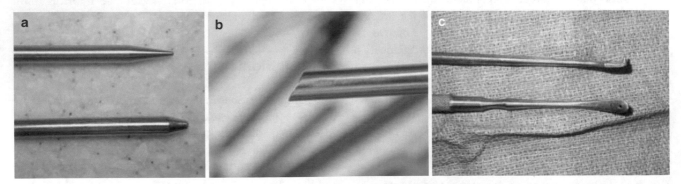

Fig. 67.2 (**a**, **b**) Trocars and nonfenestrated cannulae used for elbow arthroscopy. The use of switching sticks over which a cannula can be threaded is preferable to the customary trocar/cannula combination because there is less soft-tissue drag and, thus, it is easier to enter the

joint. (**c**) A hook retractor that has been ground and modified to fit through a small cannula and a Freer elevator with a hole drilled through the end for passing sutures

risk of neurovascular injury by minimizing the number of passes through tissues.

We also find it useful to have special instruments available such as cannulated screws, a small Freer elevator with a hole drilled in the end for passing sutures, modified skin hooks, and 28-gauge stainless steel wire to help in reducing, holding fragments, and passing sutures (see Fig. 67.2). A variety of graspers, forceps, shavers, and burrs should be available.

Portal Placement

Precautions

Because the elbow is highly constrained, it is necessary to place multiple portals to access and see all parts of the joint [7]. Anatomic studies have demonstrated that flexion of the elbow to 90° minimizes the proximity of the critical neurovascular structures [8–11]. Therefore, all portals should be established from this position. Distention of the capsule further displaces these structures away from arthroscopic instruments. Portals should be made close of the capsular insertion on the supracondylar ridge, to prevent entrapping capsular tissue between the portal and the humerus. Doing so would decrease the joint volume and compromise exposure [12, 13]. Lastly, observing standard technique, a small incision should be used to incise the skin only (no stab incisions). Next, blunt dissection should be performed through the subcutaneous tissue and down to the level of the capsule. This helps to minimize the risk to the surrounding structures by displacing them out of the proposed path prior to trocar insertion. All trocars should use blunt tips.

Standard Anteromedial Portal

This portal is located 2 cm distal and 2 cm anterior to the medial epicondyle (Fig. 67.3). The arthroscope should be aimed toward the coronoid fossa (not anteriorly), passing through the common flexor origin, posterior to the median nerve and brachial artery, which are protected by the brachialis muscle [3, 9, 10]. This portal allows an excellent view of the entire anterior compartment of the joint, in particular the radiocapitellar joint, coronoid, and trochlea. Pronation and supination will allow a full 260° arc of visibility of the radial head [8]. From this portal, the coronoid process may obstruct the proximal radioulnar joint articulation. Furthermore, the medial ulnohumeral articulation is difficult to see. This portal affords access to the anteromedial coronoid and may be useful, in conjunction with the proximal anteromedial portal, for coronoid reduction and fixation.

The structure at greatest risk is the medial antebrachial cutaneous nerve; it is an average 1 mm away from the trocar and demonstrates considerable variability [8]. The median nerve is an average 7–14 mm away.

Proximal Anteromedial Portal

This portal is often used as the starting point in elbow arthroscopy and offers an optimal view of the entire anterior compartment. It is made 2 cm proximal and 1 cm anterior to the medial epicondyle to avoid injury to ulnar nerve (see Fig. 67.3) [11, 14, 15]. When making the portal, a blunt trocar should be used to pierce the flexor pronator mass. The trocar should be slid along the anterior surface of the humerus, aimed toward the radial head [11, 15]. During this approach, the structure most at risk with this portal is the medial antebrachial cutaneous nerve.

Standard Anterolateral Portal

Originally described by Andrews and Carson as 3 cm distal and 1 cm anterior to the lateral epicondyle, this portal is very close to the neurovascular structures and is not recommended (see Fig. 67.3) [3]. Similar, less risky visualization has been described via other portals.

Proximal Anterolateral Portal

Located 2 cm proximal and 1–2 cm anterior to the lateral epicondyle, this portal permits a consistent view of the radiocapitellar joint and the medial side of the joint (see Fig. 67.3) [16, 17]. To access this portal, the trocar should be directed toward the center of the joint while in contact with the anterior humerus. Because the posterior branch of the lateral antebrachial cutaneous nerve and radial nerve are a safe distance away, this portal has been advocated as a good starting point in elbow arthroscopy [10, 17].

Posterior Radiocapitellar "Soft-Spot" Portal

This portal is commonly referred to as the "soft spot" and is located in the center of the triangle created by the lateral epicondyle, olecranon, and radial head (see Fig. 67.3). It can be used for visualization of the posterior radiocapitellar and ulnohumeral joints and for distention [18]. The risk of this portal is that the minimal distance between the capsule and the skin increases the risk of fluid extravasation into surrounding soft tissues. Therefore, it is recommended to delay placement of this portal until the procedure has begun via

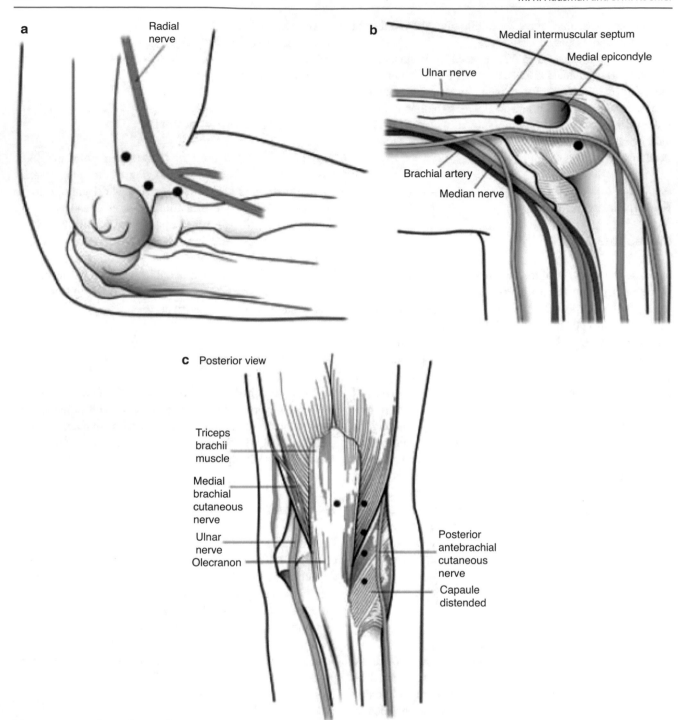

Fig. 67.3 Commonly used (**a**) lateral and (**b**) medial portals. Lateral portals include the proximal anterolateral portal, 2 cm proximal and 1 cm anterior to the lateral epicondyle; the anterior radiocapitellar portal directly anterior to the radiocapitellar joint (and closest to the radial nerve); and the posterior radiocapitellar or soft spot portal. Medially, the proximal anterolateral portal is most widely used, 2 cm proximal and anterior to the lateral epicondyle. An additional anteromedial portal can be placed 1 cm distal to the proximal anteromedial portal, but insertion is more difficult because of the more fibrous common flexor origin tendon in the more distal position. (**c**) Posteriorly, the transtriceps portal is supplemented with proximal and distal posterolateral portals for retractors and working instruments. Additional portals can be safely placed along the posterior radioulnar interval

another portal [10]. The only structures relatively at risk from this approach are the lateral antebrachial cutaneous nerve and posterior antebrachial cutaneous nerve [11, 18].

Straight Posterior (Transtriceps) Portal

The workhorse of the posterior compartment, this portal is located 3 cm proximal to the olecranon tip in the midline of the humerus between the epicondyles (see Fig. 67.3) [19]. A #11 scalpel to make a sharp stab incision into the tendon down to bone. This is safe because the ulnar nerve is palpated and the portal is made well lateral to the course of the nerve. The trocar passes through the triceps tendon and into the olecranon fossa. Complete visualization of the entire posterior compartment and gutters is easily achievable.

Proximal Posterolateral Portal

This portal is usually placed 3–4 cm proximal to the olecranon tip and just lateral to the palpable edge of the triceps tendon (see Fig. 67.3) [18]. The trocar is placed through the posterolateral capsule, just lateral to the tendon and toward the olecranon fossa. It is quite safe with the ulnar nerve and medial and posterior antebrachial cutaneous nerves. We typically use this portal as a working portal in conjunction with the straight posterior portal.

Accessory Distal Posterolateral Portal and Anterior Radiocapitellar Portal

The distal posterolateral portal (see Fig. 67.3) is used to view the posterior compartment, lateral gutter, posterior radiocapitellar joint, proximal radioulnar joint, and medial gutter while allowing the transtriceps portal to be used for a shaver or resecting forceps. A useful accessory portal is the anterior radiocapitellar portal just anterior and proximal to the joint. It should only be made under direct localization and visualization from the medial portal as it lies closest to the radial nerve. Extreme caution should be used when inserting the trocar as anterior deflection along the capsule will place the radial nerve at risk [6].

Surface Landmarks

Prior to starting, it is our practice to always mark the major topographic landmarks on the skin. We routinely mark the medial and lateral epicondyles, olecranon and proximal ulnar, radial head, radiocapitellar joint, and the path of the ulnar nerve (Fig. 67.4). We also ensure there is no ulnar subluxation present. Lastly, we mark out our proposed portals, because joint distention will distort the anatomy later in the procedure.

Order of Portal Placement

Portal placement is determined by the procedure to be done. In general, for fracture work, a proximal anteromedial portal is first established, and the lateral portals can be located with a 25-gauge needle to ensure safe, accurate placement. A posterior portal is useful for checking the posterior wall of the lateral column and the distal reduction of capitellar fractures. Coronoid fractures are fixed through anteromedial and anterolateral portals.

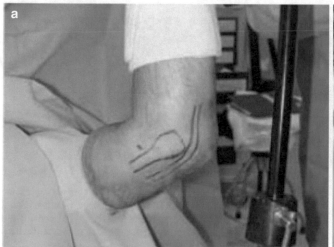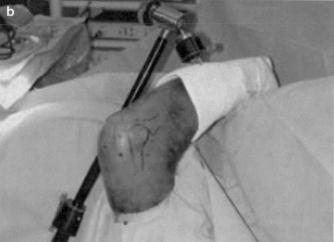

Fig. 67.4 Surface landmarks (**a**) and mapping (**b**) of all common portals prior to commencement of the surgery

Surgical Tips for Fracture Arthroscopy

1. Do not overdistend the joint. Capsular rupture has been shown to occur with a little as 20 mL [20].
2. Wait 24–36 h for clot to form (if not contraindicated).
3. Enter the joint and lavage with a 3.5 mm shaver directed posteriorly toward the humerus until the hematoma is cleared and an adequate view is established. This takes time and patience, but it is impossible to see anything until this step is completed, so be patient.
4. Leave the ulnar nerve in situ to avoid trauma and additional scarring. Furthermore, it preserves the option of later arthroscopic arthrolysis should subsequent elbow release be necessary.

Capitellum and Anterior Coronal Shear Fractures

Due to the difficulty of obtaining adequate exposure and the risks of screw placement in a hemisphere (similar to a subcapital hip fracture or slipped femoral capital epiphysis), capitellar fractures are well suited for arthroscopic treatment. These injuries frequently involve the lateral aspect of the trochlea in addition to the lateral column (Fig. 67.5) [21, 22]. Thus, the entire anterior articular surface as well as the posterior cortex of the lateral column should be inspected. This would require extensive exposure and dissection for complete visualization. However, such exposure can be accomplished arthroscopically with minimal trauma. Additionally,

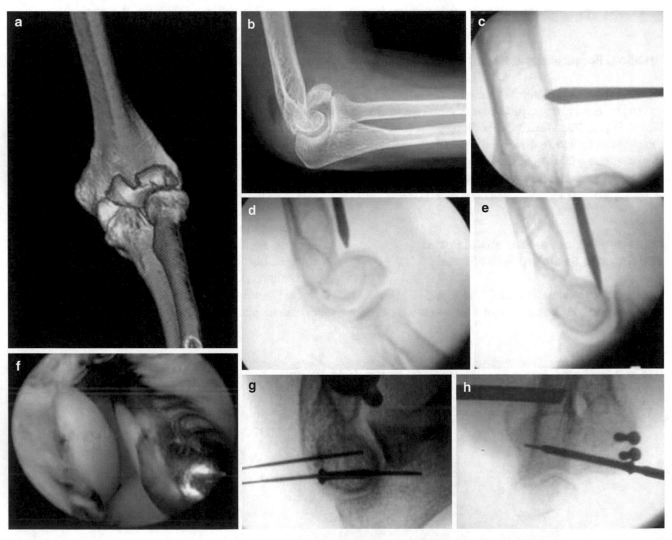

Fig. 67.5 (**a**) CT and (**b**) X-ray demonstrate an anterior coronal shear fracture involving the entire capitellum and lateral trochlea. (**c**) A "high" proximal anterolateral portal is marked out under radiologic guidance and created proximal to the fracture. (**d, e**) Extension frequently will reduce the fracture, but in this case, a complete reduction does not occur. Therefore, the trocar is used to push the fragment into an anatomic reduction. (**f**) This is confirmed with the arthroscopic view from the anterolateral portal. (**g**) Fixation is achieved with cannulated screws, again using the arthroscope to confirm optimal placement and length. (**h**) Note the use of a transcondylar screw to reinforce the fixation, permitting early use and therapy

direct visualization of the reduction is invaluable in ensuring adequate fixation, and the joint surface can be visually monitored to insure correct screw length and placement. We outline our preferred technique below, but various other techniques have been described (see Fig. 67.5) [23–25].

As previously described, the proximal anteromedial portal should be established and the hematoma evacuated from the joint. The fracture can frequently be reduced in elbow extension, but because of contact with the radial head, the fracture can redisplace when the elbow is flexed. If this occurs, then we place a trocar in the radiocapitellar joint to help the radial head "ride over" the capitellum as the elbow is flexed (much like a shoehorn is used). A trocar is then placed in a proximal anterolateral portal and is used to push and reduce the anterior coronal shear fragment. This trocar is then interposed in the radiocapitellar joint, to act as a shoehorn to prevent displacement as the elbow is flexed and allow the radial head to "ride over" the capitellum without displacing it. Once flexion more than 90° is obtained, the radial head will then help to maintain the reduction. Fluoroscopic examination will ensure that the capitellar fragment is captured by the radial head and not redisplaced.

Once reduction is achieved, the elbow should be kept flexed, maintaining the reduction. The reduction should be thoroughly visualized, both the anterior aspect of the joint and the distal humerus where there can be comminuted fragments or plastic deformation of the posterior fragment of the distal humerus that prevents a perfect reduction. We utilize a transtriceps or distal posterior lateral portal to visualize the distal humerus. When using a distal posterior lateral portal, we pass down into the lateral gutter, obtaining a view of the posterior column. It may sometimes be necessary to use the posterior radiocapitellar portal for a 3.5 mm shaver to remove debris in this area, improving visualization. The reduction of the lateral trochlear ridge can also be assessed from the posterior side, advancing the arthroscope down the lateral gutter and directing the optics proximally along the anterior humerus. Occasionally, a 70° arthroscope is helpful for this purpose.

Once an accurate reduction is achieved and confirmed, we prepare the area for fixation. Small posterior incisions are made to insert guide wires for at least two cannulated screws. If necessary, we use an anterior portal or a view from the lateral gutter with a 70° scope to observe the guide wires, thereby confirming the trajectory of the screws and assuring the proper length and position. The guide wires are advanced until just barely visible through the cartilage, and a screw 2–4 mm shorter than the measured length is selected. This process ensures that the longest possible screw is being used, instead of undersizing, which may occur when judging the screw length in a sphere on a two-dimensional radiograph. If possible, a lateral to medial transcondylar screw (2.5 or 2.7 mm) will substantially increase the strength of the fixation. Care should be taken to assess the trochlear ridge reduction if the fracture extends medially.

We prefer to start early motion. However, if there is comminution or any question about stability, then the elbow should be immobilized. We prioritize healing of the fracture over early motion, as any residual contracture can be treated with a staged arthroscopic contracture release, if necessary.

Unicondylar Fractures (AO Type B) of the Distal Humerus

A unicondylar, intra-articular distal humerus fracture is anatomically similar to a capitellar fracture or pediatric lateral condyle fracture. Triceps sparing or reflecting approaches have been advocated to avoid olecranon osteotomy. However, visualization of the articular surface is severely compromised unless a more extensive soft tissue release performed, thereby contravening the hypothetical advantage of the more limited approach. We prefer a hybrid operation. Our preference is to combine the arthroscopic view of the articular surface (the "exposure") with a combined, extracapsular medial or lateral approach to apply a plate (Fig. 67.6). Arthroscopy may then be used to confirm that articular penetration has not occurred.

Critical to the success of this operation is accurate articular reduction and reassociation of the distal articular surface to the shaft by means of a plate. Established principles of fixation should be observed [26].

Visualization and assessment of the reduction are similar to the capitellum fracture and lateral condyle fracture described above and below. However, a thicker pin (4.5 mm Steinmann pin or even biplanar pins) will be required to manipulate the larger fragment with the attached muscle origins. Once the reduction is evaluated both arthroscopically and radiographically, the fracture is temporarily fixed with the transcondylar wires or pin (our preference is a 3 mm Steinmann pin). Then, a medial or lateral midaxial incision is made for application of the plate. Because of arthroscopic-assisted reduction, no additional arthrotomy or musculotendinous dissection is required.

For a medial column fracture, the incision should be made prior to pin placement because of the proximity of the ulnar nerve, which should be identified; retracted, if necessary; and protected as the pin is inserted. When reducing a lateral column fracture, take care not to advance the pin too far medially to protect the ulnar nerve.

The plate is then applied over the K-wires or Steinmann pin in the correct position. The plate is then provisionally fixed, and a second distal transcondylar screw is placed through the plate. The initial pin can then be removed and replaced with a transcondylar screw through the plate, thus conforming to O'Driscoll's principles of distal humerus fracture fixation [26]. The remaining proximal and distal screws are then placed.

Postoperatively, we recommend that the onset of range of motion exercises should be determined by the surgeon's confidence in the strength and stability of the fixation, again prioritizing union over early motion. Restoration of lost motion is much more reliable than the treatment of avascular necrosis of the trochlea or lateral condyle.

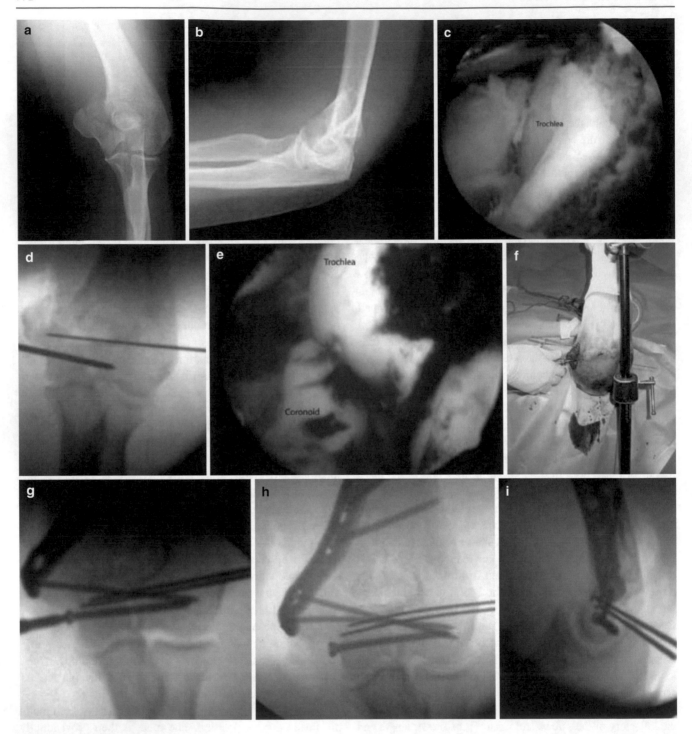

Fig. 67.6 (**a**, **b**) A comminuted medial condyle fracture as seen on X-ray. (**c**) Arthroscopically, the trochlear articular fragment is seen. (**d**, **e**) A limited medial approach is made to protect the ulnar nerve so that a heavy Steinmann pin can be inserted as a joystick to manipulate the fragment into a reduction. K-wires placed from lateral to medial temporarily stabilize the reduction, while a transcondylar screw is inserted (in a lag fashion, if necessary) to achieve an anatomic reduction. (**f**, **g**) A medial plate is applied without disturbing the flexor pronator origin. The intact lateral condyle allows an exemption from the usual "4–5" distal screw rule since the intact lateral column acts as a plate, thus achieving four distal screws that secure the articular surface to the shaft. (**h**, **i**) Reduction of a lateral column fracture involves similar steps from the lateral side

Coronoid Fractures

As we increase our understanding of the significance of coronoid fractures, the indications for repair continue to evolve. We now understand that the traditional Regan–Morrey classification type I and II coronoid fractures are frequently associated with ligament and soft-tissue injuries that can cause instability even with type I coronoid fractures [27, 28]. O'Driscoll's and Steinmann and Adams' modifications recognize the association of medial coronoid facet fractures (type II) with varus instability [29, 30]. Doornberg and Ring have demonstrated that this fracture pattern is also associated with posteromedial rotatory instability [31]. Transverse coronoid tip and anterolateral coronoid facet fractures (O'Driscoll type I)

can be associated with MCL rupture and posterolateral rotatory instability. Therefore, treatment should be determined by the presence or absence of instability and whether the instability is posterolateral or posteromedial. A medial coronoid facet fracture should not be fixed arthroscopically. Rather a buttress plate should be used to restore this important stabilizer [29]. However, coronoid transverse tip fractures and anterolateral fractures are amenable to arthroscopic reduction and fixation [32]. If there is no radial head fracture present or if the radial head is to be preserved, we prefer arthroscopic reduction and fixation of the coronoid, which thereby imparts additional stability and minimizes surgical trauma (Fig. 67.7) [33]. However, if the radial head is resected, access to the coronoid from an open, lateral approach is relatively easy.

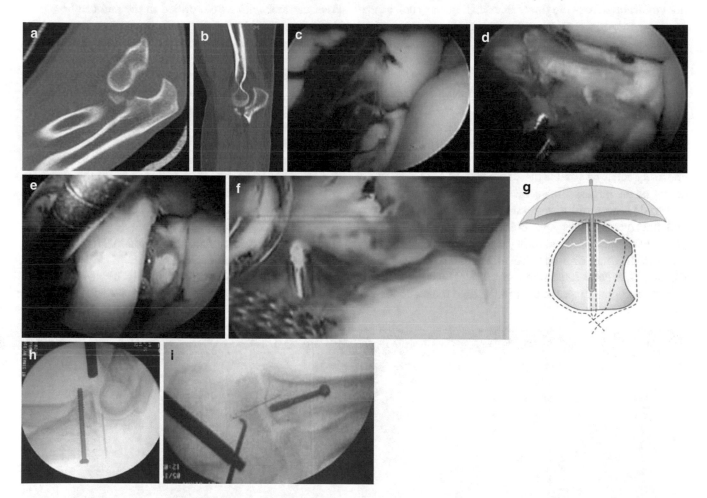

Fig. 67.7 (**a**, **b**) Preoperative CT scanning demonstrates a "terrible triad" injury with an anterior marginal fracture of the radial head, characteristic of posterolateral instability, and an O'Driscoll type I coronoid fracture. There is also anterior ulnohumeral instability, but the anteromedial facet of the coronoid is intact, signifying that posteromedial rotatory instability will not be likely if the other injuries are fixed. The radial head will be preserved in this case, limiting access to the coronoid from the lateral approach, but the anterior ulnohumeral instability is an indication for ARIF of the coronoid. (**c**) The coronoid base is visualized (with a 70° arthroscope, in this case), and (**d**) guide wires are directed from the posterior proximal ulna to the base of the coronoid. (**e**) The tip of the coronoid is then reduced, and, under arthroscopic

visualization, a guide wire and cannulated screw are placed in the coronoid from the subcutaneous border of the proximal ulna. Fluoroscopy helps determine the approximate entrance point. A second, medial hole is drilled over another guide wire for passage of a cerclage suture using a suture retriever or 28-gauge wire. (**f**, **g**) A Kevlar-reinforced suture is passed through the cannulated screw and through the second hole and then exits to the posterior border of the ulna. This further reinforcement is like an umbrella embracing the tip of the fragment. (**h**, **i**) The coronoid cerclage suture is tied after ORIF of the radial head using an arthroscopic sliding knot. The radial head fracture is then fixed through a small, lateral approach

We use standard anteromedial and anterolateral portals. Of note, if there is considerable synovitis, an anterior capsule debridement may be necessary in order to visualize the fragment. Taking the extra minutes to debride can facilitate excellent visualization. To facilitate reduction, a small modified skin hook is introduced through a cannula in the anteromedial portal to grab and reduce the coronoid fragment. Using fluoroscopy, guide wires for cannulated screws are placed through the posterior cortex of the proximal ulna just distal to the coronoid process. Two or three wires are placed to engage and temporarily fix the coronoid. They should exit just distal to the coronoid tip, angling distal posteriorly to proximal anteriorly. This way, distally directed forces on the coronoid compress, rather than distract, across the fracture. A drill guide, such as that used in anterior cruciate reconstruction surgery, can be helpful when aiming the guide wires. The arthroscope may be used to observe the correct exit point for the guide wires.

If the fragment is large enough, the placement of two partially threaded cannulated screws is preferred. We augment this repair with a cerclage loop of suture passed through the screws, which achieves a mattress suture effect. Unfortunately, most fractures will not accept two screws, and a single screw construct must be used. This screw should be placed in the center of the largest dimension of the fragment. We confirm our guide wire position and reduction with both arthroscopy and fluoroscopy. Then, we hold the coronoid fragment in place with the modified skin hook. Additional, auxiliary guide wires may also be used to temporarily stabilize the fracture. The cannulated screw guide wires are grasped with an arthroscopic grasper in the joint to hold the reduction and

prevent unintended removal of the pin while drilling with the cannulated drill.

A partially threaded 3.5 mm cannulated screw(s) is then inserted. The screw length is slightly undersized so there is a millimeter of bone between the cortex of the coronoid and the screw, thereby avoiding abrasion of the cerclage suture. We then pass our cerclage suture (Fig. 67.8). If the coronoid fracture is an anterolateral fragment, a spinal needle is placed in the soft spot, and a 28-gauge stainless steel wire is passed and extracted through the lateral portal along with the cerclage suture that has been passed through the screw. We use non-resorbable, braided suture, such as FiberWire (Arthrex, Naples, FL).

If a cerclage of the medial fragment is required, a small Freer elevator with a hole drilled in the end can be passed along the medial border of the proximal ulna. Care must be taken to remain on bone during this maneuver in order to be deep to the ulnar nerve, which lays close to the proximal ulna at the level of the coronoid. We preload this modified Freer with a 28-gauge stainless steel wire that can be used as a suture shuttle to pass the cerclage suture exiting the cannulated screw.

Our postoperative care is dictated by the presence of other injuries and the potential or presence of elbow instability. For example, posteromedial rotatory instability with an O'Driscoll type II fracture of the medial facet is difficult to stabilize. As a result, stability and healing are prioritized over motion, and many patients require a second-stage arthroscopic release to achieve full motion. However, this is preferable to persistent instability.

Type I and III injuries can usually be stabilized well enough to permit early range of motion. Weekly radiographs

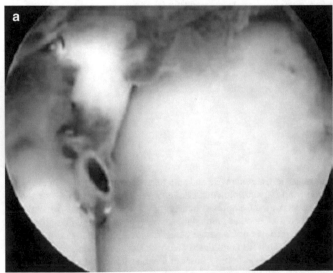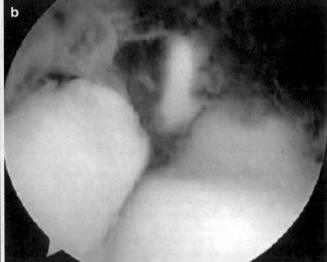

Fig. 67.8 (**a**) This case demonstrates the cerclage suture passing through the proximal radioulnar joint to secure a small anterolateral coronoid fragment. Note the vector of the suture's pull in a proximal direction, securing the fragment in a reduced position against the trochlea. (**b**) The cerclage suture (*blue*) avoids the suture anchor effect of tying to a point and effectively reduces the coronoid

are obtained to check for any signs of instability. If the radiographs demonstrate instability, a static external fixator should be applied.

Radial Head Fractures

Arthroscopic-assisted reduction and fixation of radial head fractures is described [4, 34–37]. However, this is a challenging procedure due to swelling around the injury and thus is not consistent with the principle that the arthroscopy should improve exposure, simplify the procedure, or avoid major soft tissue trauma associated with an open exposure. Since most radial head fractures can be exposed and fixed through a limited, non-destructive approach through the common extensor origin (the so-called Kaplan interval), we do not perform ARIF of the radial head.

Described methods visualize the fracture from the proximal anteromedial portal. A shaver is inserted through the proximal anterolateral portal. Reduction is accomplished with a periosteal elevator, or percutaneously placed K-wires can also be used through the fracture fragments to joystick them into appropriate position. Once reduction is achieved, these wires can be passed into the radial diaphysis to allow for cannulated headless screw placement, taking care to bury the threads beneath the articular surface to avoid impingement of the proximal radioulnar joint (Fig. 67.9). Percutaneously placed K-wires can also be used through the fracture fragments to joystick them into appropriate position (see Fig. 67.9). A soft-spot portal allows for a view of the posterior radial head. Additionally, use of the posterolateral portal has been well described as a working portal, as it allows for an optimal angle for screw entry [36, 37]. Dawson

and Inostroza have described using this arthroscopic technique to treat an angulated pediatric radial neck fracture in a child as well (Fig. 67.10) [35].

Instability

Posterolateral rotatory instability (PLRI) often results from overlooked ligamentous injury in elbow trauma [38]. For instance, as outlined above, coronoid fractures are frequently associated with elbow instability. Furthermore, the combination of an elbow dislocation, radial head fracture, and coronoid fracture (commonly referred to as the "terrible triad" in light of its notoriously poor outcome) can also result in PLRI if the damage to the lateral ligamentous complex is not recognized and treated. McKee described a standard protocol to approaching these injuries. It includes initial fixation or replacement of the radial head, fixation of the coronoid fracture, repair of the lateral collateral ligament complex, and, for residual instability, reconstruction of the medial collateral ligament and/or application of an external fixator [39].

The arthroscopic treatment of posterolateral rotatory instability of the elbow was initially described by Smith et al. in 2001 and further expanded upon by Savoie et al. in 2010 [38, 40]. In both studies, the authors provide a method for confirming the diagnosis of posterolateral rotatory instability of the elbow arthroscopically and an all arthroscopic suture plication of the complex.

First, to confirm the diagnosis, a pivot shift maneuver is performed while visualizing the anterior compartment from the proximal anteromedial portal. The radial head will be seen to sublux posteriorly in the presence of continued PLRI. In addition, the presence of a "drive-through" sign

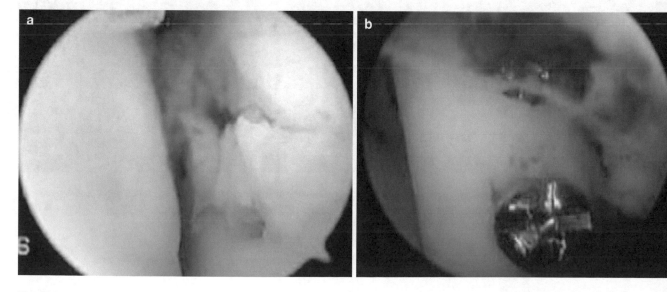

Fig. 67.9 (**a**) A view from the anteromedial portal shows a Mason type II radial head fracture after reduction and (**b**) placement of two cannulated screws

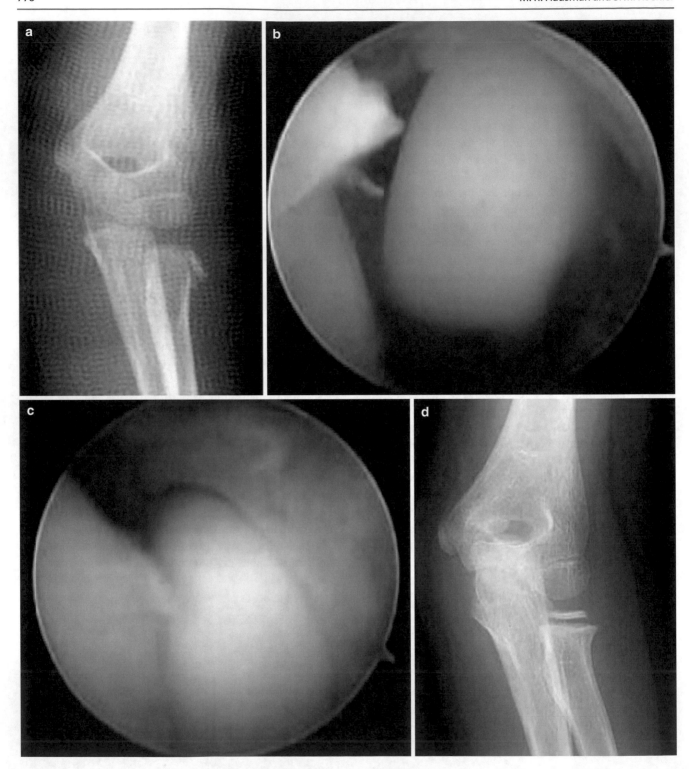

Fig. 67.10 (a) The reduction of this angulated, pediatric radial neck fracture is impeded by (b) displacement of the radial head anterolaterally into a capsular recess. (c) Following reduction, the radial head is articulating with the capitellum, and the intact periosteal sleeve stabilizes the fracture. (d) A postoperative X-ray demonstrates a good reduction

(i.e., the ability to drive the scope into the ulnohumeral joint) is present in the unstable elbow but will correct with appropriate treatment of that instability.

Arthroscopic repair of the lateral ligamentous structures involves suture plication to tighten the posterolateral capsule and the radial ulnohumeral ligament. The lateral gutter is viewed from a posterior portal. At the insertion point of the radial ulnohumeral ligament, a spinal needle is inserted into the joint. Suture is then shuttled into the joint, directly adjacent to the lateral humeral epicondyle. The two ends of the suture exit the joint through a lateral incision. As the sutures are tensioned, the lateral gutter will decrease in volume, representing tightening of the posterolateral ligamentous structures. Finally, the authors note that if a large amount of instability is found or if the ligament has avulsed from the humeral origin, a suture anchor can be placed at the isometric point of the lateral epicondyle in addition to the plication technique described [38].

In a study comparing this procedure to the classic open repair, a high rate of success was measured in both categories, suggesting this as a ready alternative to open surgery [40]. Given this, in addition to direct visualization of posterolateral subluxation of the radial head on the capitellum from the anteromedial portal, arthroscopic plication of the attenuated LUCL complex provides an effective, alternative approach to joint stabilization.

Pediatric Facture of the Lateral Condyle

The visualization of a pediatric lateral condyle fracture via the arthroscope is conceptually similar to the capitellum fractures described earlier. However, because the entire lateral column is involved, the type and trajectory of the fixation are different. Our rationale for arthroscopic assistance in these fractures is twofold. First, arthroscopy provides an excellent visualization the articular surface while avoiding extensive dissection around the lateral condyle. Thus, arthroscopy could minimize compromise of the precarious blood supply to the condyle and, hopefully, minimize the risk of avascular necrosis [41]. Second, we find arthroscopy is useful to confirm the trajectory of the fixation pins. In children whose lateral condyles are largely cartilage, this can be difficult radiographically. Lateral condyle fractures are categorized according to the Milch criteria based on where the fracture line exits in relation to the trochlear groove [42]. Reportedly, nondisplaced Milch type I fractures may be treated nonsurgically; however, we have found that truly nondisplaced fractures are extremely rare [43]. Our current treatment protocol is to arthroscopically fix displaced type I and all type II lateral condyle fractures (Fig. 67.11) [41, 44, 45].

However, if the fragment is very rotated (90° or more), then arthroscopic reduction may be difficult, and a small, open approach may be necessary.

Positioning in pediatric patients is similar to adults. A standard proximal anteromedial portal is created. As previously described, the hematoma in the joint is evacuated. Once adequate visualization is achieved, the degree and direction of displacement can be seen. A 1.6 mm (0.062 in.) K-wire can be inserted percutaneously into the lateral condylar fragment. To ensure that the pin placement is in the secondary ossification center, the arthroscope can be advanced to the trabecular bone of the secondary ossification center and the cannula placed in contact with the bone. The arthroscope is then withdrawn, and the K-wire is advanced through the cannula, into the fragment, and out the skin. As the arthroscope is reinserted in the cannula, the K-wire is withdrawn out the lateral aspect of the elbow until just the tip of the pin is seen in the secondary ossification center. Two or three 1.6 mm pins are placed under direct visualization and are used as a joystick to reduce the fragment. The pins are then alternately advanced. The reduction is inspected both under direct visualization with the arthroscope and using fluoroscopy. The pins are then trimmed and the elbow is casted.

Postoperatively, the elbow is casted 4–6 weeks until there is radiographic evidence of union and exercise is begun.

Complications

The overall complication rate from elbow arthroscopy has been reported at 6–15% [46]. This includes neurologic injury, compartment syndrome, septic arthritis, superficial infection, arthrofibrosis, thromboembolism, complex regional pain syndrome, and persistent portal drainage [13, 47–49]. The most common problem is a portal fistula, which can usually be avoided by careful closure of the portals with multiple sutures. It is also our practice to routinely prep and close drain holes after removal of the drain.

The rate of neurologic injury is cited as 0–14% [13]. Most injuries are neuropraxias and will resolve with time, but complete transection has also been seen [13]. Injury can occur with injection of local anesthetic, compression due to swelling of the joint or crushing from the instrumentation, direct trauma from trocar insertion, or laceration with a shaver. Minimizing this risk requires experience, careful attention to the anatomy and surface landmarks, and an appreciation of the special risks including distorted anatomy, contractures, rheumatoid arthritis, or heterotopic ossification. Any injury, even to cutaneous nerves, can lead to a chronic, possibly disabling condition.

Infection following elbow arthroscopy is infrequent. Superficial postoperative infections are readily treated with

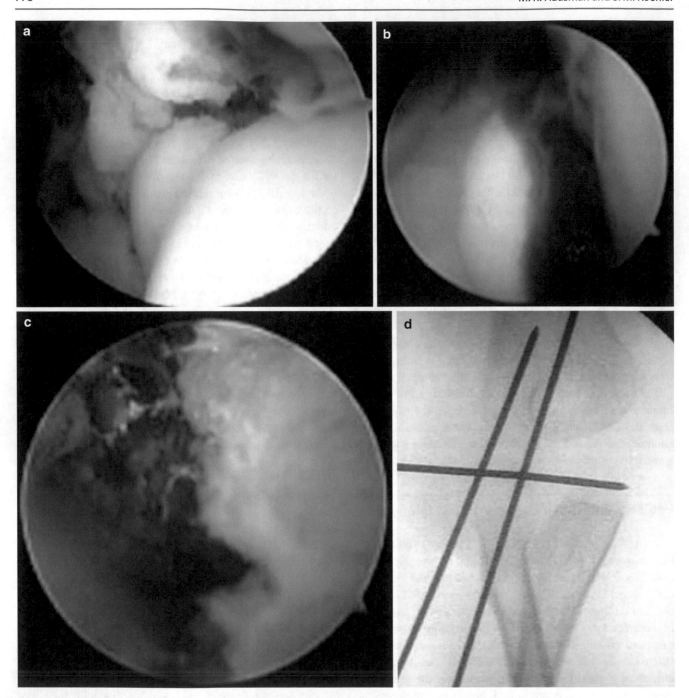

Fig. 67.11 (**a**) An arthroscopic view from the proximal anteromedial portal shows the displaced lateral condyle. (**b**) The cannula and scope are advanced up to the bone of the secondary ossification center; the arthroscope is withdrawn while holding the cannula in position; and a K-wire is advanced through the cannula into the bone. (**c**) The wire is then withdrawn from the lateral aspect of the elbow until it is just piercing the surface of the bone. (**d**) The final position of the fixation pins. Note the use of a transcondylar pin to prevent rotation in addition to the usual oblique pins

oral antibiotics. Septic arthritis has been found more commonly in patients who received intra-articular steroid injection following the procedure [13]. Steroid injections are contraindicated by fractures and ligament injuries. If steroids are used after contracture release, IV administration beginning prior to deflating the tourniquet is maximally effective.

One increasingly reported complication from elbow arthroscopy is heterotopic ossification [50]. Although a rare complication, there is some evidence that it is related to the extensiveness of the procedure [48]. The extent of the injury (e.g., "terrible triad") and recurrent instability have been implicated as negative prognostic factors [48]. Currently, we do not take any increased precautions during our arthroscopy procedures aside from warning patients of this potential complication. Some surgeons have adopted routine prophylaxis with either indomethacin or a preoperative dose of radiation prior to more-involved arthroscopic surgeries [48, 50–53]. If it does occur, the standard treatment is excision after 3 months [48].

Conclusion

While still evolving, arthroscopy has already established a role in elbow trauma management. It should only be considered a useful adjunct, however, if it facilitates the exposure or makes the reduction and fixation easier, more precise, or safer, as in avoiding inadvertent intra-articular hardware penetration. If, after initial debridement, good visualization is not achieved, arthroscopy adds no value, and the operation should be converted to a conventional open procedure. Following established arthroscopic techniques, such as using lower inflow pressures and using retractors when necessary, will avoid extravasation of fluid and swelling that would hamper a conversation to an open procedure. In the pediatric patient, arthroscopy is useful for radial neck fractures and moderately displaced lateral condyle fractures. However, if the lateral condyle fragment is spun 90°, open reduction is likely to be necessary. In the adult, arthroscopy has proven consistently helpful with capitellum and anterior coronal shear fractures. Most coronoid fractures that do not involve impaction of the medial facet can also be reduced and stabilized; however, the indications are still evolving, and if other open treatment, such as radial head arthroplasty, is required, an open approach is preferred [16, 33].

References

1. Burman MS. Arthroscopy or the direct visualization of joints, an experimental cadaver study. J Bone Joint Surg Am. 1931;VIII(4):669–95.
2. Burman MS. Arthroscopy of the elbow joint, a cadaver study. J Bone Joint Surg Am. 1932;14:349–50.
3. Andrews JR, Carson WG. Arthroscopy of the elbow. Arthroscopy. 1985;1:97–107.
4. Holt SM, Savoie FH III, Field LD, et al. Arthroscopic management of elbow trauma. Hand Clin. 2004;20:485–95.
5. Dodson CC, Nho SJ, Williams RJ 3rd, et al. Elbow arthroscopy. J Am Acad Orthop Surg. 2008;16(10):574–85.
6. Hsu JW, Gould JL, Hausman MH. The emerging role of elbow arthroscopy in chronic use injuries and fracture care. Hand Clin. 2009;25(3):305–21.
7. Ramsey ML, Naranja RJ. Diagnostic arthroscopy of the elbow. In: Baker Jr CL, Plancher KD, editors. Operative treatment of elbow injuries. New York: Springer; 2002. p. 163–9.
8. Adolfsson L. Arthroscopy of the elbow joint: a cadaveric study of portal placement. J Shoulder Elb Surg. 1994;3:53–61.
9. Lynch GJ, Meyer JF, Whipple TL, Caspari RB. Neurovascular anatomy and elbow arthroscopy: inherent risks. Arthroscopy. 1986;2:190–7.
10. Stothers K, Day B, Regan WR. Arthroscopy of the elbow: anatomy, portal sites, and a description of the proximal lateral portal. Arthroscopy. 1995;11:449–57.
11. Unlu MC, Kesmezacar H, Akgun I, Ogut T, Uzun I. Anatomic relationship between elbow arthroscopy portals and neurovascular structures in different elbow and forearm positions. J Shoulder Elb Surg. 2006;15:457–62.
12. Gallay SH, Richards RR, O'Driscoll SW. Intraarticular capacity and compliance of stiff and normal elbows. Arthroscopy. 1993;9:9–13.
13. Kelly EW, Morrey BF, O'Driscoll SW. Complications of elbow arthroscopy. J Bone Joint Surg Am. 2001;83A:25–34.
14. Poehling GG, Whipple TL, Sisco L, Goldman B. Elbow arthroscopy: a new technique. Arthroscopy. 1989;5:222–4.
15. Lindenfeld TN. Medial approach in elbow arthroscopy. Am J Sports Med. 1990;18:413–7.
16. Adams JE, Merten SM, Steinmann SP. Arthroscopic-assisted treatment of coronoid fractures. Arthroscopy. 2007;23:1060–5.
17. Field LD, Altchek DW, Warren RF, O'Brien SJ, Skyhar MJ, Wickiewicz TL. Arthroscopic anatomy of the lateral elbow: a comparison of three portals. Arthroscopy. 1994;10:602–7.
18. Baker CL Jr, Jones GL. Arthroscopy of the elbow. Am J Sports Med. 1999;27:251–64.
19. Andrews JR, Craven WM. Lesions of the posterior compartment of the elbow. Clin Sports Med. 1991;10:637–52.
20. O'Driscoll SW, Morrey BF, An KN. Intraarticular pressure and capacity of the elbow. Arthroscopy. 1990;6:100–3.
21. Ring D, Jupiter JB, Gulotta L. Articular fractures of the distal part of the humerus. J Bone Joint Surg Am. 2003;85A:232–8.
22. Guitton TG, Doornberg JN, Raaymakers EL, Ring D, Kloen P. Fractures of the capitellum and trochlea. J Bone Joint Surg Am. 2009;91A:390–7.
23. Kuriyama K, Kawanishi Y, Yamamoto K. Arthroscopic-assisted reduction and percutaneous fixation for coronal shear fractures of the distal humerus: report of two cases. J Hand Surg Am. 2010;35:1506–9.
24. Hardy P, Menguy F, Guillot S. Arthroscopic treatment of capitellum fractures of the humerus. Arthroscopy. 2002;18:422–6.
25. Mitani M, Nabeshima Y, Ozaki A, Mori H, Issei N, Fujii H, Fujioka H, Doita M. Arthroscopic reduction and percutaneous cannulated screw fixation of a capitellar fracture of the humerus: a case report. J Shoulder Elb Surg. 2009;18:e6–9.
26. O'Driscoll SW. Optimizing stability in distal humeral fracture fixation. J Shoulder Elb Surg. 2005;14(1 Suppl S):186S–94.
27. Schneeberger AG, Sadowski MM, Jacob HA. Coronoid process and radial head as posterolateral rotatory stabilizers of the elbow. J Bone Joint Surg Am. 2004;86A:975–82.
28. Closkey RF, Goode JR, Kirschenbaum D, Cody RP. The role of the coronoid process in elbow stability. A biomechanical analysis of axial loading. J Bone Joint Surg Am. 2000;82A:1749–53.
29. O'Driscoll SW, Bell DF, Morrey BF. Posterolateral rotatory instability of the elbow. J Bone Joint Surg Am. 1991;73:440–6.
30. Adams JE, Sanchez-Sotelo J, Kallina CF 4th, Morrey BF, Steinmann SP. Fractures of the coronoid: morphology based upon computer tomography scanning. J Shoulder Elb Surg. 2012;21(6):782–8.
31. Doornberg JN, Ring D. Coronoid fracture patterns. J Hand Surg Am. 2006;31:45–52.
32. Broberg MA, Morrey BF. Results of treatment of fracture-dislocations of the elbow. Clin Orthop Relat Res. 1987;216:109–19.
33. Hausman MR, Klug RA, Qureshi S, Goldstein R, Parsons BO. Arthroscopically assisted coronoid fracture fixation: a preliminary report. Clin Orthop Relat Res. 2008;466:3147–52.
34. Michels F, Pouliart N, Handelberg F. Arthroscopic management of Mason type 2 radial head fractures. Knee Surg Sports Traumatol Arthrosc. 2007;15:1244–50.

35. Dawson FA, Inostroza F. Arthroscopic reduction and percutaneous fixation of a radial neck fracture in a child. Arthroscopy. 2004;20(Suppl 2):90–3.

36. Moskal MJ, Savoie FH 3rd, Field LD. Elbow arthroscopy in trauma and reconstruction. Orthop Clin North Am. 1999;30:163–77.

37. Rolla PR, Surace MF, Bini A, Pilato G. Arthroscopic treatment of fractures of the radial head. Arthroscopy. 2006;22:233.e1–6.

38. Smith JP, Savoie FH, Field LD. Posterolateral rotatory instability of the elbow. Clin Sports Med. 2001;20(1):47–58.

39. McKee MD, Pugh DM, Wild LM, Schemitsch EH, King GJ. Standard surgical protocol to treat elbow dislocations with radial head and coronoid fractures. Surgical technique. J Bone Joint Surg Am. 2005;87(Suppl 1, Pt 1):22–32.

40. Savoie FH, O'Brien MJ, Field LD, Gurley DJ. Arthroscopic and open radial ulnohumeral ligament reconstruction for posterolateral rotatory instability of the elbow. Clin Sports Med. 2010;29(4):611–8.

41. Carro PL, Golano P, Vega J. Arthroscopic-assisted reduction and percutaneous external fixation of lateral condyle fractures of the humerus. Arthroscopy. 2007;23:1131.e1–4.

42. Milch H. Fractures and fracture dislocations of the humeral condyles. J Trauma. 1964;4:592–607.

43. Bast SC, Hoffer MM, Aval S. Nonoperative treatment for minimally and nondisplaced lateral humeral condyle fractures in children. J Pediatr Orthop. 1998;18:448–50.

44. Hausman MR, Qureshi S, Goldstein R, Langford J, Klug RA, Radomisli TE, Parsons BO. Arthroscopically-assisted treatment of pediatric lateral humeral condyle fractures. J Pediatr Orthop. 2007;27:739–42.

45. Hausman MR, Roye B. Pediatric elbow arthroscopy and reconstruction. In: Trumble TE, Budoff JE, editors. Wrist and elbow reconstruction and arthroscopy. Rosemont: American Society for Surgery of the Hand; 2006. p. 377–402.

46. Savoie FH III, Field LD. Arthrofibrosis and complications in arthroscopy of the elbow. Clin Sports Med. 2001;20:123–9.

47. Small NC. Complications in arthroscopic surgery performed by experienced arthroscopists. Arthroscopy. 1988;4:215–21.

48. Gofton WT, King GJ. Heterotopic ossification following elbow arthroscopy. Arthroscopy. 2001;17:1–5.

49. Gay DM, Raphael BS, Weiland AJ. Revision arthroscopic contracture release in the elbow resulting in an ulnar nerve transection. J Bone Joint Surg Am. 2010;92:1246–9.

50. Hughes SC, Hildebrand KA. Heterotopic ossification—a complication of elbow arthroscopy: a case report. J Shoulder Elb Surg. 2010;19:e1–5.

51. King GJ. Stiffness and ankylosis of the elbow. In: Norris TR, editor. Orthopaedic knowledge update: shoulder and elbow. Rosemont: American Academy of Orthopaedic Surgeons; 1997. p. 325–35.

52. Jupiter JB, Ring D. Fractures of the distal humerus. In: Norris TR, editor. Orthopaedic knowledge update: shoulder and elbow. Rosemont: American Academy of Orthopaedic Surgeons; 1997. p. 397–413.

53. Sodha S, Nagda SH, Sennett BJ. Heterotopic ossification in a throwing athlete after elbow arthroscopy. Arthroscopy. 2006;22:802.e1–3.

Radial Head Fractures

68

Tim Leschinger, Lars Peter Müller,
and Kilian Wegmann

Introduction

The radial head is an important stabilizer of the elbow and carries the main share of the axial load. In conjunction with the medial collateral ligament complex (MCL), it is an important secondary stabilizer against valgus stress. By preloading the lateral collateral ligament complex (LCL), it further plays an essential role in the posterolateral stabilization of the elbow joint. In order not to destabilize the joint in the event of a fracture, ligament injuries must likewise be addressed. Angle-stable, low-profile implants and suture anchors offer possible solutions even in complex situations. The reconstruction of the original radial head should be the primary goal, as it is superior to the available radial head prostheses in terms of its anatomical and biomechanical properties. In selected cases, there is the option to perform arthroscopic fracture treatment.

Indications

The classification of radial head fractures according to Mason (1952, modified according to Johnston G.W. 1962) is well established [1, 2]. It serves as guidance when determining the indication for surgery, even if it does not include accompanying injuries (e.g., ligamentous, osteochondral lesions). The choice of therapy method is influenced significantly by the type of fracture, existing accompanying injuries, the patient's personal demands, and accompanying diseases. Mason 1 fractures (joint step <2 mm) can usually be treated conservatively. Patients with Mason 1 fractures should clinically be monitored closely. If there is no significant pain relief or improvement in the range of motion within

the first 2 weeks, further diagnostics (magnetic resonance imaging; MRI) should be performed promptly to rule out any accompanying injuries (ligament lesions, interpositions).

Surgical treatment of Mason 2 fractures (joint step>2 mm, neck fractures <30° tilt) is discussed controversially [3–5]. The recommendation for treatment follows the objective to reduce the joint step and thus to prevent the development of post-traumatic osteoarthritis [4]. For some fractures of this type, there is also the option of arthroscopic treatment [6]. As with Mason 1 fractures if there is joint blockage, diagnostics (MRI) should be expanded, and if necessary, surgical treatment should follow.

Indication for surgical treatment is given in Mason 3 fractures (>3 fragments) and Mason 4 (dislocation) fractures [4, 7, 8]. The primary goal is to preserve the radial head in cases where a stable, anatomical reconstruction is possible. If reconstruction is ruled out, radial head resection remains an option if stable ligament conditions are present. However, this is rarely the case with complex multiple-fragment fractures; hence a radial head prosthesis is recommended.

The incidence of ligament injuries rises with increasing severity of the fracture and reaches up to 80% in complex fractures [9]. Treatment is possible within the context of osteosynthesis. A time window of approx. 3 to 4 weeks remains for refixation or suturing of the original ligaments. After this period, more complex ligament reconstructions (e.g., with autologous tendon transplants) are sometimes necessary.

Preoperative Planning/Contraindication

- Detailed anamnesis of the type of trauma, previous elbow/arm complaints, previous trauma or operations, and individual patient variables (handedness, occupation, sport).
- Clinical examination with obligatory assessment of the neurovascular status, detection of soft tissue injuries, and examination of further accompanying injuries.

T. Leschinger (✉) · L. P. Müller · K. Wegmann
University Hospital Cologne, Center of Orthopedic and Trauma Surgery, Cologne, Germany
e-mail: tim.leschinger@uk-koeln.de; lars.mueller@uk-koeln.de; kilian.wegmann@uk-koeln.de

© Springer Nature Switzerland AG 2022
W. B. Geissler (ed.), *Wrist and Elbow Arthroscopy with Selected Open Procedures*,
https://doi.org/10.1007/978-3-030-78881-0_68

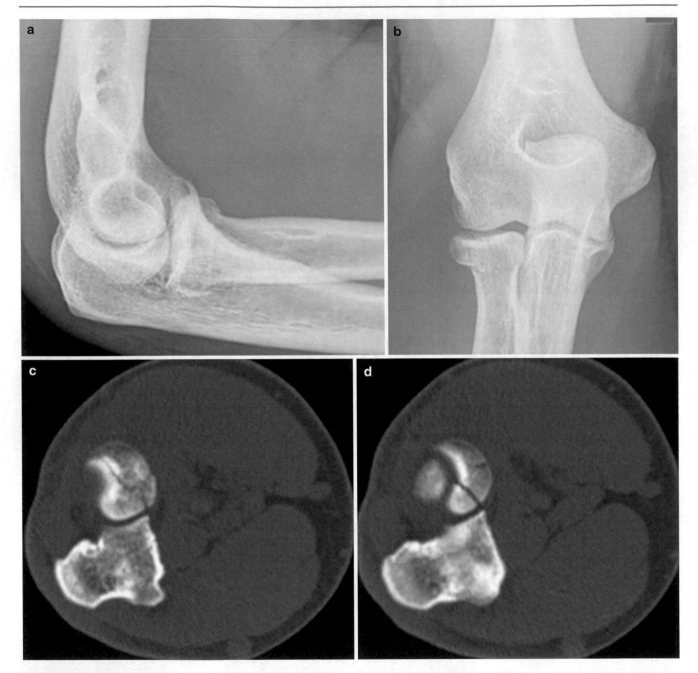

Fig. 68.1 (**a–d**) Mason 3 fracture of the radial head. Conventional X-ray of the elbow a.p. and lateral (**a–b**). The CT (axial reconstruction, **c–d**) is useful for preoperative planning and assessment of the fracture morphology

- Radiological diagnosis with conventional X-ray of the elbow a.p. and lateral view. Care should be taken to ensure that the a.p. setting is correct when the elbow is extended or that in the flexed position the X-ray tube is tilted accordingly and adjusted strictly lateral. In addition, it is often helpful to take X-ray targeting images (e.g., according to Greenspan).
- Computed tomography (CT) with coronal, sagittal, and 3D reconstruction. If the joint step height is difficult to assess, a CT (1-mm thin layer) is carried out in order to

determine the indication for surgery. In the case of complex, multi-fragment fractures, the CT is used for preoperative planning in order to clarify in advance whether alternative procedures (e.g., radial head prosthesis) may become necessary (Fig. 68.1a–d).
- MRI can be useful for assessing the extent of soft tissue injuries, the integrity of the collateral ligaments, and joint incongruences, for example, due to interposed soft tissues. MRI is also indicated in the case of prolonged healing processes, if there is a discrepancy between

radiological findings and distinct clinical findings, or if dislocation cannot be ruled out.

- Exclusion of factors that prevent surgery (infectious soft tissue changes or lesions of the soft tissue or the skin, especially in the area of entry, inoperability due to systemic disease).

Technique

Preparation/Positioning

- Check for completeness of instruments (basic instruments for osteosynthesis, 1–2 mm K-wires with drill (quick-release chuck) and special instruments for the chosen osteosynthesis (plate/screws, possibly bone anchors)
- General anesthesia (laryngeal mask/intubation anesthesia), if necessary, additive regional procedure (e.g., inter-scalene catheter)
- Single-shot antibiosis (cave: allergies)
- Positioning of the patient in the supine position with the arm placed on a radiolucent arm table. Treatment can also be performed in the side or prone position. The free positioning of the upper arm in these cases distracts the radiocapitellar articulation, which simplifies the approach to the radial head. The image intensifier can be swung into the operating field to achieve good access for radiologic evaluation.
- If necessary, placement of an upper arm blood rest (sterile)

Surgery

The skin incision begins 3 cm proximal to the lateral epicondyle and extends to the ulnar edge of the forearm, aiming approximately 7 to 10 cm distal of the olecranon. The forearm is held in pronation.

There are different options for exposing the radial head after opening of the forearm fascia. The modified Kocher approach is commonly used for radial head fracture fixation, performed between the anconeus and extensor carpi ulnaris muscular interval.

> **Tips and Tricks**
> The Kocher interval can be identified by detection of the fat strip that represents the border between the M. anconeus and the M. extensor carpi ulnaris.

The Kocher interval can be entered bluntly with the scissors, and the two muscles are separated. The anconeus muscle is pushed bluntly in dorsal direction, and the anterior extensor muscles can be dissected sharply from the joint capsule. By pronating the forearm, the deep branch of the radial nerve, which crosses the supinator muscle at the level of the radial neck, is shifted away from the incision.

> **Tips and Tricks**
> In pronation, the distance between the radial nerve and the joint line increases, so that the proximal radius can be exposed to the radial tuberosity.

The joint capsule and the annular ligament are exposed in the same sloped incision direction. The approach is anterior to the lateral ulnar collateral ligament (LUCL), palpable as a capsule reinforcement, which is spared (see Fig. 68.3a). In the trauma situation, however, it often appears damaged and detached from its original cause (see Fig. 68.6a).

If necessary, the incision can be widened proximally, and the extensor tendons from the radial epicondyle can be detached anteriorly (column approach), and the lateral collateral ligament complex (LCL) at its humeral insertion point can be detached dorsally. If both the extensor tendons and the humeral LCL attachment have been detached, the radial head can be subluxed radially. Pointed reduction forceps can be placed on the proximal part of the radial shaft for support.

The emptied fracture hematoma behind the capsule opening is removed, Langenbeck bone hooks are inserted anteriorly and posteriorly, and the joint is rinsed out and inspected. If possible, the use of Hohmann hooks on the proximal radius should be avoided in order not to compromise the deep radial branch due to uncontrolled pressure. When using the hooks, an intracapsular position has to be ensured.

When placing the radial head plate, the preparation (e.g., round raspatory) can be carried out with a pronated forearm up to the level of the radial tuberosity.

> **Tips and Tricks**
> In the case of anteriorly located fragments, which are more common in Mason II fractures [10], the Kaplan approach and the extensor digitorum communis split approach are alternatives, which allow improved access to the anterior half of the radial head, while reducing the risk of iatrogenic injury to the lateral collateral ligament complex. A preoperative CT scan can be helpful.

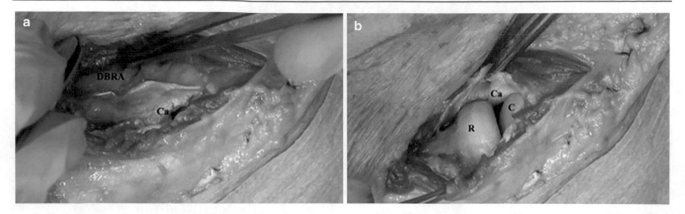

Fig. 68.2 (**a, b**) Cadaver dissection. Proximity of the deep branch of the radial nerve (DBRA) to the surgical dissection at the level of the radial head (R). Ca capsule, C capitellum

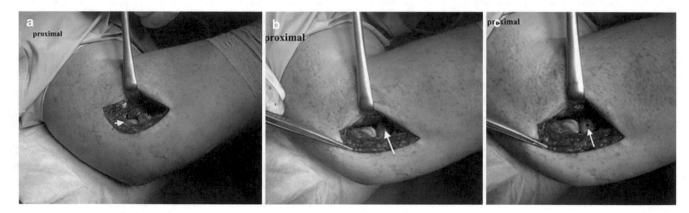

Fig. 68.3 (**a**) Approach to the radial head (R) anterior to the anterior to the LUCL (white arrow). C capitellum. (**b**) Reposition of the fracture (white arrow) and (**c**) placement of the screw below the cartilage level (white arrow)

However, extreme caution should be taken due to proximity of the deep branch of the radial nerve (DBRA) to the surgical dissection at the level of the radial head (Fig. 68.2a, b).

Repositioning in II Fractures

In Mason 2 fractures, there is a compressed anterior fragment in the most cases (anterior rim fragment). This can be deimpacted with a small chisel or elevator, and the fracture gap can be cleaned (e.g., hook, K-wire). Then, the reduction is held with a sharp reduction forceps or with a hook. K-wires can be inserted as temporary retention aids and later replaced with screws. Two screws (e.g., 2.2–3.0 mm, alternatively resorbable pins) are inserted as orthogonally as possible to the fracture gap and parallel to the joint surface in the subchondral bone. The screw heads are placed below the cartilage level. This can be achieved by using headless bone screws or milling cutters. It is important to take into account that a screw length approximately 4 mm shorter than the protrusion measurement should be chosen to place the screws on both sides of the fracture below the cartilage level (Fig. 68.3b).

> **Tips and Tricks**
> Since the average diameter of the radius head is 22 mm, the maximum screw length is usually not more than 20 mm. The screw length can already have been estimated preoperatively using a CT scan.

The correct screw length is checked under fluoroscopy in a strictly orthogonal beam path to the screw and clinically by pronation/supination with palpation and direct visualization. Any protruding screws must be replaced.

Noncomminuted two-part fractures are often suitable for arthroscopic fixation. After completing diagnostic arthroscopy, the fracture can be visualized mostly through the posterolateral or anteromedial portal with the working instruments in the direct lateral or anterolateral portal (Fig. 68.4).

Comparable to the open procedure, the fragment can usually, after sufficient debridement of the fracture hematoma,

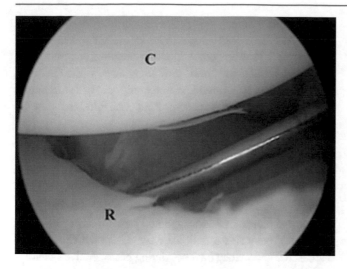

Fig. 68.4 Posterolateral view of a noncomminuted two-part fracture of the radial head (R). C capitellum

be repositioned with an elevator, and the reduction can be held either with the same elevator or alternatively with a hook. An essential and arthroscopically challenging step is the correct placement of two to three Kirschner wires (K-wires) into the radial head to facilitate temporary fixation of the fracture fragments and to serve as a guide wire for cannulated screws for definitive fixation. The wires travel up to the opposite predrilled cortex, and via a protrusion measurement, the required screw length can be determined. The K-wires are then drilled, and headless, cannulated screws (2.2 or 3.0 mm) for definitive osteosynthesis are introduced over the K-wires.

Repositioning in Mason 3 Fractures

As in Mason 2 fractures, repositioning is attempted in situ with the fracture being deimpacted. As a result, two scenarios can usually be distinguished. In the first case, a radial head fragment is firmly attached to the shaft. In this case, screw fixation may be sufficient if the remaining fragments can be attached firmly to this fragment.

In the second case, fragments are separated from the shaft so that the use of a radial head plate becomes necessary.

Fragments are deimpacted, fracture gaps are cleaned, and the fragments are repositioned one after the other to the fragment connected to the shaft. Small elevators, Kocher clamps, and sharp reduction forceps are used as aids. The fragments are temporarily transfixed with thin K-wires, and these are later exchanged for screws.

Once all fragments have been detached from the shaft, the largest fragment is taken hold of (e.g., pointed reduction forceps or Kocher clamp), repositioned against the shaft, and stabilized against the radial shaft with a K-wire, which is

inserted through the circumference of this fragment. To avoid further impediment due to the inserted K-wires, the repositioning of the further fragments and the thus necessary pronation or supination of the forearm must be taken into account when positioning the wires.

After repositioning the main fragment, further smaller fragments can be repositioned one after the other against the main fragment and the shaft and temporarily transfixed with K-wires. Thereafter, it is possible to insert interfragmentary screws subchondrally.

The thus reconstructed radial head is fixed against the shaft with a plate. During reconstruction, the physiological angulation of the radius neck of 7° to 15° must be considered. For osteosynthesis, the anatomical low-profile plates from various manufacturers are the means of choice. The use of narrow, non-angle stable T-plates is not recommended due to an increased risk of complications (material failure, pseudarthrosis).

The plates should be placed in the "safe zone." In this area, which encompasses approximately 120° to 135° of the circumference of the radial head, there is no contact with the proximal radioulnar joint during maximum pronation and supination. In maximal supination, the "safe zone" is anteroradial (Fig. 68.5a–h).

Alternatively, in the case of multi-fragment fractures, the fragments can be extirpated with subsequent on-table reconstruction. After the fragments have been screwed extra corporis, the reconstructed radial head is reinserted in toto into the joint (so-called bioprosthesis) (Fig. 68.6).

The replanted radial head is aligned with the shaft (e.g., with a Kocher clamp) and temporarily fixed against the shaft with K-wires. Finally, the plate is positioned and fixed against the shaft and the radial head in the safe zone. If the forearm is brought into maximal supination and the plate is placed as radially as possible, thus subsequent impingement of the plate at the ulna is almost impossible. K-wires can be inserted over the plate for temporary fixation and position control under the image intensifier. The plate is first fixated to the shaft with a cortex screw, which pulls the plate towards the radial shaft.

Repositioning in Mason 4 Fractures

In this type of fracture, there is also a dislocation of the radial head, e.g., in Monteggia-like lesions, transolecranon fractures dislocation, or elbow dislocations. It is therefore important to monitor and treat the accompanying injuries and to plan the incision preoperatively. If there is an accompanying injury to the proximal ulna, the fracture of the radial head can either be treated via the bony defect at the ulna or, after osteosynthesis of the ulna, possibly via the same incision (according to Boyd). Avulsions of the annular ligament, e.g., at the supinator crest bone anchors, MCL, and LCL ava-lanches, can also be treated with suture anchors (Fig. 68.7). Osteosynthesis is performed following the same principles as in the other Mason fractures.

Closure

The final wound closure is done in layers. First, the capsule and the annular ligament are potentially sutured with absorbable sutures. Some authors recommend not repairing the annular ligament to avoid postoperative stiffness. If the annular ligament at the ulna has been detached (e.g., as part of a Boyd incision), it can be reattached with suture anchors. If the extensor tendons and/or the LUCL have been detached

from the distal humerus, they are reinserted at their anatomical insertion area with transosseous sutures or suture anchors (see Fig. 68.7). The suture anchors enable knot-free refixation and, similar to rotator cuff refixation on the shoulder, can be applied in a double row technique. By using suture anchors, bulky and irritating knot convolutions can be avoided especially in slim patients.

The upper and lower arm fascia is closed with absorbable suture material. This step is important because the reconstructed fascia gives additional stability and forms the sliding layer for the muscles below.

After suturing the skin, the wound is bandaged with compresses and bandages. Plasters should be avoided, especially in the case of extensive soft tissue trauma, as otherwise tension bubbles formation may increase during postoperative swelling.

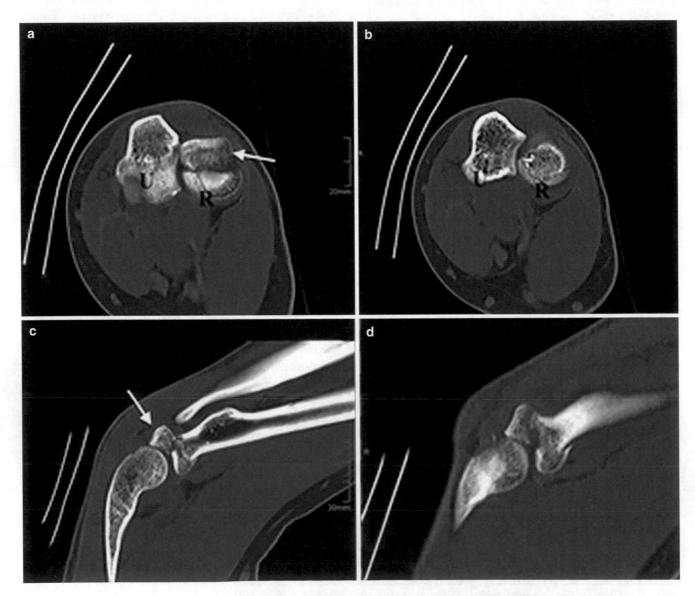

Fig. 68.5 Case presentation of a displaced Mason 3 fracture (CT scan **a–f**). In these cases for osteosynthesis, the anatomical low-profile plates from various manufacturers are the means of choice (**g, h**)

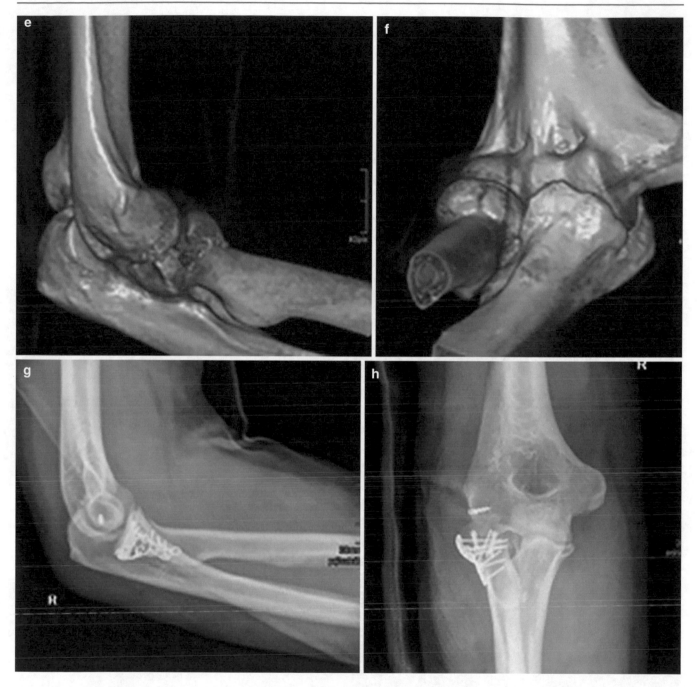

Fig. 68.5 (continued)

Postoperative Management

A fast and early functional follow-up treatment with consideration of the performed osteosynthesis and soft tissue reconstruction is desirable. In most cases, elbow ortheses until bone consolidation or ligament healing, usually for 6 weeks, are applied. These serve to stabilize the elbow against varus and valgus stress while still allowing for independent extension/flexion. However, care must be taken to ensure that the orthoses is placed correctly with its rota-

tional center being aligned at the axis of rotation of the humeral epicondyles. The range of motion can be restricted if necessary, e.g., after the ligament has been sutured; however, this is usually not necessary due to postoperative pain and swelling-related restriction in mobility. Under physiotherapeutic guidance, the arm can be used without the ortheses to practice pronation/supination in the 90° flexion position with the elbow resting.

From the sixth week onwards, the fast transition to full load is allowed. In case of additional traumatic or iatrogenic

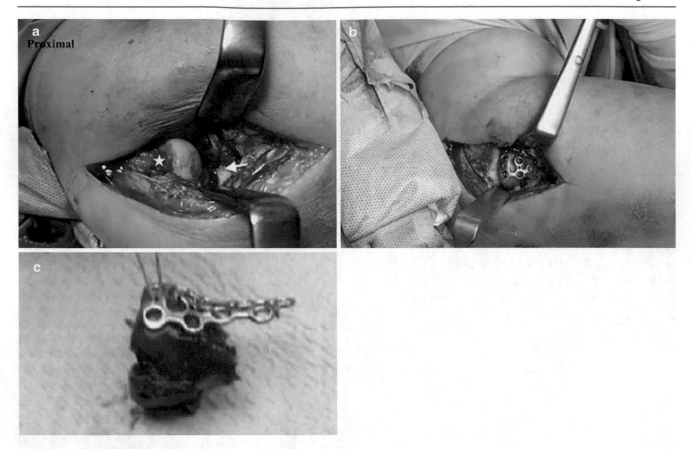

Fig. 68.6 (a–c) On-table reconstruction of a radial head fracture

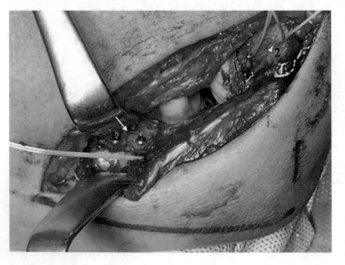

Fig. 68.7 Lateral view: Bone anchors for refixation of the LCL (1) the extensor muscles (2) and interal bracing to the ulnar insertion side (3). Additional osteosynthesis of an avulsion of the supinator crest (white arrow)

capsule ligament injuries, physical exertion is permitted after 3 months and contact sports only 6 months after the operation.

Conclusion

The radial head is an important secondary stabilizer of the elbow. The classification of radial head fractures according to Mason is well established and serves as guidance when determining the indication for surgery, even if it does not include accompanying injuries.

Mason 1

With conservative therapy, good results can be achieved in up to 95% of Mason 1 fractures. Indication for surgery is given in cases of blockages; MRI should be considered generously in cases of delayed restitution.

Mason 2

Conservative therapy for stable Mason 2 fractures leads to satisfying clinical results. However, literature suggests that surgical treatment of Mason 2 fractures produces good clinical results and lower rates of posttraumatic osteoarthritis with greater reliability than conservative treatment. Since the complication rate in the context of surgical treatment is also low, we recommend the surgical approach for this type of fracture in young and active patients. Mason 2 fractures are often suitable for arthroscopic fixation.

Mason 3 and 4

Reconstruction of the radial head should be the primary goal in these fractures. Many studies show good results with angle-stable low-profile plates, which also show lower complication rates, compared to earlier implants.

The most frequently observed complications after osteosynthesis treatment of the radial head, such as pseudarthrosis, radial head necrosis, and osteosynthesis material failure, seem to occur less frequently with newer implants.

If osteosynthesis is not possible, implantation of a radial head prosthesis is recommended. However, biomechanical studies have shown that the original radial head is superior to radial head prosthesis in terms of the area of the contact surface and maximal pressure with the capitellum. In addition, the original radial head stabilizes the elbow joint more adequately than the radial head prosthesis, especially when ligament lesions are present.

The resection of the radial head is possible if reconstruction is not an option, and the literature cites various cases of good clinical results after resection. However, resection always destabilizes the joint against valgus forces and posterolateral rotational forces and leads to a non-physiological redistribution of the axial force transmission at the ulnar column. If ligament injuries are also present, the elbow is destabilized to such an extent that osteoarthritis or discomfort in adjacent joints can quickly develop. Resection should therefore only be performed if accompanying ligament injuries can be ruled out, which is rarely the case in Mason 3 and 4 fractures.

References

1. Johnston GW. A follow-up of one hundred cases of fracture of the head of the radius with a review of the literature. Ulster Med J. 1962;31:51–6.
2. Mason ML. Some observations on fractures of the head of the radius with a review of one hundred cases. Br J Surg. 1954;42:123–32.
3. Akesson T, Herbertsson P, Josefsson PO, Hasserius R, Besjakov J, Karlsson MK. Primary nonoperative treatment of moderately displaced two-part fractures of the radial head. J Bone Joint Surg Am. 2006;88:1909–14.
4. Duckworth AD, Clement ND, Jenkins PJ, Aitken SA, Court-Brown CM, McQueen MM. The epidemiology of radial head and neck fractures. J Hand Surg Am. 2012;37:112–9.
5. Kaas L, Struijs PA, Ring D, van Dijk CN, Eygendaal D. Treatment of Mason type I radial head fractures without associated fractures or elbow dislocation: a systematic review. J Hand Surg Am. 2012;37:1416–21.
6. Michels F, Pouliart N, Handelberg F. Arthroscopic management of Mason type 2 radial head fractures. Knee Surg Sports Traumatol Arthrosc. 2007;15:1244–50.
7. Chen X, Wang SC, Cao LH, Yang GQ, Li M, Su JC. Comparison between radial head replacement and open reduction and internal fixation in clinical treatment of unstable, multi-fragmented radial head fractures. Int Orthop. 2011;35:1071–6.
8. Kaas L, van Riet RP, Vroemen JP, Eygendaal D. The epidemiology of radial head fractures. J Shoulder Elb Surg. 2010;19:520–3.
9. Itamura J, Roidis N, Mirzayan R, Vaishnav S, Learch T, Shean C. Radial head fractures: MRI evaluation of associated injuries. J Shoulder Elb Surg. 2005;14:421–4.
10. Mellema JJ, Eygendaal D, van Dijk CN, Ring D, Doornberg JN. Fracture mapping of displaced partial articular fractures of the radial head. J Shoulder Elb Surg. 2016;25:1509–16.

Olecranon Fractures

69

Andreas Harbrecht, Kilian Wegmann, and Lars P. Müller

Introduction

With a frequency of about 10%, olecranon fractures make up a significant proportion of all fractures in the upper extremity [1, 2]. Mean age is 50 years for males and 63 years for females [3]. In more than 80% of cases, simple fracture types are present, while the remaining 20% are characterized by multiple fragmentation, instability, or both in the sense of a dislocation fracture [4]. Complicated fractures are most common in direct impact trauma and increasingly in osteoporosis, which we will face more frequently in the future [5]. Laboratory studies have shown that the degree of elbow flexion at the time of direct trauma influences the resulting fracture. Radial head and coronoid fractures occur at flexion less than 80°, olecranon fractures at 90° of flexion, and distal humerus fractures at more than 110° [5, 6].

The following fracture mechanisms are possible:

- Direct impact trauma to the inflected elbow, which tends to lead to a short transverse fracture often with multiple fragmentation and soft tissue contusion
- Indirect hyperextension mechanism, which more often results in simple oblique fractures. The triceps muscle tenses the forearm and can pull the olecranon out of the ulnar condyle and fracture it.

The olecranon is characterized by a small soft tissue mantle, which is why a direct impact is often accompanied by an open fracture or at least an abrasion. This should be considered during any subsequent surgical procedure.

When treating fractures of the olecranon, it is important to understand all fracture types as joint fractures and therefore require precise X-ray analysis and understanding of the topographical anatomy and injury mechanism. Either the humeroulnar joint, the proximal radioulnar joint, or both are affected. The humeroulnar joint is a hinge joint that is well guided by the trochlea of the humerus and the incisura semilunaris ulnae. It allows a range of motion in extension and flexion of approximately 150°. The dorsal olecranon and the coronoid process neutralize cubital forces statically and thus act as a primary joint stabilizer against translational forces. These aspects illustrate the importance of the olecranon in the biomechanics of the elbow.

The incisura semilunaris ulnae has a cartilage-free zone about 5-mm wide, the "bare area" (Fig. 69.1) [7]. This bare area must be considered during osteosynthesis in order not to increase the curvature of the incisura by over compressing the cartilage surfaces during reduction. This would lead to an intra-articular malposition with consecutively reduced congruence with the trochlea (Fig. 69.2) [7, 8].

The large area medial to the midline of the ulna serves as an anterior abutment and is formed by the ulnar coronoid process. Together with the radial head, this bony part of the ulna prevents anterior dislocation in the elbow joint. The coronoid process protrudes beyond the ulna shaft not only on the cubital side but also on the medial side and forms the attachment of the medial collateral ligament at the tuberculum subliminus.

The shape of the proximal ulna is determined by a radial ("radial bow") and anterior angulation ("proximal ulna dorsal angulation," PUDA). The PUDA angle is located on average 4.5 cm distal to the tip of the olecranon and is approximately 6° (Fig. 69.3). Both its localization (3–7 cm distal to the olecranon tip) and its characteristics (0–14°) show large interindividual differences. The radial bow also varies considerably from person to person. On average, it is

A. Harbrecht (✉)
University of Cologne, Faculty of Medicine and University Hospital, Center for Orthopedic and Trauma Surgery, Cologne, Germany
e-mail: andreas.harbrecht@uk-koeln.de

K. Wegmann · L. P. Müller
University Hospital Cologne, Center of Orthopedic and Trauma Surgery, Cologne, Germany
e-mail: kilian.wegmann@uk-koeln.de; lars.mueller@uk-koeln.de

© Springer Nature Switzerland AG 2022
W. B. Geissler (ed.), *Wrist and Elbow Arthroscopy with Selected Open Procedures*,
https://doi.org/10.1007/978-3-030-78881-0_69

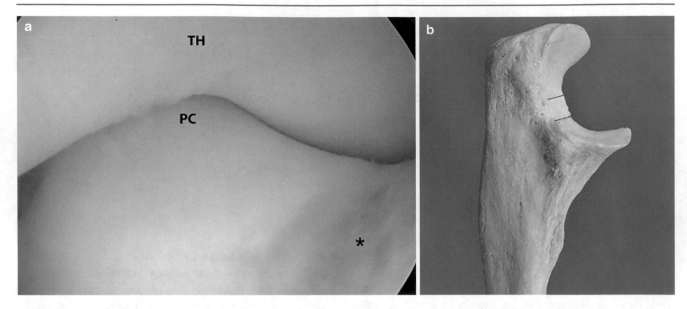

Fig. 69.1 (a) Arthroscopy of the elbow with insight into the humeroul-nar joint and presentation of the "bare area" (asterisk). PC processus coronoideus, TH trochlea humeri. (b) Macroscopic view of the proxi-mal ulna from the medial side. Red lines mark the "bare area". (Reprinted by permission from Springer Nature: Hackl et al. [8])

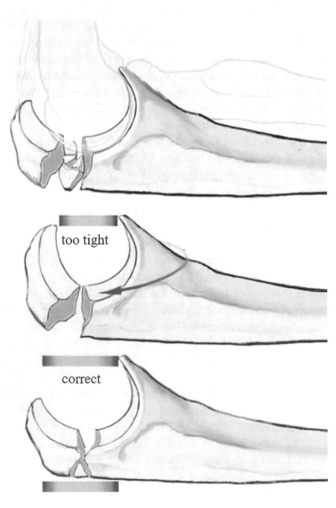

Fig. 69.2 The correct width of the incisura semilunaris ulnae is checked by fluoroscopy. (Reprinted by permission from Springer Nature: Ries et al. [32])

located about 8 cm (5.5–11.0 cm) distal to the tip of the olec-ranon and is approximately 15° (0–24°) [9–12]. Beseret al. also described an external rotation of the olecranon relative to the coronoid process of approximately 11° (2–30°) [9]. Due to the anatomical variance of the proximal ulna, the fit of dorsal plates is unreliable. Puchwein et al. were able to show in this context that varus angulation is only accounted for in a maximum of 20% of cases with available anatomi-cally contoured plates [13].

Two muscles are important to the functional anatomy of the olecranon. The triceps muscle inserts onto the posterior, proximal ulna and blends with the periosteum. It is innervated by the radial nerve and serves the elbow extension. The other one is the anconeus muscle. The lateral side of the olecranon and the proximal quarter of the posterior side of the ulnar shaft serve as the attachment of the musculus anconeus. It is innervated by the radial nerve and serves as a weak extensor of the elbow joint supporting the musculus triceps brachii. It is also involved in guiding the proximal ulna during pronation movement. As a capsule tensioner, it also prevents capsule parts from being trapped inside the elbow joint.

Intraosseous arterial perfusion is ensured at a relatively constant rate via medial branches of the ulnar artery distal to the coronoid process and two medium-sized vessels of the proximal arcade, which enter the bone via the olecranon tip. The "watershed" between these vessels is described in the bisector between the olecranon tip and coronoid tip [14].

The knowledge of this constant perfusion running in the opposite direction helps the surgeon to prepare the fracture without further damage to the vascular network and thus to maintain good biological conditions for bony consolidation [14].

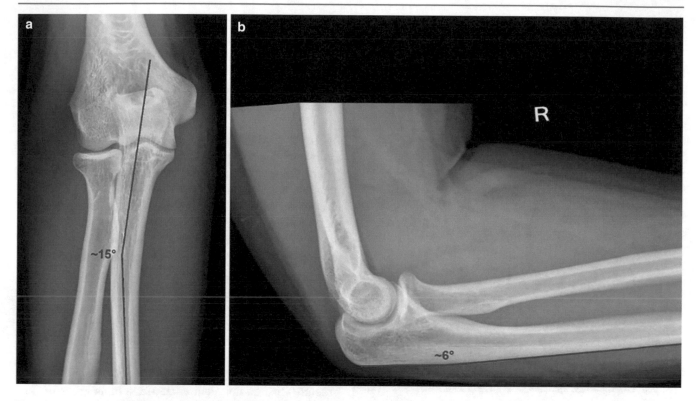

Fig. 69.3 X-rays of a right elbow. (**a**) Anteroposterior beam path showing varus angulation of the proximal ulna. (**b**) Lateral beam path showing the angle of "proximal ulna dorsal angulation" (PUDA). (Reprinted by permission from Springer Nature: Hackl et al. [8])

Patient Assessment

The mechanism of the accident must be investigated, followed by an assessment of the soft tissue conditions. Local injuries should be excluded: fractures of the coronoid, radial head fractures, Monteggia injuries, and associated distal humerus fractures. In many cases, inspection and palpation of the olecranon already indicate a fracture. Pulses on the wrist must be palpated; peripheral motor function and sensitivity must be examined and documented. Neurological deficits are not uncommon, especially in luxation fractures, and must be recorded preoperatively.

Testing of the motor function of the N. interosseus anterior as the end branch of the N. medianus can be performed quickly by active flexion in the interphalangeal joint of the thumb and in the DIP joint of the index finger. The same applies to thumb spreading and wrist and finger stretching for testing the ramus profundus of the radial nerve. If active flexion of the metacarpophalangeal joint of fingers four and five as well as the leading and spreading of the fingers can be demonstrated, the motor function of the ulnar nerve can be considered sufficiently tested and documented as intact.

Imaging

Conventional X-ray examination of the elbow joint in two planes in the a.-p. and lateral beam path is standard (Fig. 69.4). The central beam should be adjusted to the joint center. In the lateral beam path, the trochlea humeri should be shown. The radial head should be shown free, covered only by the coronoid process. A radiocapitellar (Greenspan) beam path of the radial head is useful to exclude involvement of the radial head.

A CT scan should always be obtained in cases of comminuted and or complex fractures.

A regular MRI examination is not necessary. It should only be used for specific questioning, such as concomitant cartilage lesions or complex ligamentous injuries.

Classification

Numerous classifications for olecranon fractures exist [15].

Colton developed a classification system for olecranon fractures in 1973 [16]. The Colton classification was based on fracture morphology, stability of the ulnohumeral joint, and injury mechanism. The AO classification was introduced in 1987 as a systematic method for classifying long bone fractures based on fracture line location and degree of comminution [17, 18]. This classification grouped olecranon fractures together with proximal radius fractures. Schatzker modified the AO classification from nine groups to six groups (Table 69.1). The focus is on typical fracture patterns. It considers not only the topographical classification but also the stability of the fracture and is thus an aid in deciding on the type and technique of surgical treatment [19] (Fig. 69.5).

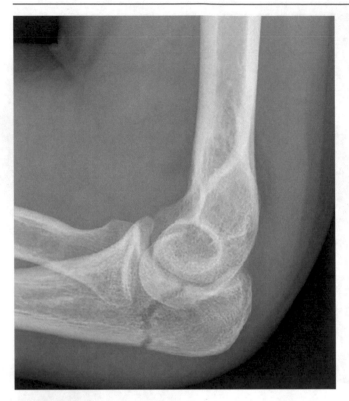

Fig. 69.4 Lateral view of an elbow with a Mayo IA fracture

Table 69.1 Schatzker classification of olecranon fractures [19]

Type	Characteristics
A	Simple transverse fracture
B	Transverse fracture with articular surface impaction
C	Intraarticular oblique fracture
D	Transverse fracture with articular surface collapse and coronoid process fracture
E	Distal oblique fracture
F	Fracture-dislocation with severe instability

Cabanela and Morrey [17] first introduced the Mayo classification in 1993 to provide a simplified classification of olecranon fractures based on fracture comminution, displacement, and stability of the ulnohumeral joint (Fig. 69.6). There are three groups, each of which is divided into two subgroups (Table 69.2). Fractures without dislocation belong to group 1, dislocated fractures in group 2, and dislocated with unstable trochlea in group 3. The subgroups differentiate further whether it is a simple fracture form (A) or several fragments are present (B). Although the distal oblique fractures (Schatzker type E) without joint instability do not find their own group (see Mayo IIIA), the classification is characterized by practical relevance and memorable grouping [15]. This classification will be from now on used in this chapter to discuss fracture types.

According to a study by Rommens et al., both the Schatzker and Mayo classification showed a high predictive value for the functional outcome [20].

Treatment Goals

We must distinguish between younger patients with high functional demands and older patients.

In younger patients, the anatomical reconstruction of the joint surface, the restoration of stability and strength, and the prevention of joint stiffening are of most importance. For older patients, the focus lays on minimizing morbidity and, if possible, maintaining independence. In these patients, concomitant injuries should be excluded, especially instability.

Indications

Conservative Treatment

Conservative therapy is reserved for stable, non-displaced fractures that do not require long-term immobilization and can be treated with functional therapy. The more inactive the patient is, the more generous the indication for conservative therapy can be. If active extension is possible without dislocation of the fracture, conservative treatment promises acceptable results. Frequent radiographic follow-ups are recommended to detect secondary dislocations in a timely manner. Exceptional indications for the conservative approach may also be given in the case of dislocated olecranon fractures with stable humeroulnar joint in the elderly. If a dislocation of more than 1.5 cm is present, a loss of 70% of the strength of the triceps muscle is to be expected [21]. There are indications that conservative therapy can lead to subjectively good results in geriatric patients. Especially in these patients, subjective satisfaction differs significantly from objective joint mobility and the radiological result of the treatment. Satisfactory results without pain can be achieved in up to 50% of the elderly, according to Parker, and 67% according to Veras del Monte with an average range of motion of 130° (extension-flexion) [22, 23]. This is all the more surprising since 9 of 12 patients radiologically showed pseudarthrosis [23]. Duckworth et al. even found 91% satisfactory results in older, less demanding patients in 2014 [24].

Immobilization of the joint, usually in a cast in 90° elbow flexion, should not last longer than 2 weeks. Passive exercise of the joint under adequate analgesic therapy should then be started. Until the 3rd week, no flexion over 90° should be performed. Pro- and supination are to be exercised freely and

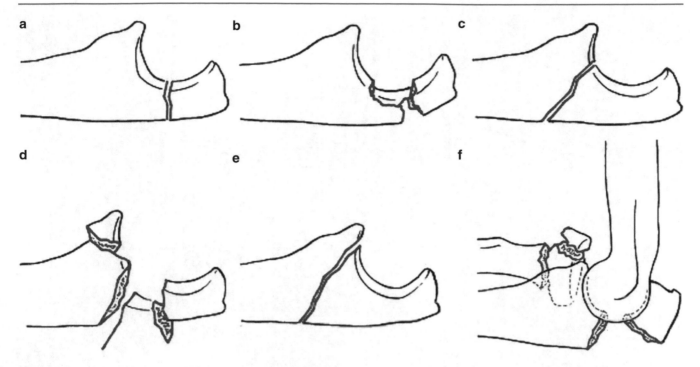

Fig. 69.5 Schatzker classification of olecranon fractures. (Reprinted by permission from Springer Nature: Gierer et al. [66])

pain adapted. After 6 weeks, active exercise should be added. Strengthening of the muscles can be initiated after 8 weeks and should end with proprioceptive exercises [3].

Operative Treatment

The indication for surgery is seen in dislocated fractures with more than 1–2 mm dislocation, loss of active extension in the elbow joint, elbow instability, as well as in failure of conservative management.

Aim of surgery is to stabilize the joint and restore the joint surface in order to minimize the risk of post-traumatic arthrosis. The traction force of the M. triceps brachii should be neutralized; the physiological joint axes should be restored. The achieved joint stability is a prerequisite for early functional follow-up treatment. In addition to the precise osteosynthesis performed, the correct choice of implant is crucial for the outcome of the surgical treatment.

There are several techniques available. Before a surgical procedure is selected, the radiographs should be carefully analyzed once again. If the fracture line runs transversely, tension band wire fixation is possible. If the fracture line runs obliquely, plate osteosynthesis is preferable. The intactness of the dorsal cortex helps additionally to indicate which procedure should be chosen. If the dorsal cortex is intact preoperatively, a tension band wire fixation can be performed. If it is comminuted, tension band wire osteosynthesis is not indicated, and plate osteosynthesis is required.

Contraindications

In young patients with an isolated olecranon fracture, there are now relevant contraindications for osteosynthesis. A stable osteosynthesis must be performed to guarantee early mobilization of the joint. Only in older patients contraindications for surgery exist. These include a high peri- and postoperative mortality risk and low patient's demands on the joint, which make a complex reconstruction with prolonged operational time an unnecessary risk.

Technique

Patient Positioning and Anesthesia

Surgery can be performed under general or regional anesthesia. With regional anesthesia and prone position, it can be very uncomfortable for the patient if a complex reconstruction of the proximal ulna requires a longer operation time. The operation can be performed in supine, lateral, or prone position. We usually prefer the prone position with the arm hanging down on a "mini-arm table" in 90° flexion in the elbow joint (Fig. 69.7). A tourniquet can be placed on the upper arm. This position is generally recommended for plate osteosyntheses and comminuted fractures. Simple fractures, planned for a tension band wiring, can be operated on in the supine position. The arm is covered so that it can be moved freely during surgery and placed on the upper body.

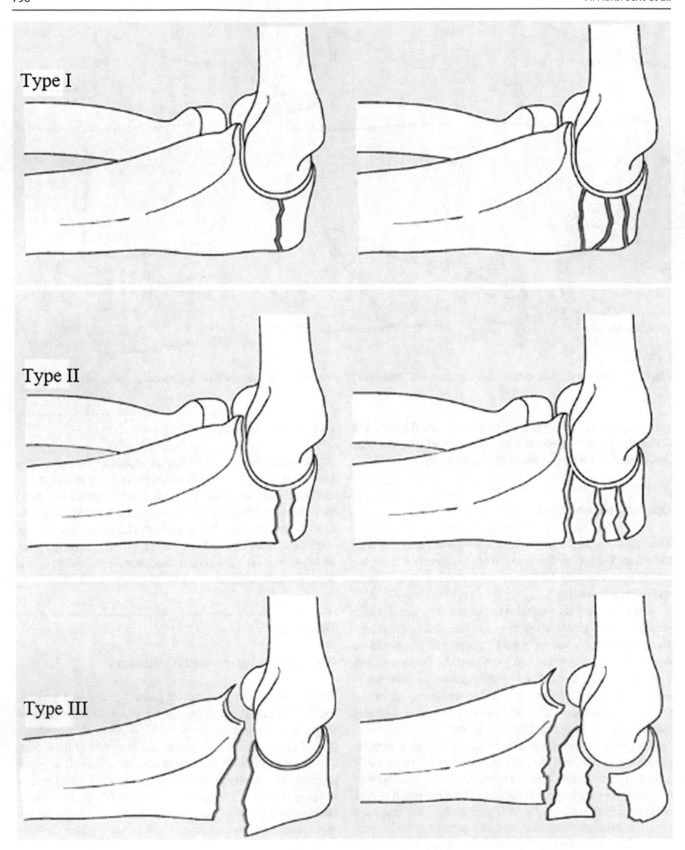

Fig. 69.6 Mayo classification of olecranon fractures. (Reprinted by permission from Springer Nature: Uhlmann et al. [67])

Table 69.2 Mayo classification of olecranon fractures [17]

Type	Characteristics	
I	Non-displaced fracture, stable joint	Fracture gap < 2 mm type A: non-comminuted type B: comminuted
II	Displaced fracture, stable joint	Fracture gap > 2–3 mm type A: non-comminuted type B: comminuted
III	Displaced fracture, accompanying lesions-instability	type A: non-comminuted type B: comminuted

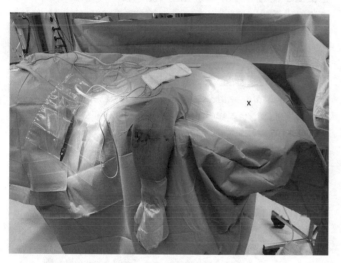

Fig. 69.7 Standard positioning of a patients' left elbow in supine position on a "mini-arm table." X indicates the patient's head

Tension Band Wire Fixation

Simple transverse fractures proximal to the olecranon midline (Mayo IA and IIA) are usually easy to stabilize and are fixed by Weber's tension band wire fixation according to traditional AO recommendations [25]. If the fracture gap exceeds the apex of the olecranon pit or oblique fractures are present, the tension band cannot trigger compression but is diverted into shear forces. The short fragment slides over the dorsal ulnar edge and shortens the olecranon joint fork.

The incision is made dorsally in the midline with a curvature radially above the tip of the olecranon. The flexor carpi ulnaris muscle is released medially; the anconeus tendon is released laterally. After reduction, the two Kirschner wires are drilled parallel directly below the joint surface at a 90° angle to the fracture line in direction of the coronoid process. The cerclage wire is passed transosseously through the ulna and guided dorsally around the drill wires and tensioned, neutralizing dislocation forces of the triceps tendon that lead to fragment dehiscence. The wires are bent 180° and

anchored intraosseously to avoid soft tissue irritation. Tensile forces are generated during movement, resulting in the transformation of these forces into compressive forces and thus compression of the fracture. Whether the described compression of the articular cortex in flexion actually occurs has not yet been clinically or experimentally proven [26]. The difficulty of tension band wiring is often underestimated and is associated with iatrogenic problems, such as insufficient implant fixation in osteoporotic bone [27]. Nevertheless, the fractures usually heal without any complications if indication and technique are correct [28].

Intramedullary Nailing

Biomechanical studies have shown that intramedullary nails in cadaveric fracture models provide less gapping at the fracture site compared to tension band wire constructs [29]. Nails are stiffer than tension band wires and were developed as low-profile devices to counteract the high metal removal rates required after olecranon fractures that were fixed by tension band wiring. Biomechanically speaking, intramedullary nailing systems offer greater fracture stability than tension band wiring [30]. There are no current clinical studies that favor their use over tension band wiring. In non-displaced fractures, there is a growing trend toward intramedullary nailing in these injuries as a low-profile implant that allows immediate mobilization. The technique requires less exposure of the bone and can be effectively used for simple and comminuted fractures of the olecranon. In a series described by Gehr and Friedl, fixation with a locking compression nail was performed in 73 patients with a mixture of simple and comminuted fractures of the olecranon. This study documented good to excellent functional results in 68 of the cases [5, 31].

Low-Profile Double-Plate Osteosynthesis

Double-plate osteosynthesis with low-profile plates offers potential advantages in lateral positioning [29, 32]. Due to the anatomical plate design and the lateral positioning, it allows bicortical and orthogonal screw fixation with respect to the direction of traction of the triceps muscle, in addition to the possibilities of angular stable fixation. This shall lead to greater primary stability [32, 33].

Approach is 3–5 cm proximal to the tip of the olecranon, starting as a dorsal skin incision above the elbow joint – in this case, the olecranon should be radially circumvented – and following distally to the dorsal edge of the ulna. The access should generally be kept as small as possible, considering the fracture pattern. To treat potential concomitant bony injuries, the approach can be widened accordingly, e.g., in injuries to the radial head or coronoid process, and the medial or lateral collateral ligament apparatus.

Afterwards, a sharp preparation of the proximal ulna can be performed with detachment of the radial and ulnar muscles. The resulting "soft tissue flaps" must be protected from excessive mechanical tension and irritation in order to ensure sufficient blood supply postoperatively and to prevent wound healing complications. The preparation of "full thickness flaps" is recommended to maintain blood supply. The ulnar nerve can be visualized and protected. This is recommended especially in complex fractures that require visualization of the medial border of the olecranon.

The fracture gap is exposed and cleaned of impacted periosteum, fracture hematoma, and cartilage/bone flakes (Fig. 69.8). If necessary, the periosteum can be minimally pushed away from the fracture margins of both fragments in order to assess the anatomical reduction that needs to be achieved. For simple fractures, the reduction result is usually referenced at the dorsal-cortical alignment. In comminuted fractures, however, it may be useful to open the fracture gap to ensure optimal reduction of all fragments. To temporally fix the reduction forceps in the ulna shaft, it is helpful to drill a radial or ulnar 2.5 mm auxiliary hole 2–3 cm distal to the fracture (Fig. 69.9). The anatomical reduction can then be achieved by grasping the proximal fragment and extending the elbow joint. An anatomical gap free reduction can be verified as described by dorsal alignment of the ulna and under fluoroscopy.

A constriction of the incisura semilunaris ulnae, which is open in the sagittal plane to the ulnar shaft axis by approximately 40° to 45° posteriorly [34], with consecutive incongruence of the humeroulnar joint compartment must be avoided. The reduction result is transfixed using one or two Kirschner wires. Ensure that the tips of the Kirschner wires do not lead into the proximal radioulnar joint. Now, the two anatomically preformed plates can be placed laterally on the olecranon. The order of plate positioning, beginning either at the radial or ulnar side, is irrelevant and should only be determined by fracture morphology. After satisfactory positioning, the implantation can start.

Depending on the soft tissue situation, it may be advisable to start drilling and screw placement in the distal part of the oblong hole after the first plate has been placed and to incise the insertion of the tendon of the triceps muscle longitudinally at the level of the proximal end of the plate, in order to have enough space to insert and sink the proximal end of the plate underneath it (Fig. 69.10). The proximal plate hole can then be filled with a locking screw that exceeds the fracture. The proximal fragment should be fitted with at least two

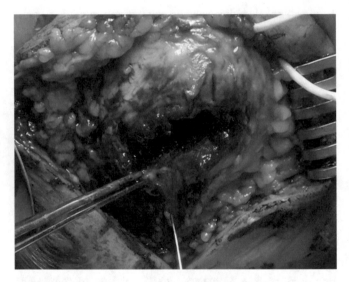

Fig. 69.8 View into the fracture site with surgical dissection of the periosteum. Yellow loop indicates the position of the ulnar nerve

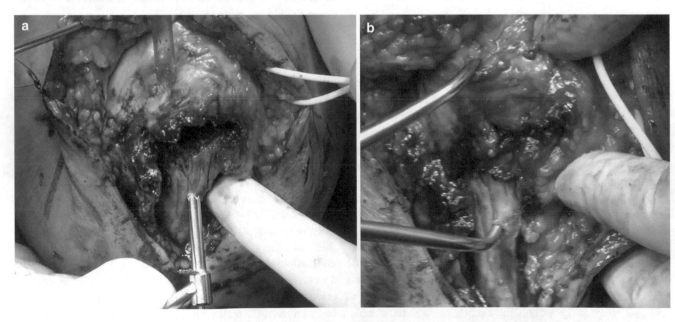

Fig. 69.9 (**a**, **b**) Drilling of the ulna shaft to prepare for a secure pressure apply through a reduction forceps. Yellow loop indicates the position of the ulnar nerve

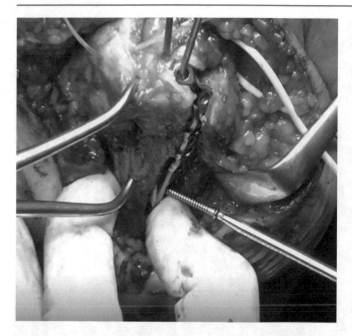

Fig. 69.10 Inserting a cortical screw into the longitudinal hole at the ulnar shaft to maintain longitudinal control of the plate. Temporary fixation of the fracture already performed by two K-wires. Yellow loop indicates the position of the ulnar nerve

locking screws. The osteosynthesis is then completed with at least two additional non-locking or locking screws in the shaft area of the ulna. Implantation of the second plate is performed in the same way. If necessary, the circular forceps can be loosened for this purpose. When the plates are in place, make sure that the most distal screws of the plates do not end at the same height of the shaft (Fig. 69.11).

An additive "off-loading triceps suture" may be useful, particularly in osteoporotic fractures [35]. The position of the ulnar nerve must be known or secured in advance. The triceps tendon is augmented 1–2 cm proximal to its insertion by a strong suture, deflected over free holes on the inserted plates and knotted over the ulna shaft (Fig. 69.12).

Singular Plate Osteosynthesis

Plate fixation was primarily used for the treatment of comminuted olecranon fractures where fixation with tension band wiring is not recommended. One-third tubular, 3.5-mm contoured limited contact dynamic compression (LC–DCP), 3.5-mm reconstruction, hook, or pre-contoured locking plates are frequently used [5, 36]. There is also the possibility of using a hook plate with prongs that impact into the displaced proximal olecranon fragment. Anatomically contoured locking plates are recent developments in olecranon

plate technology and are marketed as a superior fixation due to the angular stable design. Although good results have been achieved with the use of these plates, there is currently insufficient evidence that they are superior to other forms of plate fixation. In severely comminuted fractures, reconstruction with a one-third tubular plate may not provide sufficient strength and may lead to hardware failure [37]. The singular plates are also applied to the dorsal surface of the ulna. In this case, however, it is centrally on the ulnar edge. This is the tension side of the olecranon where the construct is biomechanically most stable. It also allows screws to be inserted into the coronoid process or along the medullary canal to provide additional stability. A 3.5-mm LC-DCP plate is adjusted to the shape of the olecranon with the bending irons at the level of the penultimate plate hole. This step is not necessary with available pre-contoured plates. To position the plate correctly close to the bone, the insertion of the triceps tendon must be split lengthwise, as described in the double-plate technique, and the proximal part of the plate must be placed against the olecranon. A possibly interfering reduction forceps is replaced by two temporarily inserted Kirschner wires. The most proximal hole of the plate is then first filled with an intramedullary screw. On the one hand, this leads to a correct plate position, as the plate presses itself against the olecranon; on the other hand, the fracture is often stabilized with this screw alone to such an extent that disturbing reduction and retention aids can be removed at this point. The osteosynthesis is completed by at least three bicortical screws in the distal fragment and at least one additional proximal screw, which is also inserted bicortically through the second plate hole proximally in the direction of the plate, analogous to the Kirschner wires of the tension band fixation. Care must be taken that screw tips do not compromise the radioulnar joint.

When using locking plates, the plate is placed on the ulna and initially attached to the shaft fragment in the shaft area with a conventional 3.5 mm screw through the longitudinal oval hole of the plate. The plate can now be moved and adjusted in the cranio-caudal direction. The fracture is then fixed in the proximal fragment with 2.7-mm screws and distally with 3.5-mm locking screws. Care must be taken to tighten the screws only to the prescribed torque, especially in osteoporotic bone.

In severe comminuted fractures, the use of plate fixation offers the additional possibility of bone grafting to support depressed joint fragments. The subcutaneous nature of the plate has led to concerns about hardware prominence. However, the incidence of symptomatic hardware protrusion is lower with plate fixation than with tension band wiring [38, 39], with 0–20% of cases requiring plate removal [5, 40, 41].

Fig. 69.11 Case 1, Mayo IIA fracture. (**a**, **b**) Preoperative X-rays in lateral and a.-p. views. (**c**, **d**) Postoperative X-rays in lateral and a.-p. views, fracture fixed with low-profile double-plates. (**e**, **f**) X-rays in lateral and a.-p. view after hardware removal

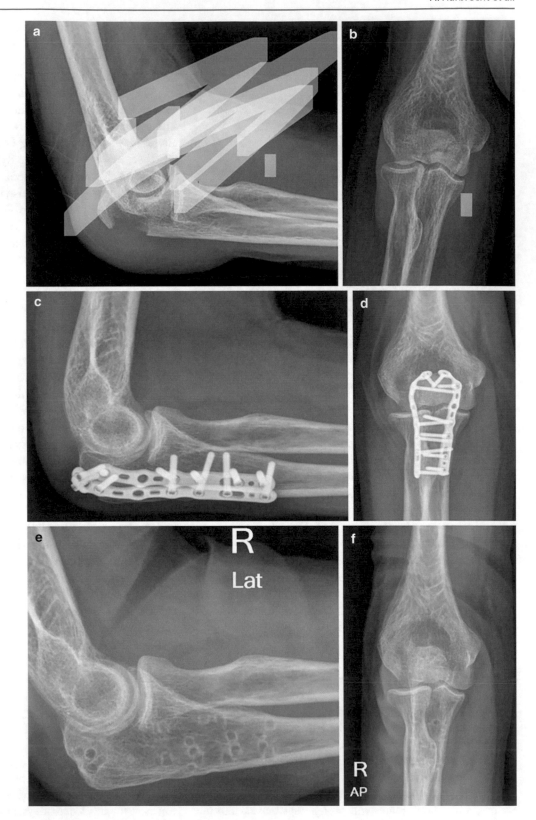

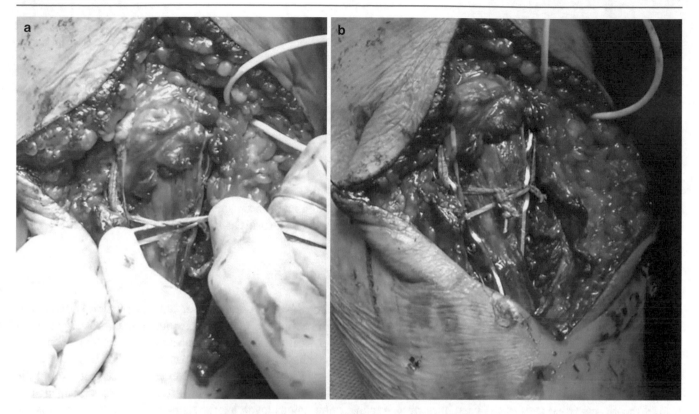

Fig. 69.12 (**a**, **b**) "Off-loading triceps suture" The triceps tendon is reinforced with two sutures proximal to its insertion, deflected over free holes on the inserted plates, and knotted over the ulna shaft. Yellow loop indicates the position of the ulnar nerve

Proximal Fragment Excision and Triceps Advancement

In elderly patients with osteoporotic bone, an extensive comminuted fracture, or a fragment too small for internal fixation, excision of the fracture fragment with triceps advancement may be a useful option. The technique has significant advantages, as it avoids the possibility of non-union and traumatic arthritis due to an irregularity of the articular surface. Fragment excision can only be performed if the coronoid, medial collateral ligament, interosseous membrane, and distal radio-ulnar joint are intact to prevent instability [37]. McKeever and Buck, who first described this technique in 1947, suggested that up to 80% of the trochlear notch can be excised without significantly affecting elbow stability [42]. Inhofe and Howard showed good or excellent results in 11 of 12 cases treated with excision of up to 70% of the trochlear notch [43]. However, Gartsman et al. reported a case of instability after resection of 75% of the trochlear notch [44], and an in vitro study by An et al. showed a linear reduction in elbow stability in more than 50% of excision [45]. One criticism of the technique is therefore that there is a possible reduction in triceps strength. Normally, the triceps tendon is sutured to the anterior edge of the ulna, creating a smooth loop for articulation with the distal humerus. An alternative position for reattaching the triceps tendon has

been suggested by DiDonna et al. in their biomechanical study, the triceps was reattached in a more posterior position, which increases the strength of the triceps compared to a more anterior attachment [46]. In general, fragment excision and triceps advancement are considered in cases where open reduction and internal fixation are unlikely to be successful. Internal fixation offers the advantage of early mobilization and bone to bone healing over long immobilization and sole suture fixation in this technique. It can, however, be used later as a salvage procedure when internal fixation fails [5].

Rehabilitation

The application of an immobilizing cast or elbow orthosis can be useful for a short time in critical soft tissue situations but should not exceed 2 weeks. This should be followed by assisted physiotherapy. The goal is an early functional physiotherapeutic exercise with free movement of the elbow joint including the adjacent joints. This can be supplemented by lymph drainage. Load baring activities and active extension against resistance should be avoided for 6 weeks. Postoperative stiffness and inactivity atrophy of the musculature should be prevented. Full load baring is permitted after radiological control with bony consolidation, usually after 3 months.

Tips and Tricks

Surgical Anatomy

The Mayo classification has a good "interobserver" and "intraobserver" agreement and is therefore the favorable classification.

Knowledge of the constant perfusion in the opposite direction helps the surgeon to prepare the fracture without further damage to the vascular network and thus maintain good biological conditions for bony consolidation. To maintain blood circulation, the preparation of "full thickness flaps" is recommended.

Tension Band Wire Fixation

A drill hole can be made at the dorsoulnar distal edge to establish secure pressure through a reduction forceps (see Fig. 69.9).

Kirschner wires should be retracted a little bit before final fixation so that they can be tucked in again when they have been bent 180° to avoid soft tissue irritation. Perform impaction of the cut proximal ends of the Kirschner wires into the olecranon.

The final osteosynthesis result should be tested intraoperatively by full flexion and extension of the elbow.

Plating

Opening the fracture site can be useful for optimal reduction of all fragments in comminuted fractures.

Special attention should be paid to intraoperative radiographs in lateral projection after preliminary reduction. The incisura semilunaris ulnae should not be over compressed but should represent a smooth anatomical surface without over compression (see Fig. 69.2). At this point, the surgeon must critically review his/her reduction result and adjust an exact lateral view in order to do so.

In comminuted unstable olecranon fractures, it may be helpful to temporarily fold away the proximal fragment and build up the reduction piece by piece onto the ulnar shaft. This means to first fix one fragment to the ulna shaft with a lost screw or Kirschner wire and finally fixing the proximal fragment with one plate, preferably two plates, according to the known technique (Fig. 69.13).

It may also be helpful to temporarily fix a larger intermediate fragment against the trochlea using a K-wire in the desired reduction position. Now the proximal fragment can be adjusted at rest, and plate osteosynthesis can be performed. The Kirschner wire is finally removed.

An "off-loading triceps suture" can be combined with osteosynthesis to reduce the risk of loss of reduction and is especially recommended in osteoporotic bones (see Fig. 69.12).

Due to the usually thin dorsal subcutaneous tissue over the olecranon, bulging nodes should be avoided.

Complications

Common complications seen after olecranon fractures are non-union, elbow stiffness, infection, ulnar neuritis, post-traumatic arthritis, and heterotopic ossification [29].

Non-union

The rate of non-union after internal fixation is about 1%, with non-union being more common in high-energy injuries [47, 48]. The most common site for ulnar nonunion is at the metadiaphyseal junction, which may be due in part to a relative lack of vascularity and in part to surgical errors [29]. Restoring the biology in these cases is a major challenge. In non-unions involving the semilunar notch, it is important to maintain its radius to avoid incongruity of the joint. Therefore, in case of bone loss, an autograft or an artificial material such as bone morphogenetic protein (BMP) must be used, together with a rigid fixation. If the blood supply is taken into account and there may be some residual bone fragments left, good results can be achieved. If the olecranon is heavily destroyed, the implantation of an elbow prosthesis remains as a salvage procedure.

Rotini et al. recommended rigid fixation and structural bone grafting and advised against a reconstructive plate (because it was not sufficiently rigid) for the treatment of 12 non-unions of the proximal third of the ulna [47]. They observed better results in patients whose non-unions were more than 5 cm distal to the tip of the olecranon, probably due to the better vascularity [29].

Papagelopoulos and Morrey reported on the treatment of 24 patients with non-unionized olecranon fractures [48]. Using the above techniques, they achieved excellent results in 12 patients, good in 4, fair in 6, and poor in 2 [5].

Elbow Stiffness

After olecranon fractures, loss of terminal extension is often expected, and patients should be advised accordingly [20]. An average loss of 10–15% compared to the contralateral side is expected, with a frequency of up to 75% [49, 50].

Infection

With regard to infection, the problem of the relatively thin soft tissue envelope becomes apparent. Infection is known to occur after open fractures rather than after closed ones. If a superficial infection occurs, the patient can be treated without implant removal. However, oral antibiotic treatment on an outpatient follow-up is not sufficient. A superficial infection can quickly develop into a deep infection due to the thin soft tissue envelope. If the infection does not subside sufficiently with intravenous treatment, surgical revision is recommended. Any devitalized tissue should be thoroughly removed, and the depth of the infection determined. In some cases, this type of treatment can at least delay the removal of the material to such an extent that bony healing occurs before the material is removed.

In severe bone infections, the material must be removed and local antibiotics must be used together with long-term antibiotic therapy and temporary stabilization of the elbow, e.g., in a fixateur. Here it is important to plan the therapy long enough and not to let impatience jeopardize the chances for a reasonable result [51].

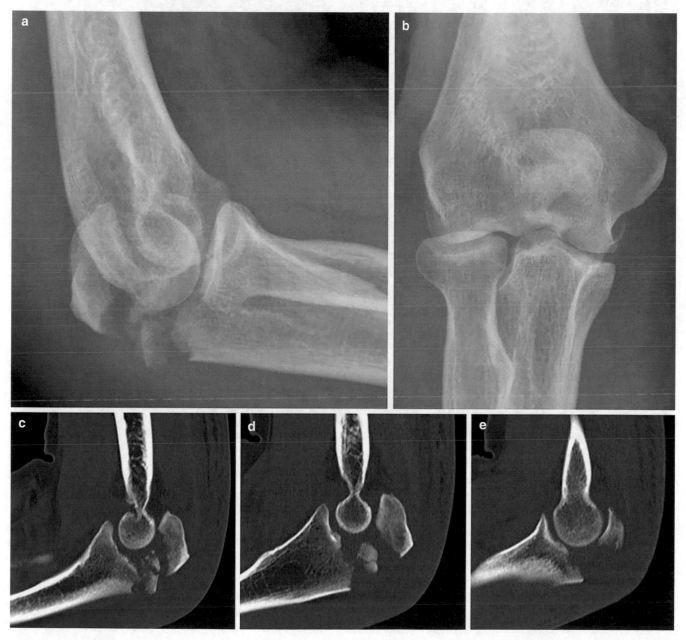

Fig. 69.13 Case 2, Mayo IIB fracture. (**a**, **b**) Preoperative X-rays in lateral an a.-p. view. (**c–e**) CT scan with sagittal reconstruction showing comminution. (**f**, **g**) Postoperative X-rays in lateral and a.-p. views, fracture fixed with low-profile double-plates and two lost Kirschner wires. (**h**, **i**) Follow-up after 3 months in lateral and a.-p. views showing increasing bony consolidation

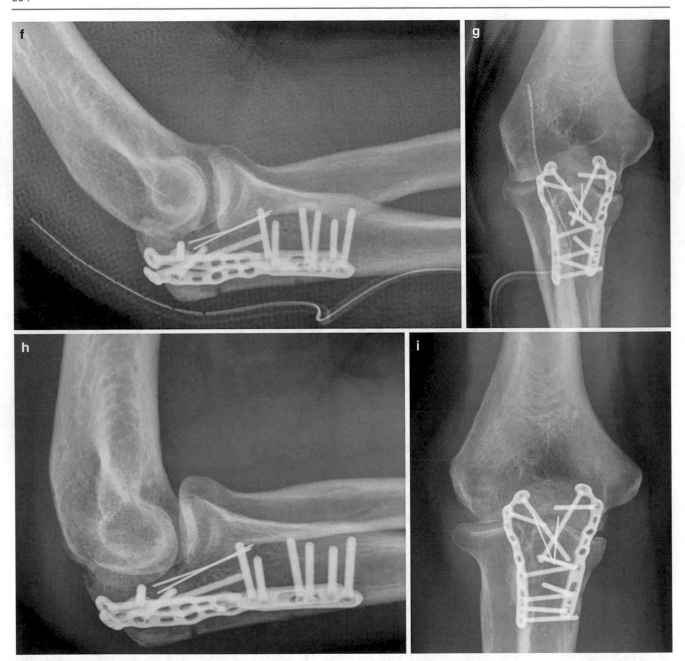

Fig. 69.13 (continued)

Ulnar Neuritis

Inflammation of the ulnar nerve is unusual and occurs in 2–12% of cases [49, 52, 53]. Observation until resolution is usually sufficient. However, ulnar neurolysis with or without transposition may be necessary if symptoms do not improve. Timing of EMG tests (electromyography) is unclear. An improvement in ulnar function is possible 3–20 months after surgery [52]. If there is significant soft tissue swelling at the time of primary osteosynthesis, it may be advisable to perform in situ neurolysis. Ulnar nerve paralysis is also associated with poor reduction of fractures, especially in medially

displaced fragments [29, 53]. Care should be taken in such fracture patterns and the ulnar nerve visualized for safety reasons.

Posttraumatic Arthritis

Rates of posttraumatic elbow arthrosis following an olecranon fracture of up to 20% have been reported. An articular step-off of 2 mm or more was associated with high chances to develop an arthrosis [54]. In a study with an average follow-up time of 4–5 years, 16 of 21 patients showed radiographic signs of osteoarthritis, with 13 showing only minor changes on X-ray and 3 showing more severe signs of arthritis. The initial fracture displacement was also associated with the development of osteoarthritis [55].

The native elbow with low grades of arthritis will function better than a prosthetic or interpositional arthroplasty and should be maintained as long as possible. If the arthrosis has become too severe, the only chance to treat those patients is total elbow replacement (TEA) [51].

Heterotopic Ossification

One study examining the rate of heterotopic ossification (HO) after elbow fractures found that rates of HO were less than 1% for isolated olecranon fractures, with only 1 in 221 fractures developing HO [56]. Based on these rates, prophylaxis against HO in isolated olecranon fractures is not recommended. Chemoprophylaxis with indomethacin may play a role in more complex injury patterns. However, there is insufficient data to make a more specific recommendation. Radiation treatment has not shown to be successful [29, 57].

Outcome

Overall, results in the treatment of olecranon fractures are good [2]. Our aim is, regardless of fracture fixation technique, bony union. The average time to union for fixation is typically 3–4 months [58]. The more unstable the fracture pattern is, the poorer long-term outcomes are [20]. Loss of terminal extension is the most common complaint after surgery, but late improvements in range of motion of up to 12° may be observed during follow-up [2, 52]. One of the longest follow-up studies available in the literature is a Swedish cohort of 45 women and 28 men who were followed up for an average of 19 years. In this cohort, 84% had open reduction and internal fixation, and 94% reported good or excellent results, with 50% of injured elbows showing radiographic signs of degeneration compared to 11% of uninjured contralateral elbows [59].

With regard to tension band wire fixation, results in 78 patients with an average follow-up of 2.76 years (range, 1.1–5.5 years) showed a non-union rate of 1.3%. In the same study, a total infection rate of 2.56% was observed [58]. Another study on tension band techniques showed an average movement arc of 116° ± 22° with an average extension loss of 15° ± 17° [55].

Regarding plating, multiple studies have shown similar good results to tension band wiring. Results of 19 patients with comminuted fractures of the olecranon treated with a locking plate showed that all healed within an average time of 4 months and had a mean range of motion of 13–136° over

a follow-up of at least 1 year. Complications included one infection and one ulnar nerve palsy, which did not resolve. Overall results showed 94% good or excellent results [60], although 19% of the patients in this study experienced extension loss of more than 30° and 56% had their hardware removed within the 2-year study window.

A Canadian study of 25 patients with a mixture of Mayo type II and III fractures treated with singular plating with a mean follow-up of 34 months showed no cases of non-union; 22 out of 25 showed good or excellent results with high patient satisfaction and low pain scores [40]. The mean values for the DASH-Score (Disabilities of the Arm, Shoulder and Hand) showed near-normal function of the upper extremities, and the results of the Short-Form 36 Health Survey showed no difference to those of comparable healthy people. The plate removal rate was 20%.

A Chinese study of interim results for comminuted and complex olecranon fractures treated with contoured plates showed an average time to union of 15 weeks, no non-unions, a mean range of motion of 14–125°, and 78.6% good or excellent results [61]. This is a slightly worse result than the results of the other studies, but this cohort was made up of more severe injuries (17 Mayo type IIB, 11 type IIIB), which are known to be associated with worse results [29].

Rochet et al. were the first to publish clinical results of the double-plate fixation technique. In their case series of 18 patients with mainly complex fracture dislocations of the proximal ulna (50% Mayo type IIIB), they reported good or excellent results in 67% of cases with a mean Broberg and Morrey score of 82 points at a mean follow-up of 30 months after double-plate fixation with two one-third cylinder tubular plates [62].

In a German study, 14 patients were evaluated after double plating with a mean follow-up of 11.7 months. The mean range of motion was 123°. Eight patients showed excellent and six cases good results. All fractures healed in time, and four patients underwent hardware removal [32].

Another study by Ellwein et al. analyzed postoperative outcome at a mean follow-up of 41 months (range: 25–61) of low-profile double plates in comparison to singular 3.5-mm LCP (locking compression plates). The double-plate group showed a range of motion of 127°, MEPS (Mayo Elbow Performance Score) of 94 and DASH of 6. A total of nine revision surgeries after double-plate osteosynthesis were recorded including seven implant removals and two misplaced intraarticular screws. The singular plate group had nine revisions with comparable good clinical results. There were no apparent clinical differences between the two treatment groups [63].

A following study by Ellwein et al. concluded in 79 patients with a mean follow-up period of 36 months (range, 24–77 months) that the rate of hardware removal owing to soft tissue irritation was not significantly reduced in the double-plating group. It was noted in 27% of patients after double-plate osteosynthesis and 38% after LCP treatment [64].

Studies regarding outcome of intramedullary nails in the treatment of olecranon fractures are scarce. In one study, 18 patients with unstable proximal ulna fractures who were followed for at least 1 year after surgery showed a range of motion within 10° of that of the contralateral elbow, no pain, and a complete return to normal activities [65]. Another study from Germany using a different intramedullary nail design reported in 68 of 73 good or excellent results in a mixed pool of simple and comminuted fractures [31].

To this date, large cohort studies comparing all available techniques for the fixation of olecranon fractures with identical fracture patterns are lacking. The surgeon must therefore adapt the advantages and disadvantages of the individual techniques to the clinical situation and develop a treatment algorithm for each fracture type.

Conclusion

Olecranon fractures make up a significant amount of upper extremity fractures. They usually occur from a fall on the elbow with direct impaction. The majority of these are simple fractures with not more than two fragments. The most common classification is the Mayo classification, which distinguishes three types with or without comminution and correlates with clinical outcome. The most common osteosynthesis techniques are tension band wire fixation for simple fractures and plate osteosynthesis with one or two plates for multifragmentary and complex fractures. Low-profile double-plate osteosynthesis combines angular stability with low buildup on the olecranon. The most frequent complication is soft tissue irritation at the elbow caused by the applied osteosynthesis, which often necessitates hardware removal.

In elderly patients, conservative therapy is also possible by means of immobilization and subsequent physiotherapeutic exercise. Especially in osteoporotic bones, a retaining osteosynthesis is difficult, and therefore, a therapy adapted to the age of such patients should be chosen. With the correctly executed technique and appropriate implant, olecranon fractures have very good clinical outcome.

References

1. Romero JM, Miran A, CH J. Complications and re-operation rate after tension-band wiring of olecranon fractures. J Orthop Sci. 2000;5(4):318–20. https://doi.org/10.1007/s007760070036.
2. Veillette CJH, Steinmann SP. Olecranon fractures. Orthop Clin N Am. 2008;39(2):229–+. https://doi.org/10.1016/j.ocl.2008.01.002.
3. Marot V, Bayle-Iniguez X, Cavaignac E, Bonnevialle N, Mansat P, Murgier J. Results of non-operative treatment of olecranon fracture in over 75-year-olds. Orthop Traumatol Surg Res. 2018;104(1):79–82. https://doi.org/10.1016/j.otsr.2017.10.015.
4. Duckworth AD, Clement ND, Jenkins PJ, Aitken SA, Court-Brown CM, McQueen MM. The epidemiology of radial head and neck fractures. J Hand Surg Am. 2012;37a(1):112–9. https://doi.org/10.1016/j.jhsa.2011.09.034.
5. Newman SD, Mauffrey C, Krikler S. Olecranon fractures. Injury. 2009;40(6):575–81. https://doi.org/10.1016/j.injury.2008.12.013.
6. Amis AA, Miller JH. The mechanisms of elbow fractures – an investigation using impact tests in-vitro. Injury. 1995;26(3):163–8. https://doi.org/10.1016/0020-1383(95)93494-3.
7. Hackl M, Lappen S, Neiss WF, Scaal M, Muller LP, Wegmann K. The bare area of the proximal ulna: An anatomical study on optimizing olecranon osteotomy. Orthopade. 2016;45(10):887–94. https://doi.org/10.1007/s00132-016-3332-z.
8. Hackl M, Rausch V, Ries C, Muller LP, Wegmann K. Olecranon fractures. Unfallchirurg. 2018;121(11):911–22. https://doi.org/10.1007/s00113-018-0567-7.
9. Beser CG, Demiryurek D, Ozsoy H, Ercakmak B, Hayran M, Kizilay O, et al. Redefining the proximal ulna anatomy. Surg Radiol Anat. 2014;36(10):1023–31. https://doi.org/10.1007/s00276-014-1340-4.
10. Grechenig W, Clement H, Pichler W, Tesch NP, Windisch G. The influence of lateral and anterior angulation of the proximal ulna on the treatment of a Monteggia fracture: an anatomical cadaver study. J Bone Joint Surg Br. 2007;89(6):836–8. https://doi.org/10.1302/0301-620X.89B6.18975.
11. Rouleau DM, Faber KJ, Athwal GS. The proximal ulna dorsal angulation: a radiographic study. J Shoulder Elb Surg. 2010;19(1):26–30. https://doi.org/10.1016/j.jse.2009.07.005.
12. Windisch G, Clement H, Grechenig W, Tesch NP, Pichler W. The anatomy of the proximal ulna. J Shoulder Elb Surg. 2007;16(5):661–6. https://doi.org/10.1016/j.jse.2006.12.008.
13. Puchwein P, Schildhauer TA, Schoffmann S, Heidari N, Windisch G, Pichler W. Three-dimensional morphometry of the proximal ulna: a comparison to currently used anatomically preshaped ulna plates. J Shoulder Elb Surg. 2012;21(8):1018–23. https://doi.org/10.1016/j.jse.2011.07.004.
14. Hardy BT, Glowczewskie F, Wright TW. Vascular anatomy of the proximal ulna. J Hand Surg Am. 2011;36a(5):808–10. https://doi.org/10.1016/j.jhsa.2011.02.011.
15. Sullivan CW, Desai K. Classifications in brief: Mayo classification of olecranon fractures. Clin Orthop Relat Res. 2019;477(4):908–10. https://doi.org/10.1097/CORR.0000000000000614.
16. Colton CL. Fractures of the olecranon in adults: classification and management. Injury. 1973;5(2):121–9. https://doi.org/10.1016/s0020-1383(73)80088-9.
17. Cabanela M, Morrey B. The elbow and its disorders. 2nd ed. Philadelphia: WB Saunders; 1993.
18. Morrey B, Sanchez-Sotelo J, Morrey M. Morrey's the elbow and its disorders. 5th ed. Philadelphia: Elsevier Inc; 2017.
19. Schatzker J. Fractures of the olecranon. In: Schatzker J, Tile M, editors. The rationale of operative fracture care. Berlin: Springer; 1987. p. 89–95.
20. Rommens PM, Kuchle R, Schneider RU, Reuter M. Olecranon fractures in adults: factors influencing outcome. Injury. 2004;35(11):1149–57. https://doi.org/10.1016/j.injury.2003.12.002.
21. Jaskulka R, Harm T. Conservative therapy of closed, dislocated fractures of the olecranon in geriatric patients. Unfallchirurg. 1991;94(8):424–9.
22. Parker MJ, Richmond PW, Andrew TA, Bewes PC. A review of displaced olecranon fractures treated conservatively. J R Coll Surg Edinb. 1990;35(6):392–4.

23. Veras Del Monte L, Sirera Vercher M, Busquets Net R, Castellanos Robles J, Carrera Calderer L, Mir BX. Conservative treatment of displaced fractures of the olecranon in the elderly. Injury. 1999;30(2):105–10. https://doi.org/10.1016/s0020-1383(98)00223-x.

24. Duckworth AD, Bugler KE, Clement ND, Court-Brown CM, McQueen MM. Nonoperative management of displaced olecranon fractures in low-demand elderly patients. J Bone Joint Surg Am. 2014;96(1):67–72. https://doi.org/10.2106/JBJS.L.01137.

25. Weber BG, Vesly H. Osteosynthese bei Olecranonfraktur. Z Unfallmed Berufskr. 1963;2:90–6.

26. Hutchinson DT, Horwitz DS, Ha G, Thomas CW, Bachus KN. Cyclic loading of olecranon fracture fixation constructs. J Bone Joint Surg Am. 2003;85a(5):831–7. https://doi.org/10.2106/00004623-200305000-00010.

27. Schneider MM, Nowak TE, Bastian L, Katthagen JC, Isenberg J, Rommens PM, et al. Tension band wiring in olecranon fractures: the myth of technical simplicity and osteosynthetical perfection. Int Orthop. 2014;38(4):847–55. https://doi.org/10.1007/s00264-013-2208-7.

28. Karlsson MK, Hasserius R, Besjakov J, Karlsson C, Josefsson PO. Comparison of tension-band and figure-of-eight wiring techniques for treatment of olecranon fractures. J Shoulder Elb Surg. 2002;11(4):377–82. https://doi.org/10.1067/mse.2002.124548.

29. Baecher N, Edwards S. Olecranon fractures. J Hand Surg Am. 2013;38(3):593–604. https://doi.org/10.1016/j.jhsa.2012.12.036.

30. Molloy S, Jasper LE, Elliott DS, Brumback RJ, Belkoff SM. Biomechanical evaluation of intramedullary nail versus tension band fixation for transverse olecranon fractures. J Orthop Trauma. 2004;18(3):170–4. https://doi.org/10.1097/00005131-200403000-00008.

31. Gehr J, Friedl W. Intramedullary locking compression nail for the treatment of an olecranon fracture. Oper Orthop Traumatol. 2006;18(3):199–213. https://doi.org/10.1007/s00064-006-1171-5.

32. Ries C, Wegmann K, Meffert RH, Muller LP, Burkhart KJ. Double-plate osteosynthesis of the proximal ulna. Oper Orthop Traumatol. 2015;27(4):342–56. https://doi.org/10.1007/s00064-014-0296-1.

33. Hackl M, Mayer K, Weber M, Staat M, van Riet R, Burkhart KJ, et al. Plate osteosynthesis of proximal ulna fractures-a biomechanical micromotion analysis. J Hand Surg Am. 2017;42(10):834 e1–7. https://doi.org/10.1016/j.jhsa.2017.05.014.

34. Leschinger T, Wegmann K, Hackl M, Müller L. Biomechanik des Ellenbogengelenks. Orthop Unfallchir Up2date. 2016;11:159–76. https://doi.org/10.1055/s-0041-108914.

35. Izzi J, Athwal GS. An off loading triceps suture for augmentation of plate fixation in comminuted osteoporotic fractures of the olecranon. J Orthop Trauma. 2012;26(1):59–61. https://doi.org/10.1097/BOT.0b013e318214e64c.

36. Lavigne G, Baratz M. Fractures of the olecranon. J Hand Surg Am. 2004;4:94–102. https://doi.org/10.1016/j.jassh.2004.02.004.

37. Hak DJ, Golladay GJ. Olecranon fractures: treatment options. J Am Acad Orthop Surg. 2000;8(4):266–75. https://doi.org/10.5435/00124635-200007000-00007.

38. Hume MC, Wiss DA. Olecranon fractures. A clinical and radiographic comparison of tension band wiring and plate fixation. Clin Orthop Relat Res. 1992;285:229–35.

39. Wolfgang G, Burke F, Bush D, Parenti J, Perry J, LaFollette B, et al. Surgical treatment of displaced olecranon fractures by tension band wiring technique. Clin Orthop Relat Res. 1987;224:192–204.

40. Bailey CS, MacDermid J, Patterson SD, King GJ. Outcome of plate fixation of olecranon fractures. J Orthop Trauma. 2001;15(8):542–8. https://doi.org/10.1097/00005131-200111000-00002.

41. Simpson NS, Goodman LA, Jupiter JB. Contoured LCDC plating of the proximal ulna. Injury. 1996;27(6):411–7. https://doi.org/10.1016/0020-1383(96)00031-9.

42. Mc KF, Buck RM. Fracture of the olecranon process of the ulna; treatment by excision of fragment and repair of triceps tendon. J Am Med Assoc. 1947;135(1):1–5. https://doi.org/10.1001/jama.1947.02890010003001.

43. Inhofe PD, Howard TC. The treatment of olecranon fractures by excision or fragments and repair of the extensor mechanism: historical review and report of 12 fractures. Orthopedics. 1993;16(12):1313–7.

44. Gartsman GM, Sculco TP, Otis JC. Operative treatment of olecranon fractures. Excision or open reduction with internal fixation. J Bone Joint Surg Am. 1981;63(5):718–21.

45. An KN, Morrey BF, Chao EY. The effect of partial removal of proximal ulna on elbow constraint. Clin Orthop Relat Res. 1986;209:270–9.

46. DiDonna ML, Fernandez JJ, Lim TH, Hastings H, Cohen MS. Partial olecranon excision: the relationship between triceps insertion site and extension strength of the elbow. J Hand Surg Am. 2003;28a(1):117–22. https://doi.org/10.1053/jhsu.2003.50036.

47. Rotini R, Antonioli D, Marinelli A, Katusic D. Surgical treatment of proximal ulna nonunion. Chir Organi Mov. 2008;91(2):65–70. https://doi.org/10.1007/s12306-007-0011-6.

48. Papagelopoulos PJ, Morrey BF. Treatment of nonunion of olecranon fractures. J Bone Joint Surg Br. 1994;76(4):627–35.

49. Sahajpal D, Wright TW. Proximal ulna fractures. J Hand Surg Am. 2009;34(2):357–62. https://doi.org/10.1016/j.jhsa.2008.12.022.

50. Rommens PM, Schneider RU, Reuter M. Functional results after operative treatment of olecranon fractures. Acta Chir Belg. 2004;104(2):191–7. https://doi.org/10.1080/00015458.2004.11679535.

51. Dyer GS, Ring D. Fractures of the proximal ulna. In: Wolfe SW, Hotchkiss RN, Pederson WC, Kozin SH, Cohen M, editors. Green's operative hand surgery. 7th ed. Philadelphia: Elsevier Inc; 2017. p. 770–85.

52. Prayson MJ, Iossi MF, Buchalter D, Vogt M, Towers J. Safe zone for anterior cortical perforation of the ulna during tension-band wire fixation: a magnetic resonance imaging analysis. J Shoulder Elb Surg. 2008;17(1):121–5. https://doi.org/10.1016/j.jse.2007.04.010.

53. Ishigaki N, Uchiyama S, Nakagawa H, Kamimura M, Miyasaka T. Ulnar nerve palsy at the elbow after surgical treatment for fractures of the olecranon. J Shoulder Elb Surg. 2004;13(1):60–5. https://doi.org/10.1016/S1058-2746(03)00220-9.

54. Macko D, Szabo RM. Complications of tension-band wiring of olecranon fractures. J Bone Joint Surg Am. 1985;67(9):1396–401.

55. van der Linden SC, van Kampen A, Jaarsma RL. K-wire position in tension-band wiring technique affects stability of wires and long-term outcome in surgical treatment of olecranon fractures. J Shoulder Elb Surg. 2012;21(3):405–11. https://doi.org/10.1016/j.jse.2011.07.022.

56. Bauer AS, Lawson BK, Bliss RL, Dyer GS. Risk factors for post-traumatic heterotopic ossification of the elbow: case-control study. J Hand Surg Am. 2012;37(7):1422-9 e1–6. https://doi.org/10.1016/j.jhsa.2012.03.013.

57. Hamid N, Ashraf N, Bosse MJ, Connor PM, Kellam JF, Sims SH, et al. Radiation therapy for heterotopic ossification prophylaxis acutely after elbow trauma: a prospective randomized study. J Bone Joint Surg Am. 2010;92(11):2032–8. https://doi.org/10.2106/JBJS.I.01435.

58. Huang TW, Wu CC, Fan KF, Tseng IC, Lee PC, Chou YC. Tension band wiring for olecranon fractures: relative stability of Kirschner wires in various configurations. J Trauma. 2010;68(1):173–6. https://doi.org/10.1097/TA.0b013e3181ad554c.

59. Karlsson MK, Hasserius R, Karlsson C, Besjakov J, Josefsson PO. Fractures of the olecranon: a 15- to 25-year followup of 73 patients. Clin Orthop Relat Res. 2002;403:205–12.

60. Buijze G, Kloen P. Clinical evaluation of locking compression plate fixation for comminuted olecranon fractures. J Bone Joint Surg Am. 2009;91(10):2416–20. https://doi.org/10.2106/JBJS.H.01419.

61. Wang YH, Tao R, Xu H, Cao Y, Zhou ZY, Xu SZ. Mid-term outcomes of contoured plating for comminuted fractures of the olecranon. Orthop Surg. 2011;3(3):176–80. https://doi.org/10.1111/j.1757-7861.2011.00139.x.

62. Rochet S, Obert L, Lepage D, Lemaire B, Leclerc G, Garbuio P. Proximal ulna comminuted fractures: fixation using a double-plating technique. Orthop Traumatol Surg. 2010;96(7):734–40. https://doi.org/10.1016/j.otsr.2010.06.003.

63. Ellwein A, Argiropoulos K, DeyHazra RO, Pastor MF, Smith T, Lill H. Clinical evaluation of double-plate osteosynthesis for olecranon fractures: a retrospective case-control study. Orthop Traumatol Surg Res. 2019;105(8):1601–6. https://doi.org/10.1016/j.otsr.2019.08.019.

64. Ellwein A, Lill H, Warnhoff M, Hackl M, Wegmann K, Muller LP, et al. Can low-profile double-plate osteosynthesis for olecranon fractures reduce implant removal? A retrospective multicenter study. J Shoulder Elb Surg. 2020;29(6):1275–81. https://doi.org/10.1016/j.jse.2020.01.091.

65. Argintar E, Cohen M, Eglseder A, Edwards S. Clinical results of olecranon fractures treated with multiplanar locked intramedullary nailing. J Orthop Trauma. 2013;27(3):140–4. https://doi.org/10.1097/BOT.0b013e318261906e.

66. Gierer P, Wichelhaus A, Rotter R. Fractures of the olecranon. Oper Orthop Traumatol. 2017;29(2):107–14. https://doi.org/10.1007/s00064-017-0490-z.

67. Uhlmann M, Barg A, Valderrabano V, Weber O, Wirtz DC, Pagenstert G. Treatment of isolated fractures of the olecranon: percutaneous double-screw fixation versus conventional tension band wiring. Unfallchirurg. 2014;117(7):614–23. https://doi.org/10.1007/s00113-013-2389-y.

Intra-articular Supracondylar Humerus Fractures

Stephan Uschok, Michael Hackl, Kilian Wegmann,
and Lars Peter Müller

Introduction

Fractures of the distal humerus are complex injuries with a low incidence of 5.7 cases per 100.000 per year [1]. As in several other fractures, the age distribution is double peaked, with the first peak for young males between 12 and 19 years of age (high energy trauma) and the second peak for older females over 80 years of age (osteoporotic fractures) [1].

Distal humerus fractures are classified by the AO/OTA classification into three types (Fig. 70.1). Extra-articular fractures are classified as type A fractures. Type B and type C fractures include intraarticular fractures with partial involvement of the articular surface (type B) or complete articular fractures (type C) and represent 60% of all distal humerus fractures.

In this chapter, intraarticular fractures extending into the supracondylar region will be discussed. These include lateral (B1) and medial (B2) fractures as well as complete articular fractures with simple or complex involvement of the supracondylar region (C1, C2, C3). Furthermore, intraarticular fractures in the sagittal plane (B3) will be discussed. Type B3 fractures are further classified according to Dubberley [2] (Fig. 70.1) into fractures of the capitellum (type I), fractures of the capitellum and the trochlea as one fragment (type II), and separated fractures of the capitellum and the trochlea (type III). Depending on the presence of a dorsal zone of comminution, all three types are classified as (a) without comminution and (b) comminuted fractures.

S. Uschok (✉) · M. Hackl · K. Wegmann · L. P. Müller
Faculty of Medicine, University of Cologne, Cologne, Germany

University Hospital Cologne, Center of Orthopedic and Trauma Surgery, Cologne, Germany
e-mail: stephan.uschok@uk-koeln.de;
kilian.wegmann@uk-koeln.de; lars.mueller@uk-koeln.de

Biplane x-ray imaging and a detailed neurovascular status are the basic diagnostics since 20% of distal humerus fractures are accompanied by nerve injuries. An additional CT scan should be performed to reveal the exact fracture pattern and, especially with 3D reconstruction, aids in surgical planning.

Indications

A surgical approach is the standard for almost all distal humerus fractures, due to inferior functional results after nonsurgical treatment.

Different procedures are available. B1-, B2-, and B3-type fractures can be approached by unilateral plate osteosynthesis and/or screw osteosynthesis. Type C fractures are treated, depending on the fracture pattern, the severity of the fracture, the age, and the functional demand of the patient, either by double-plating osteosynthesis or by arthroplasty.

Arthroplasty should be reserved for elderly, low-demand patients with non-reconstructible fractures or fractures with preexisting arthritis or deformities. In moribund patients, even in severe fractures, a nonsurgical treatment is possible (bag-of-bones) [4].

Contraindications

Nonsurgical treatment of distal humerus fractures is due to its inferior functional outcome and reserved to older, low-demand patients and patients with a high intraoperative risk profile.

Since the functional integrity of the elbow joint is an important factor in activities of daily living, the indication against a surgical procedure should be considered deeply. Furthermore, nonsurgical therapy is related to a higher risk of delayed union and non-union.

© Springer Nature Switzerland AG 2022
W. B. Geissler (ed.), *Wrist and Elbow Arthroscopy with Selected Open Procedures*,
https://doi.org/10.1007/978-3-030-78881-0_70

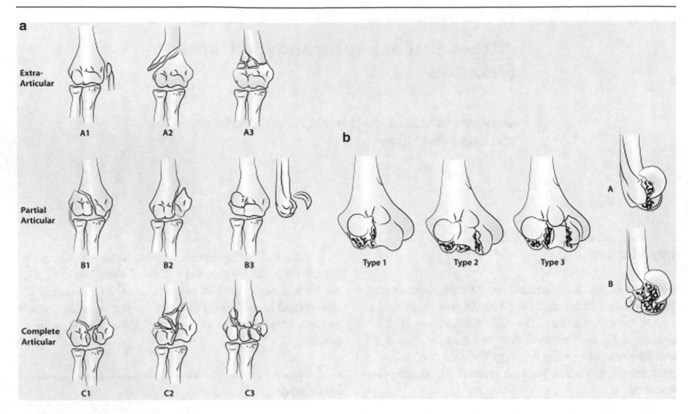

Fig. 70.1 AO classification (**a**) and Dubberley classification (**b**) of distal humerus fractures. (Permission by Dey Hazra et al. [3]. Copyright © The Author(s) 2018 Open Access. This article is distributed under the terms of the Creative Commons Attribution 4.0 International License (http://creativecommons.org/licenses/by/4.0/), which permits unrestricted use, distribution, and reproduction in any medium, provided you give appropriate credit to the original author(s) and the source, provide a link to the Creative Commons license, and indicate if changes were made)

Technique

Positioning of the Patient

Positioning of the patient depends on the fracture type and the intended surgical procedure.

Patients with a B1 or B2 fracture can be treated, using a unilateral approach. Therefore, the preferred positioning is the supine position using an arm rest. This is also the preferred positioning in patients, when a primary arthroplasty is anticipated. In these cases, an armrest is not needed; the arm is put into 90° of shoulder flexion and 90° of elbow flexion.

For type B3 and type C fractures with the intention of open reduction and internal fixation, the prone position should be preferred, since a complete visualization of the articular surface is essential in these fractures.

Surgical Approach

The preferred approach for B1 fractures and simple B3 fractures is the lateral approach.

The skin incision starts at the radial epicondyle and extends distally to the radial head. The interval between the anconeus muscle and the extensor carpi ulnaris muscle is being identified by the diverging course of muscle fibers, and after incision, a fatty streak is visible, marking the Kocher interval. The joint capsule is being visualized and incised ventrally. This leaves the lateral collateral ligament intact. If necessary, the annular ligament is split, and the bundle consisting of the annular ligament, the lateral collateral ligament, and the dorsal joint capsule is mobilized dorsally.

For better visualization, the lateral collateral ligament can be released and refixated, using bone anchors, upon closure.

For B2 fractures, the preferred approach is the medial approach described by Hotchkiss. The skin incision is placed slightly ventrally to the medial epicondyle. The extent of the incision depends on the pathology. After the skin incision, the medial intermuscular septum is visualized. The ulnar nerve is situated proximally and dorsally of the septum, next to the lateral border of the triceps muscle. The nerve should be prepared distally, through the ulnar groove to the arcade of Osbourne and proximally to the arcade of Struthers which are approximately 8 cm proximal and distal to the epicondyle. The nerve should be marked with a vessel loop, and the brachialis muscle can be mobilized off the anterior aspect of the humerus while taking care for the median nerve and the brachial artery.

For further visualization, the approach can be extended by splitting the common flexor origin.

Complex type B3 and type C fractures are addressed, using a dorsal approach.

After incision of the skin, full thickness flaps are prepared to preserve the thin soft tissue envelope of the dorsal aspect of the elbow. The ulnar nerve is situated at the medial border of the triceps muscle and is prepared proximally and distally as mentioned for the medial approach.

In most cases with a multifragmentary fracture of the articular surface, an osteotomy of the olecranon is needed for detailed visualization of the joint surface. The olecranon osteotomy is performed by sawing in a v-shaped method and completed using a chisel to avoid smooth cut surfaces and facilitating the osteosynthesis in a later step (Chevron osteotomy).

However, a triceps sparing approach, without osteotomy of the olecranon, is the preferred approach in non-reconstructible fractures where an arthroplasty is anticipated. After preparation and securing of the ulnar nerve, the triceps is mobilized medially and laterally from the distal humerus. If needed, the medial and lateral collateral ligaments and the common extensor origin and the common flexor origin are stripped from the epicondyle, for better visualization of the articular surface. This allows for a subtotal dislocation of the joint.

Osteosynthesis

In terms of osteosynthesis, an angular stable plate osteosynthesis, using preformed plates, is the standard procedure. Several implants are available.

For B1- and B2-type fractures, a unilateral osteosynthesis is sufficient. After reduction of the fracture, the reduction can be secured using two K-wires. Bending the elbow to 90° of flexion facilitates the reduction. The plate should be temporarily fixed, and intraoperative fluoroscopy ensures the correct positioning of the plate.

Type B3 fractures can be approached, depending on the fracture pattern, by screw osteosynthesis, plate osteosynthesis, or a combination of them.

For type C fractures, double-plating systems are available which can be configured in a parallel or a perpendicular arrangement. Several clinical studies could not show a differ-

ence in functional outcome between a 90° configuration and a 180° configuration, although differences in biomechanical studies have been shown [5–7]. The arrangement of the plates depends on the fracture pattern. In fractures involving a coronal shear fragment, a 90° configuration should be preferred; in low type C3 fractures, a 180° configuration should be preferred.

Reduction of type C fractures starts with the joint block. Small fragments and cortical fragments, with a risk of necrosis, should be resected. The joint block should be built up, so both columns are reduced and stable, before fixation to the diaphyseal part. Additional screw fixation aides the reduction, using screws in an immersed manner. It should be ensured that those screws do not penetrate intra-articularly.

The reconstructed joint block can afterwards be reduced to the diaphysis. The length of the implants depends on the fracture pattern. It should be ensured that the plates do not end on the same level, since this creates a rise in stress. Furthermore, it should be ensured that the plates do not overlay each other in perpendicular plate configuration. For the fixation of the joint block, as many screws as possible should be used.

In non-reconstructible fractures, arthroplasty is an option, leaving two options. Hemiarthroplasty, representing the more challenging option due to the necessity of reconstruction of the collateral ligaments. Intact or reconstructed collateral ligaments are essential for a good outcome following hemiarthroplasty. Another option is a total elbow arthroplasty, which should be reserved for elderly patients with a lower functional demand, due to the lifetime weight load limitation.

Closure

Closure begins by refixation of detached collateral ligaments. If the common extensor of flexor origin was released, it has to be reattached. The preferred method for reconstruction is by use of suture anchors.

If an olecranon osteotomy was used, an osteosynthesis has to be performed. Different methods/implants are available. The preferred method by the authors is a double-plate osteosynthesis. In selected cases, an additional triceps off-loading suture is useful to decrease the load on the osteosynthesis.

Upon closure, the ulnar nerve has to be reevaluated. Depending on the extent of the performed neurolysis, an anterior transposition is indicated. In cases with preoperative signs of ulnar nerve damage, an anterior transposition of the ulnar nerve is obligatory.

Tips and Tricks

Type B3 Fractures

Depending on the fracture pattern, there are generally two techniques for reduction and internal fixation of those fractures.

Coronal shear fractures may be reduced and internally fixed, using a direct or indirect technique. In certain cases, an arthroscopically assisted osteosynthesis is possible as well. For direct as well as indirect fixation, specialized implants are available. Cannulated, double-headed screws, where the screw head can be sunken below the articular surface level, are useful in those cases (Figs. 70.2 and 70.3).

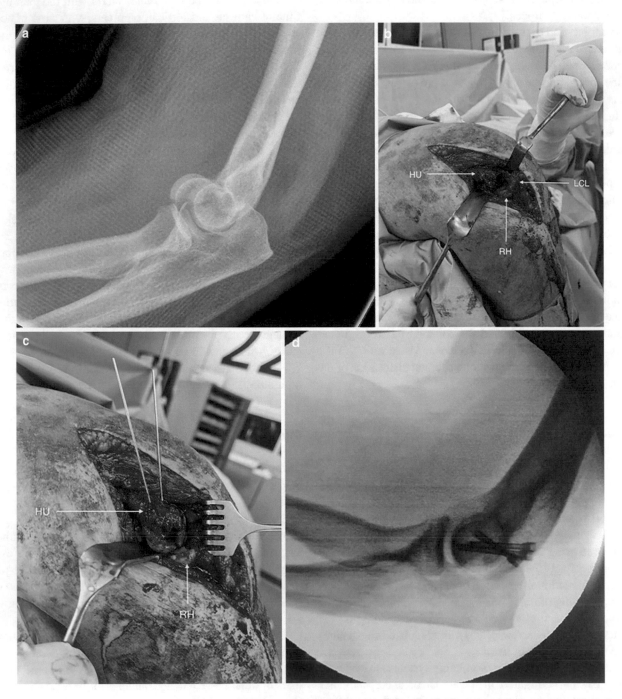

Fig. 70.2 Screw osteosynthesis of a type B3 fracture. (**a**) X-ray of a distal humerus fracture type B3 (AO classification) or type IA (Dubberley classification), (**b**) exposure of the fracture with release of the lateral collateral ligament, (**c**) temporary fixation using k-wires in an indirect technique, and (**d**) x-ray of final reconstruction using an indirect screw osteosynthesis. HU distal humerus, RH radial head, LCL lateral collateral ligament

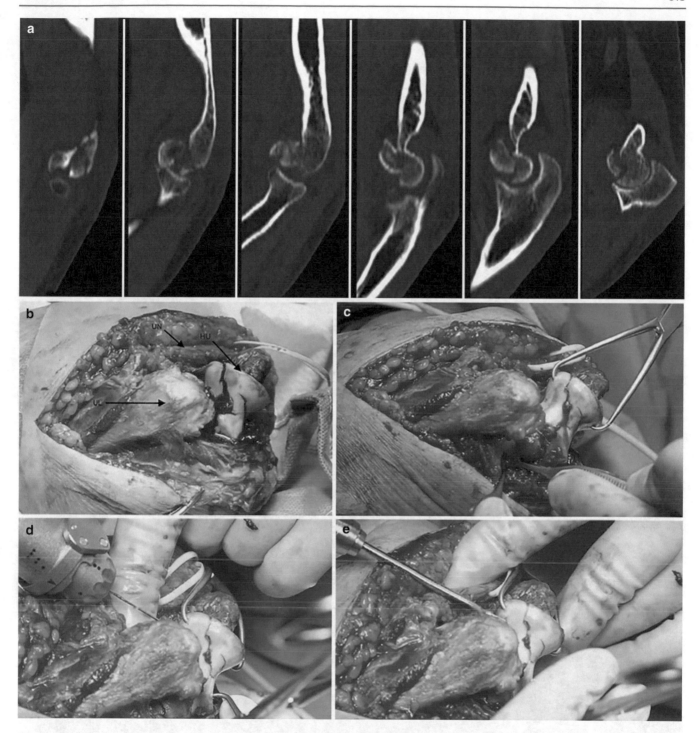

Fig. 70.3 Screw osteosynthesis of a type B3 fracture. (**a**) Sagittal CT scan of a distal humerus fracture type B3 (AO classification) or type IIIB (Dubberley classification), (**b**) exposure of the fracture, (**c**) reduction of the fracture using pointed forceps, (**d**) temporary fixation using k-wires in an indirect technique, (**e, f**) insertion of the cannulated, double-headed compression screws in an indirect and direct technique, and (**g, h**) postoperative x-ray of final reconstruction. HU distal humerus, RH radial head, UN ulnar nerve

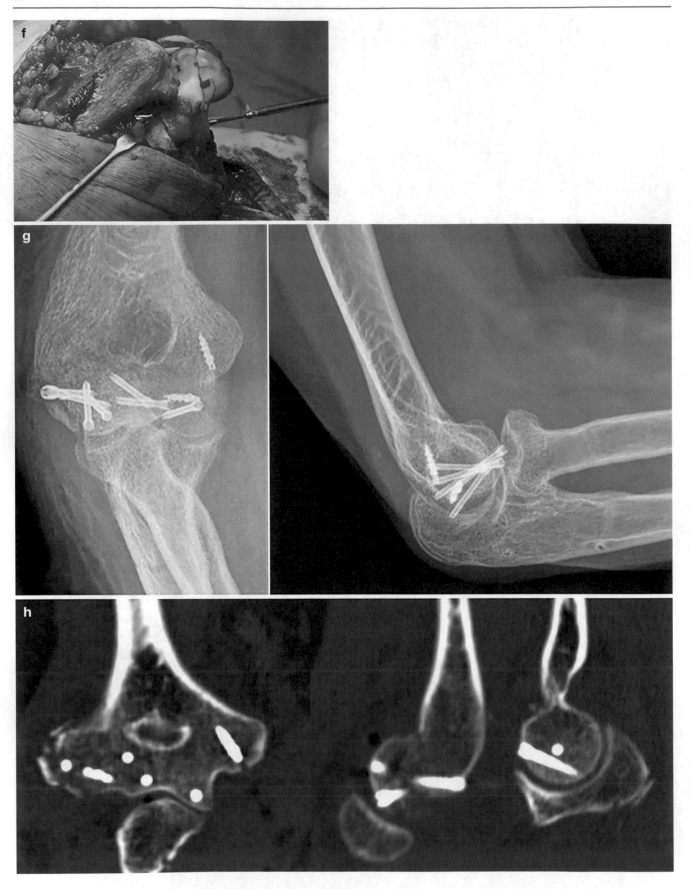

Fig. 70.3 (continued)

Type C Fractures

In type C fractures (Figs. 70.4, 70.5, and 70.6), the fracture pattern determines the surgical approach. In C1- and C2-type fractures, without comminution of the joint surface, a triceps sparing approach is possible in performing an osteosynthesis.

Even though being possible, a reconstruction of fractures with involvement of the articular surface is facilitated by the use of an olecranon osteotomy. This way, a detailed inspection of the articular surface and an anatomic reduction is possible (see Fig. 70.4b).

After performing the osteotomy, the proximal part of the olecranon with the attached triceps tendon should be wrapped into a wet gauze compress. The reconstruction begins by reconstructing the joint block in a first step using singular screws (see Fig. 70.4c). The second step involves the attach-

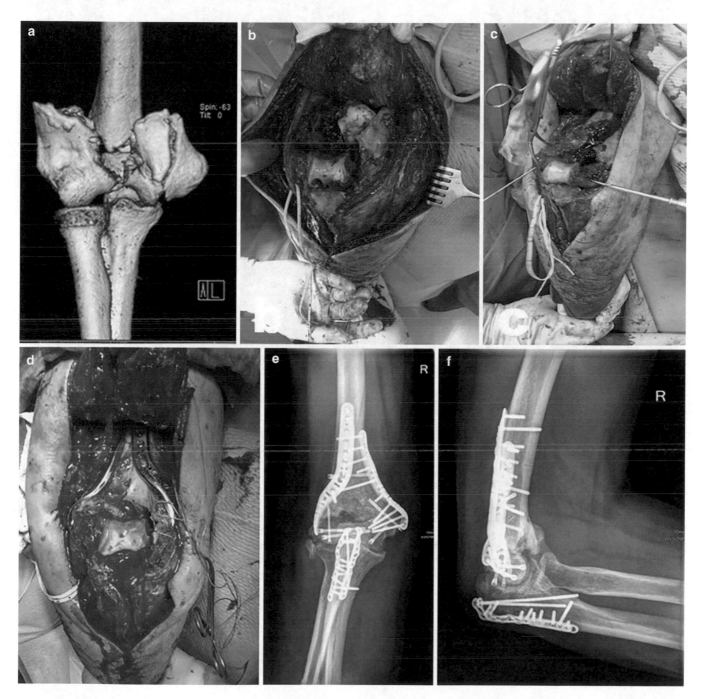

Fig. 70.4 Reconstruction of a type C fracture using screws and preformed angular stable locking plates. (**a**) 3D reconstruction of a type C3 fracture, (**b**) visualization of the fracture after performing an olecranon osteotomy, (**c**) reduction of the joint block and fixation using double headed compression screws, (**d**) reduction of the reduced joint block against the diaphysis using preformed angular stable locking plates in a 90° configuration, and (**e**, **f**) postoperative x-ray showing the reconstruction of the distal humerus and the osteosynthesis of the olecranon osteotomy using a double-plating system

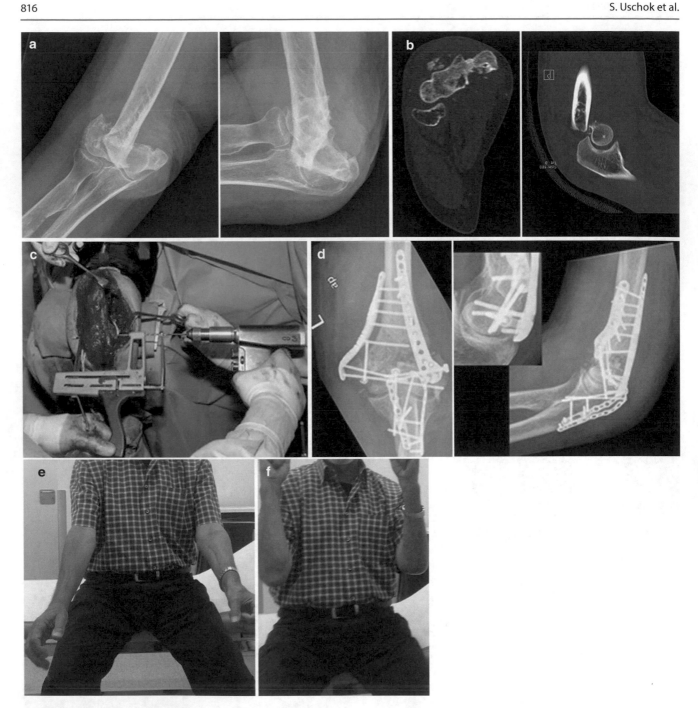

Fig. 70.5 Reconstruction of a type C fracture. (**a**, **b**) X-ray and CT scan of a type C3 fracture, (**c**) coaxial aiming device, (**d**) postoperative x-ray after double-plating osteosynthesis of a distal humerus fracture in a 90° configuration, and (**e**, **f**) functional result at 12 months follow-up

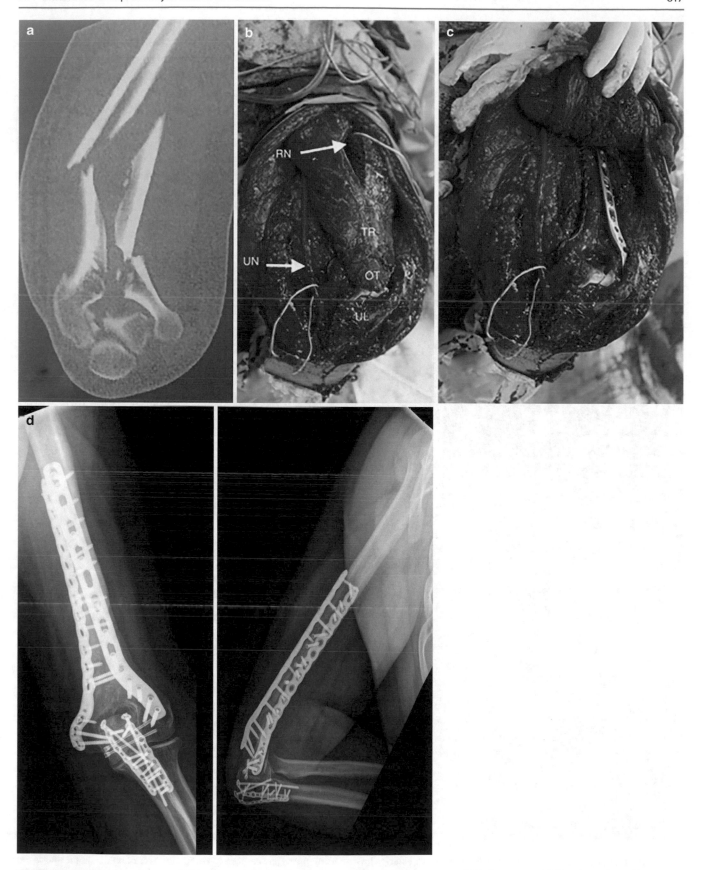

Fig. 70.6 Reconstruction of a type C fracture. (**a**) CT scan of a type C3 fracture with extension into the diaphysis, (**b**) visualization of the radial nerve, (**c**) double-plating osteosynthesis via olecranon osteotomy, and (**d**) postoperative x-ray. UN ulnar nerve, RN radial nerve, TR triceps muscle, OT olecranon tip, UL ulna

ment of the reconstructed joint block to the diaphysis using preformed plates with osteosynthesis of the olecranon osteotomy upon closure (see Fig. 70.6d–f).

Screw placement of the distal screws in double-plating osteosynthesis of the distal humerus can be facilitated by use of a coaxial aiming device (see Fig. 70.5c).

In fractures, extending into the diaphysis, special attention has to be paid to the radial nerve. The radial nerve runs on the dorsal aspect of the humerus, approximately 18 cm proximal to the epicondylar level, through the radial groove and is in close contact to the bone until 13 cm proximal to the epicondylar level, piercing through the lateral

intermuscular septum. In fractures extending into this region or rather fractures requiring an osteosynthesis with placement of the plates in this region, require a visualization of the radial nerve (see Fig. 70.6b, c). After plate placement, the level, at which the radial nerve crosses the plate, should be documented by putting it in relation to the plate holes.

In complex cases, in which a reconstruction is not possible, and an arthroplasty is anticipated, a triceps sparing approach is preferred. This approach allows for a limited evaluation of the fracture pattern, prior to implantation of an elbow prosthesis (Fig. 70.7).

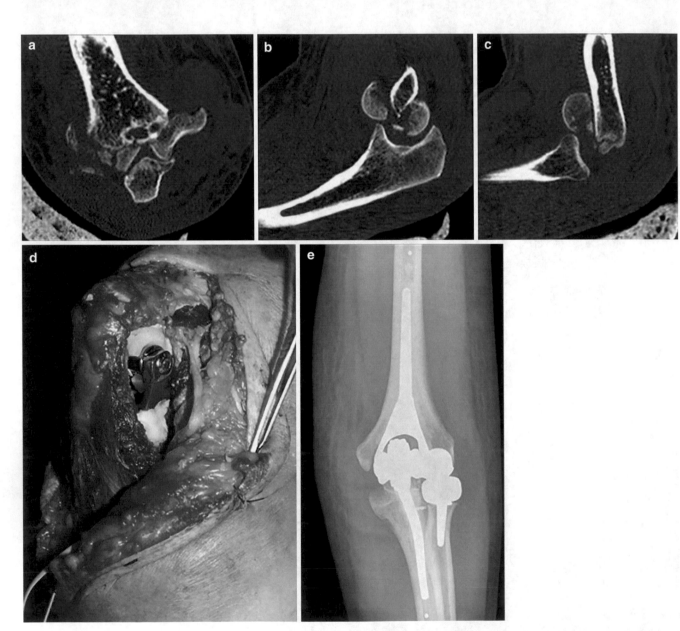

Fig. 70.7 Non-reconstructable type C3 fracture in an elderly, low-demand patient. (**a–c**) Preoperative CT scan, (**d**) medial view after implantation of a total elbow prosthesis with attached triceps tendon using a triceps sparing approach, after reduction of the prosthesis, an anterior transposition of the ulnar nerve is performed to minimize the risk of ulnar nerve irritation, and (**e**) postoperative x-ray

Conclusion

Fractures of the distal humerus are challenging, and reconstruction of those fractures should be performed in centers with upper extremity surgery.

Depending on the fracture type and fracture pattern as well as the age and demand of the patient, different procedures are available for fracture reconstruction.

An olecranon osteotomy facilitates the visualization and reduction of the fracture pattern of the articular surface but should be avoided if not necessary.

A neurolysis of the ulnar nerve should be performed to avoid nerve damage during reconstruction. In cases with preoperative ulnar nerve symptoms, an anterior transposition of the ulnar nerve is obligatory.

In cases with non-reconstructable fractures, arthroplasty is an option. This option should be reserved for elderly, low-demand patients.

References

1. Robinson CM, Hill RMF, Jacobs N, Dall G, Court-Brown CM. Adult distal humeral metaphyseal fractures: epidemiology and results of treatment. J Orthop Trauma. 2003;17(1):38–47.

2. Dubberley JH, Faber KJ, Macdermid JC, Patterson SD, King GJW. Outcome after open reduction and internal fixation of capitellar and trochlear fractures. J Bone Joint Surg Am. 2006;88(1):46–54.

3. Dey Hazra RO, Lill H, Jensen G, Imrecke J, Ellwein A. Frakturspezifische Therapiekonzepte der distalen Humerusfraktur. Obere Extremitat. 2018;13(1):23–32. https://doi.org/10.1007/s11678-018-0442-8. Springer. Epub 2018 Feb 15

4. Aitken SA, Jenkins PJ, Rymaszewski L. Revisiting the "bag of bones": functional outcome after the conservative management of a fracture of the distal humerus. Bone Joint J. 2015;97-B(8):1132–8.

5. Caravaggi P, Laratta JL, Yoon RS, De Biasio J, Ingargiola M, Frank MA, et al. Internal fixation of the distal humerus: a comprehensive biomechanical study evaluating current fixation techniques. J Orthop Trauma. 2014;28(4):222–6.

6. Zalavras CG, Vercillo MT, Jun B-J, Otarodifard K, Itamura JM, Lee TQ. Biomechanical evaluation of parallel versus orthogonal plate fixation of intra-articular distal humerus fractures. J Shoulder Elb Surg. 2011;20(1):12–20.

7. Penzkofer R, Hungerer S, Wipf F, von Oldenburg G, Augat P. Anatomical plate configuration affects mechanical performance in distal humerus fractures. Clin Biomech (Bristol, Avon). 2010;25(10):972–8.

Coronoid Fractures

Valentin Rausch, Lars Peter Müller, and Kilian Wegmann

Introduction

The ulnar articular surface consists of the olecranon and the coronoid process that together enclose the distal humerus. The coronoid process is divided into a medial and a lateral facet by a ridge that reaches the most anterior extension of the proximal ulna at the coronoid tip. With its broad surface, the coronoid process stabilizes against axial and rotational forces acting on the elbow. Under axial loading of the elbow, the coronoid process acts as a buttress against the distal humerus preventing a posterior elbow instability whereas the coronoids' anteromedial facet stabilizes the elbow joint against a posteromedial rotational instability under varus stress [1, 2]. Conversely, the coronoid process acts as a stabilizer against a posterolateral rotational instability during valgus stress. On the medial side of the coronoid process, the medial collateral ligament (MCL) inserts at the sublime tubercle, whereas the annular ligament as part of the lateral collateral ligament complex (LCLC) inserts at the lesser sigmoid notch [3, 4].

Injuries to the coronoid rarely occur in isolation but are usually part of complex injuries to the stabilizing (bony and soft tissue) structures of the elbow [5]. Common injury patterns are [1] the combination of an elbow dislocation with bony injuries to the coronoid process and the radial head which was termed the "terrible-triad" lesion of the elbow, [2] the combination of an injury to the lateral collateral ligament complex and the anteromedial facet of the coronoid process, and [3] coronoid injuries as part of complex proximal ulna fractures such as Monteggia-like lesions [6].

When treating injuries of the coronoid process, the combination of injuries to the osseous and soft-tissue stabilizers are decisive for the treatment strategy as the resulting instability of the elbow depends on the combination of the injuries. A varus and posteromedial rotational instability especially occurs if an injury of anteromedial facet is accompanied by an injury to the lateral collateral ligament complex [7, 8]. Accordingly, the coronoid becomes a more important stabilizer for a valgus and posterolateral rotational instability if the radial head is injured [9, 10].

For the classification of fractures of the coronoid process, three different classifications are available that are based on the fracture morphology or considerations with regard to the mechanism of the injury [11–13]. The Reagan and Morrey classification is solely based on the height of the fracture in relation to the total height of the coronoid in a lateral X-ray of the elbow, with fractures involving only the tip of the coronoid (type I), less than 50% of the coronoid height (type II), or >50% of the coronoids' height (type III) [11]. Adams et al. based their classification on patterns from computer tomography scanning and expanded the Regan-Morrey classification comprising transverse fractures of the coronoid process with oblique anteromedial (type 4 AM) and oblique anterolateral fractures (type 4 AL) [12]. The most comprehensive classification was described by O'Driscoll, which distinguishes between fractures of the coronoid tip, the anteromedial facet, and the coronoid base that are further divided in subtypes depending on the size and extent of the fracture fragment (Fig. 71.1) [13, 14]. We mainly use the latter in our clinical practice, since in our view the mechanism of the injury is best considered in the O'Driscoll classification.

Treatment Options

Surgical treatment of coronoid fractures is still debated, as there are only few studies with small case series on coronoid process injuries that do not allow for clear indications when

V. Rausch (✉)
BG University Hospital Bergmannsheil, Center for Orthopedic and Trauma Surgery, Bochum, Germany

L. P. Müller · K. Wegmann
University Hospital Cologne, Center of Orthopedic and Trauma Surgery, Cologne, Germany
e-mail: lars.mueller@uk-koeln.de; kilian.wegmann@uk-koeln.de

© Springer Nature Switzerland AG 2022
W. B. Geissler (ed.), *Wrist and Elbow Arthroscopy with Selected Open Procedures*,
https://doi.org/10.1007/978-3-030-78881-0_71

tip anteromedial basis

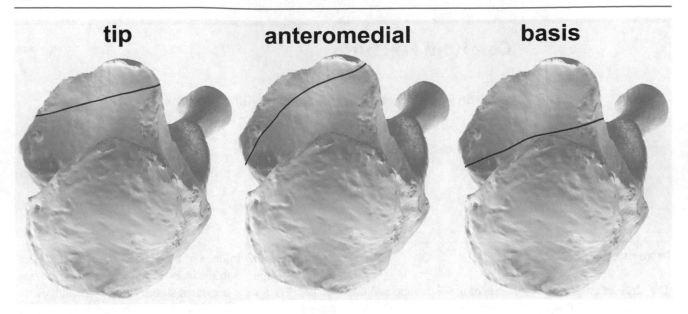

Fig. 71.1 O'Driscoll classification of coronoid process injuries. Fractures of the coronoid tip usually occur in terrible triad injuries and can be further classified in smaller (≤2 mm) or larger (>2 mm) fragments. Fractures of the anteromedial facet are located between the coronoid tip and the sublime tubercle (subtype 1) but can also include the tip (subtype 2) and the sublime tubercle (subtype 3). A fracture of the coronoid basis involves >50% of the coronoid height and is regularly associated with more complex injuries to the proximal ulna. O'Driscoll made the distinction between the subtypes whether a fracture of the olecranon was present (subtype 2) or not (subtype 1)

they should be treated surgically. Therefore, recommendations on the treatment are based on expert opinion and biomechanical studies that investigated the stability of the elbow after simulated injuries.

In general, the presence of accompanying injuries of the radial head and the adjacent soft-tissue stabilizers are crucial for the indication of operative treatment. In the absence of further bony injuries, operative treatment of large tip fractures >50% of the coronoid height is well established due to solid biomechanical studies [9]. A simultaneous radial head fracture can occur with or without a dislocation of the elbow joint. In case of a dislocation, these so-called "terrible-triad" lesions are mostly recommended for operative treatment to stabilize the elbow [15]. However, if only a small coronoid fracture <25% of the coronoid height is present and a stability of the elbow can be achieved with lateral ligament repair and reconstruction of the radial column alone, operative treatment of the coronoid process is more controversial in that a fixation of the fragment might not be necessary [16]. In the case of a simultaneous radial head fracture, we generally recommend osteosynthesis of fragments >25% of the coronoid height. The type of osteosynthesis used for these injuries and whether an arthroscopic fixation is feasible mainly depends on the size and dislocation of the fragment. Overall, only small case series on arthroscopic treatment of these coronoid fractures are available in the literature [17–22]. Several techniques are described using either cannulated screws from posterior after temporary K-wire reduction or with using an anterior cruciate ligament guide [17].

Alternative techniques include the fixation using an arthroscopic button or sutures alone [18, 19]. Lee et al. also reported good results after an all-arthroscopic treatment strategy of 24 terrible-triad injuries with osteosynthesis of the coronoid, resection, or osteosynthesis of the radial head and arthroscopic lateral ligament reconstruction [23]. In case of larger fragments, we favor one or two cannulated screws inserted posteriorly after temporary reposition of the fragments with K-wires. This osteosynthesis is well suited for arthroscopic fixation of the fragment. If a large tip fragment is only minimally displaced, the coronoid can be visualized arthroscopically, and screws are inserted in the same manner as during an open procedure. Smaller fragments can be fixated with a suture lasso technique or a suture anchor with fixation of the anterior capsule that inserts below the coronoid tip. Although suture anchors on the anterior coronoid can theoretically be inserted through small skin incisions anteriorly, we do not recommend this arthroscopically due to the proximity of the median nerve and the brachial artery although there is believed to be only a small risk to damage these structures [24].

In fractures of the coronoids' anteromedial facet, surgical stabilization is recommended for smaller fragments to avoid varus posteromedial rotatory instability, especially if these extend to the sublime tubercle, thus compromising the insertion of the medial collateral ligament [25]. However, only little evidence is available to support these recommendations. In smaller, minimally displaced fractures without signs of instability or subluxation, nonoperative treatment might therefore be considered [26]. These injuries can theoretically be addressed using cannulated screws from posterior if a large, non-comminuted fragment is present. However, these injuries usually include small rim fractures that can successfully be addressed using buttress plating that necessitates a medial open approach to the elbow. These injuries also regularly require repair of the lateral collateral ligament.

Injuries to the basis of the coronoid process regularly occur as a combination in more complex injuries to the proximal ulna such as Monteggia-like lesions or transolecranon fracture dislocations [27]. These injuries are generally addressed using a posterior approach and plate osteosynthesis.

Authors' Preferred Technique

Arthroscopic-assisted treatment of coronoid fractures is mainly limited by the location, size, and comminution of the fracture. Isolated large shear fractures are the most suitable for arthroscopic osteosynthesis, since plate osteosyntheses for more complex injuries such as comminuted fractures of the anteromedial facet cannot be used arthroscopically. Moreover, additional injuries to the radial head or the collateral ligaments are technically demanding. A significant dislocation of the coronoid process' fragment makes reduction even more difficult; therefore, arthroscopic treatment is best suited only if the fragment is minimally displaced. In cases of a terrible triad injury where a radial head fracture and reconstruction of collateral ligaments reconstruction is often planned, arthroscopic treatment is possible but technically extremely demanding, which can outweigh the advantage of the reduced surgical trauma of arthroscopic treatment. On the other hand, minimally displaced coronoid fractures without concomitant injuries do not necessarily require surgical therapy. Therefore, a strict selection of patients in whom arthroscopic refixation should be considered is necessary.

The arthroscopic treatment of coronoid fractures is routinely started with a diagnostic arthroscopy. We first apply a posterolateral portal, although an anterolateral can also be used. After the anterolateral portal is established, the anteromedial portal is created using the pass-through technique. Using the anterolateral portal, the radial head can be visualized (Fig. 71.2). This usually provides a sufficient view of the coronoid fracture. Fixation of small cartilaginous injuries is usually not feasible, and they are therefore removed (Fig. 71.3). The fracture can usually be mobilized using a raspatory, and the fracture gap can be cleared with a dissector (Fig. 71.4). Depending on the size of the coronoid fragment, one or two K-wires are then advanced percutaneously from dorsal to the fracture bed (Fig. 71.5). We recommend

inserting the K-wires angulated and ascending into the coronoid fragment to increase stability and bony contact to the definite osteosynthesis. The fracture fragment is then reduced and held, e.g., with the raspatory or an arthroscopic hook, and the K-wires are advanced through the fracture fragment (Fig. 71.6). The K-wires should not be placed too close to the joint cartilage to avoid intra-articular screw penetration. After measuring the screw length, one or two cannulated screws are inserted dorsally. We prefer partially threaded compression screws to increase interfragmentary compression of the fracture (Figs. 71.7 and 71.8).

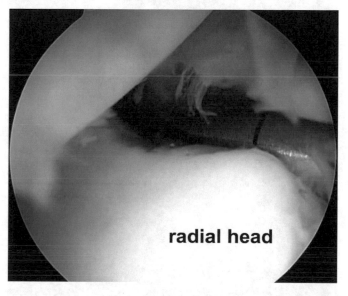

Fig. 71.2 Arthroscopic treatment of a terrible triad injury. Through the anterolateral portal, the radial head can be visualized. In this case, a small anterior cartilaginous injury of the radial head was present and was excised

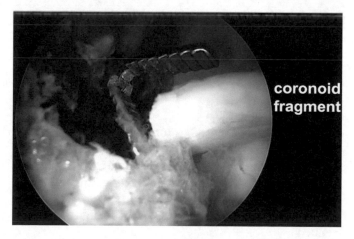

Fig. 71.3 Arthroscopy of the coronoid fracture through the anteromedial portal. Small cartilaginous flakes of the coronoid fracture are excised

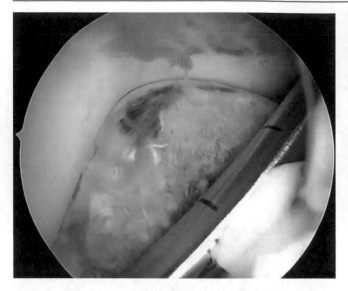

Fig. 71.4 The fracture is then cleared from interposing tissue using a dissector

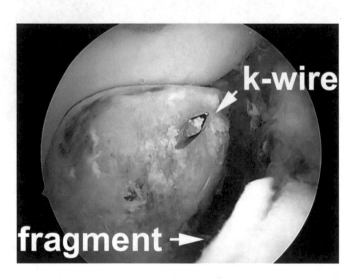

Fig. 71.5 The fractured fragment can be held using an arthroscopic grasp or a raspatorium. K-wires are introduced from posterior and advanced to the fracture

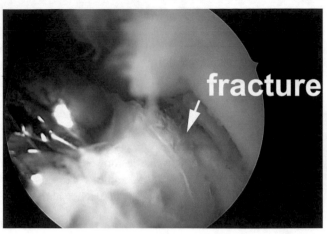

Fig. 71.6 After repositioning of the fracture, the K-wires are advanced to temporarily fixate the fracture fragment. Then, cannulated screws can be inserted from posterior

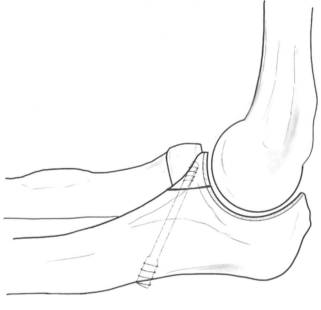

Fig. 71.7 We prefer cannulated compression screws that are angulated from distally to increase bony contact and stability of the fracture

Complications

As described above, the indication for arthroscopic treatment of coronoid fractures is decisive for the success of treatment. An instability of the elbow following these injuries should be addressed adequately, making an additional reconstruction of the collateral ligaments necessary. However, an overly aggressive therapy strategy of coronoid fractures should be avoided.

Overall, few complications have been described for the arthroscopic treatment of coronoid fractures. Reported complications include asymptomatic heterotopic ossifications,

ulnar neuropathy, persistent instability, and non-union of the fracture [17, 20]. A typical complication following fractures of the coronoid and the subsequent immobilization is an elbow stiffness. A minimally impaired elbow movement has also been reported after arthroscopic coronoid fixation, although a comparison to open fracture fixation cannot be drawn due to the small number of published cases.

A persistent instability of the elbow could indicate an overlooked primary instability after the fracture or a failed osteosynthesis. If the osteosynthesis of the coronoid (and the radial head) has healed anatomically, reconstruction of the collateral ligaments might be necessary.

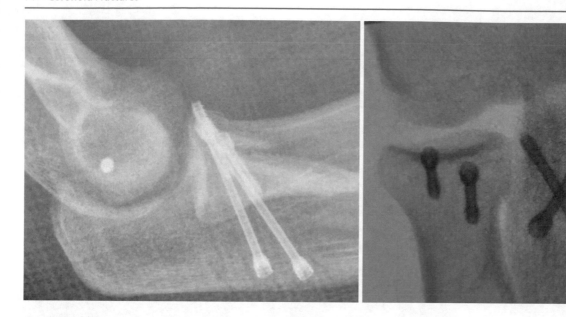

Fig. 71.8 Postoperative x-ray of an arthroscopically treated terrible triad injury. The radial head fracture was also fixated in this case using cannulated compressions screws after temporary K-wire fixation

Postoperative Considerations

In coronoid fractures without further bony injuries or instability, a high primary stability can be achieved with the screw osteosynthesis from dorsal. Therefore, we aim for an early mobilization of the elbow to avoid elbow stiffness. Typically, the patients' elbow is immobilized in a long arm cast for the first 2 weeks after surgery. To protect the elbow against varus and valgus stress, we recommend an elbow orthosis for a total of 6 weeks after surgery.

References

1. Closkey RF, Goode JR, Kirschenbaum D, Cody RP. The role of the coronoid process in elbow stability: a biomechanical analysis of axial loading. J Bone Joint Surg – Ser A. 2000;82(12):1749–53.
2. Hull JR, Owen JR, Fern SE, Wayne JS, Boardman ND. Role of the coronoid process in varus osteoarticular stability of the elbow. J Shoulder Elb Surg. 2005;14(4):441–6.
3. Hackl M, Bercher M, Wegmann K, Müller LP, Dargel J. Functional anatomy of the lateral collateral ligament of the elbow. Arch Orthop Trauma Surg. 2016;136(7):1031–7.
4. Rausch V, Wegmann S, Hackl M, Leschinger T, Neiss WF, Scaal M, et al. Insertional anatomy of the anterior medial collateral ligament on the sublime tubercle of the elbow. J Shoulder Elb Surg. 2019;28(3):555–60.
5. Adams JE, Hoskin TL, Morrey BF, Steinmann SP. Management and outcome of 103 acute fractures of the coronoid process of the ulna. J Bone Joint Surg Br. 2009;91(5):632–5.
6. O'Driscoll SW, Jupiter JB, King GJW, Hotchkiss RN, Morrey BF. The unstable elbow*†. J Bone Joint Surg. 2000;82(5):724.
7. Bellato E, Kim Y, Fitzsimmons JS, Hooke AW, Berglund LJ, Bachman DR, et al. Role of the lateral collateral ligament in posteromedial rotatory instability of the elbow. J Shoulder Elb Surg. 2017;26(9):1636–43.
8. Pollock JW, Brownhill J, Ferreira L, McDonald CP, Johnson J, King G. The effect of anteromedial facet fractures of the coronoid and lateral collateral ligament injury on elbow stability and kinematics. J Bone Joint Surg – Ser A. 2009;91(6):1448–58.
9. Hartzler RU, Llusa-Perez M, Steinmann SP, Morrey BF, Sanchez-Sotelo J. Transverse coronoid fracture: when does it have to be fixed? Clin Orthop Relat Res. 2014;472(7):2068–74.
10. Schneeberger AG, Sadowski MM, Jacob HAC. Coronoid process and radial head as posterolateral rotatory stabilizers of the elbow. J Bone Joint Surg Am. 2004;86-A(5):975–82.
11. Regan W, Morrey B. Fractures of the coronoid process of the ulna. J Bone Joint Surg Am. 1989;71(9):1348–54.
12. Adams JE, Sanchez-Sotelo J, Kallina CF, Morrey BF, Steinmann SP. Fractures of the coronoid: morphology based upon computer tomography scanning. J Shoulder Elb Surg. 2012;21(6):782–8.
13. O'Driscoll SW, Jupiter JB, Cohen MS, Ring D, Mckee MD, Driscoll SWO. Difficult elbow fractures: pearls and pitfalls. Instr Course Lect. 2003;52:113–34.
14. Sanchez-Sotelo J, O'Driscoll SW, Morrey BF. Medial oblique compression fracture of the coronoid process of the ulna. J Shoulder Elb Surg. 2005;14(1):60–4.
15. Chemama B, Bonnevialle N, Peter O, Mansat P, Bonnevialle P. Terrible triad injury of the elbow: how to improve outcomes? Orthop Traumatol Surg Res. 2010;96(2):147–54.
16. Papatheodorou LK, Rubright JH, Heim KA, Weiser RW, Sotereanos DG. Terrible triad injuries of the elbow: does the coronoid always need to be fixed? Clin Orthop Relat Res. 2014;472(7):2084–91.
17. Adams JE, Merten SM, Steinmann SP. Arthroscopic-assisted treatment of coronoid fractures. Arthrosc – J Arthrosc Relat Surg. 2007;23(10):1060–5.
18. Arrigoni P, D'Ambrosi R, Cucchi D, Nicoletti S, Guerra E. Arthroscopic fixation of coronoid process fractures through coronoid tunneling and capsular plication. Joints. 2016;4(3):153–8.
19. Hausman MR, Klug RA, Qureshi S, Goldstein R, Parsons BO. Arthroscopically assisted coronoid fracture fixation: a preliminary report. Clin Orthop Relat Res. 2008;466(12):3147–52.

20. Lee J, Yi Y, Kim JW. Arthroscopically assisted surgery for coronoid fractures. Orthopaedics. 2015;38(12):742–6.

21. Ouyang K, Wang D, Lu W, Xiong J, Xu J, Peng L, et al. Arthroscopic reduction and fixation of coronoid fractures with an exchange rod-a new technique. J Orthop Surg Res. 2017;12(1):9.

22. Shimada N, ShirakiIt K, Saita K. Arthroscopic osteosynthesis for the treatment of coronoid process fractures: a Case Reports in Orthopedics, vol. 2018, Article ID 8512963, 4 pages, 2018.

23. Lee SH, Lim KH, Kim JW. Case series of all-arthroscopic treatment for terrible triad of the elbow: indications and clinical outcomes. Arthrosc – J Arthrosc Relat Surg. 2020;36(2):431–40.

24. Arrigoni P, Cucchi D, Guerra E, Luceri F, Nicoletti S, Menon A, et al. No neurovascular damage after creation of an accessory anteromedial portal for arthroscopic reduction and fixation of coronoid fractures. Knee Surg Sports Traumatol Arthrosc. 2019;27(1):314–8.

25. Doornberg JN, Ring DC. Fracture of the anteromedial facet of the coronoid process. J Bone Joint Surg Am. 2006;88(10):2216–24.

26. Chan K, Faber KJ, King GJW, Athwal GS. Selected anteromedial coronoid fractures can be treated nonoperatively. J Shoulder Elb Surg. 2016;25(8):1251–7.

27. Strauss EJ, Tejwani NC, Preston CF, Egol KA. The posterior Monteggia lesion with associated ulnohumeral instability. J Bone Joint Surg Br. 2006;88(1):84–9.

Distal Humeral Fractures: Hemiarthroplasty

Matthew Richard Ricks, Andrew Keightley, and Adam Charles Watts

Introduction

Distal humeral fractures represent 0.5% of fractures of the adult population [1]. They often follow a bimodal pattern of distribution showing a peak in young adulthood representing high energy injury patterns and a second in the elderly denoting lower energy osteoporotic fractures [2]. Irreducible, unfixable fractures can be a surgical challenge. Non-operative treatment is an option, especially for the patient unfit for surgery or with cognitive impairment, with cast immobilisation for up to 6 weeks. However, following conservative management, poor outcomes have been reported with flexion/extension contractures, functional impairments, or painful non-unions [3–5]. Individual treatment decisions should always be based upon patient, fracture, and surgeon factors and endeavour to allow early mobilisation of the elbow to prevent the risk of stiffness. Improvements in fracture fixation and fragment-specific plating have led to an increased success in operative fixation strategies. However, achieving stable internal fixation of these fractures remains difficult due to multiple fracture planes, metaphyseal comminution, small fragment size, and bone quality [6].

With the ageing demographic in developed nations, the number of distal humerus fractures and the requirement for elbow arthroplasty procedures for trauma are increasing, but overall numbers remain low [7]. Total elbow arthroplasty can produce satisfactory outcomes for trauma and may be superior to osteosynthesis in the older population [8, 9]. However,

the use of arthroplasty comes with different complications, including aseptic loosening, osteolysis, and polyethylene wear. Distal humeral hemiarthoplasty (DHH) for the treatment of unfixable acute distal humeral fractures is an alternative solution. It has possible advantages of bone preservation, no polyethylene bearing wear, reduced humeral torque stress, no ulna component to fail, and no postoperative loading restrictions.

Indications

The primary indication for distal humeral hemiarthroplasty is an acute multi-fragmentary intra-articular fracture of the distal humerus that is not amenable to osteosynthesis in elderly patients who are suitable for surgical intervention. Some advocate total elbow arthroplasty in this population, reserving hemiarthroplasty for the younger cohort when osteosynthesis is not possible. It is a requirement of hemiarthroplasty that there is no fracture of the coronoid or radial head that will compromise elbow stability. Pre-existing painful arthrosis is an indication for total elbow arthroplasty. Open injuries would normally be managed with wound toilet and debridement and a staged arthroplasty.

The typical patient would be an active older patient. In younger patients, every attempt should be made for successful fracture fixation as there is some evidence that the outcome of hemiarthroplasty is worse in this group [7]. In the older patient with low functional demands, conservative management may be a suitable alternative.

In the setting of a failed conservative treatment or osteosynthesis with a distal humeral non-union, a hemiarthroplasty can be used. Delayed hemiarthroplasty has been associated with a reduced ROM, functional outcome scores, and an increased complication rate when compared to the use in acute fractures. This may be as a result of pre-existing joint contracture, collateral instability, or a compromised radial or ulna joint surface [10].

M. R. Ricks
Wrightington Hospital, Upper Limb Unit, Wigan, Lancashire, UK
e-mail: matthew.ricks@wwl.nhs.uk

A. Keightley
Royal Surrey Hospital, Department of Trauma and Orthopaedics, Guildford, Surrey, UK

A. C. Watts (✉)
University of Manchester, Wrightington Hospital, Upper Limb Unit, Wigan, Lancashire, UK
e-mail: adam.watts@elbowdoc.co.uk

W. B. Geissler (ed.), *Wrist and Elbow Arthroscopy with Selected Open Procedures*,
https://doi.org/10.1007/978-3-030-78881-0_72

Contraindications

Absolute contraindications to a distal humeral hemiarthroplasty are a contaminated open fracture or chronic infection. Relative contraindications include younger patients where fixation is preferred and older patients with low functional demands or comorbidities that makes surgery high risk. Olecranon fracture is not a contraindication as these can be treated successfully with osteosynthesis of the olecranon combined with a hemiarthroplasty of the elbow [11, 12]. Pre-existing painful arthritis is a contraindication to distal humeral hemiarthroplasty. Radiological signs of arthritis and arthritis of the greater sigmoid notch or radial head discovered intraoperatively in a patient without preinjury symptoms are relative contraindications; consideration may be given to conversion to total elbow arthroplasty, but these decisions have to be made on an individual basis.

Technique and Tips and Tricks

Step 1. Preoperative Planning and Patient Positioning

Preoperative planning is important when managing complex distal humeral fractures. Routinely plain radiographs and CT imaging is undertaken to allow operative planning and to understand the fracture configuration. The need for arthroplasty should be considered when there is a multifragmentary triplanar fracture, when the fracture is low on the condyles, where there is severe impaction of the articular surface or where there is insufficient subchondral bone to permit adequate fixation. An assessment of the patient's physiological fitness to withstand surgery and cognitive function to comply with postoperative rehabilitation is required.

The surgery is performed with the patient placed in a lateral decubitus position with the limb over a bolster and without the use of a tourniquet. Intravenous antibiotics are administered according to local policies, and consideration should be given to the use of intravenous tranexamic acid.

Step 2. Surgical Approach

A direct posterior midline incision is performed with full thickness elevation of skin flaps from the fascia to preserve the subcutaneous neurovascular supply. The ulnar nerve is identified proximally resting on the intramuscular septum on the medial border of triceps, and an in situ decompression is performed through the cubital tunnel and between the two heads of FCU. The nerve is not elevated from its bed to

reduce the risk of perineural adhesion or ischaemia. Care is taken to protect the nerve throughout the procedure, but no loop or sling is placed around the nerve.

A triceps on lateral paraolecranon approach is used by the authors to maintain the integrity of the extensor mechanism and to aid soft tissue balance [13]. A medial window is created using cutting diathermy through the medial border of triceps down to the medial column of the distal humerus. Retaining a small strip of triceps aponeurosis on the medial side of the window facilitates suture repair on closure (Fig. 72.1). This longitudinal window allows exposure to the medial ridge of the distal humerus and the posterior olecranon fossa. The lateral window is created using cutting diathermy through the anconeus fascia 1 cm lateral to the ridge of the proximal ulna, the fascia is elevated off the anconeus muscle to reach the ulna, and the plane between the ulna and anconeus is developed and extended proximally to split the triceps aponeurosis leaving 2/3 medial and 1/3 lateral to the split. This cuff of fascia attached to the olecranon is left to facilitate suture closure at the end of the operation as described by Stanley [14]. Figure 72.2 shows the lateral fascial tissue for the lateral approach allowing easy tissue closure. Proximally, the nerve to anconeus is at risk as it passes through the medial head of triceps from the radial groove to the anconeus muscle. The surgeon should dissect towards the midline as the exposure is extended deeper proximally to avoid this structure. The lateral column of the distal humerus, posterior capitellum, trochlea spool, and the greater sigmoid notch can be viewed through this window.

The olecranon posterior fat pad is removed, and the distal humerus fracture is examined to confirm the preoperative decision to perform hemiarthroplasty. The fracture configuration, size of fragments, and quality of bone are factors to

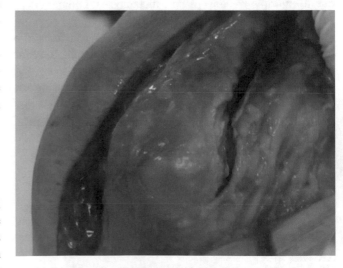

Fig. 72.1 The medial window is through the medial border of triceps. In situ decompression of the ulna nerve is undertaken, but it is not transposed out of its bed

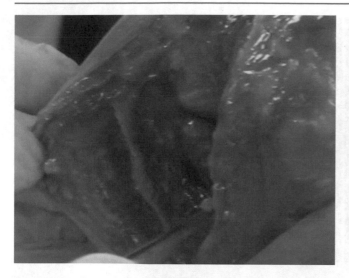

Fig. 72.2 A lateral paraolecranon approach is used between anconeus and the ulna and extending proximally to split triceps

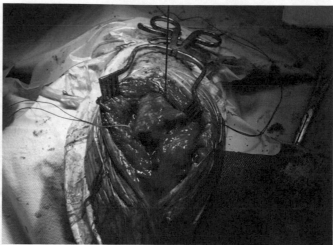

Fig. 72.4 A cerclage wire can be passed around the humeral stem to prevent fracture propagation during rasping

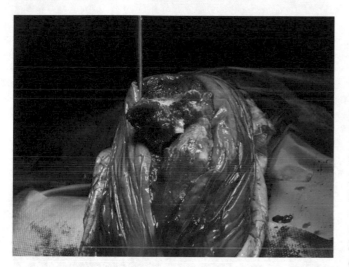

Fig. 72.3 The exposure of the distal humerus following dislocation of the elbow through the lateral window in a fracture case

help decide whether it is reconstructable. An assessment of the radial head and proximal ulnar is undertaken, and the presence of structural bone loss or moderate to severe arthritis may be an indication for total elbow arthroplasty. The distal humerus can be delivered through the lateral window for humeral preparation (Figs. 72.3 and 72.4).

Step 3. Humeral Sizing

Fragments of the humeral spool can be removed easily with a rongeur. The soft tissue attachments of the medial and lateral collateral ligaments and tendon origins on the condylar fragments are maintained. Depending on the fracture configuration, it may be necessary to trim the condylar fragments, in particular, the anterior capitellum, to fit the

prosthesis at the end of the procedure. Sizing of the implant is performed by placing a sizing spool into the greater sigmoid notch and assessing the distribution of contact with the ulna and coverage of the radial head (Fig. 72.5a, b). Size options for the spool are small, medium, large, and extralarge (Fig. 72.6). If in between sizes, the larger size is chosen as this gives better stability and reduced edge loading. Intermediate plus sizes are available that have a larger offset between the capitellum and the trochlea to give greater radial head coverage if needed [15, 16]. It is important to size correctly as an incorrectly sized prosthesis will affect stability and wear of the remaining bone stock. It is important to consider that the humeral stem size is dictated by the spool size. If the humerus is too narrow to take the correct sized stem even with reaming, it may be necessary to go down one size and to use a "plus"-sized spool.

Step 4. Humeral Preparation

If the patient has osteoporotic bone, the authors advocate using a cerclage suture or suture tape with a sliding nice knot around the distal humeral shaft to absorb hoop stresses and to prevent fracture propagation in osteoporotic bone during rasping. In the presence of thick bone, a 5-mm burr is used to gain entry to the humeral canal to allow introduction of the humeral broaches. It is important to work up through the sizes from the starting broach to the size required taking care to ensure the correct rotational alignment. The transcondylar axis is internally rotated by approximately 14 degrees relative to the flat back of the humeral shaft. Flexible reamers can be used if the canal is narrow. The cutting block is built on the humeral rasp, which is seated appropriately when the vault of the olecranon fossa is seen as a hemisphere proximal

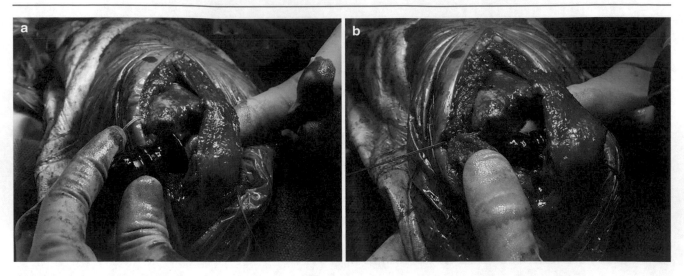

Fig. 72.5 (**a**) A sizing spool is used to determine the best implant size to use. (**b**) The spool is placed into the greater sigmoid notch to assess congruency of the trochlea spool with the notch and coverage of the radial head

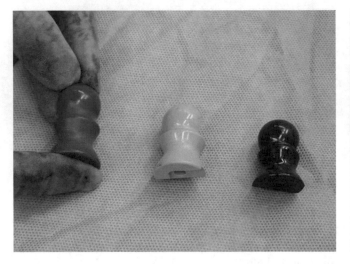

Fig. 72.6 Using the latitude system (wright medical), the anatomical spool sizes are small, medium, large, and extra-large. Between each of these is a + size that improves the ability to match the native anatomy. Illustrated here are the small (black), small + (grey), and medium (red) trial spools

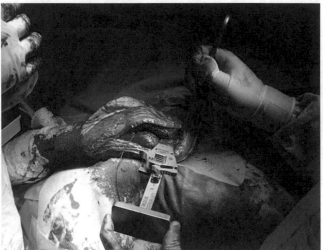

Fig. 72.7 The humeral rasp is used to assemble the cutting block

Step 5. Trial Reduction

to the cutting block (Fig. 72.7). If only an ellipse is seen, then the rasp should be removed slightly; if a roman arch is seen, it should be inserted further into the humerus (Fig. 72.8). When the rasp and cutting block are in the correct position craniocaudally and rotationally, the saw is used to cut around the cutting block with care taken not to damage any surrounding tissues. The rasp and block are removed, the cut completed, and the "gusset broach" used to create space for the internal humeral flanges.

The humeral trial is inserted, and bone graft taken from excised fragments can be chosen to fit underneath the anterior flange (Fig. 72.9). Assessment of restoration of the humeral length can be done in a number of ways, firstly by bringing the fractured condyles back into position and assessing the implant in relation to the epicondylar axis. Secondly, referencing against the native olecranon can be performed, and looking at the triceps tension to see whether the implant is at the correct length [17]. It should be difficult

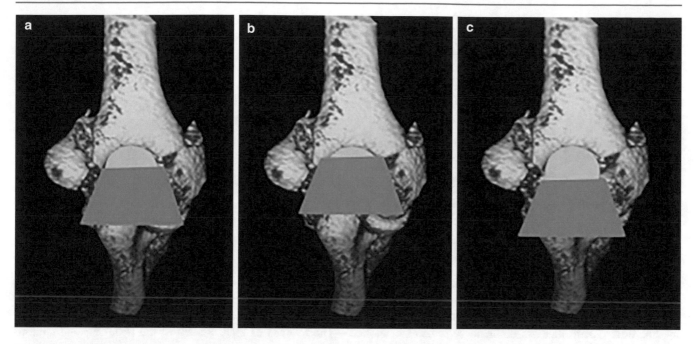

Fig. 72.8 The view of the vault of the olecranon fossa proximal to the cutting block should show a hemisphere (**a**). If it appears as an ellipse (**b**), the rasp should be backed out. If a roman arch (**c**), the rasp should be inserted further in

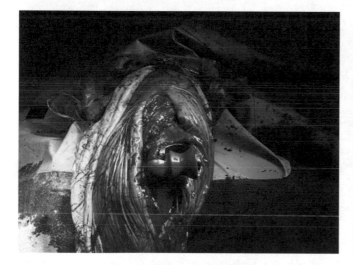

Fig. 72.9 A trial implant is inserted and trial reduction undertaken

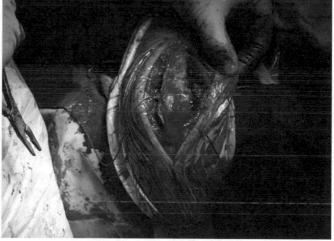

Fig. 72.10 The definitive implant is cemented in the canal and the sutures from the collateral ligaments passed through the cannulated screw of the spool

to reduce the ulna onto the end of the humerus. If it is impossible, the humeral component should be seated further into the humerus; if too easy, then the definitive implant needs to be cemented in a more distal position (Fig. 72.9).

Step 6. Cementation of Definitive Implant and Soft Tissue Repair

Cementation should be performed in a retrograde fashion using a narrow nozel cement gun. A humeral plug is used to ensure good cement pressure, and a definitive hemiartho-

plasty implant is inserted into the canal making sure the rotational alignment is correct. A no. 2 synthetic braided suture is whipped into the medial and lateral ligament complex origins, and the suture material is passed through the cannulated spool screw with a suture passer and tied to the ligament on the contralateral side (Fig. 72.10). Tightening these sutures improves the stability to the hemiarthroplasty further. It is important to assess the stability at this time. It should be impossible to dislocate the hemiarthroplasty in all positions. The extensor envelope is restored by fascial closure of the

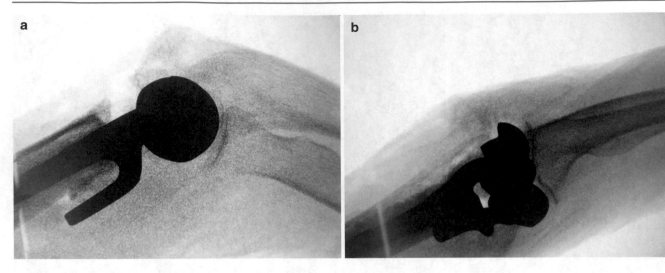

Fig. 72.11 (**a, b**) Intraoperative fluoroscopy can be used to ensure good restoration of the anatomy and reduction of the elbow joint

triceps aponeurosis on the lateral and medial side. On the medial side, ensure that the ulnar nerve remains in its bed throughout the range of movement. If it appears to be under too much tension in flexion or if it is unstable, then a subcutaneous transposition should be performed.

Additional osteosynthesis of the humeral columns is not necessary as fracture union by callus formation is usually seen. If necessary, sutures can be used to appose the fracture fragments to each other or to the yolk of the humeral implant (Fig. 72.11).

Step 8. Rehabilitation

The triceps-on approach allows you to have a congruent and intact extension complex that will allow early range of movement. This in turn will decrease the stiffness this patient group commonly find following surgery. No splints or casts are needed after surgery. A sling can be used for comfort. The patient should be encouraged to commence early active mobilisation with table slides. Strengthening can commence when range of movement is functional.

Conclusion

When faced with an un-reconstructable distal humeral fracture, distal humeral hemiarthroplasty is a reasonable option; however, the results of hemiarthroplasty compared to total elbow arthroplasty for trauma are unknown. It is vital that there is enough bone stock around the humeral stem in the metaphyseal region to provide a stable implant, but non-

union of the columns has not been shown to affect outcomes. The meticulous reattachment of the ligaments and tendons through the cannulated portion of the implant provides increased stability to the arthroplasty.

References

1. Court-Brown CM, Caesar B. Epidemiology of adult fractures: a review. Injury. 2006;37(8):691–7.
2. Robinson CM, Hill RMF, Jacobs N, Dall G, Court-Brown CM. Adult distal humeral metaphyseal fractures: epidemiology and results of treatment. J Orthop Trauma. 2003;17(1):38–47.
3. Aitken SA, Jenkins PJ, Rymaszewski L. Revisiting the 'bag of bones': functional outcome after the conservative management of a fracture of the distal humerus. Bone Joint J. 2015;97-B(8):1132–8.
4. Pidhorz L, Alligand-Perrin P, De Keating E, Fabre T, Mansat P. Distal humerus fracture in the elderly: does conservative treatment still have a role? Orthop Traumatol Surg Res. 2013;99(8):903–7.
5. Srinivasan K, Agarwal M, Matthews SJE, Giannoudis PV. Fractures of the distal humerus in the elderly: is internal fixation the treatment of choice? Clin Orthop. 2005;NA(434):222–30.
6. Clavert P, Ducrot G, Sirveaux F, Fabre T, Mansat P. Outcomes of distal humerus fractures in patients above 65 years of age treated by plate fixation. Orthop Traumatol Surg Res. 2013;99(7):771–7.
7. Palvanen M, Kannus P, Niemi S, Parkkari J. Secular trends in distal humeral fractures of elderly women. Bone. 2010;46(5):1355–8.
8. Cobb TK, Morrey BF. Total elbow arthroplasty as primary treatment for distal humeral fractures in elderly patients*. J Bone Joint Surg. 1997;79(6):826–32.
9. McKee MD, Veillette CJH, Hall JA, Schemitsch EH, Wild LM, McCormack R, et al. A multicenter, prospective, randomized, controlled trial of open reduction—internal fixation versus total elbow arthroplasty for displaced intra-articular distal humeral fractures in elderly patients. J Shoulder Elb Surg. 2009;18(1):3–12.
10. Phadnis J, Watts AC, Bain GI. Elbow hemiarthroplasty for the management of distal humeral fractures: current technique, indications and results. Shoulder Elb. 2016;8(3):171–83.

11. Nestorson J, Ekholm C, Etzner M, Adolfsson L. Hemiarthroplasty for irreparable distal humeral fractures: medium-term follow-up of 42 patients. Bone Joint J. 2015;97-B(10):1377–84.

12. Smith GCS, Hughes JS. Unreconstructable acute distal humeral fractures and their sequelae treated with distal humeral hemiarthroplasty: a two-year to eleven-year follow-up. J Shoulder Elb Surg. 2013;22(12):1710–23.

13. Studer A, Athwal GS, MacDermid JC, Faber KJ, King GJW. The lateral para-olecranon approach for total elbow arthroplasty. J Hand Surg. 2013;38(11):2219–26.e3.

14. Stanley JK, Penn DS, Wasseem M. Exposure of the head of the radius using the Wrightington approach. J Bone Joint Surg Br. 2006;88-B(9):1178–82.

15. Lapner M, Willing R, Johnson JA, King GJW. The effect of distal humeral hemiarthroplasty on articular contact of the elbow. Clin Biomech. 2014;29(5):537–44.

16. Desai SJ, Lalone E, Athwal GS, Ferreira LM, Johnson JA, King GJW. Hemiarthroplasty of the elbow: the effect of implant size on joint congruency. J Shoulder Elb Surg. 2016;25(2):297–303.

17. Phadnis J, Banerjee S, Watts AC, Little N, Hearnden A, Patel VR. Elbow hemiarthroplasty using a "triceps-on" approach for the management of acute distal humeral fractures. J Shoulder Elb Surg. 2015;24(8):1178–86.

Distal Biceps Repair

John J. Fernandez

Introduction

While the overall incidence of reported distal biceps tendon ruptures may appear low, it is likely underreported. Partially retracted tears and partial tears can make initial diagnosis elusive or difficult. Estimates on injury incidence vary from 1 to 5 cases per 100,000 patients per year which support several patient encounters per year in a general orthopedic practice [1, 2].

Patient demographic characteristics have not changed significantly over time. Distal biceps tendon ruptures are predominantly reported in the middle-age groups, with two-thirds of patients aged 35–55 years old. There is a gender incidence bias toward men as they make up over 93–95% of cases [1, 2]. Women compared to men tend to present with injury later in life, with a mean age in the mid-60s for women and mid-40s for men. Women have a relative higher proportion of partial versus complete tears. They also present with a more insidious onset rather than a single acute traumatic event compared to men. Taking these differences into account, to more properly diagnose women there must be a higher index of suspicion [3]. In addition to age and gender bias, other associated risk factors may include elevated body mass index, steroid use, and tobacco exposure [1, 2, 41].

The mechanism of injury is characteristically a single, acute event which overloads the tendon to mechanical failure. It is usually described as an eccentric load or forced hyperextension injury across the elbow during manual labor or sports. The unique nature of the distal biceps tendon and its insertion likely acts as a predisposing factor to attrition of the collagen fibers near the tendon insertion.

The anatomy of the distal biceps tendon and its insertion has been detailed, and may determine the type of surgical repair preferred or selected. The distal biceps tendon is composed of two separate tendon bundles extending from their respective heads. As the two tendon bundles travel distally, they externally rotate 90 degrees around each other before inserting onto the radius at the radial tuberosity. The insertion site is along the apex of the radial tuberosity which in 88% of individuals exists as a single ridge approximately 22 mm long and 15 mm wide [5]. The distal tendon insertion footprint is ovoid, or ribbon shaped with the short head making up approximately 60% of the area inserting distally and slightly anteriorly and the long head occupying the remaining 40% proximally and slightly posteriorly [6].

There is a relative watershed area in the blood supply near the insertion that is hypovascular. The space occupied by the distal biceps tendon between the radius and ulna is decreased by almost 50% in pronation and occupies 85% of the available space [4].

Along the lateral border of the radial tuberosity and opposite the distal tendon insertion, there can be a raised axial ridge or osteophytes of bone in 55% of individuals [7]. This combination of blood supply, anatomic factors, and local pathomechanics likely leads to attritional changes in the substance of the distal tendon and increases the risk of rupture when overloaded [8].

The diagnosis of distal biceps tendon ruptures can reliably be made with a thorough history and physical examination. The patient often relays a history of feeling or hearing a "pop" with a subsequent deformity. The amount of pain, swelling, and ecchymosis is variable. Most cases present with little if any significant pain after the first few days. A reverse "Popeye" deformity can be seen in complete ruptures secondary to distal retraction of the biceps muscle belly. If the rupture is partial or the lacertus fibrosis is intact, there may not be much deformity. A careful examination is necessary to rule out a complete rupture with an intact lacertus fibrosis masquerading as an intact tendon.

On examination, the patient typically has pain and weakness with resisted elbow flexion and particularly supination. These symptoms can be relatively nonspecific. There are other physical exam findings that may increase the sensitivity

J. J. Fernandez (✉)
Midwest Orthopaedics at Rush University, Chicago, IL, USA
e-mail: hand@rushortho.com

© Springer Nature Switzerland AG 2022
W. B. Geissler (ed.), *Wrist and Elbow Arthroscopy with Selected Open Procedures*,
https://doi.org/10.1007/978-3-030-78881-0_73

and specificity of this diagnosis. A "hook test" can be performed to assess the integrity of the tendon. If it is a partial tear or the lacertus fibrosis is intact, this test may be difficult to interpret. The clinician places the patient's shoulder in abduction with the elbow flexed to 90 degrees. In this position, the patient actively supinates the forearm, and the clinician will "hook" their finger under the lateral aspect of the distal biceps tendon if it is intact. The hook test has been found to be up to 100% sensitive and specific for complete distal biceps tendon rupture [9]. A "biceps squeeze test" can also be performed. Similar to the Thompson test for Achilles tendon rupture, the musculotendinous junction of the biceps is squeezed with the elbow at 60–80 degrees and the forearm pronated. A positive test occurs when the forearm does not supinate and implicates a distal biceps tendon tear. The biceps squeeze test is 96% sensitive for a distal biceps tendon rupture [10].

Partial rupture of the distal biceps tendon can make the diagnosis more elusive. Symptoms with partial ruptures may be relatively exertional and more sporadic in comparison to complete ruptures. The mechanism may be unknown or mild by comparison and may be insidious. Partial tearing will have a greater predilection for the long head or short head. Recent magnetic resonance imaging (MRI) analysis of partial biceps tendon ruptures has provided insight into the typical pattern of rupture and patient history. In a series of 77 patients with partial distal biceps tears, injury morphology was found to be significantly related to mechanism. The long head was involved in approximately 70% of cases with the most common injury morphology overall a partial tear of the long head with an intact short head (34%). Interestingly when subdivided by injury mechanism, traumatic ruptures were more likely to result in partial tearing of the short head (78%), whereas atraumatic ruptures were more likely to involve the long head (89%). Patients with a history of smoking were more likely to have an atraumatic mechanism [11].

Imaging is frequently unnecessary and of questionable value in patients whose history and physical examination are consistent with a complete distal biceps tendon rupture. Radiographs should be obtained but are frequently normal. In chronic cases, imaging may reveal degenerative changes of the tendon near the radial tuberosity. MRI may provide added value when the patient history and clinical examination do not correlate and to exclude alternative or additional diagnoses or to uncover partial ruptures. MRI may not be as effective in detecting partial versus complete tears. Data suggests the efficacy of MRI approaches an overall sensitivity and specificity of 92.4% and 100%, respectively, in detecting distal biceps tendon ruptures; 100% and 82.8% sensitivity and specificity, respectively, for complete tears; and 59.1% and 100% sensitivity and specificity, respectively, for partial tears [12]. Ultrasound has been described as an alternative and more cost-effective diagnostic tool [13]. This modality

rivals MRI in terms of sensitivity and specificity and may be more effective at differentiating between complete and partial tears than MRI, but is more technician dependent [14].

Indications

Treatment recommendations and indications will ultimately depend on the patient's perceived losses and future goals balanced against the intrinsic risks and cost of treatment. It is important to educate the patient on the possible outcomes of the various treatments available and their included risks and benefits.

Nonoperative Treatment

Nonoperative treatment of distal biceps tendon ruptures should always be considered and presented to the patient as a reasonable alternative. There can be a variable cosmetic deformity based on muscle mass, retraction, and future atrophy. Significant pain is unusual in the long-term follow-up but can be modest at the beginning [25].

Functional losses following distal biceps tendon ruptures are mostly attributable to deficits in supination strength (30–60%) and endurance (40–80%), flexion strength (20–30%), and endurance (30%) [17–21, 25, 27]. While these losses are measurable and fairly reproducible, several studies have demonstrated patients can have an acceptable level of satisfaction and tolerable functional loss. This may be based on patient physical demands and improvements in strength over time [22, 23, 25].

The decision to pursue nonsurgical management of distal biceps ruptures should be a shared clinical decision-making process trying to match patient expectations against possible limitations. Patients with lower functional demands or greater risks to surgery, particularly the elderly, may note a residual loss in strength and endurance to be acceptable thereby avoiding surgical treatment.

Operative Treatment

Historically, initial treatment recommendations were surgical with the first repair described in 1898. Repairs were advocated either directly to the insertion site or indirectly to the adjacent brachialis tendon. The first largest and detailed review of surgical cases was authored by Dobbie in 1941 in which he catalogued 75 cases [15]. He described the results of direct repair to the radial tuberosity compared to indirect repair to the local soft tissues. The functional results were deemed good to excellent and equivalent between both groups, but he noted an increased difficulty and relatively high complication rate associated with direct repair the tuberosity attributable to injuries of the radial nerve. It was felt that supination power was of secondary importance and could be ignored or compensated by other muscles. His conclusion was that distal biceps tendon ruptures require operative repair but that direct repair was difficult and dangerous and indirect repair to the surrounding soft tissues was recommended.

Twenty years later, Boyd and Anderson, in response to the challenges of direct repair, described a dual-incision technique exposing the radial tuberosity and repairing the tendon to a "trap door" in the bone through an incision along the posterior forearm [16]. This minimized the extent of the anterior exposure and consequently decreased the risk to the nerves. This revived the concept of direct surgical repair as a safe treatment alternative.

While diminishing the risk to nerve injury, the dual-incision technique is associated with an increased risk of synostosis and motion limiting heterotopic ossification [42, 43]. Modifications were added to the dual-incision technique to decrease these risks. Unfortunately, there have been continued reports demonstrating a significantly increased risk of synostosis and motion limiting heterotopic ossification with the dual incision technique. Most large series demonstrate this difference with some showing as much as a two- to threefold difference [44–46, 51, 53]. This can be responsible for significant morbidity including reoperation.

With the advent of newly developed anchoring devices, there was a revival in the use of the single-incision technique to repair distal biceps tendons. These devices allowed for a more limited anterior exposure, while still providing excellent strength.

The initial cortical anchoring techniques described the use of suture anchors placed into the radial tuberosity. Based on their design at the time, these anchors did not allow for creation of a socket in the radial tuberosity. They were also more difficult to secure to the tendon as these anchors had to be deployed into the bone first, after which the tendon was secured down to the anchor [54–56]. This limited the use of a more secure locking suture in the tendon.

The use of a cortical button for distal biceps tendon repair was first described by Fernandez et al. in 1997 [57]. They described using the Endobutton (Smith & Nephew, Andover MA, USA) suture anchor which was previously only used in knee reconstruction. This novel technique utilized a single-incision exposure and allowed the tendon to be fixed to the suture prior to anchoring the tendon to the tuberosity. This allowed for use of a socket in the radial tuberosity if desired. It also permitted use of more secure suture methods in the tendon itself. Since their original description, there has been a resurgence in utilizing the single-incision technique for distal biceps repair.

The approximate strength of the native intact distal biceps tendon has been shown to be 204–211 N before failure [59, 60]. The forces necessary to flex the elbow against gravity using the biceps exclusively are much lower ranging from 25 to 123 N [61]. The strength of cortical button fixation surpasses these forces and has been shown to be superior to bone tunnels, interference screws, and suture anchors making it an ideal device [58, 61]. It is recognized that suture anchors and bone tunnels also have good strength characteristics as shown clinically, but these are weaker biomechanically in comparison to cortical button constructs. A systematic review looking specifically at repair techniques revealed a significantly lower complication rate with cortical button and bone tunnel methods in comparison to suture anchors and intraosseous screws [47]. In another systematic review, cortical button fixation performed best in comparative biomechanical studies [53].

While the risk to major nerves has significantly decreased over time with the single-incision approach, there still exists a higher incidence of overall nerve injuries, mostly transient, in comparison to the dual-incision approach. There have been several large series, including meta-analysis and systematic reviews that have shown an incidence of 9–24% symptomatic involvement of the lateral antebrachial cutaneous nerve (LABCN) [44, 45, 51]. In the only prospective randomized control trial, the occurrence was as high as 40% [52]. It should be carefully noted that these injuries are almost always minor and transient and very rarely affect final outcome. The frequency of injuries to major nerves, like the posterior interosseous nerve (PIN), has been shown to be equivalent between single- and dual-incision groups in most reviews [48]. In one large series of 784 patients, the incidence of PIN injury was four times higher in the dual-incision group [49, 50].

Other criticisms of the single-incision approach are the difficulty in reattaching the distal biceps tendon to the anatomic foot print. This has been studied biomechanically in both the lab and clinically. Schmidt et al. have done work defining the anatomic footprint in detail, including the individual contributions of the short and long head bundles [6]. They have also demonstrated the differences between an anterior and anatomic insertion moment and their impact of supination forces particularly at neutral and into supination [62]. He and his group have validated the impact of the "cam" effect from the radial tuberosity on supination moment and how a defect created in the tuberosity may affect supination biomechanics [37]. The actual clinical impact of these findings appears to be less significant if not uncertain. One clinical series demonstrated a supination strength difference of 12% at neutral and 15% at 60 degrees of supination. That same series used MRI to demonstrate the differences in the tendon insertion sites. They also noted the negative pathologic changes inflicted on the supinator from the dual-incision approach. This was felt to be detrimental to supination strength [63]. In a more recent and larger series, the comparison determined a nearly 20% improvement in supination strength with the single- versus dual-incision technique. This was attributed to a more careful placement of the insertion site through the anterior approach. They felt the posterior approach was injurious to the supinator and that the tuberosity was diminished with the defect created [64].

There have been several clinical studies comparing the differences between the modified dual-incision and single-incision techniques including a prospective randomized control study [41, 52, 53, 65–67]. These have demonstrated similar long-term clinical outcomes, including return to function, satisfaction, motion, and strength. Some have shown some differences in complications rates with single-incision techniques trending higher rates of temporary neuropraxias of sensory nerves and dual-incision techniques trending higher losses in motion and motion limiting heterotopic ossification.

Our preferred method of distal biceps tendon repair utilizes a single-incision approach anchoring the tendon with a cortical button into the radial tuberosity.

Contraindications

Clinical outcomes with nonoperative treatment, while not superior to operative treatment, are relatively good. This makes the contraindications relative and dependent on individual patient characteristics and functional needs.

The functional needs of the patient need to be assessed critically. Surgical treatment should only be considered if it is felt that the expected losses in strength and endurance with nonoperative treatment will not meet the patient's functional demands.

The patient should be relatively healthy and not have significant risks with regard to wound healing, infection, and general surgical stress. The ability to cooperate with postoperative restriction, splinting, and rehabilitation is a prerequisite for surgical repair.

Patient age is not an absolute contraindication but should be considered. With advancing age, patients have a higher incidence of comorbidities. Functional demands and requirements also tend to diminish with age.

The default position for management of distal biceps tendon ruptures should begin with nonoperative treatment. Surgical treatment should only be chosen when the risk-benefit analysis is favorable for the patient.

Technique

Preparation

We recommend a supraclavicular regional anesthetic block with conscious sedation. In addition to the medical advantages, it allows for a more careful transition from anesthesia. There are reports of re-rupture occurring in the acute perioperative phase while the patient is awakening but not yet fully cooperative.

In all cases, we have a semitendinosus tendon allograft ready and available in case it is needed. We have seen cases present as acute injuries only to later find them as acute-on-chronic with a poor-quality tendon or tendon defect.

The patient is placed in a supine position with the arm on a hand table. A fluoroscopy unit should be available and positioned at the head of the table. A sterile tourniquet is utilized to allow for removal and reapplication if vascular access or repair is necessary. A thorough exsanguination after elevating the arm for several minutes is valuable as vessel identification and control is critical to success (Fig. 73.1).

Surgical Approach and Exposure

We prefer a single-incision anterior approach. This allows for an extensile exposure, if necessary, to retrieve and prepare the tendon. By becoming familiar and comfortable with

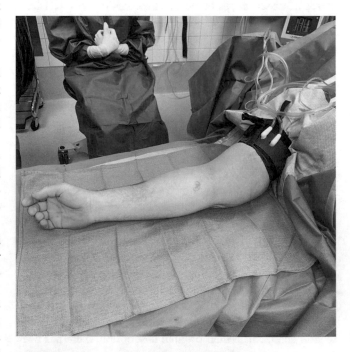

Fig. 73.1 Arm on hand table with sterile tourniquet

this approach, the surgeon will have more available options if they become necessary.

Transverse incisions have been described at both the elbow anterior flexion crease and more distally at the level of the radial tuberosity. The exposure of the radial tuberosity with a transverse incision is more limiting, and safe instrumentation with guide pins and reamers is more difficult. We find a longitudinal incision to be ideal for exposure which allows for extension proximally and distally as necessary.

Reference lines are marked first to establish the ideal position of the incision (Fig. 73.2). Fluoroscopy is used to assist in marking a line over the anterior forearm following the course of radius with the elbow held in full extension and supination (Fig. 73.3). A second line is marked crossing the first line at the apex of the radial tuberosity (Fig. 73.4). A third line is placed over the major anterior elbow flexion crease. The medial edge of the brachioradialis is palpated proximally and marked. This will feel like a "'soft spot" just radial to the anterior center of the forearm (Fig. 73.5).

A longitudinal incision is made starting 1–2 cm distal to the elbow flexion crease and along the course marked over the radius and just medial to the brachioradialis. A common misstep is to make the incision too lateral. This makes it more difficult to retract the brachioradialis during exposure of the radial tuberosity. It also places the superficial nerves at greater risk for injury from traction. The incision should almost appear to be radial to the center of the forearm. The center of the incision will include the crossed line at the radial tuberosity and extended an equal distance distally. The incision is extended distally and proximally as needed for

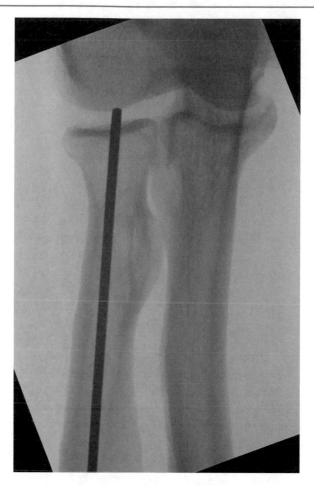

Fig. 73.3 Longitudinal line marked following radius shaft

additional exposure. In cases requiring an extensile exposure, such as chronic ruptures, the incision can be extended to the elbow flexion crease and then extended across the crease to the medial border of the biceps and brachialis and over the median nerve and brachial artery. The incision can also be extended proximally as needed particularly if the biceps needs to be mobilized.

The initial dissection should be careful and deliberate to avoid vessel bleeding and inadvertent nerve injury. There can be several large crossing veins interconnecting the basilic vein medially and the cephalic vein laterally (Fig. 73.6). These should be ligated to avoid tearing them during the exposure. While we prefer vessel clips for the deeper vessels, we recommend an absorbable, braided suture superficially. Superficial vessel clips can erode through the skin or become a foreign body irritant.

The lateral antebrachial cutaneous nerve (LABCN) must be found proximally and traced out distally (Fig. 73.7). It is easier to find the main trunk or larger branches at the most proximal extent of the wound and then trace it out distally. It will be exiting from beneath the biceps tendon laterally and proximally. As it travels distally, it will have a variable branching pattern and course. It is important to re-confirm

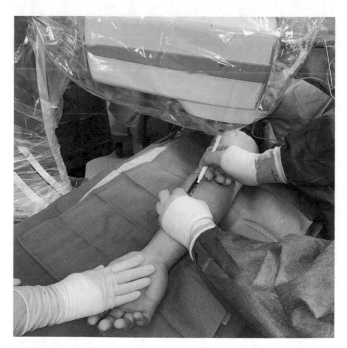

Fig. 73.2 Fluoroscopy used to help mark landmarks

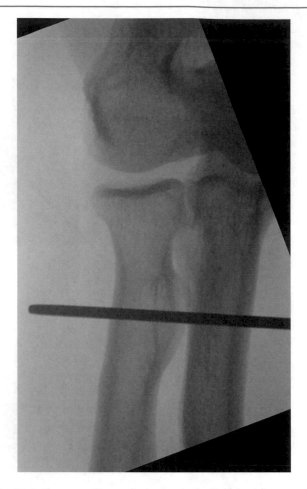

Fig. 73.4 Transverse line marked at level of radial tuberosity

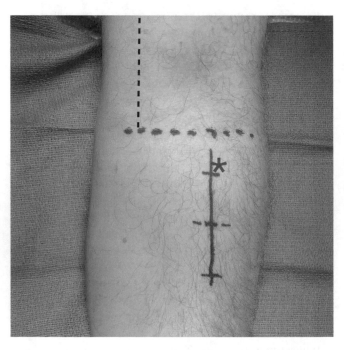

Fig. 73.5 Landmarks marked out including elbow transverse flexion crease. Black dashed line indicates extensile exposure if proximal access is needed. Asterisk indicating "soft spot" just medial to brachioradialis muscle

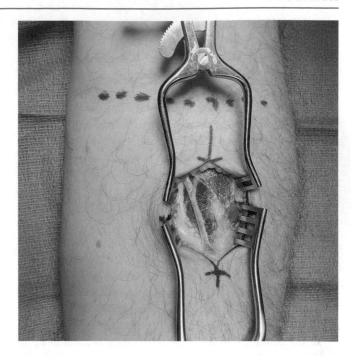

Fig. 73.6 Incision centered over radial tuberosity. Superficial veins encountered and ligated

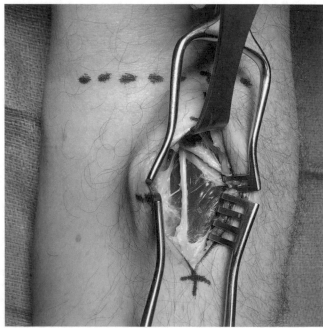

Fig. 73.7 Lateral antebrachial cutaneous nerve identified and mobilized proximally and distally to avoid injury

the course and position of the LABCN before the distal biceps tendon is repaired to assure it is not transposed lateral to the nerve.

The dissection is carried through the deep fascia. There will be perforating vessels in this area which may need to be identified and ligated. If this is a relatively acute repair, there may be ecchymosis or hematoma in the tissues and early fibrous reactive tissue. This can make dissection

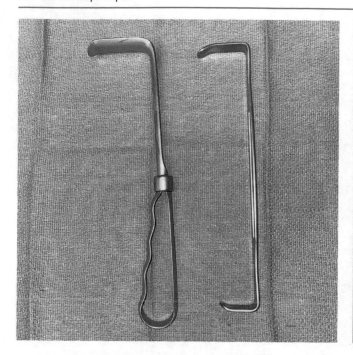

Fig. 73.8 Long, thin, direct retractors preferred for deep exposure. Avoid retractors around the lateral edge of the radius

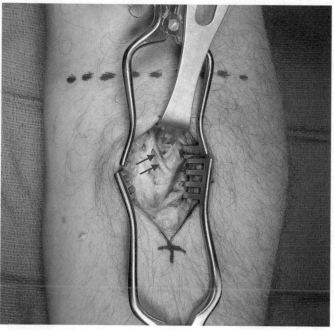

Fig. 73.9 Recurrent vessels branching off radial artery and entering brachioradialis. Blue and red arrows both indicate recurrent vessels that must be ligated

more difficult. Peanut dissector sponges work well here as they can carefully separate the vessels from the surrounding tissues. If the injury is subacute or chronic, a pseudotendon may be present. This can create confusion as it can appear like a tendon and be adherent to the surrounding tissues.

The medial margin of the brachioradialis muscle is mobilized laterally and the common flexor-pronator muscle is retracted medially both with long-angled retractors. A nasal retractor can work well as it is long and thin (Fig. 73.8). Avoid using self-retaining retractors unless superficially, as these can injure the deep vessels and lateral nerves, including the posterior interosseous nerve. Hohmann retractors around the lateral radius should be avoided for similar reasons. These can be used medially but should be avoided laterally. If used, they should be placed carefully and not retracted laterally beyond the midline of the radius.

Dissection progresses deep toward the radial tuberosity. If needed, fluoroscopy can help in reorientation. The radial artery and its recurrent vessels will now become visible (Fig. 73.9). This is one of the most critical parts of the exposure. There is usually one larger recurrent artery passing laterally or obliquely toward the brachioradialis muscle. In some cases, it is several smaller branches. The veins that accompany the arteries here form a plexus surrounding the arteries. These veins can be thin-walled and friable. The radial artery can sometimes be confused for the recurrent vessel. If there is any doubt, the exposure can be extended distally making identification easier. Vascular clips are helpful in taking down the recurrent vessels as multiple clips can

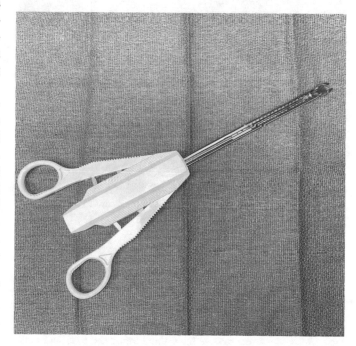

Fig. 73.10 Automatic clip applier

be applied in a small area (Fig. 73.10). Make sure to double clip the larger vessels or artery as the clips can slide or become dislodged. Appropriate sizing of the clips is important to avoid the clip from coming off or not occluding the vessel (Figs. 73.11 and 73.12). Just prior to final repair of the tendon, we recommend deflating the tourniquet to ensure hemostasis.

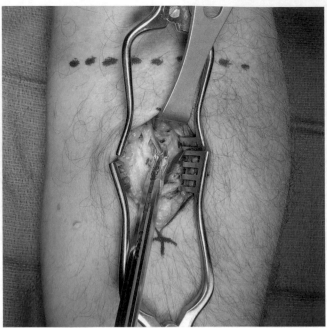

Fig. 73.11 Clipping recurrent vessels with appropriately sized clips

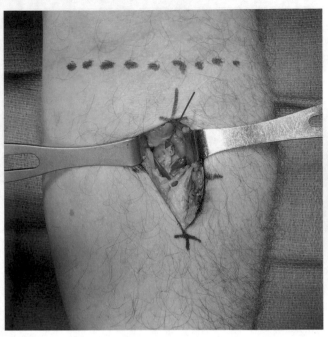

Fig. 73.13 Radial tuberosity exposed. Debride any osteophytes or residual tendon stump

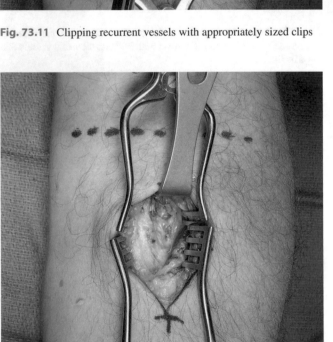

Fig. 73.12 Recurrent vessels ligated and transected to expose radial tuberosity

The radial tuberosity should now be visible (Fig. 73.13). With the forearm in full supination, the apex of the tuberosity is pointing ulnar and 40 degrees anterior [7]. Anteriorly, there is a bare area normally occupied by the bursae, and this is a good landmark to help reorient. There can be a portion of the supinator muscle that wraps around the anterior radius in

this area particularly proximally. There may be a variable amount of tendon still attached to the tuberosity. If there is an axial ridge or excrescences of bone along the anterior tuberosity, this should be debrided with a rongeur leaving the bone smooth.

If the distal tendon is partially torn, it will be visible and have a deformed, bulbous appearance. If there is a complete rupture, the lacertus fibrosis may still be intact and the tendon may be nearby. Gently placing your finger proximally along the brachialis will usually encounter the end of the tendon. It may be tangled onto itself with some early adhesions. If the end of the tendon can be felt, an Allis or Kocher clamp can be used to gently pull the tendon into the exposure.

If the tendon is not easily found, and especially in more chronic cases, a more extensile and proximal exposure may be necessary. The original incision can be extended to the transverse crease and extended medially. This allows more proximal exposure with and angled retractor. The median nerve and brachial artery now become more local to the dissection and should be anticipated. Another option is a longitudinal incision along the medial biceps avoiding the transverse crease. When the tendon is found, it is then carefully tunneled under the skin bridge into the distal and lateral exposure. The ultimate exposure is a combination in which the initial incision is extended proximally and then across the elbow flexion crease and then proximally along the medial biceps in a "step"-shaped fashion.

Preparation of the Distal Biceps Tendon

The distal biceps tendon may be encased in fibrous tissue creating a pseudotendon. This tissue must be resected to allow the tendon to be brought out to its normal length. The distal end of the tendon is resected by at least one centimeter or until healthy appearing collagen fibers are appreciated in the tendon substance (Fig. 73.14). We place the tendon end onto a wood tongue depressor and start serial sectioning similar to the way a nerve would be prepared until we feel there are sufficient healthy collagen fibers visible (Fig. 73.15). The length of the distal biceps tendon extending from the musculotendinous junction to its insertion is approximately 6 cm (63 mm ± 9.4 mm) [24]. This data can serve to guide tendon length when reconstructing the distal biceps tendon with a graft. An extensive tendon debridement can leave the tendon length short making primary repair more difficult without increasing elbow flexion. There is data describing successful repairs performed in excess of 60 degrees of flexion and in some cases 100 degrees [26].

Following the tendon debridement, the fixation suture is placed into the distal tendon (Fig. 73.16). The science of tendon repair is extensive in the field of hand surgery, and there is ample literature on best suture methods for other tendons and ligaments, including the Achilles and cruciate ligaments, respectively. These methods and principles can be extrapolated to the distal biceps tendon. The ideal suture and method would have a high peak strength, minimal deformation under cyclical loading, the ability to hold without slipping or gap-

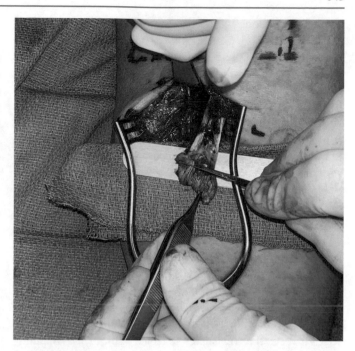

Fig. 73.15 Distal tendon resected over tongue depressor

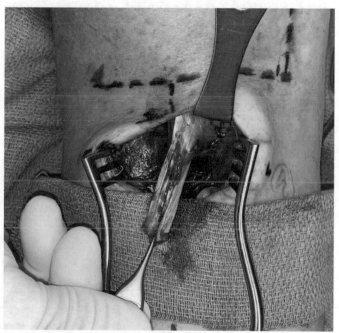

Fig. 73.16 Healthy tendon ready for suture

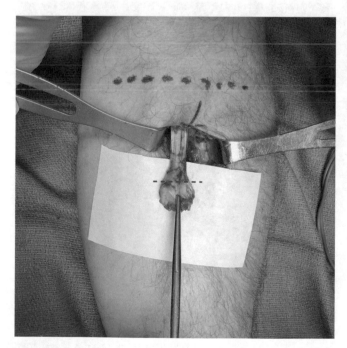

Fig. 73.14 Distal tendon demonstrating degenerative, bulbous tendon fibers

ping, good handling and knot-tying abilities, minimal bulk, and simplicity of application.

A running, locking suture is ideal as it grasps the tendon to minimize slipping and gap formation. Gap formation must be minimized as it can impede tendon healing and promote re-rupture. The Krackow suture method is arguably one of the most studied and utilized for larger tendons and ligaments. With the ability to manufacture a "loop" suture, there are other methods which can incorporate running, locking suture [28, 30, 31]. Greater than 2–3 locking loops is unnecessary as it does not add to the strength of the repair, and the additional loops can loosen over time and contribute to gapping [29]. A second suture can be added to significantly increase the load to failure [29].

An ultra-high-strength braided synthetic suture material is preferred. Polyblend suture materials show better characteristics with regard to load failure, resistance to fraying, and stretching when compared to polyester and absorbable materials. Polyblend sutures do require at least two additional throws for knotting, or six single throws, compared to polyester sutures [33, 34]. A No. 2 size suture, or equivalent, has an ideal strength-to-size property. In the polyblend material, it is superior to a No. 5 size in a polyester suture. This allows placement of multiple strands if desired without increasing bulk to the tendon. Recent developments in suture design now offer a flattened tape structure compared to the conventional round profile. This has been shown to have improved strength as well as resistance to tissue pull-out. The handling characteristics and knot strength are also improved [35, 36].

Our chosen method for suture-tendon fixation is a running, locking-loop technique with 3–4 locking loops in addition to a Bunnell suture [32]. We utilize a looped 1.3 mm SutureTape (Arthrex, Naples, FL) for suture material (Fig. 73.17). This results in four strands of ultra-high-strength suture with excellent tendon holding characteristics minimizing pull-out and gapping. This method is simple, rapid, and reproducible.

The tendon is placed through the loop. Approximately 4 cm from the end of the tendon and proximal to the loop, the straight suture-passing needle is directed from back to front (Fig. 73.18). This creates the first set of locking loops. The suture should be tensioned between throws to take any slack out of the system. The tendon is then passed through the newly created loop, and the needle is again directed back to front approximately 1 cm from the previously placed suture (Fig. 73.19). The needle is not fully advanced allowing the tip to act as a post (Fig. 73.20). The two limbs of the suture loop are then passed in opposite directions around the needle (Fig. 73.21). The needle is then advanced through the tendon creating the second set of locking loops. This is repeated two more times with the last locking loops near the end of the tendon (Figs. 73.22, 73.23, and 73.24).

A single suture can be utilized, and if this is preferred, you can then go on to the anchoring segment. We prefer to add a second suture to the construct so that one suture is used in the tension slide while the other is tied. This also creates redundancy in the repair. We prefer a Bunnell type suture placed utilizing two straight suture-passing needles (Fig. 73.25). The points of entry and exit into the tendon are staggered relative to the previously placed locking loops (Fig. 73.26). We then use a marking pen to color these two suture limbs in a way to distinguish it from other two suture limbs from the previously placed locking suture.

We perform pre-tensioning of the sutures with a manually applied and cyclical load of 90–100 N (20–25 lbs.) for approximately 10 minutes. This minimizes elongation along

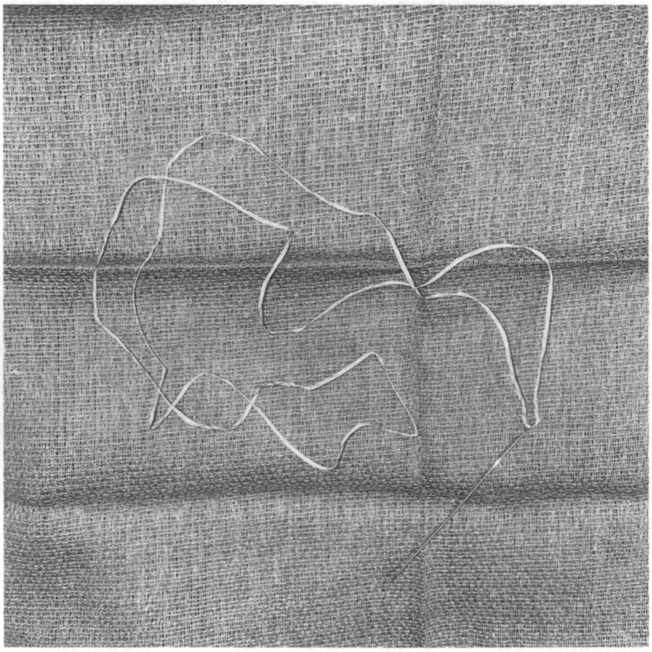

Fig. 73.17 Looped 1.3 mm SutureTape (Arthrex, Naples, FL) on a straight needle

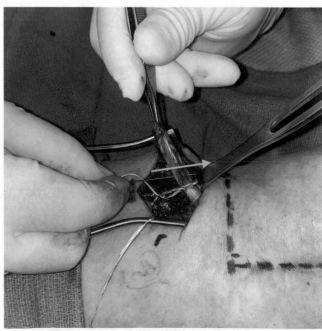

Fig. 73.18 Loop is placed around tendon with needle passed from posterior to anterior approximately 3–4 cm from tendon end. The needle should be passed proximal to the loop

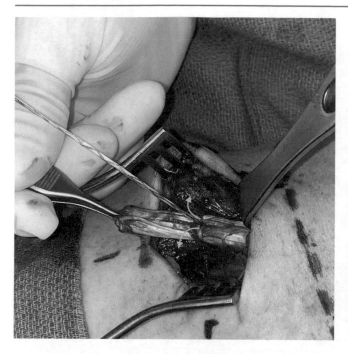

Fig. 73.19 Suture loop is opened and tendon placed through loop with needle ready to advance again from posterior to anterior

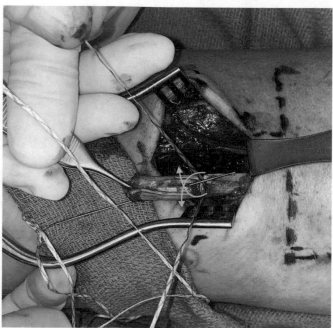

Fig. 73.21 Sutures are placed around the needle in opposite directions to create another locking loop

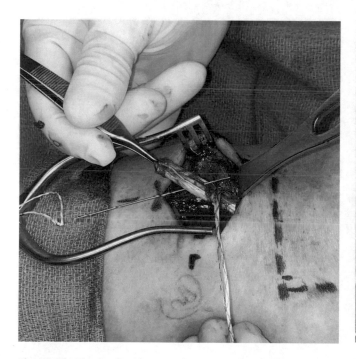

Fig. 73.20 The first locking loop is tensioned, and second pass of needle stopping short until suture is locked around the needle

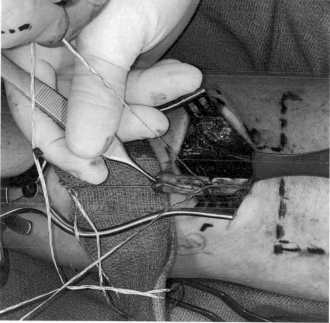

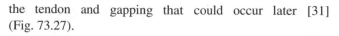

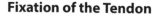

Fig. 73.22 Suture is tensioned after each locking loop is created to take slack out of system

the tendon and gapping that could occur later [31] (Fig. 73.27).

Fixation of the Tendon

We prefer anchoring the distal biceps tendon in a socket created in the radial tuberosity. There is evidence demonstrating

a 27% loss in moment arm at 60 degrees of supination incremental with loss of the tuberosity in creation of a socket [37]. It is unproven if this is clinically relevant. After distal biceps tendon repair and during cycling of forces across the repair, a variable amount of tendon-suture loosening and gapping will occur. Docking the tendon within the tuberosity will compensate for some gapping. We believe that the clinical advantages of minimizing gapping by docking the tendon

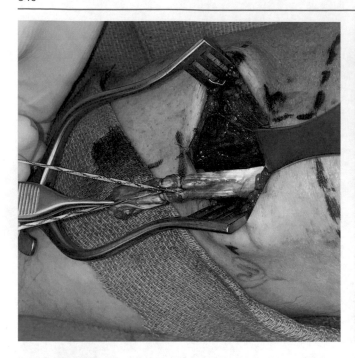

Fig. 73.23 Locking loops are repeated 3–4 times

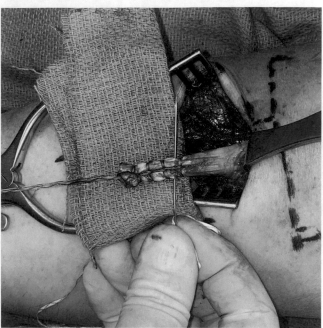

Fig. 73.25 Bunnell suture placed transversely between two most proximal locking loops

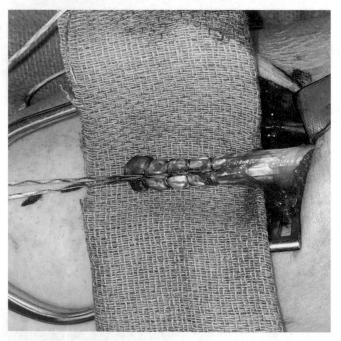

Fig. 73.24 Tendon with multiple locking loops

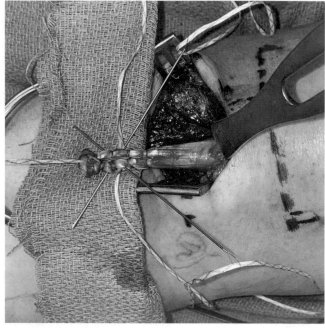

Fig. 73.26 Two straight needles used to criss-cross the suture across the tendon

outweigh the possible losses in moment arm incurred by creation of the socket.

We utilize a single cortical button on the posterior cortex of the radius for fixation of the tendon sutures. There is data revealing a difference in the moment arm contributions from the short and long head tendon bundles depending on forearm rotation [38]. There is no clinical data demonstrating an advantage in separately repairing the short and long head

tendon bundles. We therefore repair the distal biceps tendon as a single element to the insertion point. There are numerous cortical buttons available for use, many of which are specific for distal biceps tendon repair. These buttons can vary in dimension, insertion technique, and instrumentation. We prefer using the Pec button (Arthrex, Naples, FL) for fixation

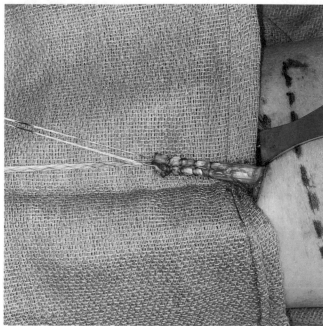

Fig. 73.27 Tendon with locking loops and Bunnell sutures exiting end of tendon and pre-tensioned now prepared for anchoring

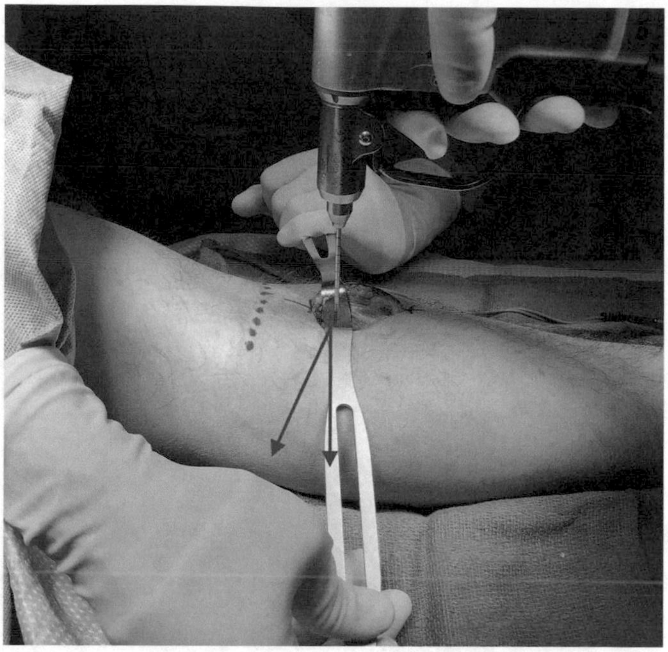

Fig. 73.28 Guide pin in radial tuberosity directed from perpendicular to up to 30 degrees posterior

as the inserter is robust and can be reset. There is also more capacity for multiple suture strands.

After the radial tuberosity is exposed, a socket is created for insertion of the tendon. We utilize cannulated end-cutting reamers. This minimizes bone debris and temperatures in comparison to a high-speed burr. While the forearm is in full supination, the guide pin for the cannulated reamer is placed as close as possible to the apex of the radial tuberosity using fluoroscopic guidance. The guide pin is directed from antero-medial to posterolateral (Figs. 73.28 and 73.29). The flexor-pronator muscles will block how far the pin and reamers can be angled. A Hohmann retractor placed medially can assist in retraction. We avoid bicortical penetration at this stage to minimize the risk to the posterior interosseous nerve. This allows the insertion point and socket to be created as ulnar as possible.

The socket is created by sequentially reaming the bone to a size accommodating the distal biceps tendon (8–9 mm). We begin with a 6 mm reamer on oscillation mode to avoid wrapping up soft tissues (Fig. 73.30). The bone at the tuberosity is relatively soft and allows the subsequent reaming to be done manually in half or full millimeter increments. We prefer this over using power as it allows us to feel the opposite cortex of the radius without penetrating it easily (Fig. 73.31).

The guide pin for the cortical button is then directed through the socket in the radial tuberosity. This should be placed with the forearm in full supination. It can be directed straight posterior, but care should be taken to avoid being too close to the edge of the tuberosity socket. With the forearm

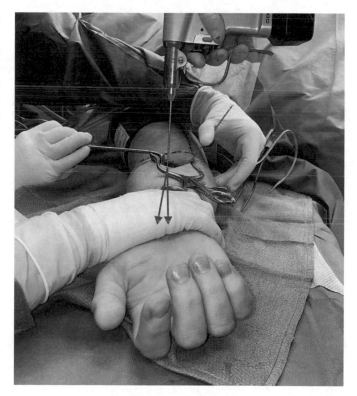

Fig. 73.29 Guide pin in radial tuberosity directed up to 10–30 degrees radial

in full supination, the posterior interosseous nerve passes laterally, 15 mm opposite the apex of the radial tuberosity. More proximally, the nerve is located more anterior. This allows the guide pin to be safely angled approximately

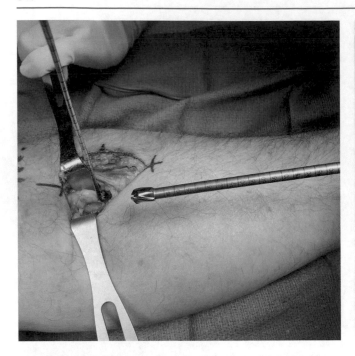

Fig. 73.30 Cannulated reamers used on oscillation to penetrate proximal cortex

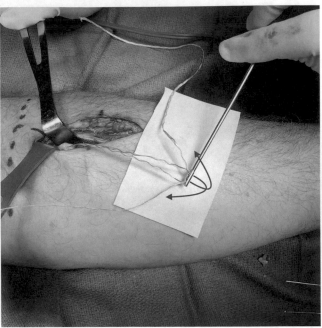

Fig. 73.32 Sutures are passed through cortical button in opposite directions

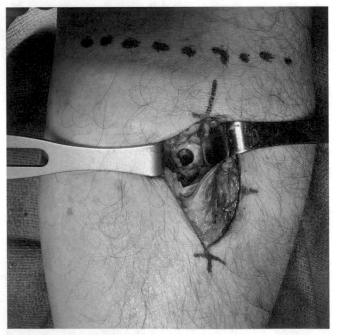

Fig. 73.31 Radial tuberosity with proximal cortex visible with larger corticotomy for tendon end and smaller hole in posterior cortex for cortical button to pass

30 degrees radial from perpendicular and 30 degrees more proximally as necessary to avoid proximity to the socket. This "safe zone" has been demonstrated through several studies [39, 64].

At this point, the tourniquet can be released to check for any significant bleeding. It is easier to control and correct

any bleeding problems before the tendon is secured. The tourniquet can be reinflated if desired to complete the repair.

The tendon sutures can be fixed to the button in two distinct ways: tension lock technique or tension slide technique. The tension lock technique ties the sutures to the button prior to passing the button. This requires estimating the distance between the button and the end of the tendon needed to "flip" the button. This depends on the cortical thickness of the bone and the distance to the first locking suture in the tendon. The tension slide technique inserts the sutures through the button but does not fix them until the button is passed through the radius (Figs. 73.32 and 73.33). After the button is anchored, the sutures are then tensioned thereby pulling the tendon into the tuberosity socket, after which the sutures are tied (Fig. 73.34). We favor the tension slide technique as it is more reproducible and reversible. This technique also allows the repair to be taken down and repeated if necessary. Whether using a tension lock or tension slide technique, the elbow should be flexed to take the tension off the sutures and allow easier advancement of the button or tendon (Figs. 73.35 and 73.36). Fluoroscopic imaging can be used to confirm placement and alignment of the button.

Wound Closure, Splint, and Medication

Irrigation is utilized throughout the operation but particularly during the preparation of the radial tuberosity. We release the tourniquet at least once prior to closure. Our preference is just before the tendon is repaired back to the bone.

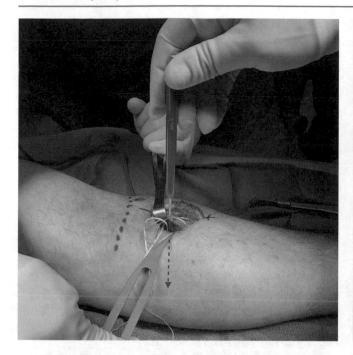

Fig. 73.33 Cortical button passed through corticotomy and through posterior cortex and locked by applying some tension to suture ends

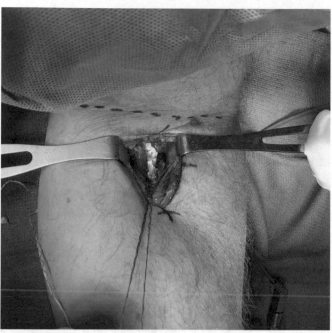

Fig. 73.35 Tension is applied to one set of sutures, while the other set is passed back through tendon with a free needle and tied. The other suture set is then similarly passed and tied

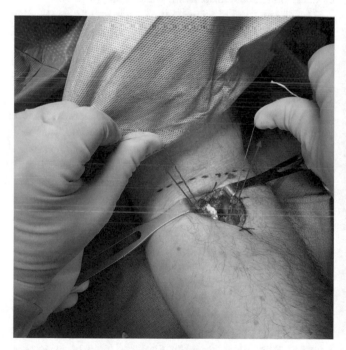

Fig. 73.34 Elbow is in flexion supination, while sutures are tensioned and tendon end is drawn into tuberosity defect

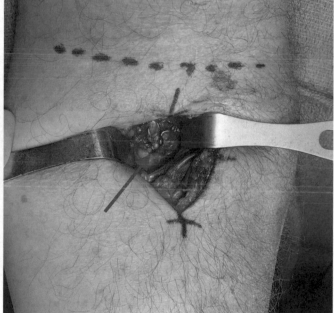

Fig. 73.36 Tendon now fixed to radial tuberosity

A deep drain is encouraged but not routinely used depending on concerns over hematoma or excess bleeding.

Wounds are closed based on preference. We use interrupted, deep, braided absorbable sutures for the subcutaneous layer followed by a running subcuticular wound closure with an absorbable monofilament suture and steri-strips.

A thick padded dressing is applied and the arm and hand are placed in a long arm splint with the elbow positioned in 90 degrees of flexion and the forearm in 45 degrees of pronation. We believe it helps to place the tendon in the radio-ulnar interspace during the early recovery. This decreases excess swelling in the end of the tendon and closes down the dead space to avoid excess bleeding and hematoma.

We try to avoid narcotics if possible and use a tiered approach to pain control. We recommend using a nonsteroidal anti-inflammatory drug for the first 2 weeks postoperatively to limit heterotopic ossification and possible synostosis. This also helps with postoperative pain and swelling. Our drug of choice is celecoxib 200 mg twice daily. This has the added benefit of being cyclooxygenase-2 selective having some protective effect on the stomach. The literature regarding prophylaxis of heterotopic ossification is most extensive in the field of total joint arthroplasty. There is no demonstrable advantage regarding the use of selective or nonselective nonsteroidal anti-inflammatories [40]. There is also no clear indication regarding how long prophylaxis should be utilized.

Postoperative Care

Patients are seen postoperatively at 7–10 days. The patient is seen by the occupational therapist and placed into a removable long-arm splint with the elbow in 90 degrees of flexion and the forearm in supination, neutral, or 45 degrees of pronation. We believe holding the forearm in mid-pronation does not compromise the safety of the repair and closes down the potential space between the radius and ulna which may limit bleeding and hematoma in that area. This position has the added benefit of being more functional with regard to light activities like keyboarding and getting dressed.

Edema modalities, including a compression sleeve, are utilized if needed. Hand strengthening with putty or gripper is utilized. No resistance or weight-bearing is allowed across the wrist or elbow. The splint can be removed for bathing and careful tasks like keyboarding and feeding. The splint must be worn to sleep or when patient may be exposed to risk of falling or unprotected contact.

Range of motion exercises are performed four time per day. Full active motion is allowed across the wrist. Extension across the elbow is allowed only with gravity and only to 40 degrees. Passive flexion is allowed at tolerated. Supination and pronation are also allowed as tolerated but only passively.

At 3 weeks postoperative, the splint is continued without change. Full elbow extension is allowed with gravity. No resistance is allowed across the elbow or forearm.

At 6 weeks postoperative, the splint is discontinued. If there is any contracture to extension or pronation-supination, gentle passive motion is allowed. Significant passive stretching, or use of dynamic or static progressive splinting, is not used until 8 weeks. Resistance across the elbow or forearm is still not allowed.

At 8 weeks postoperative, more significant passive stretching and dynamic splinting can be performed if necessary. Strengthening with resistance across the elbow and forearm begins at 5 pounds and is advanced as tolerated with full strengthening allowed at 10–12 weeks depending on comfort.

At 3–6 months postoperative, the patient is discharged to activities as tolerated without restriction. This assumes there is no significant pain and full motion has been established.

Tips and Tricks

Early timing of the surgery is likely important. Studies have demonstrated a higher incidence of complications with delay in treatment as little as 10 days from date of injury [68, 69]. This may be attributable to the collapse of the soft tissue tunnel occupied by the biceps tendon making the exposure and repair more difficult. Try to schedule these cases as a relative urgency to mitigate these problems.

Have a tendon allograft available in all cases in case it becomes needed. Cases sometimes thought to be acute may be acute on chronic necessitating a tendon graft.

The physical act of suturing the tendon and fixing it to the bone is relatively straightforward. The difficulties and complications predominantly originate from the exposure of the radial tuberosity. Detailed knowledge of the local anatomy is vital to safe exposure of the tuberosity whether utilizing a single- or dual-incision approach.

When exposing the radial tuberosity anteriorly, utilize an appropriate incision and proceed slowly to avoid unnecessary bleeding or injury to the adjacent nerves and vessels. Patients do not usually complain about the length or orientation of the incision. Whether utilizing a transverse, step-cut, or longitudinal incision, create enough exposure to minimize needed retraction of the soft tissues. This usually means using a longer incision if the exposure appears to be more difficult than anticipated.

Avoid applying self-retaining retractors or placing retractors around the lateral edge of the radius. This decreases the tension pressure along the lateral nerves. Utilize hand-held retractors that are thinner and longer at the end.

Release the tourniquet just prior to the final step of tendon fixation. This allows identification and control of excess bleeding without the tendon blocking the exposure. The tourniquet can be reinflated if desired.

Educate the patient on the details of the postoperative recovery. During the early recovery, pain is usually minimal. This may give the patient a false sense of their capabilities. Emphasize the importance of adhering to the postoperative protocol.

Conclusion

Distal biceps tendon ruptures present to orthopedic practices with an incidence making them "frequently infrequent." The indications for operative and nonoperative treatment are well-defined improving our ability to help patients make an informed decision that is individual to them. Research continues to add data that will help guide best practice with regard to treatment, particularly regarding surgical approach and choice of fixation. Outcomes with current surgical techniques are generally very good, regardless of approach or anchoring method, with a relatively low complication rate. The best surgical technique for the patient is likely the one with which the treating surgeon is most familiar. Future techniques should pursue a safe, strong, anatomic reattachment to the radial tuberosity while minimizing risk to surrounding nerves and mitigating the risk to heterotopic ossification.

References

1. Kelly MP, Perkinson SG, Ablove RH, Tueting JL. Distal biceps tendon ruptures. An epidemiological analysis using a large population database. Am J Sports Med. 2015;43:2012–7.
2. Safran MR, Graham SM. Distal biceps tendon ruptures: incidence, demographics, and the effect of smoking. Clin Orthop Relat Res. 2002;404:275–83.
3. Jockel CR, Mulieri PJ, Belsky MR, Leslie BM. Distal biceps tendon tears in women. J Shoulder Elb Surg. 2010;19:645–50.
4. Seiler JG, Parker LM, Chamberland PD, Sherbourne GM, Carpenter WA. The distal biceps tendon. Two potential mechanisms involved in it rupture: arterial supply and mechanical impingement. J Shoulder Elb Surg. 1995;4:149–56.
5. Mazzocca AD, Cohen MS, Berkson E, Nicholson G, Carofino BC, Arciero R, et al. The anatomy of the bicipital tuberosity and distal biceps tendon. J Shoulder Elb Surg. 2007;16:122–7.
6. Jarrett CD, Weir DM, Stuffmann ES, Jain S, Miller MC, Schmidt CC. Anatomic and biomechanical analysis of the short and long head components of the distal biceps tendon. J Shoulder Elb Surg. 2012;21:942–8.
7. Hutchinson HI, Gloystein D, Gillespie M. Distal biceps tendon insertion: an anatomic study. J Shoulder Elb Surg. 2008;17:342–6.
8. Davis WM, Yassine Z. An etiological factor in tear of the distal tendon of the biceps brachii. Report of two cases. J Bone Joint Surg Am. 1956;38:1365–8.
9. O'Driscoll SW, Goncalves LBJ, Dietz P. The hook test for distal biceps tendon avulsion. Am J Sports Med. 2007;35:1865–9.
10. Ruland RT, Dunbar RP, Bowen JD. The Biceps squeeze test for diagnosis of distal biceps tendon ruptures. Clin Orthop Relat Res. 2005:128–31.
11. Nicolay RW, Lawton CD, Selley RS, Johnson DJ, Vassa RR, Prescott AE, et al. Partial rupture of the distal biceps brachii tendon: a magnetic resonance imaging analysis. J Shoulder Elb Surg. 2020;29:1859–68.
12. Festa A, Mulieri PJ, Newman JS, Spitz DJ, Leslie BM. Effectiveness of magnetic resonance imaging in detecting partial and complete distal biceps tendon rupture. J Hand Surg Am. 2010;35:77–83.
13. Belli P, Costantini M, Mirk P, Leone A, Pastore G, Marano P. Sonographic diagnosis of distal biceps tendon rupture: a prospective study of 25 cases. J Ultrasound Med. 2001;20:587–95.
14. Lobo LDG, Fessell DP, Miller BS, Kelly A, Lee JY, Brandon C, et al. The role of sonography in differentiating full versus partial distal biceps tendon tears: correlation with surgical findings. Am J Roentgenol. 2013;200:158–62.
15. Dobbie RP. Avulsion of lower biceps brachii tendon: analysis of fifty-one previously unreported cases. Am J Surg. 1941;51:21.
16. Boyd HB, Anderson LD. A method for reinsertion of the distal biceps brachii tendon. J Bone Joint Surg. 1961;43:1041–3.
17. Baker BE, Bierwagen D. Rupture of the distal tendon of the biceps brachii. Operative versus non-operative treatment. J Bone Joint Surg Am. 1985;67:414–7.
18. Morrey BF, Askew LJ, An KN, Dobyns JH. Rupture of the distal tendon of the biceps brachii. A biomechanical study. J Bone Joint Surg Am. 1985;67:418–21.
19. Geaney LE, Brenneman DJ, Cote MP, Arciero RA, Mazzocca AD. Outcomes and practical information for patients choosing nonoperative treatment for distal biceps ruptures. Orthopedics. 2010;33:391.
20. Legg AJ, Stevens R, Oakes NO, Shahane SA. A comparison of non-operative vs. Endobutton repair of distal biceps ruptures. J Shoulder Elb Surg. 2016;25:341–8.
21. Nesterenki S, Domire ZJ, Morrey BF, Sanchez-Sotelo J. Elbow strength and endurance in patients with a ruptured distal biceps tendon. J Shoulder Elb Surg. 2010;19:184–9.
22. Hetsroni I, Pilz-Burstein R, Nyska M, Back Z, Barchilon V, Mann G. Avulsion of the distal biceps brachii tendon in middle-aged population: is surgical repair advisable? A comparative study of 22 patients treated with either nonoperative management or early anatomical repair. Injury. 2008;39:753–60.
23. Freeman CR, McCormick KR, Mahoney D, Baratz M, Lubahn JD. Nonoperative treatment of distal biceps tendon ruptures compared with a historical control group. J Bone Joint Surg Am. 2009;91:2329–34.
24. Walton C, Pennings A, Agur A, Elmaraghy A. A 3-dimensional anatomic study of the distal biceps tendon. Implications for surgical repair and reconstruction. Orthop J Sports Med. 2015;3:6–11.
25. Schmidt CC, Brown BT, Sawardeker PJ, DeGravelle M, Miller MC. Factors affecting supination strength after a distal biceps rupture. J Shoulder Elb Surg. 2014;23:68–75.
26. Morrey ME, Abdel MP, Sanchez-Sotelo J, Morrey BF. Primary repair of retracted distal biceps tendon rupture in extreme flexion. J Shoulder Elb Surg. 2014;23:679–85.
27. Schmidt CS, Brown BT, Qvick LM, Stacowicz RZ, Latona CR, Miller MC. Factors that determine supination strength following distal biceps repair. J Bone Joint Surg Am. 2016;98:1153–60.
28. Krackow KA, Thomas SC, Jones LC. A new stitch for ligament-tendon fixation. J Bone Joint Surg Am. 1986;68:764–6.
29. McKeon BP, Heming JF, Fulkerson J, Langeland R. The Krackow stitch: a biomechanical evaluation of changing the number of loops versus the number of sutures. Arthroscopy. 2006;22(1):33–7.
30. White KL, Camire LM, Parks BG, Corey WS, Hinton RY. Krackow locking stitch versus locking premanufactured loop stitch for soft-tissue fixation: a biomechanical study. Arthroscopy. 2010;26(12):1662–6.
31. Ostrander RV, Saper MG, Juelson TJ. A biomechanical comparison of modified Krackow and locking loop suture patterns for soft-tissue graft fixation. J Arthrosc Relat Surg. 2016;32:1384–8.
32. Mait JE, Hayes WT, Blum CL, Pivec R, Zaino CJ, Jauregui JJ, et al. A biomechanical comparison of different tendon repair techniques. J Long-Term Eff Med Implants. 2016;26:167–71.
33. Wust DM, Meyer DC, Favre P, Gerber C. Mechanical and handling properties of braided polyblend polyethelene sutures in comparison to braided polyester and monofilament polydioxanone sutures. Arthroscopy. 2006;22:1146–53.

34. Benthien RA, Aronow MS, Doran-Diaz V, Sullivan RJ, Naujoks R, Adams DJ. Cyclic loading of achilles tendon repairs: a comparison of polyster and polyblend suture. Foot Ankle Int. 2006;27:512–8.

35. Gnandt RJ, Smith JL, Nguyen-Ta K, McDonald L, LeClere LE. High-tensile strength tape versus high-tensile strength suture: a biomechanical study. Arthroscopy. 2016;32:356–63.

36. Leishman DJ, Chudik SC. Suture tape with broad full-width core versus traditional round suture with round core: a mechanical comparison. Arthroscopy. 2019;35:2461–6.

37. Schmidt CS, Brown BT, Williams BG, Rubright JH, Schmidt DL, Pic AC, et al. The importance of preserving the radial tuberosity during distal biceps repair. J Bone Joint Surg Am. 2015;97:2014–23.

38. Jarrett CD, Weir DM, Stuffmann ES, Jain S, Miller MC, et al. Anatomic and biomechanical analysis of the short and long head components of the distal biceps tendon. J Shoulder Elb Surg. 2012;21:942–8.

39. Becker D, Lopez-Marambio FA, Hammer N, Kieser D. How to avoid posterior interosseous nerve injury during single-incision distal biceps repair drilling. Clin Orthop Relat Res. 2019;477:424–31.

40. Joice M, Vasileidis GI, Amanatullah DF. Non-steroidal anti-inflammatory drugs for heterotopic ossification prophylaxis after total hip arthroplasty. Bone Joint J. 2018;100:915–22.

41. Waterman BR, Navarro-Figueroa L, Owens BD. Primary repair of traumatic distal biceps ruptures in a military population: clinical outcomes of single- versus 2-Incision technique. Arthroscopy. 2017;33:1672–8.

42. Morrey BF, Askew LJ, An KN, Dobyns JH. Rupture of the distal tendon of the biceps brachii: a biomechanical study. J Bone Joint Surg. 1985;67:418–21.

43. Failla JM, Amadio PC, Morrey BF, Beckenbaugh RD. Proximal radioulnar synostosis after repair of distal biceps brachii rupture by the two-incision technique. Clin Orthop Relat Res. 1988;253:133–6.

44. Dunphy TR, Hudson J, Batech M, Acevedo DC, Mirsaya R. Surgical treatment of distal biceps tendon ruptures. Am J Sports Med. 2017;45:3020–9.

45. Ford SE, Andersen JS, Macknet DM, Connor PM, Loeffler BJ, Gaston RG. Major complications after distal biceps tendon repairs: retrospective cohort analysis of 970 cases. J Shoulder Elb Surg. 2018;27:1898–906.

46. Amin NH, Volpi A, Lynch TS, Patel RM, Cerynik DL, Schickendantz MS, et al. Complications of distal biceps tendon repair: a meta-analysis of single-incision versus double-incision surgical technique. Orthop J Sports Med. 2016;4:1–5.

47. Beks RB, Claessen R, Oh LS, Ring D, Chen NC. Factors associated with adverse events after distal biceps tendon repair or reconstruction. J Shoulder Elb Surg. 2016;25:1229–34.

48. Nigro PT, Cain R, Mighell MA. Prognosis for recovery of posterior interosseous nerve palsy after distal biceps repair. J Shoulder Elb Surg. 2013;22:70–3.

49. Cusick MC, Cottrell BJ, Cain RA, Mighell MA. Low incidence of tendon rerupture after distal biceps repair by cortical button and interference screw. J Shoulder Elb Surg. 2014;23:1532–6.

50. Hinchey JW, Aronowitz JG, Sanchez-Sotelo J, Morrey BF. Re-rupture rate of primarily repaired distal biceps tendon injuries. J Shoulder Elb Surg. 2014;23:850–4.

51. Amarasooriya M, Bain GI, Roper T, Bryant K, Phadnis J. Complications after distal biceps tendon repair: a systematic review. Am J Sports Med. 2020;48:3103–11.

52. Grewal R, Athwal GS, MacDermid JC, Faber KJ, Drosdowech DS, El-Hawary R, et al. Single versus double-incision technique for the repair of acute distal biceps tendon ruptures. J Bone Joint Surg Am. 2012;94:1166–74.

53. Chavan PR, Duquin TR, Bisson LJ. Repair of the ruptured distal biceps tendon: a systematic review. Am J Sports Med. 2008;36:1618–24.

54. Barnes SJ, Coleman SG, Gilpin D. Repair of avulsed insertion of biceps, a new technique in four cases. J Bone Joint Surg Br. 1993;75:938–99.

55. Lintner MM, Fisher T. Repair of the distal biceps tendon using suture anchors and an anterior approach. Clin Orthop. 1996;317:114–21.

56. Strauch RJ, Michelson H, Rossenwasser MP. Repair of rupture of the distal tendon of the biceps brachii. Review of the literature and report of three cases treated with a single anterior incision and suture anchors. Am J Orthop. 1997;26:151–6.

57. Fernandez JJ, Greenberg JA, Wang T, Turner C. A new technique for repair of distal biceps tendon avulsions. American Society for Surgery of the Hand, 52nd Annual Meeting; Denver CO, September 1997.

58. Mazzocca AD, Burton KJ, Romeo AA, Santangelo S, Adams DA, Arciero RA. Biomechanical evaluation of 4 techniques of distal biceps brachii tendon repair. Am J Sports Med. 2007;35:252–8.

59. Pereira DS, Kvitne RS, Liang M, Giacobetti FB, Ebramzadeh E. Surgical repair of distal biceps tendon ruptures: a biomechanical comparison of two techniques. Am J Sports Med. 2002;30:432–6.

60. Idler CS, Montgomery WH, Lindsey DP, Badua PA, Wynee GF, Yerby SA. Distal biceps tendon repair: a biomechanical comparison of intact tendon and 2 repair techniques. Am J Sports Med. 2006;34:968–74.

61. Greenberg JA, Fernandez JJ, Wang T, Turner C. EndoButton-assisted repair of distal biceps tendon ruptures. J Shoulder Elb Surg. 2003;12:484–90.

62. Schmidt CS, Weir DM, Wong AS, Howard M, Miller MC. The effect of biceps reattachment site. J Shoulder Elb Surg. 2010;19:1157–65.

63. Schmidt CS, Brown BT, Qvick LM, Stacowicz RZ, Latona CR, Miller MC. Factors that determine supination strength following distal biceps repair. J Bone Joint Surg. 2016;98:1153–60.

64. Stockton DJ, Tobias G, Pike JM, Daneshvar P, Goetz TJ. Supination torque following single- versus double-incision repair of acute distal biceps tendon ruptures. J Shoulder Elb Surg. 2019;28:2371–8.

65. El-Hawary R, MacDermid JC, Faber KJ, Patterson SD, King GJW. Distal biceps tendon repair: comparison of surgical techniques. J Hand Surg. 2003;28A:496–502.

66. Johnson TS, Johnson DC, Shindle MK, Allen AA, Weiland AJ, Cavanaugh J, et al. One- versus two-incision technique for distal biceps tendon repair. J Hosp Spec Surg. 2008;4:117–22.

67. Watson JN, Moretti VM, Schwindel L, Hutchinson MR. Repair techniques for acute distal biceps tendon ruptures. J Bone Joint Surg Am. 2014;96:2086–90.

68. Cain RA, Nydick JA, Stein MI, Williams BD, Polikandriotis JA, Hess AV. Complications following distal biceps repair. J Hand Surg Am. 2012;37:2112–7.

69. Kelly EW, Morrey NF, O'Driscoll SW. Complications of repair of the distal biceps tendon with the modified two-incision technique. J Bone Joint Surg Am. 2000;82:1575–81.

Interposition Fascial Arthroplasty of the Elbow

74

Mark A. Dodson and William B. Geissler

Introduction

The elbow is a part of a system that enables the hand to interact with the person and their surrounding areas. Loss of motion, instability, and pain can inhibit one or all of these functions. Interposition arthroplasty has been described in the literature for over 200 years [2, 3]. It is an option for individuals with significant degenerative or inflammatory arthritis of the elbow who have failed conservative management. The goal is to improve range of motion and decrease pain in young or active patients that cannot accept the physical limitations of total arthroplasty or arthrodesis. In these patients, interpositional arthroplasty is an option. Some patients may be able to return to manual labor after this procedure. The problem in the past has been potential instability following interpositional arthroplasty. Newer techniques in surface reconstruction and ligament reconstruction have made interposition arthroplasty a useful option.

There are few options for a young patient who has elbow arthritis. While total elbow arthroplasty is a good option to improve range of motion and decrease pain, longevity of the implants and weight limitations are drawbacks. A common restriction is no lifting greater than 10 pounds with total elbow arthroplasty. The concern is elbow revision which can result in significant bone loss. If the patient has multiple revisions, it can be very challenging due to loss of bone from previous surgeries. Elbow arthrodesis is a good option for

strength, but the loss of motion is very poorly functionally tolerated. Resection arthroplasty is able to provide pain relief; however, the significant lack of stability will provide a significant functional problem. Open or arthroscopic debridement can improve pain with terminal flexion and extension and potentially improve the range of motion. This can provide short-term pain relief. While synovectomy is an option, the results can be unpredictable and are based on the amount of degenerative changes to the elbow prior to synovectomy [1].

Contraindications to fascial arthroplasty include chronic infection, joint instability, and bone loss that cannot be surgically corrected.

Surgical Technique

The patient is placed in the supine position on the operating table (Figs. 74.1, 74.2, 74.3 and 74.4). The incision is curved radially over the olecranon to preserve skin sensation. The standard dorsal approach is made to the elbow. The ulnar nerve is identified and is transposed anteriorly and will be carefully protected during the remaining part of the procedure. A triceps split approach is made retracting the tendon radially and ulnarly. Generally, the lateral collateral ligament is released hinging the elbow open on the remaining medial collateral ligament complex. A burr is used to remove any remaining articular cartilage from the olecranon (Figs. 74.5 and 74.6). The burr is used to shape and establish a congruent humeroulnar joint. Fascial grafts are then selected to cover both the distal humerus and ulnar. The author's preferred soft-tissue graft is bovine dermis xenograft, although other fascia grafts are an option.

Usually, five anchors are placed on the olecranon (Fig. 74.7). One in the center, and one in the four quadrants. The 5 × 7 bovine dermis is quadrupled on itself (approx. 4 mm) and secured in each quarter with #1 vicryl stitch (Fig. 74.8). The suture from the anchors are then placed through the graft and tied securing the graft on the olecranon.

M. A. Dodson (✉)
Hand and Upper Extremity Fellow, Department of Orthopaedic Surgery and Rehabilitation, University of Mississippi Medical Center, Jackson, MS, USA

Partner, Mid State Orthopedic and Sports Medicine Center, Alexandria, LA, USA

W. B. Geissler
Division of Hand and Upper Extremity Surgery, Section of Arthroscopic Surgery and Sports Medicine, Department of Orthopedic Surgery and Rehabilitation, University of Mississippi Medical Center, Jackson, MS, USA

© Springer Nature Switzerland AG 2022
W. B. Geissler (ed.), *Wrist and Elbow Arthroscopy with Selected Open Procedures*,
https://doi.org/10.1007/978-3-030-78881-0_74

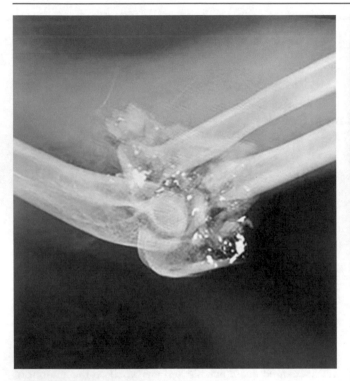

Fig. 74.1 Lateral radiograph of an extensive comminuted fracture of the proximal ulna with bone loss

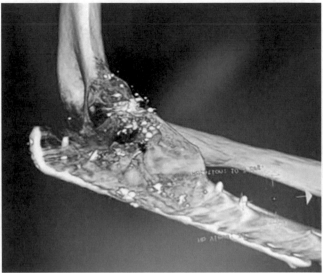

Fig. 74.3 Lateral 3D CT radiograph postoperatively showing the patient developed extensive heterotopic ossification and traumatic arthritis to the elbow

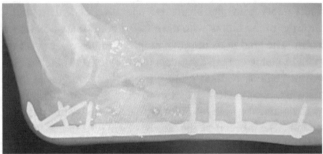

Fig. 74.4 Lateral radiograph following excision of the heterotopic ossification. The patient continued to proceed his traumatic degenerative arthritis to the elbow with severe pain and limited motion

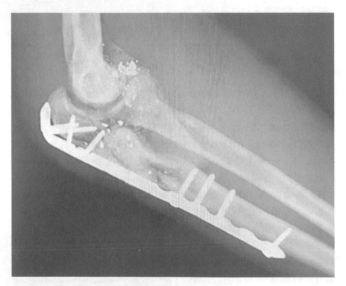

Fig. 74.2 Lateral radiograph showing anatomic restoration of the ulna following open reduction fixation. Bone cement was used to fill the bone void in this open fracture

Close attention is made to decrease any wrinkles and provide tension to the graft. It is very important that knots are tight, so that there is good contact of the graft to the exposed subchondral bone (Figs. 74.9, 74.10 and 74.11).

Attention is then focused toward the humerus (Figs. 74.12 and 74.13). Two 6 × 10 grafts are then secured with #1 vicryl. Multiple anchors are placed along the distal anterior/pos-

terior surface of the exposed distal humerus (Fig. 74.14). In addition, sutures can be placed transosseous, further securing the grafts. The grafts are tied snuggly to prevent wrinkles and provide tension to the graft on to the subchondral bone. Excess graft material is trimmed. An Arthrex 4.75 swivel lock anchor (Naples, FL) is then placed in the ulna opposite the level of the radial head (Fig. 74.15). It is important that this is drilled and tapped for the anchor to be properly inserted. The elbow is then reduced and a second anchor is drilled just anterior of the midline on the lateral epicondyle. The fiber tape is then transferred into the second anchor, which impacted into the lateral epicondyle for the internal brace. The internal brace is secured in 30° of extension when the suture is placed. This provides very secure and immediate stability to the elbow (Figs. 74.16, 74.17 and 74.18). The remaining sutures are then passed through the remaining part of the lateral collateral ligament complex to provide further stability to the joint (Fig. 74.19). The wound is irrigated and

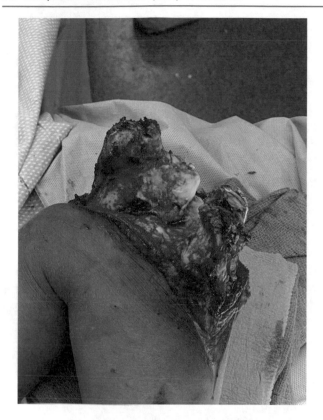

Fig. 74.5 Intraoperative photograph demonstrating the advanced traumatic arthritis of the humeroulnar joint. The ulnar collateral ligament has been released and elbows hinged open on the lateral ulna collateral ligament complex

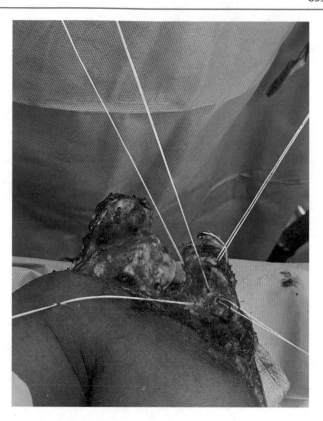

Fig. 74.7 Multiple anchors are placed in the olecranon to stabilize and hold the soft tissue graft

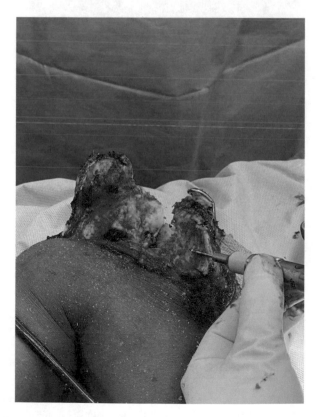

Fig. 74.6 The remaining articular cartilage is burred off the olecranon and is fashioned for the soft tissue arthroplasty

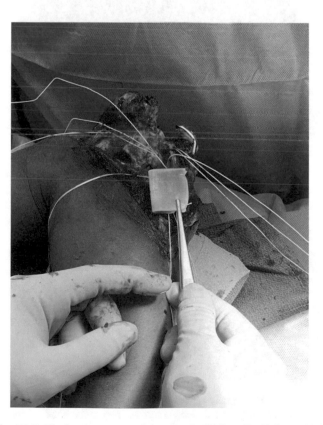

Fig. 74.8 The bovine xenograft has quadrupled on itself for a thick soft tissue covering. The sutures will be passed through the graft

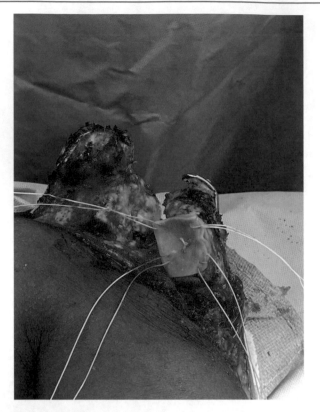

Fig. 74.9 The sutures from the anchors have been passed through the graft, and the central suture has been tied

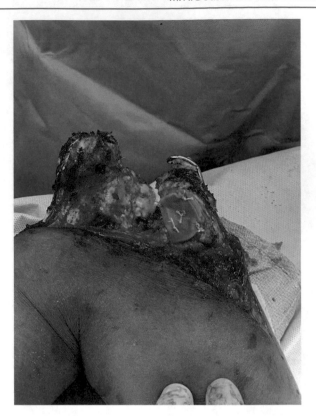

Fig. 74.11 The remaining sutures have been tied, securing the graft to the olecranon fossa

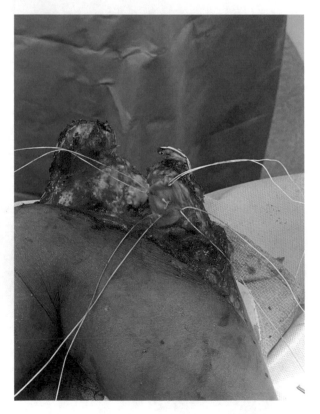

Fig. 74.10 The remaining suture anchors are tied securing the graft to the bone by covering the olecranon fossa. Note: The good tension on the graft without wrinkles

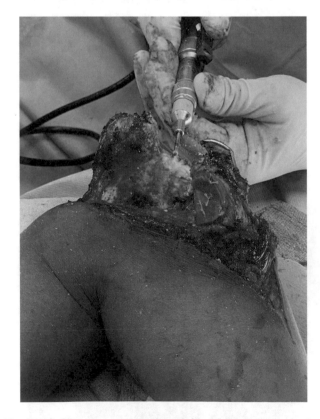

Fig. 74.12 The severe traumatic arthritis of the humerus is then returned to fashion a normal fossa for the olecranon to articulate

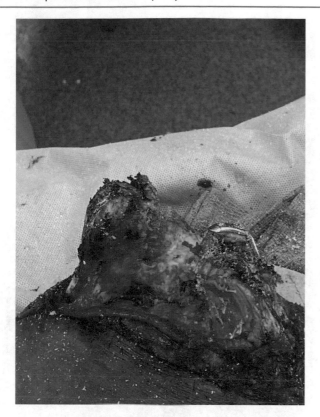

Fig. 74.13 Intraoperative photograph showing reshaping of the distal humerus in preparation for the soft tissue graft

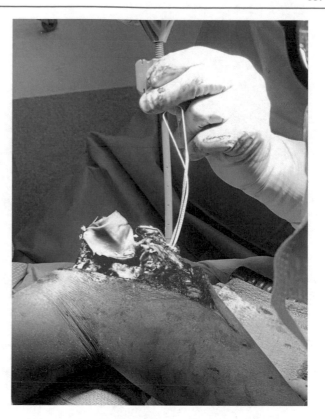

Fig. 74.15 Soft tissue graft has been stabilized by the multiple suture anchors on the distal humerus. A 4.75 Arthrex Swivel Lock Anchor (Naples, FL) is being inserted on the ulna for the internal brace to stabilize the medial side of the elbow

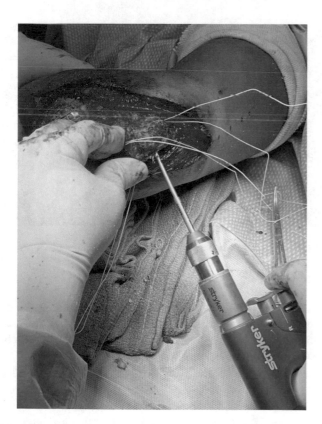

Fig. 74.14 Soft tissue sutures are then being inserted through the distal humerus to support and stabilize the soft tissue graft

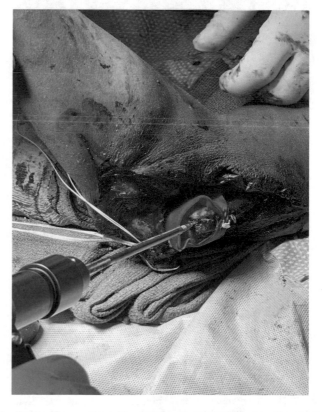

Fig. 74.16 The medial epicondyle is now being drilled to support the second Arthrex 4.75 Swivel Lock Anchor (Naples, FL) to complete the internal brace. Notice that the drill is slightly anterior to the midline

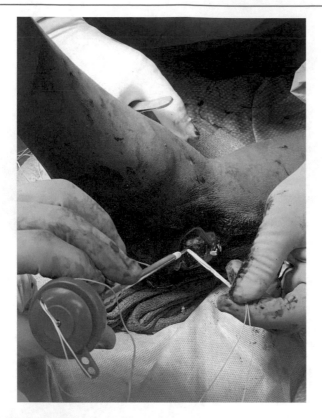

Fig. 74.17 The second anchor is being placed in the medial epicondyle to complete the internal brace

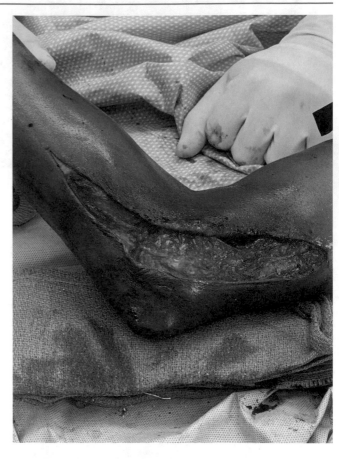

Fig. 74.19 The forearm flexion muscle mass has been reattached to the medial epicondyle for soft tissue closure

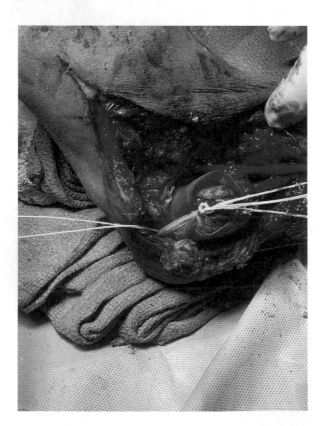

Fig. 74.18 The complete internal brace stabilizing the elbow from the medial approach. The ulnar nerve had been previously transposed submuscularly and can be seen on the anterior aspect of the humerus

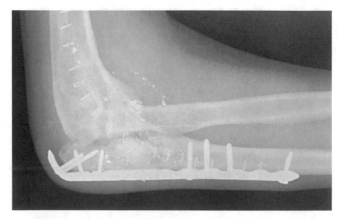

Fig. 74.20 Lateral radiograph following fascial arthroplasty to the elbow

the triceps split is closed. Reinforcement sutures #5 of ethibond are placed through transosseous holes in the olecranon through the triceps tendon in a modified Krackow stitch, reinforcing the tricep attachment on to the olecranon.

Postoperatively, the patient returns at 2 weeks, and a hinged brace set at minus 20⁻degree full extension and full flexion is used for 3 additional weeks (Fig. 74.20). At that point, the brace is stopped, and a physical therapy program for strength and range of motion is initiated. Digital range of motion exercises is initiated immediately.

Tips and Tricks

- Approach the elbow either on the medial or lateral aspect depending on the specific pathology. Release the near-sided ligament complex, and hinge the elbow open on the opposite collateral ligament.
- Shape the ulna and distal humerus into a congruent joint surface with a burr helping restore any malalignment from the severe arthritis.
- Use as many anchors as required to thoroughly stabilize the graft tissue graft onto the distal humerus and ulna. Try to secure the graft without wrinkles, and tie the knot snuggly so there is good contact between the graft and the remaining subchondral bone.
- Reduce the elbow and assess the congruency of the reduction following the soft tissue into position.
- Reconstruct the collateral ligament with an internal brace. The ligament brace is set at 30° of extension with good tension on the fiber tape.
- The remaining sutures will be then used to further repair the collateral ligament complex.

Results and Conclusions

Success of this procedure is determined by the ability of the patient to return to most of their activities of daily living. They must have a stable elbow with a functional ROM. Pain should be at an acceptable level during these activities. Good to excellent result has been reported in 26–94% of cases, though different systems have been used to evaluate this procedure [4].

Cheng and Morrey reported on distraction interposition arthroplasty in 13 patients [5]: 69% had a satisfactory relief of pain, and 62% had an excellent to good functional result at an average of 30 months.

Larson and Morrey reported in 2008 on 38 patients who had a surviving interposition arthroplasty at an average of 6 years [6]. Seven of the original 45 had undergone revision within that period. Nineteen of them rated the elbow as much better following the procedure, and 12 rated it as somewhat better. Instability was the chief reason for dissatisfaction or revision.

Larson, Adams, and Morrey reported in 2010 on patients undergoing revision fascia arthroplasty [7]. Five of the nine were satisfied with the procedure at an average of 4.7 years. The fair and poor results were related to persistent pain, instability, or stiffness.

Interposition arthroplasty of the elbow is a motion preserving procedure for patients who are not candidates for total elbow arthroplasty. It allows for the possibility of future procedures including revision facial arthroplasty or the conversion to a total elbow arthroplasty. This is one of the few salvage procedures that has the potential to significantly improve the quality of life for indicated patients.

References

1. Kroonen LT, Piper SL, Ghatan AC. Arthroscopic Management of Elbow Arthritis. J Hand Surg Am. 2017;42(8):640–50.
2. Park H, Moreau PF. Cases of excision of carious joints. Glasgow: J Scrymgeour; 1806.
3. Campbell WC. Operative orthopedics. St. Louis: C. V. Mosby; 1939. p. 390–3.
4. Papatheodorou LK, Baratz ME, Sotereanos DG. Elbow arthritis: current concepts. J Hand Surg Am. 2013;38(3).605–13.
5. Cheng SL, Morrey BF. Treatment of the mobile, painful arthritic elbow by distraction interposition arthroplasty. J Bone Joint Surg Br. 2000;82(2):233–8.
6. Larson AN, Morrey BF. Interposition arthroplasty with an Achilles tendon allograft as a salvage procedure for the elbow. J Bone Joint Surg Am. 2008;90(12):2714–23.
7. Larson AN, Adams RA, Morrey BF. Revision interposition arthroplasty of the elbow. J Bone Joint Surg Br. 2010;92(9):1273–7.

75

Mark S. Rekant

Entrapment or compressive neuropathies are common problems that typically lead to functional impairment and disability of the upper limb due to pain, altered sensation, loss of dexterity, and weakness if left untreated [1]. Cubital tunnel syndrome is used synonymously for a focal compressive neuropathy of the ulnar nerve about the medial aspect of the elbow. Cubital tunnel syndrome is a common nerve entrapment condition, affecting the upper extremity second in frequency only to entrapment of the median nerve at the wrist (carpal tunnel syndrome). Understanding the presentation of the symptoms and anatomy of the elbow is paramount for management of a patient's symptoms. Treatment for compressive ulnar neuropathy typically leads to a high level of patient satisfaction. The term *cubital tunnel syndrome* was defined in 1958 by Feindel and Stratford [2, 3], although the ability of the anatomic structures near the elbow joint to exert pressure on the ulnar nerve was known more than a century ago. In 1898, Curtis [4] performed the first published case of management of ulnar neuropathy at the elbow, which consisted of a subcutaneous anterior transposition.

Anatomy

The ulnar nerve is the terminal branch of the medial cord of the brachial plexus containing fibers from C8, T1, and, occasionally, C7. Figure 75.1 illustrates the potential sites of compression of the ulnar nerve in the region of the elbow. At the level of the insertion of the coracobrachialis muscle in the middle third of the arm, the ulnar nerve pierces the medial intermuscular septum, a site of potential compression [5], to enter the posterior compartment of the arm. At this level, the ulnar nerve lies on the anterior aspect of the medial head of the triceps, where it is joined by the superior ulnar collateral artery. The medial intermuscular septum extends from the coracobrachialis muscle proximally, where it is a thin and weak structure, to the medial humeral epicondyle, where it is a thick, distinct structure and lies medial to the brachial artery as far as the middle third of the arm.

Another potential site of compression is the arcade of Struthers [5]. This structure is found in 70% of patients, 8 cm proximal to the medial epicondyle, and extends from the medial intermuscular septum to the medial head of the triceps. The arcade of Struthers is formed by the attachments of the internal brachial ligament (a fascial extension of the cor-

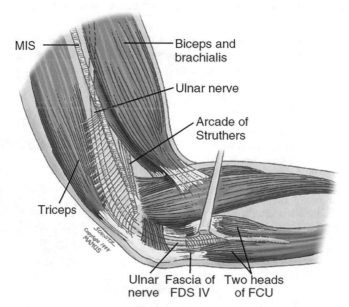

Fig. 75.1 Potential sites of compression of the ulnar nerve in the region of the elbow. *FCU* flexor carpi ulnaris, *FDS* flexor digitorum superficialis, *MIS* medial intermuscular septum. (Reprinted with permission from Rekant MS. Rehabilitation of the Hand and Upper Extremity, 7th ed. Philadelphia: Elsevier; 2021)

M. S. Rekant (✉)
Department of Orthopaedic Surgery, Philadelphia Hand to Shoulder Center, Thomas Jefferson University, Cherry Hill, NJ, USA
e-mail: msrekant@handcenters.com

© Springer Nature Switzerland AG 2022
W. B. Geissler (ed.), *Wrist and Elbow Arthroscopy with Selected Open Procedures*,
https://doi.org/10.1007/978-3-030-78881-0_75

acobrachialis tendon), the fascia and superficial muscular fibers of the medial head of the triceps, and the medial intermuscular septum.

Progressing distally, the ulnar nerve passes through the cubital tunnel. The cubital tunnel begins at the condylar groove between the medial epicondyle of the humerus and the olecranon of the ulna. The floor of the cubital tunnel is the elbow capsule and medial collateral ligament of the elbow joint. The roof is formed by the deep forearm investing fascia of the flexor carpi ulnaris (FCU) and the arcuate ligament of Osborne, also known as the cubital tunnel retinaculum [5–8]. Osborne's ligament is a 4 mm wide fibrous band that bridges from the medial epicondyle of the humerus to the medial aspect of the olecranon. Its fibers are oriented perpendicularly to the fibers of the FCU aponeurosis, which blends with its distal margin. The medial epicondyle and olecranon form the walls.

The capacity of the cubital tunnel is greatest when the elbow is in extension because the arcuate ligament is slack. Cadaveric measurements demonstrate that, as the elbow moves from extension to flexion, the distance between the medial epicondyle and the olecranon increases 5 mm for every 45 degrees of elbow flexion [9]. The shape of the tunnel changes from a round to an oval tunnel, with a 2.5 mm loss of height. The volume decreases 55% in the epicondylar canal as the shape changes with flexion. Once the nerve proceeds distal to the cubital tunnel, the ulnar nerve passes between the humeral and ulnar heads of the flexor carpi ulnaris muscle. Fibrous bands and thickened FCU fascia have been defined that compress the ulnar nerve distal to the cubital tunnel.

Sunderland [10] described the internal topography of the ulnar nerve at the medial epicondyle (Fig. 75.2). Sensory and intrinsic muscle fibers were found to be located superficially with the motor fibers to the FCU and flexor digitorum profundus deep within the nerve. The central location of these motor fibers provides protection from external forces.

Pathophysiology

Pressure can be applied to the ulnar nerve about the elbow in three ways: compression, stretch, and friction [8]. Small pressures applied to a nerve initially affect the endoneural microcirculation. The nocturnal paresthesias reported by patients stem from the increased tissue pressure and edema that occur during sleep given our body's natural diurnal fluid shifts. A critical pressure level has been reported to be 30 mm Hg within the tunnel [11]. Functional loss caused by acute compression is a result of ischemia and not of mechanical deformation [11]. Pechan and Julis [12] have measured intraneural pressure in the ulnar nerve at the cubital tunnel in cadaver experiments: The pressure was 7 mm Hg with full elbow extension and 11–24 mm Hg at 90 degrees of flexion. Werner and colleagues noted that, during elbow flexion, pressure within the tunnel increases sevenfold and can increase more than 20-fold with contraction of the flexor carpi ulnaris [13].

Experimental studies have demonstrated a progressive thickening of the external and internal epineurium as well as thickening of the perineurium. Persistent paresthesias are related to chronic alterations in the blood flow resulting from intraneural fibrosis [11, 14]. The muscle wasting and loss of two-point discrimination found in advanced nerve compression are related to loss of nerve fiber function.

Extraneural compression of longer durations (28 days) has been studied [15]. As with the short-term studies, subperineurial edema may persist even after the removal of the

Fig. 75.2 Internal topography of the ulnar nerve at the medial epicondyle. *FCU* flexor carpi ulnaris, *FDP* flexor digitorum profundus. (Reprinted with permission from Rekant MS. Rehabilitation of the Hand and Upper Extremity, 7th ed. Philadelphia: Elsevier; 2021)

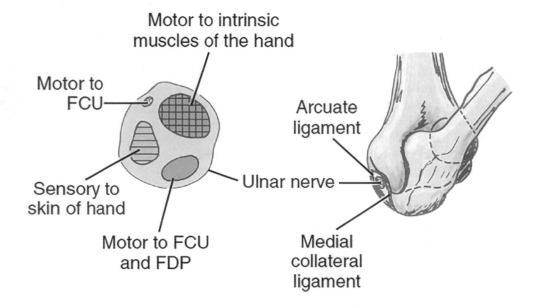

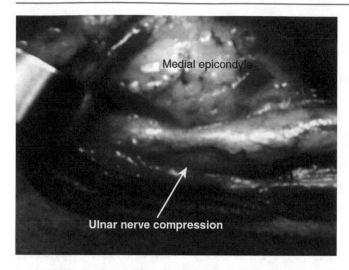

Fig. 75.3 Ulnar nerve compression at the level of the medial epicondyle

Classification

McGowan [25] provided the following classification system:

- Grade I – Mild lesions with paresthesias in the ulnar nerve distribution and a feeling of clumsiness in the affected hand; no wasting or weakness of the intrinsic muscles
- Grade II – Intermediate lesions with weak interossei and muscle wasting
- Grade III – Severe lesions with paralysis of the interossei and a marked weakness of the hand

Wadsworth [8, 26] classified the cubital tunnel syndrome on an etiologic basis: (1) acute and subacute external compression and (2) chronic internal compression caused by a space-occupying lesions or lateral shift of the ulna (injury of the capitellar physis in childhood).

Childress [17] studied 2000 ulnar nerves in 1000 normal subjects and found an incidence of 16% with subluxation of the ulnar nerve from the humeral epicondylar groove during elbow flexion. Two types of subluxation were defined: (1) the nerve moves onto the tip of the epicondyle when the elbow is flexed to or beyond 90 degrees, and (2) the nerve passes completely across and anterior to the epicondyle when the elbow is completely flexed. Approximately 75% of ulnar nerves with recurring subluxation are the first type [17].

extraneural compression. Inflammatory and fibrin deposits occur within hours, followed by proliferation of endoneurial fibroblasts and capillary endothelial cells. Fibrous tissue from endoneurial fibroblasts proliferates within several days, followed by invasion of mast cells and macrophages into the endoneurial space. Axonal degeneration is noted in nerves subjected to compression for 4 weeks.

Histologic examination of nerves at the site of compression injury reveals proliferation of the endoneurial and perineurial microvasculature, edema in the epineurial space, and fibrotic changes [4, 15, 16]. Initial changes occur in the nerve–blood barrier, followed by edema and epineurial fibrosis. Thinning of the myelin sheath then occurs at the periphery of the nerve. Axonal degeneration follows prolonged compression (Fig. 75.3). The rate and severity of these changes differ throughout the nerve, possibly because of variations in the amount of connective tissue. These pathologic changes appear to be dose-dependent, based on the duration and force of compression.

Etiology

Potential points of nerve compression or irritation include the arcade of Struthers, medial intermuscular septum, cubital tunnel at the level of the medial epicondylar groove, Osborne's ligament, as well as the fascia overlying and connecting the two heads of the FCU (see Fig. 75.1). Additional causes include subluxation of the ulnar nerve over the medial epicondyle [17], cubitus valgus, bony spurs, hypertrophied synovium, muscle anomalies [18–21], ganglia, and direct trauma.

Diagnosis

Patients with cubital tunnel syndrome often complain of sharp or aching pain along the medial aspect of the elbow, which may radiate proximally or distally [15, 27]. These patients also typically report numbness and tingling radiating into their little finger and ulnar half of the ring finger. Additional complaints may include weakness with grip and small finger usage. The term syndrome is appropriate as no two patients present with the exact same symptoms. Patient complaints vary from a vague discomfort to hypersensitivity, which is initially intermittent in nature and gradually becomes more severe and constant. Many patients report an exacerbation of their symptoms during sleep, especially with elbow flexion. Patients with longstanding neuropathy note loss of grip and pinch strength as well as loss of fine dexterity. Lastly, those with prolonged compression present with intrinsic muscle wasting and clawing secondary to ulnar nerve dysfunction [30].

Physical examination findings may include a positive percussion test (Tinel's test) over the ulnar nerve at the elbow and/or a positive cubital tunnel compression or elbow flexion test with increased nerve-related symptoms with the elbow maximally flexed. The elbow flexion test, if positive, causes reproduction or exacerbation of pain or paresthesias (or both). Evaluation should also include muscle and sensory testing, including vibratory perception and light touch with Semmes–Weinstein monofilaments.

Electrodiagnostic testing may further aid in diagnosis and treatment. Electrodiagnostic testing should include both a nerve conduction velocity study and electromyographic study. The loss of evoked sensory potential is a very sensitive indicator of altered conduction [28]. Ulnar nerve compression contributes to reduced electrical conduction velocities across the elbow of less than the typically normal 50 m/sec. Electromyographic (EMG) studies may show denervation potentials in the ulnar-innervated muscles which are consistently exhibited in cubital tunnel syndrome when nerve conduction velocity is less than 41 m/sec [29].

Roentgenographic or x-ray studies should be done to assess bony lesions that can potentially compromise the cubital tunnel leading to nerve compression.

Ultrasound imaging of the ulnar nerve at the elbow can be helpful to identify and confirm ulnar nerve compression at the elbow [34]. Ultrasound is the most commonly used imaging modality because it is inexpensive, provides high resolution, is readily available, and allows for dynamic imaging during elbow flexion. Most studies suggest that the key ultrasonographic finding is enlargement of the ulnar nerve at the site of entrapment [31–33]. As with previous studies [31–33], the ulnar nerve was enlarged in those with entrapment compared with controls.

Treatment

Nonoperative Management

Nonoperative management includes patient education, activity modification, and night orthotic positioning. The patient with intermittent symptoms, no atrophy, and mild electrodiagnostic findings may respond well to nonsurgical treatment. Despite nonoperative management, should symptoms become unremitting and increasingly symptomatic, surgical solutions exist.

Which Surgical Procedure?

Surgical options for cubital tunnel syndrome include endoscopic release, in situ decompression, medial epicondylectomy, and anterior transpositions. Unlike the limited amount of data on nonoperative therapy, a voluminous amount of information exists regarding surgical options, techniques,

and results. Dellon reviewed the literature from 1898 to 1988 and found more than 50 reports of series totaling more than 2000 patients treated for cubital tunnel syndrome. Each procedure has proponents heralding the superiority of their preferred technique. All surgical options are geared toward decompression of the ulnar nerve about the elbow's cubital tunnel. Endoscopic-assisted release allows for an extended in situ release with a markedly smaller incision and potential quicker return to function.

Endoscopic Release

The endoscopic approach to in situ decompression of the ulnar nerve is not new. Tsai and coworkers [35] used an endoscopic technique for cubital tunnel syndrome as early as 1992. Endoscopic nerve release eliminates the compression without altering medial elbow anatomy [37–39]. Ulnar nerve transposition is widely held to be not only unnecessary but also potentially deleterious [15, 18, 19] as it requires an aggressive procedure that can cause complications and jeopardize the recovery of motor and sensory function by compromising the blood supply to the nerve [3, 20–22]. Furthermore, although numerous studies showed similar clinical outcomes after transposition and in situ release, cutaneous and infectious complications were far more common after transposition [23–25]. The endoscopic technique has major advantages, which are probably related to the virtual absence of nerve dissection: rapid symptom relief, recovery of elbow function on the day after surgery, and a low risk of complications [3, 6, 15, 22, 26].

In addition, the endoscopic technique allows extensive release of the ulnar nerve, both proximally and distally. Distal release seems crucial to achieving optimal outcomes [27, 28]. According to Hoffman and Siemionow, the release should extend 10 cm distal to the medial epicondyle to minimize the risk of residual compression [29]. This goal is easily achieved using the endoscopic technique. As illustrated by several studies, endoscopic release provides good or excellent results in over 80% of patients [29, 40, 41].

Another advantage of endoscopic ulnar nerve release at the elbow may be a lower rate of neurological complications. Multiple studies evaluating surgical results after endoscopic cubital tunnel release have found no evidence of damage to the medial antebrachial cutaneous nerve of the forearm in any of the patients. The avoidance of medial antebrachial cutaneous nerve injury is a huge advantage over standard open surgical procedures utilizing a medial approach to the elbow [36, 37] where the sensory branches of this nerve are consistently injured if they are not specifically identified when performing the ulnar nerve release or transposition.

The effectiveness and safety of endoscopic cubital tunnel release was also confirmed by studies using

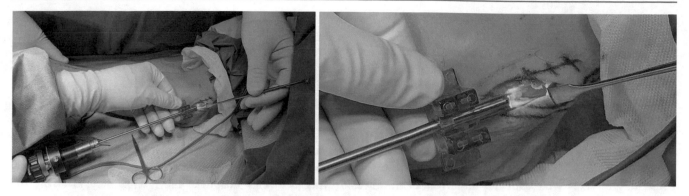

Fig. 75.4 (a, b) Endoscopic release of the ulnar nerve using the SafeView™ Soft Tissue Release system (Mission Surgical Innovations, Wayne, PA)

Fig. 75.5 Endoscopic release of the ulnar nerve using the EndoReleaseTM system (Integra). (Reprinted with permission from the Ref. [38])

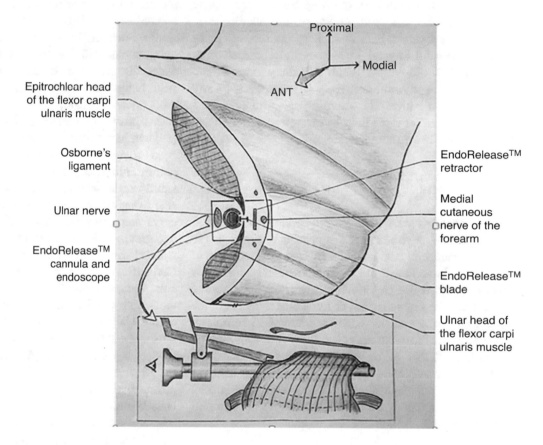

cadaver specimens [41, 42]. Gregory Bain compared endoscopic versus in situ ulnar releases in 2009. He noted less pain and higher satisfaction with endoscopic group as well as a higher complication rate in open group (11% vs. 40%). As in other studies [43, 44], the best results were obtained in the group of patients with mild and moderate preoperative symptoms. In addition to avoiding potential injury to the medial antebrachial cutaneous nerves, potential problems involving scarring, recurrence, and elbow contracture also can be avoided with an endoscopic release.

Several different surgical procedures have been described for a minimally invasive endoscopic assisted technique. My personal favorites are cannulated push cut techniques using commercially available guide systems (Segway [double-barrel design]), EndoRelease (Integra), and SafeView (Mission Surgical Innovations) (Figs. 75.4 and 75.5).

Postoperative Care

Postoperative dressing consists of a bulky soft dressing with an elastic bandage. There is no formal restriction with activity as the patient is allowed to self-modulate their activity levels based on their own symptomatology.

Results

Surgical outcomes with an endoscopic release of the ulnar nerve are on par with other described treatments such as in situ decompression, medial epicondylectomy [45–48], and anterior transpositions [54–57] with all of the methods demonstrating predictable, satisfactory results. Nerve pressure-related pain relief is dependably reported postoperatively along with other sensory symptoms showing consistent improvement. The improvement of the evoked sensory potential correlates well with the improvement in clinical symptoms [27]. Nonetheless, weakness tends to persist, and intrinsic muscular atrophy is the least likely to improve [18, 27, 41, 51]. However, those recovering from an endoscopic release tend to have less postoperative pain, smaller incision, and quicker recovery. There is little prognostic difference between successful surgical procedures, but a guarded prognosis always should be given with secondary transposition. The potential for full motor recovery after surgery is greatly reduced in those patients in whom preoperative symptoms have been present for more than 1 year or who have intrinsic muscle atrophy before surgery.

Complications

Potential complications from surgery aside from infection include postoperative stiffness, persistent soreness, nerve injury, and recurrent compression. Irritation or laceration of the posterior branches of the medial antebrachial cutaneous nerves from dissection or retraction may result in a transient or permanent loss of sensation or hypersensitivity about the medial aspect of the elbow. A postoperative flexion contracture can occur, most commonly following a submuscular transposition. Ulnar nerve subluxation may occur subsequent to either an endoscopic or in situ release, with the potential for instability following detachment of the medial collateral ligament during a medial epicondylectomy or [50] submuscular transposition.

Outcomes and Prognosis

In general, all described procedures yielded good-to-excellent results in 85–90% of patients [8, 24, 27, 49]. There is currently no consensus on the optimal operative treatment. The debate about it is highly dogmatic, with surgeons claiming excellent results for each of the treatment options. The choice of operative treatment is largely based on the surgeon's preference and experience. Several recent articles demonstrate findings indicating success with limited or simple decompression [52, 53].

Heithoff and associates [52] reviewed 12 clinical studies involving 350 patients in which a medial epicondylectomy was performed. Results were satisfactory in 72–94% of patients. Kaempffe and Farbach [60] reviewed 27 patients with partial medial epicondylectomies over an average of 13 months. Subjective improvement was noted in 93% of the cases.

In a meta-analysis by Zlowodzki and coworkers [59], comparing ulnar nerve transposition with simple decompression for the treatment of ulnar nerve compression in patients without a prior traumatic injury or surgery involving the affected elbow, no significant differences were seen in postoperative motor nerve-conduction velocities or clinical scores. This systematic review of nonrandomized studies showed simple ulnar nerve decompression to have the best results; however, the authors pointed out a potential selection bias: patients with less severe symptoms were treated more frequently with simple decompression, whereas patients with higher-grade compression syndromes were treated more often with transposition.

In a prospective randomized study, Nabhan and associates [58] compared simple decompression with anterior subcutaneous transposition in 66 patients with cubital tunnel syndrome. Thirty-two patients underwent simple decompression, and 34 underwent anterior subcutaneous transposition. No significant difference in pain, motor, and sensory deficits or nerve conduction-velocity studies was found between the two groups at 3- to 9-month follow-up. The authors recommended simple decompression of the ulnar nerve. Biggs and Curtis [61] reported on 23 in situ neurolysis and 21 submuscular transpositions. The results were equally effective, but three deep wound infections developed in the transposition group. The authors concluded that in situ release is equally effective and offers fewer complications.

Bartels and colleagues [62] reported on 75 simple decompressions and 77 anterior subcutaneous transpositions in a prospective randomized trial. The authors found no difference in clinical outcome between the two groups. The complication rate was 9.6% in the simple decompression group and 31.1% in the transposition group. The authors concluded that simple decompression was easier to perform because of reduced soft tissue dissection and the absence of muscle detachment. Additionally, simple decompression was associated with fewer complications, even in the presence of subluxation.

An earlier meta-analysis by Bartels and coworkers [63] of the literature from 1970 to 1997 revealed that simple decompression resulted in the best outcome and subcutaneous and submuscular transpositions the worst outcomes. Heithoff [64] reviewed 14 clinical studies in which a simple decompression was performed. Results were satisfactory in 75–92% of the patients.

Conclusion

Cubital tunnel syndrome is the second most common nerve compression in the upper extremity and the most prevalent at the elbow. Patients with mild symptoms may respond to non-surgical treatment. However, patients with unremitting pain, paresthesias, and potential motor weakness require surgical decompression at the point of compression with an endoscopic surgical release of the elbow providing comprehensive complete decompression of the ulnar nerve at the potential entrapment points. Outcomes are generally good and are likely to be optimal if the duration of symptoms is less than 1 year.

References

1. Campbell WW. Diagnosis and management of common compression and entrapment neuropathies. Neurol Clin. 1997;15:549.
2. Feindel W, Stratford J. Cubital tunnel compression in tardy ulnar palsy. Can Med Assoc J. 1958;78:351.
3. Feindel W, Stratford J. Cubital tunnel palsy in tardy ulnar palsy. Can Med Assoc J. 1958;1:287.
4. Curtis BF. Traumatic ulnar neuritis: transplantation of the nerve. J Nerv Ment Dis. 1898;25:480–4.
5. Spinner M. Injuries to the major branches of peripheral nerves in the forearm. 2nd ed. Philadelphia: WB Saunders; 1978.
6. Apfelbert DB, Larson SJ. Dynamic anatomy of the ulnar nerve at the elbow. Plast Reconstr Surg. 1973;51:76.
7. Osborne GV. Compression neuritis of the ulnar nerve at the elbow. Hand. 1970;2:10.
8. Wadsworth TG. The external compression syndrome of the ulnar nerve at the cubital tunnel. Clin Orthop. 1977;124:189.
9. Vanderpool DW, Chalmers J, Lamb DW, Whiston TB. Peripheral compression lesions of the ulnar nerve. J Bone Joint Surg. 1968;50B:792.
10. Sunderland S. Nerves and nerve injuries. 2nd ed. New York: Churchill Livingston; 1987. p. 728–74.
11. Lundborg G, Gelberman RH, Minteer-Convery M, Lee YF, Hargens AR. Median nerve compression in the carpal tunnel: functional response to experimentally induced controlled pressure. J Hand Surg. 1982;7:252.
12. Pechan J, Julis I. The pressure measurement in the ulnar nerve: a contribution to the pathophysiology of the cubital tunnel syndrome. J Biomech. 1975;8:75.
13. Werner C, Ohlin P, Elmqvist D. Pressures recorded in ulnar neuropathy. Acta Orthop Scand. 1985;56:404–6.
14. Mackinnon SE, Dellon AL. Experimental study of chronic nerve compression. Hand Clin. 1986;2:639.
15. Eversmann WW Jr. Compression and entrapment neuropathies of the upper extremity. J Hand Surg. 1983;8:759.
16. Eaton RG, Crowe JF, Parkes JC. Anterior transposition of the ulnar nerve using a non-compressing fasciodermal sling. J Bone Joint Surg. 1980;62A:820.
17. Childress HM. Recurrent ulnar-nerve dislocation at the elbow. Clin Orthop. 1975;108:168.
18. Dellon AL. Musculotendinous variations about the medial humeral epicondyle. J Hand Surg (Br). 1986;11:175–81.
19. Gervasio O, Zaccone C. Surgical approach to ulnar nerve compression at the elbow caused by the epitrochleoanconeus muscle and a prominent medial head of the triceps. Neurosurgery. 2008;62(3 Suppl 1):186–92.
20. LeDouble AF. Treatise on human muscular system variations and their meaning from a zoological anthropological point of view [in French]. 2nd ed. Paris: Schleicher Freres; 1897. p. 60–75.
21. Wood J. Variations in human mycology observed during the winter session of 1867-1868 at King's College, London. Proc R Soc Lond. 1868;16:483–525.
22. Hoffmann R, Siemionow M. The endoscopic management of cubital tunnel syndrome. J Hand Surg. 2006;31B:23–9.
23. Padoa E. Systematics of vertebrates. In: Padoa E, editor. Manual of comparative anatomy of vertebrates [in Italian]; 2002. p. 27–61.
24. O'Driscoll SW, Horii E, Carmichael SW, Morrey BF. The cubital tunnel and ulnar neuropathy. J Bone Joint Surg (Br). 1991;73:613–7.
25. McGowan AJ. The results of transposition of the ulnar nerve for traumatic ulnar neuritis. J Bone Joint Surg. 1950;32B:293–301.
26. Wadsworth TG. The elbow. Edinburgh: Churchill Livingstone; 1982.
27. Eversmann WW Jr. Entrapment and compression neuropathies. In: Green DP, editor. Operative hand surgery. New York: Churchill Livingstone; 1982.
28. Adelaar RS, Foster WC, McDowell C. The treatment of the cubital tunnel syndrome. J Hand Surg. 1984;9A:90.
29. Hoffmann R, Siemionow M. The endoscopic management of cubital tunnel syndrome. J Hand Surg. 2006;31B:23–9.
30. Eisen A, Danon J. The mild cubital tunnel syndrome: its natural history and indications for surgical intervention. Neurology. 1974;24:608.
31. Beekman R, Schoemaker MC, Van Der Plas JP, Van Den Berg LH, Franssen H, Wokke JH, et al. Diagnostic value of high-resolution sonography in ulnar neuropathy at the elbow. Neurology. 2004;62:767–73.
32. Beekman R, Van Der Plas JP, Uitdehaag BM, Schellens RL, Visser LH. Clinical, electrodiagnostic, and sonographic studies in ulnar neuropathy at the elbow. Muscle Nerve. 2004;30:202–8.
33. Park GY, Kim JM, Lee SM. The ultrasonographic and electrodiagnostic findings of ulnar neuropathy at the elbow. Arch Phys Med Rehabil. 2004;85:1000–5.
34. Wiesler ER, Chloros GD, Cartwright MS, Shin HW, Walker FO. Ultrasound in the diagnosis of ulnar neuropathy at the cubital tunnel. J Hand Surg [Am]. 2006;31:1088–93.
35. Tsai TM, Chen IC, Majd ME, Lim BH. Cubital tunnel release with endoscopic assistance: results of a new technique. J Hand Surg. 1999;24A:21–9.
36. Cohen G, Masmejean E. Surgical treatment of cubital tunnel syndrome. About 50 cases. e-mem Acad Natl Chir. 2008;7(4):21–30.
37. Carlier Y, Prove S, Desmoineaux P, Boisrenoult P, Beaufils P. Rev Chir Orthop Reparatrice Appar Mot. 2005;91(S8):61.
38. Marcheix PS, Vergnenegre G, Chevalier C, Hardy J, Charissoux JL, Mabit C. Endoscopic ulnar nerve release at the elbow: indications and outcomes. Orthop Traumatol Surg Res. 2016 Feb;102(1):41–5.
39. Ahcan U, Zorman P. Endoscopic decompression of the ulnar nerve at the elbow. J Hand Surg. 2007;32(8):1171–6.
40. Yoshida A, Okutsu I, Hamanaka I. Endoscopic anatomical nerve observation and minimally invasive management of cubital tunnel syndrome. J Hand Surg Eur Vol. 2009;34(1):115–20.
41. Bain GI, Bajhau A. Endoscopic release of the ulnar nerve at the elbow using the Agee device: a cadaveric study. Arthroscopy. 2005;21:691–5.
42. Mariani PP, Golano P, Adriani E, Llusà M, Camilleri G. A cadaveric study of endoscopic decompression of the cubital tunnel. Arthroscopy. 1999;15:218–22.
43. Mowlavi A, Andrews K, Lille S, Verhulst S, Zook EG, Milner S. The management of cubital tunnel syndrome: a meta-analysis of clinical studies. Plast Reconstr Surg. 2000;106:327–34.

44. Wilson DH, Krout R. Surgery of ulnar neuropathy at the elbow: 16 cases treated by decompression without transposition. Technical note. J Neurosurg. 1973;38:780–5.

45. Miller RG, Hummel EE. The cubital tunnel syndrome: treatment with simple decompression. Ann Neurol. 1980;7:567–9.

46. King T, Morgan FP. Late results of removing the medial humeral epicondyle for traumatic ulnar neuritis. J Bone Joint Surg (Br). 1959;41:51–5.

47. Froimson AI, Zahrawi F. Treatment of compression neuropathy of the ulnar nerve at the elbow by epicondylectomy and neurolysis. J Hand Surg. 1980;5:391.

48. Jones RE, Gauntt C. Medial epicondylectomy for ulnar nerve compression syndrome at the elbow. Clin Orthop. 1979;139:174.

49. King T, Morgan F. The treatment of traumatic ulnar neuritis. Aust NZ J Surg. 1950;20:33.

50. Neblett C, Ehni G. Medial epicondylectomy for ulnar palsy. J Neurosurg. 1970;32:55.

51. Craven PR Jr, Green DP. Cubital tunnel syndrome: treatment by medial epicondylectomy. J Bone Joint Surg Am. 1980;62:986–9.

52. Heithoff SJ, Millender LH, Nalebuff EA, Petruska AJ Jr. Medial epicondylectomy for the treatment of ulnar nerve compression at the elbow. J Hand Surg [Am]. 1990;15:22–9.

53. Ogata K, Shimon S, Owen J, Manske PR. Effects of compression and devascularisation on ulnar nerve function: a quantitative study of regional blood flow and nerve conduction in monkeys. J Hand Surg (Br). 1991;16:104–8.

54. Learmonth JR. A technique for transplanting the ulnar nerve. Surg Gynecol Obstet. 1943;75:792.

55. Levy DM, Apfelberg DB. Results of anterior transposition for ulnar neuropathy at the elbow. Am J Surg. 1972;123:304.

56. Mass DP, Silverberg B. Cubital tunnel syndrome: anterior transposition with epicondylar osteotomy. Orthopaedics. 1986;9:711.

57. Macnicol MF. The results of operation for ulnar neuritis. J Bone Joint Surg. 1979;61B:159.

58. Nabhan A, Ahlhelm F, Kelm J, Reith W, Schwerdtfeger K, Steudel WI. Simple decompression or subcutaneous anterior transposition of the ulnar nerve for cubital tunnel syndrome. J Hand Surg (Br). 2005;30:521–4.

59. Zlowodzki M, Chan S, Bhandari M, Kalliainen L, Schubert W. Anterior transposition compared with simple decompression for treatment of cubital tunnel syndrome. A meta-analysis of randomized, controlled trials. J Bone Joint Surg Am. 2007;89(12):2591–8.

60. Kaempffe FA, Farbach J. A modified surgical procedure for cubital tunnel syndrome: partial medial epicondylectomy. J Hand Surg [Am]. 1998;23(3):492–9.

61. Biggs M, Curtis JA. Randomized, prospective study comparing ulnar neurolysis in situ with submuscular transposition. Neurosurgery. 2006;58:296–304.

62. Bartels RH, Verhagen WI, van der Wilt GJ, Meulstee J, van Rossum LG, Grotenhuis JA. Prospective randomized controlled study comparing simple decompression versus anterior subcutaneous transposition for idiopathic neuropathy of the ulnar nerve at the elbow: part I. Neurosurgery. 2005;56:522–30.

63. Bartels RH, Menovsky T, Van Overbeeke JJ. Surgical management of ulnar nerve compression at the elbow: an analysis of the literature. J Neurosurg. 1998;89(5):522–7.

64. Heithoff SJ. Cubital tunnel syndrome does not require transposition of the ulnar nerve. J Hand Surg [Am]. 1999;24(5):898–905.

Arthroscopic Ulnar Nerve Decompression

Julie E. Adams and Scott P. Steinmann

Introduction

Patients who have conditions amenable to arthroscopic treatment, such as osteoarthritis of the elbow, rheumatoid arthritis, hemophilic arthropathy, synovitis, or other conditions, may have concomitant cubital tunnel syndrome. Additionally, it is likely that compression of the ulnar nerve at the elbow will be exacerbated following the soft tissue swelling inherent following elbow arthroscopy. Rehabilitation protocols that promote prolonged flexion and extension or repetitive cycling of elbow motion, particularly when the elbow is anesthetized by regional block, may also render the ulnar nerve vulnerable to neuritis. Although it is reasonable to make a separate medial incision to decompress the nerve either before or after the arthroscopic portion of the procedure, in some cases it is also equally reasonable to decompress the nerve arthroscopically as part of the surgical procedure. This is particularly the case in the setting of a requirement to release the posteromedial capsule, which will expose the ulnar nerve and render it especially amenable to decompression.

Indications

Indications for ulnar nerve decompression via arthroscopy include evidence of ulnar nerve compression at the elbow, typically in the setting of another concomitant reason for elbow arthroscopy. Arthroscopic ulnar nerve decompression is not our preferred technique for ulnar nerve decompression absent other arthroscopic indications.

Patients undergoing arthroscopy in general undergo a thorough neurological assessment. In addition to a good history, the results of provocative maneuvers with respect to the ulnar nerve, including Tinel's testing, cubital tunnel compression testing, and elbow flexion test, are recorded. Likewise, sensory examination, including two-point discrimination, and motor testing, such as assessment of ability to cross fingers, Wartenbergs, and strength of the first dorsal interosseous muscle, are assessed. Electrodiagnostic testing is often obtained, although it may be "normal" even in the setting of reproducible symptoms. Recent data suggest ultrasound may also be a good way to document objective evidence of ulnar nerve compression.

Most surgeons favor ulnar nerve decompression in the presence of patients who clearly demonstrate evidence of cubital tunnel syndrome by history and exam (even in the absence of objective findings on electrodiagnostic testing).

However, who undergoes ulnar nerve treatment prophylactically, without pre-extant symptoms, is a matter of ongoing discussion [1].

Contraindications

Contraindications include a subluxating ulnar nerve that may require transposition; these patients are generally better served by an open procedure. Additional contraindications include lack of surgeon familiarity or facility with arthroscopy.

Patients with medial incisions or scarring may also be better suited to an open procedure. Finally, the procedure resects the posteromedial capsule deep to the ulnar nerve, allowing the ulnar nerve to translate toward the joint and increasing the space available to the nerve medially, rather than removing the more superficial fibers of tissues that may compress the nerve. Therefore, patients with severe ulnar neuropathy

J. E. Adams (✉)
Department of Orthopedic Surgery, University of Tennessee College of Medicine – Chattanooga, Chattanooga, TN, USA

S. P. Steinmann
Department of Orthopedic Surgery, University of Tennessee College of Medicine – Chattanooga, Chattanooga, TN, USA

Mayo Clinic, Rochester, MN, USA
e-mail: steinmann.scott@mayo.edu

© Springer Nature Switzerland AG 2022
W. B. Geissler (ed.), *Wrist and Elbow Arthroscopy with Selected Open Procedures*,
https://doi.org/10.1007/978-3-030-78881-0_76

may be considered to have an open procedure to address these structures.

Technique in Detail

The authors prefer a lateral decubitus position for elbow arthroscopy, using a dedicated arm holder. The arm is prepared and draped from fingertips to axilla, and a sterile tourniquet is applied (Fig. 76.1). Arthroscopy proceeds, according to the primary pathology that needs to be addressed. Typically, these authors prefer to start arthroscopy in the anterior or posterior portion of the joint, depending on the pathology to be addressed (Figs. 76.2 and 76.3). If most of the work is required in the anterior joint, arthroscopy starts there; if most of the work is required in the posterior portion of the joint, arthroscopy starts in that portion. For the posterior arthroscopy and for ulnar nerve decompression, a direct posterior working portal and a posterolateral portal are established in the usual fashion (Fig. 76.4).

The direct posterior portal is made approximately 3 cm proximal to the tip of the olecranon, centrally,

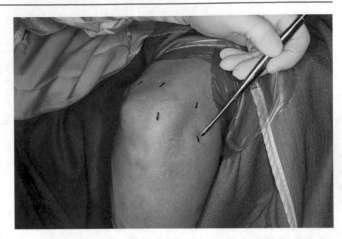

Fig. 76.2 Patient draped for elbow arthroscopy, the anterolateral portal is noted with the retractor. This is the typical starting portal for inspection of the anterior joint

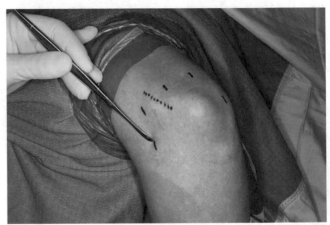

Fig. 76.3 The anteromedial portal is indicated with the probe; this is the typical starting portal on the medial side of the elbow. The ulnar nerve is marked with a dotted line

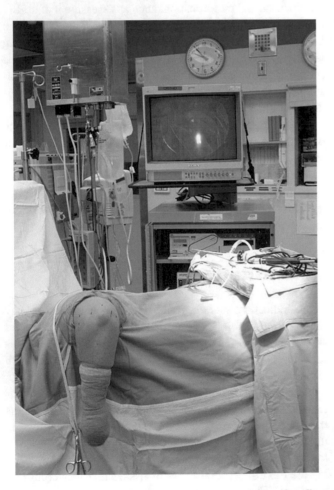

Fig. 76.1 Patient placed in the lateral decubitus position for elbow arthroscopy

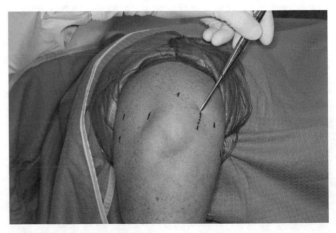

Fig. 76.4 View of the posterior portals, the ulnar nerve is identified by the probe. The direct posterior portal and posterolateral portals are seen more lateral

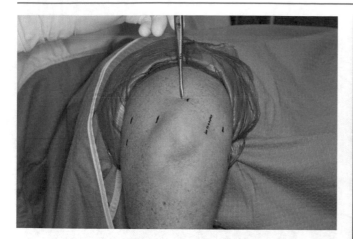

Fig. 76.5 The direct posterior portal is marked with a probe. The posterolateral portal is seen just lateral

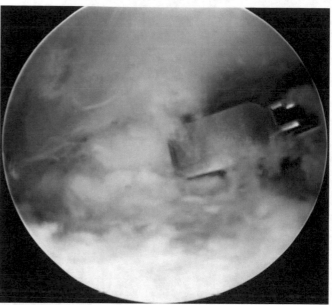

Fig. 76.6 Arthroscopic biter seen resecting the posteromedial capsule

through the triceps down to the olecranon fossa (Fig. 76.5). Shaving is necessary to remove fat and fibrous debris in order to gain a space for visualization. A radiofrequency probe may be used to facilitate this and to remove synovial tissue.

The posterolateral viewing portal is made approximately 1 cm proximal and lateral to the olecranon tip.

Direct visualization, after shaving away debris, is possible across the olecranon fossa and into the medial gutter of the joint. Under direct visualization, the shaver is used to follow into the medial gutter and to carefully expose the posteromedial aspect of the joint, the posteromedial capsule, and the medial gutter. A proximal accessory portal can also be used for placement of a blunt retractor to facilitate exposure.

Once adequate exposure of the posteromedial capsule is achieved, an arthroscopic biter is brought in to carefully and serially resect the posteromedial capsule, beginning a few cm proximal to the medial epicondylar region (Figs. 76.6 and 76.7). This continues distally down the medial gutter, until the level of the posterior portion of the anterior band of the MCL. In addition to a biter, careful use of a radiofrequency probe can be used to release the posteromedial capsule. The ulnar nerve may be visualized in the soft tissue adjacent to the resected joint capsule and is inspected to assure adequate decompression (Figs. 76.8, 76.9, and 76.10).

Following completion of the procedure, the portals are sutured and a sterile dressing applied. Postoperative rehabilitation is primarily determined by the primary procedure for which the arthroscopy is being done. Typically, full active motion is allowed on postoperative day two.

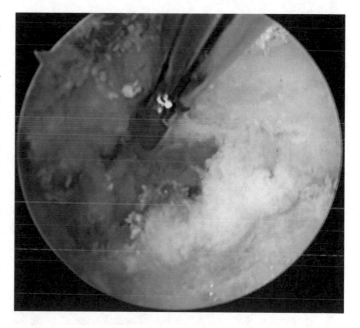

Fig. 76.7 Arthroscopic biter removing the posteromedial capsule, the ulnar nerve can be seen just to the right of the biter

Tips and Tricks

Avoid use of the arthroscopic shaver in the posterior aspect of the joint after the posteromedial capsule has been released, and the ulnar nerve is exposed to avoid inadvertent injury to

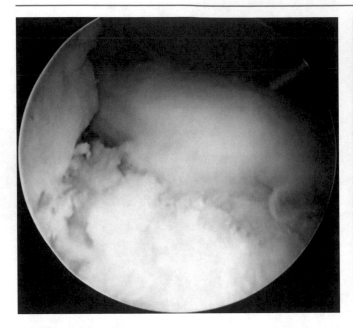

Fig. 76.8 After decompression of the ulnar nerve, the probe is seen pulling the nerve into the joint

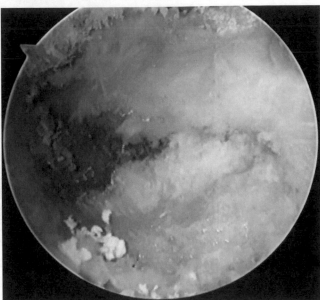

Fig. 76.10 Ulnar nerve is seen after decompression. In this case, an additional arthroscopic medial epicondulectomy was performed

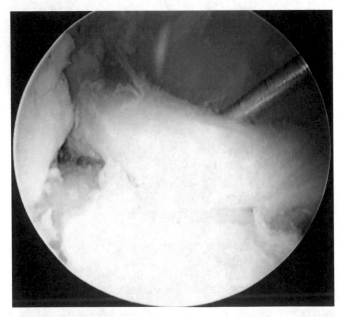

Fig. 76.9 The ulnar nerve has been decompressed, and the probe is seen holding the ulnar nerve free

the nerve. Using the direct posterior portal as the working portal and the posterolateral portal as the viewing portal is a good combination to allow resection of the posteromedial capsule.

Conclusion

Arthroscopic ulnar nerve decompression is an option for patients with mild to moderate ulnar nerve symptoms who are undergoing elbow arthroscopy for other reasons. Given that a simple in situ decompression can easily be done with a small incision, minimal simple and inexpensive equipment, easy setup and recovery, and tourniquet time of less than 10–15 min in most cases, we do not favor this procedure for patients who lack other concomitant indications for elbow arthroscopy. Most patients do well following the procedure, despite the anatomy of the procedure, which addresses deep structures which may contribute to ulnar nerve compression, rather than the more superficial structures [2].

References

1. Williams BG, Sotereanos DG, Baratz ME, Jarrett CD, Venouziou AI, Miller MC. The contracted elbow: is ulnar nerve release necessary? J Shoulder Elb Surg. 2012 Dec;21(12):1632–6. https://doi.org/10.1016/j.jse.2012.04.007. Epub 2012 Jun 26. PMID: 22743068.
2. Kovachevich R, Steinmann SP. Arthroscopic ulnar nerve decompression in the setting of elbow osteoarthritis. J Hand Surg Am. 2012 Apr;37(4):663–8. https://doi.org/10.1016/j.jhsa.2012.01.003. Epub 2012 Mar 3. PMID: 22386545.

Athletic Injuries of the Elbow

Jose Carlos Garcia Jr. and Alvaro Motta Cardoso Jr.

Introduction

Elbow injuries are common in athletes, mostly those involved in martial arts, racket sports, and overhead throwing [1–3]. Each lesion will depend on the sport's features and the devices used to perform the athletic activity. Size, weight, material properties, and additional instruments incorporated into the athletic devices are also important points to be considered.

A better treatment will depend on the biomechanics involved on each lesion and its relationship with the sport.

In this chapter, the main athletic lesions of the elbow will be addressed. For didactic purposes, the lesions will be divided by anatomic structures: ligaments, nerves, muscles and tendons, bones, and cartilage.

Ligaments

Medial Collateral Ligament (MCL)

Overhead throwing confers considerable stretch to the elbow and can cause one-of-a-kind tears. Biomechanical and clinical scientific papers have explained the causative variables in these tears and have permitted anticipation and treatment procedures to advance. Avoidance techniques, such as the checking of pitch counts, have been created to diminish the chance of harm in youthful competitors.

J. C. Garcia Jr. (✉)
Department of Orthopedic Surgery, NAEON Institute and Moriah Hospital, Sao Paulo, Brazil
e-mail: josecarlos@naeon.org.br

A. M. Cardoso Jr.
NAEON Institute, Sao Paulo, Brazil
e-mail: alvaro@naeon.org.br

Advancing surgical procedures have contributed to changes in strategies for treating certain conditions in the throwing competitor.

The MCL is of utmost importance for elbow stability. Its anterior bundle is the main stabilizer between 30° and 120° of elbow flexion. The posterior bundle contributes to stability mainly when the elbow is in a flexed position. The MCL is responsible for 54% of valgus load resistance [3].

Its tear is caused by a valgus load or during the elbow dislocation. The MCL is the foremost clinically relevant anatomic structure within the elbow of the tossing competitor. It is composed of the anterior oblique, posterior oblique, and transverse ligaments. The anterior oblique is the most grounded tendon of the complex and the foremost critical stabilizer to valgus load for throwers. Its origin is at the rotational center of the medial epicondyle, and its ulnar insertion expands distal to the sublime tubercle [4]. The anterior oblique ligament has anterior and posterior bands. Each band has a different role in different angles to resist the valgus stretch. The anterior band is tighter amid extension, and the posterior band is tight amid flexion.

The MCL gets energetic bolster from the encompassing musculature. The flexor carpi ulnaris is the essential energetic supporter to valgus stabilization of the elbow, and the flexor digitorum superficialis could be an auxiliary stabilizer [5]. These two muscles help spread the significant strengths over the elbow during the throwing.

The throwing movement makes considerable vitality and ensues strengths that are intervened by structures near the elbow. Precise speeds as high as 3000°/s have been measured at the elbow during the increasing speed stage of the throwing movement. For throwers, the MCL lesion can also be part of a continuous process of attenuation resulting in a weak ligament. The ligament can become painful, reducing the thrower's accuracy and strength, compromising performance or impeding play, even before a complete tear [6]. Elbow medial pain during the early late cocking and early acceleration phases of pitching are the most common symptoms. The moving valgus stress test

© Springer Nature Switzerland AG 2022
W. B. Geissler (ed.), *Wrist and Elbow Arthroscopy with Selected Open Procedures*,
https://doi.org/10.1007/978-3-030-78881-0_77

can be useful for determining MCL involvement [7]. Other soft tissue restraints such as capsule and flexor-pronator musculotendinous structures play a secondary but important role in preventing valgus instability during the throwing motion [3].

Maximal valgus load is reached in the acceleration phase within an elbow motion from 90° to 120° flexion to 25° extension [8]. The elbow restraint structures can resist a moment of 64 N*m and medial tensile force of 290 N [9, 10].

Since elastic properties of the MCL do not exceed 34 N*m, the other stabilizers of the elbow are critical for dodging or minimizing damage [11].

The valgus load increases stress on the others sites of the elbow. Tensile forces happen on the medial side. Shear and compressive stresses happen within the olecranon fossa as the elbow comes to extension, and compression forces happen laterally, basically at the radiocapitellar joint. A study found that sidelong contact increased 67% after the MCL was transected [12]. Understanding these strength increments the capacity to get it the connections among the conditions that happen around the elbow.

It is imperative to understand the point within the throwing movement at which pain or discomfort happens (windup, early cocking, late cocking, acceleration, deceleration, or follow through). The sorts of pitches, the number of pitches thrown per inning, and the tossing plan can also influence the athlete's performance; therefore, one ought to respect the individuality of each thrower. The curveball produces the most prominent valgus push at the elbow. The fastball and slider create the most noteworthy constraint, and the changeup creates less push on the elbow and is considered a generally secure pitch for competitors of all ages [13].

Ordinarily, the center of the examination in a throwing competitor is on the medial elbow. A tear of the MCL ordinarily happens proximally at the medial epicondyle, and edema or elevated sensibility there or along the length of the anterior oblique ligament is seen. Stress testing of the flexor-pronator mass is done. Valgus push at 0° and 30° of flexion, moreover, is regularly evaluated, but the flimsiness is regularly more unobtrusive in a tossing competitor.

The sensitivity of the moving valgus stress test is reported to be 100%, with 75% specificity [14]. A competitor with suspected MCL harm should also be evaluated for ulnar nerve pathology. Proof of nerve subluxation, a positive Tinel sign, or indications with elbow hyperflexion testing ought to be tested and noticed.

Comparative X-rays can be done with valgus stress, and its increased medial side space will strongly suggest MCL lesions. MRI is the better exam for diagnosis once it enables one to assess many pathologies around the elbow, like osteochondritis dissecans, a MCL harm, separation of the flexor-pronator mass, and attenuation of the MCL. The signal intensity on MRI can be used to anticipate rates of healing. Patients with a total or high-grade MCL tear were most likely to require surgery [15].

Ultrasonography can be a useful exam, but it lacks good scientific papers to sustain its relevance [16, 17].

Arthroscopy can also be used to diagnose the tears. With pronated forearm, elbow flexion of 60°-75°, scope is inserted trough the anterolateral portal and a valgus stress is done in order to test the ligament. One- to 2-mm joint line openings are related to partial tears and 4- to 10-mm openings to full tears [18].

Elbow ligament lesions can be disabling. These lesions are highly prevalent for Brazilian Jiu-Jitsu and other grappling martial arts [19].

The initial treatment of an MCL tear in an athlete ought to be nonsurgical. The regimen incorporates a 6-week period of rest from athletic activities as well as fortification of the flexor-pronator musculature [5]. After this treatment for those asymptomatic and presenting no signs of MCL compromise, it is suggested to optimize the sports mechanics and proprioception. For throwers, late trunk turns, less shoulder external rotation, and increased elbow flexion have been appeared to extend valgus stretch at the elbow [20]. A 42% return-to-sport rate was detailed for overhead throwers at a mean 24.5-week follow-up [21].

Surgical Reconstruction of the MCL

Surgical procedures use a medial approach. The author's preference is a medial approach through the flexor carpi ulnaris from the medial epicondyle toward the sublime tubercle of the ulna, a 7-cm incision. The graft choice will depend on the exercise demands of the patient. For very strong athletes, the semitendinosus graft can be used. A double-band palmaris longus tendon graft can also be an option.

There are several fixation methods, such as Fig. 77.8 fixation, docking technique, interference screws, and others.

The author's fixation preference is using interference screws in both sublime tubercle of the ulna and rotational center of the humerus (Fig. 77.1). This fixation is done with

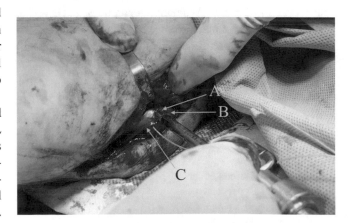

Fig. 77.1 Medial elbow. (A) Interference screw. (B) Medial epicondyle. (C) Tendon graft

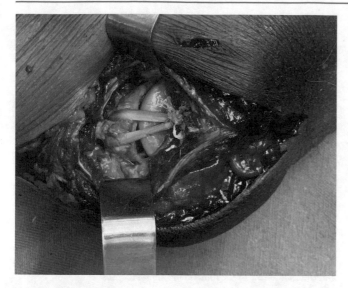

Fig. 77.2 Medial elbow. Transosseous fixation with a bone tunnel through the sublime tubercle and humeral fixation at the rotational center with interference screw

the elbow in varus stress and 60° of flexion. The ulnar nerve can be anteriorized if one understands it can be entrapped by the graft. Passing the graft through a bone tunnel within the sublime tubercle of the ulna and doing just one fixation at the rotational center of the humerus using interference screw is also an option (Fig. 77.2). The interference screw sizes are generally 5.5 × 15 mm, 4.75 × 15 mm, or 4 × 10 mm.

Hyperextension Mechanism Lesions

The most common armlock for fighters [1] presented the following sequence of events: lesion of the teres pronator at its humeral origin, MCL, and anterior capsule allowing then the elbow dislocation. After dislocation, the hyperextension continuity can even cause the brachial muscle to be torn.

The continuous arm locks have led some athletes to develop a fibrosis at the anteromedial aspect of the elbow with loss of flexion on the most affected side when compared to the contralateral side. Ulnar nerve slight symptoms are frequent in these patients, probably due to this fibrosis and tension. Anteromedial tenderness during abrupt flexion can be felt in many athletes, even those that do not mention any pain or difficulty in fight or daily activities. In the senior author's (JCG) experience, just one case needed to arthroscopically remove anterior scars. Flexor-pronator muscles are strong in these patients, and even if a lesion of MCL is present, its reconstruction is quite infrequent. Lesion of the MCL generally does not affect the sports activities of these athletes. However, if instability symptoms compromise their sports activities, MCL reconstruction can be a surgical option.

Valgus and Flexion Mechanism Lesion

This mechanism is common on the figure four armlock with grappling fighters. It presents the following sequence of events: lesion of MCL followed by the medial portion of triceps. In some cases, the lesion expands laterally and the whole triceps is torn.

Medial and central portions of the triceps have presented better strength characteristics than the lateral part [22]; therefore, patients presenting with previous triceps tendinopathy are those at risk of presenting with this instability. Indeed, the senior author has just seen this lesion in two situations, triceps tendinopathy and/or high-energy lesions.

However, the most common presentation is that just the MCL is torn. Patients in this situation are not willing to undergo a surgical procedure. For patients with complete lesions, a surgical procedure to reconstruct triceps and MCL is needed.

If triceps lesions are partial, treatment will depend on the instability and triceps residual strength.

Varus Posteromedial Rotatory Instability

The elbow stability has a substantial contribution from the osseous structures; it is markedly important in varus posteromedial instability. Coronoid is the main varus restrictor of the elbow. The coronoid oblique anteromedial fracture will occur when the trochlea impacts the medial coronoid. It is associated with the lateral collateral ligament lesion [23]. This mechanism is not so common but can be present in grappling fights due to the inverted figure four armlock.

The varus posteromedial rotatory instability grind test can be used for patients suspected of having this instability. In this test, the patient full abducts the arm away from the body and actively flexes and extends the arm. Crepitus and varus deformity are considered positive for this lesion [24].

Depending on the coronoid fracture's size, an osteosynthesis can be necessary. It can be associated with the lateral ligament reconstruction to improve stability. Indeed, the author's preference in high-demand athletes is osteosynthesis associated with lateral collateral ulnar ligament (LCUL) reconstruction using interference screws and a palmaris longus double band.

Posterolateral-Rotatory Instability of the Elbow (PLRI)

Posterolateral-rotatory instability of the elbow is caused by one of the most common mechanisms of elbow dislocation, combining slight flexion, compression, valgus, and supination. The first structure to be lesioned is the ulnar branch of the collateral lateral ligament. It acts as a restrictor to the posterior translation of the radial head in relationship to the capitellum [25].

This ligament's lesion will cause lateral elbow pain or even instability in valgus and supination with semi-extension of the elbow [25]. Some patients can also experience the posterior-lateral instability, but it is more commonly reached just under anesthesia. The posterolateral pivot-shift test, posterolateral rotatory drawer test, and chair push-up apprehension can be useful for diagnosis [24].

Lesion of the ulnar collateral lateral ligament is the first stage of O'Driscoll. It is followed by anterior and posterior capsular lesion, stage two, where the distal humerus is perched over the tip of the coronoid. The third stage is the complete elbow dislocation, compromising the MCL.

History of lateral pain after a traumatic event is a common history for this instability. Instability and/or pain when provocative tests are performed will give higher suspicion to this diagnosis. MRI can also give more details of the lesion.

The Osborn-Cotterill posterior impacted capitellum's fracture will need special attention because it can be considered for many as the elbow's Hill-Sachs, jeopardizing this articulation stability [26]. In some cases, a capitellar bone repair needs to be done before or with the ligament reconstruction [27].

Dislocation Due to the PLR Mechanism in Sports

Falling down with the elbow in semi-extension, supination, and valgus is the most important and known cause of posterolateral rotatory mechanism elbow dislocation. However, it can also happen in Olympic-style weightlifting. The Olympic-style weightlifting has two different competition lifts: snatch and the clean and jerk. The arm begins in full pronation for both lifts.

Snatch presents six phases, with the following sequence of events: first pull, transition from the first to the second pull, the second pull, turnover under the barbell, the catch phase, and rising from the squat position [28].

During the catch phase, there are combined movements on the scapular girdle and shoulder that will need an elbow supination to correct the shoulder external rotation. The catch is done with the barbell in a superior and slight posterior position in relation to the coronal plane. In this position, the elbow will be in a semi-extension position and loaded in valgus. These combinations of movements – valgus, supination, and semi-extension with excessive compressive load – will produce the posterior-lateral rotatory mechanism. Therefore, elbow dislocation can take place.

Clean and jerk presents the two phases. During the jerk phase, a catch similar to that described for the snatch is also done, with the same upper-limb characteristics [29].

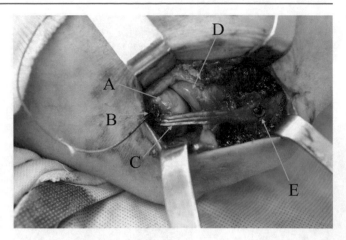

Fig. 77.3 (A) Capitellum. (B) Interference screw of the humerus. (C) Double-band palmaris Llongus autograft. (D) Radial head. (E) Interference screw of the ulna on the supinator crest

The author's preference for LCUL reconstruction is with the Kocher's approach. The graft of choice is the palmaris longus in a double-band configuration. Fixation on the supinator crest and humeral rotational center is done using interference screws (Fig. 77.3).

Nerve Entrapment Syndromes

Nerve entrapment is multifactorial. It can be associated with fibrous bands, androgen steroids abuse, trauma, deformities, and repetitive movements. Some of these situations will be pushed by athletic activities to the limit, compromising neurologic and even vascular structures. Movements involved in each sport need to be considered for diagnosing these conditions. Many times, correcting the sports gesture and adequate use of the sport devices can be the initial treatment for almost all neurologic conditions associated with sports.

Posterior Interosseous Nerve

The posterior interosseous nerve syndrome is also known as resistant tennis elbow. Indeed, it is sometimes difficult to reach the diagnosis, since this is a motor nerve and no paresthesia is associated with its entrapment syndrome. The pain is slightly anterior and distal to the lateral epicondyle. It is associated with supination movements. Resisted supination causes pain marked with the flexed instead of extended elbow. Therapeutic tests using neurotropic medications such as pregabalin can be more useful than electromyographic studies, once better peripheral neuropathic pain control has been achieved by using pregabalin [30]. Even though the dynamic electromyographic studies have high specificity and positive predictive values, they do not present sensibility

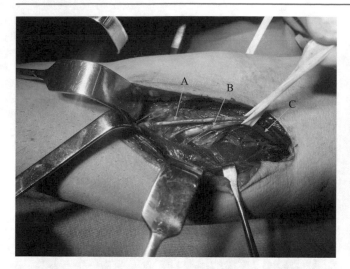

Fig. 77.4 (A) Sensitive radial nerve. (B) Posterior interosseous nerve. (C) Radial nerve

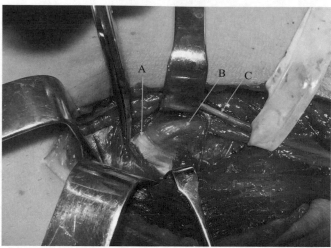

Fig. 77.5 (A) Fröse arch. (B) Posterior interosseous nerve. (C) Sensitive radial nerve

and negative predictive values high enough to achieve the diagnosis.

Movements beginning with pronation and accelerating in forced supination, as some racket sports players do, can cause this compression. In these cases, one will need to improve the sports gesture with a better balance of the shoulder movement, avoiding the overuse of forearm pronation and supination. Some sports that use the hand grip associated with forearm supination, such as Jiu Jitsu, can also present this entrapment.

Clinical treatment is based on physiotherapeutic myofascial release, stretching, and soft tissue-based management. Corticosteroids and NSAIDs can reduce local inflammation and swelling around the nerve. The author also highly recommends the use of pregabalin for treating pain associated with posterior interosseous nerve syndrome.

In refractory cases, surgical release will need to take place. One needs to be sure that the entrapment is just in the interosseous posterior nerve. If symptoms also involve the sensitive radial nerve, other possible compression regions such as the lateral head of triceps and the lateral part of the cubital fossa need to be explorated. Some cases of high bifurcation will also require an approach in the arm 4–5 cm from the lateral epicondyle.

When conservative treatment fails or the recurrence is unacceptable, the surgical procedure is necessary. In these cases, an anterior approach on the medial border of the brachioradialis is done (Fig. 77.4). The sensitive radial nerve is easily found, and any vascular alterations, such as recurrent vascular artery, fibrous bands, bursa, and synovia, need to be removed, if compressing the nerve.

The Fröse arcade and supinator are the most common compression sites, and their release is strongly recommended (Fig. 77.5).

Musculocutaneous Nerve

On the elbow, the lateral antebrachial cutaneous nerve, a sensitive branch of the musculocutaneous nerve, rises between the lateral margin of the biceps tendon and the brachialis muscle aponeurosis. An entrapment in this region is not common. Often it is due to the mechanism of resisted pronation and elbow flexion [31].

The anterolateral pain or paresthesia can be increased by direct pressure over the compression area or in forced flexion with pronated elbow.

Avoiding biceps training with the forearm pronated and full extension, at least during the treatment, are required measures. Stopping anabolic drugs abuse, for users, is also necessary. Nonsurgical management with medicines and physical therapy is the standard for treating this pathology.

For refractory cases, a release is an option. The author's preference is from antecubital fossae to proximal just lateral to the biceps. Soft tissues around the nerve and scar release associated with facial release of the brachialis are necessary (Fig. 77.6). Sometimes even a biceps triangular excision at the compression site is required.

The author did not find this biceps excision required in his experience; however, every case needs to be evaluated, and the surgeon can customize the treatment to the real necessities of every patient.

Ulnar Nerve

The ulnar nerve is located medial and posterior to the rotational center. These characteristics make this nerve mainly sensitive to valgus and flexion movements.

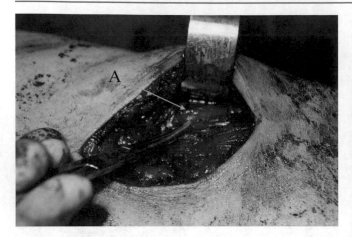

Fig. 77.6   Musculocutaneous nerve (A)

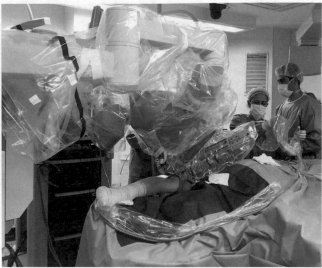

Fig. 77.7   Setup of the DaVinci® Robot on the operative field

The repetition microtrauma on throwing sports with high varus moment can cause both lesion and attenuation of the MCL. For both, the valgus can promote an ulnar nerve stretch, compromising it. Other conditions such as anconeus epitrochlearis can also be the cause of ulnar nerve entrapment, mainly in patients in which sports will cause muscular hypertrophy. One needs to take care to actually understand the correct site of compression, once the ulnar nerve can be compressed from the Strüthers arcade in the arm to the Guyon canal in the wrist. The Tinel test can be useful to elucidate the compression area. As the cubital tunnel is externally located in relationship with the rotational elbow center, the elbow flexion will tend to tension the nerve. Indeed, intraneural pressure can increase sevenfold with the elbow flexion. Thus, in cases of cubital tunnel syndrome, the elbow flexion during 30 s can reproduce paresthesia in the ulnar nerve's autogenous area, the medial part of the fourth finger, and all of the fifth finger.

Nonsurgical management with pregabalin, B-vitamin complexes and physical therapy is the standard for treating this pathology in the beginning. Surgical treatment is the next step when conservative treatment fails.

Entrapments that are secondary to other conditions will need to treat their primary cause associated with a release or anteriorization of the ulnar nerve.

For pathologies of the cubital tunnel, the best surgical option remains questionable; release or anteriorization has achieved similar effectiveness and safety [32]. Patients that have trend to nerve instability before surgery or those with secondary entrapments are better candidates for anterior transposition in the author's opinion.

Author's Preferred Treatment The nerve release can be done by open or endoscopic procedures. It is important that the release extends from the Strüthers ach to the Osborn's arch. The endoscopic release is recommended in elbows with no previous surgery and, therefore, with no previous scar tissue.

For elbows with potential scars, an open or robotic endoscopic release is an option (Fig. 77.7) [33]. In the author's opinion, endoscopic releases will present advantages mainly in less scar formation and less inflammatory reactions.

Median Nerve

The median nerve compression at the elbow is not common, being more related to anatomic variations such as Gantzer muscle, palmaris profundus, flexor carpi radialis brevis, variations of the lacertus fibrosus, supracondylar process, vascular perforation, and muscular variations [24].

Some of these anatomical variations associated with overuse can be responsible for the nerve entrapment. Initial assessment includes physical examination and X-ray studies.

The electromyographic study will often present negative results because this is essentially a dynamic condition. Physical exam will generally identify the correct entrapment site. Compression by the following structures is highly suggested in the presence of paresthesia in the median region:

- Lacertus fibrosus: Elbow-resisted flexion
- Teres pronator: Forearm-resisted pronation
- Flexor digitorum superficialis' arch: Proximal interphalangeal resisted flexion

The author suggests that each test has a duration of 30 s in order to better evaluate each possible compression site.

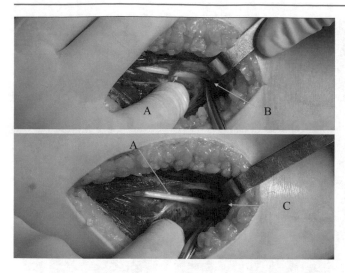

Fig. 77.8 (A) Median nerve. (B) Anomalous teres pronator. (C) Released teres pronator

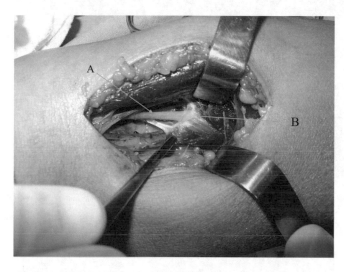

Fig. 77.9 (A) Median nerve. (B) Anomalous flexor digitorum superficialis arch

Author's Preferred Treatment An anteromedial approach following the medial border of the teres pronator is done 3–4 cm anterior to the medial epicondyle. The first structure to be found and released is the lacertus fibrosus. In sequence, one can identify near the cubital fossae the median nerve with the surrounded vascular structures. The nerve will generally pass through flexor mass in an intermuscular plan. Anatomical muscular variations can be a cause of compression, and their release is required (Fig. 77.8). The nerve is followed until it enters into the flexor digitorum superficialis' arch. This arch can be also released if one considers it can be an entrapment site (Fig. 77.9).

Muscle and Tendons

Chronic Exertional Compartment Syndrome (CECS): The "Arm Pump"

This condition can be suspected in patients with pain, commonly at the flexor mass, with worsening during activities that will require strength for gripping.

It is not an uncommon condition in competitive motorcycling, gymnastics, climbing, rowers, hockey, water skiing, kayaking, and wheelchair athletics [34].

Different degrees of compartmental syndrome will require different treatments, from rest and NSAIDs until the surgical procedures. Its suspicion is suggested in the presence of the forearm pain, loss of grip strength, and some paresthesia. These symptoms are present just during activities. Rises of 10 mmHg on intracompartmental monitoring after exercise will confirm the diagnosis [35].

Open or endoscopic fascial release is a surgical option to treat these patients [36].

Triceps

Lesions of triceps are rare, accounting for less than 1% of tendon lesions [37]. The typical lesion is avulsion from the olecranon 90%, males with 40–50 years old. They are more likely to happen in patients with triceps tendinopathies or previous partial lesions. The mechanism is eccentric contraction in maximum elongation of the muscle [24]. Changes on the tendon's architecture such as dehydration can make this structure stiffer and with a bigger elastic module. It will have a negative effect on energy dissipation, and the tendon can be torn.

When the triceps tendon is torn, a posterior deformity in the arm is apparent, with bruising and loss of elbow extension strength [38].

The "fleck sign" is commonly present in X-ray exams if there is some bone detachment; however, many times just a tendinous lesion takes place. Therefore, most of the times it is necessary to use grafts because of the tendon's poor quality and/or retraction.

Treatment needs to be personalized. If retractions are important and it is not possible to return the tendon to its original insertion, two strategies can be used:

- Fasciotomy similar to Vulpius technique. This is not recommended if the surgeon is not used to doing similar techniques. It is also not recommended for more than 5-cm distances with elbow at 90° (Fig. 77.10).
- My personal preference in large lesions is a triple autologous semitendinosus graft from the patient's knee. The

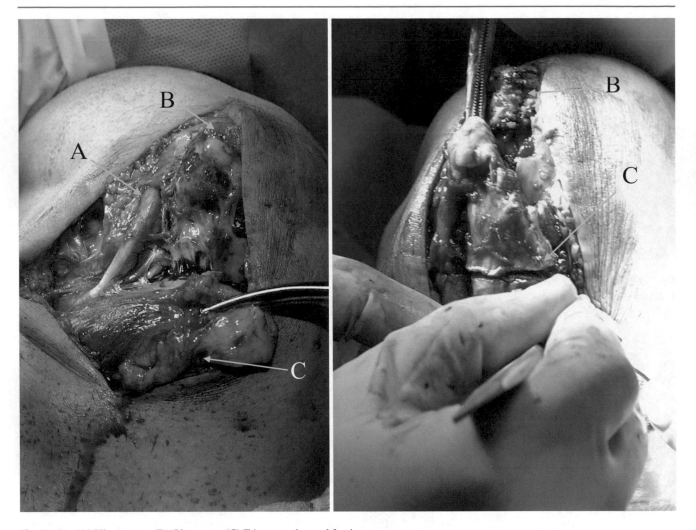

Fig. 77.10 (A) Ulnar nerve. (B) Olecranon. (C) Triceps tendon and fascia

graft passes through the olecranon by a bone tunnel and through the muscle just proximal to its myotendinous transition in an O figure. When possible, an additional tendon reinforcement is done by inserting remaining tendon into the olecranon tip in a triple semitendinosus band, Ø figure (Fig. 77.11).

- The use of cadaveric Achilles tendon graft can also be an option that can easily fit on the triceps.
- In some special cases for very high-demand athletes where it is possible to reinsert the triceps, one can make a reinforcement in O figure by using the palmaris longus associated with the triceps insertion.

A cast in semi-extension can be used in the first 3 weeks in order to better protect the sutures. Passive movements will begin 2 weeks after the surgery. Three weeks after the surgery, active movements can begin with no strength.

Biceps

Distal biceps lesions are becoming more common with time, presenting an incidence of 5:100,000 persons/year [39]. The short head of biceps inserts ulnar and distally to the long head. Lacertus fibrosus originates from the short head of biceps [40]. When this structure remains intact, it can prevent biceps retractions, making the clinical examination not so obvious. Eccentric load in a semi-flexed elbow and a biceps contraction when the elbow is forced to extend are the most common mechanisms [41].

Clinical presentation is an antecubital and cubital bruise with muscular retraction, pain, and weakness for flexion and supination. An anterior cordlike absence on the affected elbow is also a sign.

Nonsurgical treatment can be considered in elderly patients, low-demand patients, or those with no clinical con-

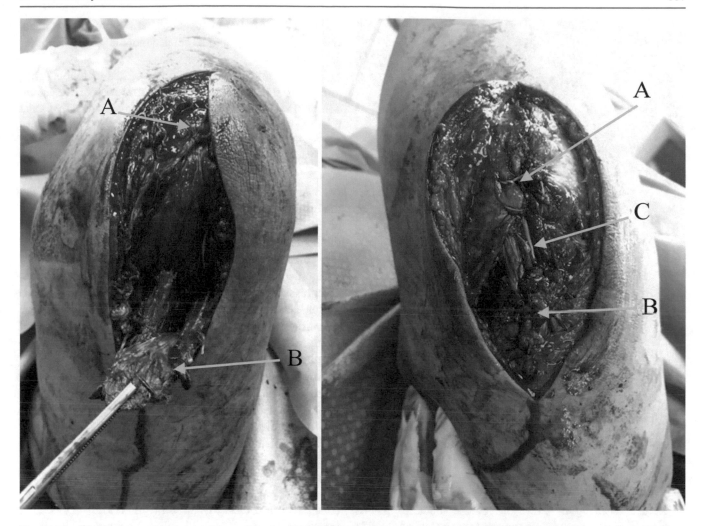

Fig. 77.11 (A) Olecranon, (B) Triceps tendon and fascia. (C) Semitendinosus grafts

ditions that will accept the arm deformity. In athletes, the surgical procedure is highly recommended.

The tendon on the bicipital tubercle can be done by two-incision or anterior approaches. The author's preference is the two-incision approach by using transosseous fixation; however, the single incision using endobutton can also be a good option (Fig. 77.12). Other fixation options are not the author's preference but also need be considered.

In chronic lesions with retractions, the use of graft is recommended (Fig. 77.13), but additional complications such as the closure of the biceps tunnel between the radius and ulna need to be considered. The only temporary radial nerve transitory palsy the author has faced was a grafted double approach.

Our institute experience is by reconstructing more than 100 distal biceps in the last 10 years. Our best results were in a two-incision approach by using transosseous fixation and single incision using endobutton. For chronic with graft, the two-incision approach was used for almost all patients.

A cast in 90° flexion can be used in the first week in order to better protect the sutures. Passive movements will begin in

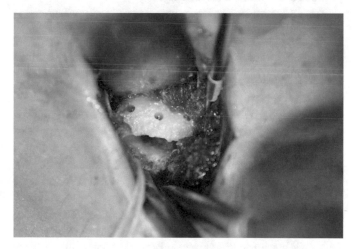

Fig. 77.12 Bone tunnels in the medial approach for transosseous distal biceps reconstruction

the following week; a sling is used. Just passive movements are allowed the second week after the surgery. In the third week after the surgery, active movements can begin with no strength.

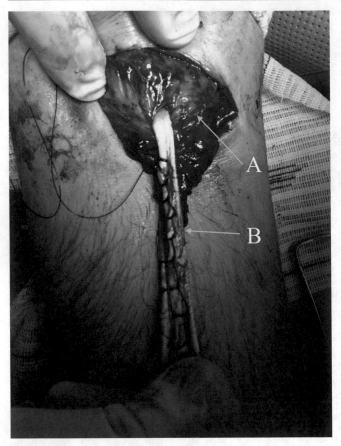

Fig. 77.13 (A) Biceps. (B) Semitendinosus graft

Return to the gym with 50% of the loads is allowed 3 months after surgery. One-hundred percent of the load is permitted 5 months after surgery.

An endoscopic approach was recently described using suture anchors.

Lateral Epicondylitis

Lateral epicondylitis could be a common source of pain on the sidelong of the elbow. This tendinopathy has a rate of 1.3% within the population between 30 and 64 years, with a peak between 45 and 54 [42]. It ordinarily influences the prevailing upper extremity and is related with a repetitive and forceful movements [43].

In spite of the fact that the lateral epicondylitis is commonly known as tennis elbow, this term is not totally justified. This tendinopathy is regularly work-related and happens in patients not playing tennis [44]; in any case, it has been assessed in 10–50% of individuals who frequently play tennis [45]. Epicondylitis is more common in male than female tennis players, unlike what happens within the common population. Lateral epicondylitis is more common than medial-sided elbow pain, with proportions allegedly extending from

4:1 to 7:1 [46]. Dominant elbow is commonly included. Intense onsets of symptoms happen more regularly in youthful competitors.

To better understand the etiology of this tendinopathy, it is basic to analyze the anatomic connections of the lateral compartment of the elbow. There are connections that exist between the extensor carpi radialis longus (ECL) and extensor carpi radialis brevis (ECRB) [47]. The extensor carpi radialis longus (ECRL) origin is muscular along the lateral supracondylar edge of the humerus. The shape of the muscle is triangular, with the summit situated proximally. Indeed, the origin of the ECRB is completely tendinous. The origin of the ECRB is found fair underneath the distal-most tip of the lateral supracondylar edge. The footprint of the tendon has a diamond shape of almost 13 × 7 mm.

Biomechanical investigation has shown that eccentric compressions of the extensor carpi radialis brevis (ECRB) muscle amid backhand tennis swings are the cause of dreary microtraumas that result in microtears within the origin of the ligament [48]. Different causes such as trauma within the lateral region of the elbow, hypovascularity, fluoroquinolone antimicrobials, and anatomic variations need also to be addressed [49–51].

Subsequently, many have shown the nature of the pathology is actually a degenerative tendinopathy. Macroscopic tearing in affiliation with the histological findings was depicted [52]. Nirschl called these histological changes "angiofibroblastic hyperplasia" [53, 54]. In his ponder, the famous gray friable tissue is characterized by disorganized collagen arrangement with juvenile fibroblastic and vascular components.

In this way, expanded rates of apoptosis and cellular autophagy have been observed in tenocytes, coming about in disruption of extracellular collagen matrix and weakening of the tendon [55]. These changes at the tendon's origin are the pathologic mending reaction to microtears caused by repetitive eccentric or concentric overburdening of the extensor muscle mass [56]. The origin of the extensor digitorum communis (EDC) is additionally involved in lateral epicondylitis [57, 58].

Patients complain of pain that emanates from the lateral epicondyle down to the lower arm, frequently related with weakness and difficulties within the handgrip. Physical examination ought to start with the cervical spine and be taken after by the whole upper extremity. The examination continues at that point to the elbow. The elbow is delicate over the lateral epicondyle and somewhat distal, into the extensor mass.

Cozen active maneuver (resisted wrist extension with the elbow in full extension and forearm in pronation) and Mills passive maneuver (maximal wrist flexion with the elbow in full extension and forearm in pronation) can worsen pain at the lateral epicondyle. The first maneuver causes agonizing eccentric contraction at the origin of the ECRB. The second maneuver places the ECRB on maximal extension, latently tensioning the muscle origin and in this way causing pain. In order to avoid the nearness of a plica, the elbow must be flexed latently with the lower arm pronated and supinated. In the event that a plica is included, the point of maximal delicacy is ordinarily found more distally and posteriorly, over the radiocapitellar joint, compared to lateral epicondylitis. Other causes of lateral-sided elbow pain can be nerve entrapments at one or more destinations, such as radial tunnel disorder or posterior interosseous nerve (PIN) disorder. Up to 5% of patients with lateral epicondylitis present radial nerve entrapment [59].

Pain evoked with resisted supination with elbow flexion or with the resisted long-finger extension (when the nerve is caught at the ECRB) can show PIN entrapment. Differential diagnosis for atraumatic lateral elbow pain may incorporate radicular cervical spine illness, radial nerve compression, intra-articular free bodies, and chondral injuries. Tumors, avascular necrosis, and osteochondritis dissecans of the capitellum, indeed on the off chance that is less common, may be considered as well.

Imaging can be performed as well. Ultrasound is additionally valuable. Frequently, times in the event that no tendon changes counting neovascularization, thinning, thickening, or tears are distinguished on ultrasound at that point an alternate conclusion ought to be looked for. MRI is frequently utilized to clarify anatomic pathology including edema within the ERCB tendon and tendinopathic changes.

A really high recovery rate can be anticipated with classic nonoperative treatment, which incorporates the following physical and recovery modalities: activity adjustment, rest, and ice. These modalities are the beginning treatment of any case of lateral epicondylopathy. The competitor ought to diminish their load intensity when side effects show with early treatment and fitting time to recuperating. The volume of training counting recurrence and intensity ought to be carefully observed and controlled on the competitor's return to court. Alterations to the way the competitor plays the game of tennis can incorporate things such as two-fisted compared to a single-fisted backhand, a more adaptable or stun retentive racquet design, lower string pressure, selecting a slower court surface, broader racquets, as well as adjust to a bigger grip.

Counterforce braces act to diminish the drive on the extensor mechanism. They are outlined to be put on the arm distal to the region of tendinopathy with the objective of moving the loading location on the tendon.

Prolotherapy is a treatment that involves the injection of sclerosing agents (mainly dextrose) into an area of painful tendinosis or osteoarthritis. It is cheap and useful for early stages of the pathology.

Coricosteroid injection has classically been one of the staples of treatment for lateral epicondylopathy. Short term is a nice option, but the results start to fade fast. Ultimately, it shows up that the dangers of injection, counting tendon tear, failure, and muscle atrophy do not outweigh the long-term benefits; however, it remains a short-term option. One needs to avoid more than 2 or 3 shots for each elbow for life.

Randomized trials have also presented worst outcomes at 1 year for steroid injected patients versus placebo and no difference between corticosteroids and physical therapy.

Injection of platelet-rich plasma (PRP) can also be a treatment option on treating the lateral epicondylopathy. The method is completed in office by drawing blood from the patient, putting the blood in a centrifuge, and reinjecting the spun down platelet products into the affected area in the patient. This procedure can be done beneath ultrasound direction to guarantee infusion straightforwardly into the tendon.

Injection of hyaluronic acid can also be used; however, its results are still controversial.

Operative Treatment

Percutaneous

A blade, regularly number 11, is embedded perpendicular to the skin front to the lateral epicondyle, at that point a 1-centimeter-long skin cut is performed. A total release of the common extensor origin is performed moving the tip of the blade anteriorly and inferiorly from the lateral epicondyle. A further displacement is at that point accomplished by the Mill's manipulation, comprising of a persuasive, full extension of the elbow with the lower arm completely pronated and the wrist and fingers held in flexion.

Open

The ERCB tendon's origin is found underneath the lateral epicondylar prominence, along a longitudinal edge, and is directed from the upper portion of the capitellum to the level of the radiohumeral joint. Its tendon runs underneath the extensor digitorum communis and its aponeurosis distally to the epicondyle. It can be effectively separated, proceeding from anterior to posterior and beginning at the intersection between the ECRL and EDC aponeurosis. The undersurface of the ECRB tendon can be raised from the ECRL muscle in oblique fashion. The aponeurosis of the EDC lies on top of the ECRB and is firmly restricted. The ECRB tendon is debrided and the epicondylar origin stripped or penetrated. The open approach leads to more prominent visualization of the operative field and the pathologic tissue; in any case, it is related with a higher frequency of complications and a longer time to return to work.

Arthroscopy

Arthroscopic release is particularly shown when a concomitant intra-articular pathology is suspected. The advantage of investigating the joint is recently expanding the indications. Patient is put in lateral decubitus position with the operative arm bolstered by an arm holder at 100° of flexion/90° of abduction at the level of the shoulder. The elbow is situated at 90° of flexion, with the lower arm hanging free from gravity. Ten milliliters of sterile saline solution are infused before setting the portals to distend the elbow joint. A proximal anteromedial portal is made 2–3 cm proximal to the medial humeral epicondyle and 1 cm front to the intramuscular septum. At that point, a 30° arthroscope is embedded into this entrance. This permits intra-articular demonstrative evaluation of the anterior compartment. The proximal anterolateral is done around 3 cm proximal and 1 cm front to the lateral epicondyle.

A retractor, pointed at the radiocapitellar joint to secure the posterior interosseous nerve, can be embedded through this portal. The instruments are introduced through the anterolateral portal, found 1.5 to 2 cm proximal and 1 cm front to the lateral epicondyle.

Lateral synovitis is debrided and the lateral capsule is released. The capsule is ordinarily intact, but every so often it is conceivable to recognize a disturbance of the basic capsule. A bipolar thermal release of the lateral soft tissues is performed. With this strategy, the capsule is first incised or released from the humerus. After the capsule is withdrawn distally, the ECRB tendon is visualized posteriorly and the ECRL can be identified more anteriorly. Once the capsule is satisfactorily resected, the ECRB origin is released from the epicondyle: starting at the top of the capitellum, the release is at that point carried posteriorly. Ordinarily, the whole ECRB withdraws distally away from the humerus. Care is taken not to release the extensor aponeurosis that lies behind the ECRB tendon. This structure can be seen as a striped background of transversely situated tendon and muscular fibers much less unmistakable than the ECRB. It is found posterior to the ECRL.

Medial Epicondylitis

Medial epicondylitis is less usual than lateral epicondylitis, and it happens mainly because of repetitive wrist flexions and forced pronation during racquet sports, overhead throwing, and golf. The main site of pain is medial elbow and gets worse when actively pronating and flexing the forearm. The diagnosis is fundamentally clinical, but ultrasonography and MRI are detailed to be valuable [60]. MRI presents signal increased about the medial epicondyle [61].

The main treatment is nonsurgical and has high rates of success. The components of a commonplace nonsurgical treatment program incorporate NSAIDs, flexibility training, ice, and guided physical treatment. Steroid infusions have

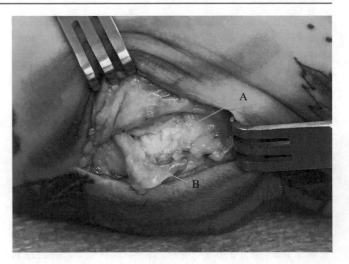

Fig. 77.14 (A) Area with degenerative tendon besides the medial epicondyle. (B) Normal tendon of the flexor pronators

moreover been utilized. The utilization of iontophoresis was found to make strides torment alleviation in a comparative scientific paper [62]. Ultrasound-guided autologous blood infusion driven to made strides scores on the visual analog and adjusted Nirschl Pain Phase scales [63].

Surgical treatment can be used as well, and the resection of the diseased tendon is done by open and miniopen (Fig. 77.14).

Bone, Cartilage, and Other Conditions

Posteromedial Impingement or Valgus Extension Overload

Valgus extension overload could be a common condition in overhead throwing athletes in which posterior and medial osteophytes encroach inside the olecranon fossa as the elbow comes to extension. An audit of 72 proficient baseball players who experienced elbow surgery found that 65% had back olecranon osteophytes [64]. Competitors regularly report posterior pain at the elbow amid ball release and as the elbow comes to extension; this can be the point at which osteophytes from the olecranon encroach inside the fossa. The athlete commonly presents with pain on extension with valgus load on examination.

When valgus stretch on the elbow is performed at 20° to 30° of flexion and the elbow is rapidly taken to extension, a positive test re-creates the torment within the posteromedial elbow. Care must be taken whether there is a concomitant MCL tear or attenuation since there is a critical relationship between these pathologies. Plain radiographs can uncover the back osteophyte.

Nonsurgical treatment starts with rest and 10–14 days of throwing limitations taken after by an interval tossing program to permit a slow return. Throwing mechanics must be adjusted amid the interval throwing program to play down push at the elbow. A longer period of rest is prescribed in the event that symptoms persist or the athlete cannot return to tossing at the prior level. Intra-articular infusion is not especially supportive in patients with posteromedial impingement and ought to not be rehashed.

Surgical treatment ought to be carefully considered.

The medial elbow supports considerable valgus forces within the tossing competitor, and engagement of the olecranon in its fossa gives auxiliary stabilization to the elbow, especially amid extension. Any laxity within the MCL may exchange push to the posteromedial olecranon and cause it to encroach on the fossa as the elbow comes to extension. This stretch initiates osteophyte growing, which at that point increments impingement by shear mass effect. Over-resection of the posteromedial olecranon can unmask or worsen symptoms of MCL damage. Twenty-five percent of proficient baseball players who experienced osteophyte extraction afterward had valgus flimsiness requiring MCL's surgery [64].

There are studies that put in check how much of the olecranon must be excised before stress is diagnosed at the MCL.

The procedure can be done in an arthroscopic or open fashion. In an open strategy, an osteotome is utilized to resect a parcel of the olecranon tip, and a parcel of the medial olecranon is removed. The arthroscopic method can be fulfilled by a posterolateral portal for seeing and a central posterior portal for working. Care must be taken to take out osteophytes and minimize resection of normal olecranon. Additional care must be taken to keep a strategic distance from ulnar nerve damage when resecting the medial angle of the osteophyte as the ulnar nerve enters the cubital tunnel. Great results have been presented in seven of nine patients who experienced arthroscopic treatment of valgus extension overload [65].

Olecranon Stress Fracture

Stress fractures of the olecranon have been depicted in javelin and other throwing athletes [66, 67]. These fractures are fundamentally portrayed as transverse or sideways, with an instrument of harm comparative to that of a valgus extension overload damage.

On physical examination, the competitor may have delicacy over the physis (if it is open), the posterior olecranon, or the posteromedial olecranon. Side effects may be evoked by forceful extension of the elbow or resisted test to triceps muscle. Regularly, the athlete has less extension than the contralateral elbow.

MRI will show edema inside the bone and permit characterization of the break line.

The treatment of an olecranon stress fracture is to some degree disputable. Nonsurgical measures require rest from tossing and conceivably brief splinting. The return to an interval tossing program is deferred until symptoms have died down and there is radiographic prove of break recuperating. As a result, throwing can be confined for as long as 6 months. Stress fractures may react to bone stimulators, but this treatment has not been well characterized.

Surgical treatment is recommended when the athlete have to come back earlier than the conservative treatment waiting time [68]. Tension band and compression screws can be used.

Persistent Olecranon Physis

It is similar to an olecranon stress fracture. The olecranon physis has two ossification centers: the posterior center is situated transverse to the longitudinal axis of the ulna and contributes to longitudinal development; a second center is more anterior at the olecranon tip, contributing to the joint surface but not to longitudinal development. These two centers combine and make a single physis that holds on until around age 14 in young ladies and age 16 in boys. This physis can end up sclerotic amid the method of closing and can be as wide as 5 mm.

Back elbow pain regularly creates pain from puberty through the late youngsters. The pain happens at terminal extension within the follow-through stage of tossing, and it can be calmed with rest.

T2-weighted MRI may present edema by the physis, but this finding is not diagnostic. Treatment begins with nonsurgical measures, counting a period of relative rest and cessation of tossing exercises. NSAIDs and ice may be utilized as required. Nonsurgical measures show up to be effective in most patients but may require as long as 4 months. The alternatives for surgical treatment incorporate open surgery (tension band or screws).

Capitellar Osteochondritis Dissecans

Osteochondritis dissecans (OCD) is a pathology of the subchondral bone that comes about the fragmentation of articular cartilage and underlying bone. It is imperative to distinguish this condition from Panner pathology, which happens in more youthful patients, is idiopathic, more often than not is self-limiting, and progresses without surgical intervention. OCD ordinarily happens at the elbow in adolescents who are high-demand, monotonous overhead throwing competitors. The pathogenesis is not totally elucidated. Hereditary components, blood supply, repetition injury, and a vulnerable epiphysis have been embroiled.

The underlying bone experiences degradation and can destabilize the overlying cartilage. Likely, a combination of components contributes to the method by which the injury is made.

Regularly, the competitor has elbow pain amid action. The pain is treacherous in onset, is soothed by rest, and advances in case the movement is proceeded.

The torment is troublesome to localize and regularly is set by the decrease of movement. The foremost common finding on examination is delicacy over the radiocapitellar joint. Crepitus can be elicited in the lateral joint with pronation and supination, and there is loss of movement of 15° to 30°. The dynamic radiocapitellar compression test can be done and elbow is completely extended, whereas the patient effectively pronates and supinates the forearm and contracts the muscles almost the elbow. A positive test reproduces the patient's pain.

X-rays can be performed. The standard AP see in full extension and lateral in 90°of flexion appear commonplace capitellar radiolucency and smoothing of the joint surface. The injury commonly happens within the anterolateral aspect of the capitellum. Within the Minami classification, a level I lesion could be a translucent cystic shadow within the center or sidelong capitellum, a level II injury includes a part line or clear zone between the injury and its subchondral bone, and free bodies are display in a level III lesion [69].

MRI has ended up as the methodology of choice for assessing these injuries. Early changes not found on plain radiographs can be identified on MRI, and the measure, area, and steadiness of the injury can be surveyed. The key to making a treatment choice is to decide whether the articular surface is intaglio and the injury is steady as seen on MRI. A fringe ring of liquid or liquid beneath the articular surface proposes an unsteady injury; these discoveries are comparative to those of an OCD injury in another zone of the body.

Nonsurgical regimens are an alternative. The treatment starts with 6 months of elbow rest without throwing movement. Anti-inflammatory solutions are utilized, and physical therapy is done to optimize movement and quality. Radiographs are surveyed at 6-week interval to guarantee that the injury is mending or is not advancing. MRI is rehashed as required at a roughly 3-month interim and compared with the first exam. An interval throwing program begins at 6 months in case of high demand competitors, if asymptomatic, and with prove of recuperating. Pitch tallies at first ought to be monitored [70]. Patients with capitellar lucency or smoothing have mending rates of 88–91% [71, 72].

A steady injury is characterized by an open capitellar development plate, localized flattening or radiolucency of the subchondral bone, and great elbow movement. In an unsteady injury, the physis is closed, with radiographic fracture and loss of elbow movement of more than 20° [73].

Surgery is performed when there is an unsteady injury or free bodies or nonsurgical treatment has failed. A few surgical strategies have been portrayed. Straightforward debridement can be successful for a contained injury including less than 50% of the capitellar surface. Microfracture or trephination of the subchondral base with a Kirschner wire moreover can be utilized after part extraction and bed preparation. Fixation of a big fragment can be accomplished through diverse strategies. A few choices exist for cartilage substitution. Mosaicplasty, osteochondral auto, and allograft can be performed as well.

Radiocapitellar Plica

Radiocapitellar plica, depicted as a cause of a snapping elbow, basically could be a hypertrophic synovial plica that snaps over the edge of the radial head as the elbow moves from flexion to extension. The differential diagnosis incorporates intra-articular free bodies, ligament lesions, lateral epicondylitis, and subluxation of the medial triceps over the medial epicondyle. A few of these conditions can be ruled out on the premise of area. The elbow examination regularly is something else generous, with soundness, full movement, and typical quality and strength. The competitor may have delicacy posterior to the lateral epicondyle and centered over the joint. Plain radiographs ordinarily are not instructive, and the plica habitually is missed on MRI.

Nonsurgical treatment can be performed, and if it fails, surgery can be needed.

Arthroscopy is done, replicating the symptoms and removing the plica.

Early range of motion is needed, and throwing is allowed from 8 weeks on.

References

1. McDonald AR, Murdock FA Jr, McDonald JA, Wolf CJ. Prevalence of injuries during Brazilian Jiu-Jitsu Training. Sports (Basel). 2017 June 12;5(2):E39.
2. Ibrahim HIH, Mohammed AE. Common injuries in racket sports: a mini review. Ortho Surg Ortho Care Int J. 2018 Mar;1(4):OOIJ.000519.
3. Wong TT, Lin DJ, Ayyala RS, Kazam JK. Elbow injuries in adult overhead athletes. AJR Am J Roentgenol. 2017 Mar;208(3):W110–20.
4. Farrow LD, Mahoney AJ, Stefancin JJ, Taljanovic MS, Sheppard JE, Schickendantz MS. Quantitative analysis of the medial ulnar collateral ligament ulnar footprint and its relationship to the ulnar sublime tubercle. Am J Sports Med. 2011;39(9):1936–41.
5. Park MC, Ahmad CS. Dynamic contributions of the flexor-pronator mass to elbow valgus stability. J Bone Joint Surg Am. 2004;86-A(10):2268–74.
6. Aibinder WR, Dines JS, Camp CL. Understanding the medial ulnar collateral ligament of the elbow: review of native ligament anatomy and function. World J Orthop. 2018 June 18;9(6):78–84.

7. O'Driscoll SW, Lawton RL, Smith AM. The "moving valgus stress test" for medial collateral ligament tears of the elbow. Am J Sports Med. 2005;33:231–9.

8. Pappas AM, Zawacki RM, Sullivan TJ. Biomechanics of baseball pitching: a preliminary report. Am J Sports Med. 1985;13:216–22.

9. Werner SL, Fleisig GS, Dillman CJ, Andrews JR. Biomechanics of the elbow during baseball pitching. J Orthop Sports Phys Ther. 1993;17:274–8.

10. Fleisig GS, Andrews JR, Dillman CJ, Escamilla RF. Kinetics of baseball pitching with implications about injury mechanisms. Am J Sports Med. 1995 Mar-Apr;23(2):233–9.

11. Ahmad CS, Lee TQ, ElAttrache NS. Biomechanical evaluation of a new ulnar collateral ligament reconstruction technique with interference screw fixation. Am J Sports Med. 2003;31(3):332–7.

12. Duggan JP Jr, Osadebe UC, Alexander JW, Noble PC, Lintner DM. The impact of ulnar collateral ligament tear and reconstruction on contact pressures in the lateral compartment of the elbow. J Shoulder Elb Surg. 2011;20(2):226–33.

13. Fleisig GS, Kingsley DS, Loftice JW, Dinnen KP, Ranganathan R, Dun S, et al. Kinetic comparison among the fastball, curveball, change-up, and slider in collegiate baseball pitchers. Am J Sports Med. 2006;34(3):423–30.

14. O'Driscoll SW, Lawton RL, Smith AM. The "moving valgus stress test" for medial collateral ligament tears of the elbow. Am J Sports Med. 2005;33(2):231–9.

15. Kim NR, Moon SG, Ko SM, Moon WJ, Choi JW, Park J. MR imaging of ulnar collateral ligament injury in baseball players: value for predicting rehabilitation outcome. Eur J Radiol. 2011;80(3):e422–6.

16. Nazarian LN, McShane JM, Ciccotti MG, O'Kane PL, Harwood MI. Dynamic US of the anterior band of the ulnar collateral ligament of the elbow in asymptomatic major league baseball pitchers. Radiology. 2003;227(1):149–54.

17. Sasaki J, Takahara M, Ogino T, Kashiwa H, Ishigaki D, Kanauchi Y. Ultrasonographic assessment of the ulnar collateral ligament and medial elbow laxity in college baseball players. J Bone Joint Surg Am. 2002;84(4):525–31.

18. Field LD, Altchek DW. Evaluation of the arthroscopic valgus instability test of the elbow. Am J Sports Med. 1996;24(2):177–81.

19. Scoggin JF, Brusovanik G, Izuka BH, Zandee van Rilland E, Geling O, Tokumura S. Assessment of injuries during Brazilian jiu-jitsu competition. Orthop J Sports Med. 2014;2(2):2325967114522184.

20. Aguinaldo AL, Chambers H. Correlation of throwing mechanics with elbow valgus load in adult baseball pitchers. Am J Sports Med. 2009;37(10):2043–8.

21. Rettig AC, Sherrill C, Snead DS, Mendler JC, Mieling P. Nonoperative treatment of ulnar collateral ligament injuries in throwing athletes. Am J Sports Med. 2001;29(1):15–7.

22. Baumfeld JA, van Riet RP, Zobitz ME, Eygendaal D, An KN, Steinmann SP. Triceps tendon properties and its potential as an autograft. J Shoulder Elb Surg. 2010 July;19(5):697–9.

23. O'Driscoll SW, Jupiter JB, Cohen MS, Ring D, McKee MD. Difficult elbow fractures: pearls and pitfalls. Instr Course Lect. 2003;52:113.

24. Morrey BF, Sanchez-Sotelo J, Morrey ME. Morrey's the elbow and its disorders. 5th ed. Philadelphia: Elsevier Health Sciences. Kindle Edition; 2019.

25. O'Driscoll SW, Bell DF, Morrey BF. Posterolateral rotatory instability of the elbow. J Bone Joint Surg Am. 1991;73:440–6.

26. Shukla DR, Thoreson AR, Fitzsimmons JS, An KN, O'Driscoll SW. The effect of capitellar impaction fractures on radiocapitellar stability. J Hand Surg [Am]. 2015;40:520.

27. de Prado-López A, León-Vaquero F, López-Castro P, Rodríguez-Echegaray C, Peces-Gonjar D, Román-Torres M, et al. Reconstruction of a traumatic lateral trochlear defect with a radial head autograft. Rev Esp Cir Ortop Traumatol. 2012;56(4):323–7.

28. Gourgoulis V, Aggelousis N, Mavromatis G, Garas A. Three-dimensional kinematic analysis of the snatch of elite Greek weight-lifters. J Sports Sci. 2000;18(8):643–52.

29. Drechsler A. The weightlifting encyclopedia: a guide to world class performance. Flushing: A is A Communications; 1998.

30. Giron I, Wajsbrot D, François T, Lemay J. Pregabalin for peripheral neuropathic pain: a multicenter enriched enrollment randomized withdrawal placebo-controlled trial. Clin J Pain. 2011;27(3):185–93.

31. Naam NH, Massoud HA. Painful entrapment of the lateral antebrachial cutaneous nerve at the elbow. J Hand Surg [Am]. 2004;29:1148–53.

32. Aldekhayel S, Govshievich A, Lee J, Tahiri Y, Luc M. Endoscopic versus open cubital tunnel release: a systematic review and meta-analysis. Hand (NY). 2016;11(1):36–44.

33. Garcia JC, Montero EFS. Endoscopic robotic decompression of the ulnar nerve at the elbow. Arthrosc Tech. 2014;3(3):e383–7.

34. Harrison JWK, Thomas P, Aster A, Wilkes G, Hayton MJ. Chronic exertional compartment syndrome of the forearm in elite rowers: a technique for mini-open fasciotomy and a report of six cases. Hand. 2013;8(4):450–3.

35. Hutchinson M. Chronic exertional compartment syndrome head to head. Br J Sports Med. 2011;45:954–5.

36. Miller EA, Cobb MA, Cobb TK. Endoscopic fascia release for forearm chronic exertional compartment syndrome: case report and surgical technique. Hand. 2017;12(5):NP58–61.

37. Anzel SH, Covey KW, Weiner AD, Lipscomb PR. Disruption of muscles and tendons. An analysis of 1,014 cases. Surgery. 1959;45:406–14.

38. Sollender JL, Rayan GM, Barden GA. Triceps tendon rupture in weight lifters. J Shoulder Elb Surg. 1998;7(2):151–3.

39. Kelly MP, Perkinson SG, Ablove RH, Tueting JL. Distal biceps tendon ruptures: an epidemiological analysis using a large population database. Am J Sports Med. 2015;43(8):2012–7.

40. Athwal GS, Steinmann SP, Rispoli DM. The distal biceps tendon: footprint and relevant clinical anatomy. J Hand Surg [Am]. 2007;32:1225–9.

41. Garcia JC, de Castro Filho CD, de Castro Mello TF, de Vasconcelos RA, Zabeu JL, Garcia JP. Isokinetic and functional evaluation of distal biceps reconstruction using the Mayo mini-double route technique. Rev Bras Ortop. 2015;47(5):581–7.

42. Sims SE, Miller K, Elfar JC, Hammert WC. Nonsurgical treatment of lateral epicondylitis: a systematic review of randomized controlled trials. Hand (NY). 2014;9(4):419–46.

43. Shiri R, Viikari-Juntura E, Varonen H, Heliövaara M. Prevalence and determinants of lateral and medial epicondylitis. A population study. Am J Epidemiol. 2006;164(11):1065–74.

44. Coonrad RW, Hooper WR. Tennis elbow: its courses, natural history, conservative and surgical management. J Bone Joint Surg Am. 1973;55:1177–82.

45. Nirschl RP. Soft-tissue injuries about the elbow. Clin Sports Med. 1986;5:637–52.

46. Gabel GT, Morrey BF. Tennis elbow. Instr Course Lect. 1998;47:165–72.

47. Cohen MS, Romeo AA. Open and arthroscopic management of lateral epicondylitis in the athlete. Hand Clin. 2009;25(3):331–8.

48. Riek S, Chapman AE, Milner T. A simulation of muscle force and internal kinematics of extensor carpi radialis brevis during backhand tennis stroke: implications for injury. Clin Biomech (Bristol, Avon). 1999;14:477–83.

49. Schneeberger AG, Masquelet AC. Arterial vascularization of the proximal extensor carpi radialis brevis tendon. Clin Orthop Relat Res. 2002;398:239–44.

50. Le Huec JC, Schaeverbeke T, Chauveaux D, Rivel J, Dehais J, Le Rebeller A. Epicondylitis after treatment with fluoroquinolone antibiotics. J Bone Joint Surg (Br). 1995;77(2):293–5.

51. Bunata RE, Brown DS, Capelo R. Anatomic factors related to the causes of tennis elbow. J Bone Joint Surg Am. 2007;89:1955–63.

52. Coonrad RW, Hooper WR. Tennis elbow: its courses, natural history, conservative and surgical management. J Bone Joint Surg Am. 1973;55:1177–82.

53. Nirschl RP. Elbow tendinosis/tennis elbow. Clin Sports Med. 1992;11:851–70.

54. Nirschl RP. Muscle and tendon trauma: tennis elbow. In: Morrey BF, editor. The elbow and its disorders. 1st ed. Philadelphia: WB Saunders; 1985. p. 537–52.

55. Chen J, Wang A, Xu J, Zheng M. In chronic lateral epicondylitis, apoptosis and autophagic cell death occur in the extensor carpi radialis brevis tendon. J Shoulder Elb Surg. 2010;19:355–62.

56. Tuite MJ, Kijowski R. Sports-related injuries of the elbow: an approach to MRI interpretation. Clin Sports Med. 2006;25(3):387–408, v.

57. Fairbank SM, Corlett RJ. The role of the extensor digitorum communis muscle in lateral epicondylitis. J Hand Surg (Br). 2002;27(5):405–9.

58. Greenbaum B, Itamura J, Vangsness CT, Tibone J, Atkinson R. Extensor carpi radialis brevis. An anatomical analysis of its origin. J Bone Joint Surg (Br). 1999;81:926–9.

59. Field LD, Savoie FH. Common elbow injuries in sport. Sports Med. 1998;26:193–205.

60. Park GY, Lee SM, Lee MY. Diagnostic value of ultrasonography for clinical medial epicondylitis. Arch Phys Med Rehabil. 2008;89(4):738–42.

61. Kijowski R, De Smet AA. Magnetic resonance imaging findings in patients with medial epicondylitis. Skelet Radiol. 2005;34(4):196–202.

62. Nirschl RP, Rodin DM, Ochiai DH, MaartmannMoe C, DEX-AHE-01-99 Study Group. Iontophoretic administration of dexamethasone sodium phosphate for acute epicondylitis: a randomized, double-blinded, placebo-controlled study. Am J Sports Med. 2003;31(2):189–95.

63. Suresh SP, Ali KE, Jones H, Connell DA. Medial epicondylitis: is ultrasound guided autologous blood injection an effective treatment? Br J Sports Med. 2006;40(11):935–9.

64. Andrews JR, Timmerman L. Outcome of elbow surgery in professional baseball players. Am J Sports Med. 1995;23(4):407–13.

65. Cohen SB, Valko C, Zoga A, Dodson CC, Ciccotti MG. Posteromedial elbow impingement: magnetic resonance imaging findings in overhead throwing athletes and results of arthroscopic treatment. Arthroscopy. 2011;27(10):1364–70.

66. Hulkko A, Orava S, Nikula P. Stress fractures of the olecranon in javelin throwers. Int J Sports Med. 1986;7(4):210–3.

67. Nuber GW, Diment MT. Olecranon stress fractures in throwers: a report of two cases and a review of the literature. Clin Orthop Relat Res. 1992;278:58–61.

68. Suzuki K, Minami A, Suenaga N, Kondoh M. Oblique stress fracture of the olecranon in baseball pitchers. J Shoulder Elb Surg. 1997;6(5):491–4.

69. Minami M, Nakashita K, Ishii S, et al. Twenty-five cases of osteochondritis dissecans of the elbow. Rinsho Seikei Geka. 1979;14(8):805–10.

70. Baker CL III, Romeo AA, Baker CL Jr. Osteochondritis dissecans of the capitellum. Am J Sports Med. 2010;38(9):1917–28.

71. Mihara K, Tsutsui H, Nishinaka N, Yamaguchi K. Nonoperative treatment for osteochondritis dissecans of the capitellum. Am J Sports Med. 2009;37(2):298–304.

72. Matsuura T, Kashiwaguchi S, Iwase T, Takeda Y, Yasui N. Conservative treatment for osteochondrosis of the humeral capitellum. Am J Sports Med. 2008;36(5):868–72.

73. Takahara M, Mura N, Sasaki J, Harada M, Ogino T. Classification, treatment, and outcome of osteochondritis dissecans of the humeral capitellum. J Bone Joint Surg Am. 2007;89(6):1205–14.

Thumb Carpometacarpal Osteoarthritis: Cutting Edge Techniques

78

William B. Geissler and Mark A. Dodson

Introduction

Thumb carpometacarpal arthritis is the second most common side of osteoarthritis in the hand [1]. The thumb carpometacarpal joint is uniquely bi-concave joint which contains two saddle shaped bones that articulate perpendicular to each other. This allows for considerable range of motion and function to the thumb. However, this joint is inherently unstable making it prone to osteoarthritis. Cooney described that 1 kg pinch at the thumb tip is amplified to a 13 kg load at the base of the thumb [2]. In patients older than 75 years, thumb carpometacarpal osteoarthritis has a radiographic prevalence in 25% in men and up to 40% in women. Osteoarthritis to the thumb carpometacarpal joint can be extremely debilitating and can lead to significantly decreased function to the hand.

Reconstruction to the thumb carpometacarpal joint is one of the most commonly performed hand surgery operations. The number of surgeries, to the thumb carpometacarpal joint, will only continue to increase as the population ages [3–7]. As seen in this textbook, there are a number of successful procedures for thumb carpometacarpal arthritis. Each procedure can be described as an arthroscopic or open partial or complete trapeziectomy with suspension of the thumb metacarpal by some type of suture device or tendon and, lastly, joint replacement.

Pyrolytic carbon is a synthetic material developed in the 1950s for the nuclear industry. It is a unique form of carbon that is created by exposing a graphite model to hydrocarbon gas at 1300 to 1500 degrees Celsius. This forms a coating of pyrolytic carbon up to 1 mm thick over the graphite substrate. It is then polished to create the final product. It is commonly known as pyrocarbon when used in medical applications. In the late 1960s, it was first used in the medical field for mechanical heart valves. In the 1970s, it was first used for metacarpal phalangeal joint replacements. Its uses have now been expanded to include arthroplasty of the wrist, elbow, shoulder, and foot [8–10].

Pyrocarbon has several characteristics that make it very desirable as a device for use in hand, wrist, and elbow surgery. Excellent wear properties with almost no particulate generation in pyrocarbon/pyrocarbon constructs. Pyrocarbon has the ability to create a surface layer of lubrication by adsorption of phospholipids. It has a modulus of elasticity similar to cortical bone, and it is bioinert with no reports of allergic reactions.

The purpose of this chapter is to describe two new, totally opposite techniques to address arthritis to the thumb carpometacarpal joint. One is a new technique for suspension of the thumb metacarpal with a lockdown device. The other technique involves a partial trapeziectomy and placement of a pyrocarbon spacer between the remaining trapezium and thumb metacarpal. Both these techniques are very new and have not been fully released on the market. The lockdown device is a simplified technique to suspend the thumb metacarpal and can be used in primary resection of the trapezium to suspend the thumb metacarpal or can be used in salvage situation. The pyrocarbon technique is particularly attractive to young patients with debilitating thumb pain who want to maintain as much pinch strength as possible compared to a resection arthroplasty.

Lockdown Thumb Metacarpal Suspension

The lockdown device is a polyester surgical mesh that was originally designed for treatment of acromioclavicular joint dislocations. With over 2000 implantations per year, and over 14,000 total implantations placed for acromioclavicular

W. B. Geissler (✉)
Division of Hand and Upper Extremity Surgery, Section of Arthroscopic Surgery and Sports Medicine, Department of Orthopedic Surgery and Rehabilitation, University of Mississippi Medical Center, Jackson, MS, USA

M. A. Dodson
Hand and Upper Extremity Fellow, Department of Orthopaedic Surgery and Rehabilitation, University of Mississippi Medical Center, Jackson, MS, USA

Partner, Mid State Orthopedic and Sports Medicine Center, Alexandria, LA, USA

© Springer Nature Switzerland AG 2022
W. B. Geissler (ed.), *Wrist and Elbow Arthroscopy with Selected Open Procedures*,
https://doi.org/10.1007/978-3-030-78881-0_78

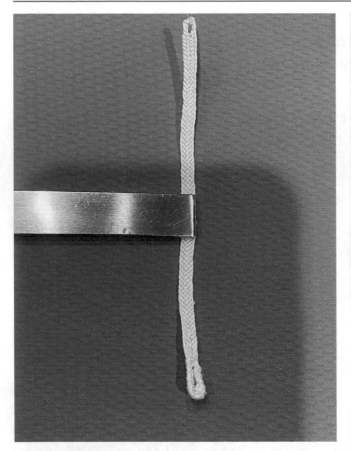

Fig. 78.1 The thumb carpometacarpal lockdown device is a synthetic mesh device that has a hard loop on one end for placement of a screw and a soft loop on the opposite in where the lockdown is passed through itself

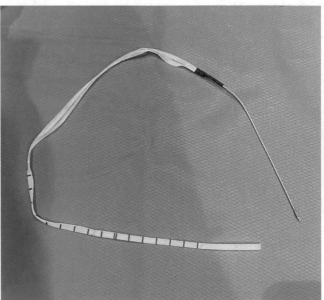

Fig. 78.2 The lockdown system has a depth gauge to measure the appropriate length of the lockdown device. One end has a flexible metal lead to help pass the depth gauge and graft across the drill holes, and the opposite end is a loop to eventually pass the lockdown device

joint instability over a 13-year period, the lockdown device has a proven track record. The lockdown device has a loop at each end. One end is a hard loop for placement of a screw and washer to secure the stabilization. The soft loop on the other end is used where the lockdown is passed through it to snug against the coracoid process. Recently, this implant has been downsized and the new technique designed to suspend the thumb metacarpal after excision of the trapezium (Fig. 78.1). The kit also contains a depth gauge with a metal lead and a loop (Fig. 78.2).

Surgical Technique

A standard dorsal incision is made over the base of the thumb carpometacarpal joint. The skin is barely incised to protect branches of the dorsal sensory branch of the radial nerve. These are identified and carefully protected. The interval between the extensor pollicis longus and extensor pollicis brevis is elevated, and the joint capsule is opened to expose the thumb carpometacarpal joint. The trapezium is then incised being carefully to protect the radial artery (Fig. 78.3).

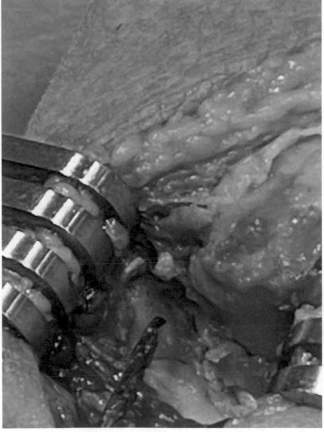

Fig. 78.3 A standard approach is made to the thumb carpometacarpal joint where the trapezium is excised. Here, the base of the thumb metacarpal can be seen and the facet of the trapezoid

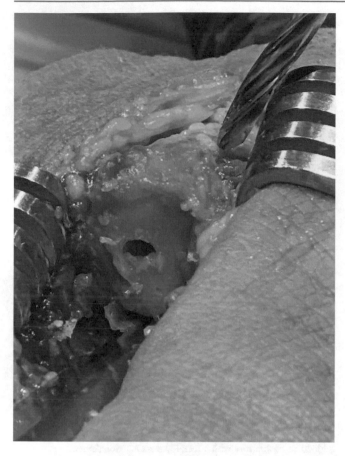

Fig. 78.4 Following excision of the trapezium, a 3.0-mm drill hole is made in the base of the thumb metacarpal

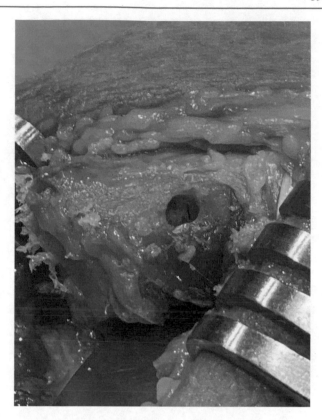

Fig. 78.5 A second 3.0-mm drill hole is made approximately 1.5–2 cm distal to the base of the thumb metacarpal on its radial aspect

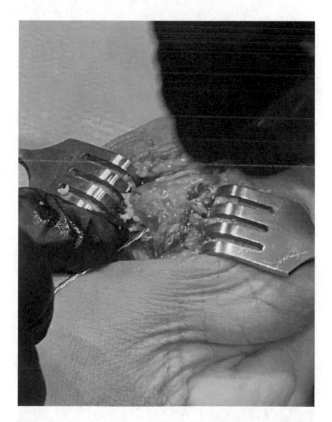

Fig. 78.6 The wire lead of the depth gauge is then passed through the base of the thumb metacarpal and exits distally through the radial base drill hole in the thumb metacarpal

A 3-mm drill hole is made in the center of the base of the thumb metacarpal (Fig. 78.4). A second 3-mm drill hole is made approximately 1.5 cm distal to the joint surface along the radial aspect of the thumb metacarpal (Fig. 78.5). The lockdown depth gauge is then placed starting at the base of the thumb metacarpal and exits out the radial aspect of the distal drill hole on the thumb metacarpal (Fig. 78.6). The depth gauge is then looped on itself (Figs. 78.7 and 78.8).

Next, a guidewire is placed through the incision at the radial base of the index metacarpal exiting the ulnar aspect of the index metacarpal. The position of the guidewire is checked under fluoroscopy. It is important that the guidewire exits along the proximal quarter or third of the index metacarpal and not too distally. If the drill hole is placed too distally, it can cause an adduction contracture to the thumb metacarpal with the lockdown device implanted. Once the ideal placement of the guidewire is confirmed under fluoroscopy, the cannulated 3-mm grill is used over the guidewire, and the bone is drilled (Fig. 78.9). The metal lead is passed through the index metacarpal from radial to ulnar (Figs. 78.10 and 78.11). The length of the lockdown thumb metacarpal suspension device is measured (Fig. 78.12). It is very important not to snug down the lockdown device which can cause impingement between the thumb and index meta-

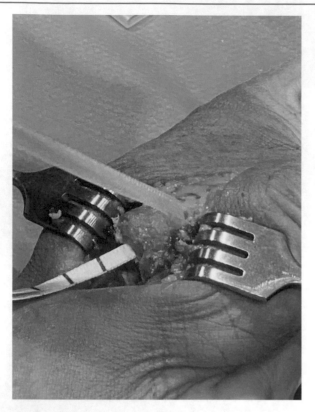

Fig. 78.7 The depth gauge is then passed through the drill holes on the thumb metacarpal from a proximal to distal direction

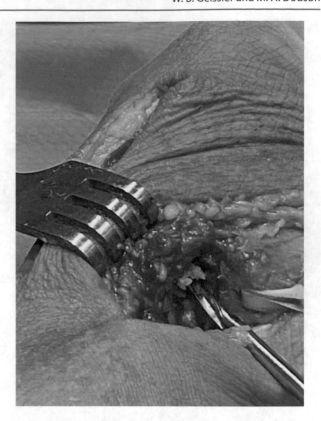

Fig. 78.9 The base of the index metacarpal is then drilled. It is important that the drill hole is not aimed too far distally so it is not to cause an adduction contracture with a lockdown suspension device

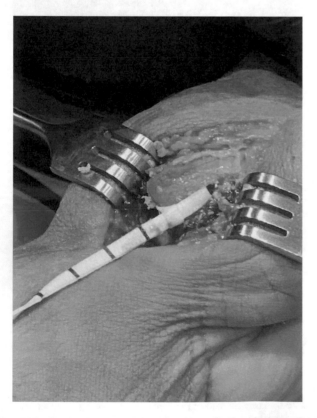

Fig. 78.8 The depth gauge is then looped on itself at the base of the thumb metacarpal

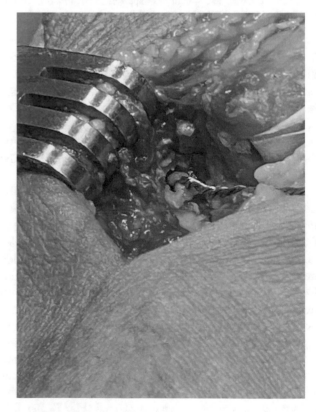

Fig. 78.10 The wire lead is then passed through the base of the index metacarpal to exit more distally or on the ulnar aspect of the index metacarpal

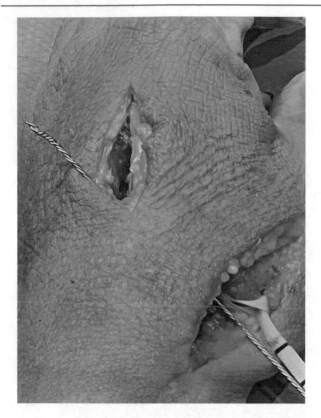

Fig. 78.11 The wire lead is then used to pass the depth gauge device across the index metacarpal

carpals. The purpose of this device is to purely suspend the thumb metacarpal from migrating proximally. The depth gauge is then pulled back out of the index metacarpal into the surgical wound. The hard knot of the selected lockdown device is then placed through the loop of the depth gauge (Figs. 78.13 and 78.14). The hard loop is then passed from proximal to distal through the thumb metacarpal as is then looped on itself through the soft loop at the base of the thumb metacarpal (Fig. 78.15). In this manner, it is going to act as a suspension device for the thumb metacarpal (Fig. 78.16). The depth gauge is reinserted through the base of the index metacarpal and is used to pull the hard loop of the lockdown through the index metacarpal. The loop should end up being at the proximal third to one-half of the index metacarpal. A 1.5-mm drill bit is then used for a 2-mm screw and washer (Fig. 78.17). Two millimeters are added to the measurement for the screw and washer to be placed on the hard loop of the device. The 2.0-mm screw and washer are then inserted through the hard loop of the lockdown device to support and suspend the thumb metacarpal (Figs. 78.18 and 78.19). Confirmation under fluoroscopy is made on successful screw placement. The joint capsule is then closed. The skin is closed and the patient is placed in a

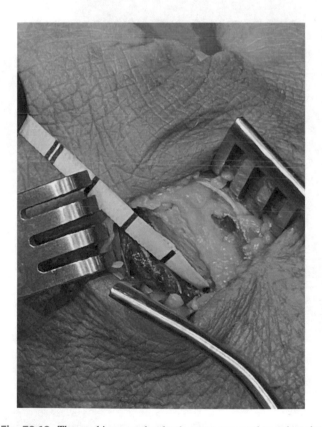

Fig. 78.12 The markings on the depth gauge are used to select the ideal length of the lockdown thumb carpometacarpal suspension device

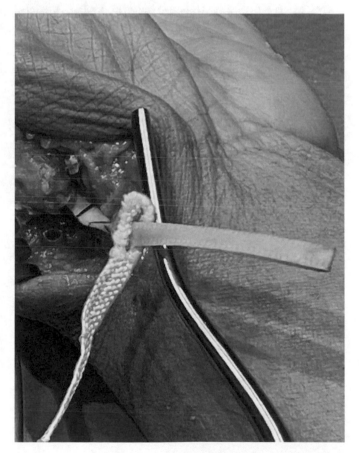

Fig. 78.13 The depth gauge is then pulled out of the index metacarpal and is then inserted into the hard loop of the lockdown device

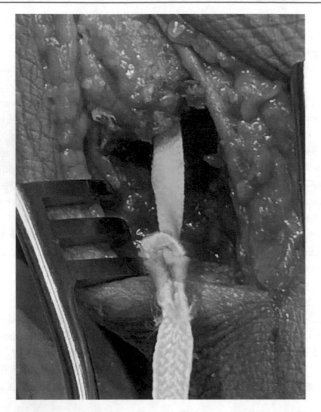

Fig. 78.14 The depth gauge is cinched around the hard loop to be used to pass the lockdown device through the thumb and index metacarpal

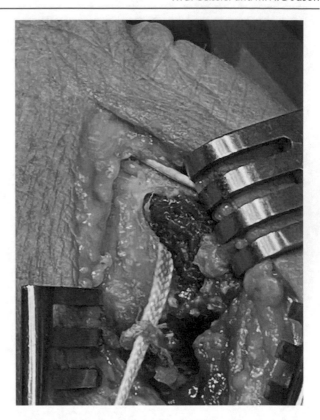

Fig. 78.16 The lockdown device is then cinched along the base of the thumb metacarpal to act as a general sling or suspension to support it

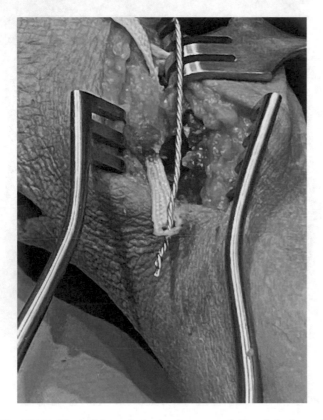

Fig. 78.15 The lockdown device has been passed through the base of the thumb metacarpal and exited distally along the radial aspect. The wire lead is then passed through the soft loop of the lockdown device

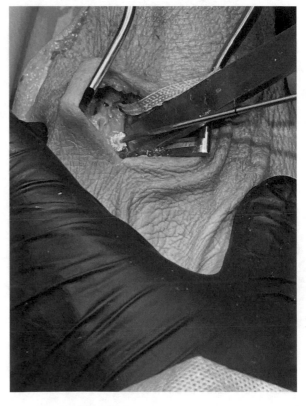

Fig. 78.17 A 1.5-mm drill is then used to drill the index metacarpal for placement of a 2.0-mm screw through the hard loop of the lockdown device

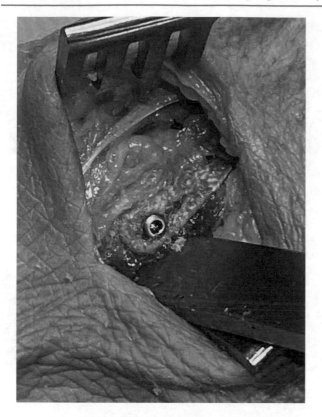

Fig. 78.18 The screw is then inserted through the hard loop into the index metacarpal

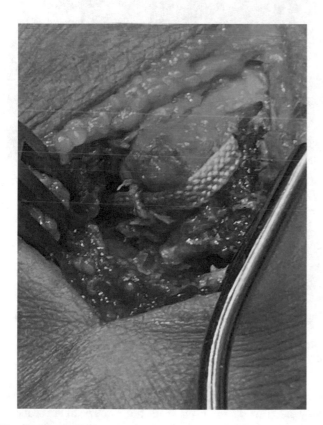

Fig. 78.19 The final construct showing the lockdown device supporting the base of the thumb metacarpal. It is important not to overtighten the lockdown device to cause impingement between the thumb and index metacarpal

thumb spica splint. The patient is placed in a thumb spica splint and returns at 2 weeks to start an active range of motion program.

Tips and Tricks

- Following incision of the skin over the thumb carpometacarpal joint, make sure to use blunt dissection to protect the dorsal sensory branch of the radial nerve. This can lead to painful neuromas and potential dystrophy if they are injured.
- Make sure there is an adequate bone bridge between the drill holes at the base of thumb metacarpal and the second more distal drill hole along the radial aspect of the thumb metacarpal for a good bone bridge. If the drill holes are placed too close together, there will be concern of the bone bridge breaking, losing support to the thumb metacarpal.
- Make sure the drill hole in the index metacarpal is not too far distal to cause an adduction contracture. The drill hole should be in the proximal quarter or third of the index metacarpal.
- When using the lockdown depth gauge, it is passed from the thumb metacarpal into the index metacarpal; do not overtighten the interval between the two metacarpals. The purpose of this device is to suspend the thumb metacarpal and not to overtighten or impinge between the two metacarpals.
- Pass the hard knot proximal to distal through the thumb metacarpal and through the soft loop of the lockdown device at the base of the thumb metacarpal. This allows for better support and suspension to the thumb metacarpal.
- Use a 2.0-mm screw that is 2 mm longer than what is measured to allow the screw and washer to be placed through the hard knot of the lockdown device and capture the opposite cortex of the index metacarpal. Confirm placement of the screw under fluoroscopy.

Ensemble CMC Is a New Pyrocarbon Implant Recommended for Use in Eaton-Glickel Stages I, II, and III

Surgical Technique

The patient is supine, and the arm is placed on a radiolucent arm board. The incision is made centered over the thumb CMC joint on the radial aspect of the thumb for approximately 3 cm in length (Fig. 78.20). The exposure to the joint is made just volar to the abductor pollicis (Fig. 78.21),

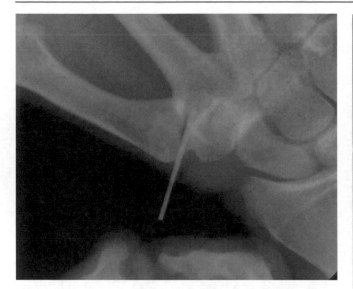

Fig. 78.20 Method for localizing CMC joint prior to incision

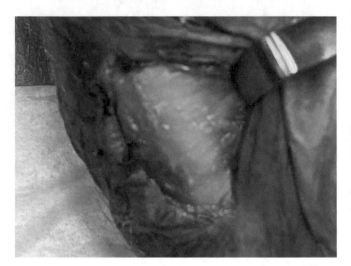

Fig. 78.21 Approach to the CMC joint should be volar to the abductor pollicis longus

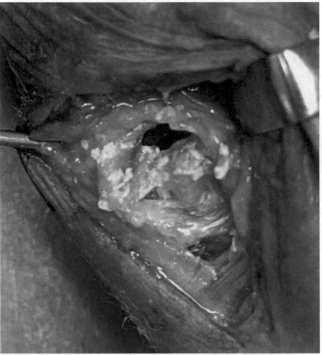

Fig. 78.22 Exposure of the CMC joint centered on the radial peak of the trapezium

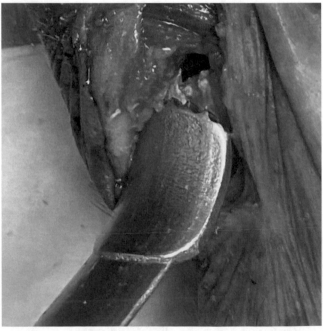

Fig. 78.23 The end rasp is used to initially establish the space for introduction of the implant

and the thenar musculature is elevated from the metacarpal. This will expose the capsule of the thumb CMC joint. A longitudinal split is made in the capsule, and it is elevated by centering on the radial peak of the trapezium in both volar and dorsal directions (Fig. 78.22). The opening should only be sufficient to allow for the placement of the largest implant. The introduction of the implants and instruments is to be centered at the radial peak of the trapezium. Osteophytes may need to be removed to allow for exposure of the joint. The end rasp (Fig. 78.23) is first placed across the base of the first metacarpal. Next the surface rasp is used to smooth osteophytes between the metacarpal and trapezium (Fig. 78.24). Only a minimum amount of bone resection should be performed. Trial implants are introduced beginning with the smallest. They should just cover

the end of the metacarpal (Fig. 78.25). Ulnar osteophytes may need to be removed from the trapezium in order to allow proper seating of the implants. The implant should be sufficiently tensioned on the preserved ligaments so that it

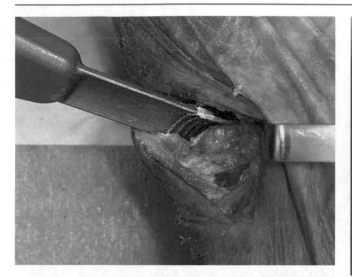

Fig. 78.24 Surface rasp is centered on the peak of the trapezium and is used to smooth osteophytes that would impede introduction of the implant

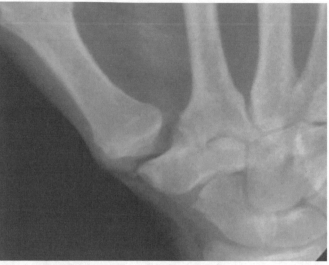

Fig. 78.26 Sizing trials and corresponding implants

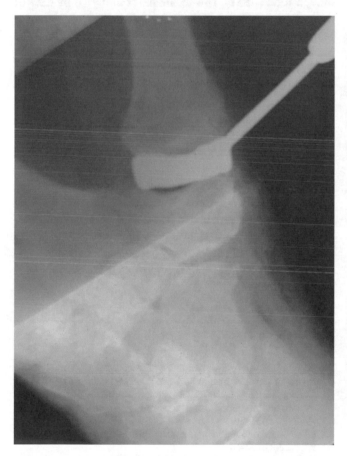

Fig. 78.25 Surface rasp positioned in the CMC joint after osteophyte removal

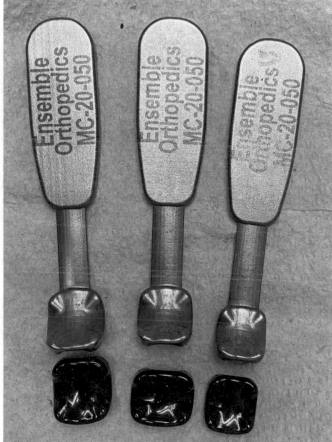

Fig. 78.27 Sizing trial in position showing appropriate placement and sizing

is stable through the arc of motion (Fig. 78.26). When the chosen implant (Fig. 78.27) is selected, it is placed in the space that has been previously prepared. Radiographs are used to assess the alignment of the metacarpal to the trape-zium (Fig. 78.28). It is then taken through a functional range of motion and should be stable (Fig. 78.29). The cap-sule is then repaired with vicryl, and skin is closed in the usual manner.

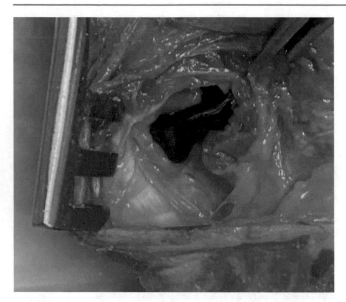

Fig. 78.29 Implant position prior to capsular closure

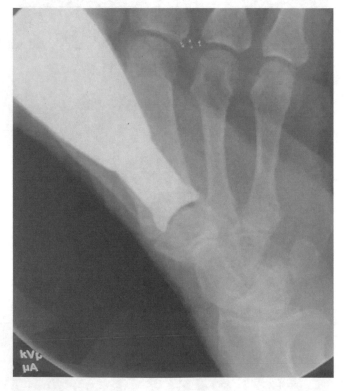

Fig. 78.28 Implant is radiolucent

Aftercare

The patient is placed in a postoperative plaster splint for 2 weeks and then in a short arm thumb spica cast for 2 weeks. At the 4-week point, the patient is then placed into a removable splint by the occupational therapist and started in gentle range of motion exercises and a strengthening program until the patient reaches 6 weeks from the date of surgery.

Tips and Tricks

- Minimal bone resection: Remove only the bone required to insert the implant and create a stable platform on the trapezium.
- Preserve the volar and dorsal ligaments of the joint. These will allow the joint to be appropriately tensioned and aid in stabilization of the implant.
- Snug or tight is much preferred over loose. A loose joint will not tighten with immobilization or K-wire fixation.
- If the joint or implant is unstable, ligament reconstruction may be required.

Discussion

One of the most widely used techniques for thumb carpal metacarpal arthritis is excision of trapezium and tendon interposition (LRTI). This technique is preferred by 62% of the active members of the Hand American Society for Surgery [11]. In this technique, the trapezium is excised, and the flexor carpi radialis tendon is harvested and used to suspend the thumb metacarpal. The suture techniques as described in this text substitute for harvesting the flexor carpal radialis to tendon to suspend the thumb metacarpal. More recently, as described, the lockdown device demonstrates a strong and secure, relatively simple method to stabilize the thumb metacarpal without depending on anchors that could pull out from the bone.

Pyrocarbon arthroplasty in early stages of thump carpal metacarpal arthritis with partial trapeziectomy has a strong potential to decrease pain and particularly still maintain adequate pinch strength. The advantage of this particular procedure is that it does not burn any bridges and can always be converted to complete trapeziectomy and suspensionplasty with other techniques.

References

1. Yao J, Park MJ. Early treatment of degenerative arthritis of the thumb carpometacarpal joint. Hand Clin. 2008;24(3):251–61. v–vi
2. Cooney WP 3rd, Chao EY. Biochemical analysis of static forces in the thumb during hand function. J Bone Joint Surg Am. 1977;59(1):27–36.
3. Glickel SZ, Gupta S. Ligament reconstruction. Hand Clin. 2006;22(2):143–51.
4. Hobby JL, Lyall HA, Meggitt BF. First metacarpal osteotomy for trapezoimetacarpal osteoarthritis. J Bone Surg Br. 1998;80(3):508–12.
5. Hartigan BJ, Stern PJ, Kiehaber TR. Thumb carpometacarpal osteoarthritis: arthrodesis compared with ligament reconstruction and tendon interposition. J Bone Joint Surg Am. 2001;83-A(10):1470–8.
6. Davis TR, Brady O, Barton NJ, Lunn PG, Burke FD. Trapeziectomy alone, with tendon interposition or with ligament reconstruction? J Hand Surg Br. 1997;22(6):689–94.

7. Burton RI, Pellegrini VD Jr. Surgical management of basal joint arthritis of the thumb. Part II. Ligament reconstruction with tendon interposition arthroplasty. J Hand Sur Am. 1986;11(3):324–32.

8. Bellemere P. Literature review: pyrocarbon implants for the hand and wrist. Hand Surg Rehab. 2018;37:129–54.

9. Cook SD, Beckenbaugh RD, Redondo J, Popich LS, Klawitter JJ, Linscheid RL. Long-term follow-up of pyrolytic carbon meta-carpophalangeal implants. J Bone Joint Surg Am. 1999;81(5):635–48.

10. van Laarhoven CMCA, Ottenhoff JSE, van Hoorn BTJA. Medium to long term follow-up after pyrocarbon disc interposition arthroplasty for treatment of CMC thumb joint arthritis. J Hand Surg Am. 2021;46(2):150.e1-e14.

11. Brunton LM, Wilgis EF. A survey to determine current practice in the surgical treatment of advanced thumb carpometacarpal osteoarthrosis. Hand (NY). 2010;5(4):415–22.

Index

© Springer Nature Switzerland AG 2022
W. B. Geissler (ed.), *Wrist and Elbow Arthroscopy with Selected Open Procedures*,
https://doi.org/10.1007/978-3-030-78881-0

Printed in the United States
by Baker & Taylor Publisher Services